Tabbner's Nursing Care

Theory and Practice

5E

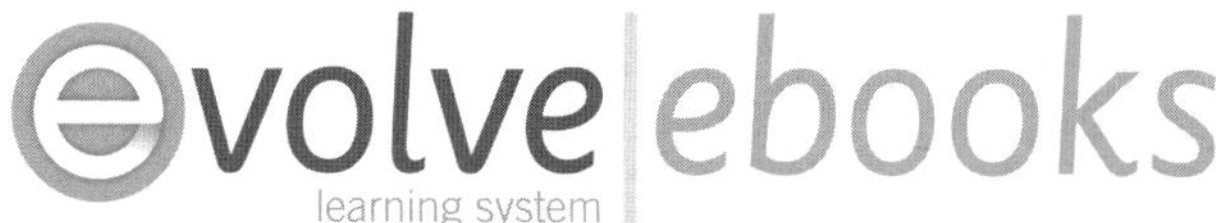
evolve
learning system
ebooks

Tabbner's Nursing Care

Theory and Practice

5E

Rita Funnell
BHlthSci (Nursing), MA (Health Studies),
RN1, RPN, Grad Cert Tertiary Education, Grad Cert Oncological Nursing
Deputy Head of School
School of Nursing and Midwifery
Victoria University, Melbourne, Vic

Gabrielle Koutoukidis
RND1, Dip App Sci (Nurs), BNurs (Mid), Adv Dip Nurs (Ed), MPH
Teaching Centre Manager
Health Science and Biotechnology Department
Holmesglen Institute, Melbourne, Vic

Karen Lawrence
RN, BA HlthSc (Nurs), GradDip (Mid), MA (HlthSc), GradDip VET
Lecturer: Acute Care
School of Nursing and Midwifery
Victoria University, Melbourne, Vic

CHURCHILL LIVINGSTONE

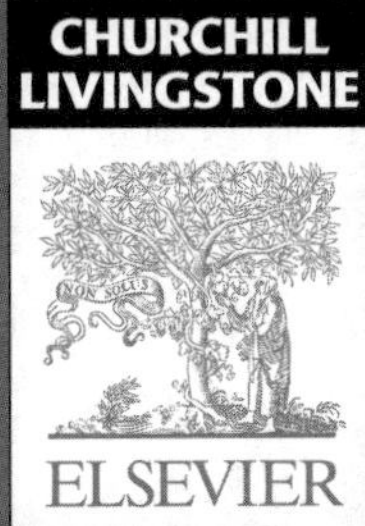

Sydney Edinburgh London New York Philadelphia St Louis Toronto

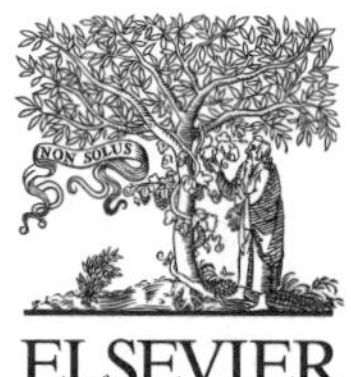

ELSEVIER

Churchill Livingstone
is an imprint of Elsevier

Elsevier Australia. ACN 001 002 357
(a division of Reed International Books Australia Pty Ltd)
Tower 1, 475 Victoria Avenue, Chatswood, NSW 2067

4th edition 2005. 3rd edition 1997. 2nd edition 1991. 1st edition 1981.

National Library of Australia Cataloguing-in-Publication Data

---

Tabbner's nursing care : theory and practice / editors, Rita Funnell, Gabrielle Koutoukidis, Karen Lawrence.

5th ed.

ISBN: 9780729538572 (pbk.)

Includes bibliographical references and index.

Nursing.

Koutoukidis, Gabrielle.
Lawrence, Karen.
Tabbner, A. R. Nursing care.

610.73

Publisher: Luisa Cecotti
Developmental Editor: Sabrina Chew
Publishing Services Manager: Helena Klijn
Editorial Coordinator: Eleanor Cant
Edited & indexed by Forsyth Publishing Services
Proofread by Tim Learner
Picture research by DW Stock Picture Library
Cover design by Trina McDonald
Internal design & typesetting by Pindar New Zealand
Printed by Ligare

CONTENTS

Unit 9 Health promotion and nursing care of the individual

Appendices

CONTRIBUTORS

The publisher and editors would like to thank all past and present contributors and reviewers. The book as it stands is the accumulated effort of many dedicated writers and nursing educators, and their invaluable work in all editions of this book is acknowledged with thanks.

Tracie Andrews, RN, BN
Director, Clinical Services,
Moreland Community Health Centre, Melbourne, Vic

Jacqui Allen, RN, BA (Hons), MPsych (Counselling)
Lecturer in Nursing, School of Nursing, Deakin University, Vic

Moya Conrick (dec), RN, RM, PhD, MC1Ed, BN, DipAppSc
Formerly Lecturer, School of Nursing,
Griffith University, Brisbane, Qld

Claudio Dellore, RPN, RN, BAppSc (Nurse Ed & Admin), GradDip (Nursing)
Quality Manager, Residential Care,
Ballarat Health Services, Ballarat, Vic

Toni Dowd, PhD, MSc, GradDipEdSt, BA, RN, Paediatric Nurs Cert
Visiting Fellow, School of Nursing, Queensland University of Technology, Qld

Anne-Katrin Eckermann, BA(Hons), MA, PhD(Anthropology)
Honorary Research Fellow, Centre for Research in Aboriginal and Multicultural Studies, University of New England, NSW

Laurel Eddy, Dip App Sci(Nursing), BN (Mid), Grad Dip CHN
Nurse Unit Manager, Benalla Home Nursing Service, Vic

Carolyn Elwin, RN, HV, MHSc (Nurse Education)
Nurse Educator, Central Coast Health,
Conjoint Senior Lecturer, Faculty of Health,
The University of Newcastle, Newcastle, NSW

Rita Funnell, BHlthSci (Nursing), MA (Health Science), RPN, Grad Cert Tert Ed, Grad Cert Oncological Nursing
Deputy Head of School, School of Nursing & Midwifery, Victoria University, Vic

Susan Gallagher, RN, RPN, RMRN, DipTeach (Nursing) BEd, MA (Ed), MRCNA, MACMHN
Senior Lecturer, School of Nursing (NSW & ACT), Faculty of Health Sciences, Australian Catholic University

Debra Griffiths, RN (Div 1), BA, LLB, LLM Legal Practitioner
Senior Lecturer, Faculty of Medicine, Nursing & Health Sciences,
Monash University, Vic

Melissa Heath, RN, Grad Cert Crit Care, BComm (Nursing, Management), Dip VET
Lecturer, Nursing, Gordon Institute of TAFE, Vic

Brigid Holroyd, MA (Education and Work) Grad Dip Educational Studies (Special Ed) Grad Cert Wound Management, RN, CM
Head Teacher, Nursing Studies, Ultimo College, Sydney Institute, TAFE, NSW

Finbar Hopkins, BHlth (Sciences) Nursing, RN, RM, RMHN Grad Dip Women's Health, MA (Women's Studies)
Course Coordinator, Bachelor of Nursing, Bachelor of Nursing/Arts, Honours, Australian Catholic University, Melbourne, Vic

Gabrielle Koutoukidis, Dip App Sci (Nurs), BNurs (Mid), Adv Dip Nurs (Ed), MPH
Teaching Centre Manager, Health Science and Biotechnology Department, Holmesglen, Vic

Gina Kruger, Master (Nursing); Grad Dip Clin Nurs Prac & Mgt (Adv Mid), Cert Mid, RN
Midwifery Lecturer, School of Nursing & Midwifery, Victoria University, Vic

Karen Lawrence, RN, BA HlthSc (Nurs), GradDip (Mid), MA (HlthSc), GradDip VET
Lecturer: Acute Care, School of Nursing & Midwifery, Victoria University, Vic

Sarah Mott, RN, RMHN, BAppSc, PhD, FRCNA, FAAG, AFCHSE, CHE
State Director, Australian College of Health Service Executives (ACHSE) NSW Branch, NSW

Allan Munro, MEd, BN, RN
Nurse Educator — Centre for Nursing and Health Education,
Ballarat Health Services, Ballarat, Vic

Nichole Orwin, Bachelor Applied Sciences, Graduate Diploma Gerontology
Private Consultant

Jenny Pitkin, RN, RM, DipAppSci (NEd), GradCertVET
Lecturer, Social and Community Studies Department, Victoria University, Melbourne, Vic

Caryl Robson, RN, BAppScAdvNsg (Nurse Ed), MEd, Cert IV in Training and Assessment
Education Consultant, Private Registered Training Organisation (RTO), Vic

Dorothy Rogers, RN, RPN, BA Hlth Sci (Nursing), CRRN, GradDipAdmin (Health), MNS
Director of Nursing — Queen Elizabeth Centre, Ballarat Health Services, Vic

Kerry Ryan, BaNsg, MA Nsg, Phd, Grad Cert Palliative Care, Grad Cert Tert Ed,
Cert IV WPAT, Recipient Bethlehem Griffiths Research Award
Senior Program Manager, School of Health, Victoria University, Vic

Sue Ryan, RN, DipAppSc (Nsg), GradDipNursingStudies (Education)
Nurse Education, Ballarat Health Services, Ballarat, Vic

Helen Sarah, RN,RM, BA, Dip Vet, Cert IV in Frontline Management
Nurse Educator, Gordon Institute of TAFE, Vic

Patricia A Sinasac, RN, BN, Adv-Dip Nurs (Ed), Grad Cert Stomal Therapy
Clinical Nurse Consultant, Stomal Therapy

Subatra Sivamalai, RN, MA Education, Grad Dip Health Science (Education)
Midwifery, Health Visitor Cert, Cert IV in Asses & Workplace Training
Co-ordinator of International/Gerontic Programs, Centre for Nursing and Health Education,
Ballarat Health Services, Vic

Sundram Sivamalai, PhD MNA BSc(Hons) DipEd RGN
Senior Lecturer, Co-ordinator — Rural Health Module,
School of Rural Health,
The University of Melbourne, Vic

Kathryn Stainton, Dip AppSc (Nursing), BN (Mid), GradDipNurs(Education), MA Hlth Sc (Nursing)
Private Consultant

Virginia Stanley, RN, CCN, BN, MHM, DipVet
Nurse Teacher, School of Applied Science,
Gordon Institute of TAFE, Vic

Michele Taylor, B Hlth Sci (Nursing), Cert IV Workplace Training & Assessment
Clinical Nurse Consultant

Jill Teschendorff, RN, RM, BAppSc, MA Hlth Sc, Cert Massage
Retired; Formerly Associated Professor of Nursing, School of Nursing & Midwifery, Victoria University, Melbourne, Vic

Adriana Tiziani, BSc (Monash), DipEd (Melbourne), M.Ed.St.(Monash), RN
Course Director, Post Graduate Studies in Wound Care,
Monash University (Parkville) Vic

Denise Tomaras, BA (Psych), DipAppSc (Orthoptics), DipEd, RN, PostGradCert (CCU)
Tender Living Care (Vic) Pty Ltd, Vic

Elizabeth Trainor, Dip Ap Sci (Nursing), Critical Care Cert, Renal Cert,
Bachelor of Educational Studies, Graduate Diploma in Nursing (Renal)
Private Consultant

Stuart Tyler, BHlthSci (Nursing), Grad Cert Tert Ed, Grad Cert Assess & Training
Acting Program Manager, School of Health, Victoria University, Vic

Sharon Ward, BHSc, PostgradDipAdvClinN (ICU) PostgradDip Midwifery
Associate Nurse Unit Manager Anaesthetics/Post Anaesthetic Care Unit,
Mercy Hospital for Women, Heidelberg, Vic

FOREWORD

This fifth edition of *Tabbner's Nursing Care* is a vital publication, particularly with the release of the HLTO7 Health Training Package, which now includes the courses leading to Enrolled Nurse qualifications in all Australian states and territories. It provides the necessary underpinning knowledge required for Enrolled Nurses from the Certificate IV and Diploma through to that required for the Advanced Diploma. It also supports the Australian Nursing and Midwifery Council (ANMC) Enrolled Nurse Competency Standards (2002) which are embedded in the course.

Over the years, to this point in time, Enrolled Nurse courses across the country have been 'ad hoc' at best. However, today we finally have a nationally accredited and recognised course for the Enrolled Nurse with a career pathway within nursing that is transportable across all health care sectors.

It is my belief this publication will greatly assist nurse educators in the delivery of a quality course for the Enrolled Nurse and play a vital role in producing a professional and highly competent Enrolled Nurse from beginning through to an advanced-practice Enrolled Nurse. At the same time it is envisaged it will lend credence, nationally and internationally, to the importance of the second-level nurse (however titled) in meeting today's ever-changing health care needs in collaboration with other sectors of nursing.

In writing the previous edition of *Tabbner's Nursing Care*, three Australian nurse educators, Rita, Gabrielle and Karen, had the courage to continue the work commenced by Nurse Ray Tabbner. Back in 1981, Nurse Tabbner recognised that second-level nurses needed enhanced educational tools to better prepare them to make their contribution to nursing.

I humbly accepted the invitation to pen this foreword in the belief that this fifth edition will provide the necessary education for Enrolled Nurses from entry to practice through to advanced practice. It is wonderful to see Nurse Ray Tabbner's work continued today and I congratulate the authors and editors of this edition.

Maryanne Craker
Secretary
National Enrolled Nurse Association

PUBLISHER'S DEDICATION

Alice Ray Tabbner
25 December 1919–13 December 1994
Ray (as she preferred to be known) Tabbner was born in Birmingham, England. After working in the St John Ambulance in World War II where she said she 'became engrossed in nursing', she completed her training as a nurse in the 1940s. She moved to Australia in 1948 and worked in a number of Sydney hospitals before settling in Melbourne.

Ray established a career in nursing education in 1953 taking on the role of Tutor at the recently established Melbourne School of Nursing. In 1954 she successfully completed her Sister Tutors Diploma through the College of Nursing Australia and remained a Tutor at the school until 1961 when she was awarded the Inaugural Nurse Scholarship in Geriatrics from Mount Royal Hospital. In consequence of receiving this award, Ray was appointed to the position of Deputy Matron of Geriatric Nursing at Mount Royal. She later established the Nursing Aides course at the Fairfield Hospital in Melbourne under the leadership of Vivian Bulwinkel, and in 1973 was appointed Deputy Director Nursing (Education), one of three executive positions at the Royal Melbourne Hospital.

An innovative educator and mentor, Ray Tabbner was one of the first nurses to call for the establishment of 'Nurse Banks' in Australia to ensure flexibility in the nursing workforce for those nurses wishing to pursue family or other interests while pursuing their chosen profession. She was also a great advocate of ongoing training to ensure nurses could maintain flexibility in their lives and return to nursing with confidence.

In 1975 she was appointed Principal Teacher at the Melbourne Nursing Aides School (later renamed Melbourne School for Enrolled Nurses), a position she occupied until 1978 when she retired to write. Originally entitled *The Handbook for Nursing Aides*, it was later renamed *Nursing Care: Theory & Practice*, and since the publication of the first edition in 1981, it has become known and loved by generations of nursing students as simply *Tabbner's*.

An article published in 1973 in the Melbourne *Sun* described her as being 'as flighty as your average banker. Her dark hair has streaks of steel grey and the creases in her dazzlingly white nurse's uniform would slice bread'. However, students from the 50s to the 70s remember her with great fondness and warmth. Ray Tabbner was said to be very approachable and a welcome relief from many 'military style' nurse educators. She taught everything from Anatomy & Physiology to Bandaging and Nursing Care and made a great impression on her students. As one student from 1955 put it, 'Everything Miss Tabbner said, I learned'.

The Tabbner name has become synonymous with Enrolled Nurse/Registered Nurse Division 2 education not only throughout Australia — the influence of her name extends via this publication to New Zealand, the United Kingdom, the Middle East, Africa and the West Indies.

The fifth edition of *Tabbner's Nursing Care* is dedicated to her memory and her contribution to nurse education.

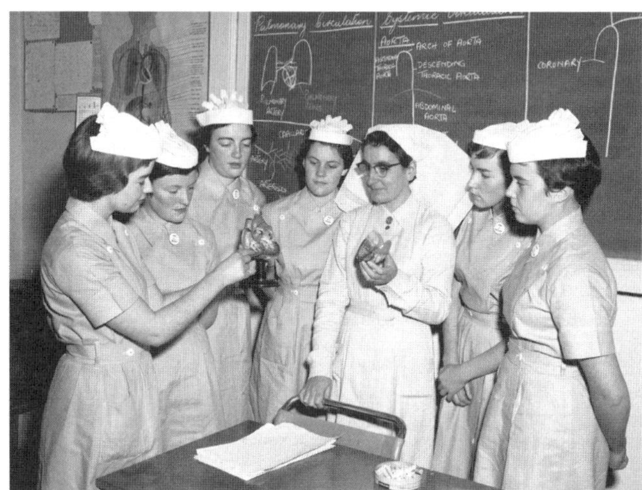

PREFACE

As the editors, we are very grateful for the enthusiastic response we had to *Tabbner's Nursing Care 4E*. We have kept the features that made it an essential resource for Enrolled Nursing students and their facilitators, such as its concise approach, language and format that are easily understood by beginning nursing students.

Tabbner's Nursing Care 5E has been thoroughly revised and builds on the strengths of the 4th edition, reflecting the changes, challenges and expansion of responsibilities in contemporary Enrolled Nurse practice. This edition is again characterised by a wellness model of nursing care. Chapters have been rationalised to ensure a logical sequencing of information and to reflect a more holistic approach to client care.

The Enrolled Nurse is a vital member of the health care team, providing client-centred nursing care which includes recognising what is normal and abnormal in assessing, intervening and evaluating individual health and functional status. Enrolled Nurses' responsibilities also include providing support and comfort, assisting with activities of daily living to enable clients to achieve their optimal level of independence, and providing for the emotional needs of clients. Where state and territory law and organisational policies allow, Enrolled Nurses may administer prescribed medicines or maintain intravenous fluids, in accordance with their educational preparation.

Enrolled Nurses are required to be information-technology literate, with specific skills in the application of health care technology. Enrolled Nurses demonstrate critical and reflective thinking skills in contributing to decision making, which includes reporting changes in health and functional status and individual client responses to health care interventions. Enrolled Nurses work as part of the health care team to advocate for and facilitate the involvement of clients, their families and significant others in planning and evaluating care and progress toward health outcomes (www.anmc.org.au). The role also requires them to act as preceptors for students and other health care workers.

Career opportunities for Enrolled Nurses are expanding and include: acute care; perioperative, emergency, intensive and coronary care; aged care; rehabilitation; community and mental health nursing, and general practice settings. In addition, Enrolled Nurses work in specialty areas such as nursing education, diabetes education, continence management, dementia management, workplace safety and wound care. There are also increasing opportunities for Enrolled Nurses to move into management positions. The following new topics have been included in this latest edition to reflect these changes:

1. National decision-making framework
2. Insertion, care and removal of indwelling catheters
3. Insertion, care and removal of nasogastric tubes
4. Venipuncture
5. Recording of an ECG
6. Tracheostomy care
7. Management of intravenous fluids and blood transfusions
8. Care of the orthopaedic client.

There is no single section dedicated to nursing older clients — rather a lifespan approach has been taken with specific care issues for older people incorporated throughout the text and in clinical interest boxes.

It should be noted that no sexism or gender-specific incidence of occupation or disease is implied by the use of pronouns relating to health care professionals, clients or others in the text. The terms 'client', 'person' and 'individual' are used interchangeably. The term 'Enrolled Nurse' is used throughout the text and is the equivalent of a Division 2 Nurse in Victoria.

SPECIAL FEATURES

The 5th edition has been carefully developed to align with the Certificate IV in Nursing and Diploma of Nursing in the HLT07 National Health Training Package for the Enrolled Nursing student. It provides a contemporary approach to nursing practice and will be an invaluable teaching resource. The text provides the theoretical knowledge on the care that clients may require in a range of health care settings and offers special features to enhance student learning of the material.

All chapters begin with:

- **Objectives** — a list of learning objectives to help the student focus on the key information in the chapter content
- **Key terms/concepts** — listed on the title page of each chapter and defined within the text
- Lived experience — vignettes taken from actual clinical situations, which can help the student understand a particular health experience from the point of view of clients, their families or nurses and other health professionals.

Each chapter ends with:

- **Review exercises** — a series of questions to test the

student's comprehension and reinforce the chapter content
- **Critical thinking exercises** — questions to stimulate the student to think critically and to solve problems
- **References and further reading** — the text is referenced to the literature and this section includes additional resource material for students with a particular interest in the chapter topic
- **Online resources** — a list of useful web links related to the chapter content.

Other features found throughout the text include:
- **Clinical interest boxes** — these include information on developmental considerations, cultural aspects of care, current research, client teaching, case studies, nursing care plans and nursing diagnoses
- **Procedural guidelines** — tables that provide a step-by-step format emphasising the use of the nursing process and including rationales for each step
- **Photographs and illustrations** — included throughout each chapter to provide clear and meaningful visual aids.

The following helpful ancillary information is provided in the appendices:
1. Standard steps for all nursing procedures
2. Units of measurement
3. Table of normal values
4. Commonly used abbreviations
5. Drug calculations.

ONLINE LEARNING SUPPLEMENTS

The 5th edition Evolve website is available at http://evolve.elsevier.com/AU/Funnell/Tabbner/ and features the following invaluable learning aids:

Instructor only

- Test bank — multiple choice questions with rationales for all chapters

Student

- Appendices
- Clinical interest boxes
- Critical thinking questions
- Image bank
- Review questions
- Web links

The redevelopment of this textbook has been an amazing journey for all of us involved in the process. It is a result of the efforts of many nursing professionals who are passionate about the education of Enrolled Nurses and the important role they play in health care settings. We appreciate their enthusiasm and support throughout the process.

Rita Funnell
Gabrielle Koutoukidis
Karen Lawrence

DEDICATIONS

To my husband, John, for his tolerance and support, to my friends and family for their interest and motivating enthusiasm, and to the team of authors and especially my co-editors with whom I have thoroughly enjoyed working.

Rita Funnell

'Let us be grateful to people who make us happy; they are the charming gardeners who make our souls blossom' — *Marcel Proust*
To my family and friends who have given me much love, support and encouragement thoughout the development of this textbook.

To the nursing students who inspired in me a passion for teaching best nursing practice.
To Rita and Karen — what a great team we make!

Gabby Koutoukidis

To my husband Gary and children Emma, Megan and Patrick — without their support, my participation in the development of this book would not have been possible.
To the co-editors, authors and the experienced team at Elsevier for all their knowledge and patience.
To the nursing students and staff at Victoria University for giving me the motivation and desire to work on something I feel so passionately about — nursing.

Karen Lawrence

STANDARD STEPS FOR NURSING PROCEDURES

REFER ALSO TO APPENDIX 1

AT THE BEGINNING OF THE PROCEDURE

- Check the order in the chart, client's nursing/medical history
- Wash your hands
- Check the client's identification
- Explain the procedure to the client
- Provide privacy
- Raise the bed to appropriate height

DURING THE PROCEDURE

- Wash hands
- Put on gloves following standard precautions
- Place on eyewear, mask and gown as appropriate
- Mentally review the step of the procedure beforehand
- Discuss the procedure with your instructor, if required
- Confirm correct facility protocols

AT THE END OF THE PROCEDURE

- Dispose of sharps appropriately
- Remove gloves and wash hands
- Make the client comfortable and inform them of how the procedure went, or of any results/values
- Restore the bed height and unit. Wash hands again
- Record and document the procedure
- Report abnormalities as required

From deWit, *Fundamental Concepts and Skills for Nursing*. Saunders, 2005; reproduced with permission.

Unit 1

The evolution of nursing

Chapter 1

NURSING: HISTORICAL, PRESENT AND FUTURE PERSPECTIVES

OBJECTIVES

- Define the key terms/concepts
- Discuss the historical development of nursing
- Explain the differences in the educational preparation of Registered Nurses (RNs) and Enrolled Nurses (ENs)
- List the four domains of Australian EN practice
- List the five characteristics of a profession and discuss how nursing demonstrates these characteristics
- Discuss the reasons nursing is in a constant state of change

KEY TERMS/CONCEPTS

Australian and New Zealand College of Mental Health Nurses Inc (ANZCMHN)
Australian Nursing and Midwifery Council (ANMC)
Australian Nursing Federation (ANF)
competency standards
Enrolled Nurse (EN)
International Council of Nurses (ICN)
National Enrolled Nurse Association (NENA)
New Zealand Nurses Organisation (NZNO)
Registered Nurse (RN)
Royal College of Nursing, Australia (RCNA)

CHAPTER FOCUS

To understand contemporary issues in nursing the student nurse needs to understand how nursing has evolved in Australia and New Zealand. This chapter includes a discussion of the history of nursing, factors influencing nursing practice, the role of the nurse in contemporary health care and professional nursing organisations. This chapter will help the student to understand and appreciate the influences of the past, present and future on modern nursing.

LIVED EXPERIENCE

Nurses these days don't look like nurses anymore. In my days we had our starched uniform with aprons, caps with colour-coded stripes to denote our status, black tights and shoes. These days most nurses wear casual slacks and blouses. They certainly look comfortable and practical but I was proud of my uniform and what it meant.

Agnes, age 70, a nurse during the 1950s

WHAT IS NURSING?

Nursing is an art and a science with a unique body of knowledge that draws from the social, the behavioural and the physical sciences. Nursing is a unique profession because it addresses responses of individuals and families to health promotion, health maintenance and health problems. There are many philosophies and definitions of nursing. Florence Nightingale defined nursing over 100 years ago as 'the act of utilising the environment of the patient to assist him in his recovery'. Nightingale considered a clean, well-ventilated and quiet environment essential for recovery. Often considered the first nurse theorist, Nightingale raised the status of nursing through education. Nurses were no longer untrained housekeepers but people educated in the care of the sick (Berman et al 2008).

Virginia Henderson was one of the first modern nurses to define nursing. The definition she posed in 1966 was adopted by the International Council of Nurses (ICN) in 1973 and still holds wide appeal to the nursing profession. Henderson defined nursing as:

> assisting the individual, sick or well, in the performance of those activities contributing to health, its recovery, promoting quality of life or to a peaceful death that the client would perform unaided if he or she had the necessary strength, will or knowledge.
>
> (Crisp & Taylor 2005: 2)

The ICN definition of nursing is now:

> Nursing encompasses autonomous and collaborative care of individuals of all ages, families, groups and communities, sick or well, and in all settings. Nursing includes the promotion of health, prevention of illness, and the care of the ill, disabled and dying people. Advocacy, promotion of a safe environment, research, participation in shaping health policy and in patient and health systems management, and education are also key nursing roles.
>
> (Brown & Edwards 2008)

Nursing also helps individuals carry out prescribed therapy, to be independent of assistance, and function to maximum potential as soon as possible (Crisp & Taylor 2005).

There are themes that are common to the many definitions of nursing (Berman et al 2008):

- nursing is caring
- nursing is an art
- nursing is a science
- nursing is client centred
- nursing is holistic
- nursing is adaptive
- nursing is concerned with health promotion, health maintenance and health restoration
- nursing is a helping profession.

In nursing, a combination of technical skill, clinical experience and theoretical knowledge is required. Historically there has been a tendency for nursing education to focus on the mastery of nursing skills. However, nursing practice is far more complex than technical skills alone. Nursing expertise is required for interpreting clinical situations and for complex decision making. It is the basis for the advancement of nursing practice and the development of nursing science. When providing nursing care, the nurse makes clinical judgments about the care needed for clients based on fact, experience and standards of care. Knowledge, expertise and lifelong learning are gained through the continual process of critical thinking (Crisp & Taylor 2005) (see Chapter 18).

RECIPIENTS OF NURSING

The recipients of nursing are sometimes called consumers, patients or clients. A consumer is defined as an individual, a group of people or a community that uses a service or commodity. Individuals who use health care products or services are consumers of health care. A patient is a person who is waiting for or undergoing medical treatment and care. Usually, people become patients when they seek assistance because of illness or for surgery. Some nurses believe that the term 'patient' implies passive acceptance of the decisions and care of health professionals, and nurses are now increasingly using the term 'client' to refer to recipients of health care. A client is a person who engages the advice or services of another who is qualified to provide this service. The health status of a client is the responsibility of the individual in collaboration with health professionals (Berman et al 2008).

HISTORICAL PERSPECTIVES

A brief history of nursing

Historical accounts of nursing reflect the dynamic and evolving nature of the profession. The word 'nurse' is derived from a Latin word meaning to nourish or cherish, and, as birth, illness, injury and death are common to all human beings, there has always been a need for someone to take on the task of caring for others. In earlier times superstition and witchcraft formed the basis of the treatment of illness, and for many centuries it was believed that sickness was a punishment for wrongdoing and that the signs of illness were evidence of the presence of evil spirits. Treatment was prescribed by witch doctors and priests and, although much of it was barbaric and caused more suffering than the illness, many old herbal remedies are still used in a modified form today. Until well into the 18th century those who suffered a mental illness were considered to be possessed by the devil and were treated with extreme cruelty.

Some of the earliest organised nursing was performed by men who staffed the hospitals founded by military religious orders during the crusades; for example, the Knights of St John of Jerusalem, the Teutonic Knights and the Knights of St Lazarus. During the 12th and 13th centuries several secular orders were active in caring for the sick, whose members included men and women. Some of the orders were the Ursulines, the Poor Clares, the Beguines and the Benedictines. Also at this time a religious order, called the Augustinian Sisters of the Hôtel Dieu, was founded in

Paris, which is the world's oldest order of nuns devoted purely to nursing.

During the 16th century, Henry VIII ordered the dissolution of the English monasteries and the confiscation of their property and enormous wealth. This meant that large numbers of sick and destitute people previously cared for by the religious orders were left to die. Workhouses were built to house the poor, many of who were sick. They lived in appalling conditions and were required to work in return for the accommodation provided. Finally, conditions in the city of London became so dreadful that Henry VIII was forced to allow hospitals such as St Bartholomew's, St Thomas's and St Mary's to be re-founded, and others to be established, after many petitions from the people of London. The hospitals were badly staffed by untrained workers, many of who were of very poor character. Patients were housed in dreary, grossly overcrowded wards.

The period from the beginning of the 18th century to the middle of the 19th century has been termed the 'Dark Ages' of nursing, during which the care of the sick and the status of the nurse reached the lowest level imaginable. The squalid conditions in hospitals and the undesirable character of those attending the sick were publicised by people such as the prison reformers, John Howard and Elizabeth Fry, and the writer, Charles Dickens, who in *Martin Chuzzlewit* created the unsavoury characters Sairy Gamp and Betsy Prig to typify the nurses of the time — criminals and women of low moral standards, uneducated and who lived and worked in appalling conditions.

In 1836, with the help of his wife a Lutheran clergyman named Theodor Fliedner established an institution called Kaiserwerth, situated near Dusseldorf in Germany. There they trained carefully selected women as deaconesses, and Kaiserwerth became famous for the high standard of training and the quality of care given to the sick. It became the centre of nurse training and received many trainees from overseas countries, some of who set up similar institutions in their own countries.

Modern nursing has evolved as a result of the influence that Kaiserwerth had on people like Elizabeth Fry, who founded the Protestant Sisters of Charity in an attempt to ensure that the sick were cared for by women of good reputation, such as Agnes Jones. Jones revolutionised conditions in the workhouses and established a school of nursing to train nurses in the care of sick people in the workhouses, and Florence Nightingale, the founder of modern nursing.

Florence Nightingale was born in 1820 during a trip made by her English parents to the Italian city of Florence, after which she was named. Her parents were wealthy and cultured and Florence received an extensive education far beyond the standard usually received by the young women of her time. She travelled widely and led the full social life common to one in her place in society but, despite this, felt unhappy and dissatisfied. She was interested in nursing but this met with strong opposition from her family and it was not until she was over 30 years of age that she was able to realise her ambition. In 1850 she spent 2 weeks at Kaiserwerth and visited again in 1851, when she was appointed as Superintendent of the 'Establishment for Gentlewomen During Illness'.

Florence Nightingale first achieved fame when, in 1854, she was asked to take a party of 38 nurses to Scutari in the Crimea. On arrival the nurses met with fierce opposition from the medical officers, who would not allow them to care for the sick and injured soldiers. Nightingale devoted her energies to improving the filthy conditions by introducing the principles of personal and communal hygiene, obtaining medical supplies, organising a good food supply, and generally establishing sanitary conditions, such as hand washing, and the importance of fresh air. Within 2–3 weeks opposition had been overcome and the nurses were invited to take over the care of the sick. To the soldiers, Nightingale became an idol and, as she brought ease and comfort to the very sick by the light of the lamp she carried at night, she became known as the 'Lady of the Lamp'.

After the Crimean War the English public raised almost £50 000 as a mark of appreciation of Nightingale's work. She used the money to establish a School of Nursing at St Thomas's Hospital in London. The first probationer nurses were admitted to the Nightingale School in June 1860 and given 1 year of training followed by 2 years of experience in the hospital. Many of these nurses became Matrons of the large hospitals in London and elsewhere. By the time Florence Nightingale died in 1910 at the age of 90, remarkable progress had been made in nursing service and education of the nurse.

HISTORY OF NURSING IN AUSTRALIA

The history of nursing in Australia is inextricably linked to our penal past. In the establishment of the original English colony at Sydney Cove, little attention was paid to the provision of care for the ill and infirm. When Sydney Hospital was opened in 1811, most nurses were convict women, with some convict men also performing nursing duties. They were provided with their keep but no wages in exchange for their labour. The nurses were frequently described as being of poor character, with drunkenness while on duty common. The first Australian lunatic asylum was opened at Tarban Creek, in Gladesville NSW, in 1811. Untrained mental attendants staffed the institution. Large numbers of disturbed people were primarily restrained as a means of control. The staff were custodians and there was virtually no emphasis on treatment.

The first trained nurses, five Irish Sisters of Charity, arrived in Sydney in 1838. The Nightingale influence was experienced in 1868, when Lucy Osburn and her four Nightingale nurses arrived. Gradually, the Nightingale principles for the care of the physically ill were adopted. Nurses were trained in practical skills such as the application of dressings, leeching and administering enemas. Of equal importance were the character traits of punctuality, cleanliness, sexual purity and, above all, obedience. A large proportion of nursing work was akin to housekeeping, dominated by domestic tasks. However, it was acknowledged that diligence and compassion were desirable characteristics in those who cared for the sick.

As scientific advances were made the recognition of the need for nursing training grew. By 1900 most of the larger Australian hospitals had three-year training programs for student nurses, with lectures delivered by medical staff. Unfortunately, because of the long hours of work, student nurses were frequently too tired to concentrate during such classes. During the 20th century the move towards professionalism would emerge and with it would come considerable conflict between the view of nursing as a vocation, which should be inherently subordinate to medicine, and the view of nursing as a profession, different from, but of equal status with, medicine.

In 1867 an Act of Parliament was passed that made it mandatory that persons showing signs of mental impairment must be sent to a lunatic asylum rather than a prison. By 1900 the mentally ill were separated from the developmentally disabled. Nursing in the mental asylum continued to be predominantly delivered by male attendants. The care continued to be custodial but medical staff provided some lectures to the attendants. The idea of employing female attendants began to receive serious consideration around this period.

The increase in training for nurses was accompanied by heightened agitation for the registration of nurses. South Australia was the first State to pass the relevant legislation in 1920. Western Australia followed in 1922, New South Wales and Victoria in 1924. The emerging sense of professionalism among nurses led to a greater focus on industrial issues. The Australian Nursing Federation held its first meeting in 1924 and through this forum the quest for greater professional recognition, increased wages and improved working conditions began — a quest that continues today (Crisp & Taylor 2005).

In 1984 the Federal Government announced full support for the transfer of nursing education into the tertiary sector. This occurred over the subsequent decade. The type of tertiary education the nurse receives will determine the level at which the nurse practises. Within Australia, there are broadly two levels of nurse. The Registered Nurse (RN) (in Victoria the term Registered Nurse Division 1 is used) is licensed to practise nursing without supervision in the fields in which they are registered. RNs are regarded as responsible and accountable for all decisions and actions taken in relation to client care. Registration requires the completion of an undergraduate degree in the higher-education or university sector. The course is generally of 3 years' duration but some programs extend over three-and-a-half or 4 years.

The Enrolled Nurse (EN) is a second-level nurse — in Victoria, the term Registered Nurse Division 2 is used. The exact nature of the scope of practice of the EN varies across states and territories, but duties are usually conducted under the direction and supervision of the RN. Entry onto the roll, or register, requires the completion of a certificate, advanced certificate or diploma (depending upon which state or territory the qualification is undertaken in), generally through the Technical and Further Education (TAFE) system or a private registered training organisation (RTO). The duration of these programs varies from 12 months to 2 years.

Traineeship

Australian state and territory governments provide financial assistance to educate ENs through programs that provide both on- and off-the-job education. EN trainees are employed by health care agencies for a period of approximately 2 years. During this time a trainee participates in a mixture of off-the-job education coordinated by an RTO, and on-the-job (workplace) experiences to develop the required competencies for enrolment with their respective state/territory nurses' board. First-level Registered Nurses provide clinical supervision and support for the trainees. RTOs and health care agencies enter written agreements specifying the responsibilities of all parties for the duration of the traineeship.

Clinical Interest Box 1.1 outlines the major milestones in Australia's nursing history.

HISTORY OF NURSING IN NEW ZEALAND

With the passing of the *Nurses Registration Act* on 12 September 1901, New Zealand became the first country to have separate legislation for the registration and regulation of nurses. The designer of the 1901 Act was a nurse, Grace Neill, who was Assistant Inspector of Hospitals. In 1899 she attended the International Council of Women's Conference in London, where nursing registration was discussed. On her return to New Zealand she worked with Dr Duncan MacGregor, the Inspector-General of Hospitals, to draft the *Nurses Registration Act*. The Act came into force in January 1902 and the register was kept by Dr MacGregor. Nurses who had already trained could apply to have their names entered. Others were to sit a State examination. The first name recorded was that of Ellen Dougherty, who had trained at Wellington Hospital in the 1880s. Within 18 months 320 nurses were registered.

The *Nurses and Midwives Registration Act 1925* and the *Nurses and Midwives Act 1945* set up statutory boards to regulate nursing. In addition to keeping the register, they could take disciplinary action against a nurse for serious misconduct. As nursing practice became more specialised, separate registers were established for maternity nurses (1925), nursing aides (1939), psychiatric nurses (1944), male nurses (1945), psychopaedic nurses (1960), community nurses (1965) and comprehensive nurses (1977). In 1977 community nurses became ENs. Midwives had separate registration from 1904 but were regulated by

CLINICAL INTEREST BOX 1.1
Major milestones in Australia's nursing history

Year	Milestone
1811	Sydney Hospital opened, Tarban Creek Asylum opened
1838	Five Irish Sisters of Charity arrived in New South Wales
1848	Opening of Yarra Bend Asylum in the Port Phillip district (later to be known as Melbourne) to enable the transfer of mentally ill prisoners from gaol
1867	Legislation was passed to ensure that mentally ill persons were sent to an asylum rather than gaol
1868	Arrival of Lucy Osburn and four Nightingale nurses. Beginning of the Nightingale influence in Australia
1885	Introduction of district nursing into Australia, based on the model developed in England
1899–1902	The Boer War years. Hundreds of female nurses volunteered but met with prejudice against female nurses in the military. A small number served in South Africa
1900	Completion of the separation of the mentally-ill and the mentally-retarded for the purposes of treatment and care
1901	Introduction of nursing registration in South Australia
1910	The formation of the Victorian Bush Nursing Association. Followed a year later by the NSW Association
1914–1918	2692 Australian nurses served in World War I, 2000 served outside Australia
1922	Introduction of nursing registration in Western Australia
1924	Introduction of nursing registration in New South Wales and Victoria
1924	First meeting of the Australian Nursing Federation held
1939–1945	One third of Australia's trained nurses volunteered for service overseas
1949	Formation of the College of Nursing Australia (now known as Royal College of Nursing, Australia)
1974	First pre-registration tertiary-based course began in Victoria. Formation of the Congress of Mental Health Nurses (now known as the Australian and New Zealand College of Mental Health Nurses)
1978	Release of the document "Goals in Nursing Education" was a joint policy statement of the College of Nursing Australia, The Royal Australian Nursing Federation, the Florence Nightingale Committee and the New South Wales College of Nursing
1979	The Royal Australian Nursing Federation joined the Australian Council of Trade Unions
1980	Formation of the National Florence Nightingale Memorial Committee, to provide postgraduate courses for nurses
1981	The first International Council of Nursing Conference in Australia
1984	The federal government announced full support for the transfer of nursing education into the tertiary sector. The anti-strike clause was removed from the constitution of the RANF
1985	The first nurses' strike in Australia occurred in Victoria
1989	The first pre-registration programs for psychiatric nursing and intellectual disability nursing commenced in the tertiary sector in Victoria
1992	The Australian Nursing and Midwifery Council (ANMC) Inc forms to ensure a national approach to the regulation and practice of nursing
1993	Transfer of basic nursing education to the tertiary sector is complete across Australia. Registered Nurses can now study at graduate diploma, Masters degree and PhD level
1996	National Enrolled Nurse Association (NENA) was formed to: • Provide a voice in the decision making of the EN role • Work towards national consistency in EN curriculum • Increase the awareness, value and profile of ENs • Support local/regional/State groups in pursuing issues
2000	Establishment of the ANMC national competency standards for the Registered Nurse
2001	Memorandum of Cooperation signed, linking the ANMC and the Nursing Council of New Zealand to work closely together on nurse regulatory issues of common interest
2002	Development of a code of ethics for nursing in Australia under the auspices of the ANMC, Australian Nursing Federation and Royal College of Nursing Australia
2002	Establishment of the ANMC national competency standards for the EN
2003	Establishment of nursing and nursing education taskforce to drive major nursing education and workforce reforms in Australia
2003	Development of a code of conduct for nurses in Australia, which states a declared position in relation to the standards of behaviour that can be expected of each nurse
2003	The ANMC and the Nursing Council of New Zealand launched its ground-breaking research project, which will see the development of Competency Standards For Nurse Practitioners in Australia and New Zealand
2006	The ANMC released Competency Standards for Nurse Practitioners

(Continued)

CLINICAL INTEREST BOX 1.1 — cont'd Major milestones in Australia's nursing history	
2006	COAG agreed to the Productivity Commission's recommendation for national registration standards for health professionals
2007	ANMC released 'A national framework for the development of decision-making tools for nursing and midwifery practice'
(Crisp & Taylor 2005; the Australian Nursing and Midwifery Council Inc [www.anmc.org.au]; and the Australian Nursing Federation (1999) The ANF celebrates 75 years. *Australian Nursing Journal* 6(8): 14–21 [anf.org.au/nena])	

the same statutory body as nurses. With the introduction of the *Nurses Act 1971* this body became the Nursing Council of New Zealand. The 1901 Act ushered in a century of control, discipline and regulation but also confirmed nursing's standing as a profession and as a vital part of the health system of a new country.

ROLES AND FUNCTIONS OF THE NURSE

Contemporary nursing requires that the nurse possess knowledge and skills in a variety of areas. In the past the principal role of nurses was to provide care and comfort as they carried out specific nursing functions. Changes in nursing have expanded the role of nurses to include increased emphasis on health promotion and illness prevention, as well as concern for the client as a whole. The contemporary nurse functions in the interrelated roles of caregiver, clinical and ethical decision maker, client advocate, case manager, rehabilitator, comforter, communicator and teacher/educator.

Caregiver

As caregiver the nurse helps the client regain health through the healing process. The nurse addresses the holistic care needs of the client, including measures to restore emotional, spiritual and social wellbeing. The caregiver helps the client and family to set goals and meet those goals with a minimal cost of time and energy (Crisp & Taylor 2005).

Clinical and ethical decision maker

To provide effective care the nurse uses critical-thinking and problem-solving skills throughout the nursing process. In providing care the nurse collaborates with the client and family and other health care professionals (Crisp & Taylor 2005).

Client advocate

In the role of client advocate the nurse protects the client's human and legal rights and provides assistance in asserting those rights if the need arises. The nurse advocates for the client, keeping in mind their religious and cultural differences (Crisp & Taylor 2005).

Case manager

As case manager the nurse coordinates the activities of other members of the health care team, such as social workers, physiotherapists and occupational therapists, when managing client care. The role of the case manager is to review the care being provided to the client, to consult with other health care professionals when their expertise is required, and to prepare the client for discharge (Crisp & Taylor 2005).

Rehabilitator

Rehabilitation is the process by which individuals return to maximal levels of functioning after illness, accidents or other disabling events. Rehabilitative and restorative care activity ranges from teaching clients to walk with crutches to helping clients cope with lifestyle changes often associated with chronic illness (Crisp & Taylor 2005).

Comforter

The role of comforter — caring for the client as a person — is a traditional and historical one in nursing. While carrying out nursing activities, nurses can provide comfort by demonstrating care for the client as an individual with unique feelings and needs.

Communicator

The role of communicator is central to all the other nursing roles. Nursing involves communication with clients, families, others of significance to the client, other nurses and health care professionals, resource persons and the community. Without clear communication it is impossible to give care effectively, make decisions with clients and families, protect clients from threats to wellbeing, coordinate and manage client care, assist the client in rehabilitation, offer comfort or teach (Crisp & Taylor 2005).

Teacher/educator

As a teacher the nurse explains concepts and facts about health to clients, demonstrates procedures such as self-care activities, determines if the client fully understands, reinforces learning or client behaviour and evaluates progress in learning (Crisp & Taylor 2005).

Career roles

Because of the increasing educational opportunities for nurses, the growth of nursing as a profession, and a greater concern for job enrichment, the nursing profession offers expanded roles and a wide range of career opportunities. Examples of career roles include nurse educators, advanced practice nurses; for example, clinical nurse specialists, nurse practitioners, nursing management and administration and nursing researchers (Crisp & Taylor 2005).

THE HEALTH TEAM

In most practice settings the nurse works with other health professionals to provide total care for clients. The health team is spoken of as being multidisciplinary, meaning that it is made up of people with education and expertise in a variety of different aspects of client care. The most important members of the team are the client and others of significance to them, such as their family. The rest of the team, which varies according to the needs of the individual, is made up of medical officers and nurses, physiotherapists, occupational therapists, social workers, speech therapists, dieticians, chaplains, nursing assistant/personal care attendant and other paramedical personnel. Teams may be formed within the team, such as the nursing team or the medical team, to ensure that complex care plans are adequately carried out.

The success of teamwork in any situation depends on a range of factors including:

- Every member of the team needs to have a true appreciation of the skills and qualities of every other member, and of the interrelationships of all team members
- There must be a common goal, and all team members should be involved in planning the methods to be used to achieve that goal
- Good communications are essential so that every person is aware of their role and is aware of any changes that occur
- The team leader is important and is responsible for coordinating the efforts of individual members of the team and for organising regular reviews of progress.

Because nurses have the greatest opportunity to interact with all the other professionals in the health care team, they often have the role of coordinating and integrating services within a managed care system.

THE REGISTERED NURSE (RN)

The RN demonstrates competence in the provision of nursing care as specified by the registering authority's licence to practice, educational preparation, relevant legislation, standards and codes, and context of care. The RN practices independently and interdependently assuming accountability and responsibility for their own actions and delegation of care to ENs and health care workers. The role of the RN includes promotion and maintenance of health and prevention of illness for individual/s with physical or mental illness, disabilities and/or rehabilitation needs as well as alleviation of pain and suffering at the end stage of life.

The RN assesses, plans, implements and evaluates nursing care in collaboration with individual/s and the multidisciplinary health care team so as to achieve goals and health outcomes. The RN takes a leadership role in the coordination of nursing and health care within and across different care contexts to facilitate optimal health outcomes. This includes appropriate referral to, and consultation with, other relevant health professionals, service providers and community support services.

The RN also contributes to quality health care through lifelong learning and professional development of herself/himself and others, research data generation, clinical supervision and development of policy and clinical practice guidelines (ANMC 2006). Clinical Interest Box 1.2 lists the settings that RNs and ENs are working in.

THE ENROLLED NURSE (EN)

The EN is an associate to the RN and must demonstrate educational preparation and competence in the provision of client-centred care, as specified by the registering authority's licence to practise. EN practice requires the EN to work under the direction and supervision of the RN, as stipulated by the relevant nurse registering authority. At all times ENs retain responsibility for their actions and remain accountable in providing delegated nursing care.

EN responsibilities in the provision of client-centred nursing care include recognising what is normal and abnormal in assessing, intervening and evaluating individual health and functional status. The EN monitors the impact of nursing care and maintains ongoing communication with the RN regarding the health and functional status of clients. ENs' responsibilities also include providing support and comfort, assisting with activities of daily living to enable clients to achieve their optimal level of independence and providing for emotional needs of clients. Where state/territory law and organisational policy allows, ENs may administer prescribed medicines or maintain intravenous fluids, in accordance with their educational preparation. Whereas ENs traditionally worked in the field of aged care, they are now prepared for practice in acute care, mental health, rehabilitation and community nursing.

ENs are required to be information-technology literate, with specific skills in the application of health care technology. ENs demonstrate critical and reflective thinking skills in contributing to decision making, which includes

CLINICAL INTEREST BOX 1.2
Areas of clinical practice for registered and enrolled nurses

In Australia in 2003, nursing workplaces/settings were listed in the following way by the Australian Institute of Health and Welfare (AIHW): hospital (including psychiatric hospital), residential aged care service, community health centre, rural hospital and health service/multipurpose service, doctors' rooms/medical practice, day procedure centre, mental health facility, tertiary education institution, development disability service, school, hospice, and other, which would include industry and private home care.

(Brown & Edwards 2008)

reporting changes in health and functional status and individual client responses to health care interventions. ENs work as a part of the health care team to advocate for and facilitate the involvement of clients, their families and others of significance to clients in planning and evaluating care and progress towards health outcomes (www.anmc.org.au).

NURSING PRACTICE — AUSTRALIAN NURSING AND MIDWIFERY COUNCIL COMPETENCIES FOR THE EN

To ensure that nurses continue to practise at a high standard that ensures safety of the public, the Australian Nursing and Midwifery Council (ANMC) developed the National Competency Standards for the Registered Nurse (1998) (www.anmc.org.au) and reviewed the National Competency Standards for the Enrolled Nurse in 2002 (www.anmc.org.au). Standards of nursing practice are developed and established from a basis of strong scientific research and the advice of clinical experts. Standards of nursing practice serve as objective guidelines for the provision of nursing care and as a means to evaluate that care. They provide a method to ensure that clients receive high-quality individualised care, to ensure that nurses know what is necessary to provide expert nursing care and to ensure that measures are in place to determine that the care meets specific standards.

Educational institutions can recommend students for registration only if they have demonstrated the required competencies. After registration or enrolment it becomes the responsibility of the individual nurse to ensure that this level of competency is maintained. It is the responsibility of the employing health facility to provide continuing education to ensure that competency standards are not only maintained but further developed (Crisp & Taylor 2005). The responsibilities included in the competency standards are illustrative of the types of core activities that an EN would be expected to undertake on entry to practice. All ENs have a responsibility for ongoing professional development to maintain an up-to-date knowledge base and skill level.

The *Competency Standards* document (2002) (www.anmc.org.au) was developed to reflect four domains of EN practice: professional and ethical practice, critical thinking and analysis, management of care and enabling. There are 10 competencies and each competency contains several elements. The elements enable measurement of whether or not the competency has been attained by an EN on entry to practice. Clinical Interest Box 1.3 outlines these 10 competencies.

Doctor Patricia Benner's seminal research, *From Novice to Expert*, explores how nurses progress in the development of expertise to explain the domains of nursing practice. Clinical Interest Box 1.4 outlines the development of nursing expertise.

SCOPE OF PRACTICE

The ANMC in April 2007 released 'A national framework for the development of decision-making tools for nursing and midwifery practice' (www.anmc.org.au). Figure 1.1 is the ANMC *Nursing Practice Decision Flowchart.* According to the ANMC, the scope of practice of an individual nurse

CLINICAL INTEREST BOX 1.3
ANMC competency standards for the enrolled nurse (2002)

Professional and ethical practice

Competency Unit 1. Functions in accordance with legislation, policies and procedures affecting enrolled nursing practice

Competency elements

1.1 Demonstrates knowledge of legislation and common law pertinent to enrolled nursing practice.
1.2 Demonstrates knowledge of organisational policies and procedures pertinent to enrolled nursing practice.
1.3 Fulfils the duty of care in the course of enrolled nursing practice.
1.4 Acts to ensure safe outcomes for individuals and groups by recognising and reporting the potential for harm.
1.5 Reports practices that may breach legislation, policies and procedures relating to nursing practice to the appropriate person.

Competency Unit 2. Conducts nursing practice in a way that can be ethically justified

Competency elements

2.1 Acts in accordance with the nursing profession's codes.
2.2 Demonstrates an understanding of the implications of these codes for enrolled nursing practice.

Competency Unit 3. Conducts nursing practice in a way that respects the rights of individuals and groups

Competency elements

3.1 Practises in accordance with organisational policies relevant to individual/group rights in the health care context.
3.2 Demonstrates an understanding of the rights of individuals/groups in the health care setting.
3.3 Liaises with others to ensure that the rights of individuals/groups are maintained.
3.4 Demonstrates respect for the values, customs, spiritual beliefs and practices of individuals and groups.
3.5 Liaises with others to ensure that the spiritual, emotional and cultural needs of individuals/groups are met.
3.6 Contributes to the provision of relevant health care information to individuals and groups.

is that which the individual is educated, authorised and competent to perform. To practise within the full scope of practice of the profession may require individuals to update or increase their knowledge, skills or competence. However the actual scope of practice is influenced by the:

- context in which the nurse practises

CLINICAL INTEREST BOX 1.3 — cont'd
ANMC competency standards for the enrolled nurse (2002)

Competency Unit 4. Accepts accountability and responsibility for own actions within enrolled nursing practice
Competency elements
4.1 Recognises own level of competence.
4.2 Recognises the differences in accountability and responsibility between RNs, ENs and unregulated care workers.
4.3 Differentiates the responsibility and accountability of the RN and EN in the delegation of nursing care.

Critical thinking and analysis
Competency Unit 5. Demonstrates critical thinking in the conduct of enrolled nursing practice
Competency elements
5.1 Uses nursing standards to assess own performance.
5.2 Recognises the need for and participates in continuing self/professional development.
5.3 Recognises the need for care of self.

Management of care
Competency Unit 6. Contributes to the formulation of care plans in collaboration with the RN
Competency elements
6.1 Accurately collects and reports data regarding the health and functional status of individuals and groups.
6.2 Participates with the RN and individuals and groups in identifying expected health care outcomes.
6.3 Participates with the RN in evaluation of progress of individuals and groups towards expected outcomes and reformulation of care plans.

Competency Unit 7. Manages nursing care of individuals and groups within the scope of enrolled nursing practice
Competency elements
7.1 Implements planned nursing care to achieve identified outcomes.
7.2 Recognises and reports changes in the health and functional status of individuals/groups to the RN.
7.3 Ensures communication, reporting and documentation are timely and accurate.
7.4 Organises workload to facilitate planned nursing care for individuals and groups.

Enabling
Competency Unit 8. Contributes to the promotion of safety, security and personal integrity of individuals and groups within the scope of enrolled nursing practice
Competency elements
8.1 Acts appropriately to enhance the safety of individuals and groups at all times.
8.2 Establishes, maintains and concludes effective interpersonal communication.
8.3 Applies appropriate strategies to promote the self-esteem of individuals and groups.
8.4 Acts appropriately to maintain the dignity and integrity of individuals and groups.

Competency Unit 9. Provides support and care to individuals and groups within the scope of enrolled nursing practice
Competency elements
9.1 Provides for the comfort needs of individuals and groups experiencing illness or dependence.
9.2 Collaborates with the RN and members of the health care team in the provision of nursing care to individuals and groups experiencing illness or dependence.
9.3 Contributes to the health education of individuals or groups to maintain and promote health.
9.4 Communicates with individuals and groups to enable therapeutic outcomes.

Competency Unit 10. Collaborates with members of the health care team to achieve effective health care outcomes
Competency elements
10.1 Demonstrates an understanding of the role of the EN as a member of the health care team.
10.2 Demonstrates an understanding of the role of members of the health care team in achieving health care outcomes.
10.3 Establishes and maintains collaborative relationships with members of the health care team.
10.4 Contributes to decision-making by members of the health care team.

(Australian Nursing and Midwifery Council Inc 2003, http://www.anmc.org.au)

CLINICAL INTEREST BOX 1.4
Benner's stages of nursing expertise

Stage I. Novice
No experience (nursing student). Performance is limited, inflexible and governed by context-free rules and regulations rather than experience.
Stage II. Advanced beginner
Demonstrates marginally acceptable performance. Recognises the meaningful 'aspects' of a real situation. Has experienced enough real situations to make judgements about them.
Stage III. Competent practitioner
Has 2–3 years' experience. Demonstrates organisational and planning abilities. Differentiates important factors from less important aspects of care. Coordinates multiple complex care demands.
Stage IV. Proficient practitioner
Has 3–5 years' experience. Perceives situations as wholes rather than in terms of parts, as in Stage II. Uses maxims as guides for what to consider in a situation. Has holistic understanding of the client, which improves decision making. Focuses on long-term goals.
Stage V. Expert practitioner
Performance is fluid, flexible and highly proficient. No longer requires rules, guidelines or maxims to connect an understanding of the situation to appropriate action. Demonstrates highly skilled intuitive and analytic ability in new situations. Is inclined to take certain action because 'it felt right'.

(Benner 1984)

- client health needs
- level of competence, education and qualifications of the individual nurse
- policies of the health care service provider
- legislation (Brown & Edwards 2008).

If nursing is responsive to individual, group and community needs for a health care service, then it follows that scope of practice will be relatively fluid in order to accommodate the public need for flexibility and diversity in the provision of nursing services. In order to gauge their scope of practice nurses are required to know the law regulating and relating to nursing practice and to have a realistic appreciation of their knowledge and skills (Brown & Edwards 2008).

NURSING — THE PROFESSION

Nursing is not simply a collection of specific skills, and the nurse is not simply a person trained to perform specific tasks. Nursing is a profession. No one factor absolutely differentiates a job from a profession, but the difference is important in terms of how nurses practise. When a person is said to act professionally, for example, it is implied that the person is conscientious in actions, knowledgeable in the subject and responsible to self and others. Although there is not universal agreement on a definition, a profession is generally expected to include the following characteristics:

- An extended and broad-based education of its members
- A theoretical body of knowledge leading to defined skills, abilities and norms
- The provision of a specific service
- Autonomy in decision making and practice
- The regulation of practice, both legally through legislation, and ethically through a code of ethics for practice.

The claim that nursing is a profession is not entirely unproblematic. The area of autonomy and decision making in practice is particularly controversial, especially in the light of the dependent relationship found at times between nursing and medicine. Five characteristics of a profession are worth consideration in relation to nursing. They are education, theory, service, autonomy and a code of ethics (Crisp & Taylor 2005).

EDUCATION

The education of nurses in Australia depends upon the level to which the nurse aspires. As a first-level nurse, RNs are licensed to practise nursing without supervision in the fields in which they are registered. They are regarded as responsible and accountable for all decisions and actions taken in relation to client care. Registration requires the completion of an undergraduate degree. The EN is a second-level nurse whose duties are performed generally under the direction and supervision of the RN, with entry onto the roll requiring completion of a certificate, advanced certificate or diploma program, generally through the TAFE system. The course for the EN is now contained within the National Health Training Package (2007).

Nursing is a dynamic profession, located within an ever-changing health care system and continuing education programs are essential in enabling nurses to remain current in nursing skills, knowledge, theory, and changes in health care policy and the law. Continuing education is provided in many different forms by health care institutions, educational institutions, professional and industrial bodies and an ever-increasing number of private providers.

THEORY

The practice of professional nursing and development of nursing knowledge has to some extent evolved from nursing theories. Theoretical models serve as frameworks for nursing curricula, clinical practice and research. Nursing theories are an attempt to elucidate the nature of nursing practice, the principles on which practice is based and the proper goals and functions of nursing in society. The development of nursing theory was an essential part of establishing professional status and independence. Nursing theory has clearly demonstrated that nursing, as a profession, shares a common body of knowledge with medicine. However, nursing has a different perspective, namely to care rather than to cure. This perspective provides nursing with its own set of knowledge and theoretical

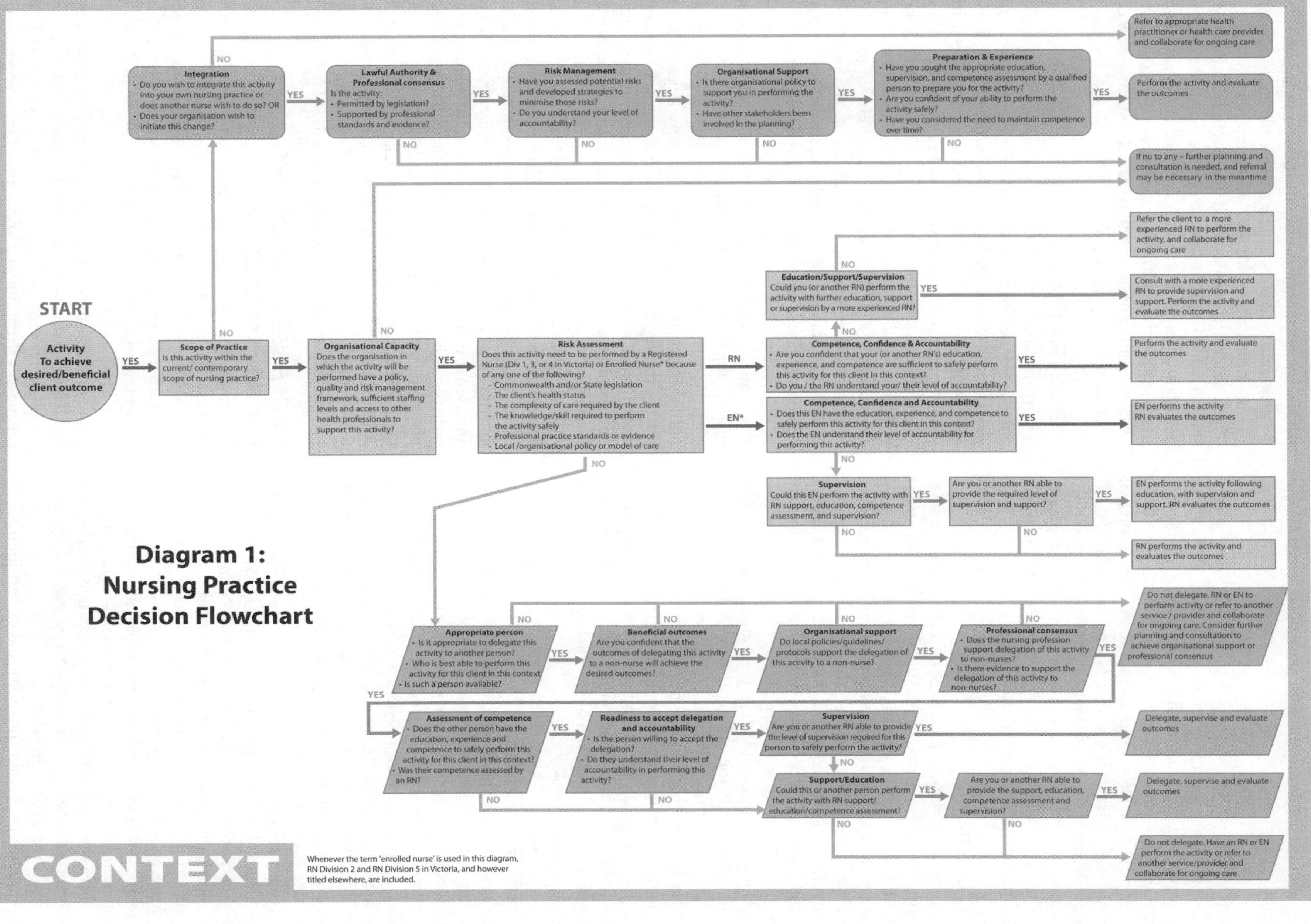

Figure 1.1 | ANMC Nursing Practice Decision Flowchart *(ANMC www.anmc.org.au)*

assumptions. Nursing theories are discussed further in Chapter 2.

SERVICE

Nursing has always been a service profession, although in the past the service was usually viewed as a charitable one largely directed towards the care of the physically ill. Nurses today need to acknowledge and value the importance of nursing care across a broad range of practice settings and with different groups of clientele. Moreover, they need to work with the client and family, individualising care, considering cultural and religious differences and providing support for the entire extended family.

AUTONOMY

Autonomy is an essential element of professional nursing. Autonomy means that a person is reasonably independent and self-governing in decision making and practice. RNs attain increased autonomy through higher levels of education, through clinical competence and in diverse practice settings. RNs are increasingly taking on independent roles in nurse-run clinics, collaborative practice and advanced-nurse practice settings. ENs also have increased autonomy in certain settings; for example, in the aged-care sector and in the community.

All nurses are accountable for the type and quality of nursing care provided. The degree to which nurses are held accountable for their actions reflects the level of education they have received, which in turn informs the degree of responsibility the nurse has in the workplace. The nursing profession regulates accountability through nursing audits and standards of practice.

CODE OF ETHICS

The need for a code of ethics was acknowledged during the Australasian Nurse Registering Authorities Conference (ANRAC) in 1990. Concern was raised that there was no clear focus on ethical behaviour for Australian nurses and that a documented code of ethics would assist in achieving this focus. The ANMC *Code of Ethics for Nurses in Australia* (ANMC 2002) comprise six value statements, each of which is further defined by several explanatory statements. The six value statements are:

1. Nurses respect individuals' needs, values, culture and vulnerability in the provision of nursing care
2. Nurses accept the rights of individuals to make informed choices in relation to their care
3. Nurses promote and uphold the provision of quality nursing care for all people
4. Nurses hold in confidence any information obtained in a professional capacity, use professional judgement where there is a need to share information for the therapeutic benefit and safety of a person and ensure that privacy is safeguarded
5. Nurses fulfil the accountability and responsibility inherent in their roles
6. Nurses value environmental ethics and a social, economic and ecologically sustainable environment that promotes health and wellbeing.

These value statements are deliberately broad to reflect the variety of nursing practice areas, and variation in populations and their health care needs. To address the more specific issues in particular areas of practice, some professional organisations have developed their own code of ethics (www.anmc.org.au).

REGISTRATION

The registration and enrolment of nurses in Australia is governed by the *Nurses Act* or *Health Professionals Registration Act* of each state or territory. In accordance with the Act each state and territory has a statutory authority with a mandate for the regulation of nursing registration. A nurse must be registered or enrolled in each and any state or territory in which they practise. The Australian *Mutual Recognition Act 1992* (Cwlth) was introduced to provide uniformity of registration across Australia. In relation to the nursing profession this Act provides the legislative framework through which a nurse registered or enrolled in one state or territory would, on application, be granted registration in a similar category in any other state or territory without undergoing further testing or examination.

In January 2006, the Australian Productivity Commission published its *Australia's Health Workforce Research Report*. One of the key workforce structure reforms recommended was to 'provide for national registration standards for health professionals and for the creation of a national registration board with supporting professional panels'. The Council of Australian Governments (COAG) agreed to the Productivity Commission's detailed recommendation but also stated that there would be further consultation with stakeholders on COAG's preferred model for the scheme. Plans towards a national regulatory scheme are in train at the time of writing and it is anticipated that the scheme will be in place by 2009. It appears to be emerging that, although there will be a national regulatory scheme, each discipline will still maintain its own regulatory authority, rather than there being one overarching national regulatory authority for all professions (Staunton & Chiarella 2008).

PROFESSIONAL NURSING ORGANISATIONS

The major professional organisation representing nursing in Australia is the Royal College of Nursing, Australia (RCNA). The RCNA has representation on several government committees and health advisory bodies. It is recognised as a key centre of influence in the health policy arena in Australia.

The Australian Nursing Federation (ANF) was established in 1924. It is the national union for nurses and the largest professional organisation in Australia. The ANF's core business is the industrial and professional representation of nurses and nursing through the activities of a national office and branches in every state and territory. ANF has an Enrolled-Nurse special interest group, the National Enrolled Nurse Association (NENA), whose mission is to promote the value of ENs and raise awareness of the EN role within the community. The National Enrolled Nurse Association also provides a forum for all ENs to participate at a national level.

Nurses in New Zealand are represented by the New Zealand Nurses Organisation (NZNO) and the Australian and New Zealand College of Mental Health Nurses Inc (ANZCMHN).

SOCIETAL INFLUENCES ON NURSING

The societal influences on nursing include developments in medical science and technology, which have impacted on the changing role and function of the nurse, and other factors such as demographic changes, cultural diversity and the consumer movement, which have also had an impact on the structure and practice of nursing.

Demographic changes

Changes that have influenced health care in recent decades include the population shift from rural areas to urban centres, increasing life span, the higher incidence of long-term illness, and increased incidence of diseases such as substance use, mental health and cancers. Nursing as a profession responds to such changes by exploring new methods for providing care, by changing educational emphasis and by establishing practice standards in new areas (Crisp & Taylor 2005).

Cultural diversity

Australia and New Zealand are multicultural societies, which means that nurses frequently encounter clients from cultures different from their own. Nurses need to be open to the challenges presented by cultural diversity and seek the information they require to provide culturally sensitive care (Crisp & Taylor 2005).

Consumer movement

The availability of information through sources such as the internet means that consumers are potentially better informed than ever before. The strength of the consumer movement is most evident in the mental health area, where pressure exerted by mental health consumers has led to initiatives such as the employment of consumer consultants within health care networks. The role of the consumer consultant is to provide support and advocacy to consumers receiving mental health services and to influence the development of policy regarding the care and treatment of consumers (Crisp & Taylor 2005).

Human rights movement

Respect for the right of all people to the optimal standard of nursing and health care is central to the philosophy of the nursing profession. This view is reflected in the code of ethics and standards of all nursing professional organisations. Nurses need to be consciously aware of personal values and where they are likely to impact on the quality of care given to a client. Where problems arise, advice or support should be requested (Crisp & Taylor 2005).

SUMMARY

The profession of nursing is in a constant state of change. The evolution of nursing has brought us to the point where there are endless opportunities to improve the health and welfare of our clients and the communities in which we live. The role of the EN and the RN has changed from that of a vocation to a role that emphasises education and professional standards, exemplified by the development of competencies for the EN and the RN and codes of ethics, as well as the national framework for decision making for nursing practice. The role of the EN is expanding and embracing new areas such as technology in health care, the administration of medications (in some Australian states and territories) and wound care procedures. The challenge for the future will be to incorporate these changes into the role of the EN while still maintaining the standards of the profession and to ensure that each nurse understands each other's roles.

REVIEW EXERCISES

1. Nursing is an art and science with a unique body of knowledge drawn from which other sciences?
2. Virginia Henderson's definition of nursing was adopted by the International Council of Nurses in 1973. Can you formulate a definition of nursing that captures its difference from other health professions?
3. In which fields of nursing are ENs educated to practise?
4. What are the four domains of EN practice in Australia as determined by the ANMC?
5. Nursing is a profession that is expected to include which characteristics?
6. Why is nursing a dynamic profession?

CRITICAL THINKING EXERCISES

1. You are an EN assigned to care for Mr Nguyen, an elderly male client in an aged-care facility. This man speaks and understands very little English and has only a minimum of personal clothing. His family visits seldom and he becomes aggressive at times; for example, sometimes he shouts out loudly and occasionally hits out with his fists. What would you include in planning this client's nursing care? Which of the 10 competencies would you need to use in nursing this client?
2. Part of your education includes experiences in different types of health care settings. What differences would you expect between nurses who practise in hospitals, long-term care facilities, and primary health care settings? Would you expect any commonalities?

REFERENCES AND FURTHER READING

Alfaro-Lefevre R (1999) , 2nd edn. WB Saunders, Philadelphia

Australian Institute of Health and Welfare (2003) *Nursing Labour Force*. AIHW, Canberra

Australian Nursing and Midwifery Council (ANMC) (2002) *Code of Ethics for Nurses in Australia*. ANMC, Canberra

—— (2003) *National Competency Standards for the Enrolled Nurse*. ANMC, Canberra

—— (2006) *National Competency Standards for the Registered Nurse*. ANMC, Canberra

Australian Nursing Federation (1999) The ANF celebrates 75 years. *Australian Nursing Journal* 6(8): 14–21

Benner P (1984) *From Novice to Expert: Excellence and Power in Clinical Nursing Practice*. Addison-Wesley Pub Co, Nursing Division, Menlo Park, California

Berman AJ, Kozier B, Snyder S (2008) *Kozier and Erbs Fundamentals of Nursing: Concepts, Process, and Practice*, 8th edn. Prentice-Hall, Upper Saddle River, New Jersey

Brown D, Edwards H (2008) *Lewis's Medical-Surgical Nursing: Assessment and Management of Clinical Problems*, 2nd edn. Mosby Elsevier Australia, Sydney

Carnevali DL, Thomas MD (1998) *Diagnostic Reasoning and Treatment Decision Making in Nursing*. JB Lippincott, Philadelphia

Crisp J, Taylor C (eds) (2005) *Potter & Perry's Fundamentals of Nursing*, 2nd edn. Elsevier Australia, Sydney

Heath HBM (1995) *Potter and Perry's Foundations in Nursing Theory and Practice*. Mosby, Turin

Keane B (1987) *Study of Mental Health Nursing in Australia*. Report to the Nursing and Health Services Workforce BrANMCh, Commonwealth Department of Health. Australian Government Publishing Service, Canberra

McCoppin B, Gardiner H (1994) *Tradition and Reality: Nursing and Politics in Australia*. Churchill Livingstone, Melbourne

Schultz B (1991) *A Tapestry of Service: The Evolution of Nursing in Australia. Volume 1: Foundation to Federation 1788–1900*. Churchill Livingstone, Melbourne

Staunton P, Chiarella M (2008) *Nursing and the Law*, 6th edn. Elsevier Australia

ONLINE RESOURCES

Australia & New Zealand College of Mental Health Nurses Inc (2003) Archives NZ, 2003. *Nursing Regulation in New Zealand 1901–2001*: www.anzcmhn.org

Australian Nursing and Midwifery Council: www.anmc.org.au

Australian Nursing Federation: www.anf.org.au

National Enrolled Nurses Association: www.anf.org.au/nena

New Zealand Nurses Organisation: www.nzno.org.nz

Royal College of Nursing Australia: www.rcna.org.au

Victoria University of Wellington: www.victoria.ac.nz/home

Chapter 2

OUTLINE OF NURSING THEORIES AND FRAMEWORKS OF CARE

OBJECTIVES

- Define the key terms/concepts
- Define nursing theory
- Explain the purpose of nursing models
- Identify the components of the nursing process
- State the importance of caring in nursing
- Discuss caring behaviours displayed by professional nurses

KEY TERMS/CONCEPTS

caring behaviours in nursing
nursing models
nursing paradigm
nursing process
nursing theory
theoretical views on caring

CHAPTER FOCUS

A study of nursing theory can help the student develop an understanding of the purpose of nursing practice. Nursing theory assists nurses to develop meaning in their approach to clients and can facilitate continuity of care. Over the last 50 years the growth of nursing as a scientific health care profession has led to the development of various philosophies and theoretical models of nursing on which nursing practice can be based. A nursing model provides the basis for the framework of nursing practice, and the direction for nursing research. Nursing theory is about what nursing means and is different from the theory taken from other disciplines that is usually the focus of the nursing classroom and specific procedures performed during clinical practicum. This chapter introduces the student to a variety of nursing theories that inform nursing practice.

LIVED EXPERIENCE

Initially, I didn't understand why we were having lectures on nursing theories. This was until our lecturer explained to us that, although most nurses have a clear idea of what nursing is, other health care professionals and the community may not understand the role of nursing. Our lecturer also explained that nursing theories provide nurses with direction and guidance for structuring professional nursing practice, education and research.

Siobhan, Enrolled Nurse student

THEORIES AND MODELS OF NURSING

Nursing, as a profession, is in the midst of change. Society is changing and nursing is affected by social forces that require a community receives a system of health care delivery that will make quality care available for all people. The demand for quality care is reflected in the philosophical belief in the dignity and value of the individual. To provide quality care, nursing must focus on the needs of both the individual and the community.

In earlier times the responsibilities of nurses were centred around sanitation measures, nutrition, hygiene and comfort, prevention of cross-infection and relief of the prime symptoms of infection. Nurses functioned not only as nurses but as housekeepers, dietitians and cleaners. Nursing has shifted from being primarily illness oriented to being a profession that is health oriented. Nurses practise in a growing variety of settings, and nursing roles continue to expand as the focus of nursing care expands. Current nursing philosophies and theoretical models reflect the trend to address the total person, in all dimensions, as an individual in interaction with the family and the community.

Nursing theories can help make sense of processes and practices. Nursing theories explain why and when nursing takes place, provide an understanding of how the practice of nursing proceeds and also assist with practice change through critique. In this way nursing theories help create an understanding of the practice of nursing, how nurses interact with clients and how nursing actions and provision of nursing care is structured (Daly et al 2006).

DEFINING THEORY AND MODEL

A *theory* is an abstract statement formulated to explain or describe the relationships among concepts or events. A nursing theory is a conceptualisation of some aspect of nursing communicated for the purpose of describing, explaining, predicting and/or prescribing nursing care. A *model* is a conceptual framework developed from a set of concepts and assumptions; it is a conceptual representation of reality. A model provides the outline for which theory provides the functions. Thus, a model represents *structure* while a theory suggests *function*. Numerous conceptual models of nursing practice have been devised, most of which:

- Are based on sound theory
- Contain implied or explicit assumptions, values and goals
- Are implemented by the nursing process.

Nursing theories serve several essential purposes, as is illustrated in Clinical Interest Box 2.1.

CLINICAL INTEREST BOX 2.1
Purposes of nursing theories and conceptual frameworks

In clinical practice:
- Assist nurses to describe, explain and predict everyday experiences
- Serve to guide assessment, intervention and evaluation of nursing care
- Provide a rationale for collecting reliable and valid data about the health status of clients, which are essential for effective decision making and implementation
- Help to establish criteria to measure the quality of nursing care
- Help build a common nursing terminology to use in communicating with other health professionals. Ideas are developed and words defined
- Enhance autonomy of nursing by defining its own independent functions

In education:
- Provide a general focus for curriculum design
- Guide curricular decision making

In research:
- Offer a framework for generating knowledge and new ideas
- Assist in discovering knowledge gaps in the specific field of study
- Offer a systematic approach to identify questions for study, select variables, interpret findings and validate nursing interventions

(Kozier et al 2004)

COMPONENTS OF NURSING THEORETICAL MODELS

Within any scientific discipline there are specific domains. A domain is the perspective and territory of the discipline and contains the subject, central concepts, values and beliefs, phenomena of interest and the central problems of the discipline. Components of a discipline's domain are described in a paradigm. A *paradigm* is a term used to denote the links to science, philosophy and theory accepted by the discipline. Nursing's paradigm directs the activity of the nursing profession and includes four links of interest — the person, health, environment/situation and nursing.

The person

Person refers to the recipient of care, including individual clients, families and the community. The person is central to the care being provided. Because the person's needs are multidimensional, it is important that nursing provide care individualised to the person's needs.

Health

Health is defined in different ways by the client, clinical setting and by the health care profession and is the goal of nursing care. The nurse is challenged to provide care based on the client's individualised level of health and health care needs at the time of health care delivery.

Environment/situation

Environment/situation includes all possible conditions affecting the client and the place in which health care needs occur. There is continuous interaction between the client and the environment. This interaction can have positive and negative effects on the person's level of health and health care needs.

Nursing

Nursing is the diagnosis and treatment of human responses to actual or potential health problems. For example, a nurse does not make a medical diagnosis of a client's heart condition but instead develops nursing diagnoses of fatigue, change in body image and altered coping mechanisms. From these nursing diagnoses, the nurse creates an individualised plan of care.

OVERVIEW OF SELECTED NURSING THEORIES

Many nursing theories have been developed in the past and many are still being developed today. The following selection of nursing theories is an historical overview that discusses nursing's four fields of interest: the person, health, environment/situation and nursing.

PEPLAU'S THEORY

In 1952 Hildegard Peplau made an attempt to analyse nursing action using an interpersonal theoretical framework. Her theory focuses on the relationships formed by people as they progress through each developmental stage. She viewed the goal of nursing as developing a relationship between the nurse and client whereby the nurse acts as resource person, counsellor, teacher and surrogate.

ABDELLAH'S THEORY

In 1960 Fay Abdellah, with her colleagues, devised a theory that emphasised the delivery of nursing care to the whole person. Using a problem-solving approach the nurse formulates a plan to help clients meet their physical, emotional, intellectual, social and spiritual needs. Abdellah identified 21 basic nursing procedures. These are to:

1. Maintain good hygiene and physical comfort
2. Achieve optimal activity, exercise, rest and sleep
3. Prevent accident, injury or other trauma and prevent the spread of infection
4. Maintain good body mechanics and prevent and correct deformities
5. Facilitate the supply of oxygen to all body cells
6. Facilitate the maintenance of nutrition to all body cells
7. Facilitate the maintenance of elimination
8. Facilitate the maintenance of fluid and electrolyte balance
9. Recognise the physiological responses of the body to disease conditions, pathological, physiological and compensatory
10. Facilitate the maintenance of regulatory mechanisms and functions
11. Facilitate the maintenance of sensory functions
12. Identify and accept positive and negative expressions, feelings and reactions
13. Identify and accept the interrelatedness of emotions and organic illness
14. Facilitate the maintenance of effective verbal and non-verbal communication
15. Facilitate the development of productive interpersonal relationships
16. Facilitate progress towards achievement of personal spiritual goals
17. Create and/or maintain a therapeutic environment
18. Facilitate awareness of self as an individual with varying physical, emotional and developmental needs
19. Accept the optimal possible goals in light of limitations — physical and emotional
20. Use community resources as an aid in resolving problems arising from illness
21. Understand the role of social problems as influencing factors in the cause of illness.

HENDERSON'S THEORY

In 1964 Virginia Henderson described the goal of nursing as helping the client to gain independence as rapidly as possible, and defined nursing as:

> assisting the individual, sick or well, in the performance of those activities contributing to health, its recovery, promoting quality of life or to a peaceful death that the client would perform unaided if he or she had the necessary strength, will or knowledge.
>
> (Crisp & Taylor 2005: 2)

Henderson identified 14 basic needs that provide a framework for nursing care. These are to:

1. Breathe normally
2. Eat and drink adequately
3. Eliminate by all avenues of elimination
4. Move and maintain a desirable position
5. Sleep and rest
6. Select suitable clothing; dress and undress
7. Maintain body temperature within normal range
8. Keep the body clean and well groomed
9. Avoid dangers in the environment
10. Communicate with others
11. Worship according to faith
12. Work at something that provides a sense of accomplishment
13. Play or participate in various forms of recreation
14. Learn, discover or satisfy the curiosity that leads to normal development and health.

(Crisp & Taylor 2005)

JOHNSON'S THEORY

In 1968 Dorothy Johnson portrayed the goal of nursing as reducing stress so that the client can recover as quickly as possible. Johnson viewed people as a collection of behavioural subsystems that interrelate to form a whole person, and her theory focuses on a person's needs in terms of the following behaviours:

- Security-seeking behaviour
- Nurturing-seeking behaviour
- Mastery of oneself and one's environment according to internalised standards of excellence
- Taking in nourishment in socially and culturally acceptable ways
- Ridding the body of waste in socially and culturally acceptable ways
- Sexual and role identity behaviour
- Self-protective behaviour.

Johnson saw the nurse's role as identifying the client's inability to adapt to stress, and as providing the nursing care necessary to assist them in resolving problems to meet their needs.

KING'S THEORY

Imogene King (1971, cited in Crisp & Taylor 2005) viewed the goal of nursing as helping individuals and groups to attain, maintain and restore health, or to die with dignity. King saw nursing as a process of interaction between nurse and client whereby, through communication, goals are set and agreement reached on ways to achieve goals.

OREM'S THEORY

In 1973 Dorothea Orem depicted the goal of nursing as helping the client to achieve health through self-care (cited in Crisp & Taylor 2005). Orem saw nursing as a service required when individuals are unable to care for themselves, or unable to be cared for by others of significance to them; that is, when demands exceed their self-care abilities. The nurse identifies why an individual is unable to care for themself, and implements measures that assist them to meet their needs. The overall goal of nursing care is to assist the client to achieve self-care whenever possible.

ROY'S THEORY

Callister Roy viewed the goal of nursing as assisting people towards health by promoting and supporting their ability to adapt to various demands (cited in Crisp & Taylor 2005):

- Meeting basic physiological needs
- Developing a positive self-concept
- Performing social roles
- Achieving a balance between dependence and independence.

Roy saw nursing as being concerned with people as total beings, and intervening when necessary to assist them to adapt to one or more of these demands.

ROPER, LOGAN AND TIERNEY'S THEORY

Roper, Logan and Tierney (1985, cited in Crisp & Taylor 2005) viewed the goal of nursing as helping people to prevent, alleviate, solve or cope with problems related to activities of living. Their model of nursing is based on their model for living and includes five main concepts:

1. Activities of living
2. Factors affecting activities of living
3. Lifespan
4. Dependence–independence
5. The nursing process.

The activities of living, which are the focus of the model, are:

- Maintaining a safe environment
- Communicating
- Breathing
- Eating and drinking
- Eliminating
- Personal cleansing and dressing
- Controlling body temperature
- Mobilising
- Working and playing
- Expressing sexuality
- Sleeping
- Dying.

At certain times nurses help clients towards independence in the activities of living, and at other times help them to accept dependence. Factors affecting the activities of living, or individuality in the activities of living, include those that are physical, psychological, sociocultural, environmental and politico–economic. Therefore, the nurse needs to acknowledge that there are many differences in the way individuals perform the activities of living.

In this model the life span serves as a reminder that nursing is concerned with individuals of all ages, and that an individual may require nursing assistance at any stage of the life span from conception to death.

The dependence–independence continuum is included in this model to acknowledge that there are certain stages in an individual's life when they are unable to perform various activities of living independently. The continuum ranges from total dependence at one end to total independence at the other, and the concept of dependence–independence is widely used in nursing practice.

It becomes apparent when comparing various models that most include similar concepts of what constitutes nursing. Selecting a particular model of nursing practice depends on numerous factors, and health care agencies may consider several before deciding on the one they consider to be most appropriate. As nursing continues to grow as a health care profession, new philosophies of nursing and theoretical models will undoubtedly be developed (see Clinical Interest Box 2.2).

RELATIONSHIP OF THEORIES TO NURSING PROCESS

The nursing process is a tool and framework for contemporary nursing practice. It is a series of planned steps that produces a particular end result. In simple terms the nursing process is a method used to assess, plan, deliver and evaluate nursing care. Clinical Interest Box 2.3 illustrates the relationship of a couple of theories to the nursing

CLINICAL INTEREST BOX 2.2
Summary of nursing theories

Theorist	Goal of nursing	Framework for practice
Nightingale, 1860	To facilitate 'the body's reparative processes' by manipulating client's environment (Torres 1986)	Client's environment is manipulated to include appropriate noise, nutrition, hygiene, light, comfort, socialisation and hope
Peplau, 1952	To develop interaction between nurse and client (Peplau 1952)	Nursing is a significant, therapeutic, interpersonal process (Peplau 1952). Nurses participate in structuring health care systems to facilitate natural ongoing tendency of humans to develop interpersonal relationships (Marriner-Tomey & Alligood 1998)
Henderson, 1955	To work independently with other health care workers (Marriner-Tomey & Alligood 1998), assisting client in gaining independence as quickly as possible (Henderson 1964); to help client gain lacking strength (Torres 1986)	Nurses help client to perform Henderson's 14 basic needs (Henderson 1966)
Abdellah, 1960	To provide service to individuals, families and society; to be kind and caring but also intelligent, competent and technically well prepared to provide this service (Marriner-Tomey & Alligood 1998)	This theory involves Abdellah's 21 nursing procedures (Abdellah & others 1960)
Orlando, 1961	To respond to client's behaviour in terms of immediate needs; to interact with client to meet immediate needs by identifying client's behaviour, reaction of nurse, and nursing action to be taken (Torres 1986; Chinn & Kramer 1999)	Three elements — client behaviour, nurse reaction, and nurse action — comprise nursing situation (Orlando 1961)
Hall, 1962	To provide care and comfort to client during disease process (Torres 1986)	The client is composed of the following overlapping parts: person (core), pathological state and treatment (cure) and body (care). Nurse is caregiver (Marriner-Tomey & Alligood 1998; Chinn & Kramer 1999)
Wiedenbach, 1964	To assist individuals in overcoming obstacles that interfere with the ability to meet demands or needs brought about by condition, environment, situation or time (Torres 1986)	Nursing practice is related to individuals who need help because of behavioural stimulus. Clinical nursing has the following components: philosophy, purpose, practice, and art (Chinn & Kramer 1999)
Levine, 1966	To use conversation activities aimed at optimal use of client's resources	This adaptation model of human as integral whole is based on 'four conversation principles of nursing' (Levine 1973)
Johnson, 1968	To reduce stress so the client can move more easily through recovery process	This theory of basic needs focuses on seven categories of behaviour. Individual's goal is to achieve behavioural balance and steady state by adjustment and adaptation to certain forces (Johnson 1980; Torres 1986)
Rogers, 1970	To maintain and promote health, prevent illness, and care for and rehabilitate ill and disabled client through 'humanistic science of nursing' (Rogers 1970)	'Unitary man' evolves along life process. Client continuously changes and coexists with environment
Orem, 1971	To care for and help client attain total self-care	This is self-care deficit theory. Nursing care becomes necessary when client is unable to fulfil biological, psychological, developmental or social needs (Orem 1991)
King, 1971	To use communication to help client re-establish positive adaptation to environment	Nursing process is defined as dynamic interpersonal re-establish positive adaptation to process between nurse, client and health care system
Travelbee, 1971	To assist individual or family in preventing or coping with illness, regaining health, finding meaning in illness or maintaining maximal degree of health (Marriner-Tomey & Alligood 1998)	Interpersonal process is viewed as human-to-human relationship formed during illness and 'experience of suffering'

(Continued)

CLINICAL INTEREST BOX 2.2 — cont'd
Summary of nursing theories

Theorist	Goal of nursing	Framework for practice
Neuman, 1972	To assist individuals, families and groups in attaining and maintaining maximal level of total wellness by purposeful interventions	Stress reduction is goal of systems model of nursing practice (Torres 1986). Nursing actions are in primary, secondary or tertiary level of prevention
Patterson and Zderad, 1976	To respond to human needs and build humanistic nursing science (Patterson & Zderad 1976; Chinn & Kramer 1999)	Humanistic nursing requires participants to be aware of their 'uniqueness' and 'commonality' with others (Chinn & Kramer 1999)
Leininger, 1978	To provide care consistent with nursing's emerging science and knowledge with caring as central focus (Chinn & Kramer 1999)	With this transcultural care theory, caring is the central and unifying domain for nursing knowledge and practice
Roy, 1979	To identify types of demands placed on client, assess adaptation to demands and help client adapt	This adaptation model is based on the physiological, psychological, sociological and dependence–independence adaptive modes (Roy 1980)
Watson, 1979	To promote health, restore client to health, and prevent illness (Marriner-Tomey & Alligood 1998)	This theory involves philosophy and science of caring; caring is interpersonal process comprising interventions that result in meeting human needs (Torres 1986)
Parse, 1981	To focus on human being as living unity and individual's qualitative participation with health experience (Parse 1990; Marriner-Tomey & Alligood 1998)	The individual continually interacts with environment and participates in maintenance of health (Marriner-Tomey & Alligood 1998). Health is a continual, open process rather than a state of wellbeing or absence of disease (Parse 1990; Marriner-Tomey & Alligood 1998; Chinn & Kramer 1999)
Benner & Wrubel 1989	To focus on client's need for caring as a means of coping with stressors of illness (Chinn & Kramer 1999)	Caring is central to the essence of nursing. Caring creates the possibilities for coping and enables possibilities for connecting with and concern for others (Benner & Wrubel 1989)

(modified from Chinn PL & Kramer ML 2004

process. Providing the framework for nursing care, the nursing process consists of five components, each of which follows logically one after the other:

- Assessment
- Nursing diagnosis
- Planning
- Implementation
- Evaluation.

The process is adaptable to different clients and different care settings. In addition, the process offers a systematic approach to nursing practice and enhances research opportunities and is compatible with many other systems in the health care delivery system, such as computer generated care plans, patient information systems and patient acuity systems. Although the nursing process is central to the domain of nursing it is not a theory. It provides a process for the delivery of nursing care, not the knowledge component of the discipline. However, there have been attempts to build a comprehensive theory from the process and to use the nursing process in conjunction with other theories that lack a process element. (For further information on the nursing process see Chapter 19.)

THEORETICAL VIEWS ON CARING

CARING

Caring is a universal phenomenon that influences the ways in which individuals think, feel and behave in relation to one another. Caring in nursing has been studied from a variety of philosophical and ethical perspectives since the time of Florence Nightingale. Several nursing scholars have developed theories on caring because of its importance not only to the practice of nursing, but also to the existence of humankind. Caring is at the heart of a nurse's ability to work with individuals in a respectful and therapeutic way.

Caring is primary

Patricia Benner, a professor in the department of physiological nursing in the School of Nursing at the University of California, San Francisco, is an internationally noted researcher and lecturer on health, stress and coping, skill acquisition and ethics. Her work has provided the basis for new legislation and design for nursing practice and education for three states in Australia (see http://home.earthlink.net/~bennerassoc/patricia.html).

CLINICAL INTEREST BOX 2.3
Selected nursing theories and the nursing process

Orem's general theory of nursing	
Assessing	Involves collecting data about the client's capacities (knowledge, skills and motivation) to perform universal, developmental, and health-deviation self-care requisites. Determines self-care deficits
Diagnosing	Stated in terms of the client's limitations for maintaining self-care (a deficit in self-care agency)
Planning	Involves considering and designing, with the client's participation, an appropriate nursing system (wholly compensatory, partially compensatory, supportive-educative, or a mix) that will help the client achieve an optimal level of self-care (i.e. enhance the client's self-care agency)
Implementing	Assisting the client by acting for or doing for, guiding, supporting, providing a developmental environment, and teaching
Evaluating	Determining the client's level of achievement in resolving self-care deficits and in performing self-care
Roy's adaptation model	
Assessing	Involves two levels. First-level assessment includes collecting data about output behaviours related to the four adaptive modes (physiological, self-concept, role function, and interdependence modes). Second-level assessment includes collecting data about internal and external stimuli (focal, contextual or residual) that are influencing the identified behaviours
Diagnosing	Focuses on adaptation problems and uses one of three alternative methods: 1. Stating behaviours within one mode with their most relevant influencing stimuli 2. Clustering behavioural information and labelling it according to indicators of positive adaptation and a typology of common adaptation problems related to each mode. Roy provides a typology of indicators of positive adaptation and a typology of commonly recurring adaptation problems according to each of the four modes 3. Labelling a behavioural pattern when more than one mode is being affected by the same stimuli
Planning	Setting goals in terms of behaviours the client is to achieve and planning nursing interventions to promote the effectiveness of the client's coping mechanisms and adaptive behaviours
Implementing	Altering and manipulating the focal, contextual and residual stimuli by increasing, decreasing or maintaining them
Evaluating	Determining the client's output behaviours with those identified in the goals

(Kozier et al 2000)

Benner (1984; and Benner & Wrubel 1989) would quickly argue that her work on expertise in nursing practice and the central role of caring is not theory in the traditional sense. Theories are typically designed to explain, predict and describe specific phenomena. Benner does not try to predict or control phenomena but attempts to give nurses a rich, holistic understanding of nursing practice and caring through interpreting expert nurses' real stories. After hearing and analysing the stories nurses tell about their clients, Benner is able to describe the essence of excellent nursing practice, which is caring.

Caring as defined by Benner and Wrubel (1989) means that persons, events, projects and things matter to individuals. It is a word for being connected. Because caring determines what matters to a person, it describes a wide range of involvements, from parental love to friendship, from caring for one's work to caring for one's pet, to caring for and about one's clients. Caring also reveals what is stressful and the available options for coping. If something does not matter to a person, it will not likely create stress or the need for coping. Benner sees the personal concern of caring as an inherent feature of nursing practice, whereby nurses help clients to recover in the face of illness, to give meaning to that illness, and to maintain or re-establish connection. Caring makes nurses notice which interventions are successful, and this concern then guides future caring.

Caring is the essence of nursing and health

From a transcultural perspective, Madeleine Leininger (1978, cited in Crisp & Taylor 2005) describes the concept of care as the essence and central, unifying and dominant domain that distinguishes nursing from other health disciplines. Care is also an essential human need, necessary for the health and survival of all individuals. Care, unlike cure, is oriented to assisting an individual or group in improving a human condition. Acts of caring refer to the direct or indirect nurturing and skilful activities, processes and decisions that assist people in ways that are empathetic, compassionate and supportive, and that are dependent on the needs, problems and values of the individual being assisted.

Leininger's studies of numerous cultures around the world have found that care helps protect, develop, nurture and provide survival to people. Care is vital to recovery from illness and to the maintenance of healthy life practices. Leininger (1988) stresses the importance for nurses to understand both universal and non-universal folk caring and professional caring behaviours to be effective in the care of clients. For caring to achieve cure, nurses must learn those culturally specific behaviours that reflect human care processes in different cultures.

Transpersonal caring

The managed care system of health care is increasingly removed from nursing's caring values and expertise. As a result, Jean Watson (1979, 1988) describes a new consciousness that is emerging, allowing nursing to raise new questions about what it means to be a nurse, to be ill, and to be caring and healing. Rejecting the disease orientation to health care, nursing instead is beginning to embrace caring as a moral ideal and an end in and of itself. Watson's transpersonal caring theory (1988) places care before cure, with caring becoming the ethical standard by which nursing care is measured.

Caring preserves human dignity in a cure-dominated health care system. Caring encompasses a metaphysical or almost spiritual dimension. Caring–healing is communicated through the consciousness of the nurse to the person being cared for. Caring–healing consciousness can take place during a single caring moment between nurse and client. An interconnectedness forms between the one cared for and the one caring. Transpersonal caring expands the limits of openness and allows access to the higher human spirit, thus expanding human consciousness. Both the nurse and the client are influenced through the transaction, for better or for worse. Watson also argues that the human caring process has an energy field greater than that possessed by each individual. The caring–healing consciousness can promote healing and release a person's own inner power and resources.

Swanson's theory of caring

In developing her caring theory, Kristen Swanson (1991) conducted interviews with three different groups: women who had miscarried; parents and professionals in a newborn intensive care unit; and socially at-risk mothers who had received long-term public-health intervention. All groups were in a perinatal situation or context and had experienced the phenomenon of caring. Each group was asked questions regarding how caring was experienced or expressed in their situation.

Swanson's theory of caring is a composite of studies of the three different groups. The theory describes caring as consisting of five categories or processes: knowing, being with, doing for, enabling and maintaining belief. Caring is defined by Swanson as a nurturing way of relating to a valued other, towards whom one feels a personal sense of commitment and responsibility. The theory supports the claim that caring is a central nursing phenomenon but not necessarily unique to nursing practice.

NURSING AS CARING

The basic premise of Boykin and Schoenhofer's (2001) theory of nursing as caring is that all humans are caring persons and that to be human is to be called to live one's innate caring nature. Developing the full potential of expressing caring is an ideal and, for practical purposes, is a lifelong process. Grounded in these assumptions, this theory posits the focus and the aim of nursing as a discipline of knowledge and a professional service as 'nurturing persons, living caring, and growing in caring'.

When entering into a human care situation for the purpose of offering nursing, the nurse focuses on coming to know the client as a caring person, understanding how that person is 'living caring' uniquely in the moment and living their dreams and aspirations for 'growing in caring'. The aim of the nurse is to come to know and then to acknowledge, affirm, support and celebrate the nursed as a caring person. Nursing is accomplished through acting on the informed intention to care in creative ways that are personally and situationally meaningful.

Caring in nursing

It is impossible to prescribe ways that will guarantee that nurses become caring professionals. There is some disagreement as to whether caring can be taught or is more fundamentally a way of being in the world. For those who find caring a normal part of their life, caring is a product of their culture, values, experiences and relationships with others. Persons who do not experience care in their lives often find it difficult to act in caring ways. As nurses deal with health and illness in their practice they grow in the ability to care. Expert nurses understand the differences and relationships among health, illness and disease and are able to see clients in their own context, interpret their needs and offer caring acts that improve clients' health. Caring behaviours are explained as follows.

Providing presence

To provide presence (being with a client) is a valued behaviour. To provide presence is to have a person-to-person encounter that conveys a closeness and sense of security. The ability to provide presence, to be with another person in a way that acknowledges one's shared humanity, is at the core of nursing as a caring practice. When a nurse establishes presence with eye contact, body language, voice tone, listening, and a positive and encouraging attitude, it creates openness and understanding. Being able to establish presence with a client also enhances the nurse's ability to learn from the client. As a result, the nurse's ability to provide adequate and appropriate nursing care is strengthened.

Comforting

Clients face situations that can be embarrassing, frightening, painful and exhausting. Whatever the feeling or symptom, clients look to nurses to provide comfort. Comforting provides both an emotional and a physical calm. The use of touch is one comforting approach whereby the nurse reaches out to clients to communicate concern and support. Touch may involve holding a client's hand, giving a back massage or gently positioning a body part. Because touch can convey many messages it must be used with discretion.

Comforting also involves the skilful and gentle performance of a nursing procedure. Any procedure is more effective when it is administered carefully and in consideration of any client concern. Anxiety is allayed in the client if the procedure to be performed is first explained by the nurse then performed confidently, safely and successfully.

Listening

Caring involves an interpersonal interaction that is much more than two persons simply talking back and forth. In a caring relationship the nurse establishes trust and open lines of communication and listens to what the client has to say. Listening is the key because it can convey the nurse's full attention and interest. Listening to the meaning of what a client says helps create a mutual relationship.

Knowing the client

To know a client means that the nurse avoids assumptions, centres on the client, and engages in a caring relationship with the client that reveals information and cues that facilitate critical thinking and clinical judgements. Knowing the client is the core of the process by which nurses make clinical decisions. By establishing a caring relationship, the mutuality that develops helps the nurse to better know the client as a unique individual and to then choose the most appropriate and efficacious nursing therapies.

Spiritual caring

Healing is not a matter of treatments or medications, but rather a work of spirit. A person's intrinsic spirit seems to be a factor in the healing process. A person's spirit is the inner essence that is the basis of their vital life principle, and spiritual health is achieved when a person finds a balance between his or her own life values, goals and belief systems, and those of others. Research has shown a link between spirit, mind and body. A person's beliefs and expectations can and do have effects on their physical wellbeing. Establishing a caring relationship with a client involves an interconnectedness between the nurse and the client. This is the reason Watson (1979) describes the caring relationship in a spiritual sense.

Family care

People inhabit their worlds in an involved way. Each person experiences life through relationships with others. Thus, caring for a person cannot occur in isolation from that person's family. As a nurse it is important to know the family almost as thoroughly as one knows the client. The family is an important resource. Success with nursing interventions often depends on the family's willingness to share information about the client, their acceptance and understanding of therapies, whether the interventions fit with the family's daily practices and whether the family can support and deliver the therapies recommended. Caring for the family takes into consideration the context of the client's illness and the stress it imposes on all members.

SUMMARY

The aim of this chapter is to introduce the student to theories and models of nursing. An overview of the theories and models of nursing helps to demonstrate how theory can inform the way in which we view the person, health, the environment and nursing itself. This allows nurses to establish connections and meaning in nursing and facilitates continuity of care. A recurrent theme in the examination of theories of nursing is the idea of caring. Caring is highly relational. The nurse and the client enter into a relationship that is much more than one person simply 'doing tasks' for another. A mutual give and take develops as nurse and client begin to know and care for one another. Caring may seem highly invisible at times, when a nurse and client enter a relationship of respect, concern and support. The nurse's empathy and compassion become a natural part of every client encounter. However, the nurse–client relationship can become very visible when caring is absent. A nurse's disinterest or avoidance of a client's request, for example, will quickly convey an uncaring attitude. Clients can tell quickly when nurses fail to relate to them. In contrast, when caring is practised, the client senses a commitment on the part of the nurse and is willing to enter into a relationship that allows the nurse to gain an understanding of the client and their experience of illness. This allows the nurse to become a coach and partner rather than a detached provider of care service.

The utilisation and application of nursing theory (in the form of philosophies, models and theories) help nurses think critically for professional practice. Theory and research together lead to a systematic inquiry, which informs practice (Daly et al 2006).

REVIEW EXERCISES

1. What major shift in nursing towards client care has taken place in recent times?
2. What is the difference between a theory and a model?
3. What are the four links of interest in the nursing paradigm?
4. What is the purpose of the nursing process in relation to nursing theory?
5. What are the common themes in nurse theorists' views on caring?

CRITICAL THINKING EXERCISES

1. As part of your EN education you are placed in different settings for your clinical practicum. Select a nursing theory and explain how it might apply to one of these settings.
2. You are caring for a client who needs to learn to manage cardiac drugs. Describe the criteria you would use to select a nursing theory for a basis for clinical practice.

REFERENCES AND FURTHER READING

Abdellah FG, Martin A (1973) *New Directions in Patient-Centered Nursing*. Macmillan, New York

Alligood MR, Marriner-Tomey A (2002) *Nursing Theory: Utilization & Application*, 2nd edn. Mosby, St Louis

Benner P (1984) *From Novice to Expert*. Addison-Wesley, Menlo Park, California

Benner P, Wrubel J (1989) *The Primacy of Caring: Stress and Coping in Health and Illness*. Addison-Wesley, Menlo Park, California

Berman AJ, Kozier B, Snyder S (2008) *Kozier and Erbs Fundamentals of Nursing: Concepts, Process, and Practice*, 8th edn. Prentice-Hall, Upper Saddle River, New Jersey

Bolander VB (1994) *Sorensen and Luckmann's Basic Nursing: a Psychophysiologic Approach*. WB Saunders, Philadelphia

Boykin A, Schoenhofer SO (2001) *Nursing as Caring: a Model for Transforming Practice*. Jones & Bartlett Publishing, Nursing Press, Sudsbury, Massachusetts

Chinn PL, Kramer ML (2004) *Integrated knowledge development in nursing*, 6th edn. Mosby, St Louis

Crisp J, Taylor C (eds) (2005) *Potter & Perry's Fundamentals of Nursing*, 2nd edn. Elsevier Australia, Sydney

Daly J, Speedy S, Jackson D (2006) *Contexts of Nursing: An Introduction*, 2nd edn. Elsevier Australia, Sydney

Heath HBM (1995) *Potter and Perry's Foundations in Nursing Theory and Practice*. Mosby, Turin

Koch S, Garratt S (2001) *Assessing Older People*. MacLennan & Petty, Sydney

Kozier B, Erb G, Berman AJ, Burke K (2000) *Fundamentals of Nursing: Concepts, Process and Practice*, 6th edn. Prentice-Hall Inc, Upper Saddle River, NJ

Kozier B, Erb G, Berman AJ, Snyder S (2004) *Fundamentals of Nursing: Concepts, Process and Practice*, 7th edn. Prentice-Hall, Upper Saddle River, NJ

Leininger M (1988) *Care: the Essence of Nursing And Health*. Wayne State University Press, Detroit

—— (2002) *Transcultural Nursing: Concepts, Theories, and Practices*, 2nd edn. John Wiley & Sons, New York

Reed P, Crawford Shearer NB, Nicholl LH (eds) (2003) *Perspectives on nursing theory*, 4th edn. Lippincott Williams & Wilkins, Philadelphia

Riehl JP, Roy C (1980) *Conceptual Models for Nursing Practice*, 2nd edn. Appleton, New York

Rosdahl CB (ed) (2007) *Textbook of Basic Nursing*, 9th edn. Lippincott, Philadelphia

Swanson K (1991) Empirical development of a middle range theory of caring. *Nursing Resources*, May–June, 40(3): 161–6

Watson MJ (1979) *Nursing: the Philosophy and Science of Caring*. Little Brown, Boston

—— (1988) New dimensions of human caring theory. *Nursing Science Quarterly* 1: 175

ONLINE RESOURCES

Patricia Benner, Professor in the Department of Physiological Nursing in the School of Nursing at the University of California, San Francisco: http://home.earthlink.net/~bennerassoc/patricia.html

Chapter 3

LEGAL AND ETHICAL ASPECTS OF NURSING PRACTICE

OBJECTIVES

- Define the key terms/concepts
- Discuss the distinctions between criminal law and civil law
- Explain legal responsibilities and obligations of nurses
- Discuss various legal issues that arise in nursing practice
- Access, compare and contrast the *Code of Professional Conduct for Nurses in Australia* and the *Code of Ethics for Nurses in Australia*
- Discuss accountability and advocacy as related to the practice of nursing
- Discuss various ethical issues and ethical dilemmas confronted by nurses

KEY TERMS/CONCEPTS

accountability
advocacy
criminal and civil law
ethical standards
legal liability
legal responsibilities of nursing students
legislation and regulations
nursing ethics
nursing regulations
vicarious liability

CHAPTER FOCUS

The aim of this chapter is to introduce the Enrolled Nurse (EN) to some legal and ethical concepts that are relevant to the practice of nursing. While the concepts of nursing ethics are generally universal, the nurse needs to be aware that the law is different between countries and can be different between states and territories. Where the nurse resides and practises determines the legal knowledge required. Further reading on these matters is necessary for safe and competent practice.

LIVED EXPERIENCE

When we were studying the legal and ethical aspects of nursing practice I began to realise that nursing is a highly responsible job, and started to worry about what could happen if I did something wrong in the clinical field. It became clear though in the lectures that, as nurses, we work in situations that give us a privilege in working with individuals, including care of their physical and emotional needs. The laws define the boundaries of that privilege and make clear what nurses' rights and responsibilities are. I kept thinking that as long as I keep this in mind and follow these, then I would always be giving the clients I was caring for the best care within my scope of practice.

Joe, Enrolled Nurse student

LEGAL ASPECTS OF NURSING PRACTICE

In a democratic society the legal system provides a framework inside which all sections of the community interact. It establishes the rights and privileges of the individual and makes provision for enforcement of rights and redress for wrongs suffered. All citizens should be aware of their legally defined rights and responsibilities, and should have an understanding of the laws that govern their personal and professional lives. Ignorance of a law is not accepted as an excuse for violation of that law.

Nurses have legal responsibilities common to all members of the community, and also the responsibilities imposed by the nature of their work, which may be defined as responsibilities in respect of:

- The provision of safe effective nursing care
- The health of the community
- The employing authority
- The nursing profession.

The functions of the law in nursing are summarised in Clinical Interest Box 3.1.

ACTS OF PARLIAMENT

There are, in each Australian state and territory, various Acts, which are laws created by a Parliament. Acts of Parliament are commonly referred to as legislation and are often accompanied by Regulations that give directions to be followed to comply with the intent of the Act. As the Acts vary from state to state and territory, nurses are advised to become familiar with the specific Acts relevant to their place of nursing practice. Some examples of these Acts are outlined in Clinical Interest Box 3.2.

Common Law

The common law is the body of law made by judges as a result of decisions in cases that come before the courts. These decisions form precedents (principles of law) and can then be applied in like cases. This body of law is often referred to as judge-made law and is equally as important as Parliamentary-made law. Some examples include the law of consent, and the law of assault and battery.

Types of law

It is important to be aware of the distinctions between criminal and civil law. Criminal laws are concerned with offences against people and their property. The government has the power to make rules as to what constitutes minimum levels of acceptable behaviour and then seeks to control behaviour through the power of the police force by ensuring that those rules are obeyed. A violation of a criminal law is called a crime, and it is sanctioned by some form of punishment, such as payment of a fine or imprisonment. Murder, robbery, rape and kidnapping are examples of crimes regarded as offences against society as a whole.

Civil laws are concerned with the relationships between people. Such laws provide the means by which rights can be enforced and wrongs can be remedied. For example, a person found to have broken the civil law will usually be required to pay a sum of money to the person alleging personal or property loss or damage. Areas of civil law include trespass, contracts and negligence.

THE EMPLOYER

An employer, such as the board of management of a hospital, is legally responsible for the acts committed by all employees in the course of their duty. This principle of *vicarious liability* is relevant to all nurses, as it renders an employer liable for an employee's actions committed in the course of employment. While the employer is held liable, they do have the right to seek a total financial indemnity from the offending employee, for example in the case of negligence. An employer must ensure that:

- Employees possess the required qualifications, registration and level of competence
- All legal requirements are met, including valid contracts of employment
- Safety standards are observed in relation to standards of patient care, buildings and equipment.

The legal liability of the employer does not absolve a nurse from individual responsibility, and legal action can be taken against a hospital and a nurse or against a nurse as an individual.

CLINICAL INTEREST BOX 3.1
Functions of law in nursing

The law serves a number of functions in nursing:

- It provides a framework for establishing which nursing actions in the care of clients are legal
- It differentiates the nurse's responsibilities from those of other health professionals
- It helps establish the boundaries of independent nursing action
- It assists in maintaining a standard of nursing practice by making nurses accountable under the law.

(Berman et al 2008)

CLINICAL INTEREST BOX 3.2
Specific acts relevant to the nursing profession

- Drugs, Poisons and Controlled Substances Act
- Mental Health Act
- Child Protection Act (or Children and Young Persons Act)
- Human Tissue Act, or Human Tissue and Transplant Act
- Nurses Act
- Coroner's Act
- Freedom of Information Act
- Health Professions Registration Act

NURSING REGULATION

Because the control and regulation of the nursing profession in Australia is determined on a state and territory basis, each Australian state and territory has its own Nurses Act or Health Professions Registration Act and Regulations. There is a Nurses Board or Nurses Council in each of the states and territories, composed of members empowered to both register and deregister nurses. Each state or territory Act is divided into sections, each one of which deals with a specific aspect concerning registration. As each state and territory has its own Act, it is essential that nurses read a copy of the relevant legislation so that they are aware of individual state and/or territory requirements. The Nursing Council of New Zealand is responsible for the registration of all categories of New Zealand nurses.

Some states and territories now have a separate register for midwives, as new education programs mean that in some jurisdictions it is possible to become a midwife by direct entry through an undergraduate degree in midwifery. In addition, all states and territories have now enacted legislation to enable the title 'nurse practitioner' to be protected (Staunton & Chiarella 2008).

By defining the terms under which a nurse may practise in each of the categories of registration, the law protects the community by deeming the nurse who has qualified to be safe and competent to practise nursing. Nurses who do not fulfil the requirements of the relevant Nurses or Health Professions Registration Act may not practise as nurses. Currently, a practising certificate or renewal of registration must be obtained from the Nurses Board in each state or territory annually by a person who is registered or enrolled and intends to practise in any branch of nursing. The responsibility for ensuring that registration or enrolment fees are paid each year rests with the individual nurse.

Each state or territory registration body and the Nursing Council of New Zealand is empowered to deregister nurses in certain circumstances; for example, a nurse's registration or enrolment may be cancelled if they unlawfully use a registration number or if they are found guilty of misconduct or negligence in a professional respect.

AREAS OF LEGAL LIABILITY IN NURSING

The nurse has a responsibility to be aware of certain legal principles, specifically in relation to:

- Contracts
- Standards of care
- Negligence
- Defamation
- False imprisonment
- Assault and battery
- Informed consent
- Confidentiality
- Documentation; for example, of incident reports
- Acts; for example, their relevant Nurses Act
- Witnessing wills
- Coroner's court.

It is important for nurses to realise that they are legally responsible for their own actions and that, although the EN works under the supervision of a Registered Nurse (RN), this does not relieve them of personal liability. Nurses have a responsibility, to themselves and their clients, to refuse to perform an activity if:

- They are asked to do something that is beyond the legal and professional scope of his or her role
- They have not been prepared to perform a function safely
- Directions are unclear, unethical, illegal or against the policies of the health care agency.

CONTRACTS

A contract is an agreement between parties that is legally enforceable because of mutuality of agreement and obligation. A contract gives rise to rights and obligations that are protected and enforced by the law. A contract may be in writing or it may arise by implication, such as the agreement that is reached between a client and a health care agency to which they are admitted. While the client is not required to sign a document, they will have entered into a contract as to the nature and extent of their proposed treatment. Private clients enter into a contract with their medical officer.

The nurse, as an employee, enters into a contract with the employer. Arising out of this contractual relationship are certain rights and obligations relevant to both the employee and the employer, as defined in a written contract of employment. The creation of industrial awards has imposed specific provisions on employers relating to the health and safety of employees, the payment of wages and the provision of certain conditions. An industrial award is a document that sets out the wages and conditions of a particular group of employees and represents the contract of employment between the employer and the employee. A copy of each award can be obtained from the Department of Industrial Relations. Employers are required to have copies of the relevant awards available so that they are accessible to employees. Nurses have a responsibility to themselves to understand their contract of employment and their industrial award.

Nurses engaged through nursing agencies are under contract to the health agency to which they have agreed to be allocated, on starting each work shift. A nursing agency is only an employment agency even though the nurse's pay may be processed through them.

STANDARDS OF CARE

Standards of care are the guidelines by which a nurse should practise and are determined by Nurses Registration Boards or Nursing Councils, professional organisations such as the Australian Nursing and Midwifery Council (ANMC), The Royal College of Nursing Australia (RCNA) and the employing health care agency.

Each source defines standards of nursing care; for example, a Nurses Board defines the scope of nursing practice; professional organisations develop standards for nursing services in policy statements, and the employing health care agency develops written policies and protocols that detail how nurses are to perform their duties. Australian nurses are also required to adhere to the *Code of Professional Conduct for Nurses in Australia* (ANMC 2003, see Online Resources at the end of this chapter).

Nurses have a responsibility to know the standards of care they are expected to meet and to understand the importance of not undertaking tasks outside their defined role and function.

NEGLIGENCE

Negligence, in a legal sense, describes conduct that falls below the standard required by law. If a nurse gives care that does not meet accepted standards, the nurse may be held liable for negligence; for example, if the nurse's actions result in harm to a client. Like other health professionals, nurses have a duty of care to their clients and, generally, negligence means failure by a nurse to take appropriate actions to protect the safety of a client or resident. This may involve failing to do something that should have been done, or doing something that should not have been done. Examples of negligent acts that have occurred include incorrect administration of medications (e.g. the wrong medication being administered), failure to communicate important information about a client's condition, and failing to take appropriate measures so that a client has consequently sustained an injury (e.g. by falling out of bed).

A plaintiff must prove three elements to succeed in an action for negligence:

1. That the defendant owed the plaintiff a duty of care
2. That this duty of care was breached by failure to conform to the appropriate standard of care
3. That the plaintiff suffered injury as a result of the breach of duty. In this regard there must be a reasonably close causal connection between the defendant's conduct and the injury or damage to the plaintiff.

The likelihood of injury to a client, and the risk of liability, is reduced when the nurse adheres to the principles of sound nursing practice and follows the established policies relating to standards of care. Clinical Interest Box 3.3 lists examples of nursing care errors that may result in negligence claims.

DEFAMATION

The term 'defamation of character' refers to any communication, spoken or written, about an individual that injures his reputation. The term 'libel' is used when the communication is written, whereas the term 'slander' is used when the communication is spoken. With regard to nursing practice, all clients have a right to expect their privacy and confidentiality to be respected, and colleagues have a right to expect that their personal and professional reputations will not be harmed.

Nurses should therefore exercise extreme caution when discussing or documenting information relating to clients and when discussing members of staff; for example, a nurse may not be openly critical of the standard of care provided by another nurse. While recognising that, at times, such criticism may be valid, a nurse who is genuinely concerned about standards of nursing care should direct his or her concern through the proper channels, such as the department of nursing administration. Nurses should refrain from gossiping about colleagues, as this practice may lead to irreparable damage of an individual's personal or professional reputation. Nurses should avoid making

CLINICAL INTEREST BOX 3.3
Categories of negligence that result in malpractice

Failure to follow standards of care, including failure to:
- Perform a complete admission assessment or design a plan of care
- Adhere to standardised protocols or institutional policies and procedures (e.g. using an improper injection site)
- Follow medical officer's verbal or written orders.

Failure to use equipment in a responsible manner, including failure to:
- Follow the manufacturer's recommendations for operating the equipment
- Check equipment for safety prior to use
- Place equipment properly during treatment
- Learn how equipment functions.

Failure to communicate, including failure to:
- Notify a medical officer in a timely manner when conditions warrant it
- Listen to a client's complaints and act on them
- Communicate effectively with a client (e.g. inadequate or ineffective communication of discharge instructions)
- Seek higher medical authorisation for a treatment.

Failure to document, including failure to note in the client's medical record:
- A client's progress and response to treatment
- A client's injuries
- Pertinent nursing assessment information (e.g. drug allergies)
- A medical officer's medical orders
- Information on telephone conversations with medical officers, including time, content of communication between nurse and medical officer, and actions taken.

Failure to assess and monitor, including failure to:
- Complete a shift assessment
- Implement a plan of care
- Observe a client's ongoing progress
- Interpret a client's signs and symptoms.

Failure to act as a client advocate, including failure to:
- Question discharge orders when a client's condition warrants it
- Question incomplete or illegible medical orders
- Provide a safe environment.

(Berman et al 2008: 68)

statements in writing in a client's documents that may be interpreted as being of a defamatory nature. Nurses must ensure that all statements relating to a client are written in an objective rather than a subjective manner.

FALSE IMPRISONMENT

False imprisonment refers to the wrongful deprivation of a person's freedom of movement, such as restraining or detaining a person against his or her will. With regard to nursing practice, there are certain situations in which a client may need to be restrained, for example, to protect them from injury, protect others from being injured or prevent damage of property. Nurses must be aware that the application of any restraint is only performed in consultation with the client's medical officer, and then only after very careful consideration. Written authorisation by a medical officer is generally required for the application of a restraint. Apart from very specific instances, there are no powers to detain a person in a health care agency against their wishes, except when they are an involuntary patient under the Mental Health legislation. All health care agencies have a document that a client is asked to sign if they decide to leave the agency against medical advice.

ASSAULT AND BATTERY

Assault and battery are considered criminal offences as well as breaches of civil law. Although the term 'assault' is used to describe both actions, there is a distinction between the two. Assault can be described as a threat to carry out a physical action on another person, thereby causing that person to be in fear of their safety. Battery involves the direct, intentional and uninvited application of physical contact to another person's body.

With regard to nursing practice, a nurse could intentionally or unintentionally commit an act of assault if they do anything that provokes fear in a client that results in the client believing that they will be harmed. As many nursing activities involve direct physical contact with a client, there is a possibility of committing the offence of battery. The important factor in situations in which physical contact is involved is to make sure you have the client's consent.

Consent may be implied, verbal or in writing. Implied consent is frequently given in the performance of nursing activities; for example, if a nurse requests a client to hold out their arm so that they can measure their blood pressure, and they do so, then they have implied their consent to that procedure. Clients frequently give consent verbally, for example, by agreeing to have a procedure performed. Written consent provides documentary evidence that consent was given. Before any invasive procedure or surgical intervention is performed a client is requested to sign a consent form.

INFORMED CONSENT

Any consent must be valid and for consent to be valid it must be voluntarily and freely given. Also, consent is only valid when the person giving it has the legal capacity to do so, when it is specific, and when the consent given is informed. Legal capacity to give consent is determined by age and the person's mental and intellectual function, as legally consent can only be given by a competent adult. Consent must be specific; that is, it must cover the precise nature of the procedure to be performed. Informed consent means that a client should be given adequate information about, and understand, the procedure to which he or she is consenting. The client giving consent should understand the risks and benefits involved as well as understanding the actual procedure. It is the responsibility of the medical officer to provide the client with an adequate explanation of any proposed medical or surgical treatment, and it is the responsibility of the nurse to provide adequate information to the client about any nursing procedure to be performed.

It is important to note that the client has the right to withhold or withdraw consent at any time but they must be informed about any detrimental consequences of refusal. If either situation arises, the event must be reported immediately to the nurse in charge and documented.

In some circumstances when it is difficult to obtain consent, for example if the client is unconscious, consent can be obtained from someone legally authorised to give consent on behalf of the client. If the situation arises that the client requires emergency treatment and it is impossible to obtain consent from the client or authorised person, the overriding duty of care that arises in such emergency situations negates the need for consent on the grounds of necessity. Alternatively, consent would be implied. See Chapter 4 for further detail on informed consent.

CONFIDENTIALITY

Nurses have an ethical obligation not to disclose confidential information acquired about clients in their care, except when such disclosure occurs during the course of their professional duties. Information that may be classified as confidential may be anything related to a client's condition, treatment being given, the prognosis, or anything relevant to a client's private life. Disclosure of such information may lead to legal action against the health care agency. The requirement for nurses to observe a duty of confidentiality is spelt out in the ANMC *Code of Professional Conduct for Nurses in Australia* (2003) and *Code of Ethics for Nurses in Australia* (2002) (Staunton & Chiarella 2008). (For the ANMC website see Online Resources at the end of this chapter.)

Information communicated in a client's nursing and medical records must be kept confidential and, therefore, nurses are responsible for protecting records from unauthorised readers. A client's right to privacy must be respected and their affairs must not be discussed with other clients, with non-professional staff or with members of the general public. Discretion should be used by nurses during their off-duty hours and they should avoid careless chatter about the health care agency, any of the clients or staff members. If approached at any time by a representative of an organisation, press, radio or television, a nurse should refrain from giving information but should refer the enquiry to the administrative section or other appropriate department of the health care agency.

DOCUMENTATION

In the course of their work a nurse is required to document information about clients on nursing care plans, progress notes and flow charts. A client's records may be required in legal proceedings, for example, as evidence in a case where negligence has been alleged. Therefore, in addition to ensuring that any information is recorded accurately and concisely for the purpose of communication between members of the health team, accurate detailing of all relevant information is necessary to provide adequate explanation to a court of law. If a client's records are required in legal proceedings they will be subject to very close scrutiny by lawyers.

Staunton and Chiarella (2008) indicate several important points regarding records:

- Reports should be accurate, brief and complete
- Reports should be legibly written
- Reports should be objectively written
- Entries in reports should be made at the time a relevant incident occurs, or as soon as possible after the incident
- Abbreviations should not be used in reports unless they are accepted within the health care organisation and there is a policy acknowledging this or widely acknowledged medical abbreviations
- If medical terminology is used in reports, the nurse should be sure of the exact meaning, otherwise it could prove misleading
- Any errors made in recording should be dealt with by drawing a line through the incorrect entry and initialling it before continuing
- No entry concerning the client's treatment should be made in the client's record on behalf of another nurse
- All reports need to be dated and signed

To reduce the risk of an incorrect entry being made:

- Don't make an entry in a client's record before checking the name on the record
- Don't make an entry in a client's record by identifying room or bed number only
- Make sure the client's name and identifying number is on every sheet of the client's record before making an entry on the sheet
- Avoid wherever possible making notes concerning a client on loose paper for rewriting later into the client's notes
- No entry concerning the client's treatment should be made in a client's record on behalf of another nurse.

REPORTING OF ADVERSE EVENTS AND CLINICAL INCIDENTS

Nurses have an ethical and legal responsibility to report any accidents or incidents that occur within a health care agency. A written report must be made immediately after an accident or incident occurs in which a client, a visitor or a member of staff was involved, even when no injuries appear to have been sustained or the incident seems trivial. Most health care agencies have special forms for this purpose. Reporting of adverse events and clinical incidents provide a source of information to improve the quality of care and to evaluate the effectiveness of policies.

There is always a possibility that the 'aggrieved person' may take legal action, in which case the written report becomes a very important document. The information included in the report must be factual, clear, concise and objective. Personal opinions must not be included, and care must be taken to avoid using terms that could be misinterpreted. For further details on documentation and reporting skills, see Chapter 20. Examples of adverse events that may be reported are listed in Clinical Interest Box 3.4

Witnessing wills

A client wishing to make a will should be given all the assistance required but it is policy in most health care agencies that nurses may not act as witnesses.

CORONER'S COURT

A coroner's court is presided over by a magistrate, called a coroner, whose main function is to detect unlawful homicide. A coroner is required to investigate any death that was unexpected, or if the person died in unusual or violent circumstances. An inquest into a death may be conducted as long as several years after the event occurred and, in the case of an inquest arising out of a client's death in a health care agency, a nurse may be called upon to give evidence. If this situation arises, nurses are advised to seek legal advice before giving a statement to the police or appearing in court. The health care agency through which the nurse is employed will generally ensure that he or she is represented by the agency's legal representatives. Alternatively, a nurse can be represented by the professional nursing organisation of which they are a member.

LEGAL RESPONSIBILITIES OF NURSING STUDENTS

Clients are entitled to expect to receive a safe standard of care, regardless of whether the care is delivered by a registered or student nurse. However, if students were not allowed to touch clients they would never be able to learn nursing skills properly. For this reason, those involved in the education and supervision of students, and the students themselves, all carry the responsibility for ensuring that students are properly supervised and are never put into a situation where the client's wellbeing might be at risk in

CLINICAL INTEREST BOX 3.4
Examples of adverse events that may be reported

Medication or IV fluids
Prescribing, administration, dispensing, labelling, delivery problem, wrong route, underdose etc.
Medical devices, equipment or property
Poorly designed, unsafe, incorrect/difficult to use, unintentional removal of wound drain etc.
Pressure ulcers
Acts of aggression
Verbal or physical, punching a person, a hole in a door, threats, swearing etc.
Behaviour and human performance
Self harm, absconding, suicide etc.
Buildings, fittings, fixtures and surrounds
Inadequate function, unsafe floor surface, shower water pressure/temperature too high etc.
Nutrition
Fed when fasting, diet not requested, problem with meal or food preparation or delivery etc.
Documentation
Illegible handwriting, electronic documentation, poorly worded.
Clinical management
Unintended injury during procedure, insufficient hand-over, delay in diagnosis, inadequate universal precautions etc.
Hospital-acquired infection
MRSA, VRE, ESBL, Parasites etc.
Falls
Oxygen/gases/vapours
Not prescribed, administered, incorrect gas/rate/frequency/route/concentration etc.
Hazards
Biological, chemical, radiation etc.
Organisation management/services
Bed allocation, staffing shortages, inadequate supervision, after-hours delays, nonavailability of supplies etc.
Security
Confidential breaches, theft, insufficient security staff, no ID badges etc.
Accidents
Patient spills hot drinks, skin tears of unknown origin etc.

South Australian Department of Health (Staunton & Chiarella 2008: 202–3)

any way. When students undertake a new procedure, they should have had previous practice in the nursing laboratories and should be carefully supervised by an experienced and competent nurse, either from their tertiary education institution or from the clinical environment in which the student is placed.

Many student nurses find work as assistants in nursing when not attending classes; however, it is important to recognise that, while such employment will undoubtedly provide valuable experience in interpersonal skills and basic nursing care, the student is employed as an unqualified member of staff, and must not take on responsibilities outside the scope of that employment or their education just because it is possible to do so by virtue of their educational program. In such a situation, the employing authority whose staff assigns such work to students may be liable for any adverse events that occur because of the delegation, as may the students themselves if they have practised outside the scope of their employment (Crisp & Taylor 2005).

ETHICS AND MORALITY

A nurse is a member of a multidisciplinary health team and, as such, has responsibilities that will vary according to the composition of the team and the status of the individual nurse. The primary concern of the health team must be the provision of the very best standard of client care and, to achieve this, it is necessary for all team members to respect the abilities and functions of their co-workers and observe *ethical standards*.

Professional groups each have a code of ethics that consists of standards of conduct that members of the group are expected to follow. Ethics may be defined as a set of moral principles that imply a commitment unrelated to monetary reward or prestige and are derived from a system of values and beliefs concerned with rights and obligations. Ethics is concerned with ascribing moral values to, or passing moral judgement on, such things as people, situations or actions. Ethics is also concerned with the justification of such ascriptions (see Clinical Interest Box 3.5).

In the course of practice nurses are frequently confronted by ethical issues and ethical dilemmas. Consequently, conflict may arise over philosophies, personal values and professional responsibility. It is most important that nurses have an understanding of their own values and some understanding of how ethical problems may be resolved without compromising personal values.

VALUES

A value is a belief about the worth of a particular idea or behaviour, or something an individual views as desirable or important. Values are acquired or learned initially in childhood, from the family and other significant people and experience. Values become part of a person during their socialisation and reflect their personal needs, the society and culture in which they live, and the people to whom they relate. Values influence the way a person interacts with others and the decisions they make.

Personal values motivate and guide a person's behaviour and it is important to recognise that each person's set of values is unique. No two individuals give equal importance to the same values. Some people have very few specific values while others have many. People may value such things as honesty, skill, justice, privacy, friendship, material goods, physical wellbeing, knowledge, talent, wealth, courage and creativity.

Considering values becomes important when a person has to take a stand for that which he or she values. Moral

CLINICAL INTEREST BOX 3.5
Ethical principlism

The theory of ethical principlism is one of the more popular ethical theories used today when considering ethical issues in nursing and health care. Ethical principlism is the view that ethical decision making and problem solving is best undertaken by appealing to sound moral principles. The principles most commonly used are:

Autonomy

Autonomy refers to a person's independent ability to decide. Applied in nursing and health care contexts, the principle of autonomy imposes on health care professionals a moral obligation to respect a client's choices regarding recommended medical treatment and associated care.

Non-maleficence

Non-maleficence is to avoid harm or hurt. Applied in nursing and health care contexts, the principle of non-maleficence would provide justification for condemning any act that unjustly injures an individual or causes them to suffer an otherwise avoidable harm.

Beneficence

The principle of beneficence is to act for the benefit of others; that is, to promote their welfare and wellbeing. Beneficent acts can include care, compassion, empathy, sympathy and kindness.

Justice

Justice can be conceptualised in many ways, such as mercy, harmony, equality and fairness. Of pertinence to health care are the conceptualisations of justice as fairness and as an equal distribution of benefits and burdens.

(Potter & Perry, 2008: 314)

or ethical dilemmas occur in health care when choices have to be made that involve putting one set of values against another. Morals relate to specific values and principles to which a person is committed, and a moral belief is a conviction that something is absolutely right or wrong. For example, some people believe that abortion is absolutely wrong in all circumstances.

NURSING ETHICS

The nursing profession has its own code of ethics, which is a statement about expected standards of behaviour and which is used to guide ethically sound professional nursing conduct and practice. The International Council of Nurses (ICN) formulated an *International Code of Nursing Ethics* (1973) outlining the nurse's responsibilities to individuals, to society, to nursing practice, to co-workers and to the nursing profession.

Recognising the ever-changing conditions in nursing practice and the need for guidance and education relating to ethical decision making, a *Code of Ethics for Nurses in Australia* was established in 1993. This was developed under the auspices of the Australian Nursing and Midwifery Council (formerly the Australian Nursing Council Inc), the Royal College of Nursing Australia and the Australian Nursing Federation. The purpose of developing the code of ethics (cited in Gray & Pratt 1995) was to:

- Identify the fundamental moral commitments of the profession
- Provide nurses with a basis for self- and professional reflection and a guide to ethical practice
- Indicate to the community the values that nurses hold.

The code of ethics is not a set of rules, but a guide for nurses to base their professional decision making upon. (For the Australian Nursing and Midwifery Council (ANMC 2002) revised value statements, see Chapter 1.) Society expects professional people such as nurses to behave with integrity, dignity, competence and compassion. *The International Code of Nursing Ethics*, *The Code of Ethics for Nurses in Australia* and the New Zealand Nurses Association *Code of Ethics* provide nurses with guidelines to assume personal responsibility for providing a standard of excellence in clinical practice. Every nurse is responsible for determining and implementing desirable standards of nursing practice and for following ethical standards in their professional conduct and in the care they deliver. The nurse has a responsibility to participate actively in developing a body of professional knowledge and the skills necessary to promote safe and effective nursing care.

Individual nurses assume responsibility for performing specific activities related to the care of clients; that is, nurses are responsible for their own actions. It is, therefore, essential that all nurses understand the scope of functions and duties associated with their role. *Accountability* means that nurses are responsible, legally and professionally, to themselves, to their clients, to their employing institution and to the nursing profession. Whenever nurses deliver nursing care to clients, they must be able to answer for their own actions — no one else is accountable for their actions. Accountability means that a nurse must assume responsibility to report any behaviour that endangers a client's safety, that they provide clients with adequate information about their care, that they maintain high ethical standards in their own practice, and that they follow the policies and guidelines developed by their employing institution and their professional organisation to promote the delivery of safe and effective nursing care. The regulatory authorities can refer to the various Codes to guide them when they are considering situations of alleged misconduct.

ETHICAL AND MORAL ISSUES

Ethical questions and moral dilemmas arise in numerous areas of medical and nursing practice and may require nurses to be involved in resolving them. Clinical Interest Box 3.6 lists just some of the common ethical issues currently facing the health care team.

Ethical decision making

Often, solving an ethical dilemma may seem almost impossible, but using the standards stated in a code of ethics helps the nurse to view such problems objectively (see Clinical Interest Box 3.7). When an ethical decision is to be made, the following factors must be considered:

- The ethical dilemma must be recognised and defined
- All the facts relevant to the issue and to the individuals involved must be obtained
- The people involved in making a decision must understand the relevant moral rules and principles involved and be able to apply them in an appropriate manner
- Proper evaluation must be made of possible solutions to the problem and of the strategies to be implemented.

Moral dilemmas will continue to occur in health care as long as choices have to be made that involve putting one set of values against another. It is therefore important that nurses keep themselves informed and are involved in discussions and debates about ethical issues and dilemmas so that they are able to make ethical decisions in an informed way rather than on a purely emotional basis.

CLINICAL INTEREST BOX 3.6
COMMON ETHICAL ISSUES

- Genetic engineering
- Artificial fertilisation
- Contraception
- Therapeutic abortion
- Child abuse
- Artificially prolonging life
- Voluntary euthanasia
- 'Not for resuscitation' orders
- Selective non-treatment
- Informed consent
- Withholding information
- Refusal of treatment
- Quality versus quantity of life
- Organ transplantation
- Dying with dignity
- Non-therapeutic research
- Conflict of values and beliefs between members of the health team

CLINICAL INTEREST BOX 3.7
Examples of nurses' obligations in ethical decisions

- Maximise the client's wellbeing
- Balance the client's need for autonomy with family members' responsibilities for the client's wellbeing
- Support each family member and enhance the family support system
- Carry out hospital policies
- Protect other clients' wellbeing
- Protect the nurse's own standards of care

(Berman et al 2008)

ADVOCACY

In a nursing context, advocacy means that the nurse acts for and on behalf of the client. To act as an advocate for a client the nurse must ensure that the client is provided with adequate and accurate information relating to their care, and the nurse must support the client in any informed decisions they make about their care. In this way the nurse meets the ethical requirement of honouring a client's right to self-determination. Nursing ethics involves respecting a client's right to:

- Be informed
- Make decisions and choices
- Confidentiality
- Privacy and dignity
- Hold their own ethical and religious beliefs.

All nurses have a responsibility to ensure that, in relation to nursing practice, the client is assured of safe and competent care and that their rights will be protected.

SUMMARY

Nursing is practised within certain legal constraints and ethical considerations that promote safe and effective care. While the *International Code of Nursing Ethics*, the *Code of Ethics for Nurses in Australia*, the *Code of Professional Conduct for Nurses in Australia* and the New Zealand Nurses Association *Code of Ethics* provide frameworks to promote excellence in clinical practice, every nurse is responsible for determining and implementing desirable legal responsibilities and obligations and standards of practice, and for following ethical standards in their professional capacity. All RNs have a responsibility to promote safe and competent client care.

REVIEW EXERCISES

1. To whom do nurses have responsibilities imposed by the nature of their work?
2. What is the difference between criminal and civil law?
3. Under what circumstances may a nurse be disqualified or deregistered from practising as a nurse?
4. Standards of care are guidelines by which a nurse should practise. Who determines these standards?
5. Name three elements a plaintiff must prove to succeed in an action of negligence.
6. What is meant by defamation of character and how may a nurse avoid being charged with such an offence?
7. With whom do nurses consult regarding consideration of restraining a client?
8. What is the distinction between assault and battery?
9. Under what conditions is consent for a medical procedure considered valid?
10. What is considered confidential information about a client?
11. What may happen to a nurse who discloses confidential information about a client in their care?
12. List nine important points to remember when documenting clients' records.

13. What type of information is not acceptable in an adverse event/clinical incident report?

CRITICAL THINKING EXERCISES

1. Mrs Kyte is a woman you are giving nursing care to. You know from her medical records and your handover report that she has been diagnosed with terminal cancer. You are told she does not know about her condition and her family do not want her to know. What do you say when Mrs Kyte asks you if she is dying? Why do you give this reply?
2. Mr Andrews, 80, was admitted for gall bladder surgery and is recuperating. On the day that the doctor allows him to walk down the corridor with assistance, he asks you to help him do so. Mr Andrews has thromboembolic disease (TED) stockings on and he has slippers in his locker. You get Mr Andrews out of bed and assist him to walk down the corridor, which has a newly buffed linoleum floor. You forget to put on his slippers, although you knew about them. While walking down the hall, you turn to look out of the window at a commotion in the car park. As you are looking, Mr Andrews' feet slip from under him and he falls to the floor, breaking his hip. Identify the elements of negligence and use this case to apply those elements.
3. You are arriving at work and are in a crowded elevator. The conversation in the elevator revolves around a nursing college student who was admitted during the night with a drug overdose. You realise that you know the student. How has the student's right to confidentiality been breached? What are your actions?

REFERENCES AND FURTHER READING

Berman AJ, Kozier B, Snyder S (2008) *Kozier and Erbs Fundamentals of Nursing: Concepts, Process, and Practice*, 8th edn. Prentice-Hall, Upper Saddle River, New Jersey

Campbell AV (1984) *Moral Dilemmas in Medicine*. Churchill Livingstone, Edinburgh

Crisp J, Taylor C (eds) (2005) *Potter & Perry's Fundamentals of Nursing*, 2nd edn. Elsevier Australia, Sydney

Crisp J, Taylor C (eds) (2008) *Potter & Perry's Fundamentals of Nursing*, 3rd edn. Elsevier Australia, Sydney

Forrester K, Griffiths D (2005) *Essentials of Law for Health Professionals*, 2nd edn. Elsevier Australia, Sydney

Fry ST, Johnstone M-J (2002) *Ethics in Nursing Practice: A Guide to Ethical Decision Making*. Blackwell Science, Oxford, UK

Gray G, Pratt R (eds) (1995) *Issues in Australian Nursing*. Churchill Livingstone, Melbourne

International Council of Nurses (1973) *ICN Code for Nurses: Ethical Concepts Applied to Nursing*. Imprimeris Populaires, Geneva

Johnstone M-J (2004) *Bioethics: a Nursing Perspective*, 4th edn. Elsevier Australia, Sydney

Lanham D (1993) *Taming Death by Law*. Longman, Melbourne

MacFarlane PJM (2000) *Health Law: Commentary and Materials*, 3rd edn. Federation Press, Sydney

New Zealand Nurses Association (1988) *Code of Ethics*. NZNA, Wellington

Potter PA, Perry AG (2008) *Fundamentals of Nursing*, 7th edn. Elsevier Mosby, St Louis

Staunton PJ, Chiarella M (2008) *Nursing and the Law*, 6th edn. Elsevier Australia, Sydney

ONLINE RESOURCES

Australian Nursing and Midwifery Council (ANMC) (2002). *Code of Ethics for Nurses in Australia*: www.anmc.org.au

Australian Nursing and Midwifery Council (ANMC) (2003). *Code of Professional Conduct for Nurses in Australia*: www.anmc.org.au

Chapter 4

NURSING RESEARCH

OBJECTIVES

- Define the key terms/concepts
- Define nursing research
- Explain the importance of research in nursing
- Compare the various ways to acquire knowledge
- Understand the basic differences between qualitative and quantitative approaches in research
- Outline the steps in conducting research
- Describe the way research, education and practice relate to each other
- Identify the importance of critical thinking and critical reading when undertaking a research project
- Discuss the importance of informed consent and ethics in relation to research
- Define evidence-based practice
- Explain how Enrolled Nurses (ENs) can participate in nursing research
- Identify future trends in nursing research

KEY TERMS/CONCEPTS

data analysis
data collection
ethical principles
hypothesis
informed consent
nursing research
qualitative research
quantitative research
reliability
research design
research problem
research question
validity
variables

CHAPTER FOCUS

Nursing theory and education are recognised as the main contributors to the development of an accountable and professional nurse in the health care environment. Research is also recognised by health care professionals as being equally important in influencing practice by informing decisions about the delivery of care to clients and their families. Today's evidence-based nursing practice integrates education, theory, practice and the findings from research to provide quality health care. Nurses are also acknowledging the need to develop skills in critically appraising research literature to enable consideration of its application to clinical practice (Beanland et al 2004).

The purpose of this chapter is to enable Enrolled Nurses (ENs) to develop an appreciation of the significance of research to them as nurse practitioners. It introduces the principles of nursing research, basic components of a research proposal, guidelines to critiquing a research article, and an overview of both qualitative and quantitative research.

LIVED EXPERIENCE

I always thought that research was something that academics did working in universities or laboratories. But I got excited when we started learning about evidence-based research in class, as I can now see how to use it in the clinical area and I also know that I will be giving the very latest nursing care to clients in my care.

Melissa, Enrolled Nurse student

NURSING RESEARCH

The term 'research' refers to a systematic way of studying or examining issues so that the knowledge about that issue is validated. It requires an understanding of the existing knowledge about the issue so that new knowledge can be developed. There are many words and terms specifically related to research referred to in this chapter, which are covered in Table 4.1 (later in the chapter).

Nursing research involves a systematic search for and validation of knowledge about issues important to the nursing profession and links theory, education and practice. Nursing research is important for:

- Validating nursing as a profession
- Documenting the effectiveness of nursing interventions
- Providing a scientific knowledge base for practice
- Demonstrating accountability for the profession.

Research-based or evidence-based practice is essential if the nursing profession is to deliver safe, effective and efficient care.

The ultimate goal of nursing is to provide evidence-based care that promotes quality outcomes for clients, families, health care providers and the health care system. Burns and Grove (2004) describe evidence-based practice as involving the use of collective research findings in:

- Promoting the understanding of clients' and families' experiences with health and illness
- Implementing effective nursing interventions to promote client health
- Providing quality, cost-effective care within the health care system.

EVIDENCE-BASED PRACTICE

Evidence-based nursing is a clinical activity based on the belief that decisions about the delivery of care to clients should be informed by the best available and current scientific evidence (Beanland et al 2004). Another definition of evidence-based practice is that it is a process within which clinical decisions are made by practitioners using the best available research evidence, their clinical expertise and client preferences, with consideration also of available and finite resources (Schneider et al 2007). The five steps universally accepted as being necessary for evidence-based practice are presented in Clinical Interest Box 4.1. Clinical Interest Box 4.2 explains evidence-based practice.

CLINICAL INTEREST BOX 4.1
Steps in evidence-based practice

1. Ask a focused question.
2. Assess appropriate evidence.
3. Appraise evidence for validity, impact and precision.
4. Apply evidence accounting for patient values/ preferences, clinical and policy issues.
5. Audit your practice/personal skills.

(Source: Jackson et al 2006; Sackett et al 2000 as modified in Schneider et al 2007: 305)

CLINICAL INTEREST BOX 4.2
Evidence-Based Practice

What Is Evidence-Based Practice?

A process of:

- synthesising research evidence
- designing clinical practice guidelines
- implementing practice changes
- evaluating outcomes

Why Do We Need Evidence-Based Practice?

- Rapid increase in amount of information
- Rapid increase in healthcare costs
- Determination of efficient and effective healthcare practices
- Increased emphasis on performance and outcome standards

Where Is Evidence Found?

- Published research
- Systematic reviews (e.g. Cochrane Collaboration; available: http://www.cochrane.org/)*
- Special collections of EBP resources (e.g. The Joanna Briggs Institute; available: http://www.joannabriggs.edu.au)

*Descriptions can be found at this website, but access to systematic reviews is by subscription only.
(Brown et al 2008: 13)

THE EVOLUTION OF NURSING RESEARCH

As early as 1854, Florence Nightingale demonstrated the importance of research in the delivery of nursing care. When Nightingale arrived in the Crimea in 1854, she found the military hospital barracks overcrowded, filthy and lacking in food, drugs and essential medical supplies. Men were dying from starvation and diseases such as cholera and typhus because of these conditions. By systematically collecting, organising and reporting data, Nightingale was able to implement sanitary reforms and prove a significant reduction in mortality rates. This is considered to be the first nursing research study (Kozier et al 2007).

Research was slow to develop in nursing, with little formal research carried out by nurses until the late 1940s. Nursing schools evolved from military and religious roots and stressed order and obedience. Training was viewed as an apprenticeship, with long hours, and nurses had little say in their own training or work. Only when nursing began to move towards advanced education and affiliation with university settings did nursing research begin to emerge. This move began in the USA. In the 1960s and 1970s the number of nurses with advanced degrees and research skills increased and the push for doctoral preparation in nursing began. Nurses began to turn to nursing care and clinical practice to provide questions for research. Nursing theories evolved that attempted to describe and explain the practice of nursing and these theories began to be tested by nurse researchers. Practice-related research flourished and by the end of the 1970s two new research journals were launched in the USA to handle the nursing research explosion (Borbasi et al 2004).

In Australia and New Zealand, nursing research awareness remained relatively low until nursing moved into the tertiary education sector in the 1970s and 1980s. This move was accompanied by a major increase in the level of research activity, which was directed at educational, disciplinary or professional issues, and research into other disciplinary areas of relevance to nursing. It is only recently that research education delivered to nurses in Australia and New Zealand has begun to prepare nurses to understand the relationship between research evidence and nursing practice, and how to go about incorporating research findings into practice (Crisp & Taylor 2005). Some ideas that have been tested and demonstrated to be useful in practice are: moist wound healing; pressure-relieving devices for the prevention of pressure ulcers; client information to improve self care and healthy lifestyles; communication with people who are dying; and nutritional support of older people in hospital (Brown et al 2008).

THE FUTURE OF NURSING RESEARCH

The value of research studies that increase understanding of clinical phenomena and provide direction for defining programs of research is well recognised and flourishing in Australia and New Zealand. Nurse researchers and nurse leaders are visibly involved at the national level, participating in policy making, representing nursing on expert panels and organisations such as the National Health and Medical Research Council (NHMRC) and lobbying for funding (Beanland et al 2004).

Magnet Hospitals are emerging in both Australia and New Zealand. The concept of a 'Magnet Hospital' is to develop and sustain an environment where nursing- and midwifery-related evidence-based practice and practice change are more likely to occur. Magnet Hospitals aim to provide a commitment to staff development and training, effective systems for implementing and evaluating quality-based treatment and care, and sustainable long term resourcing (Schneider et al 2007).

Borbasi et al (2004) state that, with the development of a national organisation for nursing research, research priorities in the 21st century are likely to be directed at nursing practice and that there will be an increased emphasis on building on the results of completed studies. They also believe that there will also be a greater emphasis on finding ways to utilise the results of nursing research in the course of day-to-day practice.

RESEARCH METHODS

Nursing research focuses on the full range of human experiences and responses and is directed towards helping well individuals improve their health status and stay healthy, as well as assisting clients who are sick or disabled by an illness to maintain or improve their health (Crisp & Taylor 2005).

The major factor that affects whether a nursing researcher uses systematic, controlled methods for studying events or problems is the extent to which he or she wishes to study the way that characteristics or variables (see Table 4.1) are different, or the way that one variable is predictive of (causally associated with) another. These studies are well organised and follow a specific procedure to enable other researchers to reproduce the study or examine the evidence and achieve the same outcomes. To guide the design of a research study, nurse researchers may create a hypothesis or statement about what they expect to see before conducting the study (Crisp & Taylor 2005).

Nurse researchers use many methods because nurses are interested in acquiring knowledge about a wide range of human needs and responses to health problems. For example, a different research method may be used by a nursing researcher interested in developing a deeper understanding of a phenomenon and how it may be experienced by clients, such as helping women deal with the consequences of incontinence after childbirth. Most methods used are either quantitative or qualitative in nature (Crisp & Taylor 2005).

QUANTITATIVE METHODS

Quantitative research methods involve the use of numbers and statistical analysis. This is a process used to gather and analyse information that has been measured by an 'instrument', such as a questionnaire, and converted to numerical data. Quantitative nursing research is the investigation of nursing phenomena that lend themselves to a precise measurement, such as pain severity, rate of wound healing, etc (Crisp & Taylor 2005). Box 4.1 describes different ways of using quantitative methods.

In quantitative research, the researcher changes one set of variables and observes the outcome or its influence on other variables. Variables are changeable qualities, such as characteristics of people or situations that can change or vary for many reasons. Temperature, pulse, respiration, blood pressure, height and weight are examples of variables.

The variable that the researcher controls or manipulates is called the independent variable. The variable that varies or changes because of this is called the dependent variable. For example, consider the statement: 'Sitting upright in bed does not make breathing easy in a client with asthma'. The independent variable relates to sitting the client in different positions, such as lying flat, semi-recumbent, lateral and upright positions. This is the variable the researcher can manipulate to study its influence on the dependent variable. The dependent variable is the measurement of breathing.

QUALITATIVE METHODS

Qualitative research is used to describe information obtained in a non-numerical form, such as data obtained

TABLE 4.1 | Common research terms

Term	Definition
Bias	Any influence that may alter the outcomes of a research study
Clinical nursing research	Nursing research that has a direct impact on nursing interventions with clients
Data	Measurable bits of information collected for the purpose of analysis
Data collection	Gathering of information necessary to address the research problem
Deductive reasoning	Logical system of thinking that starts with the whole and breaks it down into its component parts
Dependent variable	A variable that is affected by the action of the independent variable
Ethics committee	Committee responsible for review of research proposals to ensure that human subjects are protected from harm
Hypothesis	Statement of a predicted relationship or difference between two or more variables. A hypothesis contains at least one independent and one dependent variable
Independent variable	A variable that causes a change in the dependent variable
Inductive reasoning	Logical system of thinking that begins with the component parts and builds them into a whole
Informed consent	An agreement by a research subject to participate voluntarily in a study after being fully informed about the study and the risks and benefits of participation
Instrument	Device or technique used to collect data in a research study, e.g., questionnaires or interviews
Literature review	A critical summary of available theoretical and research literature on the selected research topic. It places the research problem for a particular study in the context of what is currently known about the topic
Nursing research	Research usually conducted by nurses to generate knowledge that informs and develops the discipline and practice of nursing
Population	All known subjects that possess a common characteristic of interest to a researcher
Problem statement	A statement that describes the purpose of a research study, identifies key concepts and sets study limits
Qualitative research	Used to examine subjective human experiences by using non-statistical methods of analysis
Quantitative research	The systematic process used to gather and statistically analyse information that has been measured by an instrument and converted to numerical data
Reliability	Characteristic of a good instrument; the assessed degree of consistency and dependability
Research	A systematic process using both inductive and deductive reasoning to confirm and refine existing knowledge and to build new knowledge
Research design	The overall plan for collecting data in a research study
Research process	An orderly series of phrases identifying steps that allow the researcher to move from asking a question to finding an answer
Research question	Use of an interrogative format to identify the variables to be studied and possible relationships or differences between those variables
Sample	A subset of a population selected to participate in a research study
Validity	A characteristic of a good instrument; the extent of an instrument's ability to measure what it states it will measure
Variable	A concept, characteristic or trait that varies within an identified population in a research study

(Borbasi et al 2008)

from interviews. Qualitative nursing research is the investigation of phenomena that are not easily quantified or categorised, in which inductive reasoning is used to develop generalisations or theories from specific observations or interviews (Crisp & Taylor 2005). See Box 4.2 for the different ways of using qualitative methods.

Qualitative researchers may wish to examine individual lives and their stories and behaviour, organisations and their functioning, or cultures and their interactions and social movement. As the study methodology embraces the examination of subjective phenomena, these findings are only considered to be representative of a particular person or group of people, and in a particular setting, and not reflective of other people or other settings (Borbasi et al 2004).

There are strengths in both quantitative and qualitative approaches. The quantitative approach can support a theory or argue to disprove it, and can be very useful, for example, when hospitals or governments want to introduce policy changes. The qualitative approach, by contrast, has a human focus and allows researchers to know their subjects and collect information about attitudes and satisfaction levels that are vital to improve care provided by nurses.

Box 4.1 | Types of research that use quantitative methods

CORRELATIONAL RESEARCH
Studies that explore the patterns of interrelationships among variables of interest, without any active intervention by the researcher. Correlational methods are used in testing predictive relationships among variables, for testing models or theories that seek to explain complex patterns of relationships, and for testing the most effective and efficient means of achieving positive health outcomes.

DESCRIPTIVE RESEARCH
Studies in which the aim is to accurately portray characteristics of individuals, situations or groups and the frequency with which certain events or characteristics occur. The major goal of this form of research is simply to describe what is seen in order to identify variables that may be of interest in future investigations.

EXPERIMENTAL OR QUASI-EXPERIMENTAL RESEARCH
Studies in which the investigator controls the independent variable and randomly assigns subjects to different conditions. The major goal of this research is to determine causal relationships among the variables through a controlled investigation in which only the independent variable can be the cause of changes in the dependent variable.

EXPLORATORY RESEARCH
Studies designed to develop or refine the dimensions of phenomena or to develop or refine a hypothesis about the relationships among phenomena. The major goal of this research is to explore what is seen in order to identify relationships among variables that might be of interest in future investigations.

EVALUATION RESEARCH
Studies that test how well a program, practice or policy is working. The major goal of this form of research is determining the success of a program. This type of research can determine specifically why a program was successful. When programs are unsuccessful, evaluation research can assist in identifying problems with the program, why it was not successful or even barriers to implementation of programs.

SURVEY RESEARCH
Studies designed to obtain information from populations regarding prevalence, distribution and interrelation of variables within the study population. They may be conducted for the general purposes of obtaining information about practices, opinions, attitudes and other characteristics of individuals. The major goal of this form of research is simple description or the accumulation of a large amount of data to describe the population being studied, as well as the topic of study.

(Crisp & Taylor 2005)

THE RESEARCH PROCESS

There are several steps in conducting either quantitative or qualitative research.

Box 4.2 | Types of research that use qualitative methods

ACTION RESEARCH
Studies that attempt to make qualitative research more humanistic, holistic and relevant to the lives of human beings. The major goal of this research is working in collaboration with participants in a manner that brings about desired change(s).

CRITICAL SOCIAL RESEARCH
Studies that empower individuals involved in this research by attempting to confront unjust power structures within a specific context or society. The major goal of this research is the challenging of dominant constructions of reality and the societal structures that maintain the status quo and determine allocation of power and resources.

DESCRIPTIVE RESEARCH
Studies in which the objective is to accurately portray characteristics of individuals, situations or groups and the frequency with which certain events or characteristics occur. The major goal of this research is to describe what is seen in order to detect phenomena that might be of interest in future research.

EXPLORATORY RESEARCH
Studies designed to develop or refine the dimensions of phenomena or to develop or refine a hypothesis about the relationships among phenomena. The major goal of this research is to explore what is seen in order to identify relationships among phenomena that might be of interest in future research.

HISTORICAL RESEARCH
Systematic studies designed to establish facts and relationships concerning past events. The major goal of this research may be either a descriptive account of what occurred and the facts surrounding the event(s), or a critical approach may be taken in which the researchers challenge the dominant interpretations of facts.

INTERPRETATIVE RESEARCH
Studies in which human experience is investigated to generate deeper understanding of the phenomena of interest. The major goal of this research is the exploration of the numerous ways human beings experience the complex world in which they live.

(Crisp & Taylor 2005)

STEP 1. THE RESEARCH PROBLEM

The research problem is refined through a process that proceeds from identifying a general idea of interest to defining a specific topic. A preliminary literature review reveals related factors that appear critical to the research topic. The significance of the research problem must be identified in terms of its potential contribution to clients, nurses and the medical community (Beanland et al 2004). Choosing the topic of interest may develop from:

- Discussing an issue of common interest with a colleague
- Reading about an issue in a journal, text or newspaper
- An aspect of practice being introduced for the first time

- An aspect of practice that may have been observed but needs to be validated
- Areas of work that may need to change
- Wanting to repeat a study that has already been conducted, to check the results.

STEP 2. THE PURPOSE

The purpose of the study states the aims or goals that the investigator hopes to achieve with the research. It also suggests the way in which the researcher sought to study the problem.

STEP 3. LITERATURE REVIEW

The overall purpose of conducting a review of the literature is to develop a strong knowledge base to carry out research and other consumer research activities in the educational and clinical practice settings. It is a broad, comprehensive, in-depth, systematic and critical review of scholarly publications, unpublished scholarly print materials, audiovisual materials and personal communications (Beanland et al 2004).

The literature review provides a way of checking what has already been studied in relation to the proposed study. It can also provide an understanding of the procedures, methods of analysis and variables that can influence the study (see Box 4.3).

How to search successfully for information

To conduct a successful search for information about a particular subject, the researcher needs to define the topic of interest, select appropriate search resources and selectively review and evaluate the materials produced by a search (Borbasi et al 2004). A search is conducted using indexes, abstracts and catalogues to find information about specific subjects. Books tend to give standard accepted information and practices. They provide good baseline data on a subject. Journals, however, provide more current information than books. They report changing trends and practices.

Several electronic indexes are used for nursing journals (Box 4.4), including the Cumulative Index to Nursing and Allied Health Literature (CINAHL), Index Medicus (a comprehensive index of peer-reviewed medical journals compiled by the US National Library of Medicine) and its online counterpart, MEDLINE (Medical Literature Analysis and Retrieval System [MEDLARS] online). Each index has a primary area of focus and advantages and limits. Electronic databases operate with a special vocabulary. However, the computer helps the researcher to define the preferred terms to use in a search. It is important to make the search as precise as possible; if there are several key terms, they should be used. Other limits such as gender, age and/or time factors, should also be set. Ask for assistance from the librarian if there is difficulty finding information. Many professional information sources are also available on the internet, where there is access to a wide variety of databases, client and nursing education resources, as well as some nursing journals (see Online Resources at the end of this chapter).

Critical thinking and critical reading skills

When an article on the research topic is found, the next step is to use critical thinking and reading skills. Critical thinking is the rational examination of ideas, inferences, assumptions, principles, arguments, conclusions, issues, statements, beliefs and actions. The reader needs to actively look for statements that are unsupported (Beanland et al 2004). Refer to Boxes 4.5 and 4.6.

Critical reading involves the following stages.

Preliminary understanding. This is quickly reviewing a source to gain a broad overview of its content. Skimming through the article enables the reader to make a preliminary judgment about the value of a source and to determine

Box 4.3 | Overall purpose of a literature review

- Determines what is known and not known about a subject, concept or problem.
- Determines gaps, consistencies and inconsistencies in the literature about a subject, concept or problem.
- Discovers unanswered questions about a subject, concept or problem.
- Discovers conceptual traditions used to examine problems.
- Uncovers a new practice intervention(s) or provides evidence for current practice intervention(s).
- Generates useful research questions and hypotheses for the discipline.
- Describes the strengths and weaknesses of designs or methods of enquiry and instruments used in earlier works.
- Determines an appropriate research design or method (instruments, data collection and analysis methods) for answering the research question(s).
- Determines the need for replication of a well-designed study or refinement of a study.
- Promotes development of new or revised practice protocols, policies and projects or activities related to nursing practice and to the discipline.

(Schneider et al 2007)

Box 4.4 | Examples of nursing research journals

- *Australian Journal of Advanced Nursing*
- *Journal of Advanced Nursing*
- *Nursing Research*
- *Research in Nursing and Health*
- *Applied Nursing Research*
- *Nursing Science Quarterly*
- *Journal of Nursing Scholarship*
- *International Journal of Nursing Studies*
- *Nursing Outlook*
- *Journal of Nursing Education*

(Borbasi et al 2008; Berman et al 2008)

Box 4.5 | Highlights of critical thinking and critical reading strategies

- Read primary research articles from peer-reviewed journals.
- Read secondary research (critique/response/commentary) articles from peer-reviewed journals.
- Photocopy or print copies and make notations directly on the copy.
- While reading articles:
  - keep a research text and a dictionary by your side
  - review the chapters in a research text on the various steps of the research process, criteria used to critique, unfamiliar terms and so on
  - list key variables at the top of the article
  - highlight or underline new terms, unfamiliar vocabulary and significant sentences
  - look up the definitions of new terms and write them on the article photocopy and review old and new terms before subsequent readings
  - highlight or underline identified steps of the research process
  - identify the main idea or theme of the article — state it in your own words in one or two sentences
  - continue to clarify terms that may be unclear on subsequent readings
  - make sure you understand the main points of each reported step of the research process you identified before you critique the article.
- Determine how well the study meets the critiquing criteria:
  - ask fellow students to analyse the same study using the same criteria and compare results
  - consult faculty members about your evaluation of the study.
- Type a one-page summary and critical review of each study:
  - cite bibliographic information of the reference at the top of the summary according to relevant reference style (e.g. the American Psychological Association, Harvard, Vancouver)
  - briefly summarise each reported research step in your own words
  - briefly describe strengths and weaknesses in your own words (bibliographical databases allow you to write a narrative for each paper reviewed).

(Schneider et al 2007)

Box 4.6 | Critiquing criteria

The following guidelines can be used as a guide in critiquing an article.

- Is it easy to read and understand; that is, no jargon or obscure phraseology?
- Is the topic important and relevant?
- Have the definitions, key terms and concepts been explained clearly?
- In the background to the study, is there enough information in the introduction to set the scene? Has the purpose of the study been identified?
- How did they conduct the study; that is, what is the methodology?
  - Is there evidence of reliability and validity?
  - How were the subjects selected?
  - Are they a large or small group?
- What did the researchers find, and are the methods of analysis appropriate?
- Do the discussions and recommendations relate to study? Are the author's claims justified by the data? Were the suggestions made based on personal views and not on data? Are the recommendations based on reported findings?
- Is the language used understandable?
- Is the visual material (e.g. graphs, tables, charts) easy to follow and clearly marked?
- Comment on the study's strengths as well as its weaknesses
- Justify criticisms; offer a rationale for how a different approach could have solved a problem
- Try to be objective; try to avoid being overly critical of a study because of a personal lack of interest in the topic
- Is the report or study written in an objective style or are the author's biases and viewpoints apparent?
- Does the author include a reference for every citation made in the text, so that readers can refer to earlier work on the topic?
- Check the credibility of the author
- Check the year of publication — whether it is recent or old.

(Beanland et al 2004; Burns & Grove 2004; Borbasi et al 2004)

whether it is a primary or secondary source (Burns & Grove 2004). A primary source is written by an individual(s) who developed the theory or conducted the research. A secondary source is written by an individual(s) other than the one who developed the theory or conducted the research (Beanland et al 2004).

Comprehending understanding. This requires that the source be read carefully, with the focus on understanding major concepts and the logical flow of ideas within the source. On a photocopy of the article, highlight the content considered to be important (Burns & Grove 2004).

Analysis understanding. Through analysis, the value of a source can be determined for a particular study. Analysis takes place in two stages. The first stage involves critiquing individual studies, which includes identifying relevant content. The second stage of analysis involves making comparisons among studies. This analysis allows a critique of the existing body of knowledge in relation to the research problem. According to Burns and Grove (2004), this helps to determine:

- Theoretical formulations that have been used to explain how the variables in the problem influence one another
- What methodologies have been used to study the problem
- Any methodological flaws in previous studies
- What is known about the problem

- What the most critical gaps in the knowledge base are.

Synthesis understanding. This involves clarifying the meaning obtained from the source as a whole. The meanings obtained from all sources are combined, or clustered, to determine the current knowledge of the research problem. This forms the basis of the review of literature for research study (Burns & Grove 2004).

STEP 4. THEORETICAL FRAMEWORK OR CONCEPTUAL FRAMEWORK

A theoretical framework uses a theory or theories to form a foundation or frame of reference for the research study. A theoretical framework helps the researcher explain or predict study outcomes and link these to the existing body of knowledge. Not all research studies use a theoretical framework, as sometimes a theory is not available if the area of research is new. A conceptual framework is a loosely related collection of concepts that have not yet been tested (Borbasi et al 2004).

STEP 5. HYPOTHESIS/RESEARCH QUESTIONS

When research questions are used, the purpose of the study is descriptive or exploratory and a theoretical framework is rarely identified. Research questions identify the variables to be studied and possible relationships or differences between those variables.

A hypothesis tries to predict the relationships between variables and the expected outcomes of the study. The researcher makes educated guesses based on the review of the literature and the theoretical framework. The results of the research study will either support or refute the hypotheses established (Borbasi et al 2004).

STEP 6. RESEARCH DESIGN

The research design is the overall plan that guides the way the study is conducted and analysed. The research question determines the approach to be used in the design. The design of the study must be able to answer the question posed by the researcher. Determining the appropriate design is also accomplished through the theoretical framework and review of the literature.

Certain key aspects should be considered in a study design. They include:

- Intervention: if there are interventions in the study, they should be part of the design. The study should say what the interventions are, e.g., giving certain medication. What will be the procedure for the intervention? What will be the intensity of the intervention? How long will the duration of the intervention be? Who will perform it?
- Comparisons: in some studies, when making comparisons the design must clearly state what the central issue of the study is
- Extraneous variables: the researcher must mention in the design what measures will be taken to control the extraneous variables (the factors that influence the issue under study)
- Timing of data collection: the design should indicate when the data will be collected in relation to other steps of the research process
- Research location: the design must clearly specify the location for data collection
- Communication with the study participants
- In the research design, information given to participants must be clearly identified. When, what and how much information will be provided about the study to the participants?

STEP 7. SAMPLE TYPE AND SIZE

Once the research design has been established, the subjects and the setting are then considered. The subjects of interest for a research study are known as a population. These subjects possess certain common characteristics or traits that identify them as a part of the population. Populations are usually large, so the researcher chooses a part, or sample, of the population to make the study more feasible. Subjects are selected using a sampling process. The characteristics of the sample population must closely resemble the characteristics of the population as a whole. If this occurs, the study results can be applied to the whole population (Borbasi et al 2004).

STEP 8. LEGAL AND ETHICAL ISSUES

One of the primary concerns in research is to protect the subjects from any harm, discomfort, duress or coercion. Ethics approval is normally required before any type of data are collected that involves humans. If there is more than one agency involved in the study, the researcher must obtain ethical approval, from each agency. Various agencies will have their own ethical guidelines (see Box 4.7). In Australia one of the peak bodies for research is the NHMRC (www.health.gov.au/nhmrc), who have a *National Statement on Ethical Conduct in Research Involving Humans, 1999*. Research involving Aboriginal and Torres Strait Islander peoples is considered to require particular attention to ethical issues and is governed by separate guidelines (*NHMRC Guidelines on Ethical Matters in Aboriginal and Torres Strait Islander Health Research 1991*) (Borbasi et al 2004).

When undertaking research while working in a health care facility, ENs would normally seek ethics approval from the hospital or health care facility's ethics committee. The three ethical standards that must be adhered to are beneficence, justice and respect for persons (Borbasi et al 2004) (see Chapter 3 for further explanation of these terms). Protection regarding storage, retrieval and destruction of data and all issues of confidentiality should be clearly explained for ethical approval of the study.

In New Zealand, there is considerable emphasis on ensuring that all research meets ethical standards and

Box 4.7 | The broad role of human research ethics committees

- Risks to participants are minimised.
- Risks to participants are reasonable in relation to anticipated benefits, if any, and the importance of the knowledge that may reasonably be expected to result.
- Selection of participants is equitable.
- Informed consent will be sought.
- Informed consent will be appropriately documented.
- Adequate provision is made for monitoring the research to ensure the safety of participants.
- Appropriate provisions are made to protect the privacy of participants and the confidentiality of data.
- When vulnerable subjects are involved, appropriate additional safeguards are included to protect their rights and welfare.

Potter and Perry 2005 (Data from Code of Federal Regulations: Protection of human subjects, 45CFR46 (1983, revised as of March 1993), Washington, DC, 1993, U.S. Department of Health and Human Services.)

particular effort is made to ensure that the interests of vulnerable groups are not compromised. As part of the Treaty of Waitangi, Māori cultural and ethical values are protected. The Health Research Council of New Zealand provides guidelines on ethics in health research at www.hrc.govt.nz (Borbasi et al 2004).

The NHMRC requires that all institutions involved in conducting research on humans or animals establish a relevant institutional ethics committee. This group reviews all studies conducted in the institution to ensure that ethical principles are observed, and determines the risk status of all research projects.

Informed consent

Study participants, or their guardians in cases of children or people with cognitive impairment, should be fully informed about the study with regard to its risks, benefits and costs. Crisp and Taylor (2005) state that research subjects should be:

- Given full and complete information about the purpose of the study, procedures, data collection, potential harm and benefits, and alternative methods of treatment
- Capable of fully understanding the research and implications of participation
- Able to voluntarily consent or decline to participate in the study
- Able to understand how confidentiality or anonymity is maintained.

Study subjects should also be guaranteed that there will be no repercussions to their health in any way from their treatment or care or in the case of their withdrawal from the study, and that there will be no breach of their confidential information. Confidentiality guarantees that any information provided by the subject will not be reported in any manner that identifies the subject, and will not be made accessible to individuals outside the research team. Anonymity must occur when even the researcher cannot link the subject to the data. Subjects should also be offered the opportunity to raise any concerns about the study at any stage of the study research.

STEP 9. INSTRUMENTS OR MEASUREMENT TOOLS

To examine the proposed research questions or hypotheses, the researcher must be able to collect measurable data on the variables. Data are collected using an 'instrument'. Data to be collected are usually physiological, behavioural or psychological in nature. Physical measurements could include using sphygmomanometers, electrocardiogram (ECG) machines, glucometers and thermometers. Behavioural data are generally collected through observation. Psychological measurements are used to collect data about knowledge, feelings and attitudes. These variables cannot be directly observed, so instruments such as questionnaires or interviews are used.

STEP 10. VALIDITY AND RELIABILITY

A good instrument is one that is valid and reliable. A valid instrument measures what it is supposed to measure, and a reliable instrument measures the variable consistently, dependably and accurately. Instruments used in research studies should be evaluated for reliability and validity before use in a study (Borbasi et al 2004).

STEP 11. DATA COLLECTION PROCEDURE

The researcher puts the design into action and carries out the prescribed procedures. Treatments are conducted, instruments are administered and data generated and recorded. Data must be collected in an ideal manner so that they capture the concept that is being researched in a way that is relevant, credible, accurate, unbiased and sensitive. Any small change to an aspect of data collection can influence the study and interfere with its integrity. After the data are collected, the researcher organises it into an appropriate form for analysis.

STEP 12. DATA ANALYSIS

Analysis of the data occurs to answer the research questions or to see whether the hypothesis was true. In the qualitative approach, the analysis will begin almost immediately when data collection begins whereas, in the quantitative approach, all data has to be collected first before the analysis begins. The other difference is that the qualitative data has a lot of narratives and there is no systematic rule for analysing it. The absence of systematic analytical procedures makes it difficult for researchers to argue the case for validity. The absence of universally well-defined procedures makes qualitative study difficult to be replicated.

In the quantitative approach, statistical analysis enables the researcher to reduce, summarise, organise and give meaning to the data. Descriptive statistics are used to describe the specific characteristics of the data, such as how many cases fall into a particular category of measurement, typical values and the degree of interrelationship or correlation among measurements. Examples of descriptive statistics include averages and frequencies.

STEP 13. RESULTS

The researcher presents the data, either qualitative (in narrative form) or quantitative (results of descriptive and inferential statistical tests). The findings should be presented in a clear, logical and concise way that answers the research questions or hypotheses. All results should be reported, whether or not they support the aim of the study. Tables and figures may be used to illustrate and summarise data for presentation (Beanland et al 2004).

STEP 14. DISCUSSION OF FINDINGS AND NEW FINDINGS

In the interpretation of the results, the researcher draws together the theoretical framework and makes interpretations based on the findings and theory. Both supported and non-supported results should be interpreted. If the results are not supported, the researcher should discuss the results, reflecting on the theory, as well as possible problems with the methods, procedures, design and analysis (Beanland et al 2004).

STEP 15. IMPLICATIONS, LIMITATIONS AND RECOMMENDATIONS

Once the findings are stated and discussed, the researcher then makes further recommendations for further research. Recommendations provide the consumer with suggestions regarding the study's application to practice, theory and future research. The researcher also discusses any problems or limitations encountered while conducting the study. Identifying limitations informs future researchers so they do not repeat them when conducting a similar study.

STEP 16. REFERENCES

All references that are cited in the article or research study are included at the end of a paper. The reference list supports the material presented by identifying sources in a manner that the reader can then follow up to obtain these references for their own use or for any clarification.

STEP 17. COMMUNICATING RESEARCH RESULTS

Sharing the research findings can occur through several ways, such as presenting a paper or poster at conferences or seminars at local, national and international levels; or publication of articles in nursing research or specialty journals and reports, which leads to wider circulation of the study and research findings.

PROPOSAL WRITING FOR RESEARCH APPROVAL

A research proposal is a written plan identifying the major elements of a study, such as the research problem, purpose, framework, and an outline of the methods and procedures for conducting the study. A proposal is a formal way for communicating ideas about a proposed study to receive approval for conducting the study and to seek funding. Seeking approval for the conduct or funding of a study involves submission of a research proposal to a selected group for review and, in many situations, verbally defending that proposal (Burns & Grove 2004).

WRITING A RESEARCH PROPOSAL

The ideas in a research proposal must logically build on each other to justify or defend a study. The depth of a proposal is determined by the guidelines developed by schools of nursing, funding agencies and institutions where research is conducted. Guidelines provide specific directions for developing a proposal and should be followed explicitly. Content considered to be critical in a proposal are:

- The background and significance of the research problem
- Purpose
- Framework
- Research objectives, questions or hypotheses
- Methodology or research design
- Research production plans (data collection and analysis plan, personnel, schedule and budget).

Essential sub-components of these critical elements of a research proposal include:

- Statement of the problem. This needs to:
    - be specific enough to be solved
    - be in the form of a question or declaration statement. For example, if the study were about neglect of oral hygiene in nursing homes, the question might be 'What is the impact of poor oral hygiene on residents in nursing homes?'
    - provide the background of the problem, such as how the problem came to be recognised and factors that contributed to the problem.
- Significance or importance of the problem:
    - includes the implications or possible applications of the knowledge that would be gained through the study.
- The research hypothesis (where appropriate), which should be:
    - reasonable
    - consistent with known facts or theories
    - stated in such a way that it can be tested and found to be probably true or false
    - stated in clear, simple terms.
- Assumptions and definitions:
    - all unusual terms that could be misinterpreted need to be defined
    - variables considered in the study should be defined.

- Review of related literature:
  - a brief summary of previous research and writings of recognised experts is included to provide evidence that the researchers are familiar with what is known and with what is still unknown and untested.
- An outline of the research procedure, which should include:
  - research design: a brief description of proposed mode of study
  - sampling protocol: population to be sampled, approximate sample size, characteristics and type of sample
  - specification of the proposed data gathering techniques (the actual instrument need not be included). Indicate only the data-gathering procedures, conditions for context of data collection and the time frame for data collection
  - analysis of data and methods to be used
  - projected timetable for various steps of the research
  - limitations and weaknesses of the study, as recognised by the researchers.
- Proposed budget:
  - include all necessary items and estimated costs.

A copy is typed for submission and should be free from errors in spelling, punctuation or grammar. A well designed proposal is the first step to conducting a worthwhile research project.

CONTENT OF A STUDENT PROPOSAL

Student researchers develop proposals to communicate their research projects to the faculty, members of the university, and agency research review committees. The content of a student proposal usually requires much detail and the proposed study is discussed in the future tense of what will be done in conducting the research (Burns & Grove 2004). Boxes 4.8 to 4.10 present guidelines for quantitative and qualitative student research proposals and an example of a completed submission.

Box 4.8 | Quantitative research proposal guidelines for students

INTRODUCTION
- Background and significance of problem
- Statement of the problem and statement of the purpose
- Review of relevant literature
- Framework
- Development of a framework
- Formulation of objectives, questions or hypotheses
- Methods and procedures
- Description of research design
- Identification of population and sample
- Selection of a setting
- Presentation of ethical considerations
- Selection of measurement methods
- Plan for data collection
- Plan for data analysis
- Identification of limitations
- Discussion of communication of findings
- Presentation of a study budget and timetable

REFERENCES

APPENDICES

(Burns & Grove 2005)

HOW IS RESEARCH UTILISED IN PRACTICE?

Research utilisation refers to translating the knowledge that has been generated by research into clinical practice. The ultimate goal is to formalise research utilisation to promote research-based policies, procedures and clinical practice

Box 4.9 | Qualitative research proposal guidelines for students

A qualitative research proposal might include some content similar to that of a quantitative proposal, but the guidelines are usually more flexible and abstract to accommodate the still-emerging design of the study.

INTRODUCTION
- Identification of the phenomenon to be studied
- The study purpose and type of qualitative study
- Study question or aims
- Discussion of the significance of the study

RESEARCH PARADIGM
- Identification of the research paradigm for the type of qualitative study to be conducted
- Description of the philosophical correlates of the research paradigm
- Explanation of research assumptions

RESEARCH METHODS
- Researchers' credentials for conducting a particular type of qualitative study
- Identification of the research method for the study
- Selection of site and population
- The researchers' role
- Ethical considerations
- The data collection process
- Data analysis techniques
- Plan to document the research process during the study

PRELIMINARY FINDINGS, LIMITATIONS AND PLANS FOR COMMUNICATING THE STUDY RESULTS
- Summary and relevant reference literature
- Identification of biases and previous experiences with research problem
- Disclosure of anticipated findings, hypotheses and hunches
- Discussion of how procedures will remain open to unexpected information
- Discussion of limitations of study
- Identification of a plan for communicating findings

REFERENCES

APPENDICES

(Burns & Grove 2005)

Box 4.10 | An example of a research proposal

STUDENT NURSE RETENTION AND ATTRITION IN A TAFE SETTING

Investigator: Gabrielle Koutoukidis

INTRODUCTION

The purpose of this descriptive study is to examine factors that contribute to the retention and attrition of students enrolled in the Certificate IV in Health (Nursing) at the Health Services Unit, Victoria University.

Factors that may impact on the issue of retention and attrition are identified and include work conflicts, personal problems, academic factors, being under-prepared versus being prepared for study, demographic factors and financial factors. The study will examine whether these factors differentiate between those who stay enrolled and those who leave the TAFE Nursing course.

A number of strategies and interventions to reduce attrition and increase retention of students have been introduced by the Health Services Unit over the past 5 years. These strategies are examined in terms of their effectiveness.

BACKGROUND TO STUDY

Focus groups and questionnaires conducted in 1997 within the Certificate IV in Health (Nursing) course at Victoria University revealed that students experienced stress in relation to study skills, time management, coping with social and family roles, economic and financial issues. Students' inability to manage these stresses created difficulties in terms of their progression through successful completion of the course.

The Unit conducted a further study in 1997 that was quasi-experimental in design, with a non-equivalent control group to examine the effectiveness of various strategies to address the above issues. In this study the experimental group participated in an orientation program. This program aimed to provide them with knowledge about resources available on campus to assist them both academically with study and time-management skills and psychosocially with strategies and resources to cope with stress. Both groups were resurveyed 8–10 weeks later to compare their perception of stress and their level of skill, knowledge and ability to access resources available to support them. The stress reported by the experimental group was less than that of the control group.

This study made particular recommendations and from one of these has evolved an integrated 8-week timetabled academic skills assistance program to directly support students in the development of the academic skills necessary for successful completion of the course. Preliminary evaluation of this program indicates that students who attended this program had higher marks and higher course completion rates compared with students in past years, when there was no academic skills assistance program timetabled.

LITERATURE REVIEW

Much has been written on the attrition and retention of students in courses. McGrath and Braunstein (1997) state that causes of attrition vary and that the strategies designed to reduce it produce different results at different institutions. They recommended that administrators and faculty use surveys and focus groups to evaluate the effectiveness of the existing programs and strategies, and conduct semesterly and yearly statistical analyses to establish and measure strategic goals. They also recommended that college and university administrators and faculty should work together to conduct their own research regarding the retention of students rather than rely too heavily on findings in the related literature.

Conklin (1997), McGrath and Braunstein (1997) and Fralick (1993) state that work conflicts, personal problems, financial problems, demographic and social issues, health problems and child care difficulties are the major factors that lead to high attrition rates in courses. Fralick (1993) stated that research has shown that the most critical factor in student retention is a caring attitude by staff — in addition to orientation and advising, faculty and staff can contribute to student retention by developing advisement linkages with students through campus organisations, campus activities or college work–study programs.

FRAMEWORK

Aim

To explore the reasons why students decide to either leave or stay and complete the TAFE Nursing course.

Objectives

- To identify factors that contributed to student retention in the TAFE Nursing course.
- To identify factors that contributed to student attrition in the TAFE Nursing course.
- To recommend appropriate strategies for increasing retention within the TAFE Nursing course.

METHODOLOGY

Design

This study will have a comparative descriptive survey design using questionnaires. Two questionnaires have been developed: one for students who voluntarily decide to leave the Certificate IV in Health (Nursing) course (colour-coded green [Appendix 1]); and a second questionnaire for students who complete the Certificate IV in Health (Nursing) course (colour-coded white [Appendix 2]).

The questionnaires are colour-coded to enable easy identification of the two different questionnaires when collating the data.

A comparative descriptive design examines differences in variables in two or more groups that occur naturally in the setting (Burns & Grove 1987: 244).

guidelines (Borbasi et al 2004). However, there are many barriers to translating research into practice. Borbasi et al (2004) list:

- Resistance to change
- Insufficient time and resources to implement changes to practice
- Lack of supportive infrastructure
- Lack of research skills, including an inability to critique
- Lack of professional autonomy to effect change
- Inability to access and engage with research findings.

Box 4.11 lists further barriers to research utilisation.

Box 4.10 | An example of a research proposal — cont'd

Questionnaires were selected as the instrument because there is less opportunity for bias than in an interview (Burns & Grove 1987: 311). Other advantages of a questionnaire include that subjects feel a greater sense of anonymity, that the format is standard for all subjects and is not dependent on the mood of the interviewer, and that a greater amount of data over a broad range of topics may be collected (Brink & Wood 1988: 148).

A cover letter will accompany the questionnaire, explaining the purpose of the study, the name of the researcher and the approximate amount of time that will be required to complete the form (Burns & Grove 1987: 313) (Appendix 3). The letter will be printed on Curtin University of Technology letterhead to add authenticity to the questionnaire.

A pilot test of the questionnaire will be performed with a small random sample of trainee students enrolled in the Certificate IV in Health (Nursing) course, who will be completing the course in July 2001. This is to determine the clarity of questions, effectiveness of instructions, completeness of response tests, time required to complete the questionnaire and successfulness of data collection techniques (Burns & Grove 1987: 313). In a pilot test the subjects and techniques should be as similar to those planned for the large study as possible (Burns & Grove 1987: 313). This is the reason that the trainee students were chosen, and also because they will not be included in the study.

To ensure content validity, the questionnaire will also be submitted for review by three lecturers at Victoria University who are involved in nursing education and who are experts in developing questionnaires (Brink et al 1988: 169).

Subjects

The population for this study will be all students (male and female) who enrolled full-time and part-time in the Certificate IV in Health (Nursing) course in February 2001 (about 200 students). Both students who decide to leave the course voluntarily and students who successfully complete the course will be invited to participate in this study.

Data collection

Stage 1. Questionnaires will be posted to the students, both full time and part time, who decided to voluntarily leave the course. A return envelope for the completed questionnaire will be included, with a return date indicated. These questionnaires will be posted when the students withdraw from the course. This mailing will start in July 2001 and continue until November 2001.

For the students who decide to complete the course, questionnaires will be administered during a class in the last week of the course in November 2001. A box will be placed in the student administration building at Sunbury Campus for students to return the questionnaires. Questionnaires will be collected daily for 1 week from this box.

Stage 2. To examine the variables that may have contributed to the retention and attrition rates of these TAFE nursing students. These may include work conflicts, personal problems, academic factors, being under-prepared versus being prepared for study, demographic factors and financial factors.

Data analysis

Content analysis will be performed to extract meaning from open-ended questions in the questionnaire (Burns & Grove 1987: 311). The categories derived from content analysis will be cross-tabulated with demographic data to examine the relationships between variables. Descriptive statistics will be used to describe sample characteristics that arise from the demographic data collected. The relationships between sample characteristics and data categories will be tested using Chi-square analysis (Brink et al 1988: 267). Qualitative and quantitative analysis will also be performed on the data to examine the factors that contributed to the attrition and retention rates.

Ethics

Only students enrolled in the Certificate IV in Health (Nursing) course in February 2001 will be selected for the purpose of this study. Participation is on a voluntary basis.
Participants will be informed of the purpose of the questionnaire via a cover letter, which will explain that all the information on the questionnaires will be collected anonymously. Anonymity will also be maintained through the fact that the names and addresses of participants will not be collected (Brink et al 1988: 194). A consent form will not be required, as by completing the questionnaire, which has minimal or no risk attached to it, the participant is indicating consent (Burns & Grove 1987: 353).

Confidentiality and anonymity can be further guaranteed, as the data that will be collected from the student database of the university will not include student identification numbers or names. No names will be linked to the data obtained on the questionnaires. In the data analysis, the data will be group-analysed so that individuals cannot be identified by their responses (Burns & Grove 1987: 344), thus providing further safeguards for anonymity.

Data collected will be stored in a locked file for 5 years, as per recommendations from the NHMRC Statement on Human Experimentation.

Budget

Budget items	Cost per item	Total cost	Funded by
Printing costs	2500 pages @ 0.10 cents per page	$ 250.00	Workplace & researcher
Supplies		$ 400.00	Workplace & researcher
Postage	60 sent @ 45 cents each	$ 27.00	Workplace
Return envelopes	60 sent @ 45 cents each	$ 27.00	Workplace
Travel costs (if researcher needs to fly to Perth for consultation)		$ 1000.00	Researcher
		TOTAL: $ 1704.00	

(Continued)

Box 4.10 | An example of a research proposal — cont'd

Timetable

Tasks to be performed	Performer of task	Completion of task
1. Develop questionnaire for students who voluntarily leave	Researcher	April 2001
2. Develop questionnaire for students who complete the course	Researcher	April 2001
3. Submit proposal to University School of Public Health Graduate Studies Committee	Researcher	June 2001
4. Submit proposal to Ethics committee at Victoria University	Researcher	June 2001
5. Pilot the questionnaire		
6. Collect data	Researcher	June 2001
7. Analyse data	Researcher	July – November 2001
8. Interpret results	Researcher	July – November 2001
9. Submit dissertation	Researcher	July – November 2001
	Researcher	December 2001

REFERENCES

Brink, P.J. and Wood, M.J. (1988). *Basic Steps in Planning Nursing Research: From Question to Proposal*. USA: Jones and Bartlett Publishers, Inc.
Burns, N. and Grove, S. (1987). *The Practice of Nursing Research: Conduct, Critique And Utilisation*. Philadelphia: W.B. Saunders Company.
Conklin, K.A. (1997). Course attrition: A 5-year perspective on why students drop classes. *Community College Journal of Research & Practice*, 21(8): 753–59.
Fralick, M.A. (1993). College success: A study of positive and negative attrition. *Community College Review*, 20(5): 29–39.
McGrath, M.M and Braunstein, A. (1997). The prediction of freshman attrition: An examination of the importance of certain demographic factors. *College Student Journal*, 31(3): 396–408.

APPENDICES

(The appendices are the two questionnaires and cover letter, not included here)

(Koutoukidis 2001)

Box 4.11 | Other barriers to research utilisation

THE RESEARCH ITSELF
- Poorly designed and/or implemented research
- Research not replicated
- Relevant literature not compiled in one place
- Poorly supported results
- Poorly implemented or written statistical analysis

PRACTISING NURSES
- Isolation from knowledgeable colleagues
- Nurses too new on the job to implement new ideas
- Lack of authority to implement changes

ORGANISATIONAL SETTINGS
- No support of nursing research findings
- Changes in the health care environment
- Acuity rate
- Degree of nursing shortage
- Financial constraints to implement change

THE NURSING PROFESSION
- Limited research-based journals
- Limited federal funding for nursing research
- Poor communication between practitioners and researchers
- Shortage of appropriate role models

(Crisp & Taylor 2005 (Data from: Polit DF, Hungler BP (1999) *Nursing research: principles and methods*, 6th edn. JB Lippincott, Philadelphia; Walsh M (1997) Barriers to research utilization and evidence-based practice, in A & E nursing. *Emerg Nurse* 5 (2): 24; and Carroll DL et al (1997) Barriers and facilitators to the utilization of nursing research. *Clin Nurse Spec* 11 (5): 207)

APPROACHES TO RESEARCH UTILISATION

According to Borbasi et al (2004), after a research study has been located and surveyed, it must be determined:

- Whether it is relevant to the clinical area (see Box 4.12)
- Whether the results have merit and are applicable to the area of work and clients (see Box 4.13)
- How to implement any relevant or applicable results (see Box 4.14).

Box 4.12 | Criteria for determining clinical relevance of a study

- Is the study a clinical study?
- Are the participants in the study similar to the clients in a particular clinical setting?
- Is the setting used in the study similar to the clinical setting the nurse is working in?
- Is the problem being studied one seen in the clinical area?
- Do the study findings address issues that nursing has the power to change? Do they affect the activities of daily living? Do they have ramifications for client comfort and wellbeing?
- Are the study findings helpful to the clinical routine? Do they add to the nurses' knowledge base?

(Borbasi et al 2008)

Box 4.13 | Criteria for determining clinical merit of a study

- Are the key elements of the study easily identified?
- Are the steps of the research process followed?
- Are ideas concisely and comprehensively identified?
- Are sampling methods clearly described? Are they appropriate to the study?
- Do the results make sense?
- Do quantitative studies use reliable and valid instruments?
- Do qualitative studies address issues of auditability, transferability and credibility of data?
- In qualitative studies, does the final picture of the phenomena under study flow logically from the data?
- In quantitative studies, does the discussion section clearly identify whom the results could be applied to? Are the findings clearly tied to existing knowledge?
- Have other studies been done that address the identified problem?

If the answer to any of these questions is no, then the merit might need further consideration.

(Borbasi et al 2008)

Box 4.14 | Criteria for determining implementation possibilities for a study

- Who will be affected and in what numbers?
- What are the advantages of implementation?
- What are the risks of implementation?
- What are the risks of no implementation?
- Do the advantages outweigh the risks?
- How complex is the change?
- How much will it cost?
- Who will be affected by the change besides nurses?
- What are the tangible observable outcomes of the implementation?

(Borbasi et al 2008)

THE ENROLLED NURSE AND NURSING RESEARCH

There are opportunities for ENs to have an active participation with nursing research (Clinical Interest Box 4.3). ENs may come across some research findings that can be very pertinent to their practice, and may intend to introduce the findings into their professional practice; for example, the 'new' way of managing wound care. The EN may feel that the introduction of a research idea that they have critically read has relevance to their practice.

Apart from utilising research findings into the practice settings, ENs have the opportunity to participate in nursing research activity, for example, by supporting the research team with data collection and data entry.

CLINICAL INTEREST BOX 4.3
Example of practical application of research

At a staff meeting where cost effectiveness was being discussed, an EN reported that she had read an article indicating that a particular dressing used for pressure ulcers was more cost effective than the current dressing they were using on the facility. Another nurse said that the other articles they had on file indicated that the dressing they were currently using was more effective in the treatment of pressure ulcers. The nursing team agreed that there was a conflict in the data and began a literature review to help them find more and current information to resolve the discrepancy in the findings (adapted from Beanland et al 2004).

Enrolled nurses can also participate and attend conferences. The National Enrolled Nurse Association (NENA) promotes the value of ENs and raises awareness of ENs' role within the community, while providing a forum for all ENs to participate at a national level. Check NENA's website (www.anf.org.au/nena) for information on upcoming conferences.

SUMMARY

Nursing research improves the practice of nursing and raises the standards for the profession. Involvement in nursing research takes place in designing studies, being part of a research team, collecting data, using research findings to change clinical practice, improving client outcomes and maintaining the cost of health care. Promoting research and research utilisation in practice increases the scientific knowledge base for nursing practice.

With the scope of practice constantly expanding for nurses, it is of importance that ENs are familiar with research process, so that they can continue to provide quality care to their clients. This chapter introduced some broad aspects of nursing research and its relevance to ENs.

REVIEW EXERCISES

1. Provide a brief explanation of why research is important for the nursing profession.
2. Explain the basic steps in conducting nursing research.
3. List three differences between qualitative and quantitative research approaches.
4. Why are ethics important in nursing research?

CRITICAL THINKING EXERCISES

1. If a researcher wanted to determine the most effective treatment for healing a pressure ulcer, what type of research method should be used for the study?
2. Identify some possible areas for nursing research that arise from your clinical practice rotations. How might nursing research improve your practice in these areas?

REFERENCES AND FURTHER READING

Beanland C, Schneider Z, LoBiondo-Wood G, Haber J (2004) *Nursing Research: Methods, Critical Appraisal and Utilisation*, 2nd edn. Mosby, Sydney

Berman AJ, Snyder S, Kozier B, Erb B (2008) *Kozier and Erbs Fundamentals of Nursing: Concepts, Process, and Practice*, 8th edn. Prentice-Hall, Upper Saddle River, NJ

Borbasi S, Jackson D, Langford RW (2004) *Navigating the Maze of Nursing Research: An Interactive Learning Adventure*. Elsevier Australia, Sydney

Borbasi S, Jackson D, Langford RW (2008) *Navigating the Maze of Nursing research*, 2nd edn. Elsevier Australia, Sydney: 104–6

Brown D, Edwards H (2008) *Lewis's Medical-Surgical Nursing: Assessment and Management of Clinical Problems*, 2nd edn. Mosby Elsevier Australia, Sydney

Burns N, Grove S (2004) *The Practice of Nursing Research: Conduct, Critique and Utilization*, 5th edn. WB Saunders, Philadelphia

Crisp J, Taylor C (2005) *Potter & Perry's Fundamentals of Nursing*, 2nd edn. Elsevier Australia, Sydney: 739–42, 1348, 1351

Koutoukidis G (2001) *Student Nurse Retention and Attrition in a TAFE Setting*. Dissertation proposal, Master of Public Health, Curtin University of Technology, WA

National Health and Medical Research Council (NHMRC) (1999) *National Statement on Ethical Conduct in Research Involving Humans, 1999*. NHMRC, Commonwealth Government of Australia, National Capital Printers, Canberra

—— (1991) *Guidelines on Ethical Matters in Aboriginal and Torres Strait Islander Health Research 1991*. NHMRC, Commonwealth Government of Australia, National Capital Printers, Canberra

Schneider Z, Elliot D, LoBiondo-Wood G, Haber J (2007) *Nursing Research: Methods, Critical Appraisal and Utilisation*, 3rd edn. Mosby, Sydney

ONLINE RESOURCES

American Association of Colleges of Nursing: www.aacn.nche.edu

Australian Nursing and Midwifery Council: www.anmc.org.au

Australian Nursing Federation: www.anf.org.au

Health Research Council of New Zealand, guidelines on ethics in health research: www.hrc.govt.nz

Kingston University/St George's Hospital Medical School, London: www.healthcare.ac.uk

National Enrolled Nurse Association (NENA): www.anf.org.au/nena

National Institute of Nursing Research: www.nih.gov/ninr/about.html

National Health and Medical Research Council (NHMRC): www.health.gov.au/nhmrc

New Zealand Nursing Council: www.nursingcouncil.org.nz

Royal College of Nursing Australia: www.rcna.org.au

The University of British Columbia Library: www.library.ubc.ca

Unit 2

The health care environment

Chapter 5

SYSTEMS OF HEALTH CARE DELIVERY

OBJECTIVES

- Define the key terms/concepts
- Identify areas of health in which the Commonwealth Government (Australia) plays a leadership role
- State which levels of government (Australian) are primarily responsible for the delivery and management of public health services
- State which levels of government (Australian and New Zealand) finance and regulate aged-care services
- Discuss the life expectancy of Australian citizens
- State the major employers of allied health and paramedical professionals
- State two main forms of Australia's aged-care system
- State the aim of the Australian National Health Care funding system
- State the aims of the Australian Pharmaceutical Benefit Scheme (PBS)
- Discuss issues relating to the Medicare levy in Australia
- Differentiate between primary, secondary and tertiary health care services
- List the health professional groups who comprise the health care team
- State who has a direct role in providing quality health care

KEY TERMS/CONCEPTS

alternative or complementary systems
Australian Council on Healthcare Standards (ACHS)
Commonwealth (Federal) Government
Evaluation and Quality Improvement Program (EQuIP)
Medicare
nurses and health policy reform
Pharmaceutical Benefits Scheme (PBS)
preventative, primary and tertiary health care settings
private health insurance
private sector health services
specialist medical officers
Total Quality Management (TQM)

CHAPTER FOCUS

To assist in meeting the health care needs of individuals, the nurse requires an understanding of the health care system. This chapter gives an outline of the Australian and New Zealand health care systems and focuses on health care economics as well as identifying health care settings, health care providers and services. Further focus is given to factors affecting health care delivery, the reasons for quality improvement and explanation of accreditation of health care organisations.

LIVED EXPERIENCE

When I had surgery to my hip in the 1960s I was in the hospital for about 6 weeks and had to stay in bed for most of the time. My neighbour has just had her hip done and she was told by the nurses to get up on the second day after the operation, and she was sent home about 2 weeks later. She is lucky because I hated having to stay in the hospital for such a long time away from my family.

Greta, aged 92

THE AUSTRALIAN HEALTH CARE SYSTEM

Australia has a land mass roughly the same size as Western Europe or the USA (excluding Alaska). Settlement of Australia by people now known as Aboriginal and Torres Strait Islander peoples, or Indigenous Australians, occurred some tens of thousands of years ago (Commonwealth Department of Health and Ageing 2003). Settlement by people from Great Britain and subsequently other countries began in 1788, resulting in the present day population of about 20 million, with a diversity of ethnic backgrounds. About 80% of the population lives in cities (Australian Bureau of Statistics [ABS] 2006). There are large regions that have only small scattered settlements or are unpopulated. Australia is a developed country with a generally high standard of living.

SYSTEM OF GOVERNMENT

In the 19th century, Australia was governed as a collection of British colonies. Since 1901 Australia has been an independent nation, with a federal system of government that originated from the British Government and law. The Constitution established a Commonwealth (Federal) Government, giving its parliament powers in specified fields. Each of the six states and two territories within the Commonwealth has a parliament; in the states these parliaments have powers in all areas not specified in the Constitution as Commonwealth powers. The Commonwealth, state and territory governments operate on the Westminster system, in which the political party or coalition with the majority of elected members in the lower house of the parliament forms the government (not all state and territory parliaments have an upper house). Ministers with executive powers are drawn from these elected members of government in either lower or upper houses. Within states there are local governments such as municipal and shire councils.

GOVERNMENTS, THE PRIVATE SECTOR AND HEALTH

Originally the only Commonwealth health power was in quarantine matters. However, in 1946 the Constitution was amended to enable the Commonwealth to provide health benefits and services, without altering the existing powers of the states. Consequently the two levels of government have overlapping responsibilities in this field. The Commonwealth currently has a leadership role in policy making and national issues such as public health, research and national information management.

The states and territories are primarily responsible for the delivery and management of public health services and for maintaining direct relationships with most health care providers. This includes the regulation of health professionals. The states and territories provide public acute and psychiatric hospital services and a wide range of community and public health services. These include school health, dental health, maternal and child health and environmental health programs.

The state and territory governments directly fund a broad range of health services. The Commonwealth funds most medical services out of hospital, and most health research. The Commonwealth, states and territories jointly fund public hospitals and community care for older people and those with disabilities.

All levels of government (including consumers and the non-government sectors) have some role in funding, administering or providing care for older people. Residential aged care is financed and regulated by the Commonwealth Government and provided mainly by the non-government sector (by religious, charitable and for-profit providers). Currently, the Commonwealth, states and territories jointly fund and administer community care such as delivered meals, home help and transport (Figure 5.1).

There is a large and vigorous private sector in health service and the Commonwealth Government considers that strong private sector involvement in health services provision and financing is essential to the viability of the Australian health system. For this reason the Commonwealth Government provides a 30% subsidy to people who acquire private health insurance and has introduced additional arrangements to foster lifelong participation in private health insurance.

Private health insurance can cover private and public hospital charges (public hospitals charge only clients who elect to be private clients so they can be treated by the doctors of their choice) and a portion of medical fees for inpatient services. Private insurance can also cover allied health and paramedical services (such as physiotherapist and podiatrist services) and some aids and appliances such as spectacles. Non-government, religious and charitable organisations play a significant role in health services, public health and health insurance.

HEALTH STATUS

The average age of people in Australia and New Zealand is increasing. The number of Australians and New Zealanders over age 65 is increasing more rapidly than that of the general population. It is predicted that ageing populations will demand more health care and financial resources, such as Medicare. Older people are more likely to have complex medical and health care needs, including multiple chronic conditions that may compromise their ability to remain independent. Physical and functional problems, dementia, fixed incomes and limited family or community support can put older people at an increased need for social and health care assistance (Brown et al 2008). In 2003, total life expectancy at birth was 77.8 years for Australian males and 82.8 years for females (Australian Institute of Health and Welfare [AIHW] 2006). The median age of the New Zealand population is rising, as a result, the number of deaths at older ages is increasing. Half of the male deaths in 2000–2002 occurred at ages 75 years and over, while

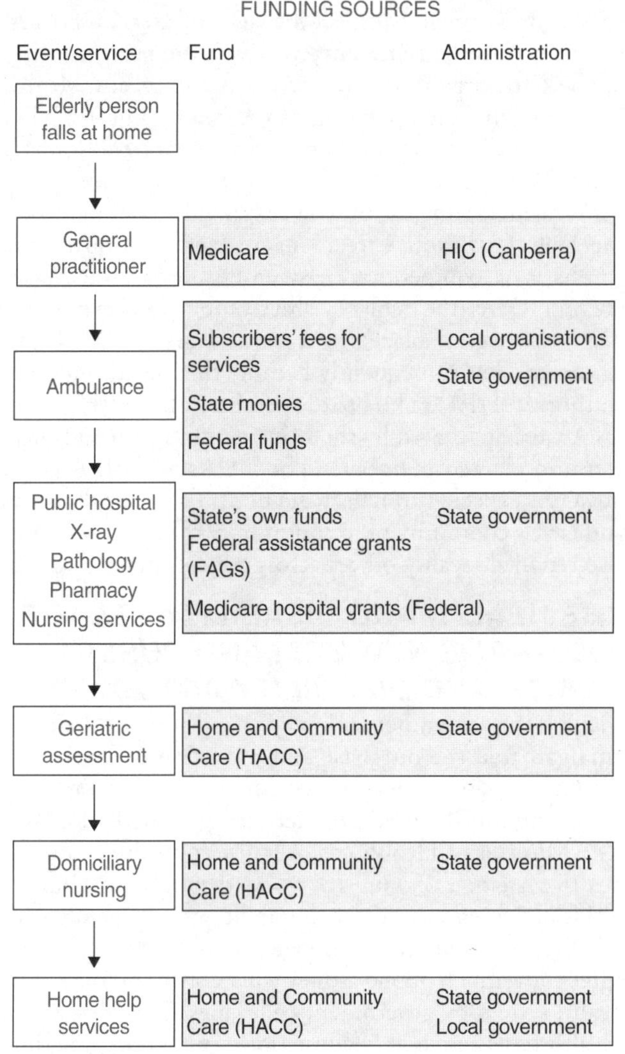

Figure 5.1 | Tiers of government health care funding
(Crisp and Taylor 2005 (Data from Clinton M, Schwiewe D: Management in the Australian health care industry 2e, with permission, Pearson Education Australia. Copyright 1998)

half of the female deaths occurred at ages 81 years and over (Statistics New Zealand, www2.stats.govt.nz).

HEALTH SERVICES DELIVERY

As indicated above, a mix of public and private sector providers deliver health services. The quality of health care provided is high in both sectors. Most medical officers are self-employed. A small proportion consists of salaried employees of Commonwealth, state or local governments. Salaried specialist medical officers in public hospitals often have rights to treat some clients in these hospitals as private clients, charging fees to those clients and usually contributing some of their fee income to the hospital. Other medical officers may contract with public hospitals to provide medical services. There are many independent pathology and diagnostic-imaging services operated by medical officers. For some allied health and paramedical professions there is a significant proportion self-employed; others are mainly employed by state and local government health organisations.

Public hospitals include facilities established by governments and hospitals, which were originally established by religious or charitable bodies but are now directly funded by government. A small number of hospitals are built and managed by private firms providing public hospital services under arrangements with state governments. Most acute-care beds and emergency outpatient clinics are in public hospitals. Large urban public hospitals provide most of the more complex types of hospital care such as intensive care, major surgery, organ transplants, renal dialysis and specialist outpatient clinics.

Private hospitals are owned by for-profit or not-for-profit organisations such as large corporate operators, religious operators and private health insurance funds. In the past, private hospitals tended to provide less complex non-emergency care, such as simple elective surgery. However, some private hospitals are increasingly providing complex high-technology services. Separate centres for same-day surgery and other non-inpatient operating-room procedures are found mostly in the private sector. Many public hospitals provide such services on the same site as inpatient care.

Specialised mental health care in the public sector is provided in separate psychiatric hospitals, general hospitals and community-based settings. Historically, mental health services have operated separately to mainstream health services, but the Commonwealth, state and territory governments are currently working under the National Mental Health Strategy to mainstream mental health services. Other key reforms taking place under the strategy focus on replacing separate psychiatric hospitals with community-based and general hospital services, and integrating mental health care into different settings.

Australia's aged-care system is structured around two main forms of care delivery: residential (accommodation and various levels of nursing and/or personal care) and community care (ranging from delivered meals, home help and transport to intensive coordinated care packages for people who otherwise would need residential care). Residential services are mainly in the non-government sector, about half being operated by religious and charitable organisations. Both public and non-government (mostly religious and charitable) sector organisations provide community care services under the Home and Community Care Program.

Medicines or pharmaceuticals prescribed by medical officers and dispensed in the community by independent private sector pharmacies are directly subsidised by the Commonwealth Pharmaceutical Benefits Scheme (PBS). Public hospitals provide medicines to inpatients free of charge and do not attract PBS subsidies. Non-prescription medicines are available from pharmacies and in some cases other suppliers such as supermarkets. The importing and supply of medicines and medical devices is regulated by the Commonwealth Therapeutic Goods Administration (TGA) to ensure the quality, safety and effectiveness of the products.

Some innovative solutions to health issues have arisen out of Australia's unique history and needs. Notable among these are:

- The Royal Flying Doctor Service which delivers care to remote areas by aircraft
- The Aboriginal and Torres Strait Islander people's community-controlled health services, which aim to meet the special needs of Indigenous Australians
- Regional health services, through which community-identified priorities for health and aged-care services in rural and remote areas are met through a flexible mix of Commonwealth- and state-funded services.

The Australian Red Cross receives Commonwealth, state and territory government funding to operate Australia's blood donation system and to coordinate matching of donors and recipients for organ transplants.

THE HEALTH AND DISABILITY SECTOR IN NEW ZEALAND

Eighty-five per cent of people in New Zealand are concentrated in urban areas. The main ethnic groups are European, Māori, Pacific Islander and Asian. As in many Western countries, a large proportion of the population is slowly growing older. It is projected that in 2031, 22% of the population will be aged 65 or over, compared with only 12% in 1988. Māori and Pacific Islander populations show a younger population structure, with roughly twice the proportion of children under 15 compared with the rest of the population.

The organisation of health and disability support services within New Zealand has gone through several changes within the last two decades. These have ranged from a 'purchaser–provider' market-oriented model in place at the beginning of the 1990s, to the more community-oriented model implemented in 2001. At the beginning of the 1990s, Area Health Boards (AHBs) were responsible for the provision of public health, secondary and community care services. AHBs did not provide preventative care services, although preventative care was subsidised by the government. AHBs were introduced under the *Area Health Boards Act 1983*. The first AHB was established in Northland in 1984 and by 1989 the country was covered by 14 AHBs.

The *Health and Disability Services Act 1993* introduced a system that separated out the purchasing of health care services from organisations that provided services. Responsibility for the purchasing of services lay with four Regional Health Authorities (RHAs). These RHAs contracted with providers of services in both the primary and the secondary care sectors. The RHAs did not have elected representatives on their boards although they did have a commitment to reflect the views of users of services. Election of these representatives was the responsibility of the fifth organisation, known as the Public Health Commission. The operation of the health and disability sector at this time reflected an international trend towards market-based systems.

While retaining the purchaser–provider split in health, the 1996 Coalition Agreement on Health removed the emphasis on competition between hospitals. In addition, the four RHAs (the Public Health Commission having been dissolved) were replaced by a single Transitional Health Authority that subsequently became the Health Funding Authority (HFA). The board members of the RHAs and HFA were appointed by the Minister of Health and there were no elected members. The RHAs and HFA were, however, expected to reflect the needs of users of services and have a commitment to community consultation. They also retained locality offices across the country.

THE HEALTH AND DISABILITY SECTOR 2000 — THE NEW ZEALAND *PUBLIC HEALTH AND DISABILITY ACT 2000*

In 2000 the government initiated change in the sector that amalgamated the purchase and provision of services in the same organisations and decentralised decision making to community-focused District Health Boards (DHBs). The Minister of Health has overall responsibility for the health system. The Minister works through the Ministry of Health to enter into accountability arrangements with DHBs, determines the health and disability strategies, and agrees how much public money will be spent on the public health system by government colleagues. The Ministry of Health has a range of key functions, including providing policy advice to the Minister of Health on all aspects of the health and disability sector, acting as the Minister's agent and providing a link between the Minister of Health and DHBs (and other health organisations), and providing general ministerial servicing functions.

Central government provides broad guidelines on what services the DHBs must provide, and national priorities have been identified in the New Zealand Health Strategy. Services can be purchased from a range of providers, including public hospitals, non-profit health agencies or private organisations. Funding is allocated to DHBs using a weighted population-based funding formula. Service providers (acute hospitals and most public health units) come under the wing of DHBs, while general practitioners (GPs), rest homes and midwives are independent and are contracted to supply services by DHBs or the Ministry of Health. Overall, there are about 80 public hospital facilities in New Zealand and a large number of privately operated aged-care facilities.

THE NEW ZEALAND HEALTH STRATEGY

Following extensive public consultation, the first New Zealand Health Strategy was launched in December 2000.

It places particular emphasis on improving population outcomes and reducing disparities between all New Zealanders, including Māori and Pacific Islander peoples.

THE NEW ZEALAND DISABILITY STRATEGY

Alongside the New Zealand Health Strategy, the *New Zealand Public Health and Disability Act 2000* also required the development of a New Zealand Disability Strategy. After extensive consultation, the first New Zealand Disability Strategy was launched in April 2001 to guide action to promote a more inclusive society. It is an intersectoral document, with relevance across the whole of the public sector in New Zealand.

This strategy presents a vision of a society that values lives of individuals with disabilities and continually enhances their full participation in society. The strategy acknowledges that disability is not something that people have, but rather that disability is a process that happens when one group of people create barriers by designing a world only for their way of living, taking no account of the impairments other people have. For example, restaurants or movie theatres without access for wheelchairs, sports events that do not cater for people with sensory (hearing, vision) or functional (upper or lower limb) impairment.

FINANCING OF THE HEALTH SYSTEM AND EXPENDITURE ON SERVICES

The cornerstone of New Zealand's health system is public finance (through taxes) of most health services with access to those services based upon need. In addition to taxes there are two other sources of finance for health services:

- Private health insurance: individuals may be covered by health insurance that may pay for a variety of treatments
- Out-of-pocket payments: payments made directly by individuals for health care services. Most health care in New Zealand is provided free of charge; the one exception to this is preventative care, for which a fee-for-service system exists. In addition, people may also use private health services if they wish. Private insurance in New Zealand does not cover rehabilitation or long term mental health services (Brown et al 2008).

THE HEALTH AND DISABILITY SUPPORT WORKFORCE

A competent adaptable health and disability support workforce is a crucial ingredient for quality health and disability support services. By international standards, the New Zealand health and disability support workforce is highly skilled and knowledgeable and well equipped to provide the wide range of technical and complex health services available. DHBs are the largest employer of health professionals in the public sector. Medical officers and other primary health care providers, rest homes and private hospitals are all private providers who may well receive public funding for services delivery.

INCREASING NUMBER OF HEALTH PROFESSIONALS

Over the last decade in New Zealand there has been a general increase in the number of health professionals. However, as with all statistics, interpretation needs to take into account a range of factors, the number currently working including those working part time and the type of nursing work undertaken. As at March 2008, there were 40 928 registered nurses; 3209 enrolled nurses; 157 nurse assistants and 45 nurse practitioners who had qualified for and purchased an annual practising certificate for 2008 (Nursing Council of New Zealand 2008).

HEALTH CARE ECONOMICS

THE NATIONAL HEALTH CARE FUNDING SYSTEM

The aim of the Australian national health care funding system is to give universal access to health care while allowing choice for individuals through a substantial private sector involvement in delivery and financing. The major part of the national health care system is called Medicare. Medicare provides high-quality health care, which is both affordable and accessible to all Australians, often provided free of charge at the point of care. It is financed largely from general taxation revenue, which includes a Medicare levy based on a person's taxable income. Commonwealth funding for Medicare is mainly provided as:

- Subsidies for prescribed medicines (with a safety net providing free medicines for the chronically ill) and free or subsidised treatment by practitioners such as medical officers, participating optometrists or dentists (specified services only)
- Substantial grants to state and territory governments to contribute to the costs of providing access to public hospitals at no cost to clients
- Specific-purpose grants to state and territory governments and other bodies.

In addition, Commonwealth general-purpose funding grants to state and territory governments flow partly to health services. State and territory governments supplement Medicare funding with their own revenues, mainly for funding public hospitals.

Some categories of Australians, such as members of the armed forces and veterans, are covered by additional special arrangements while remaining eligible for mainstream Medicare coverage. Some injuries and illnesses are covered by other forms of financing: for example, compulsory workers compensation insurance covers work-related injuries and illnesses, and injuries from motor vehicle accidents may be covered by compulsory third-party motor vehicle insurance.

Residential aged care is financed by the Commonwealth Government by means of subsidies paid to service providers, based on the level and type of care needed by the individual. Residents may pay daily care fees and accommodation payments related to the level of care, with special provisions for residents who have difficulty paying these charges. The Commonwealth decides the allocation of new residential care places by an annual regional population-based planning process, inviting providers to bid to provide the new places.

Community care services for older citizens and people with disabilities are jointly funded by the Commonwealth, state and territory governments, contributing according to their needs. Community care clients pay different fees for services depending on the type of service and the client's capacity to pay. The Commonwealth funds intensive community care packages of coordinated care to enable older adults who might otherwise require low-level residential services to continue living at home.

Medicare covers people residing in Australia who are Australian citizens, New Zealand citizens or holders of permanent visas. Some visitors and temporary residents, from countries with which Australia has made reciprocal health care agreements, are eligible for Medicare with some restrictions.

HOSPITAL CARE UNDER MEDICARE

All people eligible for Medicare are entitled to a choice of:

- Free accommodation, and medical, nursing and other care as public clients in state- or territory-owned hospitals, designated non-government religious and charitable hospitals, or in private hospitals that have made arrangements with governments to care for public clients; or
- Treatment as private clients in public or private hospitals, with some assistance from governments.

State and territory governments are responsible, under agreements with the Commonwealth Government, for ensuring that services are adequate to meet public patient entitlements and are available to all people eligible for Medicare. This component of Medicare is funded jointly by the Commonwealth Government and state and territory governments under the Australian Health Care Agreements.

On admission to public hospitals, clients may choose to be public (Medicare) clients or private clients. If they choose to be public clients they receive free medical and allied health or paramedical care from medical officers nominated by the hospitals, as well as free accommodation, meals and other health services while in hospital. Medicare-eligible clients who choose to be private clients in public hospitals are charged fees by medical officers and are charged by the hospital for hospital care, usually at a rate less than the full cost of providing these services. If the client holds private insurance this will usually cover all or nearly all of the charges of a public hospital. Medicare pays benefits subsidising part of the cost of medical officers' fees, and private insurance pays an additional amount towards medical officers' fees.

Private insurance benefits can also contribute to payment of the costs of allied health or paramedical and other costs (for example, surgically implanted prostheses) incurred as part of the hospital stay. Clients may choose to be treated in a private hospital. Private clients in private hospitals are charged fees by doctors and some allied health or paramedical staff and are billed by the hospital for accommodation, nursing care and other hospital services, such as use of operating theatres. If the client holds private insurance it will contribute to these costs. If the client is eligible for Medicare as a permanent resident of Australia, the medical officers' fees generally attract Medicare benefits.

PRIVATE SPECIALIST MEDICAL OFFICERS' SERVICES UNDER MEDICARE

For some kinds of medical services, Medicare requires the service to be provided by a medical officer who has been formally recognised as a specialist, and that another medical officer has referred the client to the specialist. If these requirements are not met, either no benefit is payable or the benefit is lower.

For most pathology and diagnostic-imaging services, Medicare benefits are paid only when another medical officer has referred the patient to the medical officer providing the pathology or imaging service. These requirements are in place to constrain costs by removing financial incentives to obtain unnecessary specialist services. As a consequence, most access to specialist medical services is on referral from medical officers (primary practitioners, or family doctors).

Medicines and pharmaceuticals

The PBS aims to provide all Medicare-eligible persons with access to effective and necessary prescription medications at a reasonable cost to the clients and to the nation. The PBS provides subsidies for about 600 kinds of drugs in nearly 1500 formulations, which means that clients can obtain reasonably priced medicines for most medical conditions. Additional drugs are added when assessed as meeting safety, quality, effectiveness and cost-effectiveness criteria.

Pharmaceutical benefits are paid as cash transfers direct to around 4800 approved community pharmacies who dispense PBS medications on a claims reimbursement basis. The PBS also provides other forms of assistance to improve affordable access to medicines, for example, specific funding for public hospitals for certain high-cost drugs, such as immunosuppressants used in transplantation.

Under the PBS all eligible persons fall into one of two categories, which determines the amount the client contributes and the amount of subsidy paid:

1. The concessional category — people who receive

certain pensions, benefits or cards administered by Family and Community Services (FACS) or the Department of Veterans' Affairs (DVA), or who meet certain criteria for being declared to be disadvantaged

2. The general category.

General clients pay the cost of dispensed medicines up to a maximum amount per item. When the dispensed price of a drug is above that maximum, general clients pay that amount and the PBS pays the balance up to the listed price. If the prescription involves a more costly but equivalent brand, the subsidy may be limited to the lower-cost brand (the minimum pricing policy).

Concessional clients pay a smaller amount per item than general clients do, and the PBS pays the balance up to the listed price. This is also subject to the minimum pricing policy. Pharmacists must check clients' entitlement cards before providing medicines at the concessional rates.

SPECIFIC FEDERAL GOVERNMENT GRANTS FOR HEALTH CARE SERVICES

Under Medicare the Commonwealth Government provides a range of grants to government and non-government bodies to achieve specific health care objectives. These include:

- The provision of services to special-needs groups such as people in rural and remote areas, Aboriginal and Torres Strait Islander peoples, and people with mental illness
- Funding of medical services that involve the use of expensive equipment, for example, the capital component of radiotherapy services performed on specific approved equipment
- Improving general medical practitioner and associated services.

THE MEDICARE LEVY

When Medicare began in 1984, the Medicare levy was introduced as a supplement to other taxation revenue to enable the Commonwealth Government to meet the additional costs of providing the same level of care for the whole population. The previous system focused on subsidies for health care groups with low incomes.

Medicare levy revenue provides the equivalent of only about 27% of Commonwealth funding for Medicare. Medicare is funded by a range of taxes such as income tax, taxes on sales of goods and services, and non-tax revenue, which together form consolidated revenue. Parliament appropriates funds for most government programs from consolidated revenue. The Medicare levy is paid by individuals at a basic rate of 1.5% of taxable income above certain income thresholds. Taxpayers on high incomes who do not have private health insurance pay an additional 1% of taxable income as part of the levy.

PRIVATE HEALTH INSURANCE

Private health insurance is an important component of funding of health care in Australia, providing about 11% of total national health care funding. For insured people it provides added benefits such as choice of doctor, choice of hospital and choice of timing of procedure. Private insurance can also assist with meeting the costs of private sector services not covered by Medicare, such as dental, optical, physiotherapist and podiatrist services.

The Commonwealth regulates insurance offered by registered health insurance organisations to ensure that the principle of community rating is maintained. Community rating means that health funds must charge everyone the same premium regardless of their health status or claims history. This ensures that private health insurance is open to a wide range of people in the community and that the aged and chronically ill are not priced out of private health insurance. To support community rating, a system of reinsurance redistributes the costs of claims for the elderly and those in hospital for an extended period across all private health insurance funds. This ensures that health funds with a high proportion of these higher-cost members are not disadvantaged. There are over 40 private health insurance funds registered by the Commonwealth. Most of these are open to everyone but some only offer cover to restricted groups such as employees of a particular firm.

To ensure a balance between the public and private health sectors in Australia the Commonwealth Government has introduced measures to address the affordability, stability and attractiveness of private health insurance. These measures are designed to encourage people to take out private health insurance and decrease the pressure on the public system. For example, the Commonwealth Government introduced a 30% rebate on private health insurance in January 1999.

Another initiative introduced by the government is Lifetime Health Cover. Lifetime Health Cover is a new system of private health insurance designed to encourage people to take out hospital cover early in life and maintain their cover. People who join a health fund before they turn 31 years of age and who stay in private health insurance will pay a lower premium throughout their lives relative to people who delay joining, regardless of their health status. People over age 30 will face a 2% increase in premiums over the base rate for every year they delay joining.

The benefit is that in the medium to longer term the rate of premium increases will be slowed by discouraging 'hit and run' behaviour (in which someone joins a health fund just before requiring treatment and then leaves soon after) and by improving the overall health of the membership of private health insurance funds so that the rate of claiming is reduced.

CONSULTATION AND ADMINISTRATION IN THE HEALTH CARE SYSTEM

In the field of health, the peak consultative body between Commonwealth, state and territory governments is the Australian Health Ministers' Conference (AHMC). The major health funding agreements are bilateral agreements between the Commonwealth and each state and territory, with the broad parameters being agreed multilaterally by the AHMC. Strategic public health and other partnerships are negotiated in similar ways. There are subordinate bodies in which officials represent Commonwealth, state and territory health departments.

The National Health and Medical Research Council (NHMRC) is funded by the Commonwealth Government but is independent. It advises governments, other organisations and health workers on a wide range of health matters and allocates substantial medical research funds provided by the Commonwealth. The Council's membership includes representatives of the major stakeholders in the health system, appointed from the public and private sectors. In addition to its peak council, the NHMRC has several ongoing committees and ad hoc working groups. The main ongoing committees are the National Health Advisory Committee, the Australian Health Ethics Committee, the Research Committee, which oversees most Commonwealth medical research funding, and the Strategic Research Development Committee.

The Commonwealth Department of Health and Ageing advises the Commonwealth Minister for Health and Ageing and the Minister for Aged Care. The Health Insurance Commission and its Medicare offices administer enrolment in Medicare, claims for Medicare benefits, pharmaceutical benefits and a range of other Commonwealth programs. The states and territories have varying arrangements for advising their Ministers and for administering public hospital and other health care programs (Commonwealth Department of Health and Ageing 2003).

HEALTH CARE SETTINGS

The health care industry involves a wide range of services that are provided by numerous systems and agencies. Health care services may be broadly classified as those that provide:

- Preventative care: health promotion and disease prevention
- Primary care: diagnosis and treatment
- Tertiary care: rehabilitation.

While the traditional medical care system provides all three types of services, many people are looking towards alternative or complementary systems of therapy, such as chiropractic services, osteopathy, homeopathy, acupuncture, reflexology or massage. Increasingly, people are choosing one or more of the less traditional approaches to health care. A person may choose an alternative or complementary system of health care for numerous reasons. One reason often given is the inability to obtain traditional health services in the way in which a person desires them and at the time they need them. For example, a person may be dissatisfied because of:

- Long waiting hours
- Lack of availability of health professionals
- Impersonality of care given
- Increasing costs of medical care
- Lack of comprehensiveness and continuity of care.

While it should be appreciated that every person has the right to choose a particular system of health care, the nurse is more likely to work within a traditional setting.

The health care delivery system in Australia and New Zealand is varied and includes:

- Health promotion programs
- Illness prevention programs
- Public and private hospitals
- Specialty hospitals
- Rehabilitation services
- Community-based agencies
- Clinics and outpatient services
- Voluntary agencies
- Hospices
- Self-help groups.

PREVENTATIVE CARE

Preventative care comprises health-promotion and illness-prevention activities. Settings for preventative care include community clinics, private homes, schools, industries and doctors' offices.

PRIMARY CARE

Primary care (the diagnosis and treatment of illness) takes place in medical officers' rooms, hospitals, clinics, outpatient services, home health agencies and various community agencies such as drug rehabilitation centres. Day care centres and surgical centres offering one-day admissions offer people an alternative to hospitalisation. Use of home health care is increasing for many reasons, such as earlier discharge from hospital and the development of support systems that enable people with chronic illnesses, such as renal failure, to remain at home. In addition to home nursing care, people may use a range of other services such as meals on wheels or home help. Home care offers an alternative to hospitalisation, a family-centred approach and continuity of care. Refer to Chapter 6 for additional information on primary care.

TERTIARY CARE

Rehabilitation, or long-term care, is provided by rehabilitation centres, some hospitals, extended care facilities, hospices and nursing homes. Rehabilitation also takes place in the individual's home through services provided by home nursing agencies. Figure 5.2 illustrates the various models of health care.

PROVIDERS OF HEALTH CARE

The health care team is defined as a group of health professionals working together to provide health care. The health team is comprised of doctors, nurses and allied health professionals, such as physiotherapists, occupational therapists, speech pathologists, dietitians, pharmacists and social workers.

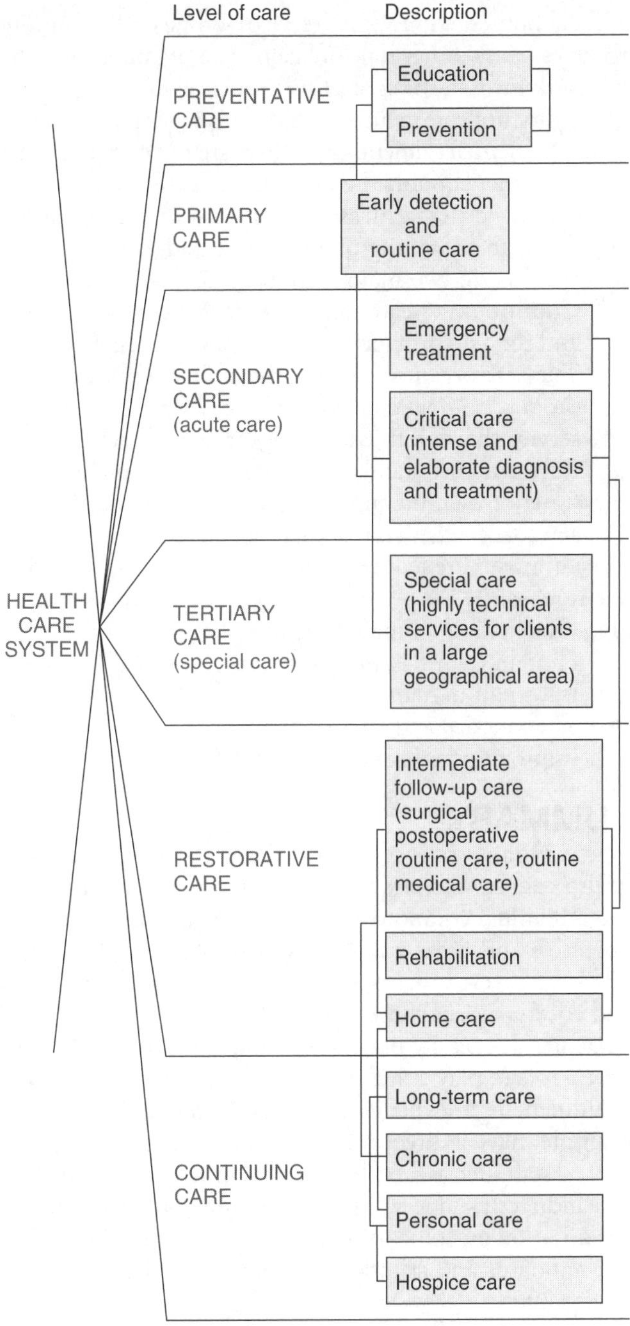

Figure 5.2 | Spectrum of health services delivery *(modified from Potter & Perry 2005 [As modified from Cambridge Research Institute: Trends affecting the U.S. health care system, 262, Health Planning Information Series, Human Resources Administration, Public Health Service, Department of Health, Education, and Welfare, Washington, DC; 1976, revised and updated 1992, US Government Printing Office.])*

FACTORS AFFECTING HEALTH CARE DELIVERY

In the past the emphasis in health care was on the diagnosis and treatment of disease; however, in recent decades the emphasis has shifted to health promotion and disease prevention. This shift in emphasis has occurred for a variety of reasons, such as consumer influences, economic and political influences and technological changes.

The health care delivery system has become more sensitive to the needs of the consumer and the community. Generally people are now more knowledgeable about health and the importance of illness prevention and are prepared to assume some responsibility for their own health. Consequently, health care services have responded by initiating and implementing a variety of health promotion programs.

The rapidly escalating costs of health care and the inability of large numbers of people to pay for health services has led to many changes in the delivery of health care. People are discharged from hospitals much earlier and, consequently, there is a greater need for more home care agencies. Health care services are required to match the economic resources available against the wants and needs of a community.

People of lower economic status frequently defer seeking health services or have to face long waiting periods before they can obtain a hospital bed for non-urgent health problems or elective surgery. Conversely, people with adequate financial resources or private health insurance are generally able to obtain the health care they require as soon as needed.

Political decisions, such as health care legislation, also influence how health care is provided. Nurses are becoming increasingly aware of the role they can play in influencing the restructuring of the health care system, such as advising local and state governments about specific health issues. Nurses, as a body, are able to exert political pressure to influence health policy reform so that the health care system responds to the needs of society as a whole.

Advances in medical technology have resulted in new and sophisticated equipment and procedures coming into use, and research has led to new treatments for life-threatening diseases. The development of sophisticated life-support equipment, and procedures such as implants and transplants, has undoubtedly saved the lives of many people. At the same time, however, technological advances have created numerous ethical dilemmas. There is much debate about the ethics of channelling vast sums of money into specific programs that benefit a relatively small percentage of the population, for example organ transplant procedures, at the expense of the health needs of the majority. Health care providers must consider the consequences of this scientific and technological explosion, for example the quality of the life being saved.

QUALITY IMPROVEMENT AND ACCREDITATION OF HEALTH CARE ORGANISATIONS

Health care organisations have a responsibility for providing quality care to clients and their families, as well as to the general community. Health care providers are therefore accountable for the outcome of care and the services provided. Quality control maintenance systems seek to ensure that specified levels of excellence are met. In the health care context quality assurance is defined as a formal process whereby the quality and appropriateness of client care and/or departmental performances are documented and evaluated by the professional group responsible.

Standards of practice are essential to this process and must be identified from the outset so that objective measurement of quality can be achieved. Attempts to provide clients with an environment that is both safe and conducive to a speedy recovery have resulted in the introduction of Total Quality Management (TQM) to the daily work practices of nurses. TQM is an approach that challenges the status quo and asserts that everything an organisation does, and how it does it, can be improved. TQM is an overall management system that views quality as all-encompassing. The system is data based and highlights cause-and-effect relationships that are acted on to produce outputs that meet or exceed client expectations.

In 1994 the Australian Council on Healthcare Standards (ACHS) issued a statement called the Charter for Change, which indicated how the council wished to function in the future. During 1995–96 a Charter for Change team was formed to consult with the health care industry. Together these groups developed a program called the Evaluation and Quality Improvement Program (EQuIP) as the approach to achieving the proposed changes. The philosophy of continuing improvement is the fundamental premise of EQuIP and naturally applies to the program itself. During 1996 key organisations acted as pilot sites for EQuIP and since then a broad range of health care organisations across Australia have embraced the program.

By providing appropriate management tools, including industry-approved standards, and by focusing on outcomes, EQuIP assists health care organisations to continuously improve their performance to provide the highest quality care to the community. It was introduced as an accreditation program for health care agencies in 1997 and is now recognised both nationally and internationally as a leader in the accreditation process. Accreditation by the ACHS involves a clinical review of management and outcomes of care as well as utilisation review of administrative and service departments. After an organisation-wide survey, an organisation may be awarded ACHS accreditation, based on the surveyor's report. In some circumstances accreditation is awarded on the condition that certain recommendations are incorporated within a specific time frame. If an organisation does not meet a significant proportion of the accepted standards then accreditation is not awarded. The public is regularly informed of accredited organisations.

The ACHS standards are unique in Australia in that they were developed in consultation with the health care industry and encompass health care organisations in their entirety. The standards apply to hospitals, day surgery units, nursing homes, community services, home or community agencies or any other type of health care organisation. The standards form the basis of EQuIP and provide a framework for quality improvement in health care organisation. They focus on essential elements of quality care and organisational functions that support the provision of care.

The standards address the issues considered most important in providing quality and safe health care and are organised in two main sections. These are:

1. Continuum of care standards, which cover the care and services provided to consumers and clients. They are organised so that they follow the care process from when a consumer or client accesses a service through to when they leave the service
2. Infrastructure standards, which cover the main functions within an organisation that are needed to support the delivery of quality and safe care.

The infrastructure standards are arranged into the following five functions:

1. Leadership and management
2. Human resources management
3. Information management
4. Safe practice and environment
5. Improving performance (ACHS 2003).

SUMMARY

The standards reflect the outcomes required if quality health care services are to be delivered. Criteria that form the individual components of the standards must be both objective and measurable to provide scope and indicate key structures, processes and outcomes. The standards and criteria reflect contemporary best practice. They must be achievable, easily understood and measurable. All staff have a role to play either directly or indirectly in providing or influencing the quality of care. Clinical service staff, for example, have a direct role in providing care, while non-clinical staff such as food services personnel influence quality care indirectly. All services and departments of a health care organisation must incorporate the principles that lie within the standards and criteria to become accredited (Crisp & Taylor 2005).

REVIEW EXERCISES

1. What are the different primary responsibilities of the Australian Commonwealth and state and territory governments in relation to health services?
2. Which levels of Australian government have a role in funding, administering and providing care for older people?
3. Which group of Australians have a record of poor health status?
4. What model of health care was implemented by the New Zealand Ministry of Health in the year 2001?
5. In New Zealand, what two sources of finance for health services are there in addition to taxation?
6. How is the Australian Medicare system financed?

7. What two categories of payment exist under the Australian PBS?
8. Identify the differences between the three levels of health care services.
9. What shift has occurred in recent decades regarding health care delivery?
10. What system or software is used in your workplace or place of last clinical practicum to ensure TQM?

CRITICAL THINKING EXERCISE

Mrs Luscombe, 62, is on an aged pension. She was recently in a car accident, suffering a fractured right leg and bruised ribs. She hopes to return to an independent lifestyle as soon as possible. Her nursing care needs have primarily involved pain management, skin care around her cast and physiotherapy. She will continue to wear her leg cast for about six weeks. What level of health care will Mrs Luscombe require before returning home?

REFERENCES AND FURTHER READING

Australian Bureau of Statistics (ABS) (2006) *Census QuickStats: Australia*. Online. Available: http://www.censusdata.abs [accessed 24 April 2008]

Australian Council on Healthcare Standards (2003) Online. Available: www.achs.org.au [accessed 24 April 2008]

Australian Institute of Health and Welfare (2006) *Life expectancy and disability in Australia 1988–2003*. Canberra

Commonwealth Department of Health and Ageing (2003). Online. Available: www.health.gov.au [accessed 24 April 2008]

Brown D, Edwards H (2008) *Lewis's Medical–Surgical Nursing: Assessment and Management of Clinical Problems*, 2nd edn. Elsevier Australia, Sydney

Crisp J, Taylor C (eds) (2005) *Potter & Perry's Fundamentals of Nursing*, 2nd edn. Elsevier Australia, Sydney

New Zealand Ministry of Health (2003) *New Zealand Health and Disability Sector Overview*. Online. Available: www.moh.govt.nz [accessed 24 April 2008]

Nursing Council of New Zealand 2008 Statistics. Online. Available: www.nursingcouncil.org.nz [accessed 24 April 2008]

Potter PA, Perry AG (2005) *Fundamentals of Nursing*, 6th edn. Elsevier Mosby, St Louis

ONLINE RESOURCES

Statistics New Zealand: www2.stats.govt.nz

Nursing Council of New Zealand: www.nursingcouncil.org.nz

Australian Council on Healthcare Standards: www.achs.org.au

Chapter 6

HEALTH PROMOTION AND EDUCATION

OBJECTIVES

- Define the key terms/concepts
- Discuss the concept of health promotion and the inception of the *Ottawa Charter for Health Promotion*
- Describe the benefits of early recognition and treatment of disease
- Become familiar with the different types of health promotion programs
- Discuss the role of the nurse in health promotion
- Facilitate client education
- Utilise the nursing process in health promotion

KEY TERMS/CONCEPTS

Declaration of Alma-Ata
disease
health
health belief model
health education
health promotion
nursing process
Primary Health Care
The *Jakarta Declaration*
The *Ottawa Charter for Health Promotion*
World Health Organization (WHO)

CHAPTER FOCUS

Owing to technological developments and medical and scientific achievements over the last century, the world's population is generally living longer and healthier lives. However, major disparities in health still exist for some of the world's population, with some countries still experiencing high morbidity and mortality rates. In recognition of these disparities in world health, the World Health Organization (WHO) began its work towards achieving health for all the world's population. Health promotion and education provide the key to minimising or eliminating disparities in world health and play fundamental roles in achieving the goals and objectives as determined by WHO. By raising the level of health awareness and providing health education for both the individual and the community, nurses play a vital role in health promotion.

LIVED EXPERIENCE

I have been trying to quit smoking by myself for years without any success until I joined the QUIT program run by the community health centre. I was able to give up a 30-year habit and feel so much better for that. I would not have been successful if it had not been for the support of the community health nurse and the other participants.

Brian, ex-smoker who used to smoke about two packets a day

HEALTH

Health is generally understood to be an absence of disease or illness. The WHO defines health as 'a state of complete physical, mental and social wellbeing and not merely the absence of disease or infirmity' (WHO 1978). WHO's definition of health is holistic in that it considers physical, psychological, cultural and social factors. According to WHO, 'health depends on our ability to understand and manage the interaction between human activities and the physical and biological environment' (WHO 1992: 409). Good health is a major resource for social, economic and personal development and an important dimension of quality of life. An understanding of what constitutes 'good' health may vary from one person to another. Political, economic, social, cultural, environmental, behavioural and biological variables can all have an impact on health. Health, then, may be defined according to circumstances, context and perceptions, and experiences, which may vary between individuals and between communities.

MAINTAINING HEALTH

Maintaining health requires achieving a balance of all aspects of life. Factors such as age, sex, family relationships, cultural influences and economic status may have an impact on achieving that balance. Several models have been developed to provide nurses with frameworks to assist people to achieve optimal health. The most common model was developed in the 1940s by Abraham Maslow. He believed that a person's motivations and behaviour are formed by attempting to meet their basic needs. Maslow defined basic human needs as physiological needs, safety and security, love and belongingness, self-esteem and self-actualisation. Maslow's 'Hierarchy of Needs' model (Figure 6.1) emphasises that some needs are more basic than others and that the more basic needs need to be met before consideration of higher needs. Nurses need to recognise each client's individuality and own value system, which will impact on prioritisation of needs.

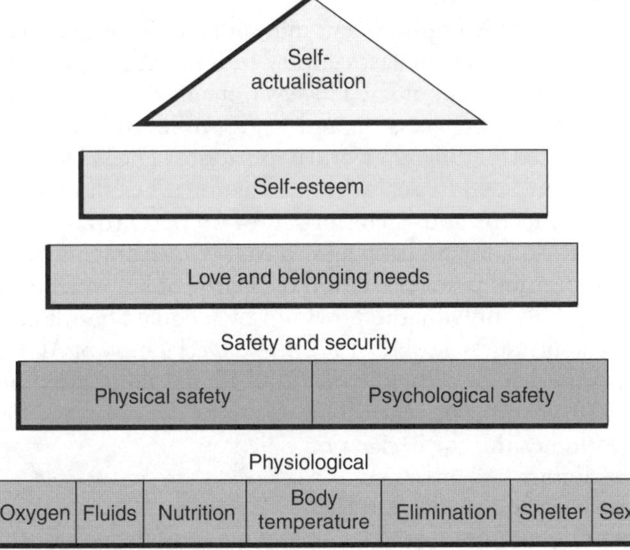

Figure 6.1 | Maslow's Hierarchy of Needs *(redrawn from Maslow AH (1970)* Motivation and Personality. *Prentice Hall, Upper Saddle River, New Jersey)*

Many factors affect individual definitions of health. Definitions vary according to an individual's previous experiences, expectations of self, age and sociocultural influences. A person's definition of health influences behaviour related to health and illness. By understanding clients' perceptions of health and illness, nurses can provide more meaningful assistance to help them gain or attain a state of health (Berman et al 2007).

ILL-HEALTH AND DISEASE

Ill-health or illness may be described as an abnormal event in which aspects of a person's social, physical, emotional or intellectual condition are impaired. Illness is not simply the presence of a disease process; rather, it is directly related to the total person and their environment and culture. Disease may be defined as a disturbance in structure and/or function of any aspect of a person. Diseases may be classified according to their cause, the way in which they are acquired, or according to the body system affected.

COMMUNITY HEALTH

Community health occurs when there is a commitment by the community to work towards achieving the health and wellbeing of individuals, families and groups. This does not necessarily mean the community needs a vast number of medical services or an array of healthy lifestyle gurus and experts. Rather, healthy communities are those that feel empowered to shape their own destiny. They enjoy broad participation in health policies and in decisions that affect daily life; members of healthy communities are able to feel they have some control over the design and sustainability of the community's current and future potential. In short, they feel a sense of commonality or cohesion with others, which becomes beneficial for all members of the community (Hertzman 2001).

EARLY RECOGNITION AND DETECTION OF DISEASE

Health care services recognise the need to focus on health rather than illness; therefore the emphasis is on health promotion and illness prevention at an individual and community level. Health promotion and illness prevention have become an important focus of health care for several reasons; for example, there are still no cures for many diseases, health care costs are rising rapidly, and the community is more aware of the value of health maintenance. Advancements in technology and scientific and medical achievements have led to the development of advanced diagnostic equipment. The early detection and recognition of the contributing factors that influence health and illness can prevent the spread of disease at both an individual and a community level. An example is the free breast-screening programs for women aged over 50 to detect tumours early and significantly reduce the need for radical surgery and improve recovery rates.

FACTORS INFLUENCING HEALTH AND ILLNESS

A person's health status depends on many personal, social and environmental factors, including:

- Lifestyle: whether the person engages in behaviours that promote health, such as exercise, or contribute to ill-health, such as smoking
- Time and place: for example, the colds and flu of winter, heart disease and diabetes being more prevalent in some countries than others
- Age: the elderly and the very young can be more susceptible to some diseases than others
- Gender: certain diseases may more commonly affect individuals of one gender, for example, the incidence of mesothelioma is higher in males
- Race: specific diseases are more common in particular ethnic or racial groups; for example, people of Mediterranean origin are more affected by thalassaemia than others
- Environment: exposure to harmful substances, such as people exposed to asbestos being at risk of developing mesothelioma
- Availability and effectiveness of health promotion programs
- Education and cognitive ability to be able to read and understand health promotion messages
- Finance: money to buy food and warm or protective clothing — poverty is a significant indicator of low social health status.

HEALTH PROMOTION

Health promotion is the process of enabling people to increase their control over, and to improve, their health. To reach a state of complete physical, mental and social wellbeing an individual or group must be able to identify and realise aspirations, satisfy needs and change or cope with the environment. Health is therefore seen as a resource of everyday life, not the objective of living. Health is a positive concept emphasising social and personal resources as well as physical capacities. Therefore, health promotion is not just the responsibility of the health sector but goes beyond healthy lifestyles to wellbeing (WHO 1986). As opposed to illness prevention activities, which aim to protect the client from actual or potential threats to health, health promotion aims to help people maintain their present level of health or increase control over, and improve, their health.

The concepts of health promotion and illness prevention are closely related (Clinical Interest Box 6.1). Nurses focus on health promotion and illness prevention when providing health care, which assists clients to maintain good health and improve health, as well as providing care after illness has occurred. Health promotion activities can be passive or active. Active health promotion activities require the client to be motivated to adopt a specific health program such as giving up smoking. Passive health promotion occurs when the client benefits from the activities of others without necessarily acting themselves, such as in the fluoridation of drinking water.

CLINICAL INTEREST BOX 6.1
Health promotion and illness prevention

Primary health-promotion practices and illness-prevention practices aim to avoid or delay occurrence of a specific disease or disorder. Examples include:

- Obtaining immunisations
- Maintaining ideal body weight
- Wearing seatbelts or safety helmets
- Minimal exposure to the sun, wearing hats and applying sunscreen when out of doors
- Consuming minimal or no alcohol when driving.

Secondary health-promotion practices and illness-prevention practices consist of steps to aid early diagnosis and prompt intervention in disease, shortening the disease process. Examples include:

- Having regular Papanicolaou (Pap) smears or prostate-specific antigen (PSA) tests
- Performing monthly breast or testicular examinations
- Regular glaucoma testing
- Bone density tests
- Brushing teeth and getting regular dental check-ups.

Tertiary health-promotion practices and illness-prevention practices consist of rehabilitation measures after the disease or disorder has been stabilised and treating existing diseases or disorders. Examples include:

- Cardiac rehabilitation
- Recovery from joint-replacement surgery
- Learning to walk with a prosthesis after amputation
- Learning to walk after a stroke
- Complying with treatment programs for chronic diseases such as arthritis or asthma.

A dynamic improvement in health and life expectancy has occurred in the last century in line with significant advances in technology. However, major disparities and inequalities in access to, and equity in, better health is recognised for different world populations. The WHO was set up in 1948 to deal with international health matters and concerns and is comprised of 192 countries. This worldwide organisation agreed that 'Governments have a responsibility for the health of their peoples, which can be fulfilled only by the provision of adequate health and social measures' (WHO 1992). The Declaration of Alma-Ata (health for all by the year 2000) came about after the 1978 WHO conference. This was to be the milestone for world health. The declaration called for:

- Equity
- Fundamental human rights
- Community participation and maximal community self-reliance
- Use of socially acceptable technology
- Health promotion and disease prevention

- Involvement of government departments other than health departments
- Political action
- Cooperation between countries
- Reduction of money spent on armaments, to increase funds for 'Primary Health Care'
- World peace.

These principles from the *Declaration of Alma-Ata* provide the underpinning concepts for 'Primary Health Care'. Primary Health Care is essential care based on practical, scientifically sound and socially acceptable methods and technology, made universally accessible to people and families in the community through their full participation and at a cost that the community and country can afford to maintain at every stage of their development, in the spirit of self-reliance and self-determination (WHO 1978).

Primary Health Care focuses on social justice, equity, community participation, socially acceptable and affordable technology, the provision of services on the basis of the needs of the population, health education and work to improve the root causes of ill-health. It emphasises working with people to enable them to make decisions about their needs and how best to address them. These guiding principles of Primary Health Care should be applied throughout the health system and adopted by all health workers (Wass 2000).

To distinguish between other often misconstrued concepts of Primary Health Care, and to understand exactly what Primary Health Care is, Wass (2000) provides an explanation of what Primary Health Care is not:

- Primary Health Care is not primary medical care or primary care. This is medical care provided for people at their first point of contact with the health system, provided in the outpatients' section of a hospital, or by a general medical practitioner
- Primary Health Care is also not primary nursing, as this is a system of nursing in which an individual nurse takes primary responsibility for specific clients. Primary Health Care is not just community-based health care. The Primary Health Care approach has implications throughout the entire health system
- Primary Health Care is applicable to all countries of the world, not just developing countries, and consequently cannot be referred to as simply Third World health care.

MODELS OF HEALTH PROMOTION

Various models of health promotion have been developed by nurses to provide conceptual frameworks for identifying a client's health behaviour and beliefs. A client's health beliefs may stem from many factors, including health perception, demographics and personality type. Tannahill's model, for example, shows health promotion as being made up of three areas: prevention, health protection and health education (Downie et al 1996). Beattie's model (1991), which is useful for charting ethical and political tensions, can be used as a planning tool. This model has four approaches to health promotion: health persuasion, personal counselling, community development and legislative action for health.

The Health–Illness Continuum Model

This model describes the relationship between health and illness and provides a method of identifying a client's level of health (see Chapter 8). This model is valuable when comparing a client's present health status with their previous level of health and for then setting nursing goals and objectives to promote a future level of health (Crisp & Taylor 2005).

The Health Belief Model

The health belief model (see Chapter 8) is one of the most widely used conceptual health promotion models and was developed to assist in understanding health behaviour. This model can be effective in developing health education strategies and can also be a useful framework for designing change strategies.

PREREQUISITES FOR HEALTH

The fundamental conditions and resources for health are peace, shelter, education, food, income, a stable ecosystem, sustainable resources, social justice and equity. To work effectively, improving health requires a secure foundation in these basic prerequisites. The *Ottawa Charter for Health Promotion* (Clinical Interest Box 6.2) highlights the need for health workers to be effective in advocacy, enabling and mediation to enable people to gain greater control over their lives (WHO 1986).

ADVOCACY

Good health is a major resource for social, economic and personal development and an important dimension of quality of life. Political, economic, cultural, environmental, behavioural and biological factors can all favour health or be harmful to it. Health promotion action aims at making these conditions favourable through advocacy for health.

CLINICAL INTEREST BOX 6.2
The *Ottawa Charter for Health Promotion*

As a response to growing expectations for a new public health movement around the world, the first International Conference on Health Promotion was held in Ottawa, Canada in November 1986. The outcome of this Conference presented a charter for action to achieve 'Health for All' by the year 2000 and beyond. This charter is known as the *Ottawa Charter for Health Promotion*.

The charter states that actions to promote health require:

- building healthy public policy
- creating environments that support healthy living
- strengthening community action
- helping people develop their skills
- reorienting the health care system.

ENABLING

Health promotion focuses on achieving equity in health. Health promotion action aims at reducing differences in current health. The charter states that 'People cannot achieve their fullest health potential unless they are able to take control of those things which determine their health. This must apply equally to women and men' (WHO 1986).

MEDIATION

The prerequisites and prospects for health cannot be ensured by the health sector alone. More importantly, health promotion demands coordinated action by all concerned: by governments, health and other social and economic sectors, non-governmental and voluntary organisations, local authorities, industry and the media. People in all walks of life are involved as individuals, families and communities. Professional and social groups and health personnel have a major responsibility to mediate between differing interests in society for the pursuit of health. Health promotion strategies and programs should be adapted to the local needs and possibilities of individual countries and regions to take into account differing social, cultural and economic systems.

Unlike previous public health approaches, the new public health movement recognises the broader issues of health promotion and the need for governments and health bodies to work collaboratively. It further recognises the need to increase community control and to consider the importance of people's environments as determinants of health. Subsequent international conferences have expanded on these fundamental issues.

Australian Government policy on health activity began in the mid 1980s. In 1986 the Better Health Commission formulated Australia's response to the goal of Health for All by 2000. *The Health for all Australians* report represents the beginning of Australia's commitment to health goals and targets, carried through in several subsequent documents, including *Health Goals and Targets for Australian Children and Youth* (Child, Adolescent and Family Health Service 1992), *Goals and Targets for Australia's Health in the Year 2000 and Beyond* (Nutbeam et al 1993) and *Better Health Outcomes for Australians* (Commonwealth Department of Human Services and Health 1994).

DETERMINANTS OF HEALTH

Many factors could potentially determine our health. In 2000, the WHO developed 10 social determinants of health: the social gradient, stress, early development, work, unemployment, social support, social exclusion, addiction, food and transport. Talbot and Verrinder (2005) describe a further set of determinants for health: peace, shelter, education, social security, social relations, empowerment of women, a stable ecosystem, sustainable resource use, social justice, respect for human rights and equity. All of these factors will raise or lower health and they can have a positive or negative impact on people (Brown et al 2008).

The health and quality of life of most Australians compares well with the rest of the world, although there are some significant differences in population subgroups. 'Poor socioeconomic status is the single biggest determinant of ill-health and death in Australia' (Australian Health Ministers 1992). This is reflected in statistics of sudden infant death syndrome, accidental drowning, motor vehicle accidents, other accidents, suicide, cardiovascular disease, respiratory disease and cancers.

Gender is also a significant determinant of health chances in Australia. Mortality rates for males are higher than those for females. Men are also less inclined to seek medical assistance.

Ethnicity is another determinant of health in Australia. While many migrants have better health on arrival than the average Australian because of the requirement of the immigration process, this advantage disappears the longer they have been in Australia because of a decline in job opportunities, different health habits from their country of origin and a lack of social support.

Aboriginal and Torres Strait Islander people

Aboriginal and Torres Strait Islander people experience higher infant mortality (three times higher than for other Australians) and a hospitalisation rate 50% higher than other Australians. Life expectancy for Aboriginal children born in 1998–2000 is 19 to 21 years less than for other Australians (Talbot & Verrinder 2005). In 1989 a *National Aboriginal Health Strategy* was produced (National Aboriginal Health Strategy Working Party 1989), which identified both key issues and potential solutions to some of the major Aboriginal health issues. The strategy emphasises the structural basis of Aboriginal health, recognising the link between Aboriginal health, land rights and domination of Aboriginal people by non-Aboriginal culture. Further, the strategy argues for Aboriginal community control of health services and research into issues related to Aboriginal people and their health. Although considered to be a valuable contribution, this strategy was evaluated five years after its release and was deemed to have been ineffectively implemented, possibly due to under-funding (Wass 2000).

GOALS AND TARGETS FOR AUSTRALIA'S HEALTH IN THE 21st CENTURY

The areas of health targeted by Australian health policies focus on preventable mortality and morbidity and include:

- Cardiovascular disease
- Preventable cancer
- Injury
- Communicable diseases
- HIV/AIDS
- Sexually transmitted infections
- Maternal health problems and disorders

- Physical impairment and disability
- Developmental disability and oral health.

Focus is also on healthy lifestyles and risk factors such as:

- Diet and nutrition
- Overweight and obesity
- Physical activity
- High blood cholesterol
- High blood pressure
- Smoking
- Alcohol misuse
- Illicit drug use
- Quality use of medicines
- Healthy sexuality
- Reproductive health
- Sun protection
- Oral hygiene
- Safety behaviours
- Immunisation
- Mental health.

Other targeted areas include health literacy and health skills, such as life skills and coping, safety skills and first aid, self-help and self-care, social support and promoting healthy environments such as the physical environment, transport, housing, home and community infrastructure, work and the workplace, schools and health care settings.

Health promotion programs include activities such as:

- Education with a view to prevention
- Promotion of food supply and proper nutrition
- Provision of an adequate supply of safe water and basic sanitation
- Provision of maternal and child health care, including family planning
- Immunisation programs
- Prevention and control of major infectious diseases
- Appropriate treatment of common diseases and injury
- Provision of essential drugs.

Other health programs are designed to address and focus on the targeted areas such as healthy lifestyles and known risk factors, health skills programs and healthy environments.

THE JAKARTA DECLARATION ON HEALTH PROMOTION INTO THE 21ST CENTURY (WHO 1997)

The *Jakarta Declaration* provides the strategies and guiding principles for health promotion to take us into the 21st century and builds on the *Ottawa Charter for Health Promotion*. The guiding principles are to:

- Promote social responsibility for health
- Increase investments for health development
- Consolidate and expand partnerships for health
- Increase community capacity and empower the individual
- Secure an infrastructure for health promotion.

The focus is still on Primary Health Care and social justice and emphasis remains on community empowerment.

THE ROLE OF THE NURSE IN HEALTH PROMOTION

The role of the nurse in promoting health can be multi-layered. It is important for all nurses to work within the confines of their scope of training and practice. For some nurses, health promotion may become simply a way of working that is client centred and holistic. To others it may be a set of more defined activities, including assessing health needs and providing information. An awareness of public health issues and factors that influence health status is an expectation of nurses.

Nurses can make a contribution to the health and social wellbeing of their individual clients by:

- Recognising there is a role for the nurse in the promotion of health and self-care
- Participating in providing health promotion interventions
- Being aware of the key health and social factors to be considered when carrying out an assessment of individual needs
- Being aware of the contributions of other professionals to assessment and intervention.

Nurses can adopt a positive perspective to health promotion when nursing in the community by:

- Recognising that clients are individuals within the group with specific needs
- Participating in health promotion activities
- Maintaining cultural awareness and sensitivity
- Learning and gaining knowledge about the community
- Empowering the community
- Networking and building on resources and partnerships
- Developing and improving personal skills required for practice.

If public health or health promotion is to be a central concept in nurses' work, then nurses' role-perception, skills, knowledge and attitude to health promotion will have a vital impact on the success or failure of health promotion activities.

HEALTH EDUCATION

Health education is linked to health promotion because the purpose of health education is to promote the presence of conditions that assist people in creating health, that is, enhancing conditions for personal and community health (Brown et al 2008). Health education can be defined as 'any combination of learning experiences designed to facilitate voluntary actions conducive to health' (Green & Kreuter 1991). Health education can be any planned educational intervention people can voluntarily take that aims to look after their health or the health of others. Ewles and Simnett (1985) broadly describe the dimensions of health education to be:

- Concerned with the whole person, encompassing physical, mental, social, emotional, spiritual and societal aspects

- A lifelong process from birth to death, helping people to change and adapt at all stages
- Concerned with people at all points of health and illness, from the completely healthy to the chronically sick and handicapped, to maximise each person's potential for healthy living
- Directed towards individuals, families, groups and whole communities
- Concerned with helping people to help themselves and with helping people to work towards creating healthier conditions for everybody 'making healthy choices easier choices'
- Involved in formal and informal teaching and learning using a variety of methods
- Concerned with a range of goals, including giving information, attitude change, behaviour change and social change.

Health education involves working with individuals, communities and society and may be guided by the principles of Primary Health Care. If nurses are to influence the health of individuals and communities, they need to be clear about what factors contribute to people's health and ill-health. There is also a role for the individual to take responsibility for their own health, and a clear role for communities and government in tackling the root causes of ill-health:

> The prerequisites and prospects for health cannot be ensured by the health sector alone. More importantly, health promotion demands coordinated action by all concerned: by governments, by health and other social and economic sectors, by non-governmental and voluntary organisations, by local authorities, by industry and by the media. People in all walks of life are involved as individuals, families and countries. Professional and social groups and health personnel have a major responsibility to mediate between differing interests in society for the pursuit of health.
>
> (WHO 1986)

Understanding how people report health problems or adopt particular health behaviours is a first step to planning for health improvement. The nurse needs to consider how and to what extent they can involve their clients in planning their own health care. Nurses may be involved in:

- Advice and information giving
- Formal and informal education and training
- Needs assessment
- Supporting people and helping people understand their condition or diagnosis
- Policy development and contributing to health improvement programs
- Community development and social action projects
- Research and raising health awareness.

Whether working with groups or individuals, certain skills are required to enable the nurse to facilitate health promotion and education. Nurses need to be clear and unambiguous. Nurses need to be non-judgmental, updated with current knowledge and informed of scope of practice, and need to try to attain an understanding of the client's concerns and position. Effective communication skills such as using open-ended questions, listening, recognising any cultural implications, body language and concise history taking and documentation will facilitate this process. When educational advice is being offered the nurse needs to check whether the client understands both the message and the language. Written material may support the interpersonal communication. The nurse often needs to be aware of other factors, such as the views of significant people in the client's life and the individual's own self-esteem that could influence the communication process. Establishing trust and rapport and having interpersonal skills will ensure effective communication.

The challenge for nurses is how and when to provide health education information. If a client has specific learning needs about health promotion, risk reduction or management of a health problem it is useful to develop and implement a teaching plan with the client. A teaching plan includes assessment of the client's ability, need and readiness to learn with identification of problems that can be resolved with teaching. The nurse then determines objectives with the client, delivers educational interventions and evaluates the effectiveness of the teaching. Clinical Interest Box 6.3 lists the principles to guide effective teaching and learning.

There are some stressors that detract from the effectiveness of the teaching effort. The stressors, including the strategies to help manage or overcome them, are outlined in Clinical Interest Box 6.4.

THE NURSING PROCESS IN HEALTH PROMOTION AND HEALTH EDUCATION

Essentially, the nursing process is a series of planned steps that produce a particular end result. Specifically, the nursing process is a modified scientific method of systematic problem solving. In simple terms the nursing process is a method used to assess, plan, deliver and evaluate nursing care. The process of nursing, or scientific method of problem solving, remains the same whether the nursing care provided is a simple measure or a sequence of complicated nursing activities, and can be adapted to individuals or communities.

Providing the framework for nursing care, the nursing process consists of five components, each of which follows logically one after the other:

- Assessment
- Nursing diagnosis
- Planning
- Implementation
- Evaluation.

It is important for the nurse to recognise that the process is ongoing and cyclical in that each step relies on the step preceding and the step following. For a more detailed account of the components of the nursing process refer to Chapter 19.

CLINICAL INTEREST BOX 6.3
Principles to guide effective teaching and learning

Principles	Teaching implications for the nurse
Allow the learner to direct the learning process.	Active participation is paramount. Learning is most likely to occur if learner sets the goals. Learners need to have their say, use initiative, experiment and find out what works for them. Identify which teaching technique is best for each learner. The nurse is a facilitator to direct the learner to resources.
Get to know other people's perspectives.	Understand the background and ideas of other people. Build new knowledge on past experience.
Be aware of the context of people's lives.	Centre the learning experience on real-life situations of the learner. Readiness and motivation to learn are high when facing new tasks.
Build on what people already know.	Identify where it is easiest for the learner to begin learning. Provide new material at a pace that is appropriate for the learner. Treat mistakes as an opportunity to learn.
Planned achievements need to be realistic.	Set realistic achievable goals. Find out what it is that the learner wants to know.
Take account of all levels of learning.	Consider whether there is a need for knowledge development, attitudes and values clarification or behaviour change and skills development.
Present information in logical steps.	Provide a logical sequence, whereby complex ideas are built on smaller ones.

(Talbot & Verrinder 2005, as modified in Brown & Edwards 2008)

CLINICAL INTEREST BOX 6.4
Strategies to help manage or overcome nurse–teacher stressors

Stressor	Approaches
Lack of time	Preplan. Set realistic goals. Use time with patient efficiently, using all possible opportunities for teaching, such as when bathing or changing a dressing. Break teaching and practice into small time periods. Advocate for time for patient teaching. Carefully document what was taught and the time spent teaching in order to emphasise that it is a primary role of nursing and that it takes time.
Lack of knowledge	Broaden knowledge base. Read, study, ask questions. Screen teaching materials, participate in other teaching sessions, observe more experienced nurse–teachers, attend classes.
Disagreement with patient	Establish agreed-on, written goals. Develop a plan and discuss with patient before teaching begins. Introduce a role model to help illustrate therapeutic expectations. Enlist the aid of family and significant others. Revise expectations; learn to be satisfied with small achievements.
Powerlessness, frustration	Recognise personal reaction to stress. Develop a support system. Rely on friends and family for positive encouragement. Network with other nurses, health professionals and community leaders to change the situation. Become proactive in legislative processes affecting healthcare delivery.

(Brown & Edwards 2008, as adapted from Lewis 2004)

It is essential to revise and update any plan of care continually to meet a client's changing needs. By using the nursing process each individual's specific needs are addressed, any problems are identified and a care plan is developed and implemented to meet those needs. The effectiveness of any care given is continuously evaluated in terms of the individual's needs.

The nursing process provides an ideal framework to achieve health promotion and education for individual clients as well as groups or communities. The overall objectives for health promotion activities can be varied to:

- Include the prevention of disease
- Ensure that people are well informed and able to make choices
- Change behaviour
- Help people acquire skills and confidence to take greater control over the factors influencing their health
- Change policies and environments to facilitate healthy choices
- Address the determinants of health, such as poverty, housing and community life.

During the assessment phase of a community's needs the principles of the nursing process remain the same. During data collection in this instance it will need to be considered that there may be many stakeholders, and research may need to be undertaken to obtain a profile of the community, which takes into account the environment, policy, available services and resources, housing, finances and perhaps cultural considerations. Key questions to ask during the assessment phase are included in Clinical Interest Box 6.5.

After collecting the data the nurse is able to identify

the problem or areas of need and is then able to make a nursing diagnosis based on these findings. Many health agencies use the diagnostic categories accepted by the North American Nursing Diagnosis Association (NANDA). These diagnostic categories are used to differentiate between an 'actual' or 'potential' health problem. For example, in Clinical Interest Box 6.6 the nurse may make the diagnosis for Mary of 'actual knowledge deficit related to recent medical diagnosis of diabetes', if it becomes apparent that Mary does not understand the implications of her current dietary habits and the need to make some changes. Once this has been determined the nurse is then able to plan the care needed for Mary to optimise activities to ensure health promotion.

Planning the care for Mary is the next phase. Planning involves setting goals, establishing priorities and determining nursing interventions to achieve the goals. This will require determining specific interventions aimed at achieving the ultimate goal for health promotion. There may be several levels of intervention, including individual one-on-one medical officer–client counselling on dietary changes, to specialist diabetes education services. Some important questions to consider are:

- Have the issues clearly been defined?
- Who are the key stakeholders?
- What has been tried before?
- Are the goals that have been set achievable and realistic?

The principles of the nursing process can again be adapted during the planning phase of health promotion activities at the community level. The above questions will provide a guide for the nurse and practitioner to ensure that objectives and aims of the program are being met.

Implementation means putting the nursing plan into action (nursing interventions) and is the actual performance of the activities that have been selected to help the client

CLINICAL INTEREST BOX 6.5
Assessment of characteristics that affect client teaching

Characteristics and Key Questions

Physical

- What are the patient's age and sex?
- Is the patient acutely ill?
- Is the patient fatigued? In pain?
- What is the primary diagnosis?
- Are there additional diagnoses?
- What is the patient's current mental status?
- What is the patient's hearing ability? Visual ability? Motor ability?
- What drugs does the patient take? Do they affect learning?

Psychological

- Does the patient appear anxious, afraid, depressed, defensive?
- Is the patient in a state of denial?
- What is the patient's level of self-efficacy?

Sociocultural

- Is the patient employed?
- What is the patient's present or past occupation?
- How does the patient describe his or her financial status?
- What is the patient's educational experience and reading ability?
- What is the patient's living arrangement?
- Does the patient have family or close friends?
- What are the patient's beliefs regarding his or her illness or treatment?
- What is the patient's cultural/ethnic identity?
- Is proposed teaching consistent with the patient's cultural values?

Educational

- What does the patient already know?
- What does the patient think is most important to learn first?
- What prior learning experiences establish a frame of reference for current learning needs?
- What has the patient's healthcare provider told the patient about the health problem?
- Is the patient ready to change behaviour or learn?
- Can the patient identify behaviours/habits that would make the problem better or worse?
- How does the patient learn best? Through reading, listening, doing things?
- In what kind of environment does the patient learn best? Formal classroom? Informal setting, such as home or office? Alone or among peers?

(Brown et al 2008, as adapted from Lewis 2004)

CLINICAL INTEREST BOX 6.6
Subjective and objective assessment

Mary, 52, has recently been diagnosed with type 2 diabetes mellitus. She states, 'I have always loved my food — in many ways it is my only enjoyment in life and now my doctor says I have to give up all the things I love to eat. I am finding it just too hard on the diet he has given me and I think I'll just give up.'

The nurse observes that Mary does not appear to have altered her lifestyle, as she eats constantly, and there are several chocolate wrappers on the bench.

Health promotion should start from the existing knowledge and beliefs of the client. To plan the individual care needed for Mary and to begin the nursing process, it will be helpful for the nurse to first determine Mary's health beliefs and her understanding of the diagnosis she has been given. This will require building up trust and obtaining a detailed social and medical history. This phase of the nursing process is the assessment phase and basically requires the gathering of subjective and objective data.

Subjective data are the client's, or other significant person's, perceptions, ideas and sensations about a health problem; for example, Mary has stated that she is finding it too hard and wants to give up. Objective data are the information observed or measured by the nurse; for example, the nurse has observed that Mary does not appear to have altered her lifestyle, she eats constantly and there are several chocolate wrappers on the bench.

achieve the set goals. The client's needs (either the individual or the community) are reassessed continuously during the implementation stage so that any new needs can be identified and so that the nursing plan can be modified or adapted. Techniques to enhance the teaching process with adults are presented in Clinical Interest Box 6.7.

After the planned nursing interventions have been implemented, the nurse must then evaluate the results to determine whether the interventions were effective. Evaluation is the process of determining the extent to which the set goals or objectives have been achieved, and enables the nurse to monitor the effectiveness of the care plan. Whether the plan was a success or not is determined by comparing the client's response to the nursing interventions within the set goals and set time frame. Evaluation also enables the nurse or practitioner to identify any new health care problems experienced by the individual client or the community.

SUMMARY

The WHO, which comprises 192 countries, was set up in 1948 to deal with international health. Major disparities and inequalities in access and equity to better health for the world population led to the *Declaration of Alma-Ata* (Health for All by the year 2000), which came about after the 1978 WHO Conference. The principles developed from the *Declaration of Alma-Ata* provide the underpinning concepts for Primary Health Care.

The first International Conference on Health Promotion was held in Ottawa, Canada in November 1986. The outcome of this conference presented a charter for action to achieve Health for All by the year 2000 and beyond. This charter is known as the *Ottawa Charter for Health Promotion*.

Health promotion and education provide the key to minimising or eliminating disparities in world health and play fundamental roles in achieving the goals and objectives as determined by the WHO. Political, economic, social, cultural, environmental, behavioural and biological factors can all have an impact on health. Health, then, may be defined according to circumstances, context and perceptions and experiences, which may vary between individuals and between communities.

By raising the level of health awareness and by providing health education, for both the individual and the community, nurses play a vital role in health promotion.

CLINICAL INTEREST BOX 6.7
Techniques to enhance client learning

- Keep the physical environment relaxed and non-threatening.
- Maintain a respectful, warm and enthusiastic attitude.
- Let the patient's expressed needs direct what information is provided.
- Focus on 'must-know' information, saving 'nice-to-know' information if time allows.
- Involve the patient and family in the process; emphasise active participation.
- Be aware of and take into consideration the patient's previous experiences.
- Emphasise the relevance of the information to the patient's lifestyle and suggest how it may provide an immediate solution to a problem.
- Schedule and pace learning experiences according to the patient's needs and abilities.
- Individualise the teaching plan, even if standardised plans are used.
- Emphasise helping the patient to learn and not just transmitting subject matter.
- Review written materials with the patient.
- Remember that simple is best.
- Ask for frequent feedback.
- Affirm progress with rewards valued by the patient to reinforce desired behaviours.

(Brown et al 2008: 59, as adapted in Lewis 2004)

REVIEW EXERCISES

1. What is meant by Primary Health Care?
2. Explain the difference between health promotion and illness prevention.
3. What is the role of the nurse in health promotion?

CRITICAL THINKING EXERCISE

Mr Smith is a 79-year-old man who you are visiting in the community. He has chronic obstructive airways disease (COAD) and requires oxygen in the home. You have recently learnt that he is secretly smoking when his wife leaves the house to do the shopping.

1. Develop a set of health promotion education strategies or interventions that would assist this client with COAD.
2. How would you evaluate your strategies?

REFERENCES AND FURTHER READING

Alcorso C, Schofield T (1991) The *National Non-English Speaking Background Women's Health Strategy*. Australian Government Publishing Service, Canberra

Anderson I (1997) The National Aboriginal Health Strategy. In: Gardener H (ed.), *Health Policy in Australia*. Oxford University Press, Melbourne

Australian Health Ministers (1992) *Enough to Make you Sick: How Income and Environment Affect Health*. National Health Strategy, Research Paper No. 1, September 1992: 10. Australian Government Publishing Service, Canberra

—— (1995) *National Mental Health Policy*, 2nd edn. Australian Government Publishing Service, Canberra

Australian Institute of Health and Welfare (2003) *Health expenditure Australia 2001–02*. AIHW, Canberra. Online. Available: www.aihw.gov.au/publications/index.cfm/title/10043 [accessed 24 April 2008]

Beattie A (1991) Knowledge and Control in Health Promotion: a Test Case for Social Policy and Social Theory. In: Gabe J, Calnan M, Bury M (eds), *The Sociology of the Health Service*. Routledge, London

Berman AJ, Kozier B, Snyder S (2007) *Kozier and Erbs Fundamentals of Nursing: Concepts, Process, and Practice*, 8th edn. Prentice-Hall, Upper Saddle River, New Jersey

Brown D, Edwards H (2008) *Lewis's Medical-Surgical Nursing: Assessment and Management of Clinical Problems*, 2nd edn. Elsevier Australia, Sydney

Child, Adolescent and Family Health Service (1992) *Health Goals and Targets for Australian Children and Youth*. Online. Available: www.dhs.vic.gov.au/health/healthstatus/publications/hyv.htm [accessed 24 April 2008]

Commonwealth Department of Human Services and Health (1994) *Better Health Outcomes for Australians: National Goals, Targets and Strategies for Better Health Outcomes in the Next Century*. Australian Government Publishing Service, Canberra

Crisp J, Taylor C (eds) (2005) *Potter & Perry's Fundamentals of Nursing*, 2nd edn. Elsevier Australia, Sydney

Downie RS, Tannahill C, Tannahill A (1996) *Health Promotion: Models and Values*, 2nd edn. Oxford University Press, Oxford

Ewles L, Simnett I (1985) *Promoting Health: A Practical Guide to Health Education*. John Wiley and Sons, Chichester, UK

Green LW, Kreuter MW (1991) *Health Promotion Planning: an Educational and Environmental Approach*. Mayfield, Mountain View, California

Hertzman C (2001) Health and human society. *American Scientist*; 89(6): 538–44

Maslow AH (1970) *Motivation and Personality*. Prentice Hall, Upper Saddle River, New Jersey

McMurray A (2006) *Community Health and Wellness: a Socioecological Approach*, 3rd edn. Mosby, Sydney

National Aboriginal Health Strategy Working Party (1989) *A National Aboriginal Health Strategy*. Department of Aboriginal Affairs, Canberra

National Centre for Epidemiology and Population Health (NCEPH) (1991) The Role of Primary Health Care in Health Promotion in Australia. Monograph Series: *Building a Picture Primary Health Care*, Sub-Set 1. Department of Community Services and Health, Canberra

National Rural Health Policy Forum (1999) *Healthy Horizons: A Framework for Improving the Health of Rural, Regional and Remote Australians*. National Rural Health Policy Forum and National Rural Health Alliance, for the Australian Health Minister's Conference, Canberra: 9

Nutbeam D, Wise M, Bauman A et al (1993) *Goals and Targets for Australia's Health in the Year 2000 and Beyond*. Department of Public Health, University of Sydney, Sydney

Spradley BW, Allender JA (2002) *Community Health Nursing: Concepts and Practice*, 5th edn. Lippincott, Philadelphia

Talbot L, Verrinder G (2005) *Promoting Health: The Primary Health Care Approach*, 3rd edn. Elsevier Australia

Wass A (2000) *Promoting Health: The Primary Health Care Approach*, 2nd edn. Harcourt Australia, Sydney

World Health Organization (WHO) (1978) *Declaration of Alma-Ata*. WHO, Geneva. (Reproduced in *World Health*, August/September 1988: 16–17.)

—— (1986) *The Ottawa Charter for Health Promotion*. WHO, Geneva

—— (1992) *Primary Health Care Reviews Guidelines and Methods*. WHO, Geneva

ONLINE RESOURCES

World Health Organization (WHO): www.who.int/en

Chapter 7

COMMUNITY-BASED CARE

OBJECTIVES

- Define the key terms/concepts
- Explain the wide variety of settings in which community-based health care occurs
- Explain the difference between the role of community health nurses and community-based nurses
- List the range of people who may require community nursing services
- Explain the philosophy of community nursing
- State the aim of community nursing
- Explain the funding for community-based care

KEY TERMS/CONCEPTS

care coordination
community health nursing roles
community nursing
community-based health care
community-based nursing roles
continuity of care
empowerment
independence

CHAPTER FOCUS

There has been a gradual change in Australian health care policies, with an increased focus on community-based health care. These changes have occurred as a result of public health policies aimed at maintaining health and preventing illness, a consumer push for more health care options, earlier discharge from acute hospitals and containment of costs.

This chapter aims to explain the roles of community nurses and the relevance of community assessment. It also clarifies the roles of two types of community nurses: community health nurses, caring for populations, communities, families and individuals; and community-based nurses, who care predominantly for individuals and families. Community-based nursing is discussed in more detail, covering its philosophy, aims, types of clients and aspects of care. The nursing process and its application in community nursing is also discussed.

LIVED EXPERIENCE

I really wanted to stay in my own home, I did not want to go into care but I had many health problems, was not able to shower myself or go shopping for groceries any more. When the district nurses started visiting it was such a relief. They help me with my medications and they have organised for people to help me shower, to help with cleaning the house, getting my shopping and paying my bills.

Mavis 78, new home-based care client

COMMUNITY-BASED HEALTH CARE

Community-based health services are provided in a wide variety of settings, including community health centres, workplaces, family and child health centres, schools, universities, day care centres, alcohol and drug rehabilitation centres, mental health centres, in homes and on the streets for homeless people. For example, mental health nurses may meet with homeless clients in the street or in a squat.

Community-based health services are involved with health promotion, health education, maintenance of wellbeing, coordination and continuity of care within the community. Community-based health care works within the framework of Primary Health Care or essential health care (Chapter 6), with its focus on increasing access to basic health care, promotion of wellbeing and the prevention of illness, relying on the client being an active partner in care and not just the care recipient.

Many community-based health services are provided at community centres and in the home. As well as community nurses there are many other health care workers who provide community-based health care, both in centres and in people's homes. Some of these include occupational therapists, physiotherapists, social workers, dietitians, general practitioners, home care workers, volunteers, personal carers and home maintenance workers. Collaborative working relationships between health care workers, institutions and agencies are essential for providing coordinated care for clients in the community.

Community health care workers have more limited access to the range of health workers than health care workers in many inpatient settings. Therefore their roles and partnerships with other health care workers extend beyond their immediate work environment. An awareness of the contributions other workers make and the development of a plan of care in consultation with the client is very important in achieving client outcomes.

THE HEALTH OF A COMMUNITY

The role of the community nurse is determined by the needs of the community they work in. One role of the community nurse is to improve the health of the community. To promote health and encourage changes in health practices, it is necessary to have an understanding of the community. This involves knowing the structure, population and the social systems of the community. The structure of a community includes its boundaries, types of housing, economy, the physical environment, water supply and sanitation.

Knowing the population involves identifying age and sex distributions, growth trends, population density, educational levels, and cultural and religious groups. The social systems of a community include the local government, education, communication, welfare, and health and transport systems.

The community nurse needs to undertake a community assessment before determining the community's needs. A community assessment provides an understanding of the community's environment. This incorporates the structure, population and social system of the community. There are several ways of achieving this. The community nurse can make observations of the structure of the community by travelling around the community and meeting with the local people. Statistical data can be collected from sources such as the Australian Bureau of Statistics, local government, existing databases, reports by other agencies and routine service data. To gather information on the social systems, the community nurse could visit agencies such as schools, health care facilities and local government departments.

Sensitivity to community perspectives is important. The initial step is to get to know the community well by seeking out community members and finding out their views on health and their perceived needs. It is vital to involve the community members in this process. The community may be more likely to support any activities for change if they are involved in the identification of the issues, the gathering of data and the plan of action.

In completing a community assessment the nurse should ensure the focus is not solely on identifying problems. The nurse should also look at the strengths and capacity for further development that exist within the community.

COMMUNITY HEALTH NURSING

A broad definition of the community health nurse is one who practises with a working knowledge of the community, its health care services, networks of care providers and other resources to give holistic, coordinated care to promote wellbeing. The community health nurse role is continuing and comprehensive and is focused on nursing and health care for populations, communities, families and individuals. It is directed towards all age groups and includes health education, health promotion, health assessment and maintenance of health.

The role of the community health nurse is diverse and continually developing. A community health nurse may be employed as:

- Community health nurse in a community health centre
- Occupational health nurse
- Women's health nurse
- School nurse.

The community health nurse liaises with many institutions, organisations, agencies and a wider range of professional disciplines than hospital or institutional-based nurses. The community health nurse also works with the community over a period of time, and therefore has increased opportunities to provide continuing education and ongoing health promotion.

Empowerment is an important issue in community health nursing and is about improving community and client control over issues affecting them. The community health nurse can create a climate for empowerment by enabling access to information and resources, as well as helping communities and clients reach decisions that are appropriate for them. The focus is on community and client choice and autonomy, allowing communities and clients to make their own informed decisions.

The community health nurse has a wide community focus as well as providing nursing care to families and individuals while the community-based nurse focuses their care on individuals and families. The community health nurse is often involved with health promotion and illness prevention as well as the treatment of illness. One of their aims is to improve the health and wellbeing of the people in the community through group work providing health education and health promotion.

The community health nurse needs to be socially responsive, becoming an active part of the community, knowing its members, their needs and the community's resources to establish effective health promotion and disease prevention programs. The community health nurse needs to assess and plan for care that is equitable, accessible, culturally sensitive and that empowers the community and its members for self-determined health care. It is important for all community health nurses to understand the lived experience of the people for whom they care and to understand community health programs available to members of the community.

Examples of community health programs are:

- Sexual health clinics — clinical and educative services dealing with all matters relating to sexual and reproductive health, including testing for, and treatment of, sexually transmitted infections, pregnancy testing and Pap smears
- Older persons' services such as Wanders on Wheels, which is a social outing for housebound older people that gives them an opportunity to visit interesting places and meet people
- Support groups such as diabetes family support groups for people with diabetes, their siblings, family and friends
- Ongoing men's support groups, for men with problems of violence, threatening behaviour or needing anger management
- Women's domestic violence support groups, for women who currently or in the past have experienced violent relationships
- The chronic illness peer-support program (ChIPS). This is an informal support group for young people with a chronic illness, set up by the Royal Children's Hospital in Melbourne in 1992.

COMMUNITY-BASED NURSING

Community nurses who provide community-based nursing provide care predominantly to individuals and families and include: generalist district nurses and specialist district nurses such as palliative care nurses, mental health nurses, wound care nurses and drug and alcohol nurses. Community-based nursing services are provided by hospitals, local or state/territory government agencies, not-for-profit organisations, church organisations or private agencies. Their primary work is in clients' homes.

Community-based nursing services comprise continuing nursing care, which may be preventive, curative, rehabilitative, supportive or palliative. They may provide a range of programs, including district nursing, palliative care, hospital-in-the-home and post-acute care. These programs may have different forms of funding. On occasion, the client may need care from more than one program. When this occurs more than one program may be provided at the same time.

The philosophy of community-based nursing is to promote wellbeing and independence, enabling clients to remain in their own homes. To achieve this, the community-based nurse provides skilled nursing care, education, information on techniques to increase levels of independence, and referral to other services. The aim of the community-based nurse is to assist clients towards achieving their optimal level of independence.

People who may require community nursing services include those who:

- Have been discharged from hospital and require continued nursing assistance, for example, to change wound dressings, administer medications, or to care for a stoma/ostomy (an artificial opening formed when a part of the small or large bowel is brought out onto the abdomen)
- Require special acute care involving the use of advanced technology, such as peripherally inserted central lines or other intravenous infusions for antibiotics
- Require continued assessment of their physical or mental state and/or their ability to manage at home
- Require instruction in techniques to help them attain or maintain independence, for example, how to monitor blood glucose or administer medications by injection
- Require emotional support as part of their nursing care; for example, to recover from, or adjust to, an acute or chronic illness
- Require care and support after the birth of a baby, for example, health assessment of both the mother and the baby, or advice on aspects of baby care
- Are experiencing a terminal illness. Palliative care programs enable individuals to remain at home for as long as they wish, or as long as is possible. The community-based nurse assists in this process in various ways, such as implementing measures to control symptoms and promote comfort, administering medications and providing support for the family (for medications see Chapter 28 and for palliative care see Chapter 43)
- Require assistance to arrange for other community support services, such as personal care, home help, meals on wheels or respite care.

ASPECTS OF COMMUNITY-BASED NURSING CARE

Aspects of community-based nursing care include:

- Recognising the individual's right to autonomy and confidentiality, and understanding the legal implications of nursing practice within the home. Community-based nurses must always remember that they are a visitor in a person's home and can therefore only implement actions at the person's request. It is essential that the nurse obtain a person's informed consent before carrying out any nursing activities. A situation may also arise where a person refuses to allow the community-based nurse to enter their home, or asks the nurse to leave. If such an event occurs the nurse must respect the individual's wishes, otherwise they may be guilty of infringing the law of trespass
- Being non-judgmental. Community-based nurses need to be aware of their own standards and values and avoid imposing these on others. Nurses may often be required to provide nursing care in homes that are vastly different from their own in terms of cleanliness, tidiness and available facilities
- Being flexible and adaptable. A community-based nurse is required to deliver nursing care in physical environments that differ vastly from the hospital environment. Equipment may have to be organised that is appropriate for the home situation
- Having highly developed assessment skills to assess not only the client but also the family needs. The client's environment also needs assessing to ensure a safe environment for the client and the nurse. For example, the installation of a hand-held shower, rails and a shower chair may be necessary to provide hygiene assistance safely
- *Care coordination* for clients, involving liaison, advocacy, care planning and referral. On admission to hospital and before discharge, community-based nurses communicate with hospital staff to assist in the continuity of client care. Acting as an advocate for the client in some situations, liaising with general practitioners and other health care workers, may be appropriate
- Having knowledge of the vast range of community resources to enable appropriate referrals for clients to services such as home help, meals on wheels, home handymen, diabetes educators, continence nurses, support groups, respite services, services to assist with shopping and banking, schemes that provide funding support, case management, advocacy, activity groups or community transport (Clinical Interest Box 7.1).

CLINICAL INTEREST BOX 7.1
Home-based care

Rebecca is a Division 2 nurse who works in a community-based nursing service. In a typical day Rebecca sees 10–15 clients in their homes. The activities she is involved in include hygiene assistance, wound care, monitoring blood glucose levels and assisting clients with the application of compression stockings.

Rebecca is responsible for organising her own day, which starts at the office base with a handover and ends there with time allowed to debrief with the coordinator and other staff. Rebecca's days are not often the same and she finds herself regularly involved in providing education and emotional support to clients and carers as well as information on other services that are available in the community.

SECURITY ISSUES IN HOME CARE

Community-based nurses function independently in a variety of unfamiliar home settings and situations. Their clients include a diverse population that encompasses all ages, a variety of health problems and families of different structures and cultural backgrounds. In their daily routine, for example, they might be required to visit clients living in a neighbourhood where the crime rate is high. This might pose additional safety concerns. Nurses should have a pre-established mechanism with the agency they are working for to signal for help if need arises, for example, having a pre-programmed emergency number in their phone, carrying a personal alarm device or ensuring that there is someone else with them when they visit the client.

CASE MANAGEMENT

Case management, a major component of community care, is another approach to providing care to clients in the community. Case management is a delivery of care that coordinates and links various health care and social services to clients and their families who have complex health needs that involve ongoing care. Generally, a case manager is appointed when a client is under a case management program. The case manager works together with nurses and other health care professionals to provide collaborative care This care includes planning, assessing needs and coordinating, implementing and evaluating care for the client in their own home. It is a service provided to the individual client and carers. Case managers can be nurses, social workers or any other appropriate health professional.

Key responsibilities of case managers are:

- Assessing clients and their homes and communities
- Coordinating and planning client care
- Collaborating with other health professionals
- Monitoring clients' progress
- Evaluating client outcomes.

Case management may also involve managing a client's care across a continuum of hospital or respite settings and the community. For example, where a client with dementia is admitted to hospital and has a community case manager, the case manager may liaise with staff in the acute assessment ward to coordinate the client's discharge back to the community.

Some hospitals or inpatient facilities may appoint one of their own staff on a short-term basis as a case manager to assist the person to return to the community. When the client is discharged the same case manager may refer the client to community-based nursing or other services as necessary to sustain and support the client's health status. This case manager may visit the client at home to ensure that continuity of care is maintained.

THE NURSING PROCESS AND COMMUNITY NURSING

The nursing process is used in community health and community-based nursing, as in most other areas of nursing. As a logical framework for nursing care, the steps of assessment, nursing diagnosis, planning, implementation and evaluation are particularly useful for clients receiving long-term care, which is often the case in community nursing.

Nurses working in the home setting have the opportunity to observe clients in their own environment, enabling a more holistic assessment. The focus on client choice and autonomy means that clients and families are encouraged to participate actively in the nursing process. As a result, the client and their family may be more proactive in the implementation phase, significantly contributing to the success of the care plan as they work towards their own goals.

ASSESSMENT

Community nursing assessments involve getting to know the client, their family, their environment and lifestyles. It involves a needs assessment as well as risk identification. The aim of the assessment is to assist the client and/or family to identify actual or potential problems, leading to a nursing diagnosis.

It includes information on:

- Physical assessment and health history
- Psychosocial assessment (education, ethnicity, emotional supports)
- Family dynamics
- Social situation (ability to manage finances, access to resources, housing, transportation)
- Functional abilities (mobility, functions related to activities of daily living)
- Client and family values, attitudes to health and services.

PLANNING

Community nursing care is client focused, with expected outcomes being identified. After expected outcomes are defined, goals to achieve these need to be set by the client in consultation with the nurse, and family when appropriate. Goals may be short or long term. Clinical pathways, care plans including each particular step in care as determined by scientific studies and expert opinion, may be used to ensure that clinical care is standardised and of a high quality while at the same time allowing for individualised care to be undertaken.

Community nurses may consider referrals to other providers as part of their care plan in order to ensure that the client's care needs are met by the most appropriate practitioner or service. If clients and family members are to undertake care themselves, education may be necessary to enable them to provide safe appropriate care. To promote empowerment it is vital that clients and family participate in care planning and in decisions regarding all services and practitioners who will provide care.

IMPLEMENTATION

Implementation of the care plan requires care coordination by the community nurse. Care may be provided by the client, family, nurse or other health care workers. The nursing role in the implementation phase is based on promoting independence. This involves teaching skills and techniques to clients and/or their families to use in their activities of daily living, and attending to clinical care as required. Delivery of clinical nursing care in the home follows the same principles for care given in the hospital, but may require some adaptation of practical nursing skills; for example, using an aseptic technique to perform a wound dressing without a dressing trolley.

Teaching opportunities abound in community nursing and it is important that nurses make use of these opportunities.

EVALUATION

Evaluation should be a continual process that occurs during every visit with the client, family or with a community group. If changes occur in health conditions, care plans are updated. If the client or family is unable to continue participating in the care themselves, needs are reassessed. Carers often provide full care 24 hours a day 7 days a week and may be very involved in implementing community nursing care plans. Community nurses evaluate carers and their need for support as caring is extremely demanding. Other forms of assistance, support and respite options should be discussed regularly to reduce carer strain.

The care plan may require changing for several reasons: goals may have been achieved; the client may achieve independence with care; new information may become available indicating a change in goals is needed; resources may no longer be available; or the client's condition may be deteriorating. Documentation of assessment, nursing diagnosis, goals, care plan, interventions and evaluation is vital to ensure continuity of care and to produce evidence of effective care.

SUMMARY

There is a gradual transition of health care provision from traditional acute hospitals to care in the community. Community-based health care provides a wide range of services designed to promote health, prevent illness and restore health. One of the main aims of community-based care is to provide a continuum of care as clients move from one level of care to another. Community nurses must be competent collaborators, educators, client advocates, change agents and researchers. Their work is centred on health promotion and health education activities with individuals, families or groups in the community.

REVIEW EXERCISES

1. List the settings in which community-based health care is provided.
2. What is the philosophy of community-based nursing?
3. What do community-based nurses aim to achieve for clients?
4. List some of the people who may require community nursing services.
5. How is the nursing process different in the home setting?
6. What is a primary consideration when planning care in the home?

CRITICAL THINKING EXERCISES

1. Mr Shift, 52, has emphysema and diabetes, and often visits the community health centre. He is homeless and spends his nights sleeping in the park. Sometimes he drops in at the local Salvation Army centre for food. What interventions would you consider to improve Mr Shift's health and quality of life?
2. Consider the community where you live. What is this community's profile and resources? What are its strengths and weaknesses? Identify two health issues that require attention.

REFERENCES AND FURTHER READING

Baum F (2008) *The New Public Health: an Australian Perspective*. Oxford University Press, Melbourne

Berman AJ, Snyder S, Kozier B, Erb B (2008) *Kozier and Erbs Fundamentals of Nursing. Concepts, Process and Practice*, 8th edn. Prentice-Hall, Upper Saddle River, New Jersey

Commonwealth Department of Veteran Affairs (2007) *Guidelines for the Provision of Community Nursing Care*. Australian Government Publishing Service, Canberra

Cox S (2000) Improving communication between care settings. *Professional Nurse* 15(4): 267–71

Creech C, Phillips P (2001) Community nursing practice: spending wisely to cut the costs of health care. *ACCNS Journal for Community Nurses* 6(1): 16–17

Elliot P (2002) The advanced nurse practitioner role in the community. *ACCNS Journal for Community Nurses* 7(3): 13–14

McMurray A (2007) *Community Health and Wellness: a Sociological Approach*. Harcourt Australia, Sydney

Miles G (2000) Clinical pathways: the care link between primary health services. *Australian Journal Primary Health Interchange* 6(3-4): 84–90

Montalto M (2002) *Hospital in the Home: Principles and Practice.* ArtWords, Ivanhoe, Vic

Potter PA, Perry AG (2007) *Basic Nursing: Essentials for Practice*, 6th edn. Mosby, St Louis

Smith J (2002) The changing face of community and district nursing. *Australian Health Review* 25(3): 131–33

St John W, Kelerher H (2007) *Community Nursing Practice: Theory, Skills and Issues.* Allen & Unwin, Sydney

World Health Organization (WHO) (1978) *Alma-Ata Primary Health Care*. WHO, Geneva

ONLINE RESOURCES

Department of Veterans' Affairs: www.dva.gov.au

Royal District Nursing Service (South Australia): www.rdns.org.au

Royal District Nursing Service (Victoria): www.rdns.com.au

Chapter 8

HEALTH AND WELLNESS

OBJECTIVES

- Define the key terms/concepts
- Explore the concepts of health and wellness in relation to both scientific data and personal experience
- Gain an overview of models of health and wellness
- Recognise the variables influencing health beliefs and practices
- Plan nursing interventions that support changes commensurate with the beliefs and values of the family unit

KEY TERMS/CONCEPTS

determinants of health
holistic
homeostasis
indices of health

CHAPTER FOCUS

This chapter provides an overview of health and wellness as distinct from the absence of disease. It provides a focus for nurses from which to view the family as a whole, recognising the interrelationship of society, culture and family on the health beliefs and behaviours of the individual. From this perspective nurses may facilitate their client's understanding of the interplay between social, psychological and biomedical components of their ill-health, and the client's own role in a multidisciplinary approach to their care while encouraging ownership of and responsibility for lifestyle change.

LIVED EXPERIENCE

I don't see myself as a person with a disability. I had my right leg chopped off because of my diabetes and was fitted with an artificial leg. Everybody was so worried that I might not be able to return to my normal farming lifestyle. I proved them all wrong — with some modifications I was able to drive in my special four-wheel bike to the paddocks and feed my cattle and tend to my farming duties. I am back to my old self.

James, 53-year-old farmer, after below-knee amputation of his right leg

CONCEPTS OF HEALTH AND WELLNESS

Concepts of health and wellness are based on both objective scientific measurements derived from large and varied population studies, as well as the subjective experience of individuals who describe themselves as being well or healthy. Scientific data provide information related to the *determinants of health* that include biological factors, health beliefs and behaviours as well as socioeconomic and environmental conditions accounting for health trends across societies and cultures. Studies of healthy people also contribute to what is referred to as *indices of health*, such as the body mass index (BMI). The BMI provides guidelines for healthy weight ranges as well as therapeutic ranges for blood cholesterol and blood sugar (see online Appendix 7: Height & weight/nutrition).

Such data have also provided a foundation for government-funded health screening and health promotion campaigns to raise public awareness of the interplay between lifestyle, nutrition, environmental health risks and disease. An example of such a program can be seen in the After School Care Nutrition Program encouraging children to become familiar with healthy food choices while raising parents' awareness of the link between poor nutrition and obesity in school-age children and the rising incidence of type 1 diabetes in adolescents.

Health and wellbeing are integral elements of each person's identity and, as such, influence actual and potential interactions with every aspect of life. The World Health Organization (WHO) promotes a positive concept of health, with defining characteristics that capture the many interrelated determinants of health as well as the importance of cultural and spiritual beliefs on health outcomes (WHO 1992). The WHO has actively supported a societal shift from focusing on illness to focusing on health, recognising that personal concepts of health are derived initially from family norms and values relating to health. For example, a child whose parents openly enjoy smoking cigarettes while denying any link with respiratory disease will share that belief until such a time that other events challenge those beliefs. Personal concepts of health are also shaped by geographical location, socioeconomic status and social structures, all of which influence and support family norms related to diet and lifestyle as well as health care access.

As children mature the values they ascribe to their health may be challenged by new information, role models outside their family of origin and by personal experience. Personal values also influence health behaviours, and a young person who prizes physical fitness may pay more attention to diet and exercise than a person in the middle years of life who attaches importance to being not ill. Older people may value health in relation to their functionality, or their ability to do things, and in enjoying life even in the presence of disease rather than focusing on the pathology of ageing.

To complete this broad overview of health and illness it is important to recognise the interrelatedness of physical and mental wellbeing as well as the interplay of both internal and external factors on each individual's state of health. Each system and subsystem within the human body continuously exchanges information to maintain a steady state or homeostasis in the face of actual or perceived change. When these adjustment processes fail to maintain an adequate physiological balance, disease or illness may result. Responses to both internal and external challenges to homeostasis vary according to the magnitude of the challenge and the emotional readiness of each individual to cope with change. Nutritional status, age, pre-existing disease and social support also influence individual responses; thus, different dimensions of wellbeing are infinitely related and linked in the socio-physical dimensions of health (see Clinical Interest Box 8.1).

MODELS OF HEALTH AND WELLNESS

A model is a symbolic representation of a complex issue such as health and provides a framework for understanding

CLINICAL INTEREST BOX 8.1
Health and wellness

Health is defined not only by the absence of disease but also includes the importance of psycho-social wellbeing, including the ability to make and maintain healthy relationships, to cope with daily stresses and to remain generally optimistic and motivated. This can be seen in the following example.

Mrs N, 89, lives on her own since her husband's death many years ago. Although she is almost blind from macular degeneration, she pursues an active lifestyle, walking her dog for at least 30 minutes every morning and participating in the administration of a day-care program for the elderly, even though many of the program participants are younger than she is.

Mrs N has evidence of rheumatoid arthritis in her hands, as well as loss of height from pronounced scoliosis of the spine, and often experiences pain from these deformities. She will often reflect on her sadness at no longer being able to knit, sew or read, as well as being annoyed with the clumsiness caused by her inflamed and disfigured finger joints.

However, while her body has a certain frailty that comes with advanced age, her voice is vibrant as she speaks animatedly to her neighbour who has come to visit. As she prepares fresh vegetables for her dinner, the smell of freshly cooked scones for the day centre pervades the kitchen. What sets Mrs N apart from many others her age is her philosophy on life — her commitment to reach beyond her physical limitations by actively contributing to her community. She has embraced the opportunities available through the use of audio tapes that substitute for letter writing, as well as being able to listen to 'talking' books. Mrs N maintains an interest in world affairs and keeps in touch with her daughter, grandchildren and, lately, her great grandchildren, all of who live overseas.

and guidance. Models are developed from research studies that identify constant factors pertaining to an issue, with recognition of links to other factors that shape or influence the outcome. Models of health can, for example, be used to predict health needs and outcomes in relation to health-related behaviours. They may also facilitate nurses' understanding of clients' care requirements in relation to their health beliefs and practices.

Nurses' work has traditionally been influenced by Western medical models of health that focus on the organic nature and cause of mental and physical disease rather than the influence of internal and external variables on the health of the whole person. This medical diagnostic-centred model is potentially disrespectful of the individual's health beliefs and may disregard the internal and external variables that shape the social, psychological and behavioural influences on health outcomes.

Contemporary nursing care delivery is guided by a *holistic* model of health, which encompasses a broader reference to both traditional and non-traditional therapies and acknowledges the interplay of physical, psychological and spiritual dimensions on the client's health. This model is client centred, respecting the individual's health care beliefs and actively including the client, family and carers in health care planning. Ideally, this holistic model of health care delivery encourages clients to take responsibility for their behaviour in relation to health and illness, empowering them to assume a greater control over culturally appropriate health care options.

The health–illness continuum model of health assists nurses to recognise individuals' states of health and wellness as a position on a continuum that ranges from a high level of wellness at one end to severe illness at the other (Figure 8.1).

This continuum represents mental and physical functionality based on vision, hearing, speech, mobility, dexterity, cognition, emotion, pain or discomfort. The health–illness continuum model can also represent the level of individual risk for disease or illness in relation to age, socioeconomic status, cultural beliefs and geographical location. By placing high risk at one end of the continuum and low risk at the other, the comparison of age with risk of infectious childhood diseases such as mumps or rubella identifies young children as being at high risk. Population statistics identify a greater risk associated with car accidents for young people between the ages of 16 and 26. Risk factors for infant mortality are related to socioeconomic status and geographical location, while the risk factors associated with tropical diseases such as malaria are far greater for people living near the equator. Cultural and religious beliefs related to health practices may prohibit groups of people from the benefits of specific care options, thus increasing their associated risk factors. A continuum does not provide us with an absolute measure, but by identifying their position on the continuum people can be encouraged to see a comparison between current and previous health states, or their position in relation to specific risk factors.

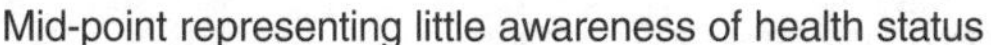

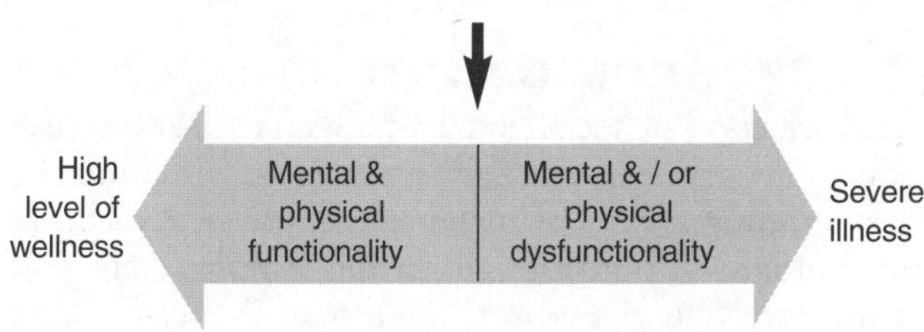

Figure 8.1 | Health–illness continuum model of health *(Elwin 2003)*

The health belief model (Crisp & Taylor 2005) demonstrates the link between people's beliefs about health and their health-related behaviours or health practices. Health beliefs can be defined as the concepts or ideas about health that the individual believes as true. Health practices can be defined as the activities or behaviours that the individual will engage in as a result of, or in line with, their beliefs about health. Many health practices can become unconscious habits, such as cleaning teeth before going to bed, and for most people health beliefs are grounded in family health beliefs, values and practices. Family health beliefs usually reflect the dominant societal attitudes to health at that time.

Further information or experiences may either support these beliefs or contribute to a change. This model identifies two factors that influence change in health-related behaviours: personal readiness for change, and the strength of the stimulus. Readiness for change may be related to an event such as health breakdown or a close encounter with death, or it may arise from dissatisfaction with personal states of health. The strength of the stimulus for change is directly related to the individual's perception of personal vulnerability to death or disease and it is precisely at this time that health education is most effective in the short term. This model may be best understood through the scenario in Clinical Interest Box 8.2.

Barriers to changing health-related behaviours include personal and financial cost to the individual, stated or anticipated family disapproval and low expectation of personal benefit related to the intended change. By recognising the subjective nature of perceived threats to health and the influence of family and cultural beliefs about health practices, the health belief model can offer nurses a guide for client readiness to change. It also assists the nurse to identify the optimal time for health education and in relation to the probability of the individual making a commitment to change.

VARIABLES INFLUENCING HEALTH BELIEFS AND PRACTICES

For each individual, health is a complex and inconsistent state, subject to change. The forces that influence change in health status arise from within the individual as well as the

CLINICAL INTEREST BOX 8.2
Application of the health belief model

Tom is a 50-year-old married man who has noticed a change in his personal level of fitness over the last few years. He acknowledged a gradual weight gain when his clothes were no longer comfortable and he began using the lift to his office because he became breathless when climbing a flight of stairs.

Related health beliefs

Tom believes that weight gain is inevitable with advancing years because both his parents had become much heavier as they aged. Both Tom and his wife smoked cigarettes but were undeterred by the health warnings on the cigarette packets because no one in their family developed lung cancer or heart disease.

Health-related event

Tom was forced to walk up stairs to his office when the lift was out of order. He was breathless from the exertion and experienced heaviness in his chest. His secretary called an ambulance and Tom was subsequently diagnosed with a myocardial infarction.

Stimulus to change health behaviours

Tom made a good recovery but the experience had frightened him. He paid attention to the health education sessions for clients in the cardiac step-down unit and sought advice about diet, exercise and cigarette smoking.

Strength of the stimulus

Tom never forgot the pain in his chest and his fear of dying. He stopped smoking and gradually increased his level of fitness with the support of the cardiac rehabilitation team. His wife was scared Tom was going to die and supported him throughout his illness and rehabilitation. She cut back her cigarette smoking and didn't smoke in front of Tom but was unable to 'kick the habit'. Tom's parents were very supportive but thought they were too old to change their health behaviours.

social and physical environments in which people live, the infrastructure for access to health care and the expectations of health that are common to that society. Internal factors include physical and intellectual development and emotional states as well as strength of character and ability to cope with change. Healthy psychological development may also be supported by spiritual beliefs and values, which bring hope and meaning to life. These internal factors cannot be separated from external factors, including socioeconomic status, cultural or family norms and values, as well as wider global influences. Figure 8.2 shows the interactions between the variety of factors that can affect health. An overview of the interrelationship of these influences on health outcomes is explored in this section.

PHYSICAL DEVELOPMENT

At birth a baby's health depends initially on fetal development and gestational age, genetic make-up and, finally, a healthy birth weight. These variables are largely related to maternal health and diet, which in turn are influenced by socioeconomic status of the family as well as cultural norms. As the children grow, their health status will be influenced by exposure to disease and their immune status. Undeniably, health beliefs and behaviours play a large part in disease prevention, for example, acceptance or rejection of immunisation schedules, and housing and sanitary conditions. Diet and exercise play an important role in further biological and psychosocial development, as do the health behaviours that are modelled by family members, for example, taking a drug, resting or massaging to relieve headache. Physical development and the experience of health cannot be separated from the society in which the individual lives, the physical body being one with the psychosocial body and the forces that shape it.

INTELLECTUAL DEVELOPMENT

For people to take responsibility for their health behaviours they must fully understand the relationship between health risks and health behaviours. Information about health can be accessed through libraries and health and medical centres, but more than ever, electronic information informs lifestyle choices. However, the ability to critically appraise this wealth of information and to make informed choices about health practices depends on many factors, for example, cognitive development, access to adequate education and family values related to academic success, and positive and negative personal health experiences.

EMOTIONAL DEVELOPMENT

Adult mental health is largely influenced through appropriate parental attachments in the early years of infant life and sets the stage for the development of behavioural self-regulation. Early relationships and active social interactions have a far-reaching effect on personality development as well as the ability to form appropriate emotional relationships as an adult. Most importantly, positive emotional experiences in early childhood influence the individual's adaptive capacities to meet the many demands of adulthood, including emotional stress and occasions of physical illness. The interrelationship of emotional and cognitive function with activation of the immune system relates to the individual's ability to heal from both biological and psychological trauma. The body's physiological response to perceived stressful events is also initiated by the brain. The release of neurochemicals sets off a cascade of physiological reactions assisting well-balanced individuals to cope with a wide range of stress and anxiety without compromising their health beliefs and practices.

SOCIOECONOMIC FACTORS

The interaction of social and economic factors on health beliefs and practices are far reaching and include the compounding effects of social status, physical location and standard of housing; education, employment and income levels; marital status, stability of the relationship and caretaker responsibilities; private health insurance and access to, and use of, health care and information.

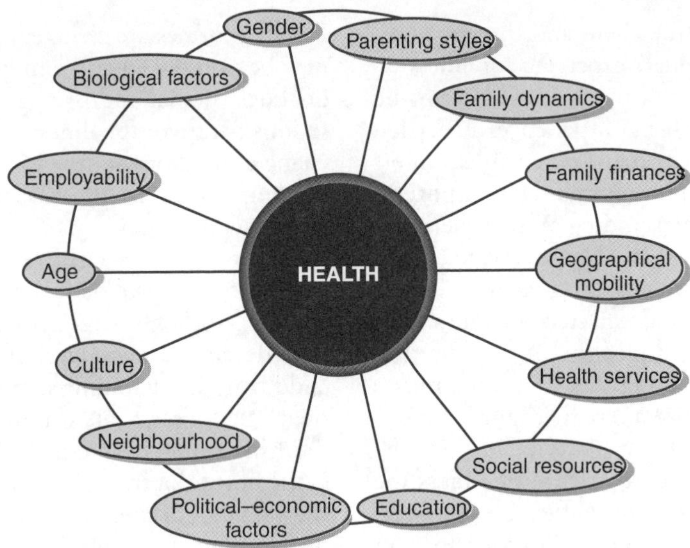

Figure 8.2 | Interactions between factors that can affect health *(McMurray 2007)*

Levels of education influence people's use of health-related information, while social status in the community largely influences the ways that families define health and how and when they seek medical aid, including the use of health screening services. The effects of these factors on health is evidenced through the increased probability of people with lower levels of education and income engaging in health-risk behaviours such as smoking cigarettes, abusing alcohol or leading a sedentary lifestyle, with associated health problems related to excess body weight and obesity.

Patterns of illness differ between people of different cultures and social classes and in Australia the health status of Aboriginal people is typically worse than that of the general population. This is partly due to the influence of Western cultures and diseases on their traditional lifestyle but is also adversely affected by a constellation of socioeconomic factors including geographic location in remote areas with under-resourced and inappropriate health care services.

FAMILY HEALTH PRACTICES

Family patterns, rituals and routines have a considerable influence on children's learned behaviours in relation to health behaviour and practices and these are often perpetuated into adulthood. Family attitudes, values and behaviours set the standard for how family members care for each other, the type of diet that is provided on a regular basis and the use of exercise both as a family activity and as a health routine. Family values also influence the use of, and compliance with, health promotion activities such as children's immunisation schedules, age-appropriate health screening practices and conformity with road and vehicle safety regulations. Information about family health values and routines are important for nurses planning health care interventions or health education. The introduction or promotion of different health care practices must be commensurate with family values and lifestyle if they are to have a positive and lasting effect. Clinical Interest Box 8.3 lists examples of healthy lifestyle choices, and Clinical Interest Box 8.4 is an example of a family's health beliefs.

NURSING AND ILLNESS

The focus of nursing care in the 21st century has largely shifted from an ill-health medical model to include client-centred holistic care and health promotion, using theory and research as a basis for practice. Nursing has moved from being disease oriented to caring for the whole person with an illness, emphasising the importance of preserving and maintaining health. This approach respects the client's perspective as valid and important and diminishes the nurse's

CLINICAL INTEREST BOX 8.3
Examples of healthy lifestyle choices

- Regular exercise
- Avoiding alcohol abuse and smoking
- Regular self breast examination
- Seatbelt use
- Bike helmet use
- Weight control

CLINICAL INTEREST BOX 8.4
Health beliefs

I remember my grandmother and mother applying turmeric paste, which is used for cooking in many Asian cuisines, on cuts and wounds. They used to tell me it was an ancient remedy and they believed turmeric had many therapeutic values. I still use this traditional method of wound management with my children when they come home with cuts and bruises from the playground and I have found that it is the cheapest, safest and most effective antiseptic cream you can get — straight out of the pantry.

(Meera, mother of four young children)

assumed right to 'know for' the client and thereby make judgements about the individual's experience of illness.

Although illness as such is not disease, it can be understood as including the client's experiences associated with acute or chronic illness such as pain, personal discomfort and embarrassment, fear and powerlessness. It is important for nurses to establish an understanding of the beliefs that surround a person's illness experience by listening to clients' stories of declining health, precipitating factors, beliefs about cause, issues of concern and expected outcomes. This places the nurse in a privileged position of confidant(e), educator and guide and by valuing these dialogues nurses can encourage clients to examine alternatives and solutions to their health care issues.

Whether clients have an acute or chronic illness the experience may have left them feeling vulnerable or powerless. When clients are actively encouraged to participate in their care management as well as to examine the implications of their diet and lifestyle on their future health outcomes, they effectively form a power-sharing partnership with the nurse. This in turn has the potential to improve their psychological wellbeing, reduce their stress and promote wellness.

IMPACT OF ACUTE AND CHRONIC ILLNESS ON CLIENT AND FAMILY

As patterns of mortality in Australia and the Western world change from the infectious epidemics in earlier centuries to long-term degenerative diseases of the present day, treatment therapies and health care provision have also changed. Modern technology and critical-care medicine facilitate many clients' recovery from trauma and acute episodes of illness, but shorter hospital stays and the provision of services that support ongoing care in the home can represent a crisis not only for the client, but also for all members of the family. The effects of illness on families and clients vary in relation to the severity of the disease, the age of the client and other family members as well as the ability of each to cope with the exigencies of treatment therapies, personal stress and changes to family dynamics.

While many people can look forward to a longer and generally healthier life, the structure of present-day family units has changed. It does not as frequently include members of the extended family, such as grandparents, who would have traditionally provided care for other members during periods of illness. The family unit, which now more often includes single parents or same sex couples, or which has been remoulded through divorce and remarriage, can be defined as an interactive system with established roles and functions for each member. Changes for one family member will set off a succession of changes because of the evolving and interdependent nature of family relationships. This situation becomes more complex in the event of chronic illness, when the sick role becomes the focus of attention and other family members must incorporate elements of responsibility into their previously established roles. Family routines are changed; previously important events may be overlooked and family members may be in a state of shock, denial and/or anger when informed about the serious nature of the illness. The mood in the family may change from hope for the future to despondency and may be compounded in some situations by financial difficulties or impact on carers.

Parents of sick children often display controlling and overprotective behaviours as an expression of their anxiety, although parents of chronically ill children may have developed some level of expertise in managing their child's care, often finding some solace and empowerment in their role. Adolescents who live with disabling conditions resulting from chronic diseases such as asthma, diabetes, cystic fibrosis or juvenile arthritis must cope not only with the demands of their illness but also with social and sexual development, completion of secondary education and entry to tertiary education or finding a position in the workforce. Just as these young people are seeking some level of independence from their family, their parents may express reluctance to loosen their ties, having shaped their lives to accommodate the demands of their illness.

SUMMARY

The care-giving role can place an enormous burden on the family's physical, psychological and financial resources. As family members attempt to make sense of the situation in the early stages of the disease, they may be best supported with clear, relevant information to facilitate coping strategies. Further support and management strategies may be negotiated relevant to the disease progression, type of care required and the age of the client, and may include involvement in established support groups for people in similar situations. Families who face the consequences of end-stage chronic or malignant disease may experience a stage of acceptance and adjustment, aided perhaps by their need for emotional support from family and friends as well as spiritual support from their religious community. As the client's health continues to deteriorate, the whole focus of support will be to reduce pain and discomfort while assisting both the client and family members to come to terms with the change in family roles and the importance of grieving before the surviving family members can regain a maximum level of function and wellbeing.

REVIEW EXERCISES

1. Identify at least three events that might influence change in a client's health behaviours.
2. Identify potential barriers to changes in health behaviours.
3. How might the family roles and dynamics change in the event of a mother of young children being diagnosed with breast cancer? How would the family roles and dynamics differ if this same diagnosis was made for the paternal grandmother rather than the mother of this family?

CRITICAL THINKING EXERCISE

Review the following statements. Identify at least two underlying assumptions for each sentence and rephrase them to better reflect your perception of the truth about these statements.

Old people don't expect to be healthy.

Young people cope better with illness than old people.

Nurses have to make allowances for the health habits of people from other countries.

REFERENCES AND FURTHER READING

Craven RF, Hirnle CJ (2003) *Fundamentals of Nursing. Human Health and Function*, 4th edn. Lippincott, Philadelphia

Crisp J, Taylor C (eds) (2005) *Potter & Perry's Fundamentals of Nursing*, 2nd edn. Elsevier Australia, Sydney

deWit SC (2001) *Fundamental Concepts and Skills for Nursing*. WB Saunders, Philadelphia

McMurray A (2007) *Community Health and Wellness: A Sociological Approach*, 3rd edn. Elsevier Australia

World Health Organization (WHO) (1992) Health promotion in developing countries: a call for action. *American Journal of Health Promotion*, 6(3): 174

ONLINE RESOURCES

MultiLingual Health Education (Canada's multi-language resource of high-quality translated information, for professional health-care providers and their clients): www.multilingual-health-education.net

Yahoo Health Education Directory: www.//health.yahoo.com

Unit 3

Cultural diversity and nursing practice

Chapter 9

CULTURAL DIVERSITY IN AUSTRALIA AND NEW ZEALAND

OBJECTIVES

- Define the key terms listed
- Define culture and ethnicity, and explain their influence on health
- Describe the level of cultural diversity in Australia and New Zealand
- Discover the processes underlying colonisation and their implications for health care
- Explore one's own attitudes, beliefs, behaviours and power and how these affect nursing practice
- Describe basic principles that underlie competence in nursing across cultures

KEY TERMS/CONCEPTS

adaptation
assimilation
cultural safety
culture
culture conflict
culture contact
culture shock
ethnicity and ethnocentrism
power
prejudice
racism
stereotyping
structural violence
systemic bias
transcultural nursing

CHAPTER FOCUS

Australia and New Zealand are multicultural societies, populated by culturally diverse people. This chapter examines the nature of cultural diversity with special emphasis on concepts such as culture and ethnicity, multiculturalism and associated processes of stereotyping, discrimination and structural violence. It explores the role of culture on people's perceptions of health and illness and the importance of power and culture shock in relationships between clients and health care providers. The chapter encourages nurses to review the literature on cross-cultural nursing and to reflect on their own position within society in order to begin to develop culturally safe practice.

LIVED EXPERIENCE

My father was hospitalised with dementia at the age of 87. We found a nursing home, which claimed to cater to the needs of 'ethnic' clients and, indeed, was owned by the Ethnic Community Council. We were surprised that my father, who always enjoyed his food, seemed to be losing weight rapidly. Concerned, my sister and I visited him at lunchtime to see what he was eating, and how — we found him refusing to be fed coleslaw, much to the distress of the nurse. She did not realise that a man of his culture, and his generation, believed that raw cabbage should be fed to rabbits and pigs, but not people.

personal communication to A-K Eckermann, 1991

CULTURAL DIVERSITY IN AUSTRALIA AND NEW ZEALAND

Indigenous Australia was marked by cultural diversity long Before Cook (BC, as the late Oodgeroo Noonuccal used to say). Some 500 different Indigenous language groups occupied the whole of the continent (Berndt & Berndt 1988) and lived in well-defined socioeconomic, political, land-owning units (Elkin 1964). The situation was a little different in New Zealand (Aotearoa). Polynesian people settled the islands between 250 and 1150CE (Belich 1996). Known as Māori, they adhered to common cultural traditions, although there were some dialectic differences between the groups (Rice 1992).

Australia and New Zealand were both colonised by the British. However, significant differences marked this process in the two countries.

In the late 18th century the British Crown claimed the continent of Australia as *terra nullius*; that is, unoccupied/empty and therefore open to settlement/annexation (see McGraw 1995; Reynolds 1987, 1989; Lippmann 1999). As a result, Indigenous Australians experienced dispossession and dislocation. For almost 200 years, governments created special laws and policies, which treated them as 'non-human' and controlled every aspect of their lives, including marriage, employment, education, recreation and religion. Today it could be argued that these policies and laws were intrinsically racist and abused Indigenous human rights by segregating, assimilating and controlling the minorities (see the work of Reynolds 1987; Broome 2001). This history has left its mark on Australian attitudes towards the country's traditional owners as well as the life chances of today's Indigenous Australians (see Saggers & Gray 1991; National Inquiry into the Separation of Aboriginal and Torres Strait Islander Children from their Families 1997; Tatz 2001; Dowd et al 2005).

In New Zealand, or Aotearoa, on the other hand, Britain recognised that it had to negotiate with sovereign, independent Māori groups (Orange 1987; Belich 1996). Perhaps, this was because the colonists could identify social structures and hierarchical power relations, marked by tribes, clans, chiefs and councils, not so very different from their own. In 1840 the British Crown signed the Treaty of Waitangi with Māori representatives of many of the multiple iwi (tribes) and hapu (sub-tribes) of New Zealand in order to ensure that further British settlement could take place. The Treaty of Waitangi was meant to safeguard Māoris' existing property and citizenship rights (Durie 1994). This treaty and the passage of the *Waitangi Tribunal Act* of 1975 ensured that Māori claims for reparations could be dealt with legally. It ensured that New Zealand has had a very different colonial experience to that of Australia (Pearson 1996). Today, the Treaty of Waitangi and the *Waitangi Tribunal Act* offer a way to address some of the consequences of colonisation. They also provide a set of principles, outlined in the New Zealand Royal Commission of Social Policy, Volume II, 1988, to guide interactions with Māori people. These are the principle of partnership, the principle of participation and the principle of protection. Nevertheless, the process of Māori colonisation has resulted in structural inequality and widespread institutional racism, which have led to poverty and the breakdown of Māori social structure, culture, language, life chances and health (Walker 1990).

At the turn of the 20th Century, Australia and New Zealand essentially consisted of two kinds of populations — immigrants who were largely from Britain, and Indigenous peoples. Indeed, Australia ensured that its immigrants would, preferably, be of northern European descent by enacting the White Australia Policy after Federation. The policy was not repealed until 1973 (Eckermann et al 2006).

Today, Australian and New Zealand societies are composed of peoples from many cultures. As Eckermann et al (2008) have pointed out, roughly 22.5% of the Australian population has been born overseas and speaks a language other than English at home (Australian Bureau of Statistics [ABS] 2004). The background of immigrants has, however, changed over the years. Julian (2004) points out that since the 1980s, much more emphasis has been placed on skilled and business migration. Further, during the 1990s, Australia instigated a quota for refugees. Such refugees tended to originate from the latest sources of conflict. Thus:

> ... refugees have also arrived in waves from different parts of the globe ... During the 1970s, the majority of refugees came from South-East Asian countries such as Vietnam, Cambodia and Laos: in the 1980s many came from Central American countries such as Chile and El Salvador: and more recently, since 1991, they have come predominantly from the former Yugoslavia, the Middle East and the Horn of Africa.
>
> (Julian 2004: 103)

Indigenous Australians constitute 2.4% of the total population in Australia (ABS 2004). The proportion of immigrants from Asia who annually migrate to Australia is now approaching the proportion from Britain and Ireland (Jupp 2002). In New Zealand, Māori people constitute 14.2% of the total population; 1 in 15 New Zealanders is of Asian descent, and 19.5% of the population has been born overseas (Statistics New Zealand 2003) — the majority of these have come from the United Kingdom and Ireland or the Pacific (including Australia). New Zealand's consistent refugee policy has seen an increase in the number of refugees accepted into the country from Eastern Europe, Indochina and Africa (Statistics New Zealand 2001).

However, cultural diversity in Australia and, to a lesser degree, New Zealand has not led to structural diversity. English remains the dominant language, and both countries' major institutions, including health, are mono-cultural. They are modelled on Britain.

This is the context in which health care providers are

expected to practise. They *will* encounter clients, their immediate and at times extended families, who belong to cultural groups different from their own. Consequently clients' beliefs and values may appear, or indeed be, at odds with their own, the practices of Western medicine and nursing philosophies. How nurses respond to their clients' beliefs and behaviours will determine how effective they will be in caring for and promoting their clients' wellness.

It is consequently important that health professionals understand concepts such as culture and ethnicity, monoculturalism, biculturalism and multiculturalism. They need to understand the impact of culture contact and culture clash on health and health perceptions if they are to provide the best possible health care for the individual as well as the community.

To begin the process of understanding, this chapter will firstly consider how culture, class, ethnicity and adaptation perpetuate cultural traditions and preferred ways of learning, thinking and interacting. All of these will, of course, influence people's attitudes to health.

WHAT IS CULTURE?

There have been many definitions of *culture* over the past 150 years dating back to the work of Tylor (1871) which all seem to emphasise:

> … that culture is learned, shared and complex. Its patterns are interrelated to make a living, breathing tapestry that works to satisfy different groups' needs. Cultures are continually adapting, comprised of beliefs, values, attitudes, language, patterns of thought and communication, religion and knowledge as well as tools and technology.
>
> (Eckermann 1995: 2)

Over the years, writers have attempted to identify some of the more important aspects of culture which impact on people, their rules for operating, beliefs and values, history and tradition. Figure 9.1 sets out diagrammatically some of the many influences identified as shaping cultures and individuals within cultures.

Figure 9.1 illustrates that socioeconomic, religious, political, historical and natural environments shape cultural values, beliefs, traditions and patterns of decision making. People learn about what is right and wrong, good and bad, important and unimportant; that is, their values, through socialisation, education and enculturation processes; from their families/friends/peers; through schools and training; and by contact with other groups. However, the environments in which individuals operate will influence their language, ethnicity and class and shape their preferred styles of interacting, learning and identity. These styles determine what motivates them to interact, with whom they prefer to interact and in what way.

An understanding of the relationship between culture, environment and thought is important to nurses who must deal with their own preferred styles of interaction, thinking and learning as well as with those of their clients. However, it is important to remember that individuals are not simply products of their cultures. Consequently, nurses and their clients respond to, initiate and adapt to change in their environments.

This process of adaptation is important. Eckermann et al (2006) cite Bennett (1969:19) who defines adaptation as the 'problem solving, creative, or coping element in human behaviour that permits a dynamic approach to environment [and culture]'.

Because cultures do not exist in a vacuum, people adapt on the basis of the particular social group with whom they share a distinct organisation, continuity and identity. Eckermann et al (2006) have argued that this group is not only 'cultural' — it is also based on socioeconomic–political characteristics; that is, *social class*. Individuals from different social classes are afforded different opportunities — they

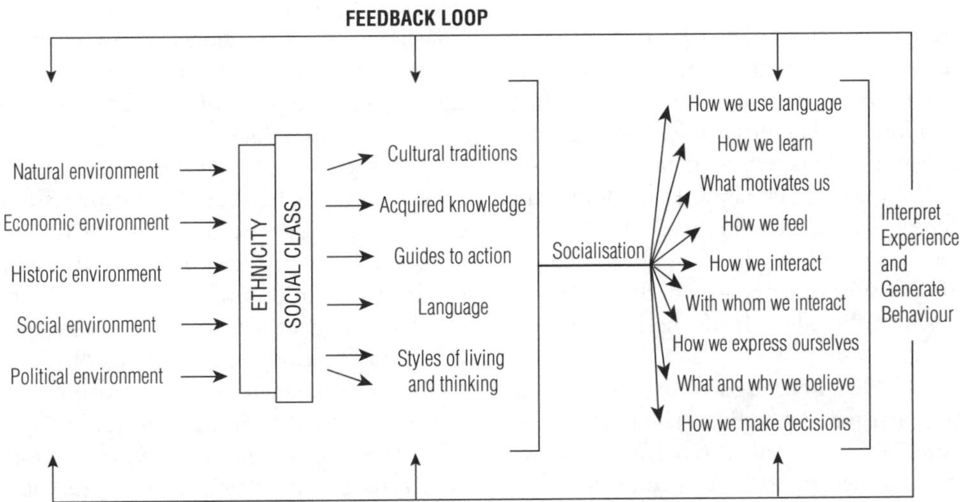

Figure 9.1 | The interrelationship of culture and environment *(Eckermann et al 2006)*

Box 9.1 | Considering personal culture

Remember, we all belong to more than one culture. I am a German Australian. I was transported to Australia by my middle-class German, bilingual parents. I was expected to gain a scholarship and to attend university. So — how many cultures can you identity? German? Immigrant? Middle class?

At university I studied to become an anthropologist. I was particularly influenced by my teachers to become interested in cultural differences in education and health — another culture?

Look at yourself — how many cultures, personal and professional, have influenced you?

have access to varying levels of power, are permitted varying levels of input into decision-making processes and their power to change their life circumstances for the better vary greatly. Indeed Spencer and Inkeles (1976: 222–3) argue that:

> One life chance can determine another, and vice versa. If being born into a wealthy family affects significantly the chance that one will be able to acquire an advanced education, this advanced education itself largely determines an individual's occupational level.
>
> In turn, one's job helps determine how much wealth one can amass ... Both wealth and education will probably help to determine the level of health a person will maintain ...

Everyone belongs to at least one culture; that is, culture of origin. Many are also members of the culture(s) of their profession(s). They will also belong to a social class. In Australia and New Zealand there are many minority groups, groups which share cultural traditions different from the mainstream, but which belong to the same class as members of the mainstream do. Box 9.1 asks nurses to consider their own group membership.

In what way, then does culture and class differ from *ethnicity*?

Some writers (e.g. Leininger 1978, 1995) believe that ethnicity and culture are different. They maintain that ethnicity relates to a group's identity, history, language, nationality and religion, while culture refers to a group's shared and learned values and beliefs, which guide action, thinking and decision making. The approach adopted in this chapter is different. As outlined in Figure 9.1, ethnicity and culture are considered part of the same thing. People cannot separate their environments — whether these be historical, religious or political — from their values and beliefs.

Eckermann et al (2006), have argued that 'ethnic' has come to mean 'minority' and has been used largely to eliminate labels such as 'race'. Social scientists (see the work of Gould 1998, for example) have become aware of how inaccurate the concept 'race' is in terms of defining or categorising anyone, and how destructively it has seeped into people's perceptions of others and their treatment of those who basically 'look different'. Consequently, 'ethnicity' has become the less emotive categorisation, and in Australia the term 'ethnics' has taken over from labels such as 'migrants', 'wogs' or 'reffos'.

By using such a label, even a neutral one, however, there is a tendency for people to express the dichotomy of 'them' and 'us'. Our 'in-group' are 'us' — *they*, the strangers, are the 'ethnics'. That leads to some confusion because, basically, everyone is 'ethnic'. All people belong to specific groups that follow distinctive and diverse cultural, social and linguistic traditions with which they identify on a very personal level; that is, everyone possesses 'ethnicity'.

Members of ethnic groups also belong to a variety of classes, because no single ethnic group fits neatly into one specific class. Consequently, both class and ethnicity affect people's life chances — and their health — which is the reason why ethnicity has been specified as yet another 'filter' which affects the way people interpret, experience and generate behaviour, as outlined in Figure 9.1.

HOW DOES CULTURE INFLUENCE HEALTH?

If different cultures have different values and beliefs, preferred ways of interacting, living and thinking, then they will have different perceptions of 'health'.

Holistic definitions such as that of the World Health Organization (WHO), or of the National Aboriginal and Islander Health Organisation (NAIHO), emphasise the link between culture and health when they stress that health concerns 'not just the physical wellbeing of the individual but the social, emotional and cultural wellbeing of the whole community' (NAIHO 1982: 2). A similar viewpoint in New Zealand focuses on the synergy between people and the wider social, cultural, economic, political and physical environment (Durie 2001).

Lay and professional health behaviours and care practices are generally based on particular values and beliefs about health and the causes of illness and disease. Consequently, how people feel pain, how they interpret *wellness* '... will all depend on a person's beliefs and value systems which are learned within a particular society and within a number of cultural contexts' (Kanitsaki 1992: 2).

Despite the fact that health care providers know and accept that health beliefs and practices vary between cultures, and despite the fact that they tend to support a holistic view of health and wellness, the biomedical model of health dominates in Australia and New Zealand and has the most legitimacy, both socially and politically (Macdonald, in Davis & Dew 1999).

Nurses' understanding of health and illness is influenced by their socialisation into the professional culture of nursing. Their training and the values and behaviours they accept as appropriate to their profession — that is, the professional culture of nursing — provides the blueprint for determining the definition of health and associated values, beliefs and practices. It is undoubtedly dominated by the biomedical ideology. Andrews (2003: 73–4) suggests that nurses often assume that their clients share their professional symbols and knowledge, assumptions and beliefs, and that they can speak and understand the same language. This can obviously lead to enormous misunderstandings.

Consequently, turn to Box 9.2 and reflect on your own attitudes, values, beliefs, practices and traditions acquired through the culture of nursing.

It would be tempting to present health care providers with a whole range of culture-specific health beliefs; for example, many Asian people believe that ill-health is caused by the imbalance between Yin and Yang while some Aboriginal people believe that illness is a form of punishment delivered by an outside agent or the spiritual world. There are a number of texts which will help nurses to learn more about culture-specific beliefs (e.g. D'Avanzo's 2008 *Pocket Guide to Cultural Assessment*). It is not the purpose of this chapter to replicate such work. Instead it focuses on developing a better understanding of the forces that shape cross-cultural situations. Working across cultures can be marked by suspicion, fear and self-doubt from both the nurse's point of view and that of the client. Culture clash and culture conflict may arise.

CULTURE CLASH AND CULTURE CONFLICT

If nurses are to develop appropriate skills to work across cultures, they need to understand the processes, which shape the way differences within and between groups are evaluated. Eckermann et al (2006) have argued that perceptions of differences depend on a number of complex interrelated factors such as ethnocentrism, stereotypes, prejudice, discrimination, power and powerlessness. Matsumoto and Juang (2004: 63) define ethnocentrism as follows:

> We define ethnocentrism as the tendency to view the world through one's own cultural filters… it follows that just about everyone in the world is ethnocentric. That is, everyone learns a certain way of behaving, and in doing so learns a certain way of perceiving and interpreting the behaviour of others. This way of perceiving and making interpretations of others is a normal consequence of growing up in a society. In this sense, ethnocentrism per se is neither bad nor good; it merely reflects the state of affairs — that we all have our cultural filters on when we perceive others.

The problem is that the 'other' becomes less good, or dangerous, or strange. A stranger in a small town is 'other', a person from another country is a foreigner or 'other', a poor person is the 'other' to the privileged. 'Otherness' may also be assigned to a whole range of human characteristics — gender and sexual orientation, religious or spiritual belief, ethnic origin or migrant experience, age or generation, or disability.

When ethnocentrism is mixed with power, then powerful systems or professions (which believe they are the best, or know what's best) are able to suppress the less powerful.

Stereotypes are over-generalisations (see Allport 1982). They, too, are part of human life and thinking because people are encouraged, from an early age, to categorise the things around them. For example, it is possible to categorise an object as 'table' — whether it has four legs or one, it makes no difference. Consequently, over-generalisations always deprive the 'object' of individuality. As a result, when stereotypes are applied to people, they develop into 'mindsets' (whether these are positive or negative) which deny individual talents and abilities; for example, all southern Europeans are hot blooded.

Prejudices or prejudgments are the positive or negative attitudes people develop around the stereotypes they have about the 'other'. Prejudices are based on half-truths, myths, rumours and over-generalisation, which are invested with a good deal of emotion. As a result, prejudices become quite resistant to change. Prejudices in their turn can lead to discrimination.

Discrimination is the acting out of prejudice, the active speaking or acting against those who are different from 'us'. But discrimination can also take the form of providing, or not providing, a service to an individual or family because it is assumed that the professional 'knows what's best for them'. So discrimination can take the form of acts of commission as well as omission.

It is easy to get caught in the progression from ethnocentrism to stereotypes to prejudice to discrimination. It is easy to make faulty assumptions and to treat people as stereotypes if they are seen as different and 'strange'. This problem is perpetuated by family, friends and colleagues as well as the media, who reflect a certain image of other groups.

The world is experiencing a particularly stressful period in this first part of the 21st century — mutual fear of 'the other' has been escalated by the 11 September 2001 terrorist acts in New York, the Bali bombings in 2002, the continuing war in the Middle East and political assassination in Pakistan in 2007. It would be naïve to assume that these events do not affect attitudes and beliefs; that is,

Box 9.2 | Reflection on attitudes, values, beliefs, practices and traditions acquired through nursing

Please reflect on:

- your personal definitions of health
- the client's definition of health
- whose definitions have been legitimised (by law and by society)
- the implications of this for nursing practice and health care
- the consequences for clients, especially people from different cultural backgrounds.

stereotypes about Muslim immigrants and asylum seekers, or, indeed, the feelings of members of such minorities about themselves and mainstream society generally. As with other types of societal attitudes and beliefs, these stereotypes may influence interactions in many aspects of life, including hospitals, clinics and community health settings. Consequently it is important to be constantly vigilant when it is claimed that *all* Germans, Aboriginal people or Italians do this, or think that.

Obviously, our attitudes towards 'the other' — that is, people who are little known — would make no difference at all, if they were never encountered. However, when those who are prejudiced and hold stereotypes about the 'other' do have contact and belong to a powerful group, such as service providers, then their attitudes and beliefs can have a major impact on the people who are stereotyped. The issue of power, then, becomes extremely important. One way of understanding power comes from the work of the sociologist Max Weber (Bendix 1966), who identified three kinds of power: political, economic and social power.

1. Political power is found in formal government policy/legislation as well as informal control and influence in the political process, and influence over public opinion. So, political power rests with politicians, at all levels of government. However, those who can influence government and public opinion — the large corporations, unions, powerful lobbies (e.g. the Australian Medical Association [AMA] or The Right To Life group) — they too have access to political power. Most people have some access to power through voting, writing letters to the editor, taking part in protests and so on. Some people don't have access to even such a small amount of power — they are effectively excluded from the political process by poor educational standards, geographic or personal isolation or lack of citizenship.
2. Economic power is generated by income, wealth, access to credit, control of employment, and control of wages and prices. So, most people will never be able to control employment or wages or prices (though some corporations, such as the stock market, as well as employers and unions can), but they will have a reasonable income and be able to generate some credit. Of course a large number of people don't have access to either.
3. Social power or social status is evident in access to political/economic power and how the community evaluates these. Most everyone categorises themself or others into one class or another — Jimmy Barnes sings 'I'm a working class man' — others are clearly identified with the middle class because of their employment and education — similarly people talk about 'blue collar', 'managerial', 'executive', 'professional'. Importantly, individuals put different values on these labels, because those who have 'higher' positions will have greater access to money, influence and decision making.

Many writers agree that those who have power are able to maintain it because of the way in which the system is structured. Indeed, those who have limited access to power and self-determination are subjected to *systemic bias*. Systemic bias is a commonly recognised term that was first introduced by Savitch (1975). He defined systemic bias as:

> ... the prerequisites necessary for access to the political system and effective performance in it. That is, the more pressure a group can muster, the better able it is to shift policies towards its objectives. Essential prerequisites for such participation are organisational and communication skills which in turn require money, commitment of personnel, a trained staff, propaganda apparatus, and the like.
>
> (Savitch 1975: 8)

To influence or change the system people have to have money, education and educated staff, access to the media and the communication skills to effectively use the media in order to persuade others that the cause is good. Thus the system itself, controlled by those who already have power within it, maintains the power because those not 'in the know' do not understand the rules, regulations, norms and values, or do not possess the resources that provide access to the system.

Consider health. To access or influence this system, one must first understand it. That is fairly unlikely, unless the person has had some health training. Consequently most clients offer themselves up to the health system without knowing what is really happening to them, and become completely powerless and dependent on 'those in the know' to advise and treat (Moodie 1973; Eckermann et al 2006). Even within the health system (i.e. among the people 'in the know') there are hierarchies of power and influence. Reflect on power structures in Box 9.3.

Systemic bias, then, effectively excludes some sections of society from accessing and participating in decision making. This not only leads to entrenched patterns of domination and dependence, as has been argued above, but it also may result in structural violence.

Following Galtung (1995), Eckermann et al (2006) define *structural violence* as the violence within the social system that disadvantages some groups to the point

Box 9.3 | Reflection on power structures

Consider the power structures in a hospital, a community health clinic and a private practice. Who makes major decisions about staff, client intervention and expenditure? Who has the highest status in the system? Who earns the most? Now think about informal power — who is most likely to influence the decision making?

that their differential life chances are clearly reflected in population statistics.

Structural violence can take three forms (Eckermann et al 2006: 64):

1. Physical violence, reflected in mortality/morbidity rates and life expectancy
2. Psychological violence, evident in substance abuse, alienation, suicides
3. Systemic frustration, expressed as interference with self-determination.

These forms of violence can be measurable over time. Consider Indigenous infant mortality. In Australia it remains twice as high as that in other groups. Further, Indigenous life expectancy persistently remains at least 15 years below that of other Australians (AMA 2002), and Māori life expectancy is 10 years below that of other New Zealanders (New Zealand Ministry of Health 2003). We can say with certainty that members of these groups are experiencing structural violence. Similarly, if sections of society are exposed to chronic poverty, then it can be argued that they are experiencing structural violence — violence inherent in the social system which limits their physical, as well as their psychological, life chances. It is important for health care providers to understand the pressures that poverty exerts on individuals and their families/communities as well as the underlying structures that create and maintain poverty.

Eckermann et al (2006) have pointed out that often, when poverty is discussed, the *people* and their lifestyles are examined rather than the *system* in which they live. There has been a great deal of literature since the 1950s that examines the values, attitudes and beliefs common among 'the poor' or 'the lower classes'. The 'blame' for poverty is firmly placed on the shoulders of those who suffer from poverty and their persistent adherence to behaviours and traditions that maintain their poverty. This research has been strongly criticised by Ryan (1976) in his book *Blaming the Victim*. Even today we have retained the 19th century distinction between the 'deserving' and the 'undeserving' poor in our social security systems and our attitudes towards people who are chronically unemployed. The 'deserving' poor are those who don't drink, gamble, make debts and try to find a job — the 'undeserving' poor are the 'bludgers' that the system has to control by checking that they go to job interviews, keep their house clean and don't let friends, lovers or relatives share their accommodation without permission from the housing authority. In the 1970s these attitudes caused most young Aboriginal men with whom Eckermann worked in South-West Queensland to refuse to 'go on the dole' when station work in the region dried up because of structural changes in the rural economy of the region (Eckermann 1979). They did not want to be labelled 'bludgers'. Similarly, since the 1980s, most unemployed Aboriginal men and women preferred to work for the dole under the Community Development Employment Program (CDEP) — decades before this scheme was introduced to the mainstream — simply to escape the control of social service departments and to maintain a measure of self esteem (Eckermann et al 2000).

THE INFLUENCE OF CULTURE SHOCK

When people who are culturally different, and who may also be poor, come into contact with the prevailing, powerful health system, they experience culture shock. We can define culture shock as:

> … that feeling of uneasiness, anxiety and stress which arises when suddenly all our familiar cues, language, interpersonal relationships, tastes and actions appear to be out of place, suspect or even inappropriate and we must reassess our behaviours in the light of foreign expectations.
>
> (Eckermann 1994: 220)

Generally we accept that travellers or immigrants may experience culture shock when they first arrive in another country. However, culture shock may persist for many years, depending on how different the new environment is, how traumatic the experience of emigration was, and how well individuals feel accepted in the new environment.

> A loss of familiar signs and symbols including words, gestures, facial expressions, customs or norms (Szustaczek & White 2001) can result in confusion, disorientation, misunderstandings, conflict, stress and anxiety …
>
> (Eckermann et al 2006: 105)

Such anxieties become even more pressing when someone is ill or has to be hospitalised. Hospitalisation will almost inevitably cause serious stress and fear for many groups. Such stress and fear is exaggerated when people are unfamiliar with the language, as well as the language, culture, rules and regulations of the institution (Brink & Saunders 1976: 1343).

Brink & Saunders (1976) originally identified five major stressors, which characterised culture shock — communication, attitudes and beliefs, customs and behaviours, isolation, and mechanical factors. Eckermann et al (2006: 110) have extended these stressors to include compliance. It is possible to visualise these stressors as a cycle of potential discomfort as outlined in Figure 9.2

It is useful to examine each of these in more detail.

Communication is a vital part of caring — good communication reassures, directs, supports and motivates. Medical language and jargon can, however, alienate those who do not have a health background. Further, the tone, pace and pattern of speech may confuse those for whom English is not their first language. Further, non-verbal communication — body language, eye contact, personal space or touch — may vary significantly between client and caregiver. It is impossible to know all about how to best communicate across cultures, however, a start towards good communication is to show respect. Another, is to use interpreters. Note that Stein-Parbury (2005) provides some useful hints about how to use interpreters

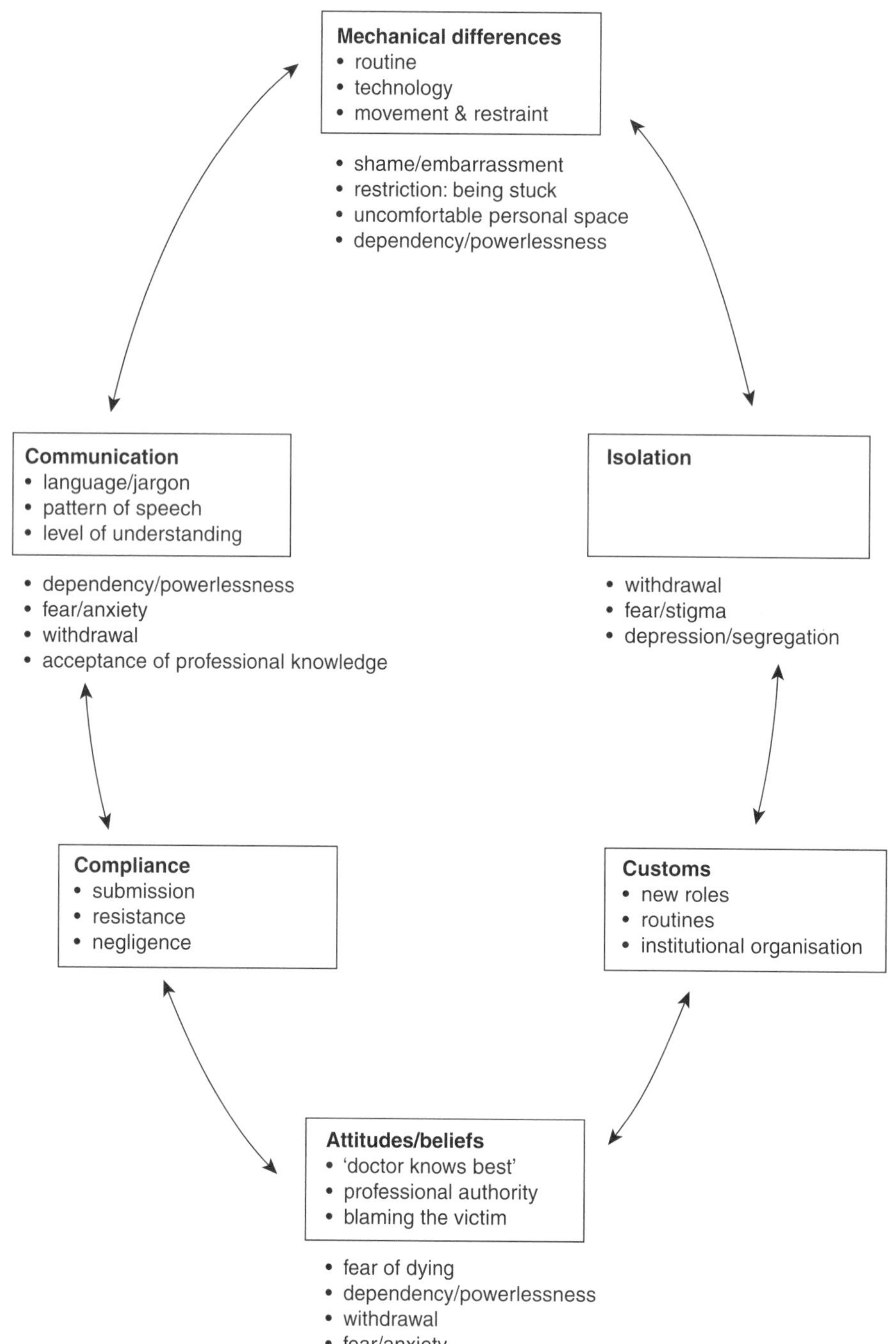

Figure 9.2 | Stressors and culture shock *(Eckermann et al 2006)*

effectively. Lack of effective communication will cause shame, embarrassment, dependency/powerlessness, anxiety, fear and withdrawal. Clinical interest Box 9.1 provides some examples of miscommunication.

The fear and anxiety generated by *isolation* is self-evident. If an individual is the only person of 'his/her kind' — who looks and talks differently — and who is far from his/her family and friends, isolation can affect their physical and psychological wellbeing.

Customs related to the hospital and medical procedures ensure that the client takes on a new, dependent role. This may be the first time a client has ever been dependent on another, and particularly a woman, for basic care.

Related to the system's customs are *mechanical differences*. Clients are restrained in beds/wards; medical technology is frightening and alienating, and daily routines (e.g. a cup of tea at 5 a.m., dinner at 4.30 p.m.) are foreign. All of these may lead to dependence and powerlessness, which in turn may reinforce shame and embarrassment.

Attitudes and beliefs, held by both staff and clients, can

CLINICAL INTEREST BOX 9.1
Examples of miscommunication

1. Consider the following scenario.

A young nurse delivers medication to an elderly European woman. She is cheerful and obliging, making sure the client has fresh water and that her pillows are fluffed up. 'There you go, dearie', she says in a loud voice, 'this will fix you right up, lovey'. The client withdraws and will not respond to any further communication. What happened? The nurse was caring and cheerful — why did the client withdraw? Perhaps the elderly lady was offended by the familiarity of address? Perhaps she didn't think it polite to be spoken to in a loud voice? Speaking loudly to a person because they are elderly and you assume that they may be deaf, speaking loudly because you assume that someone doesn't understand English, and the use of disrespectful terms of address can all cause offence.

2. Always remember that we bring our own preconceptions to an interaction.

I remember visiting an elderly Aboriginal lady who had been hospitalised after a severe stroke. She had lost the power of speech, but not her desire to communicate. The nursing staff, with the best of intentions, trying to be as culturally sensitive as possible, asked me which Aboriginal language my friend was speaking, and how they might get someone to interpret. My friend was not speaking an Aboriginal language, she was trying to communicate through the disability caused by the stroke. So, the presupposition that she was a non-English speaker was in fact a stereotype that, for a while, hindered communication.

(personal experience, A-K Eckermann 2008)

3. Recognising the importance of interpreters.

A Greek man, with limited English skills and expressing himself only in Greek, was admitted into hospital by his family during the Christmas period, following the death of his daughter just before Christmas. From his behaviour he was diagnosed as depressed with the potential for suicide. His depressed state became worse after hospitalisation and medical intervention. Because a qualified interpreter could not be accessed to help improve communication and enable the man to fully express why he was demonstrating such behaviour, a staff member took the initiative to make inquiries of a Greek welfare agency. The staff member discovered that it is the required custom for this man to mourn his daughter's death (in quite an emotional manner) for 40 days. It would be culturally inappropriate for him not to do so. The staff member brought this to the attention of the treatment team and an interpreter was accessed to assist in discussing the man's behaviour about this mourning ritual. Clarity was reached and the man was discharged shortly afterwards so that he could complete the culturally required grieving process.

(personal communication 9 August 1996, Maree Minter, NESB Liaison Officer, cited in Dowd & Eckermann, 1998, reproduced with permission)

Tips for using interpreters

Some tips about working with interpreters. Try to avoid family members, particularly children. Try not to use ancillary staff as interpreters — first of all they may not have the necessary skills to translate medical information and secondly you may be breaching confidentiality. Always speak directly to the client, not the interpreter. At times, even with the best intentions, we turn to the English speaker who may have brought the client into the surgery when we are asking questions — this can be extremely demeaning to the client. Whenever possible it is advisable to seek assistance from professional interpreters.

also generate stress and anxiety. Many Aboriginal people, for example, believe that hospitalisation will lead to death. So, they are scared and anxious when they are admitted. Staff bring their own attitudes and beliefs about people from different cultures to the interaction. They certainly, and rightly, have a strong belief in their professional knowledge. However this strong belief can easily overshadow the client and 'informed consent' may not always be informed.

Finally, all of the above stressors influence clients' *compliance*. People may agree but have no idea to what they are agreeing. They may refuse treatment overtly or covertly, they may abscond or suffer extreme depression.

Nurses are in a position of power when they interact with clients. They are the professionals, supported by a professional culture, language, traditions and customs which are a shorthand way of ensuring efficiency and effectiveness for those 'in the know', but which effectively and efficiently exclude those who 'do not know'. Their language, tone of voice and body language, rightly or wrongly, convey attitudes and prejudices, indicate concern or lack of it, and generate frustration and anger as well as trust and cooperation. These situations are amplified when the nurse and client do not share a similar language, a common frame of understanding, compatible expectations and perceptions — in short, a similar cultural background.

Nursing has been grappling with these issues and awareness of the influence of culture on care has been enhanced by the work of Leininger (1978, 1995) in transcultural nursing and Ramsden (1993, 2002) in cultural safety.

TRANSCULTURAL NURSING

According to Leininger (2002: 12), transcultural nursing is based on competent care which is appropriate to the client's beliefs, values and worldview in order to provide 'beneficial and satisfying health care, or to help them with difficult life situations, disabilities, or death'.

Leininger (2001), consequently, maintains that nurses need to understand the cultures of those for whom they care in order to predict their health needs.

According to Leininger, (1978, 1983, 1991, 1995, 1996, 2001, 2002) five general tenets underlie transcultural nursing:

1. Cultural differences and similarities exist in all cultures
2. Every culture has a system of care, which can be discovered, understood and used by the nurse to provide culturally meaningful care to the client
3. Nurses should be encouraged to discover and learn about cultural differences
4. In order to assist people of diverse or similar cultural backgrounds, nurses need to discover and use three models of operations:
   - preserve and maintain people's culture care
   - accommodate or negotiate people's culture care
   - restructure and re-pattern culture care strategies
5. All people would benefit from appropriate culture care.

A group of dedicated cross-cultural nurse researchers in Australia have used Leininger's (1978, 2002) theory as a guide to acquire culture-specific knowledge and understanding about particular cultural groups and to help them to provide culturally appropriate care (Leininger 2002: 6). Omeri (1997), an Iranian Australian, has used the theoretical framework to discover what care means to Iranian immigrants in New South Wales. Similarly, Nahas and Amasheh (1999: 38) adopted the theory to explain the meanings and expressions of postpartum depression for caring among Jordanian Australians. Further, Lim, Downie and Nathan (2004) explored the levels of theoretical and practical knowledge required by nursing students to develop appropriate levels of self-efficacy in order to practise in today's multicultural Australian health system.

Essentially transcultural nursing advocates are learning as much as possible about clients from other cultures in order to provide culturally appropriate care.

Although transcultural nursing has clearly been acknowledged in Australia as an important area of nursing practice, its development has been slow (Leininger 2002: 193). Nevertheless, it is incorporated into a growing number of nursing curricula, and transcultural nursing courses have been established at a number of universities.

CULTURAL SAFETY

A somewhat different emphasis characterises the work of Irihapeti Ramsden (1946–2003). She developed the idea of *cultural safety* in Aotearoa (New Zealand) after a first-year Māori nursing student asked: 'You people talk about legal safety, ethical safety, safety in clinical practice and a safe knowledge base, but what about cultural safety?'(Ramsden 2002: 1).

Cultural safety differs in many ways from transcultural nursing, due in part to the history of its inception and its theoretical bases. As Ramsden (2002) points out, cultural safety does not ask nurses to discover the cultural dimensions of any culture apart from their own. It does not believe that nurses could, or even should, gain an insider's understanding of any culture other than their own. It does not focus on cultural systems of care; it does not refer to culturally appropriate care. Instead, the focus is on the client's experience as the determinant of effective nursing care.

Due to Ramsden and others' work, The Nursing Council of New Zealand (1996: 9) has adopted cultural safety as part of its core curriculum. It defines cultural safety as:

> The effective nursing of a person/family from another culture by a nurse who has undertaken a process of reflection on his/her own cultural identity and recognises the impact of the nurse's culture on own nursing practice. Unsafe cultural practice is any action which diminishes, demeans or disempowers the cultural identity and wellbeing of an individual.

Cultural safety, according to Ramsden (2002), centres on the way power influences society and its members' life chances. Consequently it is about nurses' personal, professional and institutional power and how it is managed to serve people. It is also about trust and the way trust is constructed personally, culturally and institutionally.

The focus is on the nurse as a cultural bearer and power holder. Consequently, as Ramsden (2002) points out, cultural safety became concerned with issues of power and prejudice rather than particular aspects of Māori cultures.

Importantly, through Ramsden's work, the emphasis changed from the nurse's assessment of practice in terms of the client's needs to the *client's* assessment of the service/level of care. This change in emphasis has meant that 'cultural safety is an outcome of nursing and midwifery education that *enables safe service to be defined by those who receive the service*' (Nursing Council of New Zealand 1996: 40, emphasis added).

Consequently, the nurse's ability to establish and maintain trust with the client is an essential prerequisite to negotiating and delivering culturally safe care. Further, cultural safety is concerned with the transfer of power between health care providers and those receiving the service (Cooney 1994). Thus, Ramsden (2002) points out that nurses need to become aware of the level of distrust which will mark their interactions with Indigenous clients and clients from minority groups. Such distrust is based on a history of oppression.

It is suggested that cultural safety is relevant not only to New Zealand but also to Australia as a colonial nation. Indeed, the Council of Aboriginal and Torres Strait Islander Nurses (2003) has endorsed the model. Colonisation has typically been associated with all kinds of violence against Indigenous (i.e. powerless) people (Galtung 1975). Consequently, 'any action which *diminishes, demeans or disempowers* the cultural identity and well being of an individual' (The Nursing Council of New Zealand 2005: 4, emphasis added) is culturally *unsafe*. Conversely, those actions which *reinforce respect, responsibility and are regardful of difference* are likely to support cultural *safety* (Ramsden 2002).

COMPETENCE IN NURSING ACROSS CULTURES

Transcultural nursing and cultural safety have generated much of the debate about culturally appropriate care and have encouraged dialogue about how to transform the theories into practice.

The importance of cultural competence in nursing, among other disciplines, is generally attributed to the rapidly changing and diversified demography of nations (see Salimbene 1999; Tervalon & Murray-Garcia 1998; Galambos 2003). Yet, following Ramsden (1993, 2002), the authors argue that all health care professionals (as well as other professional groups) are required to be culturally safe because whenever they are interacting with a client they are entering a bicultural relationship.

Cultural competence, then, is part of the nurse's ability to provide effective and appropriate care. The Australian *National Review of Nursing Education: Multicultural Nursing Education* (Eisenbruch 2000: 4) cites a number of definitions of cultural competence derived from a range of sources. These include:

> Cultural competence is a set of congruent behaviours, attitudes, and policies that come together in a system or agency or among professionals that enable effective interactions in a cross-cultural framework … (Cross et al 1989)
>
> Cultural competency is the ability of individuals and systems to respond respectfully and effectively to people of all cultures, classes, races, ethnic backgrounds and religions in a manner that recognises, affirms, and values the cultural differences and similarities and the worth of individuals, families, and communities and protects and preserves the dignity of each. (Seattle County Department of Public Health 1994)
>
> … the ability to identify and challenge one's own cultural assumptions, the ability to see the world through culturally different lenses, to analyse and respond to the 'cultural scene' and 'social dramas' in ways that are culturally and psychologically meaningful, for client and professional alike, and the ability to turn such thinking into praxis, providing meaningful, satisfying and competent care. (Maureen Fitzgerald 1999, University of Sydney)

Many of the elements of these definitions are reflected in the *Code of Ethics for Nurses in Australia* (Australian Nursing & Midwifery Council [ANMC] 2002) and the *Code of Professional Conduct for Nurses in Australia* (ANMC 2003). Thus, nurses are expected to respect individual needs, values, culture and vulnerability.

Further, it seems that the profession is moving towards a definition of cultural competence that incorporates many of the features of transcultural nursing as well as cultural safety. Thus Salimbene (1999) defines cultural competence as a *process* whereby thoughts, attitudes and actions progress through five stages: recognition of ethnocentrism; awareness and sensitivity towards cultural and linguistic differences; development of attitudes and actions based on cultural relativism; acquisition of culture-specific knowledge; and:

> the acquisition of skills and strategies to identify cultural differences and to know how to deal with them in a way that both meets the patient's needs and expectations and satisfies the nurse's and institution's standards of quality care.
>
> (Salimbene 1999: 5)

Eckermann et al (2006) further indicate that a number of processes enhance the ability to provide competent care. These include:

- Reflecting on self, one's own culture and profession, power imbalances, attitudes and beliefs about 'the other'
- Enhancing communication skills and drawing on the skills of interpreters
- Understanding of the influence of power imbalances on 'the other'
- Developing trust
- Negotiating knowledge
- Negotiating outcomes
- Understanding the influence of culture shock.

SUMMARY

This chapter has explored the relationship between culture and health care, beliefs and actions. It has focused on understanding of culture, ethnicity and class as well as related issues of power and powerlessness, processes and practices for enhancing appropriate care, and the pitfalls nurses may encounter in developing cultural competence. Appropriate care is based on one-to-one relationships and is the basis of all nursing care. There are no checklists and no magic formula that will ensure that nurses cater for the holistic needs of clients. There is, however, a range of strategies that will enhance nurses' 'striving' (Spence 2001) for best practice within culturally diverse environments, including *reflection of self*, one's own culture and profession, power imbalances, attitudes and beliefs about 'the other'; understanding of the influence of power imbalances on 'the other'; enhancing communication skills and drawing on the skills of interpreters; development of trust; negotiating knowledge; negotiating outcomes; and understanding the influence of culture shock.

REVIEW EXERCISES

1. Define what culture means to you.
2. Write down at least three cultures to which you belong — these may be religious or spiritual cultures, one or more ethnicities, your professional culture, your age-related generation, your gender and so on.
3. Write down as many norms or rules you can think of that are part of the cultures you have identified with.
4. In your work as a nurse, reflect on the reasons you do the things you do. For example, if one of your actions is to encourage the people you serve to eat a healthy diet, what does your culture include in and exclude from a healthy

diet? Is your understanding of a healthy diet the same as that of your clients? What is the value of a healthy diet? This should help you to find out about the beliefs and values of practice.

5. Identify the main stressors of culture shock — what can you do to ease some of these stressors?
6. Define power.
7. What are the barriers to effective communication across cultures?
8. Describe the basic principles of transcultural nursing.
9. Define cultural safety.

CRITICAL THINKING EXERCISES

1. How would you react to the following statement: 'personally I can't see that there should be anything ... colour of skin, creed ... shouldn't make any difference ... ' (Dowd 1985: 257). What are the principles that underlie the belief that 'everyone should be treated the same'? How appropriate are these principles when caring for clients with different needs?
2. Describe the differences between nursing a client regardful of (taking into consideration) his or her cultural difference as opposed to treating all clients in the same way. Think — where does the notion of being 'regardful' of cultural difference come from? What does it mean in terms of reflection, trust and respect? How can these principles be built into nursing practice?

REFERENCES AND FURTHER READING

Allport G (1982) *The nature of prejudice*. Anchor Books, New York

Andrews MM, Boyle JS (2003) *Transcultural Concepts in Nursing Care*, 4th edn. Lippincott Williams and Wilkins, Philadelphia

Australian Bureau of Statistics (ABS) (2001) Census 2002. Online. Available: www.abs.gov.au/ausstats/abs@.nsf/ausstatshome?openview [accessed January 2004]

—— (2002) *National Aboriginal and Torres Strait Islander Social Survey*. Online. Available: www.abs.gov.au/AUSSTATS/ans@.nsf/DetailsPage/4714.02002?OpenDocument [accessed June 2007]

—— (2004) *Social Trends*. Online. Available: www.abs.gov.au/AUSSTATS/abs@.nsf2f762f95845417aeca25706c00834efa/D701 [accessed June 2007]

Australian Medical Association (2002) *Indigenous Health Has Flatlined for 10 Years*. Online. Available: www.ama.com.au/web.nsf/doc/WEEN-5GHAGB [accessed January 2004]

Australian Nursing & Midwifery Council (ANMC) (2002) *Code of Ethics for Nurses in Australia*. Online. Available: www.anci.org.au./02standards/codes.php [accessed January 2004]

—— (2003) *Code of Professional Conduct for Nurses in Australia*. Online. Available: www.anci.org.au/02standards/codes.php [accessed January 2004]

Belich J (1996) *Making Peoples: a History of the New Zealanders from Polynesian Settlement to the End of the Nineteenth Century*. Allen Lane and Penguin, London and Auckland

Bendix R (1966) *Max Weber: an Intellectual Portrait*. Methuen, London

Bennett JW (1969) *Northern Plainsmen, Adaptive Strategy and Agrarian Life*. Aldine Publishing Company, Chicago

Berndt RM, Berndt CH (1988) *The world of the First Australians, Aboriginal Traditional Life: Past and Present*. Aboriginal Studies Press, Canberra

Brink PJ, Saunders JM (1976) Culture shock: theoretical and applied. In Brink PJ (ed) *Transcultural Nursing: a Book of Readings*. Prentice-Hall, Toronto

Broome R (2001) *Aboriginal Australians*. Allen and Unwin, Sydney

Cooney C (1994) A comparative analysis of cultural safety. *Nursing Praxis in New Zealand* 9(1): 6–12

Council of Aboriginal and Torres Strait Islander Nurses (2003) *Recommendations to Develop Strategies for the Recruitment and Retention of Indigenous People in Nursing*. Online. Available: www.indiginet.com.au/catsin/recruitment.html [accessed 18 April 2008]

D'Avanzo C (2008) *Mosby's Pocket Guide to Cultural Assessment*. Elsevier Australia. Sydney

Davis P, Dew K (eds) (1999) *Health and Society in Aotearoa New Zealand*. Oxford University Press, Melbourne

Dowd LT (1985) The need for understanding. A case study of Aboriginal and non-Aboriginal perspectives on health care. Unpublished Master's Thesis. University of California, San Francisco

Dowd LT, Eckermann, A-K, Jeffs L (2005) Culture and Ethnicity. In: Crisp J, Taylor C (eds), *Potter & Perry's Fundamentals of Nursing*, 2nd edn. Elsevier Australia, Sydney

Durie M (1994) *Whaiora Māori Health Development*. Oxford University Press, Auckland

—— (2001) *Māori Ora the Dynamics of Māori Health*. Oxford University Press, Melbourne

Eckermann A-K (1979) Employment patterns among Aboriginal people in South-West Queensland. *Australian Economic Papers*. December pp 362–83

—— (1994) *One Classroom, Many Cultures*. Allen and Unwin, Sydney

—— (1995) *Introduction to Traditional Aboriginal Society*. University of New England Press, Armidale

Eckermann A-K, Dowd LT, Chong E, Nixon L, Gray R, Johnson S (2006) *Binang Goonj: Bridging Cultures in Aboriginal Health*, 2nd edn. Elsevier Australia, Sydney

Eckermann A-K, Dowd LT, Jeffs L (2008) Culture and Ethnicity. In: Crisp J, Taylor C (eds), *Potter and Perry's Fundamentals of Nursing*, 3rd edn. Elsevier Australia, Sydney, Chapter 8

Eckermann A-K, Dowd LT, Johnson SM (2000) Review of youth allowance in rural and remote Indigenous communities. Report submitted to the Department of Family and Community Services. University of New England, Armidale pp 227

Eckermann A-K, Dowd LT, Martin M, Nixon L, Gray, R, Chong E (1998) *Binang Goonj: Bridging Cultures in Aboriginal Health Facilitator's Guide*. University of New England Press, Armidale

Eisenbruch M (2000) *National Review of Nursing Education: Multicultural Nursing Education*. Higher Education Division, Department of Education, Training and Youth Affairs, Canberra. Online. Available: www. dest.gov.au/highered/nursing/pubs [accessed January 2004]

Elkin AP (1964) *The Australian Aborigines*, 4th edn. Angus and Robertson, Sydney

Encel S, Berry M (eds) (1987) *Selected Readings in Australian Society: an Anthology*. Longman Cheshire, Melbourne

Galambos CM (2003) Moving cultural diversity towards cultural competence in health care. *Health and Social Work* 28 (1): 3

Galtung J (1975) *Peace: Research, Education and Action*. Eijers, Copenhagen

—— (1995) Violence, peace and peace research. In: Salla M, Tonetto W, Martinez E (eds), *Essays on Peace: Paradigms for Global Order*. Central Queensland University Press. Rockhampton

Gould SJ (1998) *The Mismeasure of Man*. Penguin, New York

Inkeles A (1976) *Foundations of Modern Sociology*. Prentice Hall, Englewood Cliffs NJ

Julian R (2004) Migrant and refugee health. In: Grbich C (ed), *Health in Australia: Sociological Concepts and Issues*. Pearson Longman, Sydney

Jupp J (2002) *From White Australia to Woomera: The Story of Australian Immigration*. Cambridge University Press, Cambridge

Kanitsaki O (1992) *Transcultural Nursing: an Introductory Teaching Package for Lecturers and Teachers*. School of Nursing, Lincoln Faculty of Health Sciences. La Trobe University, Melbourne

Leininger MM (1978) *Transcultural Nursing: Concepts, Theories, and Practices*. John Wiley & Sons, New York

—— (1983) Cultural care: an essential goal for nursing and health care. *Am Assoc Nephrol Nurses and Technicians (AANNT) Journal* 10(5): 11

—— (1995) *Transcultural Nursing: Concepts, Theories, and Practices*, 2nd edn. McGraw-Hill, New York

—— (1996) Culture care theory, research, and practice. *Nurs Sci Q* 9 (2):71

—— (2002) Transcultural nursing and globalization of health care: importance, focus and historical aspects. In: Leininger M, McFarland MR (eds), *Transcultural Nursing: Concepts, Theories, Research and Practice*, 3rd edn. McGraw-Hill, New York

—— (ed) (1991) *Culture Care Diversity and Universality: a Theory of Nursing*. National League for Nursing Press, New York

—— (ed) (2001) *Culture Care Diversity and Universality: a Theory of Nursing*, 2nd edn. National League for Nursing Press, New York

Lim J, Downie J, Nathan P (2004) Nursing Students' self-efficacy in providing transcultural care. *Nursing Education Today* 24(6): 428–34

Lippmann L (1999) *Generations of Resistance, Mabo and Justice*. Longman, Melbourne

Matsumoto D, Juang L (2004) *Culture and Psychology*, 3rd edn. Thomson/Wadsworth, Belmont CA

McGraw A (1995) *Contested Ground: Australian Aborigines Under the British Crown*. Allen and Unwin, Sydney

Moodie PM (1973) *Aboriginal Health.* Australian University Press, Canberra

Nahas V, Amasheh N (1999) Culture care meanings and experiences of postpartum depression among women: a transcultural study, *J Transcult Nurs* 10: 37

National Aboriginal and Islander Health Organisation (NAIHO) (1 October 1982) *Philosophy of the Community Controlled Health Services*. Unpublished discussion paper, NAIHO. Online. Available: www.health.gov.au/oatsih/strategy/ [accessed January 2004]

National Inquiry into the Separation of Aboriginal and Torres Strait Islander Children from their Families (1997) *Bringing them Home*. Australian Government Printing Service, Canberra

New Zealand Ministry of Health (July 2003) *Decades of Disparity: Ethnic Mortality Trends in New Zealand 1980–1999,* Public Health Intelligence Occasional Bulletin Number 16, Wellington

Nursing Council of New Zealand (1996) *Guidelines for Cultural Safety in Nursing and Midwifery Education*. Nursing Council of New Zealand, Wellington. Online. Available: www.nursingcouncil.org.nz [accessed January 2004]

—— (1999) *Competencies for Entry to the Register of Nurses*. Nursing Council of New Zealand, Wellington. Online. Available: www.nursingcouncil.org.nz/culturalsafety.pdf [accessed January 2004]

—— (2005) *Registered Nurse in Clinical Practice Competency Requirements: Nursing Council of New Zealand, Wellington*. Online. Available: www.nursingcouncil.org.nz/practitioner.html [accessed December 2007]

Omeri A (1997) Culture care of Iranian immigrants in New South Wales, Australia: sharing transcultural nursing knowledge. *J Transcult Nurs* 8(2): 5

—— (2002) Reflections on Australia and transcultural nursing in the new millennium. In: Leininger M, McFarland MR (eds) *Transcultural Nursing: Concepts, Theories, Research and Practice*, 3rd edn. McGraw-Hill, New York

Orange C (1987) *The Treaty of Waitangi*. Allen & Unwin/Port Nicholson Press, Wellington

Pearson D (1996) Crossing ethnic thresholds: multiculturalisms in comparative perspective. In Spoonley P, Macpherson C, Pearson D (eds) *Nga Patai Racism and Ethnic Relations in Aotearoa/New Zealand*. The Dunmore Press, Palmerston North

Ramsden IM (1993) Kawawhakaruruhau: Cultural safety in nursing education in Aotearoa (New Zealand). Paper presented at the 2nd National Transcultural Nursing Conference, Cumberland College of Health Sciences, Sydney

—— (2002) Cultural safety and nursing education in Aotearoa and Te Waipounamu, Unpublished PhD thesis, University of Wellington, Victoria. Online. Available: culturalsafety.massey.ac.nz [accessed January 2004]

Reynolds H (1987) *Frontier*. Allen and Unwin, Sydney

—— (1989) *Dispossession*. Allen and Unwin, Sydney

Rice GW (1992) *The Oxford History of New Zealand*, 2nd edn. Oxford University Press, Auckland

Ryan W (1976) *Blaming the Victim*. Vintage Books, New York

Saggers S, Gray D (1991) *Aboriginal health and society*. Allen and Unwin, Sydney

Salimbene S (1999) Cultural competence: a priority for performance improvement action. *J Nurs Care Qual* 13 (3): 23

Savitch HV (1975) The politics of deprivation. In: Rogers HR (ed) *Racism and Inequality: the Policy Alternatives*. WA Freeman, San Francisco

Spence, DG (2001) Prejudice, paradox, and possibility: nursing people from cultures other than one's own. *J Transcult Nurs* 12(2): 100

Spencer M, Inkeles A (1976) *Foundations of Modern Sociology*. Prentice Hall, Eaglewood Cliffs, NJ

Statistics New Zealand (2001) *Census Snapshot 4*, 2003. Online. Available: www.stats.govt.nz/ [accessed January 2004]

Stein-Parbury J (2005) *Patient and Person: Interpersonal Skills in Nursing*. Elsevier/Churchill Livingstone, Sydney

Szustaczek C & White J (2001) *Cross-cultural Issues*. Compiled by C Bewry (JETAA-2001). Toronto Jet Alumni Association. Online. Available: www.toronto.jetaa.ca/cms/index.php?option=com_content& task=view&id=18-13k [accessed 15 April 2008]

Tatz C (2001) *Aboriginal Suicide is Different*. Aboriginal Studies Press, Canberra

Tervalon M, Murray-Garcia J (1998) Cultural humility versus cultural competence: a critical distinction in defining physician training outcomes in multicultural education. *J Health Care for the Poor and Underserved* 9(2): 117

Walker R (1990) *Ka Whawhai Tonu Matou/Struggle Without End*. Penguin, Auckland

Chapter 10

INDIGENOUS HEALTH

OBJECTIVES

- Define the key terms/concepts
- Develop basic understanding of the cultures of Indigenous people in Australia and New Zealand before colonisation
- Gain an appreciation of the nature of colonisation in Australia and New Zealand
- Explore the effects of colonisation on Indigenous health status
- Develop an understanding of current Indigenous health status
- Describe the relationship between Indigenous health, structural violence and culture shock
- Gain an appreciation of the importance of primary health care, community control and partnerships in Indigenous health
- Explore strategies that individual nurses may employ to ensure culturally safe practice.

KEY TERMS/CONCEPTS

Aboriginal
colonisation
community control
Comprehensive Primary Health Care
cycle of poverty
cultural safety
Māori
partnership
Primary Health Care
structural violence

CHAPTER FOCUS

This chapter begins by presenting a brief overview of traditional societies in Australia and New Zealand. It then turns to exploring colonisation in the two countries and its effects on Indigenous health. It reviews current levels of disease among the Indigenous populations of Australia and New Zealand and the effects of the cycle of poverty on Aboriginal and Māori people. It is argued that current Indigenous poor health status is the result of past and present colonisation. Factors which inhibit Indigenous self-determination in health, as well as Indigenous health care initiatives, such as community controlled health services, are reviewed in order to provide guidance for culturally safe health care provision.

LIVED EXPERIENCE

I found that the most productive times in terms of getting to know people in the community and them getting to know and trust me were our trips out bush. Sometimes I was invited to go out with a family over a long weekend or for longer during bush holiday. Out there I was dependent on the local people for everything — I was certainly the guest. It was during these times that friendships were forged and trust was deepened. After a bush trip I always found that my health care job became easier — negotiation and partnership fell into place. Yet my employer never saw this type of activity as legitimate work. We used to go out bush with the diabetics where we would all learn from each other, but this had to be done in our own time.

(Remote Area Nurse 2005, in Eckermann et al 2006: 151)

INTRODUCTION

Before exploring Indigenous health in Australia and New Zealand, it is necessary to identify who will be included in the discussions. In this chapter, the term Indigenous will include the Māori of New Zealand and the Aboriginal people of Australia. In the past, 'Aboriginal' has subsumed Torres Strait Islander people — much to their distress. Please note, Torres Strait Islanders are not the same as Aboriginal people. Their situation is unique in many respects and deserves separate discussion. While it is probably acceptable to discuss Māori as a group, even the term 'Aboriginal' does not necessarily sit easily with all of the descendants of the original owners of this continent. They have always used a range of terms to denote their in-group — for example, Murri, Murdi, Koori or Goori in SE Queensland and NSW/Victoria. Many people have also become much more specific of their identity since they have begun the slow and painful process of exerting their Native Title Claims. They proudly associate with their traditional language groups.

Today Aboriginal people form 2.4% of the total Australian population (ABS 2004). In New Zealand, Māori people constitute 14.2% of the total population (Statistics New Zealand 2003). Indigenous people in Australia, then, form a tiny minority compared to those in New Zealand.

THE INDIGENOUS PAST

Aboriginal people maintain that they have inhabited the continent since time immemorial. Archaeological evidence suggests that they have lived throughout the continent for at least 50 000 and up to 120 000 years (McGraw 1995). This length of occupation makes Aboriginal peoples the longest continuous civilisations in the world. Refer back to Chapter 9 where it was argued that Australia was a multicultural society long before the coming of Europeans because the continent was occupied by up to 500 different language groups. Refer back to the definitions of culture — language is an important indicator of culture. Consequently, there were many differences between the traditional custodians of Australia. However there was also a range of similarities. For example, all Aboriginal groups were hunters and gatherers who followed a seasonal pattern of migration across their well-defined territory (see Berndt & Berndt 1988). The nations/language groups were comprised of totemic groups, which lived in family groups and were governed by Elders. The Elders were most knowledgeable about the spiritual and physical worlds. The people's behaviour was guided by the powers of spiritual forces, which came to them from the Dreaming (see Stanner 1979). The Dreaming represented their past, their present and their future and it was celebrated in ceremony, ritual and dance. These hunters and gatherers saw themselves as custodians of their country and while neighbours could fight, they never fought about land. Land alienation was unthinkable because the spirit of the land protected its custodians. 'Strangers' or visitors would be harmed unless they travelled the land with permission and knew the correct ritual to familiarise the spirits with their presence (Berndt & Berndt 1988; Elkin 1994). From all accounts (see McGraw 1995, Broome 2002), the people were healthy — their diet was rich in vegetables, grains and some protein, their hunting and gathering life style ensured that they had plenty of exercise. Indeed, when Cook first commented about the Aboriginal people he saw, he wrote that:

> . . . in reality they are far more happier than we Europeans; being wholly unacquainted not only with the superfluous but the necessary Conveniences so much sought after in Europe, they are happy in not knowing the use of them. They live in a Tranquillity which is not disturbed by the Inequality of Condition . . .
>
> (Cook in Beaglehole 1955: 399)

It would be wrong to present traditional Aboriginal societies as utopian — no doubt they were affected by natural disasters, suffered hunger and pain, illness and injustice. However, they were self-determining; they had order and security and had developed a satisfying pattern of life where food collecting would take no more than 35 hours a week (Hiatt 1970) and there was ample time for ceremony, song and dance.

Polynesian people settled in New Zealand between 250 and 1150 CE (Belich 1996). Known as Māori, the people were organised into hierarchical, land-owning clans, sub-tribes and tribes. Māori were agriculturalists and fishers as well as hunters. They tended to live in village style communities. Their society was divided into three groups — hereditary chiefs (rangatira) who had the authority to rule, commoners, members of the clan who traced descent to the founding ancestor, and slaves, who were either born into captivity or captured in war (Te Ara — The Encyclopedia of New Zealand 2007). Unlike Aboriginal people, then, Māori were a very hierarchical society, which practised warfare to acquire land as well as slaves. Sheppard (2005) believes that Māori life in traditional times was a struggle — food was scarce, there was much warfare, life expectancy was between 25 and 30 years, pneumonia and other respiratory diseases were common. Nevertheless, 'In 1769 James Cook concluded that Māori were a healthy race, remarking on the great number of elderly men . . .' (Sheppard 2005).

Both Aboriginal and Māori societies had a strong spiritual association with the land and the world around them. Aboriginal people have described the land as their mother — for Māori 'the relationship of families and sub-tribes with land and other resources was integral with Māori creation beliefs, the deeds of ancestors, and other events told in tradition' (Sheppard 2005). Further, Aboriginal and Māori people believed in the power of the spiritual world to heal and to harm. Traditional healers were revered and feared in Australia and New Zealand because of their specialised spiritual powers. This is not to say that the people were unaware of the natural causes for illness (see Reid 1982), rather, the expectation was that transgressions against the spiritual world would also be punished by ill health. Consequently traditional healers had to have knowledge of both physical and spiritual healing. Turn to Box 10.1 for an example of traditional healing practices.

COLONISATION

Australia and New Zealand were both colonised by Britain at the hight of its colonial power. In 1788, when the first Europeans settled in Australia, it was classed as terra nullius, nobody's land according to European law, because the colonisers could not see any evidence of the kinds of social organisations (e.g. settlements, government, land use) with which they were familiar. The invaders' perception of civilisation and settlement/occupancy were guided by political philosophers of the time, such as Locke, who argued that land ownership was dependent on working the land. Land in their own countries which was not cultivated was classed as empty, common land, which could be taken by those who would cultivate it — consequently, other lands, annexed through colonisation, could be held by the Crown to be sold or leased to those who wanted to cultivate it later (Miller 1985). As a result Australia was 'discovered', annexed and settled — Aboriginal people were not even accorded the status of 'conquered people' (Gumbert 1984); the British government did not feel obliged to negotiate a treaty, and, when Cook 'claimed' Australia, the whole of the continent became Crown Land. Reflect on Box 10.2 and explore the 'mindset' which underpinned this kind of thinking.

The 'settlement' process was a little different in New Zealand. Here traders and whalers visited for decades before Britain decided to become formally involved in the government of the islands (Ministry for Culture and Heritage 2007). War raged between the Māori tribes, who had been introduced to firearms in the Musket Wars of the 1820s and 1830s. Adventurers from Britain and Australia stayed, first in small, then ever increasing, numbers. The colonial government of Australia and Britain were conscious that these elements were often lawless and attempting to organise illegal land acquisitions. Some of the Māori chiefs had petitioned the Crown for independence within the empire (Ministry for Culture and Heritage 2007). Consequently there were Indigenous forces within New Zealand, which welcomed the influence of the British. In 1840, the Treaty of Waitangi was signed.

> Māori had clear expectations of how the benefits would occur. There would be a sharing of authority, and this would enhance chiefly mana. The country would be protected from acquisition by other foreign powers. A kawana (governor) would control Europeans, especially those buying land, who were causing difficulties in some areas. The Treaty would bring settlement and more markets for Māori services that were essential to settlement, and Māori could obtain more goods and take advantage of benefits brought by Europeans. Some chiefs saw that change was inevitable. The clock could not be turned back to the period before 1840, so the treaty was seen as a way into the future.
>
> (Ministry for Culture and Heritage 2007)

The treaty certainly ceded sovereignty to Queen Victoria who was supposed to guarantee the Māori chiefs 'their land, forests, fisheries and other treasures so long as they wished to retain them (giving the Crown exclusive rights to their purchase); and granting the Māori people royal protection and the rights of British subjects' (Sheppard 2005).

Despite the fact that the Treaty of Waitangi was annulled in 1877, because it had not been legalised by an Act of Parliament, it has been officially acknowledged as the document which underpinned the nation of New Zealand (Durie 1998; Ramsden 2002). Māori, then, were accorded the status of a sovereign people at the time of colonisation, perhaps because they lived in structures with which Europeans were familiar (i.e. they were organised into groups such as clans and tribes, were ruled by chiefs and pursued agriculture). Further, they fought bloody battles against the British after the signing of the Treaty of Waitangi because of unacceptable land alienation between 1840 and 1876.

The process of colonisation in Australia was unique

Box 10.1 | Traditional healing

Professor Elkin (1977) referred to the traditional healers as Aboriginal men of high degree.

The healers are kindred to Amerindian 'men of power' and shamans. These healers are specially chosen and trained to remove the influence of sorcery and evil spirits and to restore the wellbeing of the soul or spirit. Their role is extremely important because most serious illness is thought to be brought about by loss of a vital substance from the body (soul loss), introduction of a foreign and harmful substance into the body (spirit intrusion or possession), or violation of taboos and sorcery (singing). The traditional healers usually gain the power to heal through inheritance or through special spiritual experiences. They possess a spirit called *mapanpa* which is associated with healing power.

(Devanesen 2000: 3)

Box 10.2 | 'Mindset' — reflection

After reading about the basis on which Australia was declared nobody's land — consider what that tells you about Europeans' perceptions and evaluations of different cultures.

They had no understanding yet felt that they had a right to evaluate, to measure, other cultures against their own. This habit, established in the 18th and 19th centuries, persists — we continue to evaluate others in terms of our own reference frame. It is a common, yet fairly destructive, habit and shows little understanding about the intricacies and complexities of the term 'culture'.

because the continent was annexed as belonging to nobody. Further, while Aboriginal people were actively segregated from non-Aboriginal society into reserves and missions, the policy in New Zealand was to amalgamate Māori (Ministry for Culture and Heritage 2007). In many other respects, however, colonisation had the same effect.

In both countries the first 100 years of colonisation were marked by enormous loss of Indigenous life. In Australia, Lancaster Jones (1970) estimated that between 1788 and 1947 the Indigenous population dropped between 50 and 90% (depending on the geographic region) from an estimated 300 000 at the time of colonisation. If Mulvaney's (2002) claim, that 750 000 Indigenous people occupied the continent in 1788, is correct, the loss of Indigenous life was horrific, and indicative of the many groups of traditional owners who were literally wiped out. Similarly in New Zealand, the Māori population declined by at least a third in less than a century (Durie 1998) — some believe that it declined by 50% between 1840 and 1892 alone (Te Ara — the Encyclopedia of New Zealand 2007).

Loss of Indigenous life has been attributed to warfare and introduced diseases, as well as loss of land, loss of economic independence, loss of human rights, discrimination and racism (see the work of Evans et al 1988; Reynolds 1989; Durie 1998; Lippmann 1999; or Moses 2004). The interaction of these forces is presented in Figure 10.1 below.

THE AFTERMATH OF COLONISATION

Warfare marked the struggle for land and independence between Aboriginal and non-Aboriginal people and Māori and Pakeha. In New Zealand it was recognised as war — in Australia it was called 'resistance', partly because of the way in which the country was annexed, and partly because the nature of guerrilla warfare was not yet understood by the British (see Broome 2002, Eckermann et al 2006).

Under the government policy of Protection, Aboriginal people were institutionalised in segregated reserves and missions where their lives were fully regimented and controlled. The practice has been identified as *institutional racism*; that is, racism enshrined in laws which were only applied to one sector of the Australian population and continued for 100 years in some states and territories; for example, Queensland (see Reynolds 1987, 1989, 2003; Evans et al 1988; Eckermann et al 2006). Such institutionalisation seriously affected Aboriginal people's physical, social, economic, spiritual and political welfare (see Broome 2002, Lippmann 1999). They were unable to travel, marry, bring up their children, work where they pleased, earn the same wages as non-Aboriginal workers, go to school at all or attend school beyond sixth grade, or receive pensions, unemployment benefits or child support payments. Indigenous Health statistics in Australia and New Zealand reflected government neglect and the people's despair and hopelessness following the massive culture shock of colonisation. Reflect on colonisation as culture shock in Box 10.3.

A growing number of writers (see Tatz 1999; Moses 2004) have maintained that this period of Australian colonial history was characterised by genocide. Thus Kociumbas (2004: 98–9) commented:

> What is unique about Australia is not its violence, but its apparent legality and above all its modernity. It was modern technology that made possible the pace and effectiveness

Box 10.3 | Colonisation as culture shock — reflection

Review Figure 9.2 in Chapter 9. Consider the culture shock stressors — communication, attitudes and beliefs, mechanical differences, compliance, isolation and customs.

In what ways did traditional Aboriginal societies clash with the colonists — did they speak the same language (communication), follow a similar kind of life (mechanical difference), maintain similar religions, gender roles, authority structures, family organisation or perceptions of beauty (attitudes and beliefs, compliance and customs), and — in relation to isolation — did Aboriginal groups experience shock when they were excluded from the land?

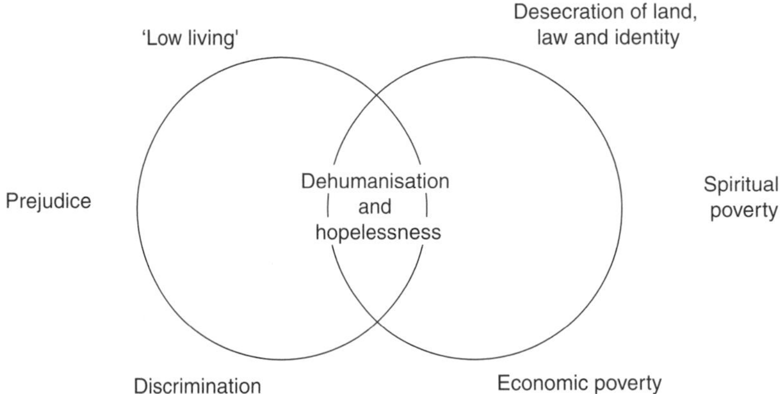

Figure 10.1 | The cumulative effects of colonisation *(reproduced with permission from Eckermann et al 2006: 19)*

> of killing, and modern law that provided the judicial niceties that condoned it. Thus it enabled minimal state involvement via visible military action, and gave carte blanche to changing groups of helpers claiming expertise in managing surviving populations where extreme surveillance did not preclude starvation, the absence of medical services, and utter neglect.

Consider Box 10.4 — this is an account of settlement life in the early 1970s — not 100 years but just one generation ago. Consider the level of surveillance which characterised Aboriginal people's lives on that settlement. Note that until the 1960s many public facilities, such as hospitals, segregated Aboriginal patients in 'Aboriginal Only' wards in most states and territories (see Dowd's 1985 account of hospitals on the east coast of NSW).

Settlements, fringe settlements on the outskirts of towns and reserves marked Aboriginal people's living conditions until the 1950s, when government policy changed from protection to assimilation and more moved into towns and cities. Because of the history of neglect and exclusion, many Aboriginal people were undereducated. Even without the barriers of racism and discrimination, many did not have the necessary education for skilled work. Consequently, Aboriginal people were among the most vulnerable in the Australian economy. Similarly, Māori people were also vulnerable, having suffered large land losses after 1840. By 1896 only 11 million acres, out of a possible 66.5 million acres, remained in Māori hands. By 1920, this was reduced to 4.7 million acres (Sheppard 2005 online). This land loss had drastic effects on the Māori economy and the ability of the Māori people to remain self-determinant.

Self-determination for Aboriginal people became Australian government policy in 1972; it changed to self-management in 1975, and it has retained that label over the past 30 years. The literature provides an extensive analysis of Australian government policies (see Lippmann 1999; Broome 2002; Eckermann et al 2006). For a brief summary consider Box 10.5. Think — why has it been necessary to develop 'Aboriginal only' policies? What effects have these policies had on Aboriginal people — have they supported or frustrated self-determination?

It is fair to say that, as a result of colonisation, many Indigenous people in Australia and New Zealand experienced chronic poverty. A simplistic definition of poverty is an absence of adequate resources. It is true that poor people have little money — and it is true that both Aboriginal and Māori people have access to lower incomes and are more likely to be dependent on social security support than other groups (see ABS 2000; Ministry of Māori development 2000). However, the situation is a good deal more complex. As Myrdal (1971) pointed out over 30 years ago, and others continue to reinforce (Cason et al 2007), people who are poor are likely to live in substandard housing, have an inadequate diet and are consequently prone to ill health. These factors will constrain their educational performance, which will limit their occupational opportunities, which will keep them in poverty. The patterns are complicated by prejudices, attitudes and values, as well as discrimination, i.e. people who live in poverty are likely to present an image, the stereotype, of 'low living' to the rest of society, which reinforces prejudice and discrimination against them. A critical social environment is likely to reinforce poor self-esteem among people who live in poverty (see Eckermann et al 2006). A visit to any housing commission estates built in the 1960s in parts of Sydney illustrates this argument — everyone 'knows' that the people there are 'social problems'. Figure 10.2 presents the relationship between these elements diagrammatically. Myrdal (1971) highlights how difficult it is to break this cycle — without

Box 10.4 | An account of settlement life in the 1970s

When I lived on an Aboriginal settlement in Queensland in the early 1970s, people got up with the siren, went to work, had lunch and stopped work with the siren. At 10pm the generator was turned off and we were all expected to go to bed so that we'd be fresh for the next day's work. To enter the settlement I had to have permission from the Director of Aboriginal Affairs and I had to report to the non-Aboriginal manager on my arrival. I had to report every time I intended to leave the settlement and report when I returned. This rule also applied to Aboriginal people who lived on the settlement or who wished to visit relatives. If a visitor was considered a 'trouble-maker' by the administration, permission was refused.

Everyone on the settlement worked — even if they swept the streets — there was no unemployment benefit or supporting parent benefit. Those 'unmarried' mothers who did not have a job would be expected to work in the dormitories, cooking or sewing, and would be paid with pocket money and food. The only pensions available were old age pensions. The settlement had attracted attention because of high infant mortality rates. The Department of Health consequently insisted that all babies be brought to the settlement clinic on a regular basis for blood and parasite, weight and height checks. If mothers did not comply, they could be fined or jailed in the settlement jail. Films or dances could only be held if the manager gave permission, gambling and drinking were prohibited. There was a boy's and a girl's dormitory for children who had been removed from their families in other parts of Queensland and who were thought to be at risk — until the 1940s all children were routinely removed from their families at age 3 and reared in the dormitories to protect them from potentially bad influences. Except for the main street, where houses were relatively good, and where all of the non-Aboriginal staff lived, houses on the settlement were virtual shacks — most did not have glass in the windows — shutters kept out the cold — the walls were not lined and few had hot water systems.

Think about this — if I was regimented in this fashion, how much more oppressive would this have been for people who called the settlement their home.

(Eckermann A-K 1971–1972, personal experience)

Box 10.5 | Aboriginal people — government policies

Government policies towards Aboriginal people may be divided into eight periods:

1. European Settlement 1788–1880s — Aborigines regarded as lowest rung in social hierarchy.
2. Segregation 1890s–1950s — strong missionary influence — 'civilising the savages'.
3. Assimilation 1950s–1960s — push for education to full citizenship.
4. Integration 1967–1972 — emphasis on choice for Aborigines.
5. Self-Determination 1972–1975 — some recognition of multicultural society, cultural diversity.
6. Self-Management Stage I 1975–1989 — Aborigines to be accountable for their decisions and manage own finances.
7. Self-Management Stage II 1989–1996 — the RCIADIC, the Mabo and Wik decisions, Native Title Legislation; increased tensions and legal actions.
8. Reconciliation or economic rationalism? — 1996 to present — review of the Stolen Generation, demise of ATSIC, increase in systemic frustrations.

(Eckermann et al 2006: 38)

a coordinated effort to address all of the elements, programs to change one element (e.g. housing) will only intensify the effects of the cycle.

The interplay of these factors has had a profound effect on Indigenous life chances today. Consequently, Dowd et al (1997: 10) have argued that:

> . . . 'diseases of civilisation' (Boyle & Andrews 1989) — genocide, dispossession, oppression, discrimination — and their aftermath reflected in unemployment, poverty and suicide, are as much illnesses as are physical diseases caused by germs, viruses or accidents.

THE HEALTH STATUS OF INDIGENOUS PEOPLE IN AUSTRALIA AND NEW ZEALAND

Australia has only become aware of the appalling status of Indigenous health since the 1960s, when Aboriginal and non-Aboriginal people came in closer contact with one another and a number of Aboriginal organisations began a concerted publicity campaign to educate the public about the state of Aboriginal affairs. In the 1960s Aboriginal infant mortality was one of the highest in the world (Moodie 1973). In the 1980s, Aboriginal infant mortality in NSW was more than twice that of others in that state. Thus:

> In 1984, Aborigines, comprising 1.2 per cent of the estimated Australian population, are estimated to be responsible for 2.6 per cent of live births, 7.6 per of still births, 5.4 per cent of neonatal deaths, 6.7 per cent of prenatal deaths, 8.2 per cent of post-natal deaths and 6.6 per cent of infant deaths.
>
> (Thompson 1985: 6)

Further, comparatively more Aboriginal people than non-Aboriginal people died in all age groups, although the difference was most marked in the age group 25–44 (National Aboriginal Health Strategy 1989). Life expectancy at the time for Aboriginal males was 22 years less than for all Australian males, while Aboriginal women's life expectancy was 15 years less than for non-Aboriginal women.

Twenty years on, and into the 21st century, nothing much has changed. Life expectancy among Aboriginal men and women continues to be up to 20 years lower than that of Australians generally, and:

> . . . mortality rates among Aboriginal people are higher in <u>all</u> age groups and five to six times higher than expected for the 34–54 years age group. Further, Aboriginal babies continue to die twice as often as non-Aboriginal babies.
>
> (Eckermann et al 2006: 54)

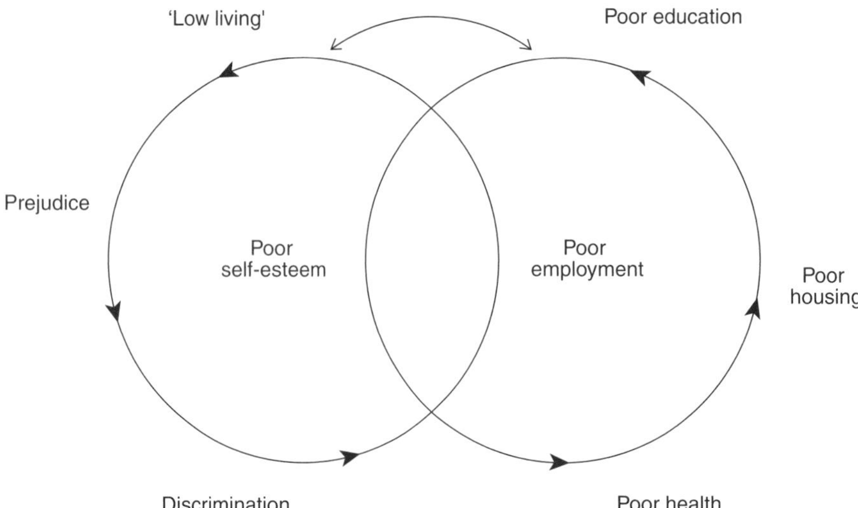

Figure 10.2 | The cycle of poverty *(reproduced with permission from Eckermann et al 2006: 45)*

As a result, the 2007 CLOSETHEGAP Report points out that the number of Aboriginal people who reach the age of 65 is lower than in Bangladesh or Nigeria. In addition, infant mortality is three times that of non-Aboriginal babies (NACCHO/Oxfam 2007: 5). By contrast, Māori mortality and morbidity rates are closing the gap; nevertheless, life expectancy is still 7.5 years below that of non-Māori and infant mortality is still about 50% higher than among non-Māori (NACCHO/Oxfam 2007).

Reflect on Chapter 9 and the influences of structural violence. Remember — the incidence of physical, structural violence can be measured over time in a group's morbidity and mortality rates. The information about Indigenous mortality rates in Australia and New Zealand affirms that both groups have consistently suffered from structural violence. The same is evident when we consider the incidents of various kinds of morbidity. Diabetes is almost 10 times as common among Aboriginal people as in the wider Australian population, and almost six times as prevalent among Māori as non-Māori people. Ischaemic heart disease is almost twice as common among Aboriginal and Māori people as it is among non-Indigenous Australians and New Zealanders and diseases of the lung and respiratory tract are two-and-a-half times more common among Indigenous people in Australia and New Zealand than the non-Indigenous populations (NACCHO/Oxfam 2007: 17).

The level of psychological, structural violence is evident in rates of suicide and incidence of mental disease as well as family violence. Although, in their report 'The Health and Wellbeing of Australia's Aboriginal and Torres Strait Islander Peoples', Edwards and Madden (2001) acknowledge that it is difficult to acquire accurate figures, they maintain that:

> . . . There are, however, hospital data which indicate that Indigenous people suffer from higher levels of many mental and behavioural disorders. In 1998–9, there were about four times as many hospital separations as expected for mental disorders resulting from psychoactive drug use. Self-harm and assault may be indicators of social and emotional distress and psychological illness in a community. Hospitalisation data show that there were many more hospital separations than expected for intentional injury in the Indigenous population.

Suicide in Aboriginal communities did not become an issue of concern until the 1980s when Aboriginal people began to demonstrate about the high rate of deaths in custody, particularly among their young men. Over the period 1980–1989, 99 Indigenous people died in custody — many of these appeared to have committed suicide. You will find their stories recorded in the publications of the Royal Commission into Aboriginal Deaths in Custody (1991). However, suicide is not only a feature of incarceration. Tatz (2001) maintains that Aboriginal suicides are at least double the rate of non-Aboriginal suicides, particularly common among young men aged 15–34, and that it may have become 'patterned, ritualised and even institutionalised, perhaps even contagious' (Tatz 2001: 102) in the rural communities he visited. Similarly, Beautrais (2003) suggests that young Māori males and females in this age group are approximately one-and-a-half times more likely to die by suicide than non-Māori young people. Further, family violence, related to substance abuse, unemployment, alienation and marginalisation, is more common among Indigenous people in Australia and New Zealand than among the non-Indigenous populations of these countries (see ABS 2004; Ministry for Social Development Te Rito 2007). In the Australian context, the recent reports on child sexual abuse in Indigenous communities are particularly disturbing. *No one* could, or should, try to argue that child abuse is part of traditional Aboriginal cultures. Ring and Wenitong (2007: 204) do, however, maintain that this crime can be related to issues associated with poverty, substance abuse and inadequate employment, as well as:

> . . . continuing inadequacies in health services for Indigenous Australians. The problem of overcrowding in houses has not been solved, and risky alcohol consumption has not abated for men and has increased for women. Imprisonment rates for adults have increased, and the gap between Indigenous and non-Indigenous juvenile detention rates has widened.

Every thinking person would agree that some sort of intervention has to take place, but what should be the nature and process of such intervention? Who should take responsibility for the intervention? Who should be held accountable?

The above discussion has demonstrated that Aboriginal and Māori people continue to suffer from varying levels of structural violence and that this situation has continued for a number of generations. Indigenous people in Australia and New Zealand have been politically active since colonisation. However, the Australian Referendum in 1967 and the establishment of the Waitangi Tribunal in 1975 could be seen as watersheds in the fight for recognition of Indigenous rights. After the Referendum, Aboriginal people were counted in the Australian census as people, rather than as part of the country's fauna and flora, and the federal government was given the right to legislate on behalf of the Indigenous minority (Lippmann 1999; Broome 2002; Eckermann et al 2006). With the establishment of the Waitangi Tribunal, Māori were provided with an accredited, formal, legal mechanism for challenging any actions, which were thought to contravene the Treaty of Waitangi and jeopardise Māori rights (Ramsden 2002). From this time on, the Indigenous people of Australia and New Zealand began the process of challenging the institutions, such as health, which were failing them. Fundamental to such failure, they argued, was the conflict of worldviews related to health.

THE MEANING OF HEALTH AND ILLNESS

Health to Indigenous people in Australia and New Zealand is a multi-dimensional concept that embraces all aspects of living and stresses the importance of survival in harmony with the environment.

Formed in Australia in 1975, the National Aboriginal and Islander Health Organisation (NAIHO) (1982: 2) states that health is:

> Not just the physical well being of the individual but the social, emotional and cultural well being of the whole community. This is a whole-of-life view and it also includes the cyclical concept of life. Health care services should strive to achieve the state where every individual is able to achieve their full potential as human beings, and thus bring about the total wellbeing of their community . . .

The core of this definition also appears in the National Aboriginal Health Strategy (1989). NAIHO was replaced in 1993 by the National Aboriginal Community Controlled Health Organisation (NACCHO), which continues to support this approach to health and its holistic approach to health care.

Similarly, Māori definitions of health are holistic and community oriented. Their models of health emphasise the interrelationship between spiritual, mental, physical and social (extended family) wellbeing (Durie 1998). Both Indigenous conceptualisations of 'health' are reflected in the World Health Organization's (WHO's) definition of health, outlined in the Alma-Ata Declaration (1978 Declaration 1) as '. . . a state of complete, physical, mental and social wellbeing, and not merely the absence of disease or infirmity, . . .'.

Such holistic definitions of health are also reflected in Indigenous people's attitudes towards sickness. Thus, Aboriginal as well as Māori people may see transgressions against spiritual powers or the rules of society as the reasons for illness. Conversely, spiritual powers may be believed to heal. For example, in the 1970s, a Wakka Wakka woman told Eckermann that when she had been hospitalised with renal failure a couple of years previously, and had not been expected to live, her deceased father and grandfather visited her and rubbed her body to take away the pain and the illness. To the surprise of hospital staff, she recovered completely.

Reflect on Chapter 9 — what is the basis of the prevailing mainstream definition of health and model of health care? Without doubt, it is a medical definition and model of care. Consider Figure 10.3 — What kinds of power imbalances are set up when a holistic model of health clashes with the medical one? What are the differences in approaches to health evident here? What are the points of potential conflict and who holds power in this interaction?

Indigenous people in Australia and New Zealand have focused on Primary Health Care (PHC) in their approach to health delivery. PHC is:

> . . . essential health care based on practical, scientifically sound and socially acceptable methods and technology made universally acceptable to individuals and families in the community through their full participation and at a cost that the community can afford to maintain at every stage of their development in the spirit of self-reliance and self-determination.
>
> (World Health Organization 1978 Article 7)

Indeed, Indigenous people in Australia and New Zealand have practised PHC since long before it was defined by the WHO.

INDIGENOUS HEALTH IN INDIGENOUS HANDS

Aboriginal people argue that their people simply do not access mainstream medical services because they feel that such services discriminate against them and make

She's sick because she didn't respect her elders
She's sick because of all the germs the mangy dogs spread around the camp

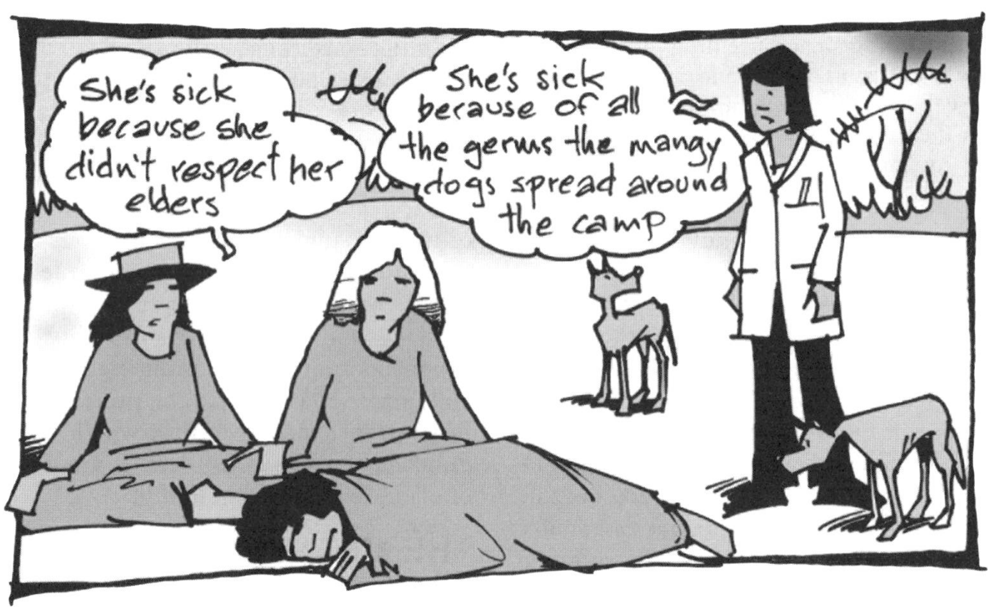

Figure 10.3 | The imbalance of power *(Eckermann et al 2006)*

no attempt to cater for their needs. As a result, they established their first medical service in Redfern in 1971. Foley (1982) points out that these services are designed by the people, for the people, according to their needs, and in harmony with their holistic view of health. Consequently the decision-making base is shifted from the medical professions to community elected boards of directors. Aboriginal Community Controlled Health Services are affiliated nationally under NACCHO.

Eckermann et al (2006: 180) have defined community control as:

- the client of that service has a large say about how the service operates;
- the community identifies its needs and then works together to address these needs;
- the community has ownership and is wholly involved in the planning and decision making;
- there is strong influence from the grassroots up;
- the community does things in its own time and at its own pace;
- accountability to the community becomes the guiding principle.

Return to Chapter 9 and review the principles and processes underlying cultural safety — identify the relationship between community control and cultural safety.

Community controlled health services have grown to 130, and are accessible to 50% of Aboriginal people (NACCHO website http://www.naccho.org.au). Such services have had a chequered history. During the 1970s, 1980s and part of the 1990s they were funded on a quarterly basis and any three-month funding allocation had to be acquitted before the service(s) received the next quarterly allocation. During the 1990s annual funding was introduced and, by the late 1990s, tri-annual funding became the rule (Eckermann et al 2006). One could ask — what does this have to do with health care? Eckermann et al (2006) maintain that successive governments believed Aboriginal organisations needed to be controlled and supervised and that this contributed to the system of funding. It, in turn, constrained Aboriginal communities' abilities to attract, develop and retain staff, plan, conduct and evaluate programs or expand services. Even today, funding for Aboriginal health is chronically short. Thus NACCHO/Oxfam (2007) point out that although funding to community controlled health services is now distributed through the Office of Aboriginal and Torres Strait Islander Health (OATSIH), and there have been significant increases:

- . . . the OATSIH budget is a relatively small portion of overall expenditure on Aboriginal and Torres Strait Islander health. The crucial shortfall is in the mainstream Medical Benefits Scheme/Pharmaceutical Benefits Scheme programs. Until Aboriginal and Torres Strait Islander peoples get their share of these programs (on a needs basis), the gap in equitable funding will not narrow. (While spending on Aboriginal and Torres Strait Islander health has increased, it hasn't done so any faster than for the rest of the population so the expenditure gap hasn't narrowed.)
- The net effect is that Australia has in effect run a system in which Aboriginal and Torres Strait Islander peoples receive a lesser level of service right across the continuum of care than the rest of the population — less on prevention, less on primary health care, less for surgery in hospital and less for rehabilitation. The apparent higher expenditure on hospital care is almost certainly less than it should be on a needs basis, given the higher illness levels
- Spending less on people with worse health is not good national policy. The Federal Government, through programs under its own direct control (i.e. Medical Benefits Scheme/Pharmaceutical Benefits Scheme, OATSIH, aged care but excluding transfer payments to the states), spends approximately $0.70 per capita on Aboriginal and Torres Strait Islander people for every $1 spent on the rest of the population

(NACCHO/Oxfam 2007: 8)

Nevertheless, most Community Controlled Health Services have achieved significant improvements in Aboriginal health. Thus NACCHO argues that if funding is allocated according to need, and if it is directed to culturally appropriate health care services, the Aboriginal health crisis could be solved. However, while this national body urges 'Indigenous Health in Indigenous Hands', it also points to the need to improve mainstream health service and to increase funding for 'the building blocks of good health such as awareness and availability of nutrition, physical activity, fresh food, healthy life style, and adequate housing' (NACCHO/Oxfam 2007: 12).

NACCHO's recommendations are not new. The organisation and its predecessor, the NAIHO, has been campaigning for appropriate health care for Indigenous Australia for a quarter of a century. Governments, however, have not been listening. Late in 1990 there was a push for community controlled health services to form partnerships with regional health authorities in order to ensure that services would not be duplicated. Some of these partnership agreements appear to have been well thought out and have proven successful (see NACCHO/Oxfam 2007); others have been little more than token (see Eckermann et al 2006). Since 2000 the Commonwealth has poured significant funds into projects, which took a 'whole of government approach' through the Council of Australian Governments (COAG). Particular COAG sites have been set up in each state and territory. The aim is to build capacity in Aboriginal communities through their partnership with state, territory, local and Commonwealth governments as well as business.

> Communities are encouraged to develop community development plans and via 'negotiation table' have the opportunity to develop a 'shared responsibility agreement and community action plan' with government. Negotiating tables are composed of community leaders and senior

> public servants. Who the community leaders might be, or how they are to be chosen, is not specified . . .
>
> (Eckermann et al 2006: 189)

Partnerships of this kind could be enormously beneficial — if the terms of the partnership are clearly and equitably defined and there is ample consultation. This is not always the case, as outlined in Box 10.6. It is clear that:

> A healthy partnership is based on trust and respect. It is not only talked about but practised. It is a two-way street — it is two or more people walking together, side by side, for a common purpose. It means backing each other up, acknowledging mutual boundaries, and taking the time to grow and learn together.
>
> (Eckermann et al 2006: 189)

Partnerships and cultural safety, then, have a lot in common: both require trust and respect. A relationship can begin with respect but trust, however, takes time.

Māori, too, are participating in partnerships with governments in order to enhance their life chances. Since they have been able to challenge established practices and processes, which have limited their rights through the Waitangi Tribunal, they have made health a treaty issue (see Durie 1998 and Ramsden 2002). It is undoubtedly true that many more Māori than Aboriginal people have participated in the health system as doctors and nurses since colonisation; perhaps because in traditional times they had access to a class of healers who were trained in a whare wanaga, a house of learning (Te Ara — The Encyclopedia of New Zealand 2007) — so the notion of formal study would not have been so very foreign to Māori. Nevertheless, Ramsden (2002) has highlighted the levels of racism and discrimination that she and many other Māori health care professionals experienced.

The 1988 New Zealand Royal Commission of Social Policy set out three principles to guide interactions between Māori and non-Māori people. These are the principle of partnership, the principle of participation and the principle of protection. On the basis of these principles a Māori health service — Te Hotu Manawa Māori (Māori heartbeat) — was set up in 1989 under the umbrella of the National Heart Foundation; it became a separate incorporated society in 1997 (http://www.tehotumanawa.org.nz/). Te Hotu Manawa Māori provides extensive national public health campaigns about nutrition, smoking, rheumatic fever and exercise. In the 1980s and 1990s, Māori held a number of important *hui*, or meetings, at which they discussed the future of Māori health and reflected on their own models of health (Ministry of Māori Development 1993–1996, Durie 1998), the influence of colonisation on their health and the need for cultural safety (Ramsden 2002). Indeed, Māori made health an issue under the Treaty of Waitangi (McKinney & Smith 2005) and were able to reach a negotiated model of health care, based on cultural safety, which became a compulsory part of the New Zealand nursing and midwifery curricula (Nursing Council of New Zealand 1996). Additionally, Māori, under the principle of partnership, formed collaborative agreements with mainstream health services to establish a range of PHC initiatives (Ministry of Māori Development 1993–1996). These have grown from 23 in 1993 to 243 in 2000–2001 (Wilson & Roberts 2005: 157). Māori, then, formed national pressure groups, rather than regional or local agreements, and their own professionals lobbied important professional bodies to achieve recognition of Māori health needs. It would, however, be wrong to assume that the level of awareness of Māori health issues among non-Māori health professionals is necessarily greater than that of non-Aboriginal health care providers about Aboriginal health. McCreanor and Nairn (2002) interviewed 25 general practitioners about Māori health and found that generally these practitioners explained:

> poor health status of Māori as a function of being Māori and so naturalise or legitimise a situation that is ethically, socially, and economically unacceptable.
>
> (McCreanor & Nairn 2002:4)

In other words, they were inclined to 'blame the victim' (Ryan 1976).

Box 10.6 | A healthy partnership?

In 2005 I visited a community in SW Queensland where two Aboriginal public servants met with the coordinator of the local Aboriginal organisation and the representative of the local council. The next day, when I attended the office, copies of a 'shared responsibility agreement' were lying on the meeting table. The coordinator had signed the agreement, without consultation with the members of the organisation or members of the wider community because it would continue funding for the local council's liaison officer who had been 'very good to us'. Some weeks later, the same Aboriginal bureaucrats visited again and informed the coordinator that he would now be expected to enrol at TAFE and complete Certificate IVs in Animal Husbandry. The coordinator was distressed because he did not want to go back to school — he had 25 years of practical knowledge of running a station and rearing livestock. I asked him to have another look at the shared responsibility agreement and we discovered that 'the community' had agreed to attend adult education courses at TAFE, and it had agreed to send their children to school regularly, as their part of the shared responsibility agreement. The Commonwealth, in turn, agreed to provide the local council with monies to continue to employ a non-Aboriginal liaison officer.

Consider:

1. What level of consultation had taken place?
2. Did the coordinator understand the terms of the agreement?
3. Was the partnership equitable?

(Eckermann A-K 2005, personal experience)

MEETING THE CHALLENGE

It appears that both Australia and New Zealand are endorsing Indigenous health policies based on Comprehensive Primary Health Care (CPHC) — as outlined in the *National Strategic*

Framework for Aboriginal and Torres Strait Islander Health (NATSIHC 2003: 17) and the Māori Health Strategy — He Korowai Oranga (Ministry of Health 2002). CPHC includes clinical services, educational/disease prevention and health improvement programs, access to all kinds of medical services as well as assistance and advocacy for communities and clients. The Australian government has committed itself to partnership and shared responsibilities, secure, long term funding, equitable access, mainstream programs which take their share of responsibility for Aboriginal health, providing resources commensurate with the problems in Aboriginal health, providing additional Indigenous services when mainstream services are inadequate, ensuring outcomes, coordination of services and developing an appropriate data base (Dwyer et al 2004: 9). The New Zealand government has committed itself to a similar partnership — however it has focused on whānau (extended family) as the centre of Māori society. Consequently the principles of partnership, participation and protection are expressed as:

> Partnership
> Working together with iwi, hapu, whānau and Māori communities to develop strategies for Māori health gain and appropriate health and disability services
>
> Participation
> Involving Māori at all levels of the sector, in decision-making, planning, development and delivery of health and disability services
>
> Protection
> Working to ensure Māori have at least the same level of health as non-Māori, and safeguarding Māori cultural concepts, values and practices
>
> (Ministry of Health 2002: 2)

This emphasis on Indigenous concepts and knowledge as well as social structures does not seem to be clearly articulated in Australian policy on Indigenous health.

As practitioners, nurses will be able to meet the challenges inherent in the health policies and the principles underlying partnerships, if they work within a framework based on respect, acknowledgement of difference and trust. In Chapter 9, Eckermann et al (2006) have outlined the cornerstones of culturally safe practice. They include:

- Reflecting on self, one's own culture and profession, power imbalances, attitudes and beliefs about 'the other'
- Enhancing communication skills and drawing on the skills of interpreters
- Understanding of the influence of power imbalances on 'the other'
- Developing trust
- Negotiating knowledge
- Negotiating outcomes
- Understanding the influence of culture shock.

Briefly consider each of these.

Reflecting on self is essential if health care providers are to understand their own society, their own attitudes and beliefs — and then take the next step and question how they have come to have the beliefs they hold dear. Ramsden (2002: 1–6) acknowledges that even as a member of a minority group operating in mainstream society:

> Unless I understood myself very well as the bearer of culturally derived attitudes such as internalised racism and social class, I could very well become the oppressor of Māori and others who were less powerful than myself.

Such reflection should help nurses to understand **the influence of power imbalances on 'the other'**. Remember, health care professionals have specialised knowledge and therefore hold power over those who do not have such knowledge. The power imbalance is accentuated by a patient's vulnerability (illness) or status in society — members of impoverished minorities generally feel less confident within the health system because of past negative experiences.

Enhancing communication skills is basic to effective health care provision. Sharing a common language is not the end to 'enhancing communication skills'. Nurses must also be aware of other people's non-verbal cues, as well as the rules and conventions associated with communication, and the acceptable behaviour or etiquette associated with communication (Furnham & Bochner 1986). Such rules may well be cultural and related to the gender and age — it takes time to find the 'right' way, however, showing respect will always help.

Trust develops when people do what they promise to do, when they are respectful of one another and show concern for one another.

Nurses are trained to acquire knowledge about clients, signs, symptoms and treatment of illnesses. They may also feel the need to learn as much as possible about other cultures in order to provide them with the best possible care. This strategy will not necessarily be successful. Knowledge about other cultures can lead nurses to believe that they know 'what's best' for an individual from that culture — it may lead to paternalism and to that client's disempowerment. It is best to **negotiate the knowledge** that clients would like to share about themselves. This can be done through the process of communication, with the help of an Indigenous colleague, and within a respectful and mutually trusting relationship.

Negotiating outcomes may be even harder — health care professionals 'know' what the best outcome is for the patient — they have been trained for many years to know. To really discuss/communicate possible outcomes and to stand back if the patient decides against what the nurse 'knows' is best is difficult. Ultimately compliance or non-compliance must be based on informed self-determination.

Culture shock has been discussed in some detail in Chapter 9, where colonisation has been identified as a massive form of culture shock. Remember that Indigenous clients are likely to suffer a double dose of culture shock in mainstream health systems — one is the system itself, the other is that it is affiliated with the power groups which have over the years discriminated against them.

Ultimately, as Johnson (1995) points out, it's so much about *what* you do but more about *how* you do it. She writes:

> Every time health care creates an atmosphere that allows people to take their own power; takes the time to have true dialogue and negotiate; takes a holistic, people–centred approach; includes cultural safety measures; fosters self-reliance; acts as a resource and values a process that leaves people feeling responsible for their own health, then it is true Primary Health Care [and culturally safe] and the way forward for the whole of Australia.
>
> Every time health care is paternalistic; does not take the time to set up true dialogue and negotiate; takes a narrow, disease-centred approach; does not take cultural safety into account; creates dependence; becomes an imposition or tries to take control, then it is prolonging the imbalance of power in our society.
>
> It is doing more harm than good, no matter how many diseases it cures.
>
> (Johnson 1995: 1)

SUMMARY

It is clear that Indigenous rates of mortality and morbidity remain unacceptably high and that they illustrate the high level of structural violence to which Indigenous communities in Australia and New Zealand are subjected. This chapter has explored Indigenous societies in Australia and New Zealand before colonisation as well as the processes of colonisation and their impact on Indigenous health. Current Indigenous health status has been examined and special attention has focused on colonisation as culture shock. Indigenous multidimensional perceptions of health have been identified and the challenges associated with providing culturally appropriate health care have been explored. It is clear that such care has to be based on principles of partnership, community control and principles underlying cultural safety. None of these principles will, however, impact on Indigenous health unless funding *according to need* is channelled into community controlled PHC providers, and mainstream services are held accountable for providing appropriate care to Indigenous people.

REVIEW EXERCISES

1. What are the differences in traditional social organisation between Aboriginal and Māori people?
2. What are the traditional Māori and Aboriginal interpretations of illness?
3. What differences are there in the colonisation processes of Australia and New Zealand?
4. What effects has colonisation had on the health of Aboriginal and Māori people?
5. Define structural violence.
6. Define poverty and its effects on Indigenous health.
7. How do Aboriginal and Māori people define health today?
8. What is meant by partnership and community control?
9. Which government policies do you think support principles of self-determination and cultural safety?
10. How can practitioners become culturally safe?

CRITICAL THINKING EXERCISE

Shattered dreams

Six young Aboriginal people from a regional town graduated as nurses and found positions at the local hospital because they wanted to stay close to their families. The Aboriginal groups of the town were delighted and often requested that one of these nurses attend to them. A few months later the shine had gone off the job for one of these young, enthusiastic nurses. She blamed herself, but during counselling it became clear that she was bearing the brunt of various forms of discrimination from other nurses. Soon after this she resigned.

Over the next 2 years — one by one — the other five Aboriginal nurses resigned for similar reasons, ranging from avoidance to blatant racism. Various attempts were made to alert the nursing hierarchy to the tragedy unfolding but the usual responses were 'they are choosing to go' or 'they just haven't got what it takes' or other 'blame the victim' statements.

Activity

1. Discuss the factors that changed the nurse from being enthusiastic to 'blaming herself' and resigning.
2. What are the tensions inherent in this scenario?
3. How could the situation have been handled differently?

REFERENCES AND FURTHER READINGS

Australian Bureau of Statistics (ABS) (2000) *Labour Force Characteristics of Indigenous Australians*, Cat No 6287.0. Online. Available: http://.nsf/0/98dada41010ea3aca2569ba007af523?OpenDocument [accessed 13 February 2004]

—— (2004) *National Aboriginal and Torres Strait Islander Social Survey 2002*. Online. Available: http://www.abs.gov.au/AUSSTATS/abs@.nsf/ProductsbyCatalogue/AD174BBF36BA93A2CA256EBB007981BA?OpenDocument [accessed January 2008]

Beaglehole JC (ed) (1955) *The Journal of Captain James Cook on His Voyage of Discovery*. Cambridge University. Press, Cambridge

Beautrais A (2003) Suicide in New Zealand I: time trends and epidemiology. *The New Zealand Medical Journal*. Online. Available: www.nzma.org.nz/journal/116-1175/460/content.pdf [accessed 16 April 2008]

Belich J (1996) *Making Peoples: a History of the New Zealanders from Polynesian Settlement to the End of the Nineteenth Century*. Allen Lane and Penguin, London and Auckland

Berndt RM, Berndt CH (1988) *The World of the First Australians, Aboriginal Traditional Life: Past and Present*. Aboriginal Studies Press, Canberra

Boyle J, Andrews M (2001) *Transcultural Concepts in Nursing Care*. Scott Foresman, Glenville IL

Broome R (2002) *Aboriginal Australians*. Allen and Unwin, Sydney

Cason B, Dunbart T, Chenhall RD, Bailie R (2007) *Social Determinants of Indigenous Health*. Allen and Unwin, Sydney

Devanesen D (2000) Traditional Aboriginal Medical Practice in the Northern Territory. Paper presented at the International

Symposium on Traditional Medicine. Awaji Island, Japan, September. Online. Available: www.nt.gov.au/. . ./comm._health/abhealth_strategy/Traditional%20Aboriginal%20Medicine%20-%20Japan%20Paper.pdf [accessed 15 April 2008]
Dowd LT (1985) The need for understanding: a case study of Aboriginal and non-Aboriginal perspectives on health care. Unpublished Masters Thesis. University of California San Francisco, San Francisco
Dowd LT, Eckermann, A-K, Johnson, S (1997) *Primary Health Care — Principles and Practice in a Cross-Cultural Setting.* University of New England, Armidale
Durie M (1998) *Whaiora: Māori Health Development*, 2nd edn. Oxford University Press, Oxford
Dwyer JK, Silborn K, Wilson G (2004) *National Strategy for Improving Health and Health Care*. Commonwealth of Australia, Canberra
Eckermann A-K, Dowd LT, Chong E, Nixon L, Gray R, Johnson, S (2006) *Binang Goonj: Bridging Cultures in Aboriginal Health*, 2nd edn. Elsevier Australia, Sydney
Edwards RW, Madden R (2001) The health and welfare of Australia's Aboriginal and Torres Strait Islander peoples. Online. Available: www. auststats.abs.gov.au/Ausstats/subscriber.nsf/0/231C5A3D2B63E9FBCA256AB800005D80/$File/47040.2001.pdf [accessed 15 April 2008]
Elkin AP (1977) *Aboriginal Men of High Degree*, 2nd edn. University of Queensland Press, Brisbane
—— (1994) *The Australian Aborigines*, 4th edn. Angus and Robertson, Sydney
Evans R, Saunders K, Cronin, K (1988) *Race Relations in Colonial Queensland: A History of Exclusion, Exploitation and Extermination*, 2nd edn. University of Queensland Press, St Lucia
Foley G (1982) Aboriginal Community Controlled Health Service: a short history. *Aboriginal Health Information Bulletin* 2(8): 13–15
Furnham A, Bochner S (1986) *Culture Shock: Psychological Reactions to Unfamiliar Environments*. Taylor & Francis, New York
Gumbert M (1984) *Neither Justice Nor Reason: a Legal and Anthropological Analysis of Aboriginal Land Rights*. University of Queensland, Brisbane
Hiatt B (1970) Woman the Gatherer. In: Gale F (ed) *Women's Role in Aboriginal Society*. Australian Institute of Aboriginal Studies, Canberra
Johnson S (1995) Primary health care or disease. Unpublished course notes
Kociumbas, J (2004) Genocide and Modernity in Colonial Australia. In: Moses AD (ed.), *Genocide and Settler Society: Frontier Violence and Stolen Indigenous Children in Australian History*. Berghahn Books, New York: 77–102
Lancaster Jones F (1970) *The Structure and Growth of Australia's Aboriginal Population*. ANU Press, Canberra
Lippmann L (1999) *Generations of Resistance: Mabo and Justice*, 3rd edn. Longman Cheshire, Melbourne
McCreanor T, Nairn R (2002) Tauiwi general practioners' talk about Māori health: interpretive repertoires. *The New Zealand Medical Journal* 115(1167). Online. Available: http://www.nzma.org.nz/journal/115-1167/272/ [accessed 16 April 2008]
McGraw A (1995) *Contested Ground: Australian Aborigines Under the British Crown*. Allen and Unwin, Sydney
McKinney C, Smith N (2005) Te Tiriki o Waitangi or The Treaty of Waitangi: what is the difference? In Wepa D (ed) *Cultural Safety in Aotearoa New Zealand*. Pearson New Zealand, Auckland: 39–57
Miller J (1985) *Koori: A Will to Win*. Angus & Robertson, Sydney
Ministry for Culture and Heritage (updated 20 Sept 2007) *Tribal Organisation — Social Rank*. Online. Available: http://www.teara.govt.nz/NewZealanders/Māori NewZealanders/Trib [accessed January 2008]
—— (updated 21 November 2007) *Signing the Treaty.* Online. Available: http://www.nzhistory.net.nz/node/2242 [accessed January 2008]
—— (updated 21 November 2007) *Governing New Zealand, Background to the Treaty*. Online. Available: http://www.nzhistory.net.nz/node/2537 [accessed January 2008]
Ministry for Social Development Te Rito (2007) *New Zealand Family Violence Prevention Strategy*. Online. Available: http://www.msd.govt.nz/publications/te-rito/ [accessed January 2008]
Ministry of Health (2002) *He Korowai Oranga — Māori Health Strategy*. Online. Available: http://www.moh.govt.nz/mhs.html [accessed 16 April 2008]
Ministry of Māori Development (2000) *Tikanga Oranga Hauora*. Online. Available: *Whakapari*: www.tpk.govt.nz/Māori / education/tohtrend.pdf [accessed January 2008]
Moodie PM (1973) *Aboriginal Health*. Australian University Press, Canberra
Moses AD (ed) (2004) *Genocide and Settler Society: Frontier Violence and Stolen Indigenous Children in Australian History*. Berghahn Books, New York
Mulvaney J (2002) Difficult to found an opinion: 1788 population estimates. In: Briscoe G, Smith L (eds), *The Aboriginal Population Revisited: 70,000 years to the present*. Aboriginal History Monograph 10. Aboriginal History, Canberra
Myrdal G (1971) The principle of circular and cumulative causation. In: Dalton E (ed) *Economic Development and Social Change, the Modernization of Village Communities*. Natural History Press, New York
NACCHO/Oxfam (2007) *CLOSETHEGAP: Solutions to the Indigenous Health Crisis Facing Australia*. Oxfam, Fitzroy
National Aboriginal and Islander Health Organisation (NAIHO) (1982) Philosophy of the community controlled health services. Unpublished NAIHO discussion paper
National Aboriginal and Torres Strait Islander Health Council (NATSIHC) (2003) *The National Strategic Framework for Aboriginal and Torres Strait Islander Health: Framework for Action by Governments*. NATSIHC, Canberra
National Aboriginal Health Strategy Working Party (1989) *National Aboriginal Health Strategy*. Department of Aboriginal Affairs, Canberra
Nursing Council of New Zealand (1996) *Guidelines for Cultural Safety in Nursing and Midwifery Education*. Nursing Council of New Zealand, Wellington
Ramsden IM (2002) Cultural safety and nursing education in Aotearoa and Te Waipounamu. Unpublished PhD thesis. University of Wellington, Victoria. Online. Available: culturalsafety.massey.ac.nz [accessed January 2004]
Rāwiri Taonui (updated 20-Sep-2007) 'Tribal organisation', Te Ara — *The Encyclopedia of New Zealand*. Online. Available: http://www.TeAra.govt.nz/NewZealanders/MāoriNewZealanders/TribalOrganisation/en [accessed January 2008]
Reid J (ed) (1982) *Body, Land and Spirit: Health and Healing in Aboriginal Society.* University of Queensland Press, St Lucia
Reynolds H (1987) *Frontier*. Allen & Unwin, Sydney
—— (1989) *Dispossessed*. Allen & Unwin, Sydney
—— (2003) *The Law of the Land*. Penguin Books, Sydney
Ring T, Wenitong M (2007) Interventions to halt child abuse in Aboriginal communities. *eMJA*, 187(4): 204–205
Royal Commission into Aboriginal Deaths in Custody

(RCIADIC) (1991) *National Reports*, vol 1–5, AGPS, Canberra

Ryan W (1976) *Blaming the Victim*. Vintage Books, New York

Sheppard DF (2005) Māori land: Māori health. Online. Available: www.abc.net.au/rural/events/ruralhealth/2005/papers/8nrhcfinalpaper00603.pdf [accessed January 2008]

Stanner WEH (1979) *White Man Got No Dreaming: Essays 1938–1973*. ANU Press, Canberra

Statistics New Zealand (2003) *2001 Census Snapshot 4*. Online. Available: www.stats.govt.nz/ [accessed January 2004]

Tatz C (1999) *Genocide in Australia*. AIATSIS, Canberra

—— (2001) *Aboriginal Suicide is Different.* AIATSIS, Canberra

Te Ara — The *Encyclopedia of New Zealand* (2007) Tribal Organisation and Social Rank: http://www.teara.govt.nz/NewZealanders/MāoriNewZealanders/Trib [accessed January 2008]

Thompson N (1985) *Aboriginal Health Status, Programs and Prospects*. Department of the Parliamentary Library, Canberra

Wepa D (ed) (2005) *Cultural Safety in Aotearoa New Zealand.* Pearson New Zealand, Auckland

Wilson D, Roberts M (2005) Māori health initiatives. In: Wepa D (ed) *Cultural Safety in Aotearoa New Zealand.* Pearson New Zealand, Auckland: 157–69

World Health Organization (WHO) (1978) Primary Health Care: Report of the International Conference on Primary Health Care, Alma Ata, USSR, 6–12 September, WHO, Geneva

Unit 4

Promoting psychosocial health in nursing practice

Chapter 11
SPIRITUALITY

OBJECTIVES

- Define key terms/concepts
- Understand the role of the nurse in spiritual caring
- Understand the different dimensions of spirituality
- Discuss the various ways that individuals express their spirituality
- Identify how the nurse might recognise that a client is experiencing spiritual pain
- Identify the attributes a nurse needs to bring to a relationship to facilitate a client's spiritual healing
- Identify five open questions the nurse could use to begin assessing a client's spirituality
- Understand how hospitalisation can impact on cultural beliefs and practices that are important to a client's spiritual health
- Identify interventions the nurse could implement to facilitate clients being able to continue to practise religious rituals and practices while in hospital
- Explain how reminiscence therapy can provide spiritual support to a resident living in an aged-care facility
- Describe factors that can foster hope in a client facing chronic or terminal illness
- Identify ways to evaluate spiritual wellbeing

KEY TERMS/CONCEPTS

generic spirituality
hope
religion
reminiscence therapy
rituals and practices
secular spirituality
spiritual healing
spiritual health
spiritual pain

CHAPTER FOCUS

A person's spirituality is connected to finding meaning and purpose in life. For some people spirituality is linked to religious beliefs, for others it is linked more to a philosophy of life. Changes in health and hospitalisation can challenge the way people perceive themselves as spiritual and may impact on the way people are able to express their spirituality. Because of their close relationships with clients, nurses are in a key position to identify spiritual concerns, but spirituality is an area that nurses may tend to avoid. This chapter provides a basic introduction to the role of the nurse in providing for spiritual needs.

LIVED EXPERIENCE

Yes, my body is a bit of a mess now. This rheumatoid arthritis makes it hard for me to get around. I hardly ever go out now but I can see my garden and the birds in the birdbath. I like to watch the clouds and the flowers and trees, all of that nurtures my spirit. But you know this is only a body and I'm not in it much of the time. I can think myself to the ocean where I can sail away with the music when I listen to Mozart or Vivaldi. Anyway, this is God's plan for me and this is only temporary.

Marjorie, age 52

DEFINING SPIRITUALITY

All people have a spiritual dimension, but spirituality is an abstract concept and therefore not easily defined. Many authors have reflected on spiritual care in nursing and have presented a range of definitions of spirituality (Greenstreet 2006; O'Brien 2007; McSherry 2006). The concept of spirituality as two dimensional is perhaps the clearest and most easily explained. Moberg and Brusek (1978) first put forward the concept that spirituality has two dimensions — vertical and horizontal. The vertical dimension relates to the way a person reaches out to a personal god, the universe or to something greater than self. The horizontal dimension refers to the way a person reaches out to, and connects with, other people and to a sense of purpose and satisfaction in life that is not entwined with religious meaning. These two dimensions transcend the physical, material world. Each person's spirituality may be more strongly linked to one of the two dimensions than the other. It may also be that an individual feels connected with only one of the two dimensions.

Either way, to be spiritually healthy, life needs to be invested with purpose and meaning. Seeking purpose and meaning may be a continuous process, sometimes lifelong (Greenstreet 2006). It may be a niggling sense of being unfulfilled that motivates the search. It is not uncommon during times of crisis, such as when facing serious loss or life-threatening illness, that a person's need to identify purpose and meaning becomes much stronger.

There is no simple answer to the question 'what is spirituality?' because a person's spirituality is intangible — a mysterious thing that cannot be isolated. It is the accumulation of everything a person is — the essence of being. Some might call this essence a person's soul. However, the word soul tends to be linked to religion, but all people are spiritual and many are spiritual without being religious (Stevens-Barnum 2003; Young & Koopsen 2005).

GENERIC SPIRITUALITY

The term 'generic spirituality' is sometimes used when referring to the spirituality of people who find meaning in life and have things in life that are sacred but not necessarily part of a specific religious tradition (Tacey 2003).

SECULAR SPIRITUALITY

The term secular is also used to describe the way people find meaning in life when their spirituality is not based on religion. Secular spirituality means making sense of questions like 'who or what am I?' and 'why am I here?' without connection to any religious underpinnings. People who have a secular spirituality may hold strong convictions that guide their concepts of right and wrong. It is these convictions rather than religious beliefs that influence the way they live their lives. These convictions encompass views about treating, and being treated by, others as someone of value and with feelings. Interacting in this positive way is viewed as a means of appreciating a person's worth and thereby acknowledging their spirituality (Smith 2002; Stein-Parbury 2005).

WAYS OF BEING SPIRITUAL

RELIGION

For some people religion is the vehicle that sustains their spirituality. For many it is satisfying because it provides clear rules about morality, a community of like-minded people and a set of rituals and practices to support their spiritual beliefs (Andrews & Boyle 2007).

There are many types of religion. Some religions are monotheistic, whereas some involve the worship of many different gods. People who follow a Christian faith, for example, believe in Jesus of Nazareth being the Messiah, or Christ, while Muslims submit to their god 'Allah'. New Zealand traditional Māori base their lives on beliefs in many gods that represent the forces of nature; two such gods are *Papa tu nuku*, the Earth Mother, and *Ranginui*, the Sky Father (Belich 2001).

Some people, including traditional Māori and Australian Aboriginal people, live a life that is permeated by a religious consciousness. For some Australian Aboriginal people this consciousness envelops a knowledge that there is a life beyond this physical world. This consciousness stems from a belief in the laws of the Dreamtime brought down by the Supreme Intelligence — the Creator. Aboriginal and Māori people have been subjected to the influences of Christianity, some choosing between Christianity and traditional spiritual beliefs, while others have chosen to engage in a mixture of the two (Tracey 2000).

A mixture of beliefs is not unusual in multicultural societies like Australia and New Zealand. Many people select parts of spiritual faiths from a range of religions, the parts of each that feel right for them in their quest to define themselves spiritually and to find meaning in life (Ferrell & Coyle 2006).

For some people religion has no bearing on their spirituality (Saucier-Lundy & Janes 2003). Atheists, for example, do not believe in the existence of God but can be very spiritual, often finding meaning in life through their work, other activities and achievements and their relationships with others.

RITUALISING

Many religions have set rituals (Mauk & Schmidt 2004). Christian denominations, for example, celebrate major life events such as birth, marriage and death, but ritual behaviour also includes many non-religious practices. Non-religious rituals can be metaphorical acts full of symbolic meaning. Setting up a room with personal belongings — things of importance like photographs, paintings and books and other treasures — can be seen as a way of exalting the spirit. When these objects are displayed, an ordinary space becomes special. English (1998) explains this as a spiritual action — a ritualising behaviour that turns the blank space into a sacred place. He suggests that many everyday behaviours, such as wearing particular clothes, getting body parts pierced or getting hair groomed in certain ways, are all rituals that express the inner spirit. He describes other actions such as going through a wedding ceremony or 'coming out' as gay as types of rituals that contribute to providing an over-arching meaning to life.

MEDITATION

Meditation is a practice that involves stillness of the body and inward reflection that, with practice, can bring about a corresponding stillness in the mind. It helps to reduce undisciplined thoughts and bring a sense of inner peace. Meditation can lead to a sense of being more in harmony with the laws of nature. It is a means of reducing stress and attaining personal growth and spiritual insights and it is possible for the calmness it induces to help a person deal with suffering and pain (O'Brien 2003; Stevens-Barnum 2003). It is an important component of Eastern culture, where philosophical traditions focus on the person as a spiritual being, with a spiritual goal. While it is predominantly an Eastern cultural practice, interest in meditation as a way to promote spiritual wellbeing is growing in Western culture.

SELF-EXPRESSION

Spiritual health is to do with finding out who you are and being that person. It is also about liking who you are. Writing or playing music, drawing or painting or writing poetry are some ways that help people find out who they are. Feeling spiritually at ease is about being happy with where you are, what you are doing in life and where you are headed (Sherwood 1997). Some people describe various activities as being spiritual. For example, a hang-glider might describe being alone in the air surrounded by beautiful sky and scenery as a spiritual experience. A deep-sea diver might feel the same about being alone in the depths of the ocean. Life experiences that provide moments of ecstasy can have a deep impact on the inner self. It can be said that such experiences are 'good for the soul', and soul tends to be viewed by some as synonymous with spirit. It is recommended that student nurses refer to the work of Kliewer and Saultz (2006) who explain differences between the soul and the spirit of a person. They provide insights into the meanings assigned to these facets of the human condition across a range of religious and cultural belief systems.

LOVING AND BEING LOVED

Part of being spiritual is about the ability to love and be loved (Maher 2005). The love can relate to that between people or to love of God. Some, but not all, people have a wonderful capacity to give and receive love. Spiritual health is enhanced when people give and receive love to their maximum capacity (English 1998; Maher 2005). For some people, being spiritual is related to having an intuitive feeling about some infinite source of energy and love.

Thus, spiritual feelings may come about through prayer, meditation, communing with nature, moments of sheer pleasure or through experiences of serious loss, pain and extreme distress. They also evolve from social and cultural influences (Andrews & Boyle 2007; O'Brien 2003).

CULTURE AND SPIRITUALITY

Social norms and cultural practices and beliefs become enmeshed into the spiritual sense of who we are and where we belong, whether or not we are conscious of it. Tradition, folklore, history, national, local and regional customs and education are all powerful influences that contribute to how people construct images of themselves. This image incorporates a spiritual dimension. When this spiritual dimension of personhood is challenged it can be the cause of psychological distress. One clear example is that of Aboriginal people, whose spiritual relationship with the land and way of living has been disrupted by white settlement. Removal from this spiritual dimension of their lives is the root of the psychological distress and social problems Aboriginal people still experience today (refer to Chapters 9 and 10).

In Australia and New Zealand many communities are made up of mixed cultural groups within which there are an assortment of traditions. The population in the communities is not static. The ebb and flow and mixing of people over time sees new ways of life emerge. There can be a blurring of boundaries between old traditions and new ways. The result is a melting pot containing the promise of new customs and cultures. The impact of cultures emerging within cultures is exciting. It has an effect on how people develop and express spiritual meanings in their lives and this will be unique to each person (Maville & Huerta 2001; Smith 2002).

SPIRITUAL HEALTH

Spiritual wellbeing can be defined as inner harmony that stems from a strong sense of satisfaction with self and with life. Spiritual health develops over time; it is a process that begins in childhood and continues throughout life (Hodges & Tod 2007). It is not static and can be challenged and changed by life events (Lewenson & Truglio-Londrigan 2007). Situations that alter a sense of self, such as ageing, grief, bereavement or illness that impacts on functioning or appearance, can disturb inner harmony and contentment (MacKinlay 2003; Shives 2007; Smith 2002). However, major life changes or challenges sometimes help people to grow more spiritual (Clinical Interest Box 11.1).

SPIRITUAL HEALTH AND PSYCHOLOGICAL WELLBEING

There are links between a person's spiritual health and their psychological wellbeing (Greenstreet 2006: Seaward 2006). The person who has not developed as a mature, psychologically strong person or who encounters significant psychological problems in life is sometimes unable to

CLINICAL INTEREST BOX 11.1
Spiritual growth

After 10 years of caring for his wife who, as a result of multiple sclerosis. has gradually become more dependent and is now quadriplegic, Jim stated: 'On reflection, I am a better person for having to care for her, I feel I am repaying her for all the years she gave to me and the kids. I feel I have given something back and I feel more satisfied within myself. Some days, even though it's hard doing everything for her, I have this inner serenity that I never ever had working at the factory. At first I was really angry but now I can see that God has done this for a purpose.'

(Funnell 1998)

CLINICAL INTEREST BOX 11.2
Spiritual pain

Conflict between beliefs and what is happening can cause a spiritual crisis. In the following case, spiritual pain is easy to recognise.

> I was brought up as a Catholic and I've always believed in God. Since I was a small child I've thought God was good, but there can't be a God, can there — what God would take a mother away from her children when they are so young? None of it was true, was it? I want to change things, forget the Church, tell the priest I don't want to be buried, I don't want that claptrap. Just put me in a box and cremate me.
>
> *(Anne, age 32, 4 weeks before she died of lung cancer)*

develop meaningful relationships (Shives 2007; Videbeck 2007). Failure to experience mutual love and concern in relationships can limit the ability to gain inner harmony and a sense of satisfaction with self and life (Videbeck 2007; Watkins 2000).

A lack of mutually caring relationships is often a feature in the lives of people needing mental health care (Videbeck 2007). Many clients in this area suffer a serious lack of inner harmony and are demoralised and dispirited. Enlightened nurses working in mental health recognise that recovery of the spirit is essential to recovery of a sense of wellbeing in these clients. The aim of care therefore encompasses the fostering of supportive relationships as well as nourishing the spirit in a variety of other ways. Some activities promoted by mental health nurses to nourish the spirits of their clients include horticultural therapy, art, music, poetry and drama therapy (Watkins 2000).

SPIRITUAL PAIN

Spiritual pain can occur when people are unable to find meaning in life or when they cannot find sources of hope, love or comfort. It can occur when a person's inner peace is disturbed, which may be caused by conflict between beliefs and what is happening to them (Olson 1997; Smith 2002).

Any life event causing loss of identity, self-esteem or control over what is happening can result in overwhelming distress or spiritual crisis (O'Brien 2007; Shives 2007; Watkins 2000). Mental illness, getting old, the onset of dementia or any illness that alters appearance or bodily function challenges a person's sense of identity and can impact negatively on self-esteem (Daniels 2004; Puddner 2000). Feelings of losing control are not uncommon, particularly in clients who suffer chronic pain, are facing unexpected disability or who are faced with a life-threatening illness. Dire circumstances often challenge a client's religious and spiritual beliefs (Clinical Interest Box 11.2). Sometimes the client's spiritual pain is clear but sometimes it is difficult to recognise and easily missed or ignored (Loseth 2002).

Recognising spiritual pain

Nurses need to be alert for themes in conversation that reflect spiritual concerns. Themes the client may focus on include feelings of:

- Unfairness (Why me?)
- Unworthiness (I'm only a burden now.)
- Hopelessness (What's the point in going on?)
- Meaninglessness (I've done nothing with my life.)
- Guilt (This is a punishment for my sins.)
- Isolation (No one can really understand.)
- Vulnerability (I don't think I will cope.)
- Abandonment (God doesn't care.)
- Anger and confusion (Why does God allow this to happen?)

(Orchard 2001; Shives 2007; Videbeck 2007)

Spiritual anxieties may be linked to the past, the present or the future. Events of the past may be the source of painful memories or feelings of guilt, such as unresolved conflict with a family member or guilt about an event such as an undisclosed extra-marital affair.

The present may give rise to feelings of isolation and anger about what is happening. For example, a client with early-onset dementia may feel very isolated when there are communication difficulties with friends and family. Angry feelings might arise as a result of the losses being suffered, such as loss of the provider role if the person was forced to leave paid work.

People may experience fear and hopelessness about the future. For example, a client who has hemiplegia and a speech deficit after a cerebrovascular accident (CVA) may fear being able to cope and may have a sense of hopelessness about living with the physical changes. Clients facing terminal illness may have a range of fears about dying and impending death (Ferrell & Coyle 2006).

Some other changes to usual behaviour may also be a sign of spiritual distress. These include:

- Agitation or restlessness
- Sleep disturbances
- Discomfort or physical pain in the absence of a physical cause
- Inconsistent and unexplained changes in mood

- Social isolation (especially rejection of people associated with spiritual heritage or religious background).

These changes can indicate psychological or physical distress, but a sad or distressed spirit can be reflected in these ways too (Carpenito-Moyet 2006). This reinforces the need for holistic assessment — all facets of health need to be assessed concurrently.

SPIRITUAL HEALING AND THE NURSE

The client in spiritual distress, possibly more than any other, needs a healing relationship. The nurse, in having the closest contact with clients, is in a privileged position, ideally placed to form healing relationships. Some of the attributes that help the nurse in developing such relationships are:

- Ability to accept the client unconditionally as a worthy person
- Genuineness
- Non-judgmental attitude
- Strong communication skills (active listening, reflection, clarification, etc)
- The ability to convey the sense of being fully focused on the client during times together
- Humility (acknowledging one's own limitations)
- Commitment (to sharing in the client's journey for a while)
- Ability to recognise one's own personal spirituality.

(Stein-Parbury 2005)

Healing relationships involve being there when a client needs support, even when it is emotionally difficult to do so, such as being with a client after her baby has died. Healing relationships involve being there and giving of oneself in a rich way that is very much more than merely 'doing for' a client. By actively sharing in the loneliness, anxiety and suffering of the client, the nurse in a healing relationship does much more than merely provide physical comfort and treatment. The nurse's presence itself touches the client's spirit by communicating personal spiritual strength, a willingness to care, to listen and to be available (Hood & Leddy 2005; O'Brien 2007; Stein-Parbury 2005).

Being with clients in this way is sometimes referred to as 'therapeutic use of self' or 'presencing'. The presence of the nurse can be important to the client during times that to nurses are everyday situations but to clients are stressful experiences (Clinical Interest Box 11.3). Presencing relates to meaningful giving of self whenever the client needs it most (Solimine 2002).

Healing relationships can be mutually beneficial. The experience of working this closely with other human beings helps nurses to discover more about themselves and moves them towards a deeper understanding of their own spirituality (Olson 1997; Watkins 2000; Ronaldson & Potter 2004).

Intervention in spiritual matters is easier for nurses who have an awareness of their own spirituality, whether it is based on religious convictions or not. It is acknowledged that nurses who reflect on their own personal spirituality and who continually monitor the meeting of their own spiritual needs are best able to understand the meaning of spiritual health. Such nurses are more comfortable in helping relationships and in dealing with clients' spiritual issues (Ronaldson 1997; Ronaldson & Potter 2004). Nurses who do not have personal awareness of their own spiritual nature are advised to take steps along the path of spiritual development. One way to start this process is for nurses to ask themselves the same questions they ask of clients when undertaking spiritual assessment. Personal spiritual awareness enables nurses to provide care that is truly holistic (Ronaldson & Potter 2004; Watkins 2000).

Help with spiritual needs can in fact be more problematic for nurses who have a strong religious faith or very strong views about particular practices, such as being strongly opposed to abortion. It may be harder for nurses with strong views to reserve judgment and to be tolerant and respectful when the practices and beliefs of clients are not compatible with their own.

All nurses need to be aware of their personal values and beliefs and be sensitive to the fact that they may inadvertently lead to assumptions about a client's wishes or needs. False assumptions can be a source of concern and may damage the spiritual wellbeing of clients.

CLINICAL INTEREST BOX 11.3
Presencing: meaningful giving of self

I was really anxious about what was causing the problem and really scared about having the tube put in to drain my urine. One nurse was doing the procedure and the other one stood at the top of the bed. I only found out later she was a student nurse. When the nurse was having trouble positioning the tube the student nurse took my hand and gave it a squeeze. She didn't say anything but her eyes and her smile were so reassuring. I never did find out her name but I was glad she was there.

(Anne Smith, age 44)

WHY NURSES MAY AVOID DEALING WITH SPIRITUAL MATTERS

Spirituality is an area of client care that many nurses may tend to avoid, perhaps because they perceive spiritual matters as too personal, or perhaps because they do not have a clear understanding of their own spirituality and feel inept. There is a tendency for some nurses to believe that the hospital chaplain or pastoral care worker should be the person to deal with spiritual issues. Referral to others may be best at times but nurses need to conduct a spiritual assessment to find out if this is so. Often the novice nurse will be in the process of developing the interpersonal skills necessary to help clients with spiritual needs. The help of others will be needed to help clients understand the meaning of illness and loss in their lives. However, sometimes the skilled empathic nurse, with or without a particular religion, is the person most able to provide

CLINICAL INTEREST BOX 11.4
The nurse and spiritual matters

The nurse may be the best person to help uplift a client's spirit:

> After the accident, when I was in the rehabilitation ward, I was so down — I knew I would never walk again. So many people came to be with me — lots of my friends, the counsellor, all my family. It was important to know they were all there for me but there was one nurse, Judy — I'll never forget her — she made so much difference. She sat and held me when I cried, and that was often then, but she never made me feel I was self-pitying. She understood, but she was also gently encouraging. She made me stronger, helped me to start feeling positive. When she went off duty she always said, 'I will pray for you, I will ask God to give you the strength to get through this'. Well, I'm not religious — never have been — but it was kind of nice, it lifted me, knowing that she cared enough to do that.
>
> *(Andrew, age 37)*

support for the client's spirit (Young & Koopsen 2005) (Clinical Interest Box 11.4).

SPIRITUALITY AND NURSING ASSESSMENT

Not every client needs help with spiritual matters but it is important to assess whether or not nursing actions are required. Holistic care entails assessing the whole range of human functioning and determining which interventions are appropriate. Clients who require help do not necessarily require direct intervention in every area assessed. They may be able to manage mobility, nutrition and hygiene without intervention. Similarly, clients do not automatically require interventions with spiritual issues. This may be one area of need that they can manage independently. Spiritual needs and beliefs are highly personal matters for many people. Nurses, pastoral care workers and other professionals must be careful not to intrude inappropriately. However, spiritual assessment is essential. If needs exist and are not identified, the client can be left without help and in serious spiritual distress.

Spiritual needs are as important to determine as any other. This may be difficult because, like some nurses, not all clients have a clear understanding of what spirituality is or of what sustains them spiritually. The following are some general questions that can help begin the exploration of spiritual matters:

- What is the purpose of your life?
- What gives your life meaning?
- What do you do to bring joy into your life?
- How is the state of your health impacting on your life? Your family? Your situation?
- What bothers you most about being ill?
- What are your sources of help? Who are the most important people in your life? Who do you turn to when you need help?
- What is the role of religion in your life?
- What religious practices are important to you?
- What sort of help do you need right now?
- How may we help?

(Boyd 2007; Sherwood 1997; O'Brien 2007)

To plan and implement care that is responsive to spiritual needs, beliefs and values need to be considered as part of assessment. Cultural, spiritual and psychological dimensions are interlinked and need to be considered together. In multicultural societies like Australia and New Zealand the range of difference in beliefs and practices is vast. In this chapter it is only possible to provide a few examples of some beliefs and practices that impact on nursing care (see Table 11.1).

These examples are included to raise awareness of difference. It is not possible here to look at all religious and cultural groups and the extensive range of beliefs and practices they encompass. It is emphasised that the beliefs and practices of migrants, refugees and Indigenous people may reflect an intermingling of traditional and Western cultural influences. Nurses need to assess the needs of each client individually. Areas where beliefs and practices vary and need to be considered in relation to nursing care include:

- Rituals and sacraments
- Diet and fasting
- Modesty needs
- Ritual ablutions and washing
- Pregnancy, labour and birth
- Abortion and contraception
- Circumcision
- Transfusions and transplants
- Care of the dying
- Care of the body after death
- Autopsies.

(Andrews & Boyle 2007; Kirkwood 1998)

(See Chapters 14 and 43 for issues concerning death and dying.)

When nurses are not sure of how to talk about or assess spiritual issues, formal assessment tools can be helpful. The Jarel Spirituality Well-Being Scale (Table 11.2) is one tool that can assist the nurse to identify the older client's spiritual strengths or areas of distress. However, use of this or a similar tool should not replace client–nurse interactions. The nurse must strive to develop excellent interpersonal skills and the ability to communicate empathically with clients on even the most personal and intimate of issues (Stein-Parbury 2005). Completion of a questionnaire does not enhance the rapport and trust between a client and nurse in the same way as honest and open communication. (Communication skills are discussed in Chapter 29.)

CARE PLANNING AND NURSING INTERVENTIONS

After assessment is completed, the client and nurse, together with family members or other carers when appropriate, plan what needs to be implemented to ensure that the

TABLE 11.1 | Beliefs and practices

Religion	Beliefs	Practices
Agnostic	Impossible to know if God exists	Specific moral values may guide behaviour
Atheist	God does not exist	
Christian (e.g. Baptist, Churches of God, Churches of Christ, Pentecostal [Assemblies of God])	May consider illness as a divine punishment or trial and that strength, coping and divine healing come through prayer and a belief in God	Some prohibit medical therapy. Feelings may be openly expressed
Buddhism	May consider illness a trial that develops the soul	May refuse treatment on holy days. Cleanliness is of great importance
Christian Science	Illness is caused by errors in thought and mind. Healing is a spiritual renewal	May oppose: drugs; IV fluid; blood transfusions; physical examination; ear, eye or blood-pressure testing; and other medical or nursing interventions
Eastern Orthodox (Greek Orthodox, Russian Orthodox, Armenian)	May oppose euthanasia and favour every effort to maintain life	Russian Orthodox males may refuse shaving
Hinduism	May minimise illness and consider it only important as it affects one's spiritual quest. Illness or injury may represent sins committed in a previous life. Reincarnation is a central belief	Self-control, self-discipline and cleanliness are emphasised
Judaism	Medical care emphasised	May oppose surgical procedures on the Sabbath (sunset Friday to sunset Saturday). May oppose shaving. May wish to wear skull cap and socks continuously, believing head and feet should be covered
Muslim	May perceive illness as God's (Allah's) will. May not show fear or doubt about illness. Expression of emotion such as anger or showing fears about pain and personal safety are seen as a weakness and may be interpreted as indicating a lack of submission to the will of Allah. Dying people should not be informed about their prognosis. It is wrong for unfamiliar men (including nurses) to touch another man's wife without permission. Male nurses and medical officers need to seek this permission	Rituals for cleanliness are important. Preparation for worship includes washing the body three times, sniffing water up the nose and washing out the mouth. Wet hands are rubbed through hair to remove dust. Devout Muslims may wish to do this 5 times a day, but exemption due to illness is possible. A jug of water is needed for cleansing of private parts after use of the toilet (it is not possible to pray without this washing).

(Kirkwood 1998; Carpenito-Moyet 2006; Patrinos & White 2001)

client's spiritual needs are met. A spiritual care plan must be centred on each individual client and include realistic short- and long-term goals.

The plan must include ways to:

- Enable the client to continue with religious and spiritual rituals and practices
- Enhance connections with people who can provide spiritual support for the client
- Facilitate activities that promote the client's inner tranquillity and sense of harmony
- Enhance the client's personal quest for meaning and self-awareness
- Promote hope.

(McIntyre & Chaplin 2001; Searle 2001)

ENABLING THE CLIENT TO CONTINUE WITH RELIGIOUS AND SPIRITUAL RITUALS AND PRACTICES

Clients who wish to continue religious practices or spiritual rituals while in hospital or other care facilities need a private and quiet environment in which to conduct them. Many care facilities have a non-denominational area set aside for this purpose. Use of this area needs to be orchestrated to fit in with what is appropriate to the client's religion, and timing will need to take account of physical care needs. The nurse also needs to ensure that workload is managed efficiently to assist the client who needs help with mobility and access.

In addition to organising visits to a designated place of worship, the nurse can promote a suitable environment for the expression of spiritual needs by:

TABLE 11.2 | Jarel Spirituality Well-Being Scale

Directions: Please circle the choice that best describes how much you agree with each statement. Circle only one answer for each statement. There is no right or wrong answer.

	Strongly Agree	Moderately Agree	Agree	Disagree	Moderately Disagree	Strongly Disagree
1. Prayer is an important part of my life.	SA	MA	A	D	MD	SD
2. I believe I have spiritual well-being.	SA	MA	A	D	MD	SD
3. As I grow older, I find myself more tolerant of others' beliefs.	SA	MA	A	D	MD	SD
4. I find meaning and purpose in my life.	SA	MA	A	D	MD	SD
5. I feel there is a close relationship between my spiritual beliefs and what I do.	SA	MA	A	D	MD	SD
6. I believe in an afterlife.	SA	MA	A	D	MD	SD
7. When I am sick I have less spiritual well-being.	SA	MA	A	D	MD	SD
8. I believe in a supreme power.	SA	MA	A	D	MD	SD
9. I am able to receive and give love to others.	SA	MA	A	D	MD	SD
10. I am satisfied with my life.	SA	MA	A	D	MD	SD
11. I set goals for myself.	SA	MA	A	D	MD	SD
12. God has little meaning in my life.	SA	MA	A	D	MD	SD
13. I am satisfied with the way I am using my abilities.	SA	MA	A	D	MD	SD
14. Prayer does not help me in making decisions.	SA	MA	A	D	MD	SD
15. I am able to appreciate differences in others.	SA	MA	A	D	MD	SD
16. I am pretty well put together.	SA	MA	A	D	MD	SD
17. I prefer that others make decisions for me.	SA	MA	A	D	MD	SD
18. I find it hard to forgive others.	SA	MA	A	D	MD	SD
19. I accept my life situations.	SA	MA	A	D	MD	SD
20. Belief in a supreme being has no part of my life.	SA	MA	A	D	MD	SD
21. I cannot accept change in my life.	SA	MA	A	D	MD	SD

FACTOR I: FAITH/BELIEF DIMENSION
(Scoring: SA = 6; SD = 1)
Item 1
Item 2
Item 3
Item 4
Item 5
Item 6
Item 8 Subscore

FACTOR II: LIFE/SELF RESPONSIBILITY
(Reverse Scoring: SA = 1; SD = 6)
Item 7
Item 12
Item 14
Item 17
Item 18
Item 20
Item 21 Subscore

TABLE 11.2 | Jarel Spirituality Well-Being Scale

FACTOR III: LIFE SATISFACTION/SELF-ACTUALISATION		
(Scoring: SA = 6; SD = 1)		
Item 9		
Item 10		
Item 11		
Item 13		
Item 15		
Item 16		
Item 19	Subscore	Total score
(Hungelmann et al, in: Ebersole & Hess 2001)		

- Closing the door or pulling curtains to provide privacy
- Planning nursing activities to allow the client uninterrupted time
- Minimising extraneous noise, e.g., televisions or radios
- Minimising interference from other clients, telephones, cleaning and other activities as much as possible.

For clients who have difficulty the nurse may need to help with such tasks as ritual washing procedures in preparation for prayer, holding rosary beads or turning pages in a prayer book. The nurse can help clients who want to pray by allowing time for them to do so; for example, before meals and before settling down to sleep at night. Clients need to know that their religious or spiritual possessions are safe while they sleep and at other times. The nurse has a role in protecting belongings such as statues, pictures, written material, clothing or other religious icons.

Religious doctrines include rules that dictate a particular lifestyle. Rules relate to various aspects of daily life, such as diet, personal hygiene and modesty. Illness and hospitalisation can make it difficult for people to observe these rules (Kirkwood 1998). The nurse has a role in helping clients to maintain practices that are of spiritual importance to them. For example, there is often a need for the nurse to work collaboratively with the client and dietitian, the aim being to ensure that meals are consistent with the client's religious practices but not detrimental to physical health or the effects of treatment.

The beliefs and values associated with religious doctrines can be a source of stress when people need to have medical or nursing interventions For example, clients who follow Judaism may oppose being shaved for surgical interventions, and nakedness is anathema to many Muslims. Muslim women are usually clothed from head to toe so that the shape of the body is not visible and they may wish their bodies to remain this way, even when in bed. Great sensitivity is needed during all care procedures and there may be particular challenges, for example, when it is required that a Muslim woman don a hospital gown for surgery (Kirkwood 1998). Patients' spiritual and religious needs are diverse. Orchard (2001) and Kirkwood (1998) provide helpful insights for nurses caring for patients of Christian, Jewish, Muslim and 'multi-faith' beliefs and practices.

Some religious and spiritual practices present significant challenges to Western medical ideas and treatments and sometimes cause ethical dilemmas for medical officers and nurses (O'Brien 2007; Stevens-Barnum 2003; Young & Koopsen 2005). For example, a client who follows the beliefs of the Jehovah's Witnesses is likely to oppose blood transfusion or organ transplantation, and some Buddhists may refuse treatment on holy days. Interventions that impinge on values and beliefs can cause spiritual distress and can be very damaging to the way clients perceive themselves as spiritual beings.

Prayer

If the nurse feels comfortable it may be helpful to pray with a client if this is requested (O'Brien 2003). The nurse should not pray with or for a client unless it is requested or permission is given. If the nurse is of a different faith it is important to ask how the client prays. For example, it would not be appropriate for a nurse to pray to Jesus with a client who is Jewish; praying to God or to the God of Abraham, Isaac and Moses would be appropriate (Carson 1989). If the nurse is not comfortable with prayer it is better to be honest about this. An alternative is perhaps to suggest a few moments silent meditation, and a referral to someone who can help with prayer.

There are some important ethical considerations concerning nurses and prayer:

- The nurse should always ask, 'Whose need is this meeting — my own or the client's?'
- The act of praying with a client should not be based on instinct that it is needed; it should always be based on careful assessment that demonstrates a spiritual need
- Prayer should never be used in a way that communicates unrealistic expectations or false hope
- Prayer should never be used as a substitute for

listening to the client or exploring issues that concern the client (Carson 1989; O'Brien 2003).

ENHANCING CONNECTIONS WITH PEOPLE WHO CAN PROVIDE SPIRITUAL SUPPORT FOR THE CLIENT

If a client wishes to have visits from the hospital chaplain or from a member of a particular religious group, the nurse will need to take the necessary steps to ensure such visits. Many health care facilities offer pastoral care services, which can be a valuable source of help for clients and staff in spiritual matters. Pastoral care services are inter-denominational and are often able to offer spiritual care across a wide range of religions, including non-Christian ones (Ronaldson & Potter 2005). The nurse has a role in facilitating meetings with any person, not just those connected to religious services, who can provide spiritual support and with whom the client wishes to spend time.

FACILITATING ACTIVITIES THAT PROMOTE INNER TRANQUILLITY AND HARMONY

The spirit can be nurtured in a variety of ways. Some clients may wish to practise the art of meditation while in hospital. The nurse may need to facilitate this by providing some physical support to help the client maintain the position normally used for meditation. The nurse may need to locate a suitably secluded place; this may be as simple as finding a quiet spot in the hospital grounds. Other clients may also value the opportunity to get outside, simply to enjoy the surroundings. Others may benefit from the provision of any peaceful environment where they can relax and read a book or listen to favourite pieces of music.

Inner tranquillity and harmony: people in residential care

People in long-term care may benefit from activities and visits to people and places that uplift the spirit, such as public or zoological gardens, or concerts and other places of entertainment. Nurses who participate in such activities can be rewarded and uplifted themselves by the positive responses that residents demonstrate when enjoying these, for some, infrequent pleasures.

Other measures can have a positive effect on the lives of older adults living in residential settings. Some aged-care facilities arrange for local school children to visit (Clinical Interest Box 11.5) and many have resident pets. In their off-duty time, some generous nurses bring their own pets and even their new babies to visit, to share their joys with the residents. These are caring interventions that can have a heartening effect on the residents' spirits.

Remembering the past can also have an uplifting effect and bring new sense to the present. *Reminiscence therapy* is characterised by deliberately and regularly encouraging people to recall positive experiences from their past (Miller 2004). The time spent with residents looking at old photographs and other memorabilia can provoke memories and images that can be shared. The time together provides companionship, and the sharing of memories allows the nurse to validate the client's life and worth. For example, saying 'I'll bet you were a good mum to those children' validates the resident's role as a mother. Validation of past experiences and achievements recognises the person as a valuable individual and raises self-esteem (Feil 2002; Miller 2004).

This acceptance by another person can also increase the resident's acceptance of self. Self-esteem and self-confidence can be further enhanced if the person is reminded of past difficulties that were overcome (Feil 2002). Reminiscing with residents enables them to make sense of their lives and connects them with those who listen. It provides the nurse with an opportunity to link with the spirit within. Positive memories and reinforcement of self-worth helps to strengthen the spirit and promotes the resident's inner serenity (Feil 2002).

CLINICAL INTEREST BOX 11.5
Lifting the spirits of aged-care residents

'I haven't any young grandchildren at all here, so I take these children as my grandchildren, and I'm not the only one — all the grandmothers here feel the same way.'
'It builds up our spirits — we're very pleased to have them coming to see us. They sit down and have a talk and read stories to us. Well, it brightens our day.'
'You sort of put your arm around them, and have a little chat with them and it is good for you because it makes you feel less lonely'.
(Older people commenting on visits from school children, Australian Broadcasting Corporation 1991)

Inner tranquillity and harmony: the role of complementary health care

A range of complementary health care techniques may help clients to achieve inner tranquillity and harmony. These include several touch-based therapies such as massage, Reiki and therapies concerned with emotions, such as relaxation, guided imagery and aromatherapy (Brydie 2005; Hood & Leddy 2005; Macnish 2001). Some nurses are implementing these therapies into their nursing practice; for example, aromatherapy and guided imagery are thought to be of considerable value in palliative care. However, nurses are advised not to implement these therapies without adequate training, safety protocols and specific management guidelines (Macnish 2001).

Inner tranquillity and harmony: specific issues for the dying

The interpersonal skills of the nurse and the ability to 'be with' clients are the most valuable tools for meeting spiritual needs, especially of those who are dying. In addition to the interpersonal skills and other interventions mentioned previously there are two specific things for the nurse to facilitate that can help the dying client achieve inner peace. The first is assisting the person to complete any unfinished business or things they wish to achieve but have not yet done. The second is ensuring that they are given permission to die if it is needed (Olson 1997).

Byock (1997) says that unfinished business often relates to interpersonal relationship issues. He suggests that the dying person may need to make one or more of five particular types of communication at the end of life to have a sense of completion. These are:

- 'I love you'
- 'I forgive you'
- 'Please forgive me'
- 'I'm sorry'
- 'Goodbye'.

These sorts of communications are necessary to be at peace with oneself and with others. They are indicative of honesty about love and the need to let go of angry feelings, grudges and the pain that stems from hurtful relationships. Forgiveness is not only important to spiritual wellbeing at the end of life, it is an important component at other times of challenge. For example, forgiveness is linked to positive adjustment to disability and loss (Solimine 2002).

Some relatives relate how it seems that loved ones struggle with the last goodbye — that they seem to need permission to go before they die. Nurses who have established a caring relationship with clients and their families will be able to gently guide relatives towards giving this permission (see Clinical Interest Box 11.6).

ENHANCING THE CLIENT'S PERSONAL QUEST FOR MEANING AND SELF-AWARENESS

By their presence in a healing relationship, confident nurses can assist clients to develop self-awareness. The interpersonal skills and personal attributes of an empathic, therapeutic nurse can help clients clarify their thoughts and feelings, clearing the way for them to make meaning out of their past and current illness experience. Nurses working in specialist areas often develop and use extra knowledge and skills that enable clients to find meaning and self-awareness. For example, a specialist nurse in a palliative care multidisciplinary team may use techniques such as breathing exercises, aromatherapy, reflexology, music and art appreciation to help clients achieve this (Searle 2001). The ultimate goal is to help clients transcend negative circumstances and achieve a sense of meaning in being alive despite the problems they face.

CLINICAL INTEREST BOX 11.6
Permission to go

I am the last of 10 children, the youngest. She was my last surviving sister. She didn't want to leave me and I didn't want her to go. But she had suffered so much and she was struggling for her breath. I think she was fighting to stay with me. The nurse said she needed to know it was OK to go. I lay down on the bed and put my arms around her. I told her I loved her and that I would be alright, that I would be with her and the others soon. I told her she should go and within a few hours she died. It was the hardest thing I ever had to do.

(Alice, age 77)

PROMOTING HOPE

Hope is inextricably linked to finding purpose in life and as such is an essential spiritual need. Without hope, people are spiritually bereft. Even when people are facing death at the end of a terminal illness, hope is essential and needs to be nurtured. Hope at this time may mean hoping to live long enough to be with a daughter on her birthday, or hope for a peaceful death or a smooth journey to an afterlife.

It has been long been recognised that hope strengthens people facing adversity (McIntyre & Chaplin 2001). While hope strengthens the ability to cope, the capacity to hope is severely challenged by many health-related conditions. For example, maintaining hope can be difficult when facing an unrelenting chronic illness. Protracted illness can create physical and mental exhaustion and engender feelings of being out of control. This can lead to stress and feelings of hopelessness. Nursing interventions that reduce physical and mental exhaustion, minimise stress and retrieve a sense of control can reignite hope. A supportive relationship and the nurse's ability to ensure physical ease are therefore vital. Keeping the client informed reduces stress and uncertainty and promotes a feeling of control (Chaplin & McIntyre 2001). Therefore the nurse who ensures that the client is provided with prompt and clear information about what is happening or likely to happen helps foster hope.

McIntyre and Chaplin (2001) interrelate three key elements to sustaining hope. These are comfort, attachment and worth (Figure 11.1). These elements are equated with physical ease, caring relationships and feeling valued. While

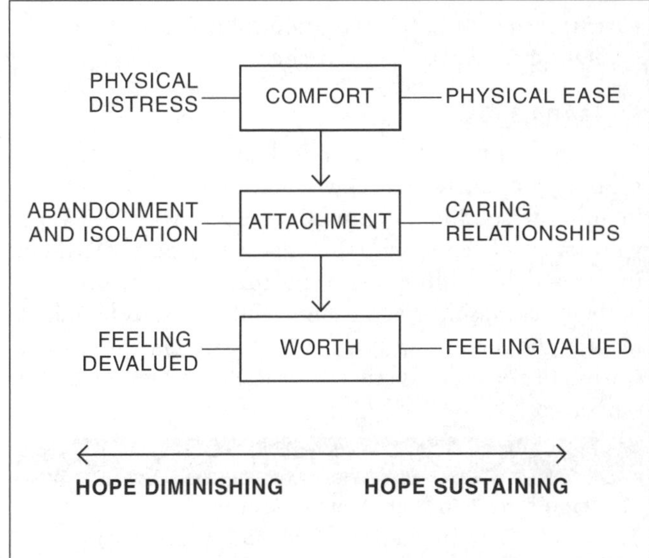

Figure 11.1 | Interrelationships of the three key elements *(modified from Kinghorn & Gaines 2007: 113)*

they have been developed from a palliative care perspective, they are also applicable to clients of all ages across many health care situations.

Nurses have an important role in fostering hope in their clients. However, some clients have the inner resources to keep themselves positive and hopeful throughout even the most challenging illness, or even when facing death. Nurses must be wary of making value judgments about those who cannot do so.

This section provided a very brief introduction to the issue of hope. Nurses are recommended to refer to the rehabilitation and palliative care literature to explore deeper understandings of this concept and its importance in nursing.

MEETING SPIRITUAL NEEDS: NURSING EVALUATION

Evaluation is a component of the nursing process that asks whether nursing interventions used were effective and the goals of care met. Only the nurse who really knows the client can evaluate spirituality effectively. This is because the client's feelings and communications more than actions are what reveal spiritual distress or spiritual wellness, and either is a matter of degree. Some of the issues the nurse needs to identify in the process of evaluation include:

- Does the client feel supported and cared about?
- Does the client express confidence in the nursing care provided?
- Does the client have a degree of self-acceptance?
- Does the client demonstrate hope in a positive future?
- Does the client have relationships with others that are spiritually sustaining?
- Does the client express pleasure in life?
- Does the client appear calm or anxious, or has anxiety reduced?
- Has the client been able to continue with religious and spiritual practices as desired?

SUMMARY

A person's spiritual dimension is not easy to identify, measure or evaluate. Nurses who communicate with clients in an understanding, compassionate and warm way and who accept all people without judgment engage with them in a way that is infused with spirituality. It is within this healing relationship that the nurse will most easily be able to identify the client's spiritual needs, implement appropriate spiritual care and, together with the client, evaluate the outcomes.

REVIEW EXERCISES

1. How is religion connected to spirituality?
2. In what ways might people who do not hold religious beliefs express their spirituality?
3. What might be the consequences if a client's spiritual concerns are not met?
4. What are the ethical considerations that a nurse should reflect on before agreeing or deciding to pray with a client?
5. What are the themes in conversation that might indicate that a client is experiencing spiritual distress?
6. What are the physical signs that indicate that a client might be experiencing spiritual distress?
7. What are the attributes a nurse requires to have to work therapeutically with clients in the area of spirituality?
8. What are some practical strategies that help make the hospital environment suitable for clients to conduct their religious rituals and practices?

CRITICAL THINKING EXERCISES

1. Mary Monahan, age 22, is a single lady who lives alone. She has been in hospital for several days after fractures to both her legs in a vehicle accident. Mary was brought up in the Catholic faith and normally attends church regularly. Before her accident she enjoyed singing in the church choir, yoga and swimming. In what ways might hospital routine, diagnostic tests, treatments and the range of nursing activities impact on Mary's spirituality? How might these impact if Mary was a practising Muslim?
2. Your client's name is Jack. He is a husband and a father of three sons, aged 7, 10 and 14. He is a member of the local football team and until now has worked as a plumber. His wife has told you their life together hasn't always been easy but it has been good. She says Jack has never really liked talking about death but, once when they did, he said he thought he would die when he was old, probably aged about 80, in his sleep, like his dad. But suddenly everything has changed. He is now lying in hospital waiting for surgery tomorrow on a brain tumour, after which he will have chemotherapy. Jack and his wife have been told the prognosis is not good, that the treatment is palliative. Part of Jack's head has been shaved, he has lost a lot of weight and is quite thin. Most of the time he lies in his bed staring into space. At other times he is agitated and can be quite aggressive in the way he speaks to you.
   a) How do you feel about approaching Jack regarding spiritual matters?
   b) If you feel at all concerned about approaching Jack regarding spiritual matters, what can you do personally to help with this difficulty?
   c) How would you set about exploring Jack's spiritual feelings?
   d) What attributes do you have that will assist you in supporting Jack through this illness experience?
   e) What other professionals could you call on to assist Jack?
   f) On what criteria would you instigate this referral?

REFERENCES AND FURTHER READING

Andrews M, Boyle JS (2007) *Transcultural Concepts in Nursing Care*, 5th edn. Lippincott Williams & Wilkins, Philadelphia

Australian Broadcasting Corporation (1991) *The Time of Your Life*. [Videotaped television documentary], ABC, Sydney

Baines P (2007) *Nurturing the Heart. Creativity, Art Therapy and Dementia*. Alzheimer's Australia. Quality Care Dementia Paper No. 3. Online. Available: http://www.alzheimers.org.au/upload/ArtTherapy.pdf [accessed 14 April 2008]

Belich J (2001) *Making Peoples: A History of the New Zealanders from Polynesian Settlement to the End of the Nineteenth Century*. University of Hawaii Press, Honolulu

Boyd MA (2007) *Psychiatric Nursing: Contemporary Practice*, 4th edn. Wolters Kluwer/Lippincott Williams and Wilkins, Amsterdam

Brydie S (2005) *Spirituality and Nursing*. Vantage Press, New York

Byock I (1997) *Dying Well*. Riverhead Books, New York

Carpenito-Moyet LJ (2006) *Nursing Diagnoses: Application to Clinical Practice*. Lippincott Williams and Wilkins, Philadelphia

Carson V (1989) *Spiritual Dimensions of Nursing Practice*. WB Saunders, Philadelphia

Chaplin J, McIntyre R (2001) Hope: an exploration of selected literature. In: Kinghorn S, Gamlin R (eds) *Palliative Nursing: Bringing Comfort and Hope*. Baillière Tindall, Edinburgh: 117–28

Daniels R (2004) *Nursing Fundamentals: Caring and Clinical Decision Making*. Thomson Delmar Learning, New York

Ebersole P, Hess P (2001) *Geriatric Nursing and Healthy Ageing*. Mosby, St Louis

English G (1998) An approach to spirituality. In: Parker J, Aranda S (eds) *Palliative Care: Explorations And Challenges*. MacLennan & Petty, Sydney

Feil N (2002) *The Validation Breakthrough. Simple Techniques for Communicating with People*. Health Professions Press, Baltimore, Maryland

Ferrell B, Coyle N (2006) *Textbook of Palliative Nursing*, 2nd edn. Oxford University Press, New York

Funnell R (1998) *For Better or Worse: Caregiving Husbands of Wives with Multiple Sclerosis*. [Unpublished Master's thesis] LaTrobe University, Melbourne

Greenstreet W (2006) *Integrating Spirituality in Health And Social Care: Perspectives and Practical Approaches*. Radcliffe Publishing, Oxford

Hodges B, Tod J (2007) *A Holistic Approach to Meeting Physical, Social and Psychological Needs*. In: Valentine F, Lowes L (eds) *Nursing Care of Children and Young People with Chronic Illness*. Blackwell, Hoboken, New Jersey

Hood LJ, Leddy SK (2005) *Leddy & Pepper's Conceptual Bases of Professional Nursing*. Lippincott Williams & Wilkins, Philadelphia

Hungelmann J, Kenkel Rossi E, Klassen L, Stollenwerk R (1987) In: Ebersole & Hess (2001) *Geriatric Nursing and Health Ageing*, Mosby, St Louis

Kinghorn S, Gaines S (2007) *Palliative Nursing, Improving End-of-Life Care*, 2nd edn. Baillière Tindall, Edinburgh

Kirkwood N (1998) *A Hospital Handbook on Multiculturalism and Religion*. Morehouse, Harrisburg, PA

Kliewer SP, Saultz JW (2006) *Healthcare and Spirituality*. Radcliffe, Abingdon, Oxfordshire

Lewenson SB, Truglio-Londrigan M (2007) *Decision-Making in Nursing: Thoughtful Approaches for Practice*. Jones & Bartlett, Sudbury, MA

Loseth D (2002) Psychosocial and spiritual care. In: Kuebler K, Berry P, Heidrich D (eds), *End of Life Care: Clinical Practice Guidelines*. WB Saunders, Philadelphia

MacKinlay E (2003) The Spiritual Dimension of Ageing. In Jewell A (ed.), *Ageing, Spirituality and Well Being*. Jessica Kingsley Publishers, Philadelphia

Macnish S (2001) Complementary therapies. In: Kinghorn S, Gamlin, R (eds), *Palliative Nursing: Bringing Comfort and Hope*. Baillière Tindall, Edinburgh

Maher P (2005) Reclaiming Spirituality in Nursing. In Andrist LC, Nicholas PK & Wolf K *A History of Nursing Ideas*. Jones & Bartlett, Sudbury, MA

Mauk KL & Schmidt NA (2004) *Spiritual Care in Nursing Practice*. Lippincott Williams & Wilkins, Philadelphia

Maville JA, Huerta CG (2001) *Health Promotion in Nursing*. Thomas Delman Learning, New York

McIntyre R, Chaplin J (2001) Hope: the heart of palliative care. In: Kinghorn S, Gamlin R (eds), *Palliative Nursing: Bringing Comfort and Hope*. Baillière Tindall, Edinburgh: 129–45

McSherry W (2006) *Making Sense of Spirituality in Nursing and Healthcare Practice: An Interactive Approach*, 2nd edn. Jessica Kingsley Publishers, Philadelphia

Miller CA (2004) *Nursing for Wellness in Older Adults: Theory & Practice*, 4th edn. Lippincott Williams & Wilkins, Philadelphia

Moberg J, Brusek P (1978) Spiritual well-being: a neglected subject in quality of life research. *Social Indicators Research* 5: 303–23

O'Brien EM (2007) *Spirituality in Nursing: Standing on Holy Ground*, 3rd edn. Jones & Bartlett, Sudbury, MA

—— (2003) *Prayer in Nursing: The Spirituality of Compassionate Caregiving*. Jones & Bartlett, Sudbury, MA

Olson M (1997) *Healing the Dying*. Delmar, Albany, New York

Orchard HC (2001) *Spirituality in Health Care Contexts*. Jessica Kingsley Publishers, Philadelphia

Patrinos D, White N (2001) Culturally competent rehabilitation care. In: Derstine J, Drayton Hargrove S (eds), *Comprehensive Rehabilitation Nursing 2001*. WB Saunders, Philadelphia

Puddner R (2000) *Nursing the Surgical Patient*. Elsevier, Sydney

Ronaldson S (1997) *Spirituality: The Heart of Nursing*. Ausmed Publications, Melbourne

Ronaldson S, Potter P (2005) Spiritual health. In: Crisp J, Taylor C (eds), *Potter & Perry's Fundamentals of Nursing*, 2nd edn. Elsevier Australia, Sydney

Saucier-Lundy K, Janes S (2003) *Essentials of Community Based Nursing*. Jones & Bartlett Publishing, Sudbury, MA

Searle C (2001) Spirituality: the professionals' and the patients' perspectives. In: Kinghorn S, Gamblin R (eds), *Palliative Nursing: Bringing Comfort and Hope*. Baillière Tindall, Edinburgh

Seaward BL (2006) *Managing Stress: Principles and Strategies for Health and Wellbeing*, 5th edn. Jones & Bartlett, Sudbury, MA

Sherwood G (1997) Developing spiritual care: the search for self. In: Roach S (ed) *Caring From the Heart: the Convergence of Caring and Spirituality*. Paulist Press, New York

Shives LR (2007) *Basic Concepts of Psychiatric-Mental Health Nursing*, 7th edn. Lippincott Williams & Wilkins, Philadelphia

Smith M (2002) Spiritual issues. In: Lugton J, Kindlen M (eds) *Palliative Care: the Nurse's Role*. Churchill Livingstone, Edinburgh: 115–39

Solimine M (2002) Spirituality. In: Hoeman S (ed.), *Rehabilitation Nursing: Process, Application and Outcomes*, 3rd edn. Mosby, St Louis

Stein-Parbury J (2005) *Patient and Person: Interpersonal Skills in Nursing*. Elsevier/Churchill Livingstone, Sydney

Stevens-Barnum B (2003) *Spirituality in Nursing: From Traditional to New Age*, 2nd edn. Springer, New York

Tacey D (2003) *Spirituality and the Prevention of Suicide*. Paper presented at the19th annual Suicide Prevention Conference, Brisbane, June. Online. Available: www.abc.net.au/religion.stories/2972766htm [accessed 15 April 2008]

Tracey R (2000) *Mixing Christianity and Aboriginal Spirituality.* Online. Available: www.exc.ca/Template/Story.asp?ID=2000090866 [accessed 14 April 2008]

Videbeck SL (2007) *Psychiatric Mental Health Nursing*, 4th edn. Lippincott Williams & Wilkins, Philadelphia

Watkins P (2000) *Mental Health Nursing: the Art of Compassionate Care.* Butterworth–Heinemann, Oxford

Young C, Koopsen C (2005) *Spirituality, Health and Healing*. Jones & Bartlett, Sudbury, MA

Chapter 12

SEXUALITY

OBJECTIVES

- Define the key terms/concepts
- Discuss the key concepts of sexual development
- Explain the terms gender identity, sexual orientation and gender dysphoria
- Understand how cultural factors impact on the expression of sexuality
- Outline psychological and physical factors that affect sexuality in males and females
- Understand the impact of disability on sexual health
- Identify and describe nursing interventions to promote the sexual health of clients in residential care
- State two primary functions of the Enrolled Nurse (EN) that promote sexual health

KEY TERMS/CONCEPTS

female circumcision
gender dysphoria
gender identity
self-concept
sexual orientation

CHAPTER FOCUS

Sexuality is a vital part of being human and therefore promoting sexual health is as important as promoting any other aspect of human functioning. Because of their working practices and relationships with clients, ENs are in an ideal situation to help clients identify sexual concerns and to facilitate them receiving specialised help when it is required.

LIVED EXPERIENCE

Physical satisfaction is not the only thing I miss — it is having someone near during the lonely nights. Sometimes I still miss sex but even more I miss having someone to touch, hold and hug.

Mavis, 79-year-old widow

WHAT IS SEXUALITY?

Each person is born with a basic drive of a sexual nature, the biological purpose of which is the reproduction of the species. Human sexuality, however, encompasses much more than the need to reproduce, as it involves the whole personality, and is influenced by physical, psychological, sociocultural and spiritual factors (Carter DeLaune & Ladner 2002; Varcarolis et al 2006; Videbeck 2007).

The physical component of human sexuality refers to the primary (genital) and secondary (e.g. breast development, hair distribution) characteristics that distinguish male from female. The psychological attributes are those expressed as a person's gender identity — their sense of knowing to which sex they belong, male or female — and their sexual behaviour. Sexual behaviour is related to biological, spiritual, social and cultural factors that influence the way a person perceives themself as a sexual being (Bristow 1997; Varcarolis et al 2006; Videbeck 2007).

Sexuality is one component of personal identity — an individual's sense of who they are — and influences the way a person thinks, behaves and interacts with others. It is a powerful component of being human, and humans adapt their sexuality to changes in their life circumstances, including changes resulting from alterations in their health.

GENDER IDENTITY, SOCIAL GENDER ROLES AND SEXUAL ORIENTATION

A person's sense of self and self-esteem is linked to expressions of sexuality and the level of comfort a person has with their own sexual orientation. Whereas gender refers to the psychological sense of being either male or female, sexual orientation refers to an enduring, romantic and sexual attraction to another person. It exists along a continuum that ranges from exclusive homosexuality to exclusive heterosexuality and includes various forms of bisexuality.

Heterosexual relationships are those between a male and a female and are the most predominant in adult humans. Homosexual relationships are those between two males or two females and are also common. People with a homosexual orientation are sometimes referred to as gay (men and women) or as lesbian (women only). Bisexual people can experience sexual and emotional attraction to members of both their own and the opposite sex.

Outside this range are transsexuals — people who have a clear and persistent feeling that they are trapped in a body with the wrong genitals. They feel they are, and were always meant to be, the opposite sex. Such a feeling often exists from early childhood and is called *gender dysphoria* (Videbeck 2007). The cause is not clearly understood but biological and social learning theories have been implicated. As they find partners whom they wish to live with or marry, transsexual people may come to desire sexual reassignment, often referred to as gender reassignment. This is hormonal and surgical treatment that aims to alter functioning and appearance as far as possible to that of the sex they believe themselves to be. Transsexuals do not consider themselves to be homosexual. The biological female who falls in love with a woman, for example, believes herself actually to be a man who loves that woman (Varcarolis et al 2006).

Being homosexual, bisexual or transsexual means that people do not conform to cultural norms for male or female behaviour; they do not fit the accepted social gender role and as a result may experience considerable stigma. Nurses who provide a warm, caring and accepting environment that allows for open and honest communication about sexuality reduce stress for clients of any sexual orientation (Shives 2007; Stein-Parbury 2005).

DEVELOPMENT OF SEXUAL ORIENTATION

Experts generally agree that sexual orientation is probably the outcome of complex interactions between biological, cognitive and environmental factors and that it is established at an early age but commonly emerges in adolescence (Perrin 2002). It is accepted that genetic and hormonal factors play a part in shaping a person's sexuality to the extent that the person has no conscious choice in the matter, but also that there are probably many combining reasons for a person's sexual orientation, which may be different for different people (Bristow 1997; Makadon 2007; Rathus et al 2007).

Societal prejudice, which sometimes includes that from family and friends, makes it very challenging for non-heterosexual people to be open and frank about their sexual orientation. Sharing such significant aspects of self is important to healthy psychological adjustment and emotional wellbeing. It has been established that the more open people can be about themselves the more likely they are to have a high self-esteem and strong interpersonal relationships (Shives 2007; Varcarolis et al 2006). Nurses have a role in educating and promoting non-judgmental attitudes towards all people in society. To achieve this nurses first need to be aware of their own attitudes, values and beliefs and be able to keep their personal prejudices to themselves when working with clients.

Sexuality can be expressed in the way someone wears their hair or clothes, their adornments and the hobbies and special interests they may have and in the way they walk and talk. Expressions of sexual orientation can be evident in patterns of physical contact and interpersonal interactions. Expression of sexuality is influenced by social and cultural norms and it is the role of nurses to understand, accept and facilitate the expression of sexuality in all clients.

CULTURAL ASPECTS OF SEXUALITY

Social and cultural rules influence what is perceived as normal within every cultural group. For example, female circumcision is a cultural and religious tradition in some African and Middle Eastern countries (Jones 2000; Hampson 2002) (Clinical Interest Box 12.1). Cultural rules, religious beliefs and other influences become an integral part of personality within members of each cultural group

CLINICAL INTEREST BOX 12.1
Cultural aspects of care

Many young girls who live in traditional Islamic and east African countries undergo female circumcision, a deeply rooted cultural and religious tradition. It is a coming-of-age ritual that ensures chastity and is seen as enhancing eligibility for marriage. There is strong opposition to female circumcision in Western countries because it is considered to be genital mutilation that reduces sexual response after puberty and is seen as a means of social control of women. There is also opposition because it results in complications such as recurrent infections, pain during intercourse, infertility and birthing difficulties.

Some immigrant families request that the procedure (of which there are different types) be performed under modern surgical conditions. Medical officers and nurses are faced with an ethical decision to participate in surgery that interferes with female sexuality or take the risk that such surgery may be performed by a non-medical person, perhaps a family member, without anaesthetic and in non-sterile conditions. There are, in any case, laws in Australia and New Zealand prohibiting female circumcision as a violation of human rights. Nurses care for affected women in a range of situations and are sometimes required to assist with care after surgical procedures to reverse female circumcision.

(Jones 2000: 262)

and have a powerful influence on the way they conduct themselves.

There is considerable diversity across cultures about the rules of sexual behaviour (Hampson 2002). For example, these rules influence:

- Dress and adornments
- The way sexual partners are found, chosen or selected
- What is acceptable during dating
- What is perceived as attractive and arousing
- Who is or is not allowed to marry and whom they will marry
- When, where and how often partners have sex
- Types of sexual activity allowed or prohibited.

(Bristow 1997; Hampson 2002; Rathus et al 2007; White 2002)

All nursing care needs to accommodate cultural diversity; however, dealing with sexual needs presents a special challenge and it is helpful for the nurse to first conduct a cultural assessment. Cultural diversity and nursing practice is the focus of Unit 3.

SEXUAL DEVELOPMENT

Growth and personality development occur as a process. Interpersonal relationships and life experiences influence the way a person's self-concept, of which sexual identity is a part, evolves. The process of sexual development begins in infancy.

SEXUAL DEVELOPMENT DURING INFANCY AND CHILDHOOD

Sexual development is the process by which a child moves through the stages of growth and development to become a mature adult sexual being, physically and psychologically. (Physical development across the lifespan is explained in Unit 5.) A sense of sexual identity is shaped by what is seen, heard and experienced. For example, gender roles and functions within the family and society are modelled and learned and this learning starts at a very early age. Sexual image begins to develop in the first few months after birth, partly because baby girls are spoken to and played with differently to baby boys, and toys and clothes are often gender specific (Perrin 2002; Sadock & Sadock 2007).

During childhood it is normal for children to experiment with the concepts of sexuality through play and fantasy as a way of expressing growing awareness and interest in their own sexuality. Early concepts of sexuality and the values attached to it are learned from role models, often parents. For example, children learn quickly what is or is not acceptable by the way parents respond to such things as undressing in the presence of others or handling their own genitals. Children who are reprimanded for nakedness or touching their genitals may develop a negative perception of their own bodies and a negative attitude towards expressing sexuality.

By age 10 most children are experiencing some of the changes of puberty. As their bodies begin to change they tend to develop a natural modesty. They are frequently curious about sex and, provided that there is an environment where sex can be spoken about comfortably, they are likely to ask many questions. Sometimes when children are in hospital and curious about their bodies they ask questions of nurses they trust. This may be an indication that information relating to sexuality or sexual matters is wanted. It is advisable for the nurse to find out what knowledge the child already has to avoid giving inappropriate answers (Carpenito-Moyet 2006). If the EN is comfortable to ask them, the questions in Clinical Interest Box 12.2 may be used by the nurse to help determine the child's knowledge and, if there seems to be anxiety, to talk about matters further.

CLINICAL INTEREST BOX 12.2
Sample questions for exploring sexuality issues with children

- What do you think the difference is between girls and boys?
- What do you know about having babies?
- How did you learn about having babies?
- It's normal for children of your age to notice changes in their bodies. Have you noticed any changes to your body?
- How do you feel about what is happening to your body?

(Carpenito-Moyet 2006)

SEXUALITY DURING ADOLESCENCE

The adolescent's need to develop a personal sense of self is strong and an adolescent will often identify with a peer group that provides an identity. It is a time of acute awareness and sensitivity to emerging sexuality and body image, when appearance, personal and sexual attractiveness and peer acceptance are of crucial importance to self-esteem and a sense of belonging (Perrin 2002; Varcarolis et al 2006; Videbeck 2007).

A positive self-concept and sense of emotional security depends significantly on the support the adolescent receives while coping with the physical and emotional changes experienced during the difficult and sometimes tumultuous transition to adulthood. Support includes allowing for privacy, the freedom to develop personal interests and new relationships, and understanding the frequent changes of mood and behaviour that commonly occur.

Particular sensitivity is needed when nursing the ill or hospitalised adolescent, because changes or threats to appearance or functioning can have a profound impact, resulting in anxiety, feelings of vulnerability and a negative impact on self-image. The nurse can help the adolescent, as any other client, by demonstrating respect, which reinforces self-worth. The nurse can show this in many ways, including by being non-judgmental, reinforcing the belief that the client is doing his best to cope, to adapt or to change and by demonstrating acceptance of the adolescent client's own perspective and feelings (Stein-Parbury 2005).

During adolescence there may be a great deal of experimentation in the expression of sexuality. Heterosexual and homosexual liaisons are common and sexual behaviour usually includes masturbation (Perrin 2002; Makadon 2007). Assurance about what is generally accepted as normal in physical and emotional development is helpful, as is open, honest and accurate information on topics such as body 'changes, sexual orientation, sexual practices, emotional responses within intimate relationships, sexually transmitted infections (STIs) and contraception. (Information about contraception and reproductive health is provided in Chapter 40.)

There are times when an EN may feel it appropriate to explore sexuality issues with an adolescent, for example, when working in sexual health clinics, adolescent mental health units and in drug and alcohol clinics. However, the EN's role is most commonly concerned with providing basic information. Information about gaining specific expertise in this is provided later in this chapter. For nurses who have the expertise and are comfortable, Clinical Interest Box 12.3 provides some sample questions to aid the exploration of sexuality issues with adolescents.

As adolescents move into adulthood they normally becomes less reliant on positive reinforcement from others as their main source of self-esteem-enhancing experiences.

CLINICAL INTEREST BOX 12.3
Sample questions for exploring sexuality issues with adolescents

- What are your parents' attitudes to sex and nudity?
- What sort of things are said about sex at home?
- What do you know about how pregnancy happens?
- What sort of birth control methods do you know about?
- What do you know about sexually transmitted infections?
- What do you know about safer sex practices?
- It is normal for people of your age to experience changes to their bodies. Is your body changing?
- How do you feel about what is happening to your body?
- At your age, some people are sexually active. What do you think about that?
- Are you sexually active?
- Do you use birth control?
- Do you practise safe sex?

(Carpenito-Moyet 2006)

SEXUALITY IN EARLY ADULTHOOD

During early adulthood people develop physically and emotionally towards sexual maturity. Individuals shape and modify their sexual image and attitudes towards sexuality, sexual relationships and behaviour. It is usual for sexual partnerships to be established and for sexual behaviour to include masturbation and sexual expression with others (Vanzelli & Duck 1996).

SEXUALITY IN ADULTHOOD

Adults have gained physical maturity and this is a time of life when many continue to explore and define emotional boundaries in relationships. It is a time when close intimate relationships are important. However, many people choose to be single and value their privacy and individuality, but this does not mean that intimacy and sexuality are not important issues for them. An adult who is comfortable in an intimate relationship is likely to have a strong sense of personal identity and feel emotionally secure, and this promotes a positive self-concept (Shives 2007; Varcarolis et al 2006; Videbeck 2007).

SEXUALITY IN THE MIDDLE YEARS

Middle age is associated with many changes, and people in their middle years may experience doubt or anxiety about their sexual attractiveness or adequacy. The term 'mid-life crisis' is sometimes used to describe a time typified by reflection on what has been achieved or not achieved; it may also be a time to contemplate stability in life or significant change (Breslin & Lucas 2003; Orshan 2006).

The major developmental change influencing sexuality for women is the onset of menopause. Some women may perceive this in a negative way and may view it as a time when maternal potential, feminine characteristics and sexual attractiveness are disappearing. Others may perceive it as a time of freedom and new challenges (Breslin & Lucas 2003; Orshan 2006). The term 'male menopause' is sometimes used to describe the changes that occur in men during this stage of the life cycle. Some men experience feelings of anxiety and depression that accompany a negative perception that their masculine virtues of strength and vigour are beginning to decline (Gould et al 2000).

In these middle years, self-image is less likely to suffer if the person has previously established a positive self-concept in relation to personal appearance and relationships with other people and is generally satisfied with life achievements (Shives 2007; Varcarolis et al 2006; Videbeck 2007).

The middle-aged person who already has a low self-image is more likely to have that esteem further reduced when the physical changes of middle age begin, such as greying hair, wrinkles, alterations to genitalia. Societal and cultural attitudes that value youth and beauty above age and experience may be a cause for anxiety in people approaching older age. If people perceive a loss of attractiveness during these years it may impact negatively on their ability to express their sexuality.

SEXUALITY IN THE OLDER ADULT

Although it is commonly believed that sexual desire diminishes with age, many older people enjoy a very healthy and active sex life (Wallace 2000). Old age for many is a time of life when the responsibilities of raising families and employment are over and there is time and freedom to enjoy sex as well as many other pleasures in life, such as hobbies and travel.

The ability to continue to enjoy an active sex life requires adaptation to the normal physical changes of ageing that include alterations to mobility, dexterity, hearing and sight. Normal physical changes also mean that older men remain capable of erection but may attain fewer orgasms, and the incidence of spontaneous erection declines (Gould et al 2000). Some men may find this a relief from unwanted or embarrassing erections during earlier years and adapt without concern to the greater need for manual stimulation from partners.

Older women may experience some discomfort due to the vaginal dryness that can accompany hormonal changes. Commercially available lubricants, pelvic floor exercises and sexual activity can help with this. It is the role of the nurse to provide helpful information that promotes the expression of sexuality (see Clinical Interest Box 12.4).

The older person may or may not desire full sexual intercourse, or it may no longer be possible, but sexuality is an important part of an individual's personality at every age (Bristow 1997; Sherman 1999b; Wallace 2005; White & Truax 2007). Sexuality and sensuality can be expressed without engaging in the act of intercourse. Touching, caressing, embracing and other verbal and non-verbal interactions are other ways of expressing these aspects of self.

ALTERATIONS TO SEXUAL HEALTH

Ideally, sex, whether full sexual intercourse or an alternative, is a satisfying act that moves through three stages: desire, arousal and orgasm (Person 1999). The need for sexual satisfaction varies considerably. Some people may desire sexual satisfaction daily, others once or twice a week or monthly, while others may have very little sexual desire at all. For some the amount of sexual activity may be a response to cultural norms or peer pressure, during adolescence, for example. Problems usually only arise if a person is dissatisfied; for example, if they wish to have increased libido (desire) or wish to engage in sexual activity more often than is possible. The reasons for dissatisfaction may be psychosocial or physical or a combination of both and can occur at any age and in the absence of complications of illness, accident or disability.

Psychosocial factors affecting *both* male and female expressions of sexuality include:

- Low self-esteem, poor sexual image of self
- Absence of a partner or lack of attraction to, or dislike of, a partner
- Fear of pain or inflicting harm (e.g. to a sick or pregnant partner)
- Fear of pregnancy or STIs
- Fear of coming to harm (e.g., a client with cardiac problems fearing heart attack)
- Concerns about privacy or confidentiality
- Religious or cultural prohibitions
- Performance anxiety
- Past traumatic sexual experiences
- Guilt (e.g. infidelity)
- Stress
- Excessive use of drugs or alcohol.

Common physical problems for women that affect sexual expression include:

- Diminished lubrication

CLINICAL INTEREST BOX 12.4
Jean's experience

Some nights, even when he was so sick with the cancer, he still wanted me. I worried it would hurt him and I was so tired caring for him that I seemed to be dry all the time, so we didn't do it. It was Nancy, the nurse who came to shower him — she made the difference. She organised respite care one afternoon a week so I could have a break. Then she talked to us about safe positions for him and told us about the lubricants I could buy. It was so comforting being able to please him and love him like that almost right until the end and I feel good now because I know it was comforting for him too.

(Jean, age 67, 3 months after her husband died)

Sample nursing diagnosis for Jean

- Sexual dysfunction related to discomfort related to lack of vaginal lubrication
- Decreased sexual activity related to fear of hurting her partner
- Decreased sexual desire related to fatigue

Goal of care

- Jean will express improved satisfaction with sexual relationship with husband within 2 weeks

- Dyspareunia (painful intercourse)
- Vaginismus (painful spasms of the vagina that make penetration impossible)
- Inability to achieve orgasm.

Common physical problems for men that affect sexual expression include:

- Inability to gain or sustain an erection long enough for penetration or sexual satisfaction
- Premature ejaculation
- Inability to ejaculate during sexual penetration.

(Long et al 1995; Person 1999; Porst & Buvat 2006; Videbeck 2007)

Sometimes problems can occur even when the sexual act is problem free and satisfying; for example, unwanted pregnancy or infertility can cause distress. (Reproductive health is discussed in Chapter 40.)

ILLNESS, INJURY AND DISABILITY AFFECTING SEXUALITY

The range of clients who are susceptible to alteration in sexual functioning is broad. It includes clients who have neurological damage due to illnesses such as Parkinson's disease or multiple sclerosis (MS) or to the effects of cerebrovascular accident (CVA) or spinal injury. These clients may have difficulties with the mechanics of sexual activity, they may experience symptoms such as problems with lubrication, erectile ability or decreased sensation affecting desire, arousal and/or orgasm. They may also experience cramping or spasms, bowel or bladder problems, pain or fatigue (MS Society of Australia 2008). Others may have anaemia, diabetes, peripheral vascular disease, respiratory disorders or cancer. Clients may have had accidents resulting in burns or amputations. Some may have a sexually transmitted infection (STI) or may have been sexually abused.

Any of these clients may feel concerned about altered body image or suffer depression and anxiety, all of which can interfere with the expression of sexuality. Inevitably, nurses will encounter clients needing help in this area. Some clients may be so ill that any form of sexual activity is impossible; others may desire to express their sexual needs. Admission to hospital or other places providing care does not necessarily mean that sexual needs are suppressed.

PROMOTING SEXUAL HEALTH IN CLIENTS WITH INTELLECTUAL IMPAIRMENT

There is strong support in the health care field that, rather than be segregated, people with intellectual or learning disabilities should be able to participate in every aspect of human experience within the general community (policy of inclusion). Nurses working in the field of intellectual disability in the community, day care centres or in residential facilities are encouraged to consider the importance of relationships in the lives of their clients from the perspective that sexual and personal relationships are one of the most treasured parts of a person's life (Oakes 2003).

In the past, strong controls have been exerted by health professionals in regard to the sexuality of people with intellectual impairment. Either they have failed to acknowledge sexual needs or have seriously interfered with the ability of clients to gain fulfilment (e.g., programs of enforced sterilisation) (Oakes 2003). The issues that arise from the move towards inclusion and normalcy are extensive and cannot be addressed in this chapter. They include the issues of choice, decision making, consent and human rights affecting desire of individuals to marry, desire for parenthood, and protection needs related to pregnancy and STIs (Gates 2006).

People with intellectual impairment can and do become parents and often need the support of nurses and other health professionals with this. It is a primary role for nurses to encourage relationships and promote sexual fulfilment for clients with intellectual disabilities by educating, advocating and facilitating.

DISINHIBITED EXPRESSIONS OF SEXUALITY

Clients who have alteration in cognitive abilities such as is associated with dementia, people with acquired brain injury (ABI), and those who have serious chronic mental illness or intellectual impairment, may sometimes be disinhibited in the way they express their sexuality. This means that they may behave in a variety of ways ranging from making inappropriate verbal suggestions to taking clothes off or masturbating in public. A quiet calm response is usually the most successful, followed by assisting them to a private place whenever possible. Nurses working with clients who demonstrate uninhibited behaviours need written policy guidelines for addressing ways to manage expressions of sexuality by their clients without infringing on their rights or sense of wellbeing (Alzheimer's Australia 2006a, 2006b; Sherman 1999b; Walker-Hirsch 2007).

PROMOTING THE SEXUAL HEALTH OF OLDER CLIENTS IN RESIDENTIAL CARE SETTINGS

Older adults adjust to many changes, such as the loss of a partner, retirement and the loss of social roles, the loss of friends, the loss of physical health and sometimes the loss of independence. Some have to adjust to the loss of their own homes. Nurses have a responsibility to ensure that the ability to express sexuality and sensuality is not an additional loss when a person moves into a residential care facility (Wallace 2000; Sherman 1999b; White 2002).

Expressions of sexuality and sensuality are important in maintaining a person's sense of self at every age, but this is not always supported in residential care. Historically in residential care settings there has been a focus on bodily functions and care, a lack of client privacy and oppressive staff attitudes towards sexual expression by residents. Although more recently this issue has been talked about, the problems are pervasive and have not yet been resolved in many residential care facilities. They remain problematic even in relation to the needs of the heterosexual population, and very little has been done towards addressing issues for clients with alternative sexuality needs (Maclean 2002; White 2002).

Nurses have an important role in helping clients to meet sexuality and intimacy needs, and this must be considered as an inclusive part of a resident's lifestyle. Nurses can help residents maintain a positive self-image and express themselves as sexual beings by:

- Accepting and promoting that expressions of sexuality are normal
- Providing privacy when a resident's sexual partner visits
- Advocating that shared accommodation and double beds be available for couples if that is what both partners desire
- Avoiding and advocating against staff talking or joking about a resident's sexual activity (e.g. masturbation)
- Providing and respecting privacy (e.g. knocking before entering a resident's room)
- Encouraging touch, hugs, etc, when appropriate
- Ensuring that clients are well groomed
- Encouraging use of perfume and adornments
- Complimenting residents on their appearance.

(Hill 2002; Ebersole et al 2008)

Sexuality and dementia

While some people with progressive dementia lose interest in sexual activity early in the illness, others may continue to have sexual desires and drives well into the advanced stages of the disease. Where the person with dementia is able to satisfy these needs appropriately there is no problem, but sometimes, sexual behaviour is, or is perceived as being, a problem. Sometimes actions can be perceived as sexually inappropriate when in fact the behaviour represents something unconnected to sexuality. For example, a resident who is continually touching the genital area may be sore or uncomfortable or may simply need to go to the toilet.

If behaviour is sexually motivated and inappropriate, for example, if it is being conducted publicly, the matter may be resolved and the person's dignity maintained by gently discouraging the behaviour or by redirecting the person with dementia to another activity. Some residents who have dementia may behave in a sexually inappropriate manner that is totally different to behaviour before the onset of their dementia. The underlying cause is the invisible damage to the brain caused by the illness. It can be helpful to remember that the person with dementia does not intentionally seek to embarrass or annoy others (Alzheimers Australia 2006b).

Many people who have dementia have enjoyed a satisfying sexual life at home with their partners right up until the time of admission to a residential care facility (Sherman 1999a). Providing a single room and opportunities to be together undisturbed provides valuable privacy (see Clinical Interest Box 12.5).

Sometimes residents, one or both of who may have dementia, may form relationships together. This may mean that they simply wish to spend time together, hold hands, hug or kiss. It may mean that they wish to sit, lie down together or become more intimate. This can be reassuring and comforting for both but can also cause problems in different ways. Specific problems and dilemmas arise if:

- One or both has a wife or husband but are no longer aware of their marital status because of memory impairment in dementia
- One or the other is at risk of harm or injury as a result of the relationship
- The new relationship distresses a spouse or other family members
- One client is exerting power over the other, or in any way coercing the other
- Staff are in conflict about the 'rights and wrongs' of the situation and cannot agree on how it should be managed
- Staff and relatives are in conflict about how the situation should be managed.

In such cases it is advisable for the health care facility to have a clear formulated policy concerning residents and sexual behaviour. This should guide responses and can be shown to family members in cases of conflict about what should happen. A policy may indicate that if there is no evidence of overt sexual activity the rights of the residents to have a relationship will be respected; alternatively, the policy may indicate that such relationships will be deterred by close monitoring or by moving one client to another facility.

Ideally, relatives should be alerted to how the pathophysiology of dementia can lead to the possibility of such

CLINICAL INTEREST BOX 12.5
Sexuality needs of patients in residential care

Mr and Mrs Jacobs were married for over 50 years and, until her own health deteriorated, Mrs Jacobs cared for her husband at home. Despite his confusion, Mr Jacobs, who has Alzheimer's dementia, continued to desire and enjoy sexual intimacy with his wife until he was admitted to a dementia-specific residential care unit. Within a few weeks nurses reported that Mr Jacobs was often agitated and had started touching them in ways they described as 'sexual and inappropriate'. Mrs Jacobs was upset to hear about this and talked tearfully to the nurse in charge about how she had reluctantly been rejecting her husband's sexual advances when she visited because she felt embarrassed even to embrace in front of other people.

Mr Jacobs was moved from a shared to a single room and this enabled the couple to share undisturbed time together. Mr Jacobs became much less agitated and his advances towards the nurses became a very infrequent occurrence.

relationships developing and be made aware of relevant policies before loved ones are admitted to the facility. Also, before accepting employment, staff should be given time to consider such policies in relationship to their own values, attitudes and beliefs. When policies covering this issue are not in existence, nurses are advised to advocate that they be developed collaboratively with staff and be implemented as soon as possible. Clinical Interest Box 12.6 illustrates how a pre-existing policy and prior explanations affected, in a positive way, one man's response to his wife's relationship with another resident.

An extensive range of opinions and responses and many ethical and moral dilemmas surround this issue and other issues of sexuality in dementia care. Barbara Sherman has written extensively on this topic in her book *Sex, Intimacy and Aged Care*, which provides constructive ideas for nurses about dealing with older people's feelings, desires and expressions of sexuality (Sherman 1999b).

Nurses working with older clients, as with any others, need to assess interest and functioning in relation to sexuality, and plan care for each individual client. As part of assessment the nurse needs to recognise that some medications as well as the effects of dementia, other illness or disability can affect sexual activity. Antidepressants, antispasmodics, steroids, diuretics and antihypertensives, for example, can all reduce desire (Smith 1999). Depression can also affect libido and it is not uncommon for clients in residential care to experience feelings of worthlessness and depression (Bevan & Jeeawody 1998).

CLINICAL INTEREST BOX 12.6
Ian's experience

I arrived at the nursing home and saw my wife, Andrea, sitting in the dining room, in front of everyone, holding hands with a man. It was a bit of a shock even though I knew about the possibility of it happening. It had been explained to me before she was admitted that with her dementia it could happen.

They had told me that their policy, as much as possible, was to respect the rights of residents to have relationships. I spoke to one of the nurses and she said that Andrea and the man, Tom, seemed to have a gentle affection for each other and that both seemed happier since they had started spending much of their time together. She also said that Andrea sometimes called the man by my name, Ian. She explained that Andrea was most likely experiencing this new relationship as a familiar one, shared with a kind, caring man — a man just like me. I felt better when she explained how, because of the damage to her brain, Andrea no longer had the capacity to differentiate between Tom and me.

I'm still jealous, but I try to put that aside because I like to know that she is happy. I feel the nurses understand because they said to ring up when I was coming to visit. I know they make sure that when I arrive she is not with Tom — she's often walking with a nurse or in the nurses' station. She seems to be expecting me and she always greets me with a smile.

Wherever nursing care is taking place, nurses will need to assess sexuality needs, plan care and evaluate outcomes for individual clients.

IMPLEMENTING THE NURSING PROCESS

The crucial thing for nurses to recognise is that sexual needs do not disappear or become inappropriate after any change in health circumstances. No matter what the illness, injury or disability, sexual health needs to be assessed in conjunction with the client's previous attitudes, beliefs, knowledge, experiences and behaviours relating to expression of sexuality. Therefore, assessment and care planning incorporate physical, psychological, social and cultural elements. (Chapter 19 discusses these components of the nursing process.)

Nurses may find it uncomfortable asking questions about sex, sexual desires or functions with clients of any age, but this is an important component of nursing assessment and practice that tends to be neglected. It is easier for the nurse with knowledge, skill and an awareness of personal feelings about sex and sexuality to be comfortable and confident when discussing sexuality issues and avoid embarrassment. It is appropriate for the nurse to assess only those areas pertinent for the client at the time and to permit the client to decline to answer.

NURSING ASSESSMENT

When taking a nursing history it helps for the nurse to ask questions in a matter-of-fact manner and to be clear about why the questions relating to sexuality are being asked. A comfortable approach to specific issues might be, 'Sometimes people who have this illness experience some sexual changes; have you noticed any changes happening to you?' The essential element is for the nurse to establish a relationship and an environment where the client feels safe talking about sexual concerns, and to be aware that the client may not reveal the most concerning issues during the initial interview but at a later time (Stein-Parbury 2005) (Clinical Interest Box 12.7).

CARE PLANNING

Whenever possible, care planning is a collaborative activity that follows identification of nursing diagnoses. The nurse and client together develop a care plan that responds to individual needs. If appropriate, the client's sexual partner may be included in the planning. This is particularly relevant when one partner in an established relationship has alterations to bodily function or appearance; for example, the partner of a client who has an ostomy (ileostomy or colostomy) may respond negatively or with caution and this may cause a decreased desire for a sexual relationship that could be helped by professional intervention. It is one aim of care to facilitate open communication between sexual partners and between the partners and health professionals. It is this open and honest communication

CLINICAL INTEREST BOX 12.7
Jill's experience

Jill, aged 35, was diagnosed with multiple sclerosis (MS) 3 years ago. She is married to David and has a six-year-old daughter. She continues to work 2 days a week as an administration officer. Recently she fell and broke her arm and needed to stay in hospital overnight.

The nurse on night duty found Jill in the day room, unable to sleep, so she made her a drink and sat with her for a while. After some small talk about Jill's job and her daughter she asked, 'How has having MS affected your life?', and later, 'How has it affected your relationship with David?' She discovered that Jill and David were not getting on so well, mostly because they didn't have sex anymore because it was 'too difficult now'. The nurse asked, 'What has changed that makes it difficult?'

She discovered that Jill was experiencing painful cramps and spasms in her legs at night that made it impossible to get comfortable and sometimes made it difficult to separate her legs at all. Jill seemed to believe that this was part of the MS that she must accept. The nurse reassured her that cramps and spasms could be helped by medication or physiotherapy and suggested that Jill think about contacting her doctor and the Multiple Sclerosis Society for expert advice. She gave Jill a copy of the Multiple Sclerosis Society information brochure and offered to contact the society on her behalf if she wished.

Sample nursing diagnosis for Jill

- Alteration in sexual activity related to pain and discomfort

Goal of care

- Jill will seek medical advice and gain effective treatment for cramps and spasms
- Jill will gain support of experts at the Multiple Sclerosis Society
- Jill will report a decrease in painful cramps and spasms
- Jill will express improved relationship with husband and a resumption of sexual activity within 1 month.

about sexual concerns that helps clients feel positive about their sexuality even when faced with serious impairment (Schapiro 2003).

The most valuable asset a nurse can have when assessing clients and planning care related to sexuality is competent communication skills. The nurse with excellent interpersonal skills such as listening, asking open-ended questions, using silence and summarising the discussion will help clients to share feelings, concerns and information about sexuality (Stein-Parbury 2005) (Chapter 29 discusses communication skills). Nurses involved in planning care also require the following assets:

- Knowledge about genital structure, the sexual response cycle and changes in the life cycle
- Ability to be non-judgmental and not make assumptions about sexual preferences
- Confidence about their own sexuality
- Awareness of their own limitations and knowing when to refer the client to a specialist health care professional. The specialist may be another nurse, a physician, gynaecologist, urologist, endocrinologist or psychologist.

PROMOTING SEXUAL HEALTH USING THE 'PLISSIT' MODEL

The PLISSIT model developed by Annon (1976) provides guidelines for assessment and care planning related to sexual concerns of clients. This model outlines four stages of interventions used in sexual counselling and provides a useful framework for nurses.

P = permission

The first level, P, stands for the giving of permission. It acknowledges sexuality as a valid area for the nurse to assess. In the course of a nursing assessment the nurse can raise the topic of sexuality, giving the client permission to talk about sexual matters. The nurse's role is to facilitate the client being able to talk freely about sexual activities and concerns without being judged.

LI = limited information

This relates to the nurse providing basic information about sexuality and sexual functioning. ENs are able to provide basic information when they have the knowledge and confidence to respond appropriately. This may include, for example, explaining to an anxious teenage boy that frequent unwanted erections are a normal part of sexual development.

SS = specific suggestions

Specific suggestions are aimed at solving a client's problem and require knowledge and expertise. It is sometimes within the role of the EN to make a specific suggestion about a sexual concern. For example, a knowledgeable EN may elicit concerns about unwanted pregnancy and be able to suggest the use of condoms or other birth control methods.

IT = intensive therapy

This is the highest level of involvement and relates to sexual matters that require nurses to refer clients to specialist medical officers and/or sexual counsellors. For example, an EN would refer a man who was anxious about erectile dysfunction for medical and psychological assessment.

Nurses with a professional interest in developing expertise in dealing with sexuality issues can undertake one of a range of post-basic courses for health professionals. For example, Weerakoon and Wong (2003) outline an online course based on the PLISSIT model.

EVALUATION

The nurse reviews the way clients respond to interventions to determine if goals have been achieved. ENs who have gained the necessary experience and feel comfortable may facilitate open discussion about sexual concerns then relate identified needs to the Registered Nurse (RN). Appropriate specialists and supports can then be put in place. Perhaps the most important thing to acknowledge here is that healthy sexuality does not depend on being free of illness, injury or disability. Clients adapt to life changes, even the most serious of events, and adjust and adapt to new ways of achieving satisfaction. They are forced to change from what has previously been perceived as 'normal' sexual expression to other satisfying activities. For example, people with disabilities find new positions for sexual intercourse, learn how to gain satisfaction without the use of a penis, from oral or manual means, for example. They learn how to manage intercourse with urinary catheters in situ or use medication or aids such as vacuum tubes or other substitute 'erectors'. All these things take time, and success, or lack of it, is judged by the client. Evaluation is therefore client focused and only the client can define a personal definition of healthy sexuality (Schapiro 2003).

PROFESSIONAL BOUNDARIES AND SEXUALITY

INNOCENT SEXUAL ADVANCES

There are times when clients make sexual advances to nurses. Sexual advances may be due to confusion, disorientation or intellectual impairment, or they may be intentional. A client with dementia, for example, may touch the nurse's breast because he mistakes the nurse for his wife. In this case the sexual behaviour is due to mental confusion and it is appropriate for the nurse to respond quietly, calmly and firmly, without embarrassing the client. The nurse also needs to consider if there is inadvertent sexual provocation, by the use of perfume, for example. Confused clients might easily misinterpret signals. While the example used here is male client to female nurse, the advances can and do sometimes occur the other way around. The first step in the situation of any sexual advance, verbal or physical, is for the nurse to assess the mental competency of the client in relation to understanding and accountability.

Sometimes a male client may have an involuntary erection while the nurse is in his presence, which may cause embarrassment for the client and the nurse, male or female. Involuntary sexual arousal is a common and natural event. For example, adolescent boys respond with an erection to a range of emotional states including fear, anxiety, anger and pain. As the male ages he is conditioned to respond with erection only in sexual situations, although in situations of extreme fear or anxiety an adult male may respond with an erection. Involuntary erection may also occur when there is a neurological disorder such as brain damage, or it may occur in the elderly confused person. If while attending to a client he becomes sexually aroused, the nurse can tactfully ignore it, professionally make it clear that it is not unusual and not a concern, or use humour to reduce embarrassment. It would also be appropriate, particularly in the case of long-stay clients, to check whether or not care planning incorporates and adequately meets sexuality needs.

INTENTIONAL SEXUAL ADVANCES

There are instances where sexual behaviour towards the nurse is intentional. If the client is able to understand, the action is intentional and the implications understood, the nurse should address the inappropriateness of the behaviour rather than directly criticise the person. The nurse could explain: 'I feel uncomfortable about you touching me like that and it is not appropriate — please do not do it again.' Inappropriate verbal or physical behaviour, especially if it is repeated, needs to be reported to the nurse in charge and documented objectively. In situations that are not easily resolved, help should be obtained from a professional counsellor experienced in dealing with sexual matters.

THE CLIENT AND THE NURSE: SEXUAL ATTRACTION

Nurses are sometimes challenged by, and need to be aware of, the limits and boundaries of the professional nurse–client relationship. It is the responsibility of the nurse to establish clear sexual boundaries with clients. Even if there is mutual sexual attraction and the client consents to or even initiates the sexual relationship it is still considered sexual misconduct to engage in a sexual relationship with a client. Nurses tend to be at risk of overstepping sexual boundaries when they are feeling emotionally unfulfilled or when they are facing an emotional crisis. Clinical Interest Box 12.8 identifies some at-risk warning signs:

Any behaviour by a nurse that is seductive, demeaning, harassing or reasonably interpreted by a client as sexual is an abuse of the nurse–client relationship and a violation of the nurse's professional responsibility. Nurses need to be aware of when they are sexually attracted to a client and prevent moving across the professional boundary. Clinical Interest Box 12.9 lists some hints to aid in preventing this.

Professional nursing organisations such as the Nursing Councils in New Zealand and Australia and the Nurses Boards in each state and territory of Australia provide guidelines and advice concerning all professional practice boundary issues.

SUMMARY

Sexuality is a dynamic component of human life and can be affected negatively by illness and injury. The nurse is in a

CLINICAL INTEREST BOX 12.8
Sexual boundaries — are you at risk?

- Do you dress for work with a particular client in mind?
- Do you consider a particular client to be 'yours'?
- Do you feel others misunderstand or are too critical of 'your' client?
- Have you kept any secrets with this client?
- Are you guarded or do you feel defensive when questioned about your interactions?
- Have you ever flirted with this client?

CLINICAL INTEREST BOX 12.9
Sexual attraction — hints on how to avoid crossing the professional boundary

- Learn to recognise signs
- Provide a professional explanation for all aspects of client care
- Respect client dignity and privacy at all times
- Maintain clear, appropriate and professional communication at all times
- Don't discuss personal problems or any aspect of your intimate life with a client
- Admit to sexual attraction if it is a threat to your professional behaviour and request the care of the client be transferred to another nurse

prime position to promote sexual health and must be mindful of issues pertinent to those with physical, intellectual and other cognitive disorders, such as dementia. Dementia and other disorders can lead to disinhibited sexual behaviour, which requires sensitive nursing management to ensure the rights and dignity of affected clients are maintained.

The PLISSIT model of assessment and care planning provides useful guidelines for health professionals involved in assisting clients with sexuality concerns. The essentials for being competent in this area are having high-level communication skills and being comfortable talking about sex and sexual matters. It is not uncommon for nurses to experience discomfort: those who do need a plan to deal with their discomfort. The nurse who has strong communication skills and is comfortable with sexual issues will help the client to share sexual concerns and this is the first and most important step in promoting sexual health.

REVIEW EXERCISES

1. Explain the terms gender identity, sexual orientation and gender dysphoria.
2. Apart from sexual intercourse, how else can people express their sexuality?
3. Suggest six psychological factors that may negatively affect the expression of sexuality.
4. Suggest four questions you might ask of an adolescent boy when exploring sexuality.
5. Suggest an appropriate response for the nurse to make when a confused 90-year-old client with dementia touches her breasts when she is assisting him with his shower.
6. As an EN, how can you facilitate aged-care residents to express themselves as sensual or sexual beings?

CRITICAL THINKING EXERCISES

1. Consider a 24-year-old client with intellectual disability living in a residential care setting.
   a) How much time and energy is devoted to enabling this person to meet new people, make significant relationships and maintain those relationships?
   b) How does this relate to the time you spend on these issues?
   c) How does this relate to the time and energy allocated to other aspects of care?
   d) As an EN working in the unit, how could you facilitate improving this client's social contact and ability to form new relationships?
2. As an EN you are working with Mary in a short-term rehabilitation setting. Mary is recovering from a CVA that occurred 2 weeks ago. She is sharing a room with two other women. Mary is not yet able to get around without the use of a walking stick and the support of a nurse. She manages her shower and dresses herself very slowly and with some assistance. She has some difficulty with speech but is progressing with rehabilitation help from the speech therapist. She is expected to stay in the unit for at least another 4 weeks. This afternoon she is very weepy and says, 'I'm alright really, it's just that I don't sleep. I miss John so much — the bed's so lonely without him.'
   a) How would you explore this comment and Mary's feelings?
   b) What nursing interventions might you consider?
   c) How might other health professionals assist?

REFERENCES AND FURTHER READING

Alzheimer's Australia (2006a) *Intimacy and Sexual Issues*. Help Sheet. No. 2.19. Online. Available: http://www.alzheimers.org.au/upload/HS2.19.pdf [accessed 23 April 2008]

—— (2006b) *Disinhibited Behaviours*. Help Sheet. No. 5.10 Online. Available: http://www.gtp.com.au/Alzheimer/inewsfiles/Disinhibited_behavious_(English).pdf [accessed 23 April 2008]

Anderson BA (2005) *Reproductive Health*. Jones & Bartlett, Sudbury, MA

Annon JS (1976) The PLISSIT model: a proposed conceptual scheme for the behavioural treatment of sexual problems. *Journal of Sex Education and Therapy* 2: 211–15

Bevan C, Jeeawody B (1998) *Successful Ageing: Perspectives on Health and Social Construction*. Mosby, Sydney

Breslin ET, Lucas VA (2003) *Women's Health Nursing: Toward Evidence Based Practice*. Saunders, St Louis

Bristow J (1997) *Sexuality*. Routledge, New York

Capezuti EA, Zwicker D, Mezey M, Gray-Miceli D, Kluger M (eds) (2007) *Evidence-Based Geriatric Nursing Protocol for Best Practice*, 3rd edn. Springer Publishing Company, New York

Carpenito-Moyet LJ (2006) *Nursing Diagnoses: Application to Clinical Practice*. Lippincott Williams and Wilkins, Philadelphia

Carter DeLaune S, Ladner PK (2002) *Fundamentals of Nursing: Standards & Practice*.Thomas Delmar Learning, New York

Crisp J, Taylor C (eds) (2005) *Potter & Perry's Fundamentals of Nursing*, 2nd edn. Elsevier Australia, Sydney

Ebersole P, Touhy TS, Hess P, Jett K, Luggen A (2008) *Toward Healthy Ageing: Human Needs and Nursing Response*, 7th edn. Elsevier, St Louis

Gates B (2006) *Care Planning and Delivery in Intellectual Disability Nursing*. Blackwell Publishing, Ames, IN

Gould DC, Petty R, Jacobs HS (2000) For and Against — the Male Menopause. *British Medical Journal*, 320 (7238), March: 858–61

Hampson G (2002) *Practice Nurse Handbook*, 4th edn. Blackwell Publishing, Ames, IN

Harvey JH, Wenzel A, Sprecher S (2004) *The Handbook of Sexuality in Close Relationships*. Lawrence Erlbaum Associates, New York

Hill RD (2002) *Geriatric Residential Care*. Lawrence Erlbaum Associates, New York

Jones J (2000) Concern mounts over female genital mutilation. *British Medical Journal* 321 (7256), July: 262

Long BC, Phipps WJ, Cassmeyer VL (1995) *Adult Nursing: A Nursing Process Approach*. Elsevier, St Louis

Maclean D (2002) Sex a Matter of Policy? American Medical Directors' Association Newspaper, *Caring for the Ages* 3 (2) February 2002. Online. Available: www.amda.com/caring/february2002/sex.htm [accessed 16 April 2008]

Makadon HJ (2007) *The Fenway Guide to Lesbian, Gay, Bisexual and Transgender Health*. ACP Press, Philadelphia

MS Society of Australia (2008) *What are the Symptoms of MS?* Online. Available: www.msaustralia.org.au/misinformation/faqs.htm#4 [accessed 23 April 2008]

Oakes P (2003) Sexual and personal relationships. In: Gates B (ed.), *Learning Disabilities: Towards Inclusion*, 4th edn. Elsevier Science, Edinburgh

Orshan SA (2006) *Maternity, Newborn and Women's Health Nursing*. Lippincott Williams & Wilkins, Philadelphia

Perrin EC (2002) *Sexual Orientation in Child and Adolescent Health*. Springer, New York

Person ES (1999) *The Sexual Century*. Yale University Press, New Haven, Connecticut

Porst H, Buvat J (2006) *Standard Practice in Sexual Medicine*. Blackwell Publishing, Hoboken, New Jersey

Rathus SS, Nevid JS, Fichner-Rathus L (2007) *Human Sexuality in a World of Diversity*. Allyn & Bacon, New Jersey

Sadock BJ, Sadock VA (2007) *Kaplan and Sadock's Synopsis of Psychiatry*. Lippincott Williams & Wilkins, Philadelphia

Schapiro R (2003) *Sexuality and Multiple Sclerosis*. International MS Support Foundation. Online. Available: www.ms-doctors.org/Fairview_sexuality.shtml [accessed April 2004]

Sherman B (1999a) *Dementia with Dignity: a Handbook for Carers*. McGraw Hill, Sydney

—— (1999b) *Sex, Intimacy and Aged Care*. Jessica Kingsley Publishing, London

Shives LR (2007) *Basic Concepts of Psychiatric-Mental Health Nursing*. Lippincott Wilkins and Williams, Hagerstown, MD

Smith M (1999) The nurse as promoter of sexual health. In: Smith M (ed), *Rehabilitation in Adult Nursing Practice*. Churchill Livingstone, Edinburgh

Sprunk E, Alteneder R (2000) The impact of an ostomy on sexuality. *Clinical Journal of Oncology Nursing,* March–April 4(2): 85–8

Stein-Parbury J (2005) *Patient and Person: Interpersonal Skills in Nursing*. Elsevier/Churchill Livingstone, Sydney

Vanzelli N, Duck S (1995) *A Lifetime of Relationships*. Brooks/Cole, Pacific Grove, CA

Varcarolis E, Benner-Carson V, Shoemaker NC (2006) *Foundations of Psychiatric Mental Health Nursing: A Clinical Approach*. WB Saunders, Philadelphia

Videbeck SL (2007) *Psychiatric Mental-Health Nursing*, 4th edn. Lippincott Williams & Wilkins, Philadelphia

Walker-Hirsch L (2007) *The Facts of Life and More: Sexuality and Intimacy for People with Intellectual Disabilities*. Brookes/University of Michigan

Wallace M (2000) *Sexuality and Intimacy: Textbook of Gerontological Nursing*. Mosby, St. Louis

—— (2005) Sexuality. *Urological Nursing*, 25(5): 373–4 (Oct)

Weerakoon P, Wong M (2003) Sexuality education on-line for health professionals. *Electronic Journal of Human Sexuality* 6. Online. Available: www.ejhs.org/volume6/SexEd.html [accessed 23 April 2008]

White BS, Truax D (2007) *The Nurse Practitioner in Long-Term Care*. Jones and Bartlett, Sudbury, MA

White I (2002) *The Challenge of Sexuality in Healthcare*. Blackwell Publishing, Ames, IN

Chapter 13

STRESS AND ADAPTATION

OBJECTIVES

- Define the key terms/concepts
- Identify common stressors related to illness and hospitalisation
- Describe the physiological and psychological responses to stress
- Explain the stages of the general adaptation syndrome
- Outline the significance of appraisal in relation to stress
- Understand the range of factors that influence a person's ability to successfully adapt and cope with stress
- Explain the significance of defence mechanisms in stress and coping
- Identify a range of constructive and destructive coping mechanisms
- Identify a range of therapeutic tools that promote stress adaptation and coping
- Demonstrate a range of nursing skills that alleviate stress in anxious clients

KEY TERMS/CONCEPTS

anxiety
appraisal
cognitive restructuring
constructive coping mechanisms
defence mechanisms
destructive coping mechanisms
eustress
external stressor
guided imagery
homeostasis
humour
internal stressor
progressive relaxation
stress
stress adaptation

CHAPTER FOCUS

Throughout life each person is faced with situations capable of producing stress responses. There is an intricate and complex relationship between psychological and biological responses to stress and how these reactions link to physical and mental health or ill-health. The way individuals respond and adapt to stress may be quite different — what may cause a mild reaction in one person may evoke a much stronger stress response in another. Depending on the individual and the stressor, the experience of stress may be positive, negative or a mixture of both. Illness and hospitalisation can be a stressful experience for clients and families. The role of the nurse involves recognising stress and anxiety and the associated physical and psychological responses, understanding the causes and implementing holistic nursing care strategies to help clients cope with physical and emotional responses during periods of health-related stress.

LIVED EXPERIENCE

I was so anxious I couldn't stop shaking and I felt that I couldn't get my breath. I know it was only a biopsy to them, but to me it was huge. There was one nurse who noticed how distressed I was and she showed me how to breathe in and focus on relaxing my muscles as I breathed out. She did it in time with me for quite a while, until they were ready for me. Without that I don't know how I would have coped.

Joan, 52, before a breast biopsy

The art and science of nursing is based on the concept of holism. This concept is essential in understanding stress and its relationship to physical and mental health or ill-health. This is because stress and the way individuals adapt and cope is related to the interplay between environmental, cultural, spiritual, psychosocial and biological dimensions of each person. A basic concept of this chapter is therefore that each person is unique and the whole person a totality of body, mind and spirit.

DIMENSIONS OF STRESS AND STRESSORS

Stress is any emotional, physical, social, economic or other factor that requires a response or change. Stress can lead to a variety of psychological responses, the most common of which is anxiety. *Anxiety* can be defined as a feeling of apprehension, uneasiness, uncertainty or dread. The source of the anxiety may be real and easily identified or it may be a perceived threat and the person may not be able to identify the cause. Everyone experiences anxiety. It may be experienced on four different levels: mild, moderate, severe and panic level. It can be classified as normal, acute or chronic and has the potential to affect the person at a very deep level and to a point where self-esteem can be seriously eroded (Boyd 2007; Keltner et al 2006; Varcarolis 2006).

Stress can result in psychological and physiological effects, and prolonged stress can result in physical illness. This is because the immune system responds to a person's internal and external environments and, when exposed to excessive stress, becomes damaged, reducing the body's ability to combat infection and disease. Prolonged stress has been linked to many physical health problems, including migraine headaches, allergies, asthma, gastric ulceration and other disorders of the digestive tract. Scientists explain the physical manifestations of prolonged stress as being related to chemical, hormonal and cellular changes (deWit 2005; Rice 2000).

A *stressor* is the stimulus that precipitates stress. Stressors can be classified as physical or psychological. Physical stressors include bodily trauma such as injury or surgery, blood loss, pain, infection and illness. Psychological stressors can be defined as any stimuli that the person interprets as challenging, demanding or threatening. These are usually events and circumstances that demand a change or response. Psychological stressors relate to situations that result in emotional tension; for example, interpersonal conflict such as might occur with divorce, personal loss such as the death of a loved one, and changes in family or social role such as might arise from redundancy, retirement or illness.

Stressors can also be classified as internal or external. *Internal stressors* arise from within the person. They include hunger, thirst, fatigue, fever and the effects of pregnancy or menopause. Internal stressors also include strong emotions such as embarrassment, shame or guilt. *External stressors* are those that originate outside a person and include environmental conditions such as exposure to overly high or low temperatures, overcrowding, noise and, of course, the traumatic effects of accidents or natural disasters such as fires, floods, hurricanes and earthquakes. External stressors also include issues such as peer group pressure, social isolation and the demands of study, family or work (deWit 2005; Watkins 2001).

A stressor may be perceived as positive, negative or a mixture of both. Many situations are both demanding and stressful, evoking mixed responses; a new job can be challenging and stressful but at the same time a positive and personally rewarding experience; the stress of a looming exam or competitive event can be very stressful but the stimulus also provides high levels of motivating energy that leads to positive outcomes (Varcarolis 2006; Stuart & Laraia 2004; Shives 2007).

Different people may respond to the same stressor in totally different ways. For example a footballer faced with the prospect of scoring the winning goal after the final siren has sounded may perceive this as a challenge, a chance to shine — and may well do so. Another might perceive this situation as a major threat to self-esteem — fear of performing badly may cause his body to feel like jelly, which may result in poor performance. Despite differences in individual responses to stress, there are some common themes concerning what is perceived as stressful. People generally feel anxious when they perceive a loss of or threat to their:

- Health or the ability to function independently
- Self-esteem, self-respect or self-control
- Control over their life and/or loss of freedom
- Personal resources and supports (emotional, practical, financial, spiritual, social and cultural)
- Loved ones
- Ability to achieve goals, dreams or expectations (Keltner et al 2006).

Illness and hospitalisation are commonly significant stressors. Nurses frequently encounter a range of stress responses when providing care to clients. In fact, anxiety is the word most commonly used by clients to describe their emotional response to illness (Shives 2007). The nature and degree of stress a client experiences is an important component of wellbeing that is evaluated by the nurse as part of ongoing holistic nursing assessment. Some people adapt to hospitalisation, many cope successfully with illness, but others need help and support. The nurse in all areas of care, and particularly in mental health care, needs to facilitate exploration of the significance of particular stressors to each individual client.

ADAPTATION TO STRESS

A person's ability to adapt to, and cope with, stress depends on the combined aspects of the stressor itself and the characteristics of the person. Aspects of the stressor that influence the person's response relate to the nature, origin, timing and number of stressors. Specifically this relates to:

- Extent and intensity
- Duration

- Number and type of concurrent stressors
- Number of stressors within a given time period.

The way in which individual people adapt to stress may be quite different and depends on the cumulative effect of:

- Background and culture
- Needs
- Desires
- Self-concept
- Internal resources
- External supports; for example, personal relationships, access to support services, finances
- Knowledge, including past experience with similar stressors
- Skills
- Personality traits
- Maturity
- General health.

The way individuals adapt to stress is related to coping mechanisms, many of which are learned during childhood and adolescence. Coping mechanisms can be constructive (adaptive) or destructive (maladaptive). *Constructive coping mechanisms* include the ability to be flexible in response to different situations, to take responsibility, and to be independent and assertive when needed. *Destructive coping mechanisms* ward off anxiety without resolving the cause of the problem, and include defence mechanisms such as denial and repression and behaviours such as being constantly submissive. Constructive lifestyle factors include a healthy diet, exercise, effective time management and illness-prevention measures such as regular medical checks, vaccinations and breast screening. Destructive lifestyle factors include smoking, excessive consumption of alcohol and other drugs, and a sedentary lifestyle. The combination of multiple influences determine a person's ability to adapt and cope successfully with stress. Adapting to stress involves physiological and psychological responses.

PHYSIOLOGICAL ADAPTATION

Physiological adaptation to stress concerns how the central nervous system and the immune system work as an integrated whole to maintain *homeostasis*, a state of healthy balance within the body. Automatic mechanisms operate to monitor, maintain or restore a healthy state of equilibrium. These feedback mechanisms sense when there is an alteration or interruption to the norm and make adaptive responses. These processes occur continuously in response to the minor stresses of everyday life, keeping the body's internal environment constant. In the case of trauma, physical illness or prolonged stress the homeostatic responses may struggle to adapt and fail to restore normal concentrations of gases, nutrients and ions, body temperature and blood pressure to within normal limits. Medical interventions such as fluid replacement, oxygen therapy and nutritional measures can assist the process but, if unsuccessful and failure of the natural homeostatic mechanisms continues, cells die and eventually death of the person occurs.

The physiological response to acute stress is known as the fight-or-flight response. It begins when people are faced with a threat or stressful situation. When the body prepares to fight or flee, a number of changes occur. The autonomic nervous system and the neuroendocrine system combine to provide the body with the capacity to deal with the stressor. Hormones needed to adapt to the stress are secreted, muscles tense, the heart beats faster, the breathing and perspiration increase, the pupils dilate and blood sugar level increases. Once the cause of the stress is removed, homeostatic mechanisms involving the parasympathetic nervous system and decreased activity in the hypothalamus and pituitary gland return the body from its state of heightened readiness to relaxed mode (Keltner et al 2006). The fight-or-flight response is vital to defend against and tolerate danger. However, continued unresolved stress results in a chronic stress condition that impacts on the body and may produce any of a wide range of diseases and disorders. Box 13.1 indicates some of the health concerns that have been linked to stress. The body responds to stress in the same way regardless of the source of the stress and whether or not the stress is real or perceived.

Prolonged stress may also lower the threshold at which the body responds to threats, so that future stressors may trigger the physical stress response more easily. This can lead to a stress cycle whereby the person responds to relatively minor events with physical reactions and psychological fears beyond those congruent to the situation. Symptoms such as a rapid or pounding heart and rapid breathing start to become worrying, making the person even more anxious; this then reactivates the stress response, causing symptoms to become more severe. This can evolve into a cycle of stress, anxiety and more stress that ultimately causes increasingly severe or frequent episodes of high anxiety and, sometimes, negative thoughts and fears that can interfere with the person's normal lifestyle, physical and mental health (Clinical Interest Box 13.1).

A range of anxiety disorders such as panic disorder, acute stress disorder (ASD) and post-traumatic stress disorder (PTSD) has been linked to this stress cycle. Recurrent and prolonged stress causes a range of effects on mood,

Box 13.1 | Health concerns linked to stress

- Migraines
- Gastritis and gastric ulceration
- Mental problems (e.g. depression, panic disorder)
- Allergies, including eczema
- Asthma
- Ulcerative colitis
- Irritable bowel syndrome
- Crohn's disease
- Sexual dysfunction
- Eating disorders
- Cardiac disease
- Arthritis
- Cancer
- Diabetes
- Hypertension

(adapted from deWit 2005)

CLINICAL INTEREST BOX 13.1
The stressor–anxiety stress cycle

It started months ago, I don't know why. Now it is really bad. Just the thought of driving to pick my daughter up from school causes my heart to race, I get the shakes, I feel faint, sometimes I feel sick. Sometimes my heart is pounding so hard I'm sure I'm going to collapse or even die. My doctor says that won't happen, so I feel stupid, but I can't help it and these symptoms have gotten worse and worse. Now I am so anxious I never go out in the car at all. I pay for a taxi to collect my daughter from school every day.

(Sharon, 32, currently working with a therapist to gain control of her anxiety symptoms)

Box 13.2 | Common physiological effects of stress

- Abdominal pain/ distension
- Dry mouth
- Nausea/vomiting
- Dizziness
- Shakiness and tremors
- Chest discomfort
- Dyspnoea
- Hyperventilation
- Palpitations
- 'Butterflies'
- Diarrhoea
- Urinary frequency
- Faintness
- Muscle tension
- Diaphoresis
- Flushing
- Pallor
- Tachycardia

cognition and behaviour in addition to physical responses. Overwhelming stress or distress can seriously interfere with mental wellbeing and can cause the person to lose contact with what is real or not real. This may manifest with a range of effects, including disorganised and/or delusional thoughts and hallucinations.

INDICATORS OF STRESS

Stress is not easily measured but the nurse can assess and evaluate clients' subjective stress by exploring their feelings. Objective indicators may be observed in a variety of physiological, psychological, cognitive and behavioural responses. Examples of some common effects are outlined in Box 13.2. and Table 13.1.

Illness and hospitalisation and frightening medical procedures may mean that clients feel they have little control. Many people adapt successfully to the reality of what is happening to them and are able to remain optimistic and cheerful. However, individuals respond differently to the experience of illness, and high levels of anxiety and frustration at being ill or feeling neglected mean that clients may respond with irritability. This may manifest as constant complaints and criticisms or even displays of anger towards people around them, including nurses. Anxiety may also result in clients becoming withdrawn. Some may become passive and dependent on others and behave in an immature way. Some clients may become introspective and self-absorbed, showing no interest in anything other than themselves and their illness. Nurses who understand these behaviours as ways of attempting to cope with stress and anxiety continue to respond with empathy and are therefore able to promote a relationship of trust with the client. An example of a nursing diagnosis for an anxious client might be, 'Anxiety related to verbalised "fear of hospitals", as evidenced by changes in vital signs, discomfort due to diaphoresis (sweating) and client's inability to sit still, pacing and wringing hands'. A trusting relationship and effective communication skills (Chapter 29) facilitate the client being able to talk about and deal with fears and other feelings and ultimately to adapt more positively to their situation.

STRESS ADAPTATION MODELS

Two significant theoretical models concerning responses to stress are Selye's stress adaptation model and Lazarus's interactional model. An understanding of theoretical models enables the nurse to understand the mechanisms people use to adapt to stress in their lives. The ability to adapt has positive effects such as the resolution of conflicts and increased self-confidence. When people are continually unable to adapt effectively they are at risk of physical or mental ill-health and, in the worst-case scenario, death.

SELYE'S STRESS ADAPTATION MODEL

In 1950 Hans Selye published a now renowned work called *The Stress of Life*. In a later edition he defined stress as the wear and tear on the body (Selye 1976). Selye links the wear

TABLE 13.1 | Common psychological, cognitive and behavioural effects of stress

Psychological	Cognitive	Behavioural
Sadness	Confusion	Unable to sleep
Depression	Forgetfulness	Under- or over-eating
Labile mood	Inability to concentrate	Talking rapidly/loudly
Irritability	Decision making is difficult	Stammering
Quick to anger	Comprehension impaired	Inability to sit still
		Finger tapping
		Constant pulling at hair
		Constant pumping of leg up and down
		Inability to control tears

and tear on the body to chemical changes that instigate a process of adaptation.

In the 1950s Selye popularised a physiological understanding of how a person responds to stress. Selye's version of stress adaptation is that, when faced with stress, the body responds in three distinct phases: alarm reaction, stage of resistance and stage of exhaustion. These stages involve structural and chemical changes in the body that have become known as the general adaptation syndrome (GAS).

Alarm reaction

This is the initial reaction of the body to any stressor. It is a complex set of reactions between the hypothalamus, the sympathetic nervous system and the adrenal medulla. This is the fight-or-flight response referred to earlier. It creates a heightened level of alertness and mobilises the body's resources for immediate physical activity in readiness to tackle the threat. Bodily responses are designed to rapidly increase circulation, promote release of glucose for energy and decrease activity that is not essential to combat the threat.

Stage of resistance

If the cause for the stress is not removed, the body moves to this second stage of the GAS. The resistance stage provides the body with what it needs to continue fighting a stressor long after the effects of the alarm stage have fizzled out. Reactions in this stage involve the anterior pituitary gland and the adrenal cortex. The resistance reaction is slower to start than the alarm reaction but the effects are longer lasting. They serve in part to maintain the readiness created by the alarm stage, such as increased levels of glucose for energy; however, during this phase the body also begins the process of trying to return physical functioning closer to normal homeostasis.

If this stage of the GAS continues for a prolonged period of time without periods of relaxation and rest to counterbalance the stress response, sufferers become prone to fatigue, concentration lapses, irritability and lethargy. Significantly, continued release of excessive amounts of the steroid cortisol, stimulated during prolonged stress, leads to suppression of the immune response. Reduced immunity makes the body more susceptible to health problems ranging from the common cold and other infections to disorders such as headaches, gastritis, a range of intestinal disorders and cancer (Keltner et al 2006; Herlihy & Maebius 2002).

Stage of exhaustion

In this stage the body runs out of its reserve of body energy and immunity. This is the result of the inability to adapt or cope. Mental, physical and emotional resources suffer heavily. By this stage there is a significant loss of potassium ions, which interferes with the function of all body cells. Cells function less and less effectively and unless potassium depletion is reversed they will begin to die. The body experiences adrenal exhaustion, and the adrenal cortex no longer produces sufficient hormones to prevent a drop in blood glucose levels, so that eventually the body cells fail to receive adequate nutrients. The effect of a prolonged or strong resistance reaction on the body places a particularly heavy demand on the heart, blood vessels and adrenal cortex. Thus, previous health can be thought of as an indicator of a person's capacity to adapt and cope physically with stress. The inability to adapt, and the continuation of exposure to stress, results in progressive mental and physical exhaustion, illness, collapse and ultimately cardiac failure, renal failure and death.

Selye also identified that the body adapts to physical stressors at the local level, for example, when stress occurs within a single organ or area of the body. This is termed the local adaptation syndrome (LAS). It applies, for example, when a person sustains an insect bite on the foot and the body responds to the local inflammation.

Selye (1974) defined two particular concepts of stress; distress and eustress. *Distress* is described as the negative outcome that drains energy and gives rise to feelings of anxiety, confusion and depression, and creates an inner sense of helplessness and hopelessness. Mental illness is closely associated with human distress. Watkins (2001) links difficulty in adapting and coping with overwhelming distress to the distress behaviours and feelings associated with poor mental health, for example, defensive or self-harming behaviour, despair, helplessness, anger, guilt and self-loathing. *Eustress* is described as the converse effect that gives rise to positive outcomes — motivating energy, feelings of happiness and an inner sense of peace and hope.

Psychosocial changes

Although Selye did not elaborate on the psychosocial effects of stressors, psychosocial changes have been aligned with the GAS model (Table 13.2).

During the alarm stage there may be some positive psychosocial effects, such as new learning and the development or enhancement of problem-solving skills (Keltner et al 2006). During the resistance stage, problem solving and learning are more difficult than during the alarm stage; they can be achieved, but often only with help. During the resistance stage the use of defence mechanisms is increased. These are coping mechanisms that operate mostly at an unconscious level. They serve to help people resolve inner conflict, reduce fear or anxiety and protect self-esteem and personal sense of security.

Defence mechanisms (Table 13.3) help people to reduce their anxiety by denying, misinterpreting or distorting what is happening. For example, when clients are faced with information that causes overwhelming anxiety, such as a diagnosis of cancer, they may unconsciously use the mechanism of denial to protect themselves from anxiety that is not manageable at that time. Denial may take the form of refusing to talk about the diagnosis, not informing

TABLE 13.2 | Stress adaptation syndrome

Stage	Physical response	Psychosocial changes
Stage 1: Alarm reaction Mobilisation of the body's defensive forces and activation of the fight-or-flight mechanism	Noradrenaline and adrenaline are released, causing vasoconstriction, increased blood pressure and increased rate and force of cardiac contractions Hormone levels are increased The adrenal cortex enlarges Shrinkage of the thymus, spleen and lymph nodes Irritation of the gastric mucosa	Increased level of alertness Increased feelings of anxiety Task-oriented, defence-oriented, inefficient or maladaptive behaviour may occur
Stage II: Stage of resistance Optimal adaptation to stress within the person's capabilities	Hormone levels readjust Reduction in activity and size of adrenal cortex Lymph nodes return to normal size	Increased and intensified use of coping mechanisms Tendency to rely on defence-oriented behaviour Psychosomatic symptoms may develop
Stage III: Stage of exhaustion Loss of ability to resist stress because of depletion of body resources: fight, flight or immobilisation occurs	Decreased immune response with suppression of T cells and atrophy of thymus Depletion of adrenal glands and hormone production Weight loss Enlargement of lymph nodes and dysfunction of lymphatic system If exposure to the stressor continues, cardiac failure, renal failure or death may occur	Defence-oriented behaviours become exaggerated Disorganisation of thinking Disorganisation of personality Sensory stimuli may be misinterpreted, with appearance of illusion Contact with reality may be reduced and delusions and hallucinations may occur If exposure to the stressor continues, stupor or violence may occur

(Wilson & Kneisl 1996)

TABLE 13.3 | Common defence mechanisms

	Mild use	Extreme use
Repression	Man forgets wife's birthday after a marital fight	Woman is unable to enjoy sex after pushing out of her awareness a traumatic sexual incident during childhood
Displacement	Client criticises a nurse after his family fail to visit him in hospital	Child who is unable to acknowledge fear of his father becomes fearful of animals
Projection	Man who is unconsciously attracted to other women accuses his wife of flirting	Woman who has repressed an attraction towards other women refuses to socialise. She fears another woman will make homosexual advances towards her
Undoing	After flirting with her male work colleague, a woman buys her husband tickets to a show	Man with rigid and moralistic beliefs and repressed sexuality is driven to wash his hands when around attractive women to gain composure
Denial	Man reacts to news of the death of a loved one: 'No, I don't believe you. The doctor said she was fine'	Woman whose husband died 3 years ago still lays a place for him at the dinner table and talks about him in the present tense

(adapted from Varcarolis 2006)

or even lying to loved ones, and planning activities without consideration of the illness.

There are many defence mechanisms. Another common one is rationalisation. Rationalisation is justification of certain behaviours by faulty logic and by attributing motives to the behaviour that are socially acceptable. The behaviour, however, in reality is not justified. A mother who smacks her small child too hard might rationalise this behaviour by saying 'It was OK because he couldn't feel it through the nappy anyway', This rationalisation helps her to cope with feelings of concern and inadequacy about being unable to meet her own and other people's expectations of a 'good mother'. Defence mechanisms are adaptive relief behaviours used by everyone but, when overused, are reflective of self-deception and distortions of reality that are likely to interfere with personal growth and personal feelings of satisfaction.

Generally, many people manage to adapt and get through very stressful situations successfully, and their body physiology returns to normal. If not, the person moves from the resistance stage into the last stage of the GAS, the stage of exhaustion. By the exhaustion stage the emotionally overwhelming effects of continued exposure to stress may be manifesting with symptoms of serious mental disturbance. People may become totally unable to function, appear disorganised and be unable to make decisions. Thoughts and actions may become illogical and the personality altered. Orientation to reality may be seriously impaired and behaviours such as withdrawal and aggression may manifest. At this stage people do not always appear visibly anxious but the risk for suicide may be very real.

Cognitive and sociocultural stressors are thought to be among the most potent in activating the biological stress response. Social isolation and responses to grief, for example, are known risk factors for illness, especially in the elderly and the socially and economically disadvantaged. It is known that grief, in the case of the death of a spouse, increases the risk of illness and death in the surviving spouse, especially during the first 6 months after bereavement (Keltner et al 2006).

LAZARUS'S INTERACTIONAL THEORY

Lazarus does not believe that biological response models like the GAS provide a complete explanation regarding the outcomes of stress on individuals. He believes that individual people differ in their vulnerability to stress and to the way they interpret and react to particular stressors. The most significant aspect of Lazarus's (1966) theory is the concept that it is the way in which individuals interpret the stressor and their ability to cope (appraisal) that determines the effects of the stress. Individual appraisal of the situation depends on the factors mentioned earlier and include the individual's personal values, beliefs and feelings and what is viewed as important or not important to that person; for example, the stress of a job interview will generally be appraised as very high if the person desperately needs or wants the particular job.

Three types of appraisal are outlined here: primary, secondary and reappraisal. Primary appraisal relates to judgments about the specific situation made by the person. The person answers the questions: What does this mean to me? What effect will this have on me? Secondary appraisal relates to the person's assessment of how they will deal with any given situation. It involves appraisal of what might hinder coping and what personal strengths, resources and supports can be drawn upon to deal with the matter. It also involves appraisal of possible approaches or solutions to the situation faced. Reappraisal occurs after fresh or extra information has been gathered.

Lazarus advocates that the level of stress and anxiety is determined by the outcome of this appraisal; that it is connected to whether or not the person appraises the situation as manageable, as draining, or exceeding personal coping resources and endangering personal wellbeing (Lazarus & Folkman 1984). The coping strategies that individual people have developed influence how they appraise a situation and may or may not equip them to deal with particular stressors. Sometimes a person's normal coping strategies will not equip them to deal with a particular type of situation and this has negative effects; for example, a nurse who has learned to cope with conflict by being submissive is likely to find it difficult to deal with a conflict situation at work, even when it is at variance with their personal values and work ethic (Clinical Interest Box 13.2).

An understanding of theoretical models provides a basis on which nurses develop skills that help assess the impact of stress on clients, and their coping mechanisms. The nurse will need to assess the person's perception of the stressor, the current level of health and fitness, previous life experiences, social support systems and established coping mechanisms (deWit 2005). This encompasses actively listening to the client to gain understanding of the client's:

- Responses to the feelings generated by the stressor
- Perceptions of and reactions to the stressful event
- Past and current ways of coping with feelings and stressors
- Own appraisal of their coping skills, e.g., does the client perceive that their coping skills are adequate for most or all the situations previously encountered or do they perceive deficits in this area?

In addition to this type of exploration of the client's experiences, the nurse uses keen observation skills to note the client's behavioural responses. Assessing clients' stress and coping abilities is important in every area of

CLINICAL INTEREST BOX 13.2
Appraisal of established coping mechanisms

Megan has worked as an Enrolled Nurse at Silverstone Lodge for several years. New management has changed the culture of the organisation. Megan feels that staff cuts and the focus on getting tasks done quickly has seriously lowered quality of life for the clients. She is no longer able to spend time reminiscing and caring for them in special ways. She believes this to be extremely important for all the residents of this facility, especially for the many who have dementia. Megan would like to challenge the management about this situation but she does not appraise herself as having the inner resources to do so. She doesn't feel strong enough, she thinks of herself as weak because she has never been able to stand up to her dominating mother, and now a bullying husband. She is experiencing headaches and is unable to sleep because the problem at work is so stressful and appears to be insoluble.

nursing and particularly so in mental health care. Less than adequate coping skills in the past influence future vulnerability to stress and the potential for significant mental health problems such as depression, anxiety disorders and disorders of perception. The primary aims of mental health professionals include helping clients to identify current coping mechanisms, reducing the use of destructive mechanisms, strengthening constructive coping mechanisms and promoting an improved level of self-esteem.

ILLNESS AND STRESS

HOSPITALISED ADULTS

Hospitalisation means that clients are not, for the duration of their stay, able to follow their usual daily routines; for example, the diet or exercise they are used to. They often severely miss the lack of home comforts and the presence of family, friends and familiar things. They may also be stressed by an unknown diagnosis and frightened about possible pain and discomfort, potential treatments and outcomes. The nurse can help alleviate some of this anxiety by providing full and timely information. Anxiety can affect concentration and memory, so when a client is anxious it is particularly important to ascertain whether the information has been understood, to repeat it if necessary and provide written information that the client may consider later (see Chapter 29).

Clients also have to adapt to stressors such as the lack of privacy, which may include concerns about sharing a room with strangers, strangers finding out about their medical details, having to wear hospital gowns that are open down the back, exposure of private areas during surgery, investigative procedures or treatments and having health care workers barging in during toileting or bathing. The nurse can help alleviate some of these stressors by introducing newly admitted clients to those in the shared room, by being diligent about protecting confidentiality and taking practical steps to prevent unnecessary exposure (see Chapter 27). Nurses not assisting with personal care should themselves undertake not to enter the room or the area behind closed curtains without first confirming that the client is not exposed.

Some clients may be very anxious about the ability to meet religious dietary and worship, or modesty and hygiene, requirements. Those with limited spoken English are likely to be stressed about the ability to understand or be understood. A nursing assessment that carefully identifies cultural and spiritual needs is the tool that helps the nurse minimise associated stressors. Resolution might include coordinating care to allow time for prayer, adapting Western orientated hygiene methods to suit specific modesty needs and involving an interpreter (see Chapters 9 and 11).

Other stressors include the worry about family responsibilities, costs of medical treatment and perhaps loss of earnings while sick. Compounding the problem there may be an inability to sleep because of pain, discomfort, noise, a strange bed or missing the usual sleeping partner. Empathic and considerate general nursing care activities can significantly reduce these common anxieties. (Care activities relating to these stressors are explained in Chapters 34 and 35.)

A significant aspect of care related to minimising stress is establishing a relationship that demonstrates respect and empathy for the client. This includes being prepared to sit and listen to the client and facilitating the expression of fears and anxieties (see Chapter 29).

CHILDREN

It is not unusual for children to feel anxiety. Very young children often fear strangers or being left alone; preschoolers often fear imaginary creatures, animals and the dark. School-age children may experience anxiety about their own safety; for example, being very anxious during a storm. As children move towards the middle years of school and head into adolescence, anxieties tend to become more focused on performance at school, appearance and other social and health issues.

It is quite common for children to develop fears about losing their parents (separation anxiety). When this anxiety is strong, children may be diagnosed with separation anxiety disorder. Children who have separation anxiety may experience physical symptoms such as nausea, vomiting, stomach pains, palpitations, respiratory difficulty and dizziness. Separation anxiety can occur at any age. Children may follow parents around the house, needing to be constantly in very close proximity, they may refuse to go to school and may worry about being kidnapped and killed, or their parents being killed. Most children outgrow this fear but some have symptoms that recur periodically and especially when attachments are threatened or disrupted, such as at the time of hospitalisation (Fontaine & Fletcher 2002).

The nurse who is aiming to reduce stress in children is most therapeutic when able to listen actively and encourage dialogue with open questions such as, 'Tell me about what you like playing with at home'. It is best to avoid the specific question–answer format because children tend to feel uncomfortable about this and answer with very short, simple responses that give little information. Communicating effectively with children is a specific communication skill (see Chapter 29). Children are very sensitive to insincere platitudes and fake sentiments and are usually very quick at determining if a nurse is genuine and can be trusted.

Working with emotionally stressed children in the area of mental health is an area of specialty. A variety of therapies are helpful, including play therapy, art therapy and guided imagery. The goals of therapy are to:

- Establish rapport
- Help children reveal feelings they are unable to verbalise
- Enable children to act out feelings, anxieties or tension in a constructive manner

- Understand children's relationships and interactions with others of significance to them in their lives
- Teach adaptive socialisation skills
- Enhance self-esteem.

Guided imagery and children

Guided imagery is an anxiety-reducing technique that many adults find helpful. It is a form of therapy that helps clients consciously visualise positive images to lift their mood, reduce their anxiety, deal with the effects of illness or trauma or prevent illness (Hitchcock & Schubert 2002). In a simple form it can successfully be used with children to increase their coping skills and enhance their feelings of self-worth. Children usually have strong imaginations and are able to conjure up mental pictures quite easily. Guided imagery begins with a short relaxation exercise followed by general directions for the imagery (visualisation). Children may be gently guided towards mental images of heroes and heroines that help them cope, and may be able to visualise themselves and their families as happy and cheerful. They may also imagine different ways of interacting with others (Fontaine & Fletcher 2002). For example, Laura, aged 10, had frequent nightmares and was very frightened of the 'dark monster who comes in the night'. She was able to imagine herself a friend — a fire-breathing dragon. Through guided imagery she learned how to call on her dragon friend, who she called Sheba, to come and stay by her to protect her whenever she felt scared.

Hospitalised children

When time allows, it can help to reduce stress if children are able to visit the hospital and become familiar with the staff and the environment before admission. During hospitalisation a child's anxiety may be relieved by the presence of a parent or other familiar person. The child may also feel less worried if allowed to bring familiar items into hospital.

Parents often wish to stay with a child who is hospitalised, but some are not able to do so because of other family or work commitments. Parents who are unable to stay often feel guilty and stressed. The nurse who is non-judgmental and understanding of this can do much to reduce feelings of guilt with comforting statements such as, 'Don't worry, I know you have to go. I'll take good care of him. You can ring me when you can to see how he is.'

The nurse who ensures that parents are comfortable, especially those staying for long periods or overnight, is usually warmly appreciated. Ensuring that parents are provided with all the information available can help alleviate anxiety — the unknown is sometimes the most serious stressor. Many parents like to help with basic needs such as the child's hygiene, and a child may prefer and be comforted by this, but help from family members should not be assumed unless the hospital has previously discussed a shared care agreement.

Children who are hospitalised for lengthy periods have socialisation and educational needs. Most acute care hospitals catering for children have specialists who ensure that these needs are met.

ADOLESCENTS

Sometimes high levels of stress during hospitalisation can result in adolescent behaviours that challenge the nurse. The adolescent years are a time of incredible physical and psychological adjustment. The tasks of adolescence include acceptance of a changed body image, establishing independence from parents, deciding on a career pathway and adjusting to a comfortable sexual role. The adolescent may be supersensitive to recent body changes and may have concerns about body image. The threat of body exposure may be a source of great embarrassment. The nurse can help reduce adolescent stress by respecting client autonomy and valuing the client as a person, facilitating the verbalisation of fears, demonstrating sensitivity to concerns about body image, exposure and function, and providing clear explanations about all care, treatment and procedures.

Common reasons for hospitalisation in adolescence include vehicle and sporting accidents, unsuccessful suicide attempts, teenage pregnancy, sexually transmitted infections, drug abuse and depression. Anorexia nervosa and bulimia nervosa are also common but are generally treated on an outpatient basis unless severe enough to be life threatening (Shives 2007). Whatever personal views the nurse may hold about these issues, every client deserves to be cared for with compassion and without judgment.

Sometimes concerns are overwhelming for the adolescent and may result in emotional responses such as resentment, hostility or guilt. The hospitalised adolescent may become isolative, manipulative, reject hospital rules or even physical care if feelings such as fear, guilt or embarrassment are unmanageable (Clinical Interest Box 13.3).

Stressors may be lessened by supportive peer interactions. Visits from friends are important, especially when adolescents are placed on wards with only adults for company. This may help relieve anxiety about missing

CLINICAL INTEREST BOX 13.3
The link between fears and behaviour

Melanie, 15, was diagnosed with diabetes. She was resentful and hostile towards the nurse who was encouraging her to self-administer her insulin medication. Melanie stormed away, shouting and refusing the treatment altogether. A little later the nurse sat and talked with Melanie, who eventually disclosed fears about how having diabetes would affect her social life. She also revealed beliefs that the diabetes was her own fault — a punishment for promiscuous behaviour and a termination of pregnancy that she had not told her parents about. The nurse listened without judging Melanie, alleviated some of the guilt by answering questions about the onset of diabetes, and helped her to identify some ways that she might cope with the diabetes after discharge.

school, social activities or losing touch with the peer group. Sometimes the adolescent client's feelings and fears can be exacerbated because adult clients in a shared room tease or give erroneous advice or information. It should be acknowledged that while the adolescents may strive to demonstrate adult behaviour, they may be struggling with homesickness — hospitalisation is sometimes the first time young teenagers have been separated from parents or family without being with their peers (Shives 2007). Nursing interventions to address adolescent emotional responses and some of the more common behaviours are identified in Table 13.4.

OLDER ADULTS

People in the older age group frequently experience many losses and changes in a relatively short time frame. Some older people adapt effectively to the stress this causes. Many are able to plan and implement a successful transition from work to retirement. Many are able to respond positively to the challenges and find exciting and creative activities that provide a high quality of life well into old age. Others experience difficulty with the transition, the accumulative losses and changes and suffer stress overload. Nurses may be able to observe signs of this, such as unconscious repetitive actions that serve to relieve tension and stress, and, sometimes, changes to cognitive abilities. Many physical changes such as those that affect sight and hearing or mobility may occur gradually and this allows time for the process of adaptation. However, such stressors, whether slow or sudden, may compound with social losses and concerns about the future to the point where strong inner resources are needed to avert a stress crisis. Some of the stressors faced by older people include:

- Changes in body image
- Increases in rent or living costs and ability to manage financially now or in the future
- Coping with home maintenance
- Loss of driver's licence or transport independence
- Death of friends, siblings or pets
- Chronic or acute pain
- Concern about care and protection when frail and vulnerable
- Fear of losing, or loss of, mental abilities
- Fear of loneliness, dying alone, or not being found
- Fear of institutionalisation and leaving own possessions or pets
- Inheritance conflicts
- Intolerance or negative ageist attitudes demonstrated by others
- Caring for a spouse with dementia.

Anxiety and low self-esteem often occur together and particularly in older people who are ill, hospitalised or living in residential care settings. The way care is provided and the nurse's communication with clients or residents can have a highly positive effect on reducing anxiety and increasing morale. Two basic principles for minimising stress are:

TABLE 13.4 | Nursing interventions for a selection of common adolescent emotional responses and behaviours

Adolescent emotional response/behaviour	Nursing Interventions
Embarrassment	Reassure and maintain confidentiality. Provide an opportunity to talk about concerns, without family present if necessary Be alert to feelings regarding body image and need for privacy Encourage as much self-care as possible Provide for personal space and minimal body exposure during care Ensure that client has information about procedures or surgery, and expected impact on body
Homesickness	If possible, provide for home conveniences such as TV, telephone and snacks Facilitate dietary preferences when appropriate Encourage family members to bring in favourite foods, provided that they meet with any medical dietary needs Ensure client is kept informed of news from home
Fear	Accept without judgment any defences or behaviour used to retain control. Report concerns so that a person confident about broaching these matters is able to discuss with client Ensure that client is provided with detailed explanations regarding treatment, nursing care and progress
Resentment	Facilitate exploration of feelings of resentment to help identify underlying cause Encourage visits from peers and siblings, with flexible visiting hours as much as possible Coordinate care so that any school work can be continued when able Do not 'side with' parents in any criticism of the adolescent or his behaviour even if the client displays anger or hostility
(adapted from Shives 2007)	

1. Limiting change as much as possible; for example, when and where possible, have the same people provide services and care (change increases stress) (Clinical Interest Box 13.4)
2. Coordinating care and implementing any essential changes during the times when clients are best able to cope. People frequently have times of the day, month or year when they are functioning better or less stressed than others; for example, it would not be advisable to discuss changing a client's accommodation arrangements late in the evening if that is when they are most tired; it would be unwise to introduce any major changes near the anniversary of a significant bereavement.

The nurse can also help to limit the damage from the structural and chemical changes to the body and the risk of illness caused by prolonged stress by ensuring that, whenever possible, the client or resident has a highly nutritious diet (see Chapter 31), and by ensuring the provision of an environment and nursing strategies to ensure the client or resident obtains adequate rest and sleep (see Chapter 34) (Ebersole et al 2008).

Preventing and treating stress in the older person

Preventing and treating stress in the older person includes promoting self-worth, a sense of control, feelings of connectedness and hope. The nurse can facilitate feelings of self-worth by complimenting clients on their achievements and encouraging reflection on personal strengths. A sense of control can be promoted by allowing clients or residents to make decisions for themselves. For a client with dementia this may mean offering simple choices that do not confuse, for example, 'Would you like to wear this dress today?'. Simple actions such as encouraging participation in group activities, introducing clients to each other and smiling and speaking to the client that you pass in the corridor helps to foster feelings of connectedness. Providing pleasurable experiences and things to do fosters happiness and hope, even in very difficult circumstances. For example, the client who has cancer or a degenerative disorder can still enjoy the pleasures of music, a beautiful garden, the smell of roses, the company of pets, children and other social interactions.

CLINICAL INTEREST BOX 13.4
Avoiding change — regular services reduce client stress and increase ability to cope

Mavis is totally dependent now, she can't move much at all. I change her, feed her, put her to bed. I do all the cooking. I used to cope better when Joanne was our regular nurse. She came as regularly as clockwork to bath Mavis. She came at the same time every day, except weekends, for eight years. She could do it all herself, manage the lifter and everything. While she was here I could sit and have my breakfast, read the paper and relax. It was the thing that set me up for the day. Since Joanne left to have her baby we have had a constant stream of different people, for weeks now, not even always the same time of day. Mostly I have to show the new ones how to do it, help them get her into the lifter. I just get them knowing what needs doing when a different person comes. I really miss that one little bit of peaceful time in the mornings, and Mavis doesn't even bother trying to talk to them now. She used to enjoy her bath with Joanne. Now we both hate it and I don't know how much longer I can go on like this. Some days I feel like screaming and I've even thought about walking out. It's surprising what a difference that little bit of time made.

(Frank, 68, carer husband of Mavis, who has multiple sclerosis)

THE NURSE AND STRESS

Caring for others takes energy and only nurses who care for themselves can continuously provide sensitive and empathic care to clients. The emotional nature of nursing means that those working within it are likely to be more vulnerable to stress than those in other occupations (Erickson & Ritter 2001; Johnson et al 2006). The term 'nursing burnout' is used to explain an advanced form of work-related stress related to a group of symptoms that involve physical, emotional and behavioural categories. These include a depletion of physical energy and emotional exhaustion. Burnout relates to stress that has drained personal coping resources and may be caused, in part, to nurses not having adapted to their own stresses and strains constructively (Ekstedt & Fagerberg 2005). Anyone can burn out, become seriously stressed and unable to cope if work and personal commitments are overwhelming. Some actions that help nurses to adapt and cope with stress include:

- Distinguishing between what it is possible and not possible to change, and accepting the 'givens'
- Establishing a priority list of work tasks
- Mixing and balancing stressful and non-stressful activities and projects
- Setting limits, e.g., on meeting the demands of others
- Building a support system of co-workers and friends
- Allowing time to acknowledge and reflect on personal feelings
- 'Debriefing' after stressful events at work
- Recognising that it is usually possible to find alternatives and make choices
- Maintaining a healthy lifestyle; for example, diet, exercise, sleep, rest, relaxation
- Self-checking whether tasks are essential to do when busy; for example, 'What will happen if I don't wash the kitchen floor this week?'
- Recognising internal sources of stress (shoulds and oughts)
- Acknowledging at the end of the day and each week what was achieved, rather than focusing on what should or ought to have been done
- Re-examining personal values — clarifying what is or is not important in life.

THERAPEUTIC APPROACHES TO STRESS MANAGEMENT

A range of basic elements contribute to minimising client stress and anxiety. These include:

- Friendly, relaxed nurse–client and staff relationships
- Flexible treatment and care schedules
- A calm and quiet environment
- Supportive relationships with clients and their families
- Effective orientation to the ward or care facility; for example, hostel or aged-care accommodation unit
- Adequate information, with information repeated if necessary
- Active participation of clients in planning care
- Facilitating clients to express feelings and thoughts
- Promoting exercise, healthy nutrition and periods of relaxation
- Assisting clients to make correct appraisals of situations
- Assisting clients to identify effective and ineffective coping behaviours
- Raising awareness of complementary therapies that may help.

Some specific therapeutic approaches include education, cognitive behaviour therapy, medication, assertiveness training and humour.

EDUCATION

Education is an important component of nursing care. The aim is to use education to improve clients' adaptive responses to anxiety. The nurse collaborates with each individual client to determine what education might be helpful, then formulates care activities designed to increase the client's knowledge of the stressors that precipitate anxiety, and coping resources and adaptive and maladaptive responses. Goals include helping the client recognise signs and symptoms of their own anxiety, gain insights into the anxiety and cope with the threat. Education is most effective when it incorporates principles and techniques of cognitive behaviour therapy. One such technique is *self-training*. Self-training is particularly helpful for people who experience recurrent symptoms of anxiety that are more severe than is warranted by the situation, for example, clients who experience unwarranted anxiety at panic level (panic attacks).

Self-training helps clients to reduce their anxiety, first by recognising physical symptoms as being caused only by their anxiety. Then by undertaking positive 'self-talk', for example:

> I am feeling anxious about this but I can control these responses. I won't focus on my symptoms, I will just breathe slowly, relax and concentrate on finishing what I'm doing. These feelings will soon pass. I am OK. I can manage this until the symptoms stop.

Self-training helps people to regain control when anxiety threatens to become overwhelming.

COGNITIVE BEHAVIOUR THERAPY

Cognitive behaviour therapy (CBT) is based on three main treatment approaches: reducing anxiety, cognitive restructuring and learning new behaviour. The goal is to help clients develop their coping skills. It is a strong focus for therapy in the area of mental health and can be used for a variety of problems, including depression and a range of anxiety disorders. However, after the nurse has learned the principles of CBT they can be applied in any health care setting to promote healthy coping responses. CBT often incorporates teaching the client how to reduce anxiety by using progressive relaxation techniques and guided imagery. When clients have been taught these techniques they are armed with self-help tools that can provide them with a way to control their stress levels and enhance feelings of control (Morgillo-Freeman & Freeman 2005).

Cognitive restructuring

Cognitive therapy is based on the understanding that it is people's expectations and appraisal of events that determines adaptation to stress. It presupposes that behaviour can be altered by changing a person's established thoughts and beliefs. Cognitive restructuring helps clients to identify thoughts that are distorted and anxiety provoking. The aim is to help them identify, catch, stop and challenge distorted thoughts. Ultimately this helps people to appraise situations and events realistically. Table 13.5 provides examples of common cognitive distortions.

Catching and challenging thoughts is a two-stage process. The person must first learn to 'catch' the distorted thought, such as, 'I forgot to put my name on the list, I must be losing my mind, I forget everything, I'm getting more and more stupid'. After catching the thought, the person must consciously relax for 15–30 seconds. Next, the person must challenge the self-demeaning thought and examine the evidence for it: 'Do I actually forget everything? Am I really stupid? Am I going mad?' Often the answer will be reassuring, for example, 'No, I don't forget everything, I remember most things, most of the time. So, I just forgot to put my name of the list, no big deal. I am not stupid, I am just a very busy person.' The catch, stop and challenge technique usually results in more realistic thinking.

It takes practice to change what are often ingrained patterns of distorted thinking to realistic thinking, but when practised effectively, this technique becomes automatic and provides the client with a powerful self-help tool — a new coping strategy to help alleviate anxiety. The examples of CBT provided here aim to serve only as an introduction to an important therapy for anxiety and anxiety-related disorders.

MEDICATION

A variety of medications may be used to help people who are experiencing difficulty adapting to stress. They are usually prescribed only for people whose level of anxiety interferes with activities of daily living. Medications

TABLE 13.5 | Examples of common cognitive distortions

Distortion	Definition	Example
Magnification	Exaggerating or trivialising the importance of events	'I've lost my purse, which just goes to show how unreliable I am'
Perfectionism	Needing to do everything perfectly to feel good about oneself	'I'll be a failure if I don't get a high distinction in every subject'
Mind reading	Believing that one knows the thoughts of another without validation	'They probably think I'm fat and stupid'
Catastrophising	Thinking the worst about people and events	'I'd better not go on that holiday, it will probably be cold and rain all the time, there will probably be horrible people there and I probably won't even like the place'
Over-generalisation	Draws conclusions about a wide variety of things on the basis of one single event	A student who has failed an examination thinks 'I'll never pass any of my other exams this semester and I'll get kicked out of the course'
Personalisation	Relates external events to oneself when it is not justified	'My boss said our company's productivity was down this year, but I know he was really talking about me'
Dichotomous thinking	Thinking in extremes — that things are either all good or all bad	'If my husband leaves me I might as well be dead'
Arbitrary inference	Drawing a negative conclusion without supporting evidence	A young woman concludes 'My friend no longer likes me' because she did not receive a card from her on her birthday
Selective abstraction	Focusing on details but not on other relevant information	A wife believes her husband doesn't love her because he spends a lot of his time on keeping fit and working on his car, but she ignores his affectionate actions, such as the gifts he brings her and the special holiday they are planning together

(adapted from Stuart & Laraia 2004)

include benzodiazepines, which reduce anxiety and worry symptoms, and tricyclic antidepressants and monoamine oxidase inhibitors (MAOIs) that can be helpful in treating people who experience panic disorders and phobias. However, while medications tackle the symptoms of anxiety they do not help establish an understanding of the cause, nor help in developing coping strategies to alleviate the problem. If they are necessary, anti-anxiety drugs should therefore always be used in conjunction with psychosocial treatments. Recent studies demonstrate that cognitive behavioural therapy (combining relaxation exercises and cognitive restructuring), with the goal of bringing the worry process under control, is the most effective psychosocial treatment for anxiety disorders (Stuart & Laraia 2004).

ASSERTIVENESS TRAINING

Many stress states occur and linger because people react to tension in a passive (submissive) or aggressive way. The ability to be assertive helps people to be in control of situations that impact on their lives, and a sense of control reduces stress. Assertive behaviour is the honest and open communication of personal views, needs and emotions. It is neither passive nor aggressive. Assertive people do not allow others to take advantage of them and therefore are not victims. Being assertive is a non-aggressive way to remain in control without hurting others. However, it is not a simple matter to change behaviour. Learning to be assertive, when normally being passive or aggressive, takes time. It is best learned slowly over several sessions and is best taught by a competent facilitator. Some mental health nurses become excellent facilitators.

HUMOUR

It is an important part of a nurse's role to help people verbalise feelings, fears and anxieties. However, introspection is energy demanding and cannot be sustained for long periods of time. The role of the nurse is to listen to clients who need an opportunity to discuss the issues that are concerning them, some of which might be deeply important, but the nurse needs to recognise that clients frequently require relief from those sometimes very emotionally laden and distressing feelings. Humour is one way to facilitate this. Throughout life people often use humour as a way to cope with stress. Humour can and does often play an important role in maintaining a sense of normality even when people are faced with serious illness. McIntyre and Chaplin (2001) emphasise the palliative care nurse's responsibility

CLINICAL INTEREST BOX 13.5
Therapeutic care and humour

'When I had my stroke I felt like my life was finished, but the nurses were all very firm with me, pushed me to help myself dress and so on. I am so grateful now for that but what helped me more than anything at the time was two particular nurses, who both had a lovely sense of humour, so essential when life seems so grim. Their humour was never directed at me, nor did it ever make light of the seriousness of what was happening to me. What it did was help me get a sense of perspective and help me see light when otherwise things looked pretty black.'
(Rhonda, age 57)

to use humour to foster light-heartedness and normality in the lives of their clients, the reason being that a sense of normality can in turn support the client's sense of control. Maintaining a sense of control is one aspect of care that can help reduce the level of stress associated with any given situation.

Humour occurs in the general nursing area in a number of ways, including funny get-well cards, balloon flower arrangements and other cheer-up gifts. Clients often enjoy light relief from humorous books or cartoons and comedy programs on the television. Humour 'scrapbooks' can be effective and the use of visiting clowns can be helpful in lifting the spirits of seriously ill children. Nurses and clients frequently use humour to help:

- Promote comfortable and therapeutic relationships
- Relieve or release feelings of tension, anxiety, anger and aggression
- When feelings are too painful or stressful to cope with at that moment
- Facilitate the learning process.

Norman Cousins (1979) felt that humour was invaluable in coping with the stress of his chronic debilitating illness. After unsuccessful traditional medical treatment he promoted the use of funny movies, books and jokes as a somewhat controversial, but successful, method of treatment. He produced journal articles, a book and a movie that popularised fun and laughter as a therapy. Since then, humour as a form of therapy has gained validity. Clinical Interest Box 13.5 provides an example of the therapeutic use of humour. Scientists have hypothesised that laughter releases endorphins into the circulation, and endorphins are reported to lift mood (Varcarolis 2006).

Humour, however, is a diffuse 'fuzzy' sort of thing — a matter of taste and influenced by each person's culture. Therefore a level of caution is appropriate in using humour to relieve stress. Not all people have a sense of humour or share the same sense of humour, and sometimes it might not be appropriate to use humour. The nurse will need to evaluate the client's receptivity to fun and laughter — a light approach will not always work. However, if it does not feel right at one time, it may work well at another.

SUMMARY

To develop a helping relationship that promotes the delivery of effective nursing care, a nurse requires knowledge about how the experience of illness affects people of all ages. Illness is a major stressor that affects not only clients who are ill, but also those who are close to them. When stress occurs, an individual uses both physical and emotional energy to respond and adapt; they may use defence mechanisms. An understanding of the theories that explain the process of adaptation to stress, and knowledge of therapeutic approaches, will enhance the nurse's ability to care effectively for anxious, stressed clients. Nurses who work collaboratively with clients to help strengthen their capacity to cope with illness and stress may experience deep feelings of satisfaction when they are successful. To work effectively with anxious and stressed clients, nurses must be able to recognise their own levels of stress and attend to the measures that maintain their own mental and physical wellbeing.

REVIEW EXERCISES

1. Discuss the effects of hospitalisation in relation to clients and stress.
2. Define the differences between internal and external stressors.
3. Identify five aspects of a stressor that influence the ability to adapt and cope.
4. Identify 10 aspects of the individual person that influence adaptation and coping.
5. Explain the possible physiological, psychological, cognitive and behavioural effects of prolonged stress.
6. State five aspects of lifestyle that prevent or promote stress adaptation and coping.
7. Explain the purpose of defence mechanisms, identify two and provide an example of each in use.
8. Explain the difference between constructive and destructive coping mechanisms and provide an example of each.
9. Identify three emotional responses commonly experienced by hospitalised adolescent clients. Outline the nursing interventions that promote their ability to adapt and cope successfully with these feelings.
10. Outline a range of nursing skills that facilitate older clients living in residential care to adapt to the stresses of their situation.

CRITICAL THINKING EXERCISES

1. You are admitting Joanna, a 20-year-old single woman who works as an assistant in a dress shop. She lives in a house with three friends. Joanna is being admitted to a four-bed ward after being reviewed in the accident and emergency unit. She is to have an appendicectomy later today. You observe and sense Joanna's anxiety.
   a) Develop a series of questions so that you can ascertain the various stressors Joanna might be facing.

b) Develop a series of questions so that you can ascertain her stress adaptation and coping skills.
c) You identify that Joanna has not been in hospital before. She is very anxious about what has and will happen to her and, in particular, she is concerned about being with strangers. Identify nursing interventions that will assist Joanna to adapt and cope with this unexpected situation.

2. You have a budget of $200 to create a 'humour bag' for each of two hospital units in a general hospital, the children's unit (clients up to 15 years of age) and the adult medical/surgical unit (male and female mixed). The humour bags will be available for the use of clients, families and staff alike. What will you put in each and why?

REFERENCES AND FURTHER READING

Boyd MA (2007) *Psychiatric Nursing: Contemporary Practice*. Lippincott, Philadelphia

Cousins N (1979) *Anatomy of an Illness*. Bantam, New York

deWit S (2005) *Fundamental Concepts and Skills for Nursing*, 2nd edn. WB Saunders, Philadelphia

Ebersole P, Hess P, Touhy TS, Jett K, Luggen A (2008) *Toward Healthy Ageing*, 7th edn. Mosby Elsevier, St Louis

Ekstedt M, Fagerberg I (2005) Lived experiences of the time preceding burnout. *Journal of Advanced Nursing*, 49(1), 59–67

Erickson RJ, Ritter C (2001) Emotional labour, burnout, and inauthenticity: Does gender matter? *Social Psychology Quarterly* 64(2), 146–63

Fontaine K, Fletcher J (2002) *Mental Health Nursing*. Prentice Hall, Upper Saddle River, New Jersey

Gulick E (2001) Emotional distress and activities of daily living functioning in persons with multiple sclerosis. *Nursing Research* 50(3) (May/June): 147–54

Herlihy B, Maebius N (2002) *The Human Body in Health and Illness*, 2nd edn. Saunders, Philadelphia

Hitchcock JE, Schubert PE (2002) *Community Health Nursing: Caring in Action*. Thomas Delmar Learning, New York

Johnson S, Cooper G, Cartwright S, Donald I, Taylor P, Millet C (2006) The experience of work-related stress across occupations. *Journal of Managerial Psychology* 20(2), 178–87

Keltner N, Schwecke L, Bostrom C (2006) *Psychiatric Nursing*, 5th edn. Mosby Elsevier, St Louis

Lazarus RS (1966) *Psychological Stress and the Coping Process*. McGraw Hill, St Louis

Lazarus RS, Folkman S (1984) *Stress, Appraisal and Coping*. Springer, New York

McIntyre R, Chaplin J (2001) Hope: the heart of palliative care. In: Kinghorn S, Gamlin R, *Palliative Nursing: Bringing Comfort and Hope*. Baillière Tindall, Edinburgh

Morgillo-Freeman S, Freeman A (2005) *Cognitive Behavior Therapy in Nursing Practice*. Springer, New York

Potter PA, Perry AG (2006) *Basic Nursing*, 6th edn. Mosby Elsevier, St Louis

Rice VH (ed) (2000) *Handbook of Stress, Coping, and Health: Implications for Nursing Research, Theory, and Practice*. Sage Publications, Thousand Oaks, CA

Selye M (1974) *Stress Without Distress*. Lippincott, Philadelphia

—— (1976) *The Stress of Life*. McGraw Hill, New York

Shives LR (2007) *Basic Concepts of Psychiatric-Mental Health Nursing*. Lippincott Wilkins and Williams, Hagerstown, Maryland

Stuart GW, Laraia MT (2004) *Principles and Practice of Psychiatric Nursing*, 8th edn. Mosby, St Louis

Thomas LA (2003) Clinical management of stressors perceived by patients on mechanical ventilation. AACN clinical issues: advanced practice in acute & critical care. *Psychosocial Issues* 14(1): 73–81

Varcarolis E (2006) *Foundations of Psychiatric Mental Health Nursing: A Clinical Approach*. WB Saunders, Philadelphia

Watkins P (2001) *Mental Health Nursing: the Art of Compassionate Care*. Butterworth–Heinemann, Oxford, UK

Wilson H, Kneisl C (1996) *Psychiatric Nursing*, 5th edn. Addison Wesley, Menlo Park, CA

Chapter 14

LOSS, GRIEF AND DEATH

OBJECTIVES

- Define the key terms/concepts
- Identify the types of losses that may cause grief
- Identify the losses faced by an older person moving to a residential care facility
- Outline the difference between staged and cyclic theoretical models of grief
- Describe common physical and psychological responses to grief
- Assist in planning and implementing care for a client who is grieving
- Assist in planning and implementing the specific physical and psychological care required by a client who is dying
- Assist with supportive bereavement care after the death of a client

KEY TERMS/CONCEPTS

bereavement
cumulative loss
dying
grief
hospice
loss
palliative care
pastoral care

CHAPTER FOCUS

The experience of grief in response to loss is known to occur to all human beings, regardless of age, gender, beliefs or culture; ultimately, then, loss and grief, and death and dying are a part of life. Potentially life entails undergoing many losses, large or small, all of which may bring an experience of grief. The experience of grief, loss and bereavement is an individual and subjective one; hence it is intrinsically difficult to define or quantify. To assist clients and others of significance to them, the nurse requires knowledge and understanding of many aspects of loss, grief, dying, death and bereavement. Only by understanding these phenomena and coming to terms with their own feelings about them can nurses adequately support others who are experiencing loss and grief. Grief needs to be considered as a health issue because ongoing physical and mental health may be adversely affected if grief issues remain unresolved.

LIVED EXPERIENCE

It is easy to lose faith and hate the world when the people we love die; but, as someone said to me not long after Jake died: 'We are who we choose to be. We can be happy or sad. It is our choice.' This person unwittingly gave me the impetus to kick-start my life by making me think about how society views and copes with death.

Hayes-Smart 2002: 20

Grief is a normal reaction to loss. Coping with loss, particularly that of a loved one, involves moving through a complex and multidimensional process of grieving. Grief has the potential to impact on every aspect of a person's existence including the physical, social, cognitive, emotional, behavioural and spiritual aspects of everyday life (Ferrell & Coyle 2006). Two of the most important tasks that need to be achieved, in order to move successfully through the grieving process, are to accept the reality of the loss and to cope with any emotional and social effects that result.

LOSS

TYPES OF LOSS

Loss can be actual or perceived, temporary or permanent, and occurs when someone or something can no longer be seen, heard, known, felt or experienced (Box 14.1). Feelings of loss and grief can apply to many events. Losses include those that relate to:

- Treasured objects or possessions
- Relationships
- Health
- Age (lost youth)
- Status
- Lifestyle
- Independence
- Freedom
- Spiritual and cultural matters
- A sense of safety and security
- Future hopes, dreams and expectations.

Loss can be symbolic and strong when it relates to cultural and spiritual matters, for example, the loss of homeland or the effects of dispossession experienced by Indigenous people in Australia, New Zealand and other countries (Kellehear 2002). Losses can be multiple and all losses impact on self-concept (Varcarolis 2006). While grief is commonly profound when a loved one dies, profound grief often accompanies other types of loss. The perception of the degree of loss relates to the value placed by the individual on that which is no longer present. In a global sense, loss and associated grief cannot be quantified, so it cannot be generalised that one person's loss is greater or less than that of another person. The impact of loss ranges from minor to catastrophic.

Loss of an aspect of the self can be devastating and can severely affect a person's body image and self-esteem. Individuals commonly experience much grief over the loss of a body part or loss of a physiological function. They may also experience temporary or permanent changes in body image and self-esteem, as self-esteem is influenced by how personal physical characteristics and abilities are perceived.

To nurses, an event such as admission to a health care facility may seem fairly routine; however, a person who is admitted, even electively, is separated from a familiar environment and is therefore potentially experiencing a loss. If the admission is for a short time only, the effects of this loss are not likely to be great, but if a person is deprived of a known environment for an extended period, the effects of that loss can be severe. Some people experience several losses at the one time; for example, a terminally ill person may experience loss of independence, body image, social status, financial security, plans for the future and relationships. People who are ageing often face similar types of losses; in particular, older people admitted to residential care facilities are confronted with significant important losses, including leaving the family home, loss of privacy and independence, loss of a familiar lifestyle, surroundings

Box 14.1 | Examples of loss

- Separation
- Divorce
- Children leave home
- Adoption
- Death of loved ones
- Death of pets
- Abortion
- Migration
- Imprisonment
- Loss of treasured objects

Health (due to illness, injury or the ageing process)

- Body parts
  - Amputation
  - Mastectomy
- Body function
  - Mobility
  - Bladder/bowel
  - Hearing loss
  - Vision Loss
- Mental capacity
  - Memory
  - Cognitive ability
- Independence
- Appearance (illness/injury)

Status/role

- Occupation
  - Retirement
  - Retrenchment
- Financial
  - Retirement
  - Retrenchment
- Social
  - Older people may lose multiple friends to death
  - Older people may lose familiar lifestyle, possessions or pets when moved to residential care
- Cultural
  - Familiar environment
  - Homeland
  - Effects of dispossession felt by Indigenous people and refugees

CLINICAL INTEREST BOX 14.1
Cumulative losses experienced by older people moving into residential care facilities

- Freedom and independence
- Familiar environment and possessions
- Familiar diet and routine
- Company of family and friends
- Pets
- Privacy
- Status
- Financial independence and control
- Choice (e.g. when to get up, go out, eat, go to bed, what to do or what to watch on television)

These losses may compound others that commonly accompany the ageing process; for example, reduced hearing, vision, mobility and energy. They may also accompany the losses to memory and cognition associated with progressive dementia, or the losses of physical abilities and self-esteem associated with chronic neurological disorders and cerebrovascular accidents.

and belongings, loss of health and separation from loved ones (Clinical Interest Box 14.1). Adjustment to multiple losses may be difficult and grief may accumulate. (Chapter 13 provides further information concerning older adults, multiple losses, stress and adaptation.) However, it should not be forgotten that many people cope with significant loss and change throughout their lives, many adapt successfully, even when losses accumulate, and some people find they gain in confidence and are strengthened personally after coping successfully with grief (Howarth 2000).

GRIEVING RESPONSES TO LOSS

Reactions to loss are influenced by a variety of factors including:

- The stage of an individual's growth and development
- Cultural and spiritual beliefs
- Socioeconomic status
- Relationships with others of significance to them (often referred to as significant others)
- Previous loss(es) and personal coping mechanisms (Brown 2007; Cicero 2007; Cowles 1996; Walsh et al 2002).

Clinical Interest Box 14.2 illustrates how children respond to loss.

CLINICAL INTEREST BOX 14.2
The responses of children to loss

Children are unable to grieve intensely for lengthy periods of time. It is usual that they have short periods of intense grief and crying, interspersed with periods of other activities such as watching television or playing. This might appear to be denial of what has happened (e.g. death of a family member); if so it is temporary protection from the pain of reality. It may also provide time for the child to reflect on the event (e.g. death of a family member), so it is helpful and appropriate behaviour.

Some children may regress in behaviour; for example, they may revert to bed wetting or thumb sucking. Particularly school-aged children associate misdeeds with causing death and may feel they are to blame. Care involves:

- Being honest and open; for example, not saying 'Mummy has gone away' when she has died and will not be coming back
- Helping children to release sad feelings, fears and anger
- Providing reassurance that they are not to blame
- Promoting feelings of being loved, safe and secure
- Promoting acceptance of their own feelings as being normal, even though they may be strong and unfamiliar
- Promoting help from support groups that are specifically aimed at helping grieving children to express feelings; for example, via drawings, talking with other children, or sending letters to heaven.

(Olson 1997)

Reactions to loss are influenced by the type of loss experienced; for example, loss of a loved person through death usually results in deep grief. It is important to remember that people respond to loss in different ways, depending on the significance of the loss. Grief is a natural but unique response to loss. Grieving, or mourning, are normal reactions that help an individual to recover slowly from a significant loss. It is considered normal and healthy to experience intense and painful emotions relating to loss. It is also recognised that painful feelings diminish with time but may never totally disappear. After any great loss, people may return to an apparently normal life, but it is likely that they are 'different'. A person faced with a serious loss may begin to grieve before the loss actually occurs. For example, older people may experience anticipatory grief as they anticipate the lifestyle changes and losses that old age brings. The process of grieving for a dying person before death occurs is also anticipatory grief. It enables a degree of preparation and 'letting go' but, ultimately, the depth of grief is still acute when death eventually does occur (Cicero 2007; Old & Swagerty 2007).

Acute grief is a reaction that begins at the time of a loss, for example, loss of a person through sudden death, who perhaps leaves for work and does not return, or the loss of a limb as the result of an accident. Later, grief is described as still present but less acute and less overwhelming.

While people experience grief in different ways, certain patterns of grieving have been observed and documented. The concept of phases of grieving can be useful in helping the nurse to recognise and support grieving persons.

THEORETICAL FRAMEWORKS

Theorists often describe grief as a process that involves several stages or phases. The stages are identified according to descriptions of the responses commonly experienced by people as they face up to a loss. One well-known theory or model of the grieving process is that described in the late 1960s by Dr Elisabeth Kubler-Ross, a psychiatrist and renowned authority on the process of dying, who describes the grieving process as having five stages:

1. Denial and isolation
2. Anger
3. Bargaining
4. Depression
5. Acceptance.

By recognising the stages that a grieving person may experience, nurses are better able to understand what is happening and respond appropriately to that person. The grieving person may not experience every stage, or experience the different stages in any given order. Although grief may be observed to follow a logical sequence, it is not necessarily a linear process. For many people it is not simply a matter of 'moving on' if and when a previous stage is 'complete'. It is sometimes impossible to differentiate clearly between stages, as a person rarely moves neatly from one to another. Generally a person moves back and forth between the feelings of grief until final resolution or acceptance occurs.

Theorists generally have focused their work on grief associated with death and dying, but the stages they have identified can be applied to grieving individuals facing sadness from many other types of loss. Other theorists have proposed somewhat different stages to Dr Kubler-Ross, but the themes are similar. Engle (1964), for example, describes the grieving process as occurring in three stages — shock and disbelief, developing awareness, and reorganisation and restitution — while Parkes (1986) describes four stages — shock and disbelief, protest, disorganisation and reorganisation. Table 14.1 identifies some of the behaviours associated with various phases of the grieving process.

More recently, O'Nians (1993) has also described the grief process as characterised by stages of mourning, in which people shift in linear fashion from one stage to another. However, more contemporary writings on the grieving process tend to describe it as being more random than do the earlier theorists. Grief is described as cyclic, oscillating, 'coming in waves', or like walking through a maze. People often describe their grief experience as a wide and chaotic range of feelings that may come randomly, or perhaps all at once — shock, sadness, anger, guilt, depression and despair, as well as relief, hope and acceptance. Feelings are often said to be confusing, swinging forwards and backwards, with peaks and troughs of intense emotion being common. This is represented in the form of a cyclic model rather than one that is linear or staged (Shives 2007; Varcarolis 2006).

A similarity of contemporary thinking to linear models is in the outcome that, with working successfully through the grief experience, people do survive their grief and are able to re-establish themselves within their new situation. Eventually hope emerges and they find a new way to relate to their changed world.

Periods of intense grieving and mourning vary widely and it should be remembered that while some people may

TABLE 14.1 | Phases of grieving

Phase	Behaviours
Early response • Shock and disbelief • Denial • Protest	This phase is accompanied by thoughts such as 'This can't be happening, it's not true'. The individual may emotionally deny the loss that has occurred, or is about to occur, by refusing to talk about it and keeping permanently busy to avoid thinking about it. The individual may withdraw from social interactions and, if the loss relates to illness, may seek the opinion of several medical officers, hoping that the initial diagnosis was incorrect. This phase may be accompanied by physiological responses such as tachycardia, sweating, nausea and faintness.
Middle phase • Anger, bargaining, depression • Developing awareness • Despair	The person begins to realise that the loss is real and may experience thoughts such as 'Why me?, Why is this happening?, Why now?' Feelings of anger, frustration, guilt and depression may occur as they begin to realise that nothing can be done to alter the situation. The person looks for someone to blame, and anger may be displaced onto medical officers or nurses, family members or God 'Bargaining' occurs when the person tries to postpone reality by making a 'deal'; for example, with God. For example, 'I'll work hard to raise funds for the church if you just stop this from happening'. A sense of powerlessness underlies these responses. There is a sense of great loss of all things valued, especially the impending ultimate loss of 'being'
Later phase • Acceptance • Detachment • Restitution • Recovery	Acceptance involves how the individual realises the inevitability of the situation and begins to accept the loss. Depression and anger subside and the person can talk about what has or is going to happen Detachment refers to how the dying individual may gradually narrow their world by reducing visitors to close friends or family and withdrawing from everyday activities and interests Restitution refers to the formal ritualistic phase of mourning; the time when friends and family gather together for the funeral. It serves to emphasise the finality of death (Varcarolis 2006) When people are adjusting to a significant loss and 'moving on' in a positive way, they are said to be in the recovery phase. Recovery may be a long process

apparently return to normal life functioning within a few months, many people require much longer to work through their grief. Ferrell and Coyle (2006) provide an explanation of many models of grief, stressing that the task of grieving is hard work. It is expected that the grieving person may experience a wide range of feelings. Expressions of these feelings may include:

- Crying or wailing
- Withdrawal from people, work and leisure activities
- Lack of energy, interest and motivation
- Hostile behaviour
- Physical symptoms such as inability to sleep, eat or concentrate; chest pain, headaches or gastrointestinal disturbances (Boyd 2007; Cicero 2007; deWit 2005; Kaye 1996).

Box 14.2 provides a summary of some common symptoms associated with grief.

DYSFUNCTIONAL GRIEVING

Total absence of feelings normally associated with grief is believed to be an unhealthy psychological response, and unresolved grief can lead to delayed or distorted reactions. Ongoing dysfunctional emotions, and health problems can occur if grieving work is ignored or denied (Varcarolis 2006; Stuart & Laraia 2005; Boyd 2007). Clinical Interest Box 14.3 identifies some of the symptoms of dysfunctional grieving.

CLINICAL INTEREST BOX 14.3 Symptoms of dysfunctional grieving

- Constant, prolonged and severe physical and emotional symptoms lasting 2–3 months or longer
- Limited response to support
- Profound and persistent feeling of hopelessness
- Completely withdrawn or fear of being alone
- Inability to work, create or feel emotion or positive states of mind
- Maladaptive behaviours in responses to the loss, including:
  - Drug or alcohol misuse
  - Promiscuity
  - Feeling numb, dead or unreal
  - Feeling actively suicidal
  - Aggressive behaviours
  - Compulsive spending
- Recurrent nightmares, feelings of constant fear
- Compulsive re-enactments of occasions relevant to the loss
- Exhaustion resulting from lack of sleep and hyperactivity
- Prolonged feelings of depression, panic attacks
- Self-neglect

(adapted from Varcarolis 2006)

Box 14.2 | Common symptoms of grief

PHYSICAL

- Nausea
- Loss of appetite and weight loss
- Insomnia or excessive sleeping
- Shortness of breath
- Ache or pain in the chest
- Palpitations
- Fatigue
- Symptoms of the same illness the deceased person experienced

EMOTIONAL/BEHAVIOURAL

- Sadness
- Depression
- Mood swings
- Crying
- Apathy, lack of interest and motivation, inability to complete tasks
- Loneliness, sense of isolation, abandonment
- Anxiety, feelings of helplessness, restlessness, anger, guilt, irritability
- Tendency to make mistakes, clumsy and accident prone
- A need to tell and retell and remember things about the loved one and the illness/death experience

COGNITIVE

- Inability to concentrate/focus
- Inability to plan/coordinate even routine tasks
- Forgetfulness
- Confusion, disorientation, indecisiveness (particularly prominent in older people)
- Sensing the loved one's presence, hearing the voice, seeing the face, expecting the person to walk in the door

(adapted from deWit 2005)

THE TASKS OF SUCCESSFUL MOURNING

Professionals specialising in grief work may be required to promote a return to wellness in people who have not successfully achieved the tasks of mourning and are displaying symptoms of dysfunctional grieving. The tasks of successful mourning are identified as:

- Accepting the reality of the loss
- Actively working through the pain of grief
- Adjusting to an environment in which the deceased person is missing
- Restructuring the relationship (and the family's relationship) with the deceased to reinvest energy in other relationships and life pursuits (Worden 1991).

It is considered that the tasks of mourning have been completed successfully when the bereaved person can reflect and realistically remember the good and bad times of the relationship with the deceased loved one and can think about the pleasures and the disappointments without distress. This does not mean that there will not be times when sadness emerges afresh, but these will be brief and may be related to triggers that include birthdays and anniversaries. The time that it takes to complete the tasks of mourning may be harder to accomplish and take longer when a parent loses a child, as this is not in the usual scheme of things, or when death is unexpected, particularly if it has occurred by suicide or violent means such as homicide. However, as stated previously there are no rules or set time lines for grieving and mourning. The response to any loss is unique to each individual.

WORKING WITH GRIEVING PEOPLE

The person must be allowed and encouraged to talk and work through grief. To appropriately support them the nurse requires a caring, understanding empathic approach and an ability and willingness to listen. The grieving person really needs someone who is prepared to take a risk and get involved, someone who is not afraid of intensity of feeling but who will encourage the expression of it as part of healing (see Chapters 29 and 43). As nurses, we cannot grieve for the person, lessen the intensity of their feelings, or protect or shield people (even children) from the pain or the hard work of the grief experience. In caring for a grieving person the nurse needs to acknowledge the loss, facilitate the expression of thoughts and feelings, and support the person as they move through the feelings of grieving.

FACILITATING THE EXPRESSION OF FEELINGS

Encouraging a person to talk, and listening to a grieving person express feelings, are important parts of the nurse's role. A person may need to begin to resolve grief before being able to discuss personal feelings, or may be embarrassed about showing strong emotions. If a person chooses not to share feelings, the nurse must respect this decision but should make it clear that a later opportunity to talk will be possible.

A grieving person may react to loss by expressing anger. The nurse should realise that expressions of anger are usually not directed towards anyone in particular, but are the individual's way of responding to a situation. The nurse should not engage in avoidance, but encourage individuals to express their feelings appropriately, even anger. If the nurse can accept a person's right to be angry, the person will be more able to express anger and so begin to work through grief. The person's significant others may be hurt and bewildered by the expression of anger and in such a case the nurse may be able to help them by explaining that anger is one possible way of dealing with a stressful situation.

The nurse should always show a willingness to be with the grieving person when needed. It is important to communicate concern and understanding and use effective listening techniques. People are more likely to express feelings if they know that the nurse is prepared and willing to listen. Platitudes offer no support or assistance in times of grief and should be avoided (Stein-Parbury 2005). Almost everyone at some time has inadvertently uttered a platitude such as 'Don't worry', or 'I know how you feel', often because they do not know what else to say. Words are not necessarily the most important aspect of effective communication, and the individual may obtain comfort if a nurse simply sits and indicates willingness to listen attentively and not make judgments or offer advice. In some cases, the therapeutic use of touch may be appropriate, for example, placing an arm around a shoulder or simply holding a hand may enable a grieving person to express feelings. Just staying with the person and allowing them to feel and say what they need to is often the most empathic form of communication. Simply being with the person, silently, may be the most appropriate and helpful response (Stein-Parbury 2005) (see Chapter 29).

At times the nurse may feel personally unable to facilitate effective communication. Caring for a grieving person can be difficult and may evoke strong personal feelings or memories for the nurse. In such a situation, the nurse should seek advice and support, perhaps from another experienced nursing colleague proficient in dealing with grief and supporting staff through difficult and emotional situations. Some health care facilities provide grief counsellors or *pastoral care* workers, who assist those experiencing grief, including supporting the nurses who are caring for them. Nurses also require the opportunity to discuss and debrief after caring for the dying or when any sad or challenging events are experienced (Lockhart 2007).

It is understandable that inexperienced, and sometimes experienced, nurses may be uncomfortable in interacting with grieving people. Sometimes this means that nurses avoid discussing strong emotions by:

- Changing the subject when strong emotions or concerns are revealed
- Avoiding mentioning pertinent issues; for example, a client's poor prognosis, for fear of upsetting the client (when in reality the client is already upset and possibly needs to talk about concerns)
- Responding to expressed feelings with silence or turning away
- Making light of the matter, 'You're just having a bad day'
- Philosophising; for example, 'It is for the best'
- Referring; for example, 'You'll have to ask the doctor'
- Denying; for example, 'Don't worry, you'll be alright'
- Moralising; for example, 'If only you'd given up smoking'.

(See Chapters 29 and 43 for further information concerning emotional issues and therapeutic communication with clients.)

DEVELOPING SELF-AWARENESS

Nurses are advised to attend seminars and discussion groups, to refer to appropriate literature and to continually examine personal feelings and responses in relation to emotional issues that arise in the workplace. Clinical Interest Box 14.4 provides an opportunity for nurses to begin the process of developing self-awareness in relation to issues of loss, death and dying.

Although the death of any person is a stressful event and it is impossible to describe one death as being worse than another, nurses will sometimes encounter situations where

CLINICAL INTEREST BOX 14.4
Developing self-awareness

As nurses, and as individuals, it is important to become self-aware and begin to confront issues of life and death. Think about each question below, and answer briefly, but as honestly as possible. Then ask a friend to do the same and discuss your responses.

- What gives meaning to your life?
- What possessions enhance your ability to enjoy life and live productively?
- What physical ability would be most difficult for you to lose?
- What life role would it be most difficult for you to lose?
- How do you imagine you might die?
- If you were to die soon, what would you like to be written as your epitaph?
- What would you do if you were told today that you only had 3 months to live?
- What losses have you experienced (death or other)?
- How have these losses influenced your life?
- How have these losses affected your thoughts and feelings about death?
- How do you think you will manage as a nurse, in supporting people with grief and loss?

the grief of clients and relatives is totally overwhelming (Lockhart 2007). These may include the death of a baby or child, traumatic or violent death, or suicide at any life stage. It is not usually the expectation that death will occur in these ways. After the initial shock, some people may find support and comfort from self-help groups comprised of others who have experienced similar situations. It remains, however, a personal choice whether such contact and interaction is instigated by those who are grieving. As already outlined, people grieve in different ways and have different needs. A range of organisations has been formed to help meet the needs of those mourning loss. These include grief and loss workshops, support groups for children and older people, groups that specifically focus on reproductive loss, and those aimed to address the issues faced by divorced men.

DEATH AND DYING

In the course of daily activity, the nurse will have contact with people who are dying and with their significant others. As the dying individual and their significant others look to the nurse for emotional support, it is important that the nurse has examined personal feelings about, and attitudes towards, death. It is important that nurses develop their own philosophy on the subject of death and the process of dying. It cannot be assumed that it is only the elderly who die. Nurses may be faced with neonatal death, death of children and teenagers, as well as the death of adults of varying ages. To die suddenly from natural causes in old age is probably what most people would regard as appropriate, but death may come at any age or life stage, for example, parents may outlive their children, even though this is not their expectation. In addition, issues may arise related to the nature of the death — it may be sudden, or dying may occur over days, weeks or months.

ATTITUDES TOWARDS DEATH

Values, attitudes, beliefs and customs are the cultural aspects of an individual's lifestyle that influence reactions to death and expressions of grief. A personal philosophy about the meaning of death also influences a person's reactions. Religion plays an important part in the lives of many people, particularly when they are facing death, while other people may have no religious belief in a supreme being or an afterlife. Religious faith often gives meaning and hope to a person in a time of crisis. Death of a loved one, and the grief that follows, may also pre-empt an intense time of confusion and questioning of faith (see Chapters 11 and 43).

FEARS RELATED TO DEATH AND DYING

The nurse needs to understand and accept that there are a diversity of feelings and attitudes towards death and dying. A knowledge base of various religions and cultures will help the nurse to relate to an individual's spiritual needs. While some people view death as a natural event that holds no fears, many others experience great anxiety about dying and death. Common fears associated with dying and death include:

- Fear of pain and isolation while dying
- Fear of loss of dignity
- Fear of non-existence
- Fear of being buried alive
- Fear of what happens after death
- Fear of an afterlife that may not be pleasant (Kaye 1996; Olson 1997; Lugton 2002; Berger et al 2006).

A nurse needs to support dying clients in whatever feelings they may experience and endeavour to help them reach the position of accepting impending death.

A person who is facing severe loss, such as their own death, may ask the nurse difficult questions such as, 'Am I going to die?' Many nurses, understandably, may be uncomfortable about answering such questions. The type of response depends on many factors, such as:

- Has the person and/or their significant others been informed of the prognosis?
- What is the person's stage of growth and development, and their level of understanding?
- Have the significant others requested that the person's prognosis be withheld from them, and is this a reasonable request?
- Have the nurses caring for grieving persons been prepared adequately to deal with such questions?

There are no standard answers to questions that may be asked by clients who are dying, but there are several steps a nurse may take to achieve competency in this area and to gain a greater depth of understanding of the issues that surround death and dying, for example:

- Reading recommended literature, particularly in relation to the individual dying in a health care setting
- Discussing aspects of death and dying with experienced nursing colleagues and bereavement counsellors
- Attending in-services, seminars, courses or other related educational forums to broaden skills and knowledge.

Discussing death and dying is still considered by many people to be morbid or in poor taste, and Western culture generally tends to deny and defy death. The experience of grieving is perceived by many in Western culture as a personal and private matter that should go on 'behind closed doors'. It is interesting to note, however, that contemporary society's attitudes are changing somewhat. It appears to be becoming more acceptable that expressing grief is a normal and healthy response, and that even public outpouring of grief may be legitimate and therapeutic. This is evident in recent world examples, such as the public response to the death of Princess Diana, the terrorist attacks in New York and, more recently, the Bali nightclub bombings. There has also been a significant public response in the form of marches and letters saying 'sorry' for the grief still experienced by Indigenous people as a result of European colonisation (Raphael 2000).

Certain attitudes are also becoming more common. These include the acceptance and inclusion of children when families are grieving and, in particular, their participation at funerals, and the increasing use of the more positive 'celebration of life' services. Another change is society's increased acknowledgement of the grief associated with the cumulative losses encountered as old age approaches and recognition that this often raises issues slightly different to grieving in other age groups (Parkes 1997). There is also growing recognition of the losses and grief associated with refugees and with adoption (Raphael 2000).

It is only by continuing to explore and discuss these and other topics that nurses can come to understand the full range of loss and grief issues.

THE CHOICE OF WHERE TO DIE

Whenever possible, when death is predicted and expected, the dying person should be cared for in the environment of their choice. Family and significant others must also be allowed to participate in choosing the most appropriate setting. Some people choose to remain at home, while others may feel that a hospital or hospice is better able to meet their specific needs (Berger et al 2006; Ferrell & Coyle 2006; Olson 1997).

Many people express the wish to die at home, and some health care services provide personnel and equipment to enable fulfilment of this wish. A home care program may be provided by a palliative care service. *Palliative (hospice) care* is an approach or philosophy regarding the care of terminally ill people. (See Chapter 43 for specific information concerning palliative care.) The philosophies and the practices based on them relating to palliative or hospice care may be provided almost anywhere, including within a specialised hospice environment in a general hospital, such as in a palliative care unit. The trend is towards providing community-based palliative care or hospice programs, including for specialised groups, such as terminally ill babies and children.

CARE OF THE DYING

Care of the dying is one of the most challenging tasks nurses face. It can be demanding and stressful but can also be very rewarding. Although a nurse cannot control the inevitability of death, there is much that can be done to make the final stages of life as comfortable as possible for the individual and their significant others.

It is important for the nurse to recognise that a dying person is also a living person and that, as long as dying people are alive, they have the same needs as anyone else. As a result of the dying process, some of those needs assume a greater priority than others. The overall goal of care is the promotion of physical and emotional comfort and spiritual ease. Even during the dying process the individual should be helped to retain independence. When this is no longer possible, care should be provided in a manner that preserves self-esteem and dignity.

PHYSICAL CARE

The dying process is often accompanied by discomforts and problems, including breathing difficulties and alterations in nutrition, hydration, elimination, mobility and sensory perception. In addition, the dying person may experience acute or chronic pain. A nursing care plan is developed after assessing the person's needs and, while each individual may have different needs, there are some common problems and some general nursing interventions.

Impaired mobility

When ambulation is no longer possible, maintenance of good body alignment is an essential comfort measure. The client should be positioned as comfortably as desired, with bedding and pressure-relieving mattresses and devices placed to enhance comfort. Clients should be repositioned gently and anatomically correctly every 2–4 hours to promote maximum comfort and prevent muscle soreness, contractures and skin breakdown.

Breathing difficulties

The individual may experience shortness of breath and may be unable to cough or expectorate to clear the airway. When possible, the person should be nursed in an upright or semi-upright position to facilitate breathing. When this is not possible, positioning should be on the side, to prevent aspiration of secretions. Oxygen therapy and oronaso-pharyngeal suctioning may be required to ensure adequate aeration and make breathing easier.

Inadequate nutrition and hydration

The client may be unable to swallow and/or tolerate oral foods or fluids, or may need assistance with eating and drinking. If able to eat and drink, foods and beverages of choice should be provided at the times the client feels like eating. Mouth care and offering alcoholic beverages are sometimes useful measures to stimulate the appetite, although it is expected that appetite will decrease naturally as death approaches. Nausea and/or vomiting may be relieved by providing chips of ice to suck or soda water to sip, or by administering antiemetic medications. If gag or swallowing reflexes are decreased, semi-solid, soft or liquid foods should be offered. If the client cannot swallow, nasogastric feeding or intravenous therapy may be considered in some cases to prevent or relieve thirst (see Chapter 33).

Problems of elimination

Common problems experienced may include constipation, diarrhoea, impacted faeces, retention of urine and incontinence. Measures that may be implemented to prevent or alleviate these problems include:

- Laxatives to prevent constipation, if fluid or fibre intake are unable to be maintained
- Rectal suppositories to relieve constipation
- Catheterisation to relieve retention of urine
- Protective continence pads and specially designed sheets or, to a much lesser extent, external urinary drainage devices, to prevent discomfort and skin breakdown from urinary incontinence (see Chapters 34 and 35 for further information on bowel and urinary elimination)
- Maintenance of skin integrity, clean, dry bedding and an odour-free environment.

Dry mouth

The provision of a clean mouth is extremely important, particularly if the client is unable to swallow. Mouthwash or rinses are appropriate if the individual is able to expectorate. To prevent the mouth from becoming dry and coated it should be cleansed gently every 2–4 hours. A light film of lip balm should be applied to the lips to prevent skin cracking or to relieve discomfort (see Chapter 27).

Eye problems

Dryness and corneal irritation can occur as a result of decreased effectiveness of the blinking reflex. Measures to prevent or alleviate eye discomfort include cleansing the eyelids to remove crusts, instillation of artificial tears and instillation of eye lubricant ointment (see Chapters 27 and 28).

Skin breakdown

If the client is emaciated and lacks sufficient adipose tissue to support bony prominences, or is unable to move, the risk of developing decubitus ulcers is increased. To prevent breakdown, the skin should be kept clean and dry, with moisturising lotion applied to counteract any excess dryness. Pressure-relieving devices such as sheepskins or special mattresses should be used, and position changes should occur every 1–2 hours.

Pain

Pain should be assessed regularly. Appropriate supportive nursing care should be provided and analgesic medications prescribed and administered to avoid peaks and troughs of pain (see Chapter 35).

Altered sensory perceptions

The dying person may experience decreasing visual or tactile acuity. To minimise any anxiety associated with diminished sensory perception, unless contraindicated the room should be kept comfortably light and the person's personal possessions placed where they can be seen or touched. Visitors should sit close by and, if the client's vision is poor, they should tell the person who is there. Although the sense of touch may be diminished, the individual is generally able to feel the pressure of touch, so it is important to maintain physical contact.

The sense of hearing is usually not diminished, so it is important to continue to speak in a normal tone and manner. Even if the dying person appears to be unaware of surroundings, all family and personnel should assume that the person is still able to hear. Some individuals gain comfort from hearing their favourite pieces of music, and relaxation tapes may also be soothing. If the individual is unable to speak, the nurse should attempt to anticipate needs, and people should continue to make communicative attempts even though there may be no reply.

Confusion and restlessness

These states can be caused by physical discomforts such as pain, lack of sleep or retention of urine, or they may be related to medications, such as analgesics, hypnotics and antiemetics. Restlessness may be related to anxiety or fear from a variety of sources. It is important to determine the cause and implement appropriate care. If no cause can be found, or if the individual remains restless and confused, mild sedation may be prescribed.

PSYCHOLOGICAL CARE

The nurse can help to promote the individual's psychological comfort by:

- Encouraging family and friends to stay with the client if this is desired by the client. This can prevent or reduce feelings of loneliness or isolation
- Explaining all care and treatments
- Allowing expression of feelings
- Listening
- Answering questions honestly
- Providing comfort by touch, when appropriate
- Respecting wishes about extraordinary means of supporting or prolonging life

- Responding to any request for a visit from a member of the clergy
- Respecting the need for privacy when significant others are present.

The nurse is often involved in assisting the dying person's significant others. Generally the closest family members will want to be with the dying person and some may want to help with care, even though they might find this emotionally or physically difficult. The nurse can assist by:

- Helping them to learn to interact with the dying person, if they are experiencing difficulties
- Encouraging them to help with simple care measures such as assisting to eat and drink, or providing hygiene
- Providing them with privacy when they prefer to be alone with the dying person
- Ensuring that they are informed of areas within a health care facility where they can rest or obtain meals and refreshments
- Allowing them to express their feelings and fears
- Providing comfort by touch, when appropriate
- Informing them appropriately of the client's condition, and of impending death
- Enabling them to be with the client at the moment of death if this is what they wish.

SPIRITUAL CARE

The spiritual needs of dying individuals may be defined as a search for meaning or a sense of forgiveness, hope and love. Not all dying people experience all of these needs or feel them with equal intensity. The nurse should be sensitive to the spiritual needs of each person and implement actions that may help to meet those needs. Chapters 11 and 43 provide information concerning spiritual wellbeing and palliative care for the dying.

DEATH AND POST-MORTEM (AFTER DEATH) CARE

Death is precipitated by failure of one or more of the three major body systems: the central nervous system, the cardiovascular system or the respiratory system. Death may be anticipated, as in the case of a terminal illness, or it may be unexpected, for example, as the result of a road accident. When death occurs, the time is noted and a medical officer is notified as soon as possible. The death must be confirmed by a medical officer, who will issue a death certificate.

SIGNS OF IMPENDING DEATH

As a person approaches death, the following physiological changes begin to occur:

- Loss of muscle tone, which results in relaxation of the facial muscles, difficulty in swallowing, decreased peristalsis, diminished body movement and decreased urine output, with possible incontinence of urine and faeces
- Slowing of the circulation, which results in mottling and cyanosis of the extremities, and cold skin
- Changes in the vital signs: decreased blood pressure, weaker pulse and changes in breathing. The respirations may become rapid, slow, shallow or irregular. Cheyne–Stokes respirations may occur; this is a cyclic pattern of respirations that gradually become more shallow, followed by periods of apnoea (no breathing) (deWit 2005)
- Changes in sensory perception: blurred vision and impaired sense of taste and smell.

Signs of imminent death include loss of reflexes, faster and weaker pulse, noisy breathing due to accumulating secretions in the throat (sometimes called 'the death rattle') and inability to move. It is important to remember that hearing is usually the last of the senses to fail.

When the breathing ceases completely, the heart continues to beat for a very short time (a few minutes at most) and then stops. The pupils become fixed and dilated. It is at this time that death is said to have occurred, unless the client is on a ventilator. When a client is mechanically ventilated, brain death must be established to determine death (deWit 2005).

Brain death

Death may be broadly defined as the final cessation of body functions, but with the advent of modern technology and transplant procedures, a more precise definition of death has become necessary. Determination of death must be made in accordance with accepted medical standards. There are established standards for determining brain death, which can be described as irreversible cessation of total brain function, as determined by clinical examination. Two medical officers generally perform the same clinical examination, independently and at separate times. Certain conditions must be present before the examinations are performed, including that the individual's body temperature must be within normal limits, and sufficient time must have elapsed for any drugs to be excreted from the body. In most instances, before brain death can be diagnosed, the individual must meet the following specific conditions:

- Total unreceptiveness and unresponsiveness to the environment
- Absence of spontaneous movement, including breathing
- Absence of reflexes
- 'Flat' electroencephalogram (EEG).

These or similar criteria are designed to help demonstrate beyond any doubt that an individual has no cerebral activity.

EFFECTS OF DEATH ON THE BODY

After death the body undergoes a series of changes — rigor mortis, algor mortis and tissue breakdown (decomposition).

Rigor mortis

Rigor mortis (stiffening of the body) is a physiological state that begins to occur about 2–4 hours after death. The condition, which is due to lack of adenosine triphosphate (ATP) required for muscle relaxation, is characterised by rigidity of the muscles of the body. Stiffness occurs systematically through the involuntary muscles and the full process usually completes within 48 hours. As chemical activity ceases, usually within about another 96 hours, body stiffness disappears and rigor mortis passes (Crisp & Taylor 2005).

Algor mortis

Algor mortis refers to how the body cools after death. Cooling occurs at a rate of about 1°C per hour (Crisp & Taylor 2005).

Post-mortem decomposition (tissue breakdown)

Discolouration, mottling and/or a bruised appearance of the skin may become apparent, particularly in susceptible areas such as the back and buttocks. The breakdown of red blood cells releases haemoglobin, which discolours vessel walls and surrounding tissue.

Internal tissues and organs break down in the later stages of decomposition and liquefy. This occurs more rapidly in hot conditions and can cause a bacterial hazard (Crisp & Taylor 2005). When clients die at home and the weather is hot, the process can be delayed for a few hours by the use of cooling systems, fans and icepacks. This may be important and necessary if relatives need time to grieve before the body is removed from the home, or to allow time for relatives living at a distance to arrive and say their goodbyes.

IMMEDIATE CARE AFTER DEATH

When death has occurred in a health care facility and has been confirmed by a medical officer, and provided that there are no cultural or religious factors to indicate otherwise, the body is straightened as much as possible and all pillows are removed except one flat one, which is left under the head. The limbs are straightened and the arms should be placed at the sides of the body. All nursing and medical equipment, such as oxygen apparatus, is disconnected and removed from the bedside. The eyes are closed. If dentures were removed they should be replaced, provided that they fit relatively well and can give the mouth good support. It may be necessary to place a rolled towel under the jaw to prevent it from sagging. The relatives should be consulted about their wishes in relation to any jewellery present on the body. Whether any jewellery, such as a wedding ring, was removed or left in position is documented. If a ring is left on it should be taped in position to prevent dislodgement and subsequent loss. The bedside locker and wardrobe are emptied and a list is usually compiled of the individual's possessions, which are then given to the relatives, who sign to acknowledge receipt of the articles. Any items that were deposited in the agency's safe are collected, given to the relatives, and a receipt obtained.

LAST OFFICES

Last offices are commonly performed as soon as possible after the death. This term describes the preparation (or laying out) of the body for removal to a hospital mortuary or holding area. If a person dies unexpectedly, for example, postoperatively, or under suspicious circumstances (injury, accident, murder or suicide), last offices may be postponed and an autopsy performed, independently or as part of a coroner's inquest. An autopsy is a post-mortem examination that may be performed to determine the cause of death. Consent for autopsy needs to be given by the next of kin, except in a coroner's case, when no permission is needed. Special procedures must be followed in preparing the body for removal from the ward before autopsy. Generally any tubes, such as drainage or intravenous lines, are left in position, although this policy varies.

Each health care facility has its own protocol regarding last offices, and the nurse should refer to the policy manual for directions. The equipment required may be kept in each ward or distributed from a central point, and it may be known by one of several names: mortuary bundle, mortuary box or mortuary pack. In general terms, the preparation of a body involves washing, dressing, wrapping and appropriate labelling of the body.

Some cultural and religious groups have precise teachings regarding dying and death. Death is viewed in many ways, and cultural attitudes towards death can be broadly classified as accepting, denying or defying. In caring for the dying, and before death, the nurse must determine whether any special cultural or religious beliefs or practices need to be observed in relation to care of the body after death. Any specific practices that must be performed by members of a particular group should be adhered to as fully as possible. There are, for example, many different cultural and religious practices concerning how the body should be washed and prepared for burial, and who should perform these tasks; different rituals may need to be conducted; and there are different practices concerning how the body should be positioned, who should view the body and how soon after death the burial should occur (Kirkwood 1998).

If there are no specific requirements, portable screens are placed around the bed to provide privacy and dignity and last offices are carried out in a quiet respectful manner (Table 14.2). Sometimes, as a body is moved, the sound of air being expelled from body orifices may be heard. Sometimes urine or faeces, usually only in small amounts, may leak from the body. As in life, if this should happen, the nursing response is calm and professional, and the person's body is washed carefully while respecting privacy and dignity. Ideally two nurses should conduct post-mortem care but this is not always possible. A nurse who is undertaking post-mortem care for the first time is encouraged to ensure that there is a supportive experienced nurse available to assist.

TABLE 14.2 | Guidelines for post-mortem care

Review and carry out the steps in Appendix 1 before continuing with the following to prepare the client's body for transfer to the mortuary or funeral home

Action	Rationale
Assessment and preparation	
Confirm the client's identity	Ensures correct identification for transfer to mortuary/funeral home
Determine whether an autopsy is planned. Verify autopsy consent has been signed	Drainage tubes are not removed if an autopsy is planned
Determine if the family wishes to assist with caring for the body, or if they wish to view the body after the nurse has completed the preparation	Assisting with care can provide a sense of closure for family members. Viewing the body allows time to say goodbye and may promote acceptance of the reality that death has occurred
Gather equipment. Position the over-bed table ready for use	Promotes efficiency
Raise the bed to a comfortable working height	Prevents back injury/strain
Implementation	
Wash hands and don gloves	Standard precautions to protect from body fluids
Position client in supine position with one flat pillow under the head	Raising the head limits pooling of blood, which might cause discolouration of the face
Close the eyes and mouth. Replace dentures first if they are not already in situ. Place a small rolled-up towel under the chin if necessary to keep the mouth closed	Closing the eyes and mouth and supporting the chin maintains the face in the most natural position during rigor mortis
Remove jewellery and clothing. List personal items on the designated valuables list. Place items in the bag to be returned to the family, according to policy	Enables safe return of valuables to family
Cleanse all areas of the body soiled with body fluids. Place protective pads under the rectum and between the legs to protect from any leakage	After death, sphincter muscles relax, permitting contents of bladder and bowel to leak from the body
Remove all tubes (intravenous lines, catheters, nasogastric or wound-drainage tubes) unless autopsy is planned	Enhances appearance of body for family viewing
The inflated balloon should be deflated before removal of a urinary catheter. If tubes are to be left in situ, remove the drainage bag or intravenous fluid container, cut the tubing, leaving a section long enough to fold over twice and secure with an elastic band (check agency policy beforehand)	Deflating balloon in catheter prevents tissue damage on removal
Remove soiled dressings, clean wounds and redress with leak-proof dressing material. Remove any adhesive marks with appropriate solution/solvent	Improves appearance of the body
If a family member is assisting with care or coming to view the deceased person, dress the body in a clean hospital gown. The gown may be removed before wrapping the body ready for transfer to the mortuary	Dressing the body in a gown preserves dignity and is less distressing for the family than seeing the body wrapped in a shroud
Comb the hair and arrange in the client's usual style	Provides dignity in death and seeing the deceased person well groomed is supportive of family emotions
After the family leaves, place an identity tag that bears the full name of the deceased, their age, sex, religion, and time and date of death on the deceased client's ankle (or area designated by agency policy)	Ensures correct identification throughout process until funeral occurs
Position the body on the shroud and check for placement of drainage protection pads. Fold and secure the shroud according to agency procedure. Apply any other wrapping designated by agency policy, e.g. plastic body bags may be used routinely or in some circumstances, such as when client had contagious illness	Shroud covers the body and prevents unnecessary exposure

(Continued)

TABLE 14.2 | Guidelines for post-mortem care — cont'd

Action	Rationale
Attach another tag carrying the same information as the tag attached to the ankle to the outside of the shroud, where it is easily visible	Ensures correct identification
Transfer and accompany the body to the mortuary according to agency policy; for example, designated trolley, designated route. Ensure the transfer is as discreet as possible — close the doors to clients' rooms and have lift doors opened in advance. In some agencies it is policy for mortuary attendants to wrap the body. In such cases it may be policy to transport the body to the mortuary with the face uncovered	Transport to the mortuary is performed quickly and discreetly to preserve privacy and to avoid upsetting others
Document post-mortem care	Documentation provides legal proof concerning the nursing care conducted
Evaluation	
Reflect on the following: • Was the procedure carried out in a quiet, private and dignified manner? • Was the family supported effectively and helped to say goodbye to the deceased person in the manner they desired? • Were the family's cultural and religious needs effectively managed and met? • Did the deceased person appear clean, well groomed, peaceful and cared for? • Was the discomfort or distress of other clients minimised as much as was possible?	Reflection and evaluation helps determine if desired outcomes have been achieved and whether or not policies, procedures and nursing measures need to be amended
(adapted from deWit 2005: 193–4)	

If there are other people in the vicinity when a client has died, nurses should be guarded in their comments and avoid any conversation that could be distressing to others. Other clients may be upset and appreciate being taken to another area while post-mortem care is conducted. Other clients may also benefit from talking about the experience of the person's death.

When the post-mortem care is completed, the body is taken to the hospital mortuary. In some agencies, such as small residential care units that do not have a mortuary, a funeral director may remove a body directly to the funeral home. In the mortuary the body is placed in a special cooling unit to slow decomposition. Many funeral homes and mortuaries are equipped with a special viewing room so that relatives and friends may still view, or spend time with, the body if they wish, or if identification of the body is required. A nurse may be required to accompany a person to this area and in doing so should be sensitive to the fears and feelings that the person may be experiencing. It may be helpful to prepare the person by explaining that after death the body appears very pale and will feel cold when touched.

CARE OF THE BEREAVED

After death has occurred, the significant others may experience shock and disbelief, even if the individual's death was anticipated. Reactions to the death will vary from numbness and immobility, to outbursts of weeping or wailing, or may include expressions of feeling relief or comfort from the fact that their loved one is no longer suffering. The nurse should not discourage bereaved persons from expressing their grief. If the nurse is also affected by the death and feels like expressing sadness or crying with the bereaved, this is often appropriate. People who have lost someone dear to them are often touched to see that the nurse who cared for that person is also grieving.

If the significant others were not present at the moment of death they are encouraged to view the body. Even if they were present at the time of death they are encouraged to stay with the body for as long as they would like to, and to say their 'goodbyes'. Although it is a painful and sometimes frightening experience, it is believed that the bereaved are often more able to accept that death has occurred, and accept the finality of death, if they view the body of the deceased loved one (McKissock & McKissock 1998).

When a baby is stillborn or dies soon after birth, the entire family (siblings, grandparents, etc) should be given the opportunity and encouraged to spend as much time as they want with their baby. Seeing, holding and perhaps bathing and dressing their baby, and the creation of memories (naming the baby, taking photographs, keeping footprints and perhaps a lock of hair, having a funeral service) are now viewed as sources of great comfort to bereaved families (McKissock & McKissock 1998). Traditional views and practices in relation to reproductive loss, including hospital-arranged burial or disposal of the body and not encouraging parental contact, are inappropriate in most cases.

To make the experience of viewing a loved one more beneficial, the significant others should be informed of certain facts before they view the body. It is necessary to explain what to expect; for example, unless the death has occurred within the last 1–2 hours, the skin will be very pale, may be discoloured and will feel cold to touch. The bereaved should be accompanied into the room and, depending on their wishes, the nurse should either remain or leave them in privacy for as long as they wish to be there. Commonly one person, sometimes two or more people together, spend time with the deceased loved one.

When the bereaved are ready to leave the viewing room it is appropriate to direct them to an area where they can sit down and where they can be given the opportunity to discuss their response to the experience. After a death the bereaved are required to carry out various functions, such as collecting the person's belongings, informing friends and relatives and notifying a funeral director and arranging a funeral or memorial service. The nurse should inform the bereaved of the availability of support persons and groups in the community, and they should be provided with information and options, but not advice.

LEGAL AND ETHICAL ISSUES

Certain legal and ethical considerations and moral dilemmas exist in caring for dying individuals, particularly with the advent of modern technology and life-prolonging techniques. Such issues may involve:

- Living wills, Right-To-Die Acts, and advance directives (e.g. resuscitation versus non-resuscitation, or partial resuscitation)
- The individual's right to know their prognosis and to make choices regarding the implementation of life-prolonging treatment
- Euthanasia or assisted suicide: the act of ending another person's life, often known as mercy killing (but with a distinction between passive and active euthanasia). Passive euthanasia is deemed to occur when a client chooses to die by refusing treatment that might prolong life. Active euthanasia is generally defined as administering a drug or treatment to kill the client. Assisted suicide is described as making available to clients the means to end their life (such as a weapon or drug), with knowledge that suicide is their intent. Both active euthanasia and assisted suicide are considered to violate legal and ethical boundaries in Australia at present, but there is currently considerable controversy about under which circumstances euthanasia or assisted suicide might be legally, morally and ethically justified and acceptable — when outcomes may be seen as a compassionate and humane response
- Organ donation — the possibility of organ and tissue donation (kidneys, livers, hearts, lungs, corneas) may be considered by a person before their death, and given as an advance directive (currently in some areas permission can be indicated on a driver's licence) otherwise permission may be sought after death from the next of kin. Certain criteria need to be met to determine the suitability of organs for harvesting and transplantation. Donation of organs remains a personal and emotive issue, which is often broached with newly bereaved relatives and requires tactful management.

(See Chapter 3 for further information about ethical issues in nursing.)

POSITIVE ASPECTS OF GRIEF AND LOSS

The grief and loss experienced by individuals can create positive outcomes. Sometimes people report that they have gained personal strength and personal growth after surviving loss and grief. For example, after the grief of losing an emotionally deep and close relationship such as a marriage, a person may feel free to follow new pursuits. This often allows new creativity and fresh energy to emerge. As a result, people often become richer and fuller individuals, with more to give to others as a result (Howarth 2000). Society frequently benefits from a personal crisis experienced by an individual; for example, 'Mothers Against Drink Drivers' and many other advocacy groups have emerged this way (Kellehear 2002).

SUMMARY

Loss, grief, dying and death are phenomena that will be experienced by every person. To assist people experiencing such situations the nurse requires knowledge and understanding of the many and changing human responses associated with loss, grief, dying and death. Knowledge of the theoretical models of grief and mourning can promote this understanding. In addition, sensitivity to particular cultural and religious beliefs and practices is needed to provide appropriate and therapeutic care. The nurse also requires personal strength and courage to become involved with clients and relatives during the process of experiencing loss and grief. Only by understanding and coming to terms with personal feelings about these phenomena can a nurse respond appropriately to people who are experiencing them, and offer truly supportive and therapeutic care. Nurses will encounter clients and relatives experiencing loss and grief in almost every field of nursing and they are encouraged to participate in a range of activities to promote and enhance skill and knowledge to help them work effectively in this area.

REVIEW QUESTIONS

1. List 10 types of loss that are commonly part of the human experience.
2. State five common physiological and five common psychological responses common in grieving people.
3. Explain the concept of cumulative loss.
4. Explain the difference between linear and cyclic models of grieving.
5. State and explain the five stages of grief identified by Dr Elisabeth Kubler-Ross.
6. Identify five signs of impending death.
7. Identify five signs of imminent death.
8. State three clear physical signs that death has occurred.
9. Outline the nursing measures for post-mortem care of a deceased client.
10. Outline how you would provide support for bereaved relatives about to view the body of a deceased loved one.

CRITICAL THINKING EXERCISES

1. Consider some of the questions a dying person or their relatives might ask. What questions would you find particularly difficult to answer and why? Think about answers that would be appropriate.
2. Jim Dawson, 70, has rheumatoid arthritis, which interferes significantly with his mobility and movement. Until recently he lived happily with his wife, Marion, who looked after the house, and assisted him with hygiene, toileting and meals and other care when necessary. Together they enjoyed listening to music, watching old films and television dramas and watching the bird life in their small garden. Three weeks ago Marion died unexpectedly and, as there was no way that Mr Dawson could manage alone at home, and no family members able to offer enough assistance, he was admitted to hospital. He has been assessed and is now waiting for placement in a residential care facility.
   a) What sort of physical and emotional responses may he be experiencing? How can you, as an Enrolled Nurse, help Mr Dawson in relation to physical and emotional responses to loss, and preparing for a new life in the aged-care facility?
   b) What you know of residential care facilities? What factors do you think will help or hinder Mr Dawson's journey through grief and loss?

REFERENCES AND FURTHER READING

Berger AM, Shuster, JL, Von Roenn JH (2006) *Principles and Practice of Palliative Care and Supportive Oncology*. Lippincott, Wilkins and Williams, Hagerstown, MD

Boyd MA (2007) *Psychiatric Nursing: Contemporary Practice*, 3rd edn. Lippincott, Wilkins and Williams, Hagerstown, MD

Brown E (2007) *Supporting the Child and the Family in Paediatric Palliative Care*. Jessica Kingsley Publishers, London

Cicero JK (2007) *Waking Up Alone: Grief and Healing*. Author House, Bloomington, IN

Cowles K (1996) Cultural perspective of grief: an expanded concept analysis. *Journal of Advanced Nursing* 23: 287–94

Crisp J, Taylor C (eds) (2005) *Potter & Perry's Fundamentals of Nursing*, 2nd edn. Elsevier Australia, Sydney

Daly C (2005) *Transitions in Nursing: Preparing For Professional Practice*, 2nd edn. Elsevier, Sydney

deWit S (2005) *Fundamental Concepts and Skills for Nursing*, 2nd edn. WB Saunders, Philadelphia

Engle GL (1964) Grief and grieving. *American Journal of Nursing* 64: 93

Ferrell B, Coyle N (2006) *Textbook of Palliative Nursing*, 2nd edn. Oxford University Press, New York

Hayes-Smart R (2002) *No, I'm not Alright*. Axiom Publishing, Adelaide

Howarth G (2000) Dismantling the boundaries between life and death. *Mortality* 5 (20): 127–38

Kaye P (1996) *Symptom Control in Hospice and Palliative Care*. Hospice Education Institution, Essex, CT

Kellehear A (2002) Grief and loss: past, present and future. *Medical Journal of Australia* 177 (4): 176–7

Kirkwood N (1998) *A Hospital Handbook on Multiculturalism and Religion*. Morehouse, Harrisberg, Philadelphia

Kubler-Ross E (1969) *On Death and Dying: What the Dying Have to Teach Doctors, Nurses, Clergy, and Their Own Families*. Scribner, New York

Kuebler K, Berry P, Heidrich D (2002) *End of Life Care — Clinical Practice Guidelines*. WB Saunders, Philadelphia

Lockhart S J (2007) *Of Secrets, Sorrows, and Shame: Undergraduate Nurses' Experiences of Death and Dying*. Unpublished Masters Thesis. Faculty of Education: The University of Melbourne

Lugton J (2002) Support processes in palliative care. In: Lugton J, Kindlen M (eds), *Palliative Care: the Nursing Role*. Churchill Livingstone, Edinburgh

McKissock M, McKissock D (1998) *Bereavement Counselling — Guidelines for Practitioners*. The Bereavement C.A.R.E. Centre, Sydney

—— (1999) *Coping with Grief*, 3rd edn. ABC Publishing, Sydney

O'Nians R (1993) Support in grief. *Nursing Times* 89 (50): 62–4

Old, JL, Swagerty, DL (2007) *A Practical Guide to Palliative Care*. Lippincott, Wilkins and Williams, Hagerstown, MD

Olson M (1997) *Healing the Dying*. Delmar, Albany, NY

Parker J, Aranda S (1998) *Palliative Care: Explorations and Challenges*. MacLennan & Petty, Sydney

Parkes CM (1986) *Bereavement: Studies of Grief in Adult Life*, 2nd edn. International Universities Press, New York

—— (1997) Bereavement and mental health in the elderly. *Reviews in Clinical Gerontology* 7: 47–53

Raphael B (2000) Grief and loss in Australian society. In: Kellehear A (ed), *Death and Dying in Australia*. Oxford University Press, Melbourne: 116–29

Shives LR (2007) *Basic Concepts of Psychiatric-Mental Health Nursing*. Lippincott Wilkins and Williams, Hagerstown, MD

Stein-Parbury J (2005) *Patient and Person: Interpersonal Skills in Nursing*. Elsevier Australia, Sydney

Stuart G, Laraia M (2005) *Principles and Practice of Psychiatric Nursing*, 8th edn. Elsevier/Mosby, St Louis

Turner, M (2006) Talking With Children and Young People About Death and Dying. Jessica Kingsley Publishers, London

Valentine F, Lowes L (2007) *Nursing Care of Children and Young People With Chronic Illness*. Blackwell Publishing, Hoboken, NJ

Varcarolis E (2006) *Foundations of Psychiatric Mental Health Nursing: A Clinical Approach*. WB Saunders, Philadelphia

Walsh K, King M, Jones L, Tookman A, Blizard R (2002)

Spiritual beliefs may affect outcome of bereavement: prospective study. *British Medical Journal* 324: 1551

Williams C (2007) *Therapeutic Interaction In Nursing*. Jones & Bartlett Publishers, Sudbury, MA

Worden WJ (1991) *Grief Counselling and Grief Therapy*, 2nd edn. Springer, New York

ONLINE RESOURCES

National Association for Loss and Grief (Australia) Inc: www.griefaustralia.org

National Association for Loss and Grief (Victoria): www.nalagvic.org.au

Unit 5

Nursing individuals throughout the lifespan

Chapter 15

THEORIES OF GROWTH AND DEVELOPMENT: CONCEPTION THROUGH TO LATE CHILDHOOD

OBJECTIVES

- Define key terms/concepts
- Compare and discuss the various theories of development
- Compare the theories of Sigmund Freud, Erik Erikson and Jean Piaget
- State the factors that influence growth and development
- Discuss the theories in relation to nursing a child
- State the factors that influence growth and development
- Describe the major physical and psychosocial changes that occur during each stage of development
- Describe the process of conception
- Discuss the growth and development of the placenta
- Explain intrauterine growth and development of the fetus
- Discuss the transition from intrauterine to extrauterine life
- Discuss the growth and development of neonates
- Examine the growth and development from early to late childhood

KEY TERMS/CONCEPTS

cognitive development
development
embryo
emotional development
extrauterine
fetus
growth
intellectual development
intrauterine
maturation
maturational development
moral development
personality development
physical development
psychoanalytical approach
reflexes
social development
social learning

CHAPTER FOCUS

Nursing children is challenging at times, as their understanding of life changes throughout their growth and development. This chapter looks at various developmental theories, which view development as a continuous process. Growth and development are processes that begin at conception and continue through each stage of the life cycle. Human development involves biological and psychosocial components. Biological science is concerned mainly with structure and function, while the psychosocial sciences focus on the behavioural aspects of development. Nursing care of the infant and child is directed at promoting the optimal level of health for each individual. It is important for the nurse to understand that both infancy and childhood are unique phases of development and that these phases are accompanied by special needs. To understand these needs the nurse first requires knowledge of normal growth and development, beginning with conception.

LIVED EXPERIENCE

When discussing with my children what they would like to be when they grow up, Emma, age 8, said, 'A nurse like you, mummy'. Megan, age 6, said, 'An animal doctor'. I then asked my son Patrick, age 4, the same question. He thought carefully before he responded, 'I am going to be a lion'.

Karen Lawrence

Nurses care for people who are in different stages of development. A basic understanding of growth and development enables the nurse to recognise the needs of each individual and, thus, to provide appropriate care. Human growth and development are orderly processes that begin at conception and continue until death. Every person progresses through definite phases of growth and development, but the rate and behaviours of this progression vary with each individual.

Every person is a unique individual and, while growth and development are generally categorised into age stages or by using terms describing the features of an age group, categorisation does not take into account individual differences. It does, however, provide a means of describing the characteristics associated with most individuals at stages when comparative developmental changes appear. Growth and development affect the whole person and, although defined separately, overlap and are dependent on each other.

Physical growth results as cells repeatedly divide then synthesise new components, causing an increase in the number and size of cells and, consequently, an increase in the size and weight of the body or any of its parts. Growth can be measured in height and mass or by the changes in physical appearance and body functions that occur as a person grows older.

Development refers to the behavioural aspects of a person's progressive adaptation to their environment and is related to changes in psychological and social functioning.

Maturation is the process of attaining complete development and is the unfolding of full physical, emotional and intellectual capabilities. The term maturation is generally used to describe an increase in complexity that enables a person to function at a higher level.

A person's development encompasses a range of dimensions besides the physical, for example, emotional and moral development. There are several theories, or approaches, regarding growth and development of these different dimensions. This chapter discusses these approaches and their implications for nursing practice.

THEORIES OF DEVELOPMENT

Some theories view development as a continuous process that moves from the simple to the complex, while other theories view development as a process characterised by alternating periods of equilibrium and change. The various developmental theories differ in how the human being is viewed. The following section of this chapter provides the reader with an introduction to the major theories, or approaches, which are psychoanalytical, cognitive–developmental, maturational, social learning and moral. It is not the intent of this section to provide the reader with an in-depth analysis of these theories, rather to provide an overview of each approach. It is expected that the reader will consult further texts, such as Sigelman (2003) if more information is required.

FREUD'S THEORY

Sigmund Freud (1856–1939) founded the psychoanalytical approach to, or theory of, development. Freud's theory stresses the formative years of childhood as the basis for later psychoneurotic disorders, primarily through the unconscious repression of instinctual drives and sexual desires. His theory emphasises the drives of sex and aggression, which he saw as motivating much human behaviour.

According to Freud, an individual's personality is composed of the 'id', the 'ego' and the 'superego' (Sigelman 2003). The id is that part of the psyche that is the source of instinctive energy, impulses and drives. Based on the pleasure principle, it directs behaviour towards self-gratification. The ego represents the conscious self and is that part of the psyche that maintains conscious contact with reality and tempers the primitive drives of the id and the demands of the superego with the physical and social needs of society. The superego is the individual's conscience, which is formed as the result of internalisation of societal demands and restrictions (Carel 2006).

Freud's theory of development is based on a series of psychosexual stages through which a person must pass. Successful completion of each stage is necessary before the next stage can be entered without detrimental effects on future development. According to Freud, specific body areas are the primary sites for expression and achievement of needs, and these sites change from stage to stage. Table 15.1 outlines the stages of development according to Freud's theory.

ERIKSON'S THEORY

Using the psychoanalytical framework, Erik Erikson based his (1963) theory of development on the process of socialisation. He describes another series of stages of personal and social development as the 'eight ages of man', and views development as a continuous struggle for an emotional–social balance (Sugarman 2001).

According to Erikson, a person spends his whole life constructing, shaping and reshaping his personality, which is influenced by psychological, biological, social and environmental factors. Erikson identifies core problems that the individual tries to master during each stage of personality development. Progression to the next stage depends on resolution of the problem; however, no core problem is ever entirely resolved, as each new situation will

TABLE 15.1 | Developmental stages according to Freud

Stage	Age	Behaviours
Oral	0–18 months	• Uses mouth as source of satisfaction
Anal	1–3 years	• Focuses on pleasurable sensations arising from the anal region • Learns muscular control of urination and defecation • Exhibits increasing independence: learns to walk, talk, dress and undress • Learns to say 'no'
Phallic	3–6 years	• Focuses on pleasurable sensations arising from the genital region • Learns sexual identity • Perceives the parent of the same sex as a rival • Identifies with the parent of the same sex • Emergence of the superego • Develops refinement of motor and intellectual activities
Latency	6–12 years	• Enters a quiet stage: sexual development lies dormant, emotional tension eases • Experiences a normal homosexual phase • Identifies with peers and teachers • Increases intellectual capacity
Genital	12 years–adult	• Experiences reawakened sex drives • Develops secondary sex characteristics • Exhibits concern over appearance • Strives towards independence • Matures intellectually • Experiences identity crisis

present a conflict in a new form. Table 15.2 outlines the stages of development according to Erikson.

PIAGET'S THEORY

The theory of cognitive development focuses on the gradual development of cognitive processes, such as problem solving, and on the gradual development of intellectual growth. Cognitive development is the process by which a child becomes an intelligent person, acquiring knowledge and the ability to think, learn, reason and abstract.

Jean Piaget's (1952) theory of cognitive development, which deals only with cognition and does not take into account all psychosocial aspects of the personality, views development as gradual, progressive and related to age. Piaget's views are that, for learning to occur, a variety of new experiences or stimuli must exist. He believed that there are four major stages in the development of logical thinking, and that each stage builds on the accomplishments of the previous stage. Table 15.3 outlines Piaget's stages of cognitive development (Huitt & Hummel 2003).

GROWTH AND DEVELOPMENT

Growth and development are interrelated processes that are influenced by a variety of factors. The theoretical approaches outlined in this chapter, together with various other approaches, provide a framework for understanding the complexities of growth and development. Each approach emphasises different aspects of development; for example, cognitive developmentalists concentrate primarily on intellectual development, psychoanalytical theorists emphasise social and personality development, while maturational theorists focus primarily on physical growth and development (Santrock 2007).

It is important for the nurse to understand that childhood incorporates unique phases of development, and that these phases are accompanied by special needs. To care for individuals from infancy to adolescence, the nurse first requires knowledge of normal growth and development. By understanding what is normal, the nurse is more able to recognise departures from normal and, therefore, to plan and implement appropriate nursing actions.

Growth and development affect the total person and, although separately defined, growth and development overlap and are interdependent. Both occur from the moment of fertilisation until death. Growth in weight (mass) and height is variable and not uniform throughout life. The maximum rate of growth occurs before birth, in the 4th month of fetal life. Growth in height stops when maturation of the skeleton is complete. Standard growth charts are available on which measurements of growth may be periodically plotted and compared with the norm for that particular age group.

Growth and development occur in specific directions. Development is closely related to maturation of the nervous system, and occurs in the cephalocaudal direction (head to tail), which is logical; for example, motor control must be established in the brain before the neuromuscular connections required by leg and back muscles for walking develop. The second direction is from the centre of the

TABLE 15.2 | Erikson's stages of development

Stage	Age	Conflict	Behaviours
I	0–1 year	Trust versus mistrust	Develops basic trust in someone who consistently responds to needs. When needs are not met, may develop basic mistrust of others
II	1–4 years	Autonomy versus shame and doubt	Develops a sense of self-control and independence. Feelings of shame and doubt may arise if made to feel self-conscious, or when expected to be dependent in areas where not capable
III	4–8 years	Initiative versus guilt	Plans and undertakes tasks and initiates a fantasy life whereby they can work out fears and conflicts. A sense of guilt may arise if a child is made to feel that their activities or imaginings are bad
IV	8–12 years	Industry versus inferiority	Engages in tasks and activities that can be carried through to completion. Needs and wants real achievement. Feelings of inferiority or inadequacy may arise if a child believes that they cannot measure up to the standards set for them by others
V	12–20 years	Identity versus role confusion	Establishes own identity and intimate relationships. Role confusion may result if unable to solve conflicts about role in society
VI	20–30 years	Intimacy and solidarity versus isolation	Enters into intimate relationships by allowing others to share the psychosocial and physical aspects of their personality. May experience a sense of isolation if unable to become close to others
VII	30–60 years	Generativity versus self-absorption and stagnation	Establishes and guides the next generation and strives to ensure the continuation of their work and lifestyle. If unable to assume responsibility for promoting the future, may experience a sense of stagnation. As a result, becomes self-absorbed and experiences difficulty in relating to the world
VIII	60 years–death	Integrity versus despair	Strives to feel a sense of worth. A sense of integrity develops when an individual feels satisfied with past achievements. Despair arises when an individual is unable to recognise or accept their worth, or when they feel remorse for that which might have been

TABLE 15.3 | Piaget's stages of cognitive development

Stage	Age	Intellectual development
Sensorimotor	Birth–2 years	This stage of intellectual development is governed by sensations in which simple learning takes place. Problem solving is primarily trial and error, as the child progresses from reflex activity, through repetitive behaviours, to imitative behaviour. The child gradually acquires a sense that external objects have a separate and independent existence and that they exist even when they are not visible to them
Preoperational	2–7 years	During this stage the predominant characteristic is egocentricity, wherein the child considers their own viewpoint as the only one possible. Thinking is concrete and tangible and the child lacks the ability to make deductions or generalisations. Problem solving does not usually follow logical thought processes
Concrete operational	7–11 years	Thought becomes increasingly logical, and problems are solved in a systematic fashion. The child is able to consider points of view other than their own. Towards the end of this stage, the child demonstrates a greater reasoning ability
Formal operational	>11 years	Thinking is characterised by logical reasoning. The adolescent is able to think in abstract terms, draw logical conclusions and solve problems

body outwards (proximodistal); for example, infants learn to control shoulder movements before they control hand movements (Santrock 2007).

There is a sequence, order and pattern to growth and development. There are certain developmental tasks that must be accomplished during each stage. A developmental task is a set of skills and competencies specific to each developmental stage, which children must accomplish to deal effectively with their environment. Each stage lays the foundation for the next stage of development. The stages of development are:

- Prenatal (conception to birth)
- Infancy (birth to 12 months)
- Early childhood (12 months to 5 years)
- Later childhood (5 years to 12 years)
- Adolescence (12 years to about 18 years)
- Adulthood (18 years onward).

Development encompasses various aspects — motor, vision and hearing, speech and language, intellectual, emotional, personality, moral and social. Although there is an orderly pattern to the processes, the rate of growth and development varies among individuals.

CONCEPTION

Conception, formally defined as the union of a single egg and sperm (gametes), is the benchmark of the beginning of a pregnancy. This event does not occur in isolation but as a result of a series of events, including ovulation (release of the egg), union of the gametes and implantation of the embryo into the uterus. Only after all these events are successfully completed can the process of embryonic and fetal development begin (Figure 15.1 and Table 15.4).

Fertilisation of the ovum occurs in the distal third of the uterine (fallopian) tube. The fertilised ovum (zygote) develops by simple cell division as it travels to the uterus. When it reaches the uterus, it is a sphere of cells and is referred to as a morula. The morula separates into an outer (ectodermal) and an inner (endodermal) cell mass, fluid forms and fills the space between the two layers, and the structure is then referred to as a blastocyst. The outer layer of the blastocyst becomes the trophoblast and will develop

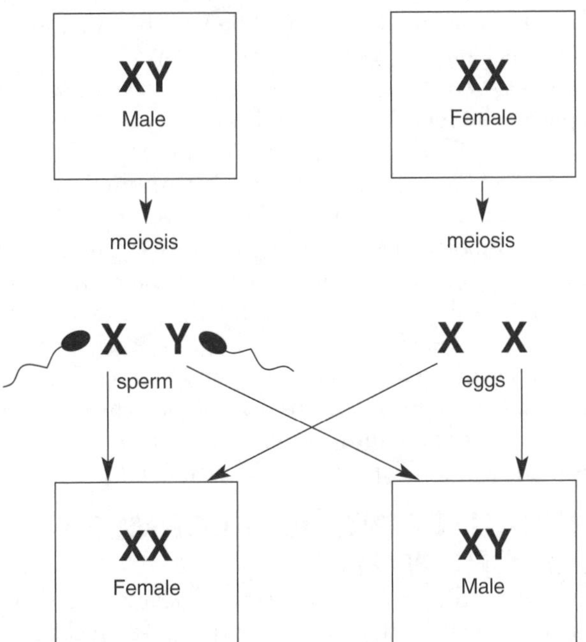

Figure 15.1 | Sex determination *(modified from Leifer 2007)*

TABLE 15.4 | Fetal growth terms

Term	Time period in fetal development
Ovum	From ovulation to conception (fertilisation)
Zygote	From conception (fertilisation) to implantation
Embryo	From implantation to 8 weeks after conception
Fetus	From 8 weeks after conception until term
(Sherblom Matteson 2001)	

into the placenta and outer membrane, while the inner layer will develop into the embryo, cord and inner membrane. Between these two layers a third layer (mesoderm) will form.

Implantation (embedding in the endometrium) occurs about 10 days after fertilisation and normally occurs in the upper body of the uterus. After implantation, the lining of the uterus grows over the blastocyst and pregnancy is established. From this stage onwards the lining of the uterus is termed the decidua (Marieb 2004).

The inner cell mass of the blastocyst differentiates into three distinct layers:

- The outer layer (ectoderm), which develops to become the skin, hair, nails, brain and nervous system
- The middle layer (mesoderm), which develops to become the circulatory, musculoskeletal and urinary systems, and most of the reproductive tract
- The inner layer (endoderm), which develops to become the intestines, internal organs, respiratory system and the germ cells of the ovaries or testes (Marieb 2004).

As development continues, a cavity appears above the ectoderm. The lining of this amniotic cavity becomes the amniotic membrane, which secretes fluid that makes up part of the 'liquor' (the fluid that surrounds the embryo). The amniotic cavity enlarges so that eventually the embryo is suspended by the umbilical cord in a closed sac (membranes) of amniotic fluid.

The embryo continues to develop until by the end of the 2nd month it resembles a human, and is called a fetus. From this stage onwards the major activities are growth and organ specialisation. By the end of 40 weeks the fetus is about 50 cm long and weighs between 2.7 and 4.1 kg (Table 15.5).

DEVELOPMENT OF THE PLACENTA, MEMBRANES, LIQUOR AND CORD

THE PLACENTA

The outer cells of the trophoblast develop projections (villi), which project into the maternal capillaries to allow the exchange of oxygen, nutrients and waste products. The villi eventually join with an area of uterine tissue to form the placenta. The placenta continues to grow throughout the pregnancy, with one surface (maternal surface) attached to

TABLE 15.5 | Embryonic and fetal growth and development

Zygote (5 weeks)	Complete sac 1 cm in diameter covered with chorionic villi. No recognisable human characteristics
Embryo (6 weeks)	Sac 2–3 cm in diameter, weight 1 g. Head enlarges, arm and leg buds forming, primitive heart beginning to function, circulation in primitive form, connections made between vessels in chorion
10 weeks	Embryo 4 cm long. External genitals appear, anal membrane breaks down, hands and feet recognisable, human form apparent
Fetus (12 weeks)	Fetus 8 cm long, weight 15 g. Fingers and toes, eyes and ears, circulation and kidneys developed, nasal septum and palate have fused, endocrine glands and nervous system begin to function
16 weeks	Fetus 16 cm long, weight 110 g. Sex easily identifiable, fingernails visible, good heartbeat, fetal movements felt. Basic development complete — the fetus now has to mature
20 weeks	Length 22 cm, weight 300 g. Vernix on skin, lanugo (fine hair) on body, eyebrows, fetus now legally viable
24 weeks	Length 30 cm, weight 600 g. Wrinkled skin, fat deposited, brain development continues
28 weeks	Length 35 cm, weight 1000 g
32 weeks	Length 42 cm, weight 1700 g. Skin red, wrinkled
36 weeks	Length 46 cm, weight 2500 g. Nails reach fingertips
40 weeks	Length 50 cm, weight 3400 g. Baby well covered with fat, skin red, not wrinkled, all organs functioning with the exception of the lungs
(modified from Bobak & Jensen 1993)	

the lining of the uterus, and the other (fetal surface) with the umbilical cord arising from its centre. The fully formed placenta is disc-shaped, about 2.5 cm thick in the centre, and weighs about 500 g. The functions of the placenta are nutritional, respiratory, excretory and hormonal (Marieb 2004).

THE MEMBRANES

The two fetal membranes — the amnion and the chorion — are derived from part of the trophoblast and attached to the placenta. The inner membrane (amnion) encloses the fetus and liquor and covers the fetal surface of the placenta and the cord. The outer membrane (chorion) is continuous with the margin of the placenta and adheres to the wall of the uterus (Marieb 2004).

LIQUOR

The liquor (amniotic fluid) is the pale straw-coloured liquid that surrounds the fetus in the amniotic sac. Derived mainly from the secretions of the cells in the amniotic membrane, liquor is 99% water plus mineral salts. The functions of liquor include protection of the fetus, and maintenance of an even intrauterine temperature (Marieb 2004).

THE UMBILICAL CORD

The umbilical cord extends from the fetal umbilicus to the fetal surface of the placenta. It contains two umbilical arteries, which transport deoxygenated blood from the fetus, and one umbilical vein, which transports oxygenated and nutrient-rich blood from the placenta to the fetus. The vessels in the cord are embedded in a thick jelly-like substance and the cord is covered by amniotic membrane. At 40 weeks of pregnancy the cord is about 1.25 cm in diameter and 60 cm long (Leifer 2007).

FETAL CIRCULATION

The fetal circulation is designed so that the major blood flow bypasses the fetal lungs. Oxygen and nutrients move from the maternal blood into the fetal blood, and fetal wastes move in the opposite direction. As blood from the umbilical vein flows towards the fetal heart, most of it bypasses the fetal liver through the ductus venosus and enters the inferior vena cava. Some of the blood entering the right atrium is shunted into the left atrium through the foramen ovale, a temporary opening in the septum between the atria. Blood that enters the right ventricle is pumped out through the pulmonary artery, where it meets the ductus arteriosus, a short vessel connecting the pulmonary artery to the aorta (see Figures 15.2 and 15.3). Because the fetal lungs are collapsed, blood enters the systemic circulation through the ductus arteriosus. The aorta transports blood to the fetal tissues and, ultimately, back to the placenta through the umbilical arteries (Marieb 2004).

INTRAUTERINE DEVELOPMENT AND GROWTH

The prenatal period is the stage of development from conception to birth, normally lasting 40 weeks. After implantation has occurred the lining of the uterus undergoes changes so that by about the 13th day after conception the

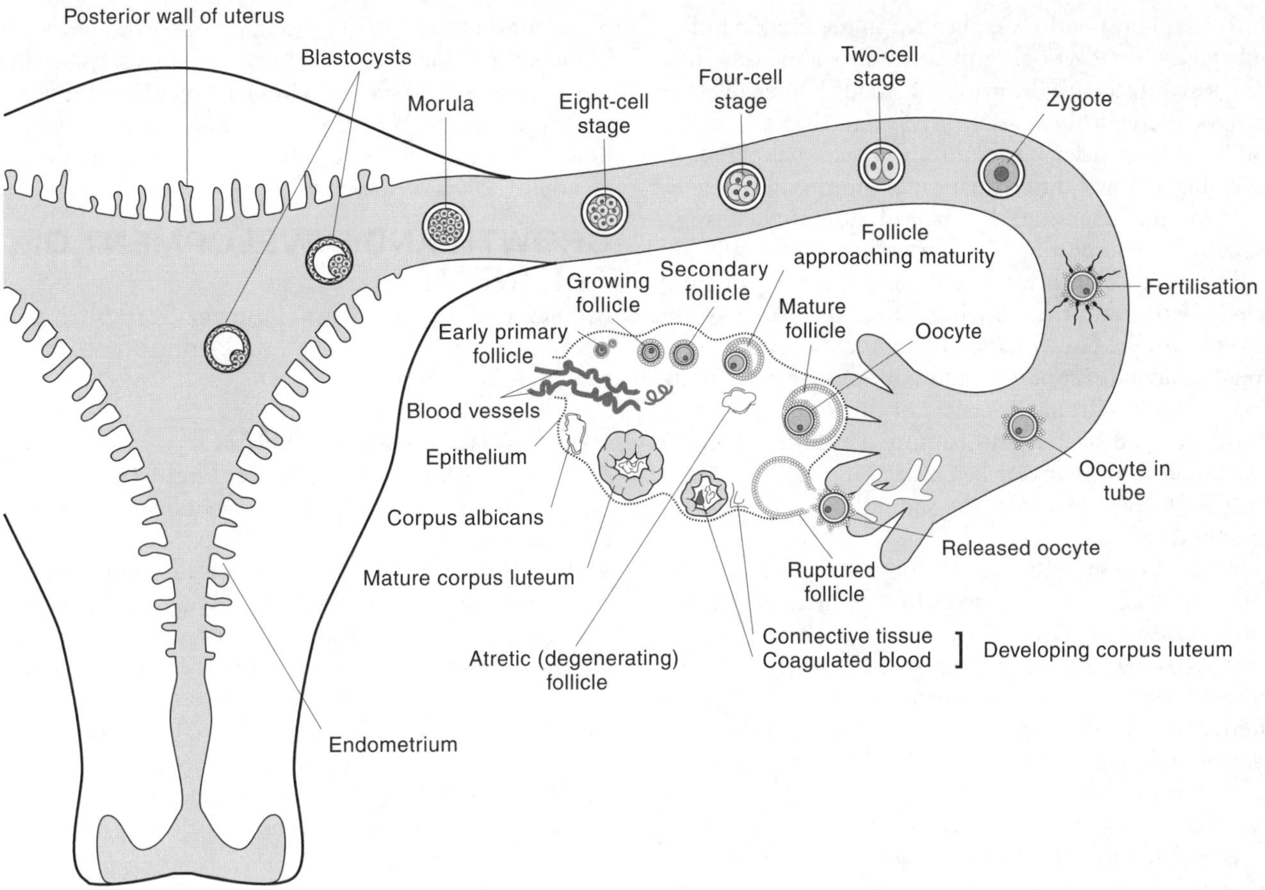

Posterior wall of uterus
Blastocysts
Morula
Eight-cell stage
Four-cell stage
Two-cell stage
Zygote
Follicle approaching maturity
Secondary follicle
Growing follicle
Early primary follicle
Mature follicle
Oocyte
Fertilisation
Blood vessels
Epithelium
Corpus albicans
Mature corpus luteum
Oocyte in tube
Released oocyte
Ruptured follicle
Atretic (degenerating) follicle
Connective tissue
Coagulated blood
Developing corpus luteum
Endometrium

Figure 15.2 | Ovulation, fertilisation and implantation *(reproduced from Leifer 2007, with permission)*

To head, neck, arms
Pulmonary trunk
Ductus arteriosus (3)
Venous blood
Unexpanded lungs (pulmonary vascular resistance therefore high)
Aorta
SVC
R
A
Placenta undertakes the functions of respiration, waste disposal, nutrition
L
A
Oxygenated blood
Ductus venosus (1)
RV
LV
IVC
Foramen ovale (2) in interatrial septum
Hypogastric (umbilical) arteries (4)
To trunk and legs

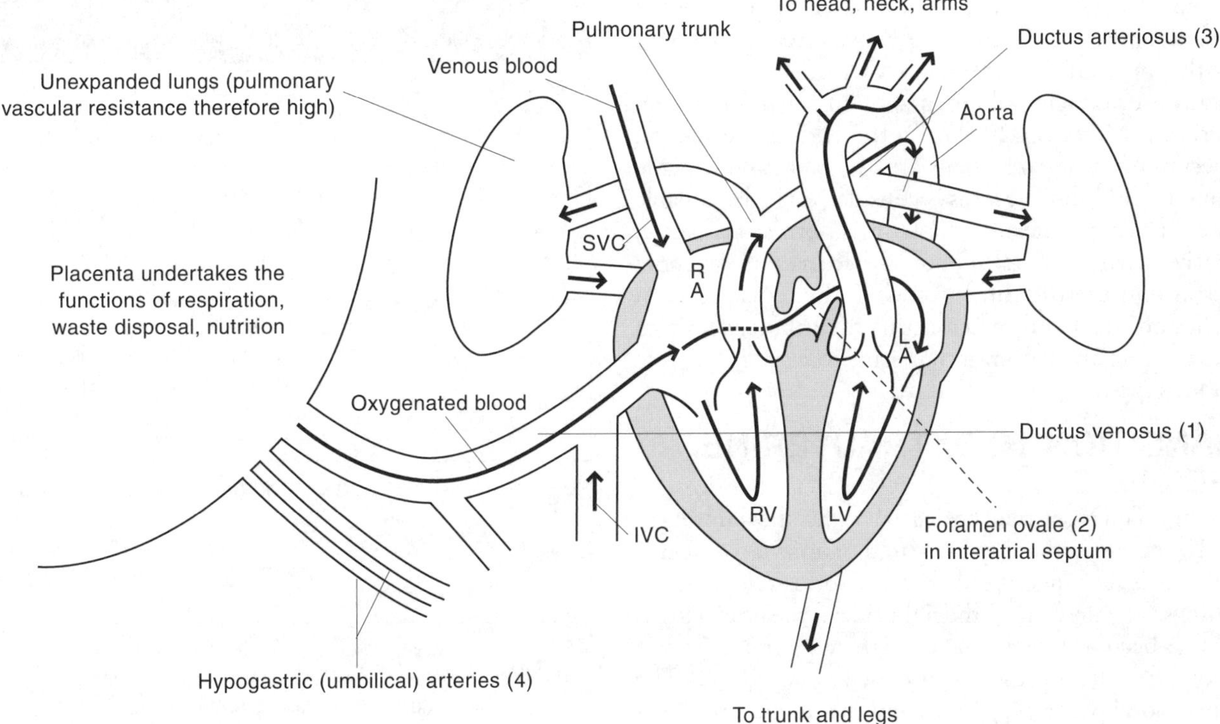

Figure 15.3 | Fetal circulation *(reproduced from Leifer 2007, with permission)*

embryo is almost entirely embedded in the uterine lining. Embryonic blood vessels grow outwards and come into intimate contact with the maternal blood. This enables the embryo, and later the fetus, to receive nutrient substances from, and to transfer wastes into, the maternal blood. As the embryo grows, differentiation of groups of cells gives rise to specific tissues and the shape of the embryo changes to gradually assume a human appearance (Leifer 2007).

By the 7th or 8th week, the developing organism is called a fetus, and the principal external features of the body are visible. Growth and development occur first in a cephalocaudal direction (head to tail), then in a proximodistal direction (from the centre of the body outwards). Thus, the head of the fetus is more developed than the legs, and arm buds appear before leg buds. Development in the limbs proceeds from the shoulders and hips to the hands and the feet.

Intrauterine growth and development occurs in three main stages, each lasting 3 months (the first, second and third trimesters). Different tissues and regions of the body mature at different rates, while growth in length and mass proceeds at a predetermined rate. Growth in length and mass depends on factors inherent in the fetus, placenta and mother. Growth and development of the fetus may be impeded by factors such as infectious agents (e.g. the rubella virus) chemical agents (e.g. ionising radiation or certain drugs), immunological factors (e.g. the Rh factor), or by nutritional factors (e.g. maternal mineral deficiency).

The first trimester of intrauterine life is the most crucial for the developing fetus, as it is during this period that the fetal cells differentiate and develop into essential organ systems. Any factors that cause interference with growth can result in extensive structural or functional alteration or congenital absence of an organ or system (Sherblom Matteson 2001). By the end of the second trimester, most organ systems are complete and capable of functioning, and the fetus is considered viable (capable of life outside the uterus). If a fetus is born at this stage, extensive environmental support is necessary to promote survival. During the third trimester, the fetus grows in length and mass and, when born, the infant is able to make the transition from intrauterine to extrauterine life without support.

TRANSITION TO EXTRAUTERINE LIFE

After the infant is born and begins to breathe, the shunting of blood from the pulmonary artery to the aorta via the ductus arteriosus is no longer needed and blood is circulated to the lungs. The pressure in the right side of the heart falls as the lungs become fully inflated and there is little resistance to blood flow. This causes the foramen ovale to close. The infant's blood oxygen level rises and the ductus arteriosus constricts and is converted to a fibrous ligament. The closure of these structures thus depends on the initiation of respiration. The cardiovascular system adapts so that blood circulation no longer bypasses the lungs, and the lungs are able to inflate, thereby enabling gaseous exchange (see Figure 15.4). When blood stops flowing through the umbilical vessels, the circulatory pattern becomes that of an adult (Bobak & Jensen 1993).

GROWTH AND DEVELOPMENT OF THE INFANT

Infancy is the stage of development from birth to 12 months. The first 28 days of extrauterine life are referred to as the neonatal period.

PHYSICAL DEVELOPMENT

At birth the spinal cord and lower brain centres are well developed and, while not capable of coordinated movement, the infant exhibits a range of reflexes:

- Eye reflexes: when a bright light is directed towards the eyes, the pupils contract; blinking is elicited when objects are brought towards the eyes
- Oral reflexes: the 'rooting' reflex is elicited when the infant's cheek contacts the mother's breast and in response to peri-oral touch. This reflex enables the infant to find a nipple in order to feed
- The Moro reflex: elicited by a sudden loud noise or movement. If this occurs the infant draws the legs up

TABLE 15.6 | Growth and development — birth to 12 months

Age	Motor, communication, manipulative and social skills
Birth to 1 month	Primitive reflexes: can suck, grasp and respond to sudden sounds. Crying patterns and 'cooing' noises
1–3 months	Holds head up when prone, holds head erect when held in a sitting position. Begins to vocalise. Smiles responsively. Distinguishes parents from others
3–5 months	Turns head towards sounds. Rolls from prone to supine. Makes sounds when spoken to, may squeal with pleasure. Clasps hands together and can hold a rattle. Begins to watch own hands. Smiles and vocalises
6–9 months	Sits with support and, later, alone. Sits up from a lying position. Crawls. Babbles and vocalises; says words like mum-mum, da-da. Picks objects up between finger and thumb. Reacts to strangers with anxiety
10–12 months	Pulls self into a standing position, may walk with support. Says single words. Obeys simple instructions. Imitates adults, e.g. will scribble with a crayon. Expresses emotion. Can hold a cup to drink

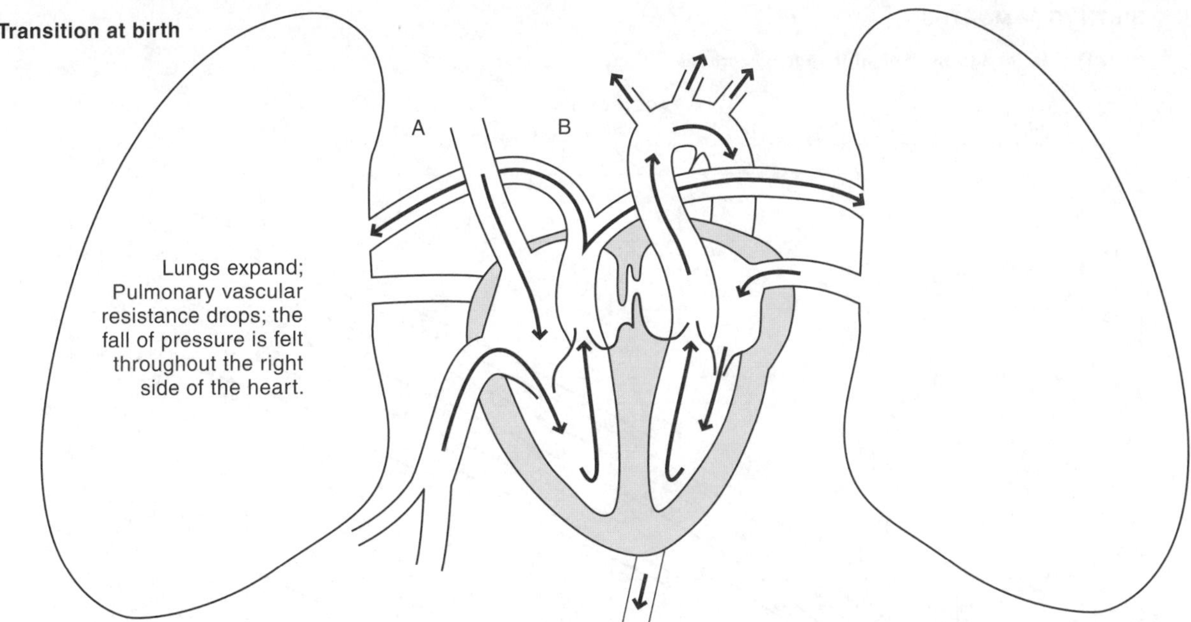

Figure 15.4 | Transition to extrauterine life

and the arms fan out and then come together towards the midline in an embrace position

- The grasp reflex: elicited when the palm is stimulated so that the fingers flex and grip the object
- The walking reflex: elicited when the infant is held upright, with the sole of his foot pressing on a firm surface. This initiates flexion and extension of the legs, simulating walking
- Tonic neck reflex: this is a postural reflex that is sometimes assumed by sleeping infants. The head is turned to one side, the arm and leg of one side are extended, and the opposite arm and leg are flexed in a 'fencing' position (Leifer 2007).

After several months these basic reflexes disappear and are gradually replaced by conditioned reflexes.

MOVEMENT

Locomotion proceeds in stages. First, the infant learns to position the head in space, then to crawl on hands and knees, later to move about while sitting upright, and, finally, to stand, balance and walk. Thus, motor development occurs in the cephalocaudal direction.

At birth an infant is about 50–55 cm long and weighs about 2.8–4.5 kg. During the first 12 months the infant increases in length by more than one-third, and mass almost triples (see Figure 15.5). As the infant grows in height and mass, internal organs also grow and develop to cope with the increasing demands made on them. Growth is influenced by hormones, especially thyroxine and growth hormone.

At birth the infant will follow a moving person with their eyes; binocular vision begins at 6 weeks and is established by 4 months. At about 6 months the infant can move the head and eyes in every direction. By 12 months they are able to recognise familiar people and objects at a distance.

Infants can hear at birth and by 1 month they are able to move their eyes towards a sound. The brain is not sufficiently developed initially for any meaning to be attached to sounds, but by 5 to 6 months the infant turns immediately to the sound of their mother's voice even when she is quite a distance away.

Speech develops from vocalising at birth and crying as a means of communication, until at 12 months the infant is able to say one or two recognisable words. With time the number of words spoken increases and they become clearer. The rate of vocabulary gain varies and is related to factors such as the amount and type of speech the infant hears (Leifer 2007).

INTELLECTUAL DEVELOPMENT

The process of acquiring intellectual skills is often referred to as cognitive development. Cognitive activities, such as reasoning, thinking and problem solving, involve two main processes — perception and conceptualisation. Perception is the sensory process by which a person obtains information about themself and their environment. Through the senses, an infant perceives many stimuli, such as pressure, pain, warmth, cold, sound, taste and visual images. Conceptualisation is the process of concept formation and is an intellectual activity that facilitates reasoning, thinking and problem solving. Concepts allow sense to be made of the information received through the senses.

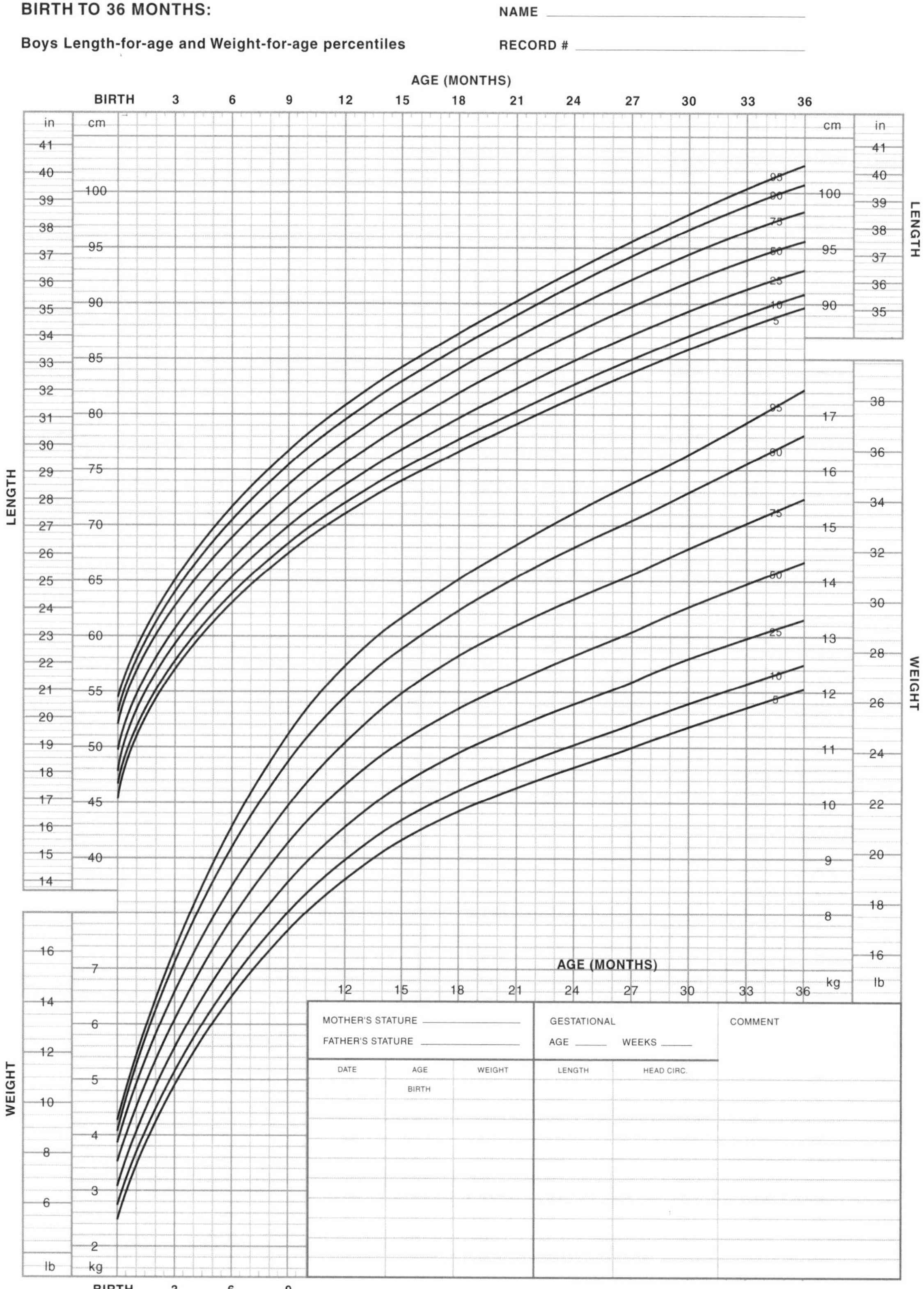

Figure 15.5 | Growth charts — newborn to infant boys *(Centers for Disease Control and Prevention: www.cdc.gov/nchs — reproduced with permission from the National Center for Health Statistics)*

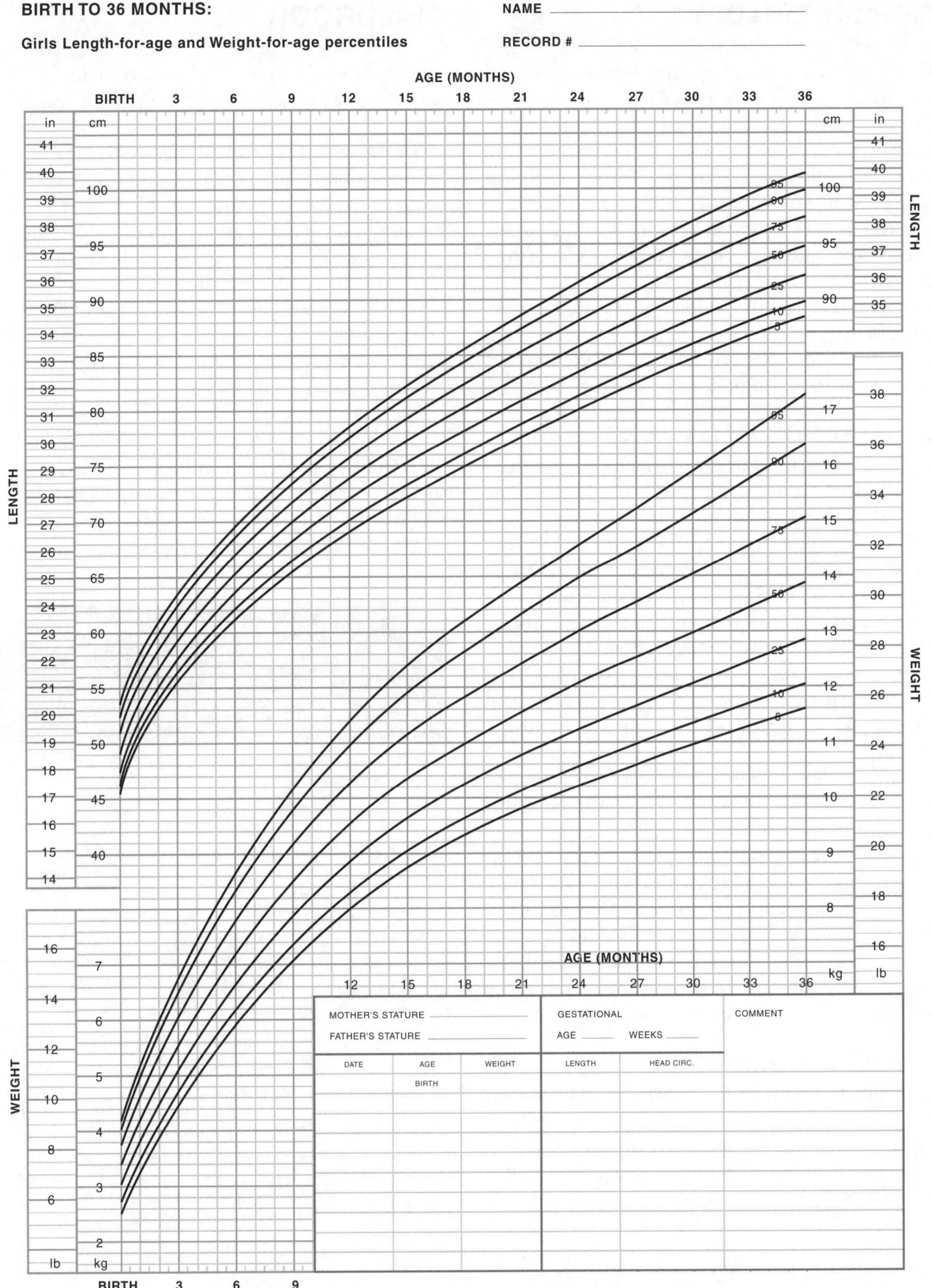
BIRTH TO 36 MONTHS:
Girls Length-for-age and Weight-for-age percentiles
NAME
RECORD #
AGE (MONTHS)
BIRTH 3 6 9 12 15 18 21 24 27 30 33 36
LENGTH
WEIGHT
in
cm
kg
lb
95
90
75
50
25
10
5
MOTHER'S STATURE
FATHER'S STATURE
GESTATIONAL AGE WEEKS
COMMENT
DATE
AGE
WEIGHT
LENGTH
HEAD CIRC.
BIRTH

EMOTIONAL DEVELOPMENT

Emotion is the term used to describe a feeling. Anger, fear, joy and sorrow are typical emotions. Emotional development depends on a variety of factors such as maturation, heredity, socialisation and the environment. Most emotional expressions appear to be learned, and emotional development is related to age. While some forms of emotional expression appear to be inborn or develop through maturation, learning is important in modifying emotional expression to conform to the patterns approved by a specific culture.

At birth infants are able to exhibit distress and pleasure; by 3–6 months they can express anger, distrust and fear; and by about 8–10 months they can exhibit anxiety, surprise, dissatisfaction, obstinacy, anticipation and frustration.

PERSONALITY DEVELOPMENT

Personality may be defined as the 'characteristic patterns of behaviour and modes of thinking that determine a person's adjustment to his environment' (Bolander 1994). An individual's personality encompasses many factors: intellectual abilities, motives, emotional reactivity, attitudes, beliefs and moral values. An infant is born with certain potentialities, the development of which depend upon maturation and experiences encountered in growing up. Therefore, personality is the product of heredity and environment, and personality development is a complicated process involving all aspects of the individual and the environment.

The theories of personality development of Sigmund Freud and Erik Erikson are outlined at the start of this chapter. Although various theories provide a simple way of looking at personality, in actuality development of personality is far more complex. Broadly, personality development can be viewed as a process that begins in infancy, continues into adulthood, and is the way in which a person relates to his environment and circumstances. Personality is shaped by inborn potential as modified by experiences that affect the person as an individual.

SOCIAL DEVELOPMENT

Social development refers to how a person learns to interact with others and begins early in an infant's life; smiling, for example, can be considered a social response. Initially a smile can be elicited in response to strangers but after about 6 months the infant's smile becomes more selective. As the infant begins to vocalise and later to speak, social interaction is increased.

The family is the first, and most important, social institution for the infant. Later on, other people become significant in a child's social network, for example, those at kindergarten and school. Social roles such as brother or sister or playmate are gradually acquired during social development in infancy. Play provides the opportunity for social development, whereby the infant learns the social expectations that accompany relationships.

CHILDHOOD

Childhood may be divided into two stages of development: early childhood (from 12 months to about age 5), and late childhood (extending from age 6 to adolescence).

PHYSICAL DEVELOPMENT

During early childhood there is a steady increase in growth so that by about 30 months the birth mass is quadrupled. Physical growth slows and stabilises during the preschool years so that by age 5 years the child is about 18.6 kg in mass and about 109 cm tall.

During the toddler years (12–24 months) chest circumference continues to increase in size and exceeds head circumference. After the 2nd year the chest circumference exceeds the abdominal measurement, the lower extremities grow and the child assumes a taller, leaner appearance.

By the end of toddlerhood most of the body systems are relatively mature. The internal structures of the ear and throat continue to be short and straight, and the lymphoid tissue of the tonsils and adenoids remains large. (These circumstances account for a high incidence of ear, throat

TABLE 15.7 | Growth chart — infant to younger child

Age	Motor, communication, manipulative and social skills
12–18 months	Walks on own, can climb stairs and onto chairs. Imitates words and has a vocabulary of 3–24 words. Turns pages, scribbles, plays with building blocks constructively. Can identify several parts of their body. Likes to play with other children
24 months	Able to run, climb, walk up and down stairs alone. Begins to put two or three words together, begins to use pronouns. Imitates adult activities, can dress himself but not do up buttons. Plays with other children
3 years	Runs confidently, jumps, can ride a tricycle. Can say his own name and sex. Listens to stories. Vocabulary of 250–800 words. Thinks egocentrically. Plays constructively. Interacts with peers
4 years	Catches a ball, can hop on one foot. Knows many letters of the alphabet and can count up to 10.
5 years	Recites and sings. Asks lots of 'why' and 'how' questions. Vocabulary of 800–1500 words. Can use scissors. Plays co-operatively with others Can skip and hop. Can identify colours. Increased vocabulary, enjoys jokes and riddles. Ties shoelaces, does up buttons. More independent. Strongly identifies with parent of the same sex

and upper respiratory tract infections during this stage of development.) In later childhood most systems are mature and can adjust to moderate stress and change.

Motor development continues rapidly during early childhood so that the toddler is able to walk up and down stairs, kick a ball, and jump. By the end of the 3rd year, most children can run well and ride a tricycle. Drawing progresses from spontaneous scribbling to drawing stick-people, circles and other recognisable objects. Improving motor skills allow more intricate manipulations during later childhood.

Towards the end of childhood, a child grows on average 2.5–5 cm/year and increases in mass by about 1.5–3 kg/year. The average 12-year-old is about 150 cm tall and weighs about 38 kg. Body proportions take on a slimmer appearance, as fat gradually diminishes and its distribution patterns change. Cardiovascular functioning is refined and stabilised so that the heart rate averages 70–90 beats/minute, ventilations average 16–18 breaths/minute, and blood pressure normalises at about 110/70 mmHg. Development of all body systems continues during middle childhood to become more efficient and adult-like in function.

Bones continue to ossify, but ossification of small and long bones is not completed during this stage of development. By about age 10, all temporary teeth have been shed and most permanent teeth have erupted.

The school-age child gains increasing control over his muscular coordination and fine motor coordination (Cameron 2002).

INTELLECTUAL DEVELOPMENT

The major cognitive achievement of early childhood is the acquisition of language, and verbal language skills are further developed with an increased vocabulary and fluency of speech.

By the beginning of the 2nd year, the child is able to think and reason, and the concepts of time, space and causality (cause and effect) begin to have meaning.

By about age 5, egocentric thinking is replaced partially by intuitive thought. The child begins to acquire the ability to use thought processes to make sense of experiences, events and actions. Piaget describes this stage of development as concrete operational. The ability to read becomes a valuable means of increasing knowledge. During the ages of 6–12 years the ability to think abstractly and to solve problems develops and improves (Mitchell & Ziegler 2007).

EMOTIONAL AND PERSONALITY DEVELOPMENT

As a child learns to be more specific in the expression of emotions, they begin to learn the effects of their own behaviour on others. New motives appear that are learned by interacting with other people. While an infant's early behaviour is largely determined by basic biological needs, such as crying when hungry, much of the later behaviour is involved with meeting psychological needs such as security, acceptance, approval and feelings of self-worth. Emotions can activate and direct behaviour in the same way as biological drives.

Relationships with others play an important role in emotional and personality development. As the child interacts with other people they learn to cope more effectively with them, and an ability to co-operate or compete with others involves a sense of accomplishment. The more positive a child feels about themself the more confident they will feel about trying for success. Every small success increases the child's self-image, and a positive self-image makes the child feel likeable and worthwhile. If a child is incapable of, or unprepared for, assuming the responsibilities associated with a sense of accomplishment, they may develop a sense of inadequacy or inferiority.

It is generally recognised that if a child's need for love and security is not met they may become insecure and unable to relate effectively to others in later life. Therefore, throughout childhood, emotional and personality development depend largely on having psychological needs met. Emotional deprivation results in developmental retardation. Young children especially do not thrive if their main carer is hostile or indifferent to them and their needs (Mitchell & Ziegler 2007).

SOCIAL DEVELOPMENT

With increasing age, social development becomes less family dominated than in infancy. Not only do the quality and quantity of contacts with other people exert an influence on the growing child, but a widening range of contacts is essential to learning and to developing a healthy personality. Each group the child becomes involved with, such as school friends, provides a social relationship of varying strength and type. One of the most important socialising agents in a child's life is the peer group with whom they explore ideas and the physical environment. Through peer relationships children learn ways in which to relate and deal with others, such as those in positions of authority.

As a child interacts with peers they become aware that there are views other than their own. As a result the child learns to persuade, bargain and co-operate to maintain friendships. The child becomes increasingly sensitive to the social norms and pressures of the peer group, and the need for peer approval becomes a powerful influence towards conformity. Peer relationships in which a child experiences love and closeness from a friend seem to be important as a foundation for close relationships in adulthood.

Although increased independence is the goal of middle to late childhood, children still feel secure knowing that there is someone, such as the parents, to implement controls and restrictions. With a secure base in a loving family, a child is able to develop self-confidence and independence (Mitchell & Ziegler 2007).

FACTORS INFLUENCING GROWTH AND DEVELOPMENT

A person's development is influenced both by genetic factors and by the environment. Genetic factors are often referred to as the natural forces that influence development, while environmental factors are referred to as the nurturing forces. It is difficult to separate the effects of 'nature' and 'nurture', as individual development is affected by the interaction between these two forces.

Another factor that influences development is maturation which is a genetically programmed sequence of physical changes that is independent of environmental circumstances. Many behavioural changes that occur in the early months of life are related to maturation of the nervous system, muscles and glands. These changes represent a continuation of the growth processes that guide the development of the fetus within the uterus. Although maturation is not controlled by the environment, it can be accelerated or impeded by the quality of the environment, and by life experiences.

GENETIC FACTORS

Genetic factors influence many aspects of a person's physical and psychosocial being. Research indicates that, as well as determining physical characteristics, genetic factors also influence parts of a person's psychological make-up, such as temperament.

The central structure of a living cell is its complement of genes, which are located on the chromosomes within the cell nucleus. Many thousands of genes are carried on the chromosomes. In humans each cell normally contains 46 chromosomes. Human sperm and ova, however, each contain 23 chromosomes. When fertilisation occurs the sperm and the ovum unite, each contributing 23 chromosomes to the zygote, making a total of 46 chromosomes in 23 pairs, which are replicated in every cell of the body as the embryo develops. Because of the high number of genes in each chromosome, some of which are 'shuffled' during replication, and because during cell division each pair of chromosomes sorts randomly into the daughter cells with respect to other pairs, it is extremely unlikely that any two human beings would ever have identical genetic make-up, even with the same parents. One exception is identical (monozygotic) twins who, having developed from the same ovum, have exactly the same chromosomes and genes (Thibodeau & Patton 2004).

The single cell formed at fertilisation is capable of multiplying and developing into a fetus, with its sex and other characteristics, such as hair and eye colour, racial characteristics and physical stature predetermined. Each person's genetic structure is unique and lifelong, so heredity affects all stages of development. While each person's capacities are inherited, the extent to which they are used in development is influenced by the environment.

ENVIRONMENTAL FACTORS

The hereditary potential a person is born with is greatly influenced by the environment they encounter. Therefore, the environmental conditions to which an infant is exposed are a major influence on development. Environment refers to the people with whom an individual has contact, the experiences they have throughout life and the physical surroundings they are exposed to.

Attachment (bonding) is the process by which the parents and infant establish a relationship. Both parents and the infant have a role to play in the attachment process, whereby each establishes emotional ties with the other. As the parent responds to the infant, the infant responds to the parent, for example by cooing or eye contact. Creating a situation in which the parent's and the infant's eyes meet in visual contact is significant in the formation of emotional ties. Research has suggested that this early social attachment provides the security necessary for infants to explore their environment, and that it forms the basis for interpersonal relationships in later years.

Failure to form an attachment to one or a few primary persons in the early years has been related to an inability to develop close personal relationships in adulthood (Sanson 2003). Early stimulation is important in providing the background necessary to cope with the environment at a later stage. Stimulation is provided by handling the infant, allowing them to move about freely and assume different positions, and by providing conditions whereby the infant receives visual and auditory stimuli, such as coloured objects, mobiles and the sounds of voices and music. Many studies have been performed that indicate that a stimulating early environment is important for later intellectual development. Conversely, too much stimulation too soon could be upsetting for an infant, who may exhibit distress at being unable to respond to multiple stimuli (Sanson 2003).

The family and peer group are the most influential forces on a person's psychosocial growth and development, as it is through these groups that an individual learns about themself, others and society.

Through its various functions, the family exerts a major influence on development. It is through the family environment that the individual first learns about self, the world and their place within a society. Initially the individual adopts the family's values and belief systems. Family functions include providing love and security, meeting the basic needs such as food and warmth, facilitating emotional and social development, and helping the individual to learn about society, roles and behaviours (Sigelman 2003).

A person's peer group exerts a major influence on development, as it is through the peer group that an individual learns skills of socialisation and different ways of interacting with others. The peer group also places demands and expectations on peers to adapt their behaviour to achieve group purposes. It is often through the peer group that a person learns about success and/or failure, receives support or rejection and learns to question thoughts and feelings.

CLINICAL INTEREST BOX 15.1
Vitamin D deficiency

In some ways, Leon Jordan is a pretty typical teenager — he doesn't get much outdoor exercise, prefers movies and video games and won't drink milk. These habits contributed to a vitamin D deficiency that may have helped weaken the 15-year-old's bones and leave him prone to fractures. Doctors say it's an often overlooked problem that may affect millions of adolescents. Often undetected and untreated, vitamin D deficiency puts them at risk for stunted growth and debilitating osteoporosis later in life. While too much sunlight is bad, ultraviolet rays also interact with chemicals in the skin to produce vitamin D and it is recommended that young people spend about 10 minutes a few times a week in the sun without sunscreen because it can block the absorption of ultraviolet rays.

Experiences, which may promote learning, enable an individual to progress developmentally through the lifespan. At each developmental stage a person must learn to master a task or skill before progressing to the next stage. Gradually individuals use their accumulated skills and experiences to develop a range of effective behaviour.

Factors within the everyday environment, such as nutrition, housing and socioeconomic status, have been found to influence development. For example, the adequacy of nutrients in the diet influences how physiological needs are met, and subsequent growth and development. When a diet is lacking in adequate nutrients, deficits in height, weight and developmental progression occur (Clinical Interest Box 15.1).

NURSING IMPLICATIONS

Nursing care of infants and children is directed towards promoting the optimal level of health for each individual. Care involves preventing disease and injury, promoting family involvement in child care, health teaching, participating in a team approach to care and implementing measures to meet the physical, emotional, social and cultural needs of each individual. Development encompasses various aspects, such as motor skills, vision and hearing, speech and language, intellect, emotions, personality, morals and social skills. (For facts about childhood obesity see Clinical Interest Box 15.2.)

CLINICAL INTEREST BOX 15.2
Childhood obesity

Facts about childhood obesity

- During the period 1985 to 1995 the level of combined overweight/obesity in Australian children more than doubled, and the level of obesity tripled in all age groups and for both sexes.
- In 1995, the percentage of overweight or obese children and adolescents aged 2–17 years was 21% for boys and 23% for girls.
- The proportion of obese girls aged 7–15 years increased considerably from 1.2% in 1985 to 5.5% in 1995.
- The number of obese boys increased from 1.4% to 4.7%.
- Obese children have a 25–50% chance of being obese as an adult and this might be as high as 78% in older obese adolescents.
- Children or adolescents who are overweight or obese are more likely in the short term to develop endocrine, gastrointestinal or certain orthopaedic problems than children of healthy weight and more likely in the longer term to develop cardiovascular disease.
- Another result of childhood obesity is social discrimination. This is associated with poor self-esteem and depression.

(NSW Department of Health 2006)

Although there is an orderly pattern to the processes, the rate of growth and development varies among individuals. Growth and development are influenced by heredity, environment, physical care, mental stimulation, personal potential and emotional security (Cameron 2002). (The characteristic stages of development in children are listed in Tables 15.1–15.3.)

PAEDIATRIC CARE

The term paediatric means of or pertaining to a child, and paediatric nursing is the area of nursing concerned with the care of infants and children. Paediatric nursing requires knowledge of normal growth and development as well as knowledge of the needs and health problems of individuals in these age groups.

The role of a paediatric nurse can be described as that of carer, coordinator, educator and emotional support and resource person. The nurse who is involved in paediatric care, together with other members of the paediatric team, needs to adopt a holistic attitude towards caring for the child and parent(s) as a family unit. Many health care facilities recognise the need for family-centred care and adopt a philosophy to meet the needs of the family as a unit.

It is important for the nurse to recognise that children are not small adults, and that their reactions are generally quite different from the adults' reactions to illness, treatment, separation from family and admission to hospital.

CHILD HEALTH SERVICES

There are a variety of child health services whose broad aims are promoting the health of infants and children, providing parental support and care for the child who is ill. Many of the services are involved in preventing ill-health and are concerned with monitoring the health of children from birth. Preventive services include child health clinics and school health services.

Child health clinics play an important role in assessing growth and development — health education; screening for physical, metabolic and neuropsychiatric disorders; and providing immunisation against infectious diseases. The child health nurse aims to develop a close relationship with the mother and newborn infant as soon as possible after the birth. Advice is provided on infant hygiene, nutrition, growth and development, and preventive health measures such as recommended immunisation schedules. The nurse counsels and supports parents, consults with a paediatrician on health problems, refers children and families for supportive care as appropriate and keeps comprehensive records. These records include information on the child's growth and development, immunisations and illnesses and are important tools for assessment and for detecting situations that require early intervention and preventive action.

School health services aim to promote health by providing health education programs, by ensuring that each child is as healthy as possible so that each may obtain the maximal benefit from educational programs; and by assisting in detecting and managing children with impairments, disabilities or learning difficulties. School health services perform routine medical services just before or soon after children enter school, and selective medical examinations during school life. The school nurse plays an important role in preventing and detecting illness and disabilities. Two of the tests performed on all children assess acuity of sight and hearing.

Child guidance clinics staffed by educational psychologists, social workers and psychiatrists are available to assess children and provide services to help children overcome any difficulties. The services assist children who show evidence of emotional instability or psychological disturbance to attain personal, social or educational readjustment.

Children with mental or physical impairments are provided for by health, education and social services. Integration in ordinary schools is promoted so that all children can receive education, irrespective of the degree of their disability. In some instances this may not be possible and it may be necessary to provide education at home or in a special school. Every effort is made to ensure that a mentally or physically impaired child can develop to their fullest potential.

NEEDS OF INFANTS AND CHILDREN

The needs of children throughout the various stages of development are both physical and psychosocial. Physical needs include the need for food, water, oxygen, elimination, warmth, safety and protection. Further information regarding the nutritional needs of children at various stages of development can be found in Chapter 31. Meal times in a hospital should be pleasant unhurried occasions and the environment should be one that enables children to enjoy meals. Psychosocial needs include the need for love and affection, security, dependence and independence, and self-development. When physical or psychosocial needs are not met, children experience disruptions to their biological, emotional, social or educational growth and development. When needs are not met there are a variety of effects on the child, such as a greater incidence of disease and accidents, failure to thrive, behavioural problems, delayed language skills, antisocial behaviour such as conflicts with the law or substance use and abuse, learning difficulties and social inadequacy.

SUMMARY

Growth and development are processes that begin at conception and continue throughout each stage of the life cycle. Growth may be defined as the physical changes that occur in a steady and orderly manner, while development relates to changes in psychological and social functioning. The stages of growth and development are generally described as being prenatal, infancy, childhood, adolescence and adulthood. Characteristic changes occur at each stage, but the pace and behaviours of growth and development vary with each individual.

To care for individuals from infancy to late childhood the nurse first requires knowledge of normal growth and development. Infancy and childhood are unique phases of development accompanied by special needs. The nurse who is working with children or adolescents needs to develop certain skills to provide a high quality of care.

During the 38 weeks after human conception, amazing growth and development occurs. Growth is referred to as the increase in number and size of cells of an organism as it increases in both length and weight. In the biological context, development is the manner in which cells differentiate into tissues and systems that perform a specific purpose. This chapter covers the intricate experiences that occur from conception through to birth and looks at the expected developmental growth of a young child.

REVIEW EXERCISES

1. There are several theories about the various stages of growth and development, particularly in regard to infants and children. Name the stages according to Freud, Erikson and Piaget.
2. State the factors that influence growth and development during all stages.
3. Define fertilisation. Where does it normally occur?
4. Explain the importance of the placenta and umbilical cord to fetal growth.
5. Outline some of the major developmental changes during fetal growth.
6. List the developmental stages of early childhood and briefly outline the changes that occur during each phase.

CRITICAL THINKING EXERCISE

1. Claire is 22 and has attended the baby health clinic for a routine 8-week check up. Claire is curious about the stages of infant development and asks, 'How is my baby doing? How long should he be and how much should he weigh now? When will he start smiling and trying to roll onto his back?'
   a) What subjective and objective data do you need before you answer?

b) What nursing diagnoses could you apply? How will you validate these?
c) What goals might be developed and how will these be prioritised?
d) What interventions might you offer?
e) How will you evaluate the effectiveness of your interventions?

2. Thomas, aged 3, is admitted to your ward for elective surgery to remove his tonsils. His weight is 35 kg and you notice on admission that he is very pale and doesn't attempt to communicate either verbally or physically with his mother or you. You ask his mother if he is normally very quiet and she tells you 'he never speaks, he just sits and watches television all day'.
   a) What physical and psychological factors may be affecting Thomas's growth and development?
   b) As a nurse, how would you educate Thomas's mother on the importance of diet and exercise for a three-year-old child?

REFERENCES AND FURTHER READING

Bobak I, Jensen M (1993) *Maternity and Gynecological Care. The Nurse and the Family*. Mosby, St Louis
Bolander VB (1994) *Sorensen and Luckmann's Basic Nursing: A Psychophysiologic Approach*. WB Saunders, Philadelphia
Cameron N (2002) *Human Growth and Development*. Academic Press, Amsterdam
Carel H (2006) *Life and Death in Freud and Heidegger*. Rodopi, Amsterdam
Crisp J, Taylor C (eds) (2005) *Potter & Perry's Fundamentals of Nursing*, 2nd edn. Elsevier Australia, Sydney
Hockenberry M, Wilson D, Winkelstein ML (eds) (2005) *Wong's Essentials of Paediatric Nursing*, 7th edn. Mosby, St Louis
Huitt W, Hummel J (2003) *Piaget's Theory of Cognitive Development*. Educational Psychology Interactive. Valdosta State University, Valdosta, GA
Leifer G (2007) *Introduction to Maternity & Pediatric Nursing*, 5th edn. WB Saunders, Philadelphia
Marieb EN (2004) *Human Anatomy & Physiology*, 6th edn. Pearson, San Francisco
Mitchell P, Ziegler F (2007) *Fundamentals of Development: the Psychology of Childhood*. Psychology Press, East Sussex
NSW Department of Health 2006 *Childhood Obesity NSW*. Online. Available: www.health.nsw.gov.au/obesity/adult/about.html [accessed 9 May 2008]
Pilliteri A (2003) *Maternal and Child Health Nursing: Care of the Childbearing and Childrearing Family*, 2nd edn. Lippincott, Philadelphia
Sanson A (2003) *Children's Health and Development. New research directions for Australia*. Australian Institute of Family Studies, Melbourne
Santrock J (2007) *Child Development*. McGraw-Hill, Boston
Sherblom Matteson P (2001) *Women's Health During the Childbearing Years*. Mosby, St Louis
Sigelman CK (2003) *An Introduction to Theories of Personalities*. L Erlbaum Associates, Mahwah, NJ
Sugarman L (2001) *Life-Span Development: Frameworks, Accounts, and Strategies*. Psychology Press, Sussex
Thibodeau GA, Patton KT (2004) *Structure and Function of the Body*, 12th edn. Mosby, St Louis

Chapter 16

GROWTH AND DEVELOPMENT: LATE CHILDHOOD THROUGH TO ADOLESCENCE

OBJECTIVES

- Define the key terms/concepts
- Describe the physical changes that occur at puberty
- Define preadolescence
- Discuss factors influencing the growth and development of the adolescent
- Describe the physiological changes that occur during adolescence
- Plan health promotion activities for a group of adolescents
- Discuss the role of the peer group during adolescence

KEY TERMS/CONCEPTS

adolescence
anorexia nervosa
bulimia nervosa
gynocomastia
menarche
oestrogen
preadolescence
puberty
pubescence
role diffusion
sexually transmitted infection (STI)
testosterone

CHAPTER FOCUS

Adolescence is the period of transition between childhood and adulthood. The nurse must have a clear understanding of the normal ranges of expected growth and development for this period, which is essential for individualising care. Adolescence is an area of care that requires specific knowledge and skills to enable the nurse to recognise health concerns when they arise and implement health promotion and preventive strategies in the appropriate context. This chapter discusses concepts of growth and development for adolescence and looks at nursing implications and health promotion for this period.

LIVED EXPERIENCE

I find it really hard to talk to her. She never seems to listen to what I am trying to say and sometimes I think it is not worth trying because she doesn't trust me to make the right choices. I want to tell her how I feel but I don't know how.

Sally, age 15

I know I don't give her enough credit for making the right choices. Even though I have taught my children to always make their own decisions and not let others make them for them, now that she is a teenager I think back to what I did without my parents knowing and I get scared of the situations she might get into.

Sally's mother

An understanding of adolescent development is essential for nurses in their daily practice. Adolescence is the period in the lifespan where the individual, previously reliant on parents and carers for values and identity, becomes independent and, in this move towards independence, attempts to create a new and personal identity. It is a time when group identity is vital, often a time of experimentation with self-image, and a time to question family values and beliefs. Adolescents are capable of abstract thought and understand many variables within a given situation. This chapter highlights the growth and development of the adolescent and how nursing knowledge of this phase can provide optimal nursing care for the adolescent when hospitalised.

PREADOLESCENCE

The transitional period between childhood and adolescence is referred to as preadolescence. It may also be referred to as late childhood, early adolescence and pubescence. Prepubescence is the period of about 2 years before puberty when the individual is developing preliminary physical changes that herald sexual maturity.

PHYSICAL DEVELOPMENT

Preadolescence physically refers to the beginning of the second skeletal growth spurt, when physical changes such as the development of female breasts and pubic hair also begins. These physical changes occur about 2 years earlier in girls than boys (Graber et al 1997).

Preadolescents have increased cognitive and social skills and are able to describe their feelings about the developmental changes they are experiencing. They can also think through the changes and become better at problem solving and achieving their goals.

In the preadolescent stage children become more social and their behavioural patterns become much less predictable. Included in this stage is experimentation with make-up by girls and an interest in music and performers that are popular with older adolescents. Interest in sexual activity develops. Preadolescents often develop friendships with adults other than their parents. They use these relationships to gather information about adults. (See Chapter 12 for more information on sexuality and the adolescent.)

ADOLESCENCE

Adolescence is the period of development from age 12 to 20 and is the stage that marks the transition from childhood to adulthood. Adolescence is a stage of development characterised by sudden physical changes and social and emotional maturing. Adolescence is frequently described as a transition period between childhood and adulthood, which begins with the gradual appearance of secondary sex characteristics and ends with cessation of body growth.

The term adolescent usually refers to psychological maturation of the person, whereas puberty refers to the point at which sexual maturity is achieved and reproduction becomes possible. Puberty mainly refers to the maturational, hormonal and growth process that occurs when the reproductive organs begin to function and the secondary sex characteristics develop. Adolescence is the period of transition between puberty and adulthood (Mitchell & Ziegler 2007).

Adolescence involves three distinct sub-phases: early adolescence (age 11–14), middle adolescence (15–17 years) and late adolescence (18–20 years).

PHYSICAL DEVELOPMENT

The physical changes of early adolescence (puberty) are primarily the result of hormonal activity. Physical changes occur rapidly in both males and females. Physical distinctions between boys and girls are determined on the basis of distinguishing characteristics: primary sex characteristics are the internal and external organs that carry out reproductive functions (ovaries, breasts, penis, uterus); secondary sex characteristics play no direct part in reproduction but are the changes that occur in the body as a result of the hormonal change (development of facial and pubic hair, changes in voice, fat deposits). Secondary sex characteristics externally differentiate males from females.

The main physical changes are:

- Increased growth rate of the skeleton and muscles
- Alteration in the distribution of muscle and fat
- Gender-specific changes, such as changes in shoulder and hip width
- Development of the reproductive system and secondary sex characteristics.

Height and weight usually increase during the prepubertal growth spurt. The final 20% to 25% of height is achieved during puberty, with most of this growth occurring in a 24–36 month period. For girls this usually begins between 8 and 14 years of age. Weight increases by 7–25 kg and height increases by 5–20 cm. Growth in height usually stops 2–2.5 years after menarche in girls. For males this growth spurt occurs between 10 and 16 years of age. Height increases by 10–30 cm and weight increases by 7–30 kg. Growth in length of the limbs and neck precedes growth in other areas. Increases in hip and chest width take place in a few months, followed by an increase in shoulder width several months later.

Growth in height usually stops at age 18–20 in boys. The individual often appears awkward and clumsy and the sequence of changes is responsible for the long-legged gawky appearance that is often seen. These changes require the adolescent to adjust their perception of their self in space as well as accepting a new body image. Fat becomes redistributed into adult proportions as height and mass increase, and the adolescent gradually assumes an adult appearance. Adolescents are concerned about physical changes that make them different from their peers, and the nurse should reassure them about normal growth curves and that their own growth patterns are normal (Green-Hernandez et al 2001).

HORMONAL CHANGES OF PUBERTY

The increase in hormonal activity during puberty leads to maturing of the body shape and achievement of fertility. All physical changes are the result of hormonal influences. Hormonal production is controlled by the anterior pituitary gland, which is in turn stimulated by the hypothalamus. The stimulation of the anterior pituitary results in the release of the gonadotrophic hormones that stimulate the gonads. As a result of this stimulation, testicular cells produce testosterone and ovarian cells produce oestrogen. These hormones contribute to the development of secondary sex characteristics and play an essential role in reproduction. The changing concentration of these hormones is also linked to problems of adolescence, such as body odour and acne (Green-Hernandez et al 2001; Clinical Interest Box 16.1).

Sexual maturation in girls

The initial indication of puberty in most girls is the appearance of breast buds. Breasts begin to develop from about age 10 (development continues until about age 17) (Figure 16.1). Around 2–6 months later, growth of pubic hair on the mons pubis begins (Figure 16.2). The initial appearance of menstruation (*menarche*) occurs about 2 years after the first pubescent changes. The normal age range of menarche is 10.5–15 years, with ovulation usually beginning 6–14 months after menarche.

Concerns about pubertal delay in girls should be considered if breasts have not started to develop by age 13 or if menarche has not occurred within 4 years of the onset of breast development (Sigelman 2003).

Sexual maturation in boys

Testicular enlargement accompanied by thinning, reddening and increased looseness of the scrotum are the first pubescent changes in boys and usually occur between age 9.5 and 14. This is often followed by the initial appearance of pubic hair. Penile enlargement begins, with continuing testicular enlargement and growth of pubic hair (Figure 16.3). Facial hair may develop along with early voice changes. *Gynocomastia*, temporary breast enlargement, and tenderness are common during mid-puberty. This breast enlargement usually disappears within 2 years. Height and weight growth occur towards the end of mid-puberty. Nocturnal emissions of seminal fluid are an indication of puberty in the male and occur spontaneously and periodically during sleep. In late puberty the testicles and penis enlarge, and the voice deepens. Axillary hair develops and facial hair extends to cover the neck.

Boys may be considered to have pubertal delay if there is no enlargement of the testes or scrotal changes by age 13.5–14 or if genital growth is not complete 4 years after enlargement of the testicles.

The physical changes that occur during adolescence are rapid and dramatic and play a significant role in psychosocial development. By understanding these hormonal changes the nurse is able to reassure and educate adolescents about their body care needs. The timing of these physical changes depends on factors such as heredity and nutrition and whether the child is a boy or girl. The sequence of pubertal growth changes (Tables 16.1 & 16.2) are the same in most individuals (Sigelman 2003).

CLINICAL INTEREST BOX 16.1
Case study: Sarah

Sarah, 11, presents crying and asking for a physical examination, as she noticed when she went to the toilet that there was blood on the toilet paper. As her nurse you know that you need to gain her trust and calm her down. You introduce yourself and let her know that you will stay with her throughout her stay. Because she has never been in a hospital, you interpret what is going on around you, using everyday language. After providing tissues and a hug, as soon as she seems calmer you ask Sarah what she knows about menstruation or 'periods'. It becomes clear to both of you that this is what is occurring and you spend time with her going over what is happening. After review by the doctor it is determined that a physical examination is not required. She asks you to contact her mother and you ring her and explain what has occurred and organise for her to come and collect her.

PHYSIOLOGICAL CHANGES

The strength and size of the heart and systolic blood pressure and blood volume increase during puberty. The pulse rate and basal heat production decrease. Boys have a higher blood volume than girls, which may be related to boys having a greater muscle mass. All formed elements of the body reach adult levels. Respiratory volume and vital capacity are increased, but respiratory rate and the basal metabolic rate decrease. As a result of increased strength and size of muscles and increased cardiac, respiratory and cardiac functioning, physiological responses to exercise change dramatically.

COGNITIVE DEVELOPMENT

Adolescents are capable of using deductive reasoning and abstract thinking and can consider the logic of a problem. This stage, known as the period of formal operations, is the highest level of intellectual development, according to Piaget (see Chapter 15). Being able to think logically about role behaviours enables adolescents to develop their own thoughts and means of expressing their identity. Intellectual development continues through formal education and the pursuit of personal interests. Without an appropriate educational environment, individuals may not reach this stage. The teenager can think abstractly and is no longer restricted to the real and actual, but can deal with the hypothetical. Adolescents are able to manipulate more than two different variables at one time. They think about what might be, whereas primary school-age children only think about what is. This allows adolescents to have more

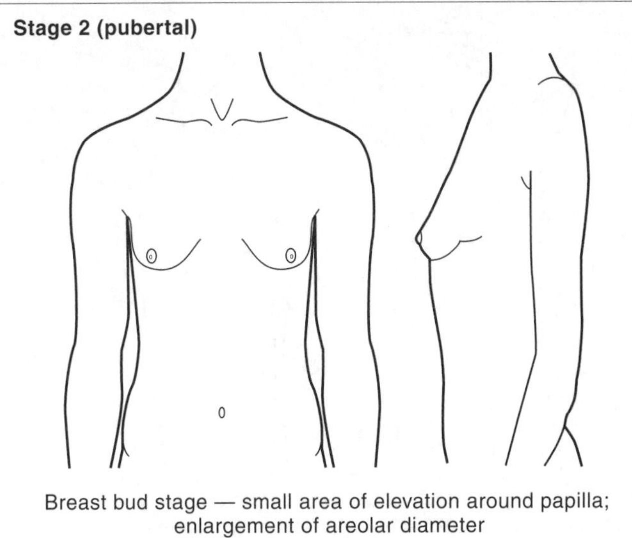

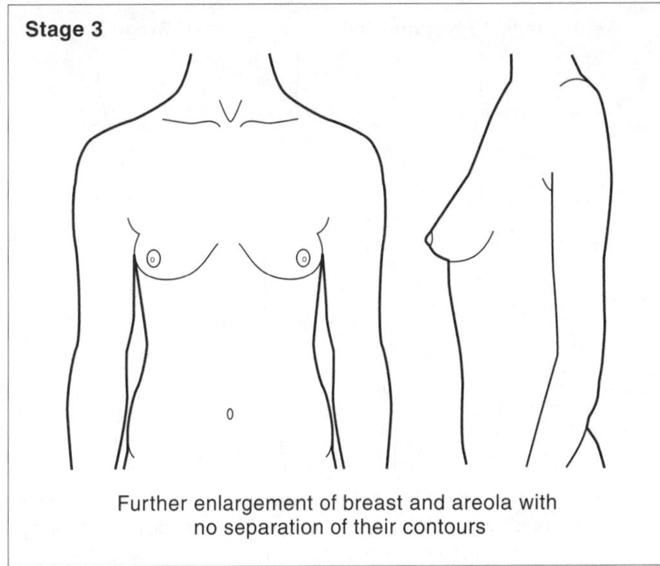

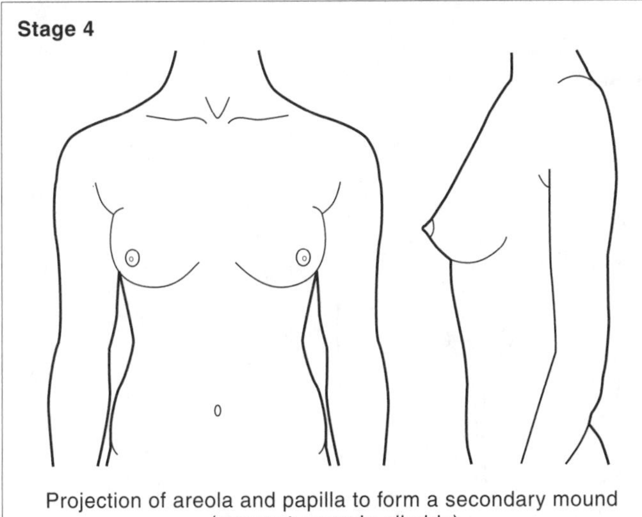

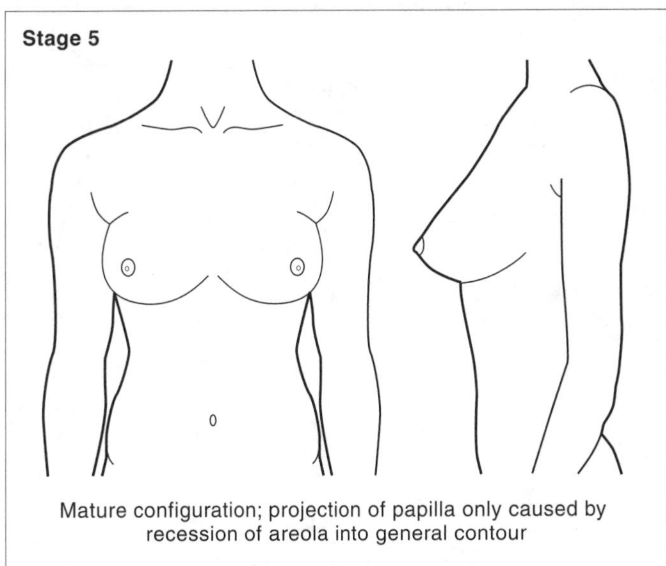

Figure 16.1 | Development of breasts in girls. Stage 1 (prepubertal elevation of papillae only) not shown *(Adapted from Hockenberry 2005 [Modified from Marshall WA, Tanner JM: Arch Dis Child 44:291, 1969; Daniel WA, Paulshock BZ: A Physician's guide to sexual maturity, Patient Care May 13, 122–124, 1979])*

skill and insight when playing board games or video games, for example.

By mid-adolescence, cognition develops an introspective quality. At this stage adolescents wonder about what others think of them and increasingly imagine the thoughts of others. They question society and its values and, although they have the ability to think as well as an adult, they do not have the experiences that an adult has on which to build. They can think about the consequences of their actions and can detect logical consistency or inconsistency in a set of statements or actions. For example, they will question a parent who swears but tries to persuade the adolescent not to use bad language.

Language development is relatively complete by adolescence, although vocabulary continues to expand. The main focus becomes the development of communication skills that can be employed effectively in various situations. Adolescents need to share thoughts, facts and feelings to parents, teachers, peers and others. The skills needed are varied. The adolescent must decide whom they will communicate with, the message they wish to share and the way they will transmit the message. For example, the way a teenager tells peers about a new relationship is not the same as the way they tell their parents (Mitchell & Ziegler 2007).

PSYCHOSOCIAL DEVELOPMENT

Adolescence is a stage of transition, a time between childhood and adulthood when the young person is seeking and learning the skills to become independent. Adolescence is often a period of emotional turmoil and insecurity, caused by the conflict between the need and desire for independence

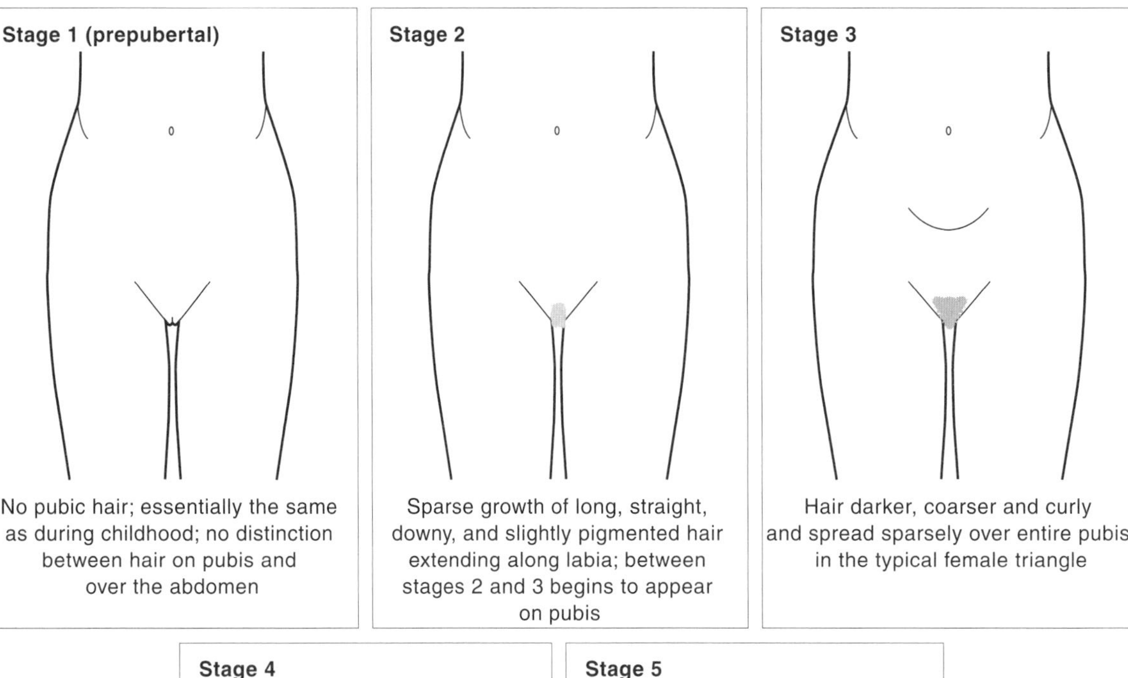

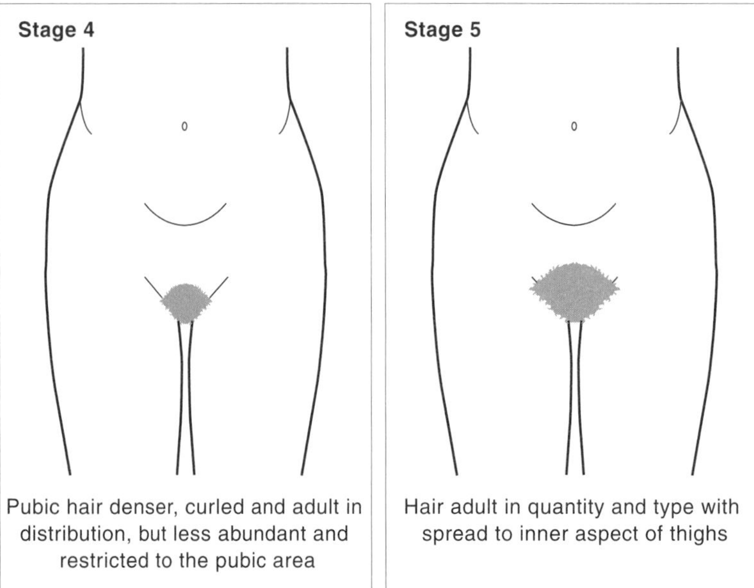

Figure 16.2 | Growth of pubic hair in girls *(Adapted from Hockenberry 2005 [Modified from Marshall WA, Tanner JM: Arch Dis Child 44:291, 1969; Daniel WA, Paulshock BZ: A Physician's guide to sexual maturity, Patient Care May 13, 122–124, 1979])*

and the need to retain dependence on others. It is a time when identity is consolidated and a time when choices about vocation and lifestyle must be made. Relationships with parents undergo change and the adolescent begins to assert individuality and a desire for independence, often by resisting adult authority and advice. The adolescent usually displays mood swings, and experiences confused emotions. In later adolescence, emotions are better controlled and more mature. However, an older adolescent is still subject to heightened emotion and their expressive behaviour reflects feelings of insecurity and indecision.

For those working with adolescents, knowledge of the theories of adolescent development is essential to obtain an understanding of the adolescent stage and the ability to recognise the tasks of adolescence. One such theory is Erikson's theory of human development (1963) which encompasses the whole of the lifespan in eight stages, each of which involves opposing crises which must be negotiated to be able to go on to the next stage. This theory recognises the period of adolescence as a time spent searching for identity. Erikson sees identity (or role) confusion as the main danger of this stage. The adolescent's search for identity involves the quest for individual, sex-role, moral and group identity (Mitchell & Ziegler 2007).

Group identity

Adolescents seek to belong to a group to feel that they belong and have status. The pressure to belong to a group

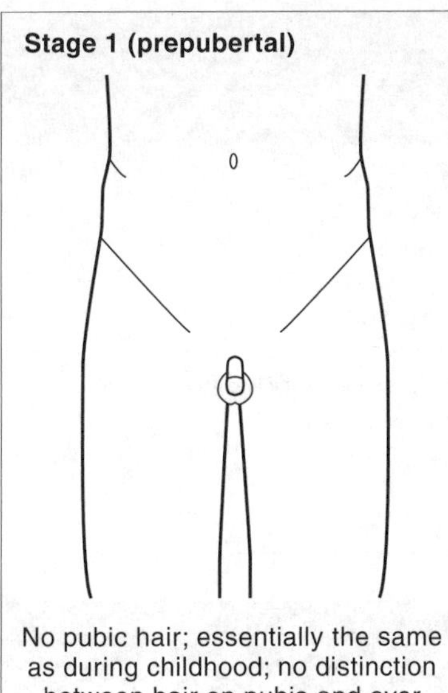

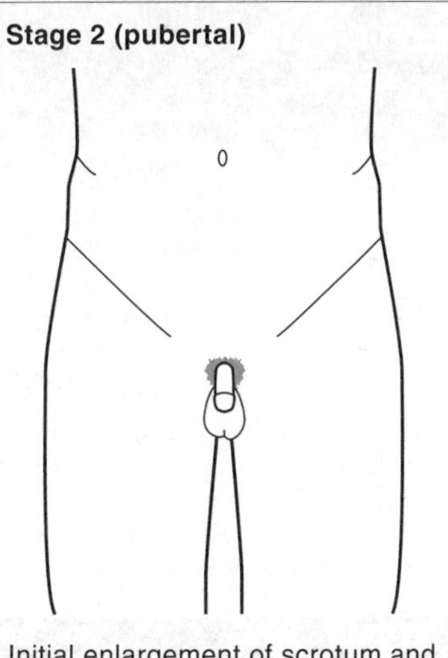

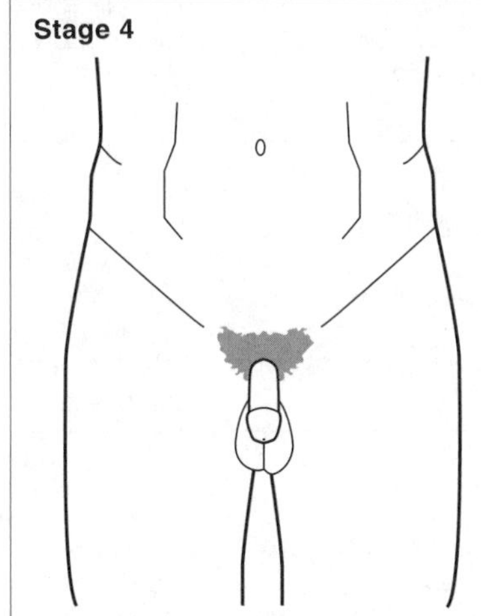
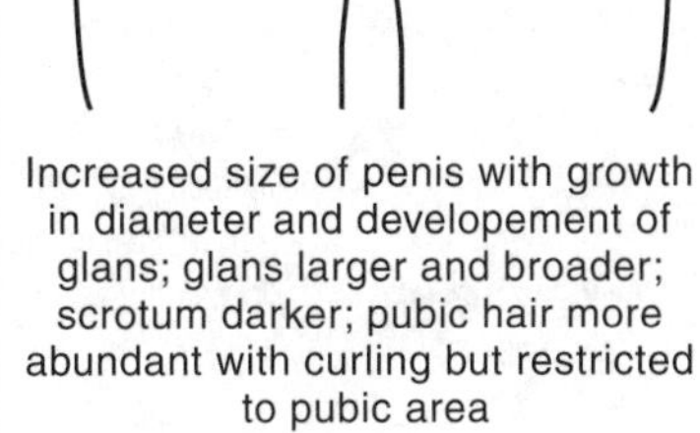

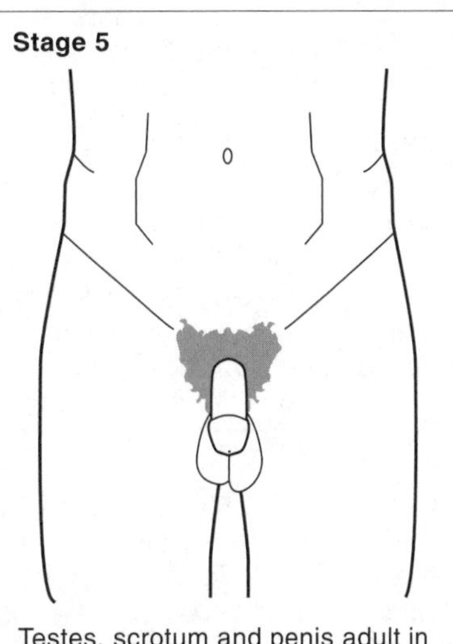

Figure 16.3 | Developmental stages of secondary sex characteristics and genital development in boys *(Adapted from Hockenberry 2005 [Modified from Marshall WA, Tanner JM: Arch Dis Child 44:291, 1969; Daniel WA, Paulshock BZ: A Physician's guide to sexual maturity, Patient Care May 13, 122–124, 1979])*

intensifies and, as the adolescent moves away from the family, the values of the peer group and their appraisal of them become increasingly important. Peer groups provide a sense of belonging, approval and the opportunity to learn acceptable behaviour. By developing close bonds with peers, adolescents are able to develop a frame of reference for their own identity.

Individual identity

A sense of identity is the individual's concept of who they are and where they are going in life. To find out who they are, adolescents must formulate standards of conduct and know what they value as important and worth doing. This fulfils their need for a sense of their own worth and importance. Adolescents need to develop their own ethical systems based on personal values. When parental views and values differ greatly from those of peers and other important figures, the possibility for conflict is great. As a result, the adolescent may experience role diffusion as they try out one role after another and may have difficulty in synthesising the different roles into a single identity. A positive identity eventually emerges after periods of confusion and adjustment, as the

TABLE 16.1 | Usual sequence of maturational changes in adolescence

Boys	Girls
Skeletal growth spurt	Skeletal growth spurt
Enlargement of testes and scrotal sac	Beginning of breast development
Appearance of pubic hair	Appearance of pubic hair
Changes in larynx and voice	Menarche
Enlargement of penis and prostate gland	Ovulation and completion of breast growth
Nocturnal emissions	Appearance of axillary hair
Growth of downy facial hair	Widening of pelvis, deposition of body fat
Appearance of axillary hair	Abrupt decrease of linear growth
Increase in shoulder width	
Deepening of voice, appearance of coarse facial hair	
Abrupt decrease of linear growth	

TABLE 16.2 | Growth and development during adolescence

Early Adolescence (11–14 years)	Middle Adolescence (14–17 years)	Late Adolescence (17–20 years)
Growth		
Rapidly accelerating growth Reaches peak velocity Secondary sex characteristics appear	Growth decelerating in girls Stature reaches 95% of adult height Secondary sex characteristics well advanced	Physically mature Structure and reproductive growth almost complete
Cognition		
Explores newfound ability for limited abstract thought Clumsy groping for new values and energies Comparison of 'normality' with peers of same sex	Developing capacity for abstract thinking Enjoys intellectual powers, often in idealistic terms Concern with philosophical, political and social problems	Established abstract thought Can perceive and act on long-range operations Able to view problems comprehensively Intellectual and functional identity established
Identity		
Preoccupied with rapid body changes Trying out of various roles Measurement of attractiveness by acceptance or rejection by peers Conformity to group norms	Modifies body image Very self-centred; increased narcissism Tendency towards inner experience and self-discovery Has a rich fantasy life Idealistic Able to perceive future implications of current behaviours and decisions; variable application	Body image and gender-role definition nearly secured Mature sexual identity Phase of consolidation of identity Stability of self-esteem Comfortable with physical growth Social roles defined and articulated
Relationships with parents		
Defining independence–dependence boundaries Strong desire to remain dependent on parents while trying to detach No major conflicts over parental control	Major conflicts over independence and control Low point in parent–child relationship Greatest push for emancipation; disengagement Final and irreversible emotional detachment from parents; mourning	Emotional and physical separation from parents completed Independence from family with less conflict Emancipation nearly secured

adolescent makes choices about the future. (See Chapter 12 for more information on sexual identity.)

Moral development (identity)

Moral development is consolidated in adolescence as the teenager moves from accepting the decisions of adults to gaining their own set of morals and values. Kohlberg (1964) explains moral development in terms of stages and, according to his theory of moral development, adolescents begin to question existing moral values and learn to make choices. The development of moral judgment depends on communication, cognitive skills and peer interaction. Not

TABLE 16.2 | Growth and development during adolescence — cont'd

Early Adolescence (11–14 years)	Middle Adolescence (14–17 years)	Late Adolescence (17–20 years)
Relationships with peers		
Seeks peer affiliations to counter instability generated by rapid change Upsurge in close idealised friendships with members of the same sex Struggle for mastery takes place within peer group	Strong need for identity to affirm self-image Behavioural standards set by peer group Acceptance by peers extremely important — fear of rejection Exploration of ability to attract opposite sex or same sex romantic partners	Peer group recedes in importance in favour of individual friendships Testing of romantic relationships against possibility of permanent alliance Relationships characterised by giving and sharing
Sexuality		
Self-exploration and evaluation Limited dating, usually group Limited intimacy	Multiple plural relationships Internal identification of heterosexual, homosexual or bisexual attractions Exploration of 'self-appeal' Feeling of 'being in love' Tentative establishment of relationships	Forms stable relationship and attachment to another Growing capacity for mutuality and reciprocity Dating as a romantic pair May publicly identify as gay, lesbian or bisexual Intimacy involves commitment rather than exploration and romanticism
Psychological health		
Wide mood swings Intense daydreaming Anger outwardly expressed with moodiness, temper outbursts and verbal insults and name-calling	Tendency towards inner experiences; more introspective Tendency to withdraw when upset or feelings are hurt Vascillation of emotions in time and range Feelings of inadequacy common; difficulty in asking for help	More constancy of emotion Anger more apt to be concealed
(Hockenberry & Wilson 2007)		

all adolescents reach the same level of moral development. Boys may have more justice-oriented responses to moral problems, while girls have been found to have more caring responses. Table 16.3 summarises the developmental behaviours of adolescents.

SOCIAL DEVELOPMENT

Social development involves an expansion of the network of social relationships and social activities. For many adolescents the peer group remains the most important social group, serving as a strong support for the adolescent and providing a sense of belonging. It provides a link between independence and autonomy. Adolescents may move away from family domination and define their identity independently of parental authority. Adolescents may want to separate from parental restraints but at the same time may be fearful of the consequences associated with independence. This process of achieving independence often involves turmoil and ambiguity as both adolescent and parent learn new roles. Conflicts can arise from almost any situation or subject. Adolescents may find themselves argumentative, critical and remote with both parents as they attempt to achieve independence from parental controls. This rejection is usually not consistent and varies with mood changes. Some research suggests that parents need to be guided towards an authoritative style of parenting in which authority is used to guide the adolescent with clear, consistent messages regarding expectations, while allowing a level of freedom appropriate to their development (Baker et al 1999). Social relationships develop outside the family, which help the adolescent identify their role in society.

RESPONSES TO PUBERTY

How the adolescent responds to the physical changes of puberty depends on the stage of development. In early adolescence some adolescents are preoccupied with the changes in their body and are very interested in their sexual organs. If the boy has not been prepared in advance by his parents he may turn to his peers for information and help. Girls find body changes difficult to adjust to and are often concerned with weight increase and associated fat deposits. This may lead them to think they are obese and lead to fad dieting. Adolescents can be concerned with whether they are

TABLE 16.3 | Developmental behaviours of adolescents

Relationships with parents
Adolescents' desires for increasing independence and autonomy and continuing need for some dependence and limit setting by parents place strain on their relationship. Effective communication and democratic parenting are best tools for meeting this challenge.

Relationships with siblings
Younger siblings rarely understand their adolescent sibling's need for privacy to think, dream and talk with peers. Adolescents often enjoy interacting with and guiding younger brothers and sisters when timing is convenient for them and they can remain in control.

Relationships with peers
Peer group is factor of critical influence to adolescents, who have increasing need for recognition and acceptance. Companionship offered by peer groups provides secure environment for individuals to try out new ideas and share similar feelings and attitudes. Adolescents often form cliques with peers from same socioeconomic group with similar interests. Cliques, which are highly exclusive, help their members, who have strong emotional bonds, develop their identities. The crowd, which is more impersonal than the clique, offers opportunities for heterosexual interaction and social activities. The crowd also maintains rigid membership requirements; clique membership is usually a prerequisite for crowd membership.

Self-concept
Formal and informal peer groups are primary force in shaping self-concept of group members. Popularity and recognition within peer group enhance self-esteem and reinforce self-concept. Total immersion in peer group may make it appear that adolescents have no original thoughts and are incapable of making decisions. Adolescents who withdraw from peers into isolation struggle with developing identity.

Fears
Fears in this age group centre around peer group acceptance, body changes, loss of self-control and emerging sexual urges. Adolescents constantly examine their bodies for changes and signs of imperfection. Any defect, real or imagined, is cause of endless worry. Adolescents' developing awareness of economic and political problems may result in fear of going to war with its resulting death and destruction.

Coping patterns
Repertoire of coping behaviours has expanded with experiences adolescents have gained from life and from developing cognitive maturity. By age 15, most use full range of defence mechanisms, including rationalisation and intellectualisation. Adolescents' problem-solving abilities have matured, and they can reason through philosophical discussions and complex situations that require abstract thinking and proposition of hypotheses. Some adolescents use avoidance coping strategies in which the problem is denied or repressed and an attempt is made to reduce tension by engaging in chemical abuse or avoiding people.

Morals
According to Kohlberg (1964), as youths approach adolescence they reach conventional level, where internalisation of expectations of their family and society begins. Initially there is considerable conformity to rules to win praise or approval from others and to avoid social disapproval or rejection; later, they seek to avoid criticism from persons of authority in institutions.

Diversional activity
Many adolescents develop special interests in certain sports and concentrate on developing maximal skills therein. Recreational activities are often determined by what is popular with peers and what can provide independence from parents (e.g., computers, cars).

Nutrition
Total nutritional needs become greater during adolescence. Girls' energy needs decrease, and their need for protein increases slightly. Iron needed by adolescents is almost twice that of adult men, and growth spurts increase calcium demand.

(modified from Crisp & Taylor 2005)

normal and will compare their body with images in the media and their peers. Early or late onset of puberty leads to higher rates of risk-taking behaviours (Graber et al 1997).

HEALTH RISKS

The major causes of morbidity and mortality in adolescents are not diseases but health-damaging behaviours related to depression, injury, violence, sexually transmitted infections (STIs) and pregnancy.

ACCIDENTS

Accidents are the greatest cause of deaths in the adolescent age group (Dolan & Holt 2000). A tendency for risk-taking behaviour together with feelings of indestructibility make adolescents particularly prone to accidents, especially those involving motor vehicles and sports.

SUICIDE

Suicide accounted for 19% of deaths among older teenagers (aged 17–19 years) in 2000, making it the second most common cause of death in that age group (Australian Bureau of Statistics [ABS] 2002). Suicide usually results from a combination of factors. The following warning signs may occur for at least a month before a suicide attempt:

- Withdrawal
- Loss of initiative
- Decreased performance at school
- Crying, sadness and loneliness

CLINICAL INTEREST BOX 16.2
Sample nursing care plan for the adolescent with anorexia nervosa

Assessment

Katie is a 15-year-old girl admitted to your ward with anorexia nervosa. Her weight has dropped to 45 kg, she exercises excessively, takes laxatives and will only eat small amounts of vegetables and fruit. She has recently broken up with her boyfriend and believes this is because she is 'fat'.

Nursing diagnosis

- Altered nutrition: less than body requirements
- Body image disturbance related to altered perception

Planning

Goals

- Client will consume nourishment adequate for weight gain
- Client will reduce energy expenditure
- Client will express perception of self in acceptable ways

Expected outcomes

- Client will show gradual weight gain
- Client participates in quiet and planned activities
- Client expresses self in acceptable ways
- Client demonstrates development of a positive body image

Intervention	Rationale
Start high-calorie diet	Adequate nourishment for gradual weight gain
Explain diet plan with client	To encourage compliance
Monitor physical activity	To evaluate if appropriate
Avoid coercive techniques	Is usually ineffective for long-term change
Encourage participation in own care	To promote a sense of control

Evaluation

- Observe client's activity
- Observe client's eating habits
- Ask client to identify healthy eating patterns

- Disturbance in sleep and appetite
- Verbalisation of suicidal thoughts
- Giving away of possessions.

The nurse needs to be able to identify precipitating events and adolescent suicide risk factors. If assessment suggests that the adolescent is at risk of suicide the nurse needs to facilitate referral to mental health professionals while helping the adolescent to focus on positive aspects of life and develop coping skills such as problem solving, anger management, conflict resolution and assertive communication.

EATING DISORDERS

Overeating or under-eating during adolescence is of concern particularly for girls, who, when they experience the normal increase in fat deposition and weight associated with the growth spurt, are more likely to resort to dieting. Anorexia nervosa is a clinical syndrome with physical and psychosocial components. People with anorexia nervosa have an intense fear of gaining weight and refuse to maintain their weight at the normal minimal weight for their age and height. Bulimia nervosa involves binge eating followed by behaviours such as induced vomiting, use of laxatives and excessive exercise to prevent weight gain. It is important to take a thorough dietary history (Field et al 2003). See Clinical Interest Box 16.2 for a sample care plan for an eating disorder.

SUBSTANCE ABUSE

Substance abuse involves the use of mood-altering substances in an attempt to create a sense of wellbeing or improve levels of performance. All adolescents are at risk of substance abuse. In 1997 alcohol accounted for 3700 deaths in people aged 15–44, while 18 200 deaths were

CLINICAL INTEREST BOX 16.3
Case study — sexual education of a young adolescent

Jane, 14, presents to hospital asking to have a pregnancy test done but begs the nurse not to contact her mother, whom she knows socially. Karen, the nurse, knows she has to maintain her professional role and act quickly to reassure Jane that what happens between them will remain confidential. Karen ensures privacy to gain a history and shows concern for Jane asking her to tell her why she thinks she is pregnant. Because Jane's explanation leads Karen to believe that she is not likely to be pregnant, she tells Jane that she is going to ask her several questions to better understand what is going on. Jane is extremely anxious so Karen starts with less sensitive questions first. She uses language that is understood by both her and Jane and clarifies terms such as 'having sex'. At the end Karen reflects on what Jane has told her and why she cannot be pregnant. She offers to call the school nurse to spend some time with Jane so she can better understand how a person becomes pregnant, and to discuss safe sex.

CLINICAL INTEREST BOX 16.4
Teaching clients about transmission of sexually transmitted infections

Objective
- Client will identify how sexually transmitted infections are transmitted

Teaching strategies
- Provide information on the transmission of sexually transmitted infections (STIs)
- Educate about the symptoms and names of STIs
- Encourage the use of condoms if sexually active
- Inform the adolescent about the consequences of sexual activity

Evaluation
- The adolescent is able to identify the common STIs, how they are transmitted and their consequences

CLINICAL INTEREST BOX 16.5
Cultural aspects of care

Aboriginal adolescents have their own set of problems and may feel alienated from both traditional Aboriginal culture and mainstream society. Health issues involve learning or emotional difficulties, accidental injuries, death from suicide, violence, teenage pregnancy and sexually transmitted infections. Alcohol and drug use is high. Poverty and limited access to health care are major factors affecting Aboriginal adolescents. Health promotion topics need to be directed towards issues identified by the adolescents. Literature needs to be culturally sensitive and in the appropriate language. Knowledge regarding health beliefs and healing practices must be assessed. The nurse needs to adopt a culturally appropriate approach to provide effective client education.

attributed to tobacco. Accidental opiate overdose accounted for 600 deaths (ABS 2000).

SEXUAL EXPERIMENTATION

Sexual experimentation during adolescence is often seen as behaviour to confirm sexual orientation. The two main consequences of sexual activity during adolescence are sexually transmitted infections (STIs) and unplanned pregnancy. A thorough sexual history should be included in any screening of adolescent health. The nurse can use the interview process to identify risk factors. Education about the ways STIs are transmitted is recommended, as most adolescents believe they are not at risk. The rate of adolescent pregnancy has fallen in Australia. This is a result of education and the availability of contraception and, in most states and territories, abortion. (See Clinical Interest Boxes 16.3 and 16.4.)

NURSING IMPLICATIONS

The nurse who is caring for an adolescent needs to recognise that this stage of development is generally a difficult one and that rebellion against rules and regulations, criticism of treatment and lack of cooperation by an adolescent may be due to a combination of an instinctive negative reaction

TABLE 16.4 | Health promotion during the adolescent period

Adolescent health concern	Health promotion
Accidents	Provide information on proper use of sports equipment Emphasise proper pedestrian behaviour Promote proper behaviour while a passenger in a vehicle Use of seatbelts Encourage attendance at driver education course, reinforce dangers of drugs when driving Teach basic rules of water safety Promote use of safe sports and recreational facilities Instruct in safe use and respect for firearms
Suicide	Be alert for signs of depression Offer suicide prevention education Teach methods to cope with a suicidal peer Promote alternatives to suicide
Substance abuse	Educate about the risks of tobacco, alcohol and drug use Screen for substance abuse
Sexually transmitted infections	Provide information about mode of transmission and symptoms Encourage use of condoms, abstinence from sexual activity Educate about the consequences of sexual activity
Nutrition	Provide information about nutritional requirements during adolescence Educate about the risks of snacking and irregular mealtimes Promote regular consumption of breakfast and a balanced diet

(modified from Crisp & Taylor 2005)

against authority, and hidden anxieties and fears. Much of the behaviour observed in the adolescent is related to the struggle for independence and the external constraints that are placed on this maturation process. (For cultural aspects of care, see Clinical Interest Box 16.5.)

HEALTH PROMOTION

Health promotion for adolescents consists mainly of teaching and guidance to avoid health-damaging behaviours and risk-taking activities. Health professionals who work with adolescents should acknowledge their increasing independence and responsibility, and try to maintain privacy and confidentiality. Health promotion during adolescence (Table 16.4) is directed towards:

- Establishing healthy habits of daily living in relation to personal care, such as vision, hearing, posture, body-piercing and sun-tanning
- Education in stress-reducing techniques
- Providing information on nutritional requirements and eating habits and behaviours
- Accident prevention in relation to vehicle-related injuries and sport injuries
- Immunisation
- Exercise and activity
- Education about sexuality and guidance on avoiding STIs and unplanned pregnancies
- Substance abuse.

The nurse needs to be aware of the prevalence of adolescent problems affecting healthy habits of daily living and must make assessments accordingly. Community and school-based health programs focus on illness prevention and health promotion. Nurses can play an important role in preventing injuries and deaths related to accidents and substance abuse.

SUMMARY

Adolescent behaviour patterns highlight the need for the nurse to understand the expected process through which an adolescent passes. Adolescents cannot be cared for wholly as adults, as they often lack the emotional maturity to cope with independence and still require the emotional support of parents or adult carers. Nurses with an understanding of adolescent phases will be able to develop an environment that provides privacy and protects independence, which will enable the adolescent to feel supported in unfamiliar surroundings.

REVIEW EXERCISES

1. Identify the three sub-phases that occur in puberty.
2. What does preadolescence refer to?
3. Summarise the weight and skeletal changes that occur during adolescence.
4. Identify the major causes of death in adolescents.
5. List the two main consequences of sexual experimentation in adolescents.
6. Define puberty.

CRITICAL THINKING EXERCISES

1. Kathryn, 14, has come to you concerned that she is not developing at the same rate as her peers. Discuss ways that you could educate Kathryn about the physical changes of puberty and the possible variations.
2. Chris is a 15-year-old boy admitted to hospital with behavioural problems. Discuss ways to identify signs of a possible suicide attempt. How could you improve his stay in hospital?

REFERENCES AND FURTHER READING

Ali N, Siktberg L (2001) Osteoporosis prevention in female adolescents: calcium intake and exercise participation. *Pediatric Nursing*, 27(2): 132–9

Australian Bureau of Statistics (ABS) (2002) *Australian Social Trends* ABS, Canberra. Online. Available: http://www.abs.gov.au [accessed 9 March 2008]

Baker JG, Rosenthal SL, Leonhardt D (1999) Relationship between perceived parental monitoring and young adolescent girls' sexual and substance use behaviours. *Journal of Paediatric Adolescent Gynaecology*, 12: 17–22 (also in Wong & Hockenberry-Eaton 2001)

Bolander VB (1994) *Sorensen and Luckmann's Basic Nursing: a Psychophysiologic Approach*. WB Saunders, Philadelphia

Busen N, Modeland V, Kouzekanani K (2001) Adolescent cigarette smoking and health risk behaviour. *Journal of Pediatric Nursing*, 16(3): 187–93

Carr-Gregg M, Shale E (2002) *Adolescence: A Guide for Parents*. Finch Publishing, Sydney

Crisp J, Taylor C (eds) (2005) *Potter & Perry's Fundamentals of Nursing*, 2nd edn. Elsevier Australia, Sydney

Dolan B, Holt L (2000) *Accident and Emergency Theory into Practice*. Baillière Tindall, Edinburgh

Erikson EH (1963) *Childhood and society*. In: Crisp J, Taylor C (eds) (2005), *Potter and Perry's Fundamentals of Nursing*, 7th edn. Elsevier Australia, Sydney

Field A, Austin SB, Taylor CB, Malspeis S, Rosner B, Rockett H, Gillman W, Colditz G (2003) Relation Between Dieting and Weight Change Among Preadolescents and Adolescents. *Pediatrics* (112)4, October, 900–6

Graber JA, Lewinsohn PM, Seeley JR, Brooks-Gunn J (1997) Is psychopathology associated with the timing of pubertal development? *Journal of the American Academy of Child and Adolescent Psychiatry* 36: 1768–75 (also in Wong and Hockenberry-Eaton 2001)

Green-Hernandez C, Singleton JK, Aronzon DZ (2001) *Primary Care Pediatrics*. Lippincott Williams & Wilkins, Philadelphia

Hockenberry M, Wilson D, Winkelstein ML (eds) (2005) *Wong's Essentials of Paediatric Nursing*, 7th edn. St Louis, Mosby

Hockenberry MJ, Wilson D (2007) *Wong's Nursing Care of Infants and Children*, 8th edn. St Louis, Mosby

Kohlberg L (1964) Development of moral character and moral ideology. In: Hoffman ML, Hoffman LNW (eds), *Review of Child Development Research*, vol 1. Russell Sage Foundation, New York

Mitchell P, Ziegler F (2007) *Fundamentals of Development: the Psychology of Childhood*. Psychology Press, East Sussex

Pilliteri A (2003) *Maternal and Child Health Nursing: Care of the Childbearing and Childrearing Family*, 2nd edn. Lippincott, Philadelphia

Sanson A (2003) *Children's Health and Development. New Research Directions for Australia*. Australian Institute of Family Studies, Melbourne

Santrock J (2007) *Child Development*. McGraw-Hill, Boston
Sigelman CK (2003) *An Introduction to Theories of Personalities*. L Erlbaum Associates, Mahwah, New Jersey
Sugarman L (2001) *Life-Span Development: Frameworks, Accounts, and Strategies*. Psychology Press, Sussex
Wong DL (2000) *Wong and Whaley's Clinical Manual of Pediatric Nursing*, 5th edn. Mosby, St Louis
Wong DL, Hockenberry-Eaton M (eds) (2001) *Wong's Essentials of Paediatric Nursing*. Mosby, St Louis

ONLINE RESOURCES

United States National Library of Medicine: www.nlm.nih.gov (links to Medline)

Chapter 17

GROWTH AND DEVELOPMENT FROM THE YOUNGER ADULT THROUGH TO THE OLDER ADULT

OBJECTIVES

- Define the key terms/concepts
- State the factors that influence growth and development
- Describe the major physical and psychological changes that occur during each stage of development

KEY TERMS/CONCEPTS

emotional development
intellectual development
physical development
social development
theories of ageing

CHAPTER FOCUS

Growth and development of the adult is divided into three stages: young adult, middle adult and older adult. Physical, intellectual, social and emotional development varies at each stage of adult life. Not only natural growth and development but also environment, social and life choices influence health issues that arise in adult life. Theories of ageing are discussed and continue to be developed.

LIVED EXPERIENCE

I didn't start running until I was 40. I wanted to get fitter, so I stopped smoking and started running. Two years later I won the South Australian veteran 5000 metre championship and the veterans' State cross-country championship. I still run 10 km every day. I'm fitter now than I was at 20 and there are lots of others the same. In my club there are men and women — many older than me — still running and still competing.

John Funnell, age 64

Early adulthood is the period of development from 19–20 years to about 45 years of age. From 46–65 years is classed as middle adulthood, while late adulthood is the period from 65 years on. Adult development involves orderly and sequential changes in characteristics and attitudes. This chapter looks at the continuation of the lifespan, looking at the growth and developmental changes that occur throughout adulthood.

EARLY ADULTHOOD

PHYSICAL DEVELOPMENT

With the exception of the major physical changes that accompany a pregnancy, physical changes are minimal during this stage of development. This is often the peak time for athletic performance, childbearing and maximum health.

INTELLECTUAL DEVELOPMENT

Formal and informal educational experiences and life experiences together with occupational opportunities increase the young adult's conceptual and problem-solving skills. Maximum memory and cognitive speed occur at this stage. Decision-making processes need to be flexible, as the young adult is constantly adjusting to changes in the home, the workplace and in personal life.

EMOTIONAL AND PERSONALITY DEVELOPMENT

Emotional development concerns adjustment to independent adult life and centres on the formation of adult relationships. Erik Erikson describes this stage of development as that between 'intimacy and solidarity' and 'isolation' (see Chapter 15). The young adult chooses to adopt one of various lifestyles whereby emotional relationships are established. Some of the choices that may need to be made include whether to marry, to become a parent, to pursue a career or to travel (Sigelman 2003).

SOCIAL DEVELOPMENT

During this stage young adults generally give more attention to occupational and social pursuits and attempt to improve their socioeconomic status. Their network of relationships provides opportunities for fulfilling a variety of social roles and entering a range of different social systems. Young adults can choose to remain within the prescribed expectations of their society or to relate to society in their own way (Sigelman 2003).

MIDDLE ADULTHOOD

PHYSICAL DEVELOPMENT

Major physiological changes occur between the ages of 45 and 65 years. Physical growth is replaced by physical degeneration, bringing about changes including:

- Decreased skin turgor
- Greying and loss of hair
- Decreased muscle mass
- Decreased range of joint motion
- Changes in the menstrual cycle preceding menopause, due to declining production of oestrogen and progesterone
- Decreased level of androgen, leading to male andropause
- Possible diminished acuity of the senses (Ebersole et al 2005).

INTELLECTUAL DEVELOPMENT

Changes in intellectual capacity are relatively uncommon, except in the presence of disease or trauma, and the middle-aged adult is able to continue learning. Some people may experience increased difficulty with concentration and retention of information.

EMOTIONAL AND PERSONALITY DEVELOPMENT

Erik Erikson describes middle adulthood as the stage characterised by 'generativity' versus self-absorption (in Sigelman 2003). Some people achieve a sense of generativity by rearing a family, others by developing careers. This is regarded as the stage when a person is interested in establishing and guiding the next generation, and one in which people strive to ensure continuation of their work and lifestyle. If an adult is unable to assume responsibility for promoting the future they may experience a sense of stagnation, become self-absorbed and be unable to relate effectively to their world (Sigelman 2003).

SOCIAL DEVELOPMENT

In middle adulthood there are likely to be many changes in a person's life, such as children moving away from home, change in career, and assuming responsibility for the care of ageing parents. Loss of a spouse or partner by divorce or death is not uncommon. Retirement will be a reality for most adults towards the end of this stage, so it is necessary to plan for the future well before the event. People generally build up a framework of leisure pursuits, hobbies, relationships and financial security in preparation for retirement (Sigelman 2003).

CARING RESPONSIBILITIES OF YOUNG AND MIDDLE ADULTS

The expanding aged population has increased the need for informal carers. Many young adults are carers to a spouse, family member or close friend. Often the middle-adult female or spouse assumes the role of principal carer. During middle-adult life people experience their parents' decline and death and their own children coming of age, marking the transition in intergenerational relationships. The people who will provide care have thus been defined as 'the sandwich generation' — traditionally those sandwiched between ageing parents who need care and/or help, and their children. This concept was expanded by Carol Abaya to include the 'club sandwich' — those in their 50s or 60s sandwiched between ageing parents, adult children and grandchildren; or those in their 30s and 40s with young children, ageing parents and grandparents (Abaya ND).

The overall effects on carers are physical, emotional and financial. Physically, health may suffer as carers place themselves at the end of the priority list for rest, meals and personal wellbeing. The influence of decreased and/or altered socialisation with family and friends, potential conflict with spouses, and decreased levels of happiness or depression are sometimes experienced by carers. Further, frustration, agitation and feelings of hostility and resentment may plague the caregiver, leading to guilt and disruption to the carer's relationships. The relationship of middle adults with their children appears to be more at risk, with alterations to expected roles. The financial burden related to medical, nursing or allied health needs can be enormous. Maintaining medications, safety, nutrition and hygiene may require assistance and incur costs.

It is recommended that carers take time out for themselves and resource or accept help from others. The role of carer is complex and influences most aspects of their lives and thus has critical implications for the health care system and professionals (Ebersole et al 2005).

GRANDPARENTS

The latter half of the last century has seen changes that influence the family unit. More women now work outside the home, divorce rates have increased, there are single-parent families, blended families, and same-sex parents in families. People move interstate or internationally for career or relationships, making distance between families a challenge.

Traditionally, grandparents were considered 'keepers of the community'. Family traditions and history were maintained by grandparents keeping and telling family stories. They represented the link between the past, present and future. The wisdom and practical knowledge of older adults are less valued today, whereas elders were once considered wise and were respected. In some cultures the value and respect of elders has been maintained, for example in some Asian or Middle-Eastern cultures.

Grandparents today may still fulfil the traditional roles, as they had anticipated; for others it can be very different. Grandparents may find themselves involved with the care of grandchildren and providing support to their adult children. Others have limited involvement owing to distance, which provides the greatest obstacle to relationships between grandparents and grandchildren. Fractured families can leave grandparents without the opportunity to maintain a relationship with the grandchildren. Visitation rights of grandparents are an issue when a marriage breaks down. The relationship of grandparents with the daughter or daughter-in-law determines the closeness. Middle-adult females usually perform keeping of 'kinship', which influences the family relations (Grigorenko & Sternberg 2001).

LATE ADULTHOOD

The last developmental stage begins when a person reaches about 65 years of age. Older adults undergo a number of changes and to understand the reasons for these changes it is necessary to have some knowledge of the various theories of ageing. There are several theories regarding the process of ageing but there are no certain conclusions as to the cause. Pathological changes due to disease should not be confused with normal ageing and it is important to make distinctions between the degenerative changes of ageing and the pathological changes superimposed on the ageing process.

Ageing is a complex process that begins at conception and ends with death. Theories of ageing include:

- Genetic theory: there is little doubt that heredity is a factor in the ageing process, and the genetic theory states that a person's lifespan is programmed within the genes. This means that an individual inherits the family's tendencies for long or short life
- Stress theory: this theory proposes that natural changes occur in the body throughout a person's lifetime and that the ability to replace worn out cells is decreased by the stresses experienced throughout life
- Cell ageing: the chemical structures of the cell and its nucleus have been studied in relation to ageing. One suggestion is that chemical errors could be incorporated in the cells of ageing tissues, which adversely affect overall cell function. There are two main theories about what is thought to take place in cells as they age and eventually die. The first suggests that the cell itself is the main cause of the ageing process, with cells having a predetermined life, while the other theory suggests that ageing affects the organisation of cells, and implies a failure of communication between cells and the environment around them
- Immunological theory: some theorists suggest that there are several cellular mechanisms capable of attacking various body tissues and that these mechanisms act more frequently in ageing
- Psychological theories: various theories state that factors other than heredity, such as lifestyle, personality and the environment, also influence a person's lifespan. These theories attempt to explain the psychosocial changes that occur with advancing age. For example, the 'disengagement theory' suggests that even under optimal personal and social circumstances, decreased physical and psychic energy characterise the latter years of the life cycle. This theory states that decreasing social involvement and activity are inevitable and necessary for successful ageing.

Therefore, while the process of ageing is complex and inevitable, there is no one theory to explain why it occurs (Grigorenko & Sternberg 2001).

PHYSICAL CHANGES

Certain physical changes are associated with ageing that are not pathological processes. They occur in all people but take place at different rates and depend on accompanying circumstances. They include:

- Loss of subcutaneous fat and collagen, leading to inelastic and wrinkled skin
- Atrophy of sweat glands, leading to skin dryness
- Osteoporosis (thinning of bone)
- Shortening of the trunk as a result of intervertebral space narrowing
- Decreased joint mobility and range of joint motion
- Decreased muscle mass and strength
- Decreased rate of voluntary or automatic reflexes
- Decreased ability to respond to multiple stimuli
- Decreased visual acuity and accommodation
- Diminished hearing acuity and pitch discrimination
- Decreased senses of smell and taste
- Increased chest rigidity, increased ventilatory rate with decreased lung expansion
- Loss of blood vessel wall elasticity and change in cardiac function; for example, diminished cardiac output
- Decreased secretion of saliva and digestive enzymes
- Diminished intestinal motility
- Decreased liver function
- Decreased renal efficiency, reduced bladder capacity and control
- Decreased breast tissue and uterine size; atrophy of vaginal epithelium
- Decreased testicular size and decreased sperm count.

While the general picture of ageing suggests a gradual diminution of system function, it should be remembered that many older adults show undiminished vigour and organ function little different from those of earlier years; for example, sexual activity can continue into the 80s and 90s (Ebersole 2001).

BEHAVIOURAL CHANGES

There is a general misconception that all older adults experience decreasing intellectual function and that learning becomes impossible. It is important to understand that structural and physiological changes occurring in the brain during the ageing process do not necessarily affect the individual's intellect. Intellectual performance improves with environmental stimuli and, if an older adult receives sufficient stimuli, cognitive function is generally retained or improved.

Emotional and personality changes may occur, particularly in respect to how older adults view themselves. Many elderly people experience social isolation for many reasons, and older people's self-esteem partially depends on whether they are accepted into social relationships and interactions. An older person may choose to reject personal interactions, preferring their own company to that of others. Some elderly people may be isolated from society because of younger people's attitudes towards, and rejection of, the aged. When society emphasises the negative aspects of ageing and rejects the positive aspects, older individuals experience a loss of self-respect, and a sense of worthlessness. Erik Erikson describes this stage of development as characterised by 'integrity versus despair' (refer to Chapter 15, Table 15.2).

Increased life expectancy has motivated the inclusion of a ninth stage of Erikson's theory for individuals 80 years plus, described as exclusivity versus rejectivity. The premise is one of a sense of either belonging or rejection by family and/or peers. The characteristics of earlier stages are experienced in reverse — mistrust versus trust, inferiority versus industry — leading to isolation and/or rejection of the individual. (For life expectancy statistics, see Clinical Interest Box 17.1.)

Many psychosocial changes occur with ageing. How a person adapts to and copes with these changes depends on many factors, such as personality and social support network. Changes may include:

- Retirement
- Loss of a lifelong partner
- Altered socioeconomic status
- Decreased independence
- Change in health status
- Change in housing and/or environment.

For some these changes can be positive, such as more time to enjoy hobbies, travel, less stress, etc. An elderly person who fears loss of control may see these and other social changes that can occur during the latter years of life as a threat. A person's need to control their environment is not diminished simply because they are becoming older. When control over what is happening to and around them is decreased, for example, after redundancy at work, older people may experience loss of self-esteem and worth. As a result, they may experience severe psychological distress, which can be reflected in physical ill-health (Sigelman 2003).

CLINICAL INTEREST BOX 17.1
Life expectancy

Between 1997 and 1999 in Australia, life expectancy at birth was 76.2 years for men and 81.8 years for women. Internationally, Australia's life expectancy is estimated to rank behind those of Japan, Switzerland, Hong Kong and Sweden by about 1–2 years; is about the same as those of France, Canada, Spain and Greece; and is higher than those of New Zealand, the UK and the USA.

Half of deaths in 1999 occurred after 77.8 years of age. This compares with the equivalent figure of 52.6 years for the Indigenous population of Australia.

SUMMARY

Growth and development are processes that begin at conception and continue throughout each stage of the life cycle. Growth may be defined as the physical changes that occur in a steady and orderly manner, while development relates to the adjustment to the changes in psychological and social functioning. The stages of adult growth and development are early adulthood, middle adulthood and older adulthood. Characteristic changes occur at each stage, but the pace and behaviours of growth and development vary with each individual.

REVIEW EXERCISES

1. Under the headings of early, middle and late adulthood, briefly outline the growth and developmental phases.
2. Using the above exercise as your guide, discuss how this knowledge would be beneficial to you as a nurse.
3. There are two main theories about what is thought to take place in cells as they age. Briefly describe both of these theories.

CRITICAL THINKING EXERCISES

1. Freud is reported as having said that love and work are the keys to success in adult life. Considering the changes to home, family and workplace from yesteryear, discuss the relevance of this statement to contemporary lifestyle.
2. In view of the 'ageing of Australia', what are the implications for future health service providers?

REFERENCES AND FURTHER READING

Abaya C (ND) *The Sandwich Generation*. Online. Available: http://www.thesandwichgeneration.com [accessed 9 March 2008]

Australian Bureau of Statistics (ABS) (2000) Looking into the Future — Australian Population Projections. *Australian Demographic Statistics, March Quarter 2000*. ABS Cat No 3101.0. ABS, Canberra

Cluning T (2001) *Ageing at Home — Practical Approaches to Community Care*. Ausmed Publications, Melbourne

Ebersole P (2001) *Geriatric Nursing and Healthy Aging*, 1st edn. Mosby, St Louis

Ebersole P, Hess P, Touhy T, Jett K (2005) *Gerontological Nursing & Healthy Aging*, 2nd edn. Elsevier Mosby, St Louis

Grigorenko E, Sternberg RJ (2001) *Family Environment and Intellectual Functioning: A Life-Span Perspective*. Lawrence Erlbaum Associates, London

Hudson R, Richmond J (2000) *Living, Dying, Caring. Life and Death in a Nursing Home*. Ausmed Publications, Melbourne

Koch S, Garratt S (2001) *Assessing older people*. MacLennan and Petty, Sydney

Nay R, Garratt S (2004) *Nursing Older People: Issues and Innovations*, 2nd edn. Churchill Livingstone, Sydney

Sigelman CK (2003) *An Introduction to Theories of Personalities*. L Erlbaum Associates, Mahwah, New Jersey

Sugarman L (2001) *Life-Span Development: Frameworks, Accounts, and Strategies*. Psychology Press, Sussex

Tabloski PA (2006) *Gerontological Nursing*. Pearson Education/ Prentice Hall, New Jersey

ONLINE RESOURCES

Useful resource for providing support: www.caregiving.com

Stress management, discussion of caregiver burnout: www.info.gov.hk/elderly/english/healthinfo/elderly/caregiverstress-e.htm

United Nations 18 principles related to aged care, New Zealand Public Policy: www.ageconcern.org.nz/advocacy_on_issues/Policy_Manifesto_1999/I-HealthCare.htm

Caregivers Bill of Rights: www.carlearbours.com/secrets.htm

The 'sandwich generation' definition, Carol Abaya: www.thesandwichgeneration.com

Ageing theories: www.infoaging.org

Health information: www.healthinsite.gov.au

General information and overview of body systems and ageing: www.e-geriatric.net

Nursing care plans: www.mcentral.com/careplans/plans

Unit 6

The nursing process

Chapter 18

CRITICAL THINKING, PROBLEM-BASED LEARNING, AND REFLECTIVE PRACTICE

OBJECTIVES

- Define the key terms/concepts
- Explain the purpose of clear language, intuition and reflection
- Contrast the traditional methods of learning with problem-based learning in nursing
- Discuss the purpose of reflective practice in nurse education
- Discuss how critical social theory can help develop the nursing profession
- Explain different writing styles that may be used for logs and journals for reflecting on practice

KEY TERMS/CONCEPTS

clear language
critical thinking
experiential learning
intuition
log keeping
problem-based learning (PBL)
reflection
reflective practice

CHAPTER FOCUS

Students are presented with a vast amount of theory that needs to be processed and retained if they are to practise safely as nurses. Some of the methods that are used to pass on this knowledge are problem based, or reflective practice models of learning, or even critical thinking as a distinct study. The main purpose of each is to integrate practice and theory to develop nurses' understanding during the learning experience, and develop thinking and learning as lifelong processes.

LIVED EXPERIENCE

So far this year I have been to two different clinical facilities. In the first one we worked as a team, and in the second one I was allocated residents to look after, as I am able to look after them totally and can plan my shift and then document in the care plan and progress notes. I feel like I can give holistic care!

Nicholas, Enrolled Nurse student

This chapter introduces student nurses to different approaches in the development of professional practice. While critical thinking, problem-based learning (PBL), and reflective practice have some components in common, they present different ways of acquiring knowledge and skills necessary for effective client care.

CRITICAL THINKING

Thinking and learning are interrelated lifelong processes. As a person selects a career path, it is important for them to become more aware and skilled in thinking. Over time, the knowledge and practical experiences gained help individuals to broaden their ability to make thoughtful observations and judgments. Critical thinking is the active, organised, cognitive and mental process used to carefully examine one's thinking and the thinking of others. It involves the use of the mind in forming conclusions, making decisions, drawing inferences and reflecting. It means taking nothing for granted. A critical thinker identifies and challenges assumptions, considers what is important in a situation, imagines and explores alternatives, applies reason and logic, and then makes informed decisions. For a new student nurse, critical thinking begins when the student seriously questions and in a continuing way tries to answer again and again: 'What do I really know about this nursing care situation and how do I know it?'

Critical thinking presupposes a certain basic level of intellectual humility (e.g. acknowledging one's own ignorance) and a commitment to think clearly, precisely and accurately and to act on the basis of genuine knowledge. When nurses direct critical thinking towards understanding and assisting clients in finding solutions to their health problems, the process becomes purposeful and goal oriented. Through critical thinking a person addresses problems, considers choices and chooses an appropriate course of action. It is clear that critical thinking requires not only cognitive and mental processing skills but a person's habit to ask questions, to remain well informed, to be honest in facing personal biases, and to be always willing to reconsider and think clearly about issues (Alfaro-LeFevre 1999).

Nurses who are good critical thinkers face problems without forming a quick, single solution and instead focus on the options of what to believe and do. This requires discipline to avoid premature decision making. Learning to think critically helps a nurse to care for clients as their advocate and to make better informed choices about their care. Critical thinking is more than just solving problems — it is an attempt to continually improve. Nurses learn to focus on preventing problems and maximising a client's potential. A critical thinker learns from each clinical experience and pursues each new opportunity with an openness and renewed purpose to excel in practice.

CLEAR LANGUAGE

An important aspect of critical thinking is the use of language. Thinking and language are closely related processes. The ability to use language is closely associated with the ability to think meaningfully. To become a critical thinker, a nurse must be able to use language precisely and clearly. When language is vague or inaccurate it reflects similar thinking. As nurses care for clients it becomes important not only to communicate clearly with clients and families but also to be able to clearly communicate findings to other health professionals. When a nurse uses incorrect terminology, jargon or vague descriptions, communication is ineffective. Critical thinking requires a framing of one's thoughts so that the focus and resultant message are clear. It is helpful to reflect on your language and consider whether what you communicate expresses an idea, position or judgment precisely and clearly (Alfaro-LeFevre 1999).

INTUITION

Expertise in nursing involves the ability to think critically about the knowledge required for a client's care and the knowledge the nurse brings to a nursing care situation. The expert nurse practises intuitively on a deep knowledge base that is applied in daily practice, and each clinical experience is a lesson for the next one. Intuition is the immediate feeling that something is so, without the benefit of conscious reasoning. It is a common experience that all people have after interacting repeatedly with their environment (Hood & Leddy 2005).

A nurse gains intuitive knowledge by learning to describe accurately in precise nursing language the common client responses in nursing care situations. However, it is important to remember that quality nursing practice does not depend solely on intuition. Just as it is critical for nurses to know what knowledge they have, it is even more critical to know what knowledge they do not have. If nurses do not recognise how much they do not know in relation to what they do know, they are endangering the health and wellbeing of their clients. Each clinical situation must be carefully thought through. Even if a nurse believes intuitively that a client is experiencing an expected change, it is important to confirm that finding through appropriate clinical observations and measurements. Thoughtful analysis of what the nurse knows, plus a review of the most current clinical data, allows the nurse to make an accurate and sound clinical decision. Prejudices, biases and failure to acknowledge one's limitations do not result in thoughtful professional practice (Hood & Leddy 2005).

REFLECTION

One important aspect of critical thinking is reflection. This is a process of thinking back or recalling an event to discover the meaning and purpose of that event. For a nurse, reflection involves thinking back on a client situation or experience to explore the information and other factors that influenced the handling of the situation. Reflection requires adequate knowledge and is necessary for self-evaluation, to review one's successes and mistakes. The process of reflection helps nurses seek and understand the relationships between concepts learned in the classroom and real-life clinical incidents. Reflection also helps the nurse judge personal performance and make judgments about standards of practice. It is a process that helps make sense out of an experience and facilitates the incorporation of the experience into the nurse's view of themself as a professional (Rolfe, Freshwater & Jasper 2002).

Engaging in reflection is very individualised. Not everyone reflects in the same way. Some people make mental pictures of the information they contemplate; some prefer quiet thought whereas others may prefer to reflect on new knowledge by discussing it with others.

Learning to be reflective takes practice. A nurse who chooses to reflect on a clinical experience must be open to new information and be able to look at the client's perspective as well as their own. Reflecting on experience reveals behaviour significant to the nurse's professional development. Through reflection the nurse recognises that the actions were either successful or unsuccessful. The next time a similar experience arises, the nurse uses approaches that were successful or revises an approach to ensure a successful outcome (Crisp & Taylor 2005).

PROBLEM-BASED LEARNING

Growing numbers of nursing faculties around the world believe that new models of education are required for nurses to develop the knowledge, skill and abilities to be critical thinkers, independent decision makers, lifelong learners, effective team members and competent users of information technologies. Problem-based learning (PBL) has emerged as the most promising approach to pursue when implementing a major shift in the philosophy, structure and process of nurse education curricula (Rideout 2001). PBL is a teaching–learning model that may take a variety of forms but which essentially places the student at the centre of the learning process and is aimed at integrating learning with practice.

In a normal lecture-based course an academic stands out front and 'teaches' students, that is, gives them information. Lecturers assume that students copy and learn from this information, which they are then able to regurgitate at examinations, as well as carry away to apply to work situations. PBL is different because it is based in the practical-work-type situation, where the onus is put on the students. Students need to identify what they need to know. Usually in small groups (about 10 students), students are given problem situations (usually case studies) and in that group students will discuss, research, process the material to work effectively, solve the problem, produce a report, and may sometimes make a verbal presentation for the benefit of other PBL student groups (Clinical Interest Box 18.1).

The clear purpose of PBL is to integrate practice and theory to produce understanding in action. With PBL, students acquire knowledge in the process of tackling contextualised situations. PBL has no prior commitment to a particular subject or discipline — it is open to taking into account whatever information or knowledge will help with the problem. This is different from other conceptions of knowledge that insist on basic foundations before tackling involved situations. Case studies as used by the students capture some of the reality of actual situations, as they generate more active involvement and enhance student learning (Feldman & Greenberg 2005).

PBL has been established successfully in some Bachelor of Nursing programs and its success may influence curricula of Enrolled Nurses in the future. In the established Bachelor programs students work in tutorial groups throughout their whole 3 or 4 years of study. Students are positioned into

CLINICAL INTEREST BOX 18.1
A problem-based learning scenario

Information for students

In groups of five, read each step carefully. Before moving on, consult with your facilitator at the end of each step.

Step 1: Preoperative assessment

Mrs Brown, 55, is admitted to the surgical ward at 0700 hours for a total abdominal hysterectomy. Her history is as follows:

- Dysmenorrhoea for 10 years
- Menorrhagia for 2 years
- Insulin-dependent diabetes mellitus since age 3
- Current medications: aspirin, medroxyprogesterone acetate (the oral contraceptive pill), Actrapid/Protophane insulin 20/80.

1. Explain each of the above mentioned medical conditions.
2. Formulate a list of questions that you would need to ask Mrs Brown.
3. Make a list of all the preoperative procedures that you may need to undertake and why you are performing them.
4. List eight potential complications (physical and psychological).

Step 2: Postoperative assessment

Mrs Brown has returned from theatre at 1530 hours. She is currently nil by mouth, has a dressing over her lower abdomen, intravenous therapy (IVT) is in progress, and she has an indwelling catheter on free drainage and antiembolitic stockings on.

1. What vital signs will you undertake and why do you perform each of these?
2. What other observations will you perform and what is the significance of your assessments?
3. What nursing care will you provide for Mrs Brown:
   - In the immediate postoperative phase?
   - Over the next 12 hours?

Step 3: Nursing care plan

Prepare a nursing care plan for Mrs Brown during the postoperative phase, including five nursing diagnoses. For each diagnosis provide:

- Three interventions
- Three rationales
- An evaluation for the diagnosis.

Step 4: Report

Prepare your case study to present to the class for further discussion.

situations in which they are the Registered Nurse and have to process that situation, working out what they need to know to function safely and competently. Students need to gather the knowledge and apply it to developing action plans or similar evidence of learning.

Within PBL, when presented with a problem or situation the students need to first ask: What do we know? What do we need to know? Where can we find this information? A student in a PBL program has deliberate placing in a workplace situation, works as a team member and develops organisational, research and communication skills. They become part of a group, develop skills to contribute to the group, deal with conflict in the group, and hence have group responsibilities. PBL facilitators give support and guidance, keeping student groups on track, and prompt, challenge student assumptions, listen, encourage and learn from students. They also help to maintain a safe environment in which students are free to express their ideas while remaining non-judgmental.

PBL focuses on organising the curricular content around problem scenarios rather than subjects and disciplines. Students engage with the complex situation presented to them and decide what information they need to learn and what skill/s they need to manage the situation effectively. While teachers still have a major role in this type of learning, it is not a didactic teaching. Rather, their role revolves around facilitating the PBL group (Feldman & Greenberg 2005).

REFLECTIVE PRACTICE

While reflection is a component of critical thinking and an essential part of PBL, reflective practice is being used as a teaching and learning model in many nurse education programs for the development of critical thinking by students. Many graduate nurses also continue to use reflective practice as a method of critical thinking for their professional development.

KNOWLEDGE

During the course of most traditionally styled nursing education programs, students are presented with three types of knowledge:

- Propositional knowledge, which is presented in lectures and is mainly concerned with theories from related disciplines such as bioscience and psychology
- Interpretive knowledge, which is presented in nursing and science laboratories as well as tutorials and is mainly concerned with the acquisition of psychomotor (hands-on) and communication skills
- Experiential knowledge, which is mainly presented as clinical practicums. Experiential knowledge is not gained only by participating in clinical practice — we learn from experience in all aspects of life. However, the reflective approach can be used as a purposeful method of teaching and learning in this setting to gain more knowledge and skills from the experience.

Box 18.1 | Examples of traditional nurse education knowledge

PROPOSITIONAL KNOWLEDGE
Attend lectures on the cardiothoracic system

INTERPRETIVE KNOWLEDGE
Practise measuring vital signs in the nursing practical laboratory

EXPERIENTIAL KNOWLEDGE
Gain clinical experience by caring for a patient with an illness

Box 18.1 gives examples of these three traditional types of knowledge.

The aims of this method of teaching and learning are to:

- Facilitate students' understanding of current practice in various settings
- Facilitate students' progression beyond that of novice in various domains of nursing practice when possible (Benner 1984)
- Encourage post-registration nurses to become autonomous agents for change by identifying and understanding things that place limitations on nursing.

REFLECTIVE SEMINARS AND CLINICAL CONFERENCES

These are held for most of the clinical practicums, usually during the last hour of each student's clinical shift. During these conferences clinical teachers encourage students to reflect on their recent experiential learning. The implications of the experiences discussed are then considered and put into practice the next time a similar experience is encountered. This process goes beyond what is normally seen as learning from experience, in that it follows a systematic sequence of activities beyond the experience itself.

MODEL OF EXPERIENTIAL LEARNING

Reflection is one of the most crucial stages in the process of gaining experiential knowledge and the teacher can assist the student in this process by using a model devised to promote reflection. The model consists of a series of stages through which the student nurse should progress, having completed an experience.

- Stage 1: Returning to the experience. During the first stage the student is encouraged to simply 'replay' the whole experience over again, describing what happened but not judging it
- Stage 2: Attending to feelings. The aim of this stage is to assist the students to get in touch with their own feelings about the experience. They should try to utilise any positive feelings they may have about it, such as the pleasure they felt at being complimented by the client. Some feelings can actually form barriers to learning, so these need to be removed by such means as laughing

about an embarrassing incident or by expressing feelings to another person. This removal of obstructing feelings is vital if learning is to take place
- Stage 3: Re-evaluating the experience. This final stage consists of a number of substages, which in essence involve the students in associating the experience with their existing ideas and feelings about a given incident or procedure, and testing for consistency between them (Quinn 2000).

Reflection needs to be practised until the student feels comfortable with each stage, and this is best accomplished by sharing the reflections with other students (Rolfe, Freshwater & Jasper 2002). Experiential learning allows each student nurse to consider some aspect of their nursing and reflect on this experience, discussing the experience with a small group to analyse and clarify it, then considering the implications for their future nursing practice. Kolb (1984) is a major promoter of experiential learning and views learning as a central process of human development.

CLINICAL INTEREST BOX 18.2
Journal entry of a Registered Nurse

One lady came in for a CTG for decreased fetal movement. I sat with her for 20 minutes and just talked to her, explaining what the graph meant. When she came into labour I was on again and she was so pleased to see me. It made me feel good to know that she had confidence in me. She had the urge to push early and I encouraged her to breathe the first few contractions. The obstetrician arrived and did a vaginal examination and the head was coming down quickly. He said to me, 'Quick, get the delivery trolley set'. I had already done that, it was good to be prepared. It made me realise I could think one step ahead. That is what I missed at the start of the year. I had no idea how to prepare ahead because I didn't know what came next. I am an organised person at work and I think ahead and plan accordingly, but at first as a student midwife I didn't have the knowledge to do that.

(Karen Lawrence, student midwife, journal entry, 7 July 1995)

LEARNING IN PRACTICE

Jean Lave, anthropologist, and Etienne Wenger, computer scientist, promote the notion of situated learning. That is, learning is fundamentally a social process and not solely in the learner's head (Lave & Wenger 1991). Wenger extended the concept and in 1999 published a further book *Communities of Practice: Learning, Meaning, and Identity*. In this book Wenger suggested that learning is becoming an urgent topic but it is not always easy to think about how to foster learning in innovative ways. Wenger continues by suggesting 'Communities of Practice' are formed by people who engage in a process of collective learning in a shared domain of human endeavour. In a nutshell: Communities of practice are groups of people who share a concern or a passion for something they do and learn how to do it better as they interact regularly. This can be applied to Nursing where as a student nurse you undertake a specified amount of time 'learning' in the clinical environment. Here the learning is exposed to a culture of learning by observing experienced nurses using a combination of different approaches in their professional practice.

LOG KEEPING

To learn experientially is to learn more about ourselves; our skills, values, beliefs and attitudes. A log assists reflection on what we do. The log, sometimes also referred to as a diary or journal, remains private to the individual (except where it has previously been announced to be a component of assessment for students) and is where nurses can note their thoughts, feelings and changing attitudes (see Clinical Interest Box 18.2). The log can aid reflection of the process of change, both as it occurs and after it has occurred. It enables nurses to look back and review their progress in the clinical setting. Also, because they are required to write in it regularly, it encourages the development of the reflective approach as a way of life (Nicklin & Kenworthy 2000).

The distinction between writing styles in keeping a record is that logs are identified as being structured and factual, diaries as being unstructured and personal, and journals as serving the purposes of both. Keeping a written record as a medium for reflection is likely to involve several types of writing.
- Journalistic — events and circumstances are factually recorded
- Analytical — attention is focused on component parts of the topic
- Ethnographic — writing is grounded in the observer's observations and experience
- Creative–therapeutic — free-flowing and spontaneous writing, often done at the height of feelings
- Introspective — the most complex type and which challenges one's own thoughts, sensory experiences, feelings and behaviour (Holly 1984).

Log keeping aids reflection for the purpose of action research for nurses at all levels, whether in education, administration or clinical practice. Nurse lecturers and clinical teachers are encouraged to keep a log themselves to challenge their own thoughts, sensory experiences, feelings and behaviour, both as teachers and in relation to their clinical practice. Action research and praxis (change through action) intentionally seek change through reflection on action. Moreover, by keeping logs themselves, lecturers and clinical teachers are able to identify any difficulties students may have with requirements of their education program.

KNOWING IN ACTION

This form of professional practice is tacit (knowing more than we can say) and spontaneously delivered without deliberation. It works as long as the particular situation falls within the boundaries of what the professional has learned to treat as normal. Knowing in action is executing some activity, recognising, deciding and adjusting without having to 'think about it' (Clinical Interest Box 18.3).

CLINICAL INTEREST BOX 18.3
Knowing in action — action present

a) 'She was frothing at the mouth, she's got no gag reflex and I just hear her gargle, and I thought, "Oh, I don't like the sound of that". She was on her back, so I quickly put her head to the side, and I thought I needed suction. Where is it, then found it and I cleaned her mouth and she was fine.'
b) 'Because I read his chart I acted the way I did. I was aware that he had a previous heart problem so, rather than leaving him there, I thought I had better stay with him and if he is developing further problems I can always ring for the Registered Nurse.'

REFLECTION IN ACTION/ACTION PRESENT

This form of professional practice questions the assumption-based structure of knowing in action. It is making sense of surprise; that is, when something fails to meet expectations. In reflection in action/action present when the professional can still make a difference to the situation at hand, their thinking serves to reshape what they are doing, while they are doing it. Reflection gives rise to on-the-spot experiment, by thinking up and trying out new actions intended to explore the newly observed phenomenon or occurrence. These new actions test tentative understanding of the situation or affirm the moves that have been invented to change things for the better.

The rethinking of some part of knowing in action leads to on-the-spot experiment and further thinking that affects what the professional does. In moment-to-moment appreciation of a process, the professional deploys a wide-ranging repertoire of images of contexts and actions. Reflection in action is a process delivered by the professional who is unable to say what they are doing. Professionals share an 'appreciative system' of the set of values, preferences and norms in terms of which they make sense of the practice situations. They formulate goals and directions for action and determine what constitutes acceptable professional conduct. When professionals respond to the indeterminate zones of practice by holding conversations about it (such as in reflective seminars), they remake part of their practice world, and thereby reveal the usually tacit process that underlies all their practice (Redmond 2004; Clinical Interest Box 18.4).

REFLECTION ON REFLECTION IN ACTION

This is 'thinking back' with reference to the sequence of operations and procedures the practitioner executes. These descriptions by professionals of knowing in action are always constructions. They are always attempting to put into explicit symbolic form a kind of intelligence that begins by being tacit and spontaneous. These descriptions include the clues observed, the rules followed, or the values, strategies and assumptions that make up the professionals' 'theories' of action. However, the procedures, rules and theories that may be included in these descriptions of reflection on reflection in action are static, as opposed to the dynamism of knowing in action or conversation on the indeterminate zones of reflection in action or action present (Clinical Interest Box 18.5).

CLINICAL INTEREST BOX 18.4
Reflection in action/action present

a) 'I thought "I can't let this client die. I've got to act quickly, she may aspirate. I've got to suck her out, I don't want her to die on me." The solution was to remove the nasogastric tube that was causing the secretions building up in her mouth and, because of her lack of gagging, she was just secreting saliva. I removed the nasogastric tube. I felt that I acted to the best of my ability and knowledge at the time and under possible stress. The only other thing I thought about doing was ringing for help, but I had the situation under control. I felt good after it, because I had done something constructive, and this woman didn't aspirate on me, which could have created further problems.'
b) 'I was thinking, "Please don't do it in front of me (arrest). I don't know what to do. I don't feel confident that I could (handle the situation)." I was sort of looking around me when I was taking his pulse, but at the same time I was looking and asking myself, "Where's the oxygen, where's the suction, where to throw the pillows, and is everything around me just in case, um . . . who's in the room?", and all those things were going through my mind. I felt good afterwards, because he didn't really arrest. It was one of the signs, it's a possibility that he might have arrested, but I decided don't panic at every little thing, take things into your own hands. I felt good about my decision to stay there with him.'

CLINICAL INTEREST BOX 18.5
Reflection on reflection in action

a) 'I've just spent the last hour or so of this shift in the "freeze" room, which is like an ICU on this particular neurosurgery ward, and I was caring for a girl of 17 who was involved in a motor car accident. She is unconscious and she's only responding to painful stimuli. She had a nasogastric tube, which she pulled out, and of course it coiled in her mouth, then she started frothing and I thought, "Oh, hang on what's going on here?", so I quickly removed her nasogastric tube and I had to suck her out because I could see her aspirating her saliva.'
b) 'I was caring for a client transferred from ICU, who had previous cardiac problems. He survived cardiac arrest and when I was looking at his charts he just woke up and said he's got a pain in the chest, and I asked him where. He showed me around the heart area and instead of calling for the Registered Nurse I started observing him more, checking his resps, taking his pulse and blood pressure and still staying with him.'

SUMMARY

Whether students are presented with problem-based or reflective practice models of learning, or even critical thinking as a distinct study, the main purpose of each is to integrate practice and theory to produce nurses with understanding in action and who develop thinking and learning as lifelong processes.

REVIEW EXERCISES

1. What is critical thinking?
2. What is intuition?
3. How does reflection help the nurse?
4. How does PBL differ from other teaching modalities?
5. Why is reflective practice being used as a teaching and learning model in many nurse education programs?
6. What are the three stages of reflection using a model of experiential learning?
7. What method of research is appropriate to initiate change in the nursing profession by Registered Nurses?
8. What does 'tacit' mean in relation to knowing in action?

CRITICAL THINKING EXERCISE

Select a recent day in clinical practice and write about any incident that happened while caring for a client, or interacting with a work colleague.

1. Describe as thoroughly as you can what you did.
2. Describe your decision-making process.
3. Describe what you were thinking when dealing with the incident.
4. Describe your strengths and weaknesses while dealing with the incident.
5. Describe what you would do differently when a similar incident occurs.
6. Describe what you gained from the incident.
7. Identify your thoughts, perceptions and feelings about the incident now while reflecting on it.

REFERENCES AND FURTHER READING

Alfaro-LeFevre R (1999) *Critical Thinking in Nursing: a Practical Application*, 2nd edn. WB Saunders, Philadelphia

Benner P (1984) *From Novice to Expert — Excellence and Power in Clinical Practice*. Addison-Wesley, Menlo Park, California

Crisp J, Taylor C (eds) (2005) *Potter & Perry's Fundamentals of Nursing*, 2nd edn. Elsevier Australia, Sydney

Facione N, Facione P (1996) Externalizing the critical thinking in knowledge development and clinical judgment. *Nursing Outlook* 44: 129

Feldman HR, Greenberg MJ (2005) *Educating Nurses for Leadership*. Springer Publishing Company, New York

Holly M (1984) *Keeping a Personal-Professional Journal*. Deakin University Press, Geelong

Hood LJ, Leddy S (2005) *Leddy & Pepper's Conceptual Bases of Professional Nursing*, 6th edn. Lippincott Williams & Wilkins, Philadelphia

Kolb DA (1984) *Experiential Learning*. Prentice Hall, Englewood Cliffs, NJ

Lave J, Wenger E (1991) *Situated Learning: Legitimate Peripheral Participation*. Cambridge University Press, Cambridge

Miller MA, Babock DE (1996) *Critical Thinking Applied to Nursing*. Mosby, St Louis

Nicklin PJ, Kenworthy N (2000) *Teaching and Assessing in Nursing Practice: An Experiential Approach*. Elsevier Australia, Sydney

Paul RW, Heaslip P (1995) Critical thinking and intuitive nursing practice. *Journal of Advanced Nursing*, 22: 40

Quinn FM (2000) *The Principles and Practice of Nurse Education*, 4th edn. Nelson Thorne, Philadelphia

Redmond B (2004) *Reflection in Action: Developing Reflective Practice in Health and Social*. Ashgate Publishing Ltd, Aldershot

Rideout E (2001) *Transforming Nursing Education Through Problem-Based Learning*. Jones and Bartlett Publishers, Boston

Rolfe G, Freshwater D, Jasper M (2002) *Critical Reflection for Nursing and the Helping Professions: A User's Guide*. Palgrave Macmillan, Basingstoke

Wenger E (1999) *Communities of Practice: Learning, Meaning, and Identity*. Cambridge University Press, Cambridge

ONLINE RESOURCES

Problem-based learning resources:

www.pbl.cqu.edu.au/content/online_resources.htm

www.pbl.vu.edu.au/InformationOnPBL.html

Chapter 19

COMPONENTS OF THE NURSING PROCESS

OBJECTIVES

- Define the key terms/concepts
- Discuss the steps used in nursing diagnosis and the use of the NANDA approved nursing diagnosis
- Examine the difference between a medical and nursing diagnosis
- Discuss the planning phase and development of nursing care plans
- Provide an overview of the nursing process
- Provide an explanation of the assessment phase, including conducting assessments requiring cultural awareness

KEY TERMS/CONCEPTS

assessment
diagnosis
evaluation
implementation
interventions
NANDA (North American Nursing Diagnosis Association)
nursing care plans
nursing process
objective data
planning
subjective data

CHAPTER FOCUS

The nursing process is a systematic problem-solving method by which nurses can plan and provide care for clients. This process enables the nurse to identify clients' actual or potential problems. The nursing process consists of five dynamic and interrelated phases: assessment, diagnosis, planning, implementation and evaluation. This chapter examines the five components of the nursing process and provides nurses with a framework for care planning, which is systematic and methodical.

LIVED EXPERIENCE

I watched my buddy nurse admit a new client today. Mrs Brown is 77 years old and is going to have surgery tomorrow. I observed how the nurse gave Mrs Brown time to settle into the ward and introduce her to the other clients in the room. We all sat down together and started to obtain Mrs Brown's nursing history. I began to see what the lecturers really meant by the nursing process — this was just the beginning.

Gabrielle, Enrolled Nurse student

Essentially the nursing process is a series of planned steps that produce a particular end result. Specifically, the nursing process is a modified scientific method of systematic problem solving. In simple terms the nursing process is a method used to assess the clients' needs and plan, deliver and evaluate nursing care. The process of nursing, or scientific method of problem solving, remains the same whether the nursing care provided is a simple measure or a sequence of complicated nursing activities.

AN OVERVIEW OF THE NURSING PROCESS

Providing the framework for nursing care, the nursing process consists of five components, each of which follows logically one after the other:

- Assessment
- Nursing diagnosis
- Planning
- Implementation
- Evaluation.

It is important for the nurse to recognise that the process is ongoing and cyclical in that each step relies on the step preceding and the step following. Figure 19.1 shows diagrammatic representation of the nursing process.

To meet clients' changing needs it is essential to revise and update any plan of care continually. Using the nursing process, each individual's specific needs are addressed, any problems are identified, and a care plan is developed and implemented to meet those needs. The effectiveness of any care given is continuously evaluated in terms of meeting clients' needs (Alfaro-LeFevre 2005).

ASSESSMENT

Nursing assessment is the process of obtaining and communicating information (data) about a client, through a variety of methods. The purpose of obtaining information is to identify areas in which nursing intervention is required. Data may be obtained from the client, from others of significance to them, from health team members, and from the client's past or present medical and nursing records. The data obtained may be either subjective or objective.

Subjective data are the client's, or other significant person's, perceptions, ideas and sensations about a health problem. For example, a client may supply information about their sensations of a painful and itching skin, and state that they feel hot. *Objective data* are the pieces of information observed or measured by the nurse. For example, the nurse may observe the presence of a rash on the client's body, and may then measure their temperature and observe that it is elevated. Methods of obtaining both subjective and objective data include the nursing history, physical examination and observation, and laboratory and diagnostic tests (Alfaro-LeFevre 2005).

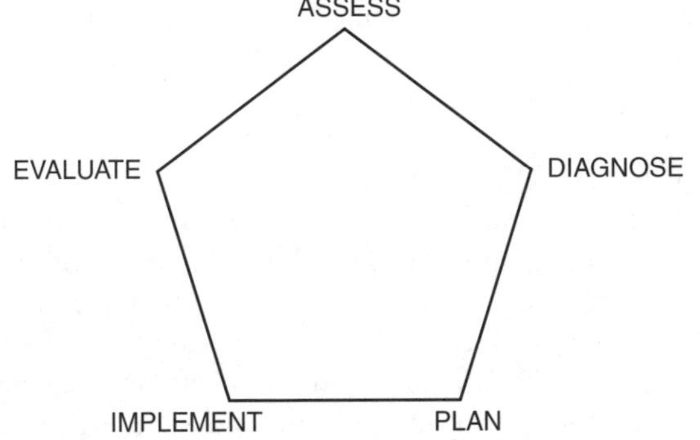

Figure 19.1 | Components of the nursing process

The nursing history

A nursing history is obtained by talking with the client and/or significant other person and is achieved by means of a structured interview. As it is essential that the information is recorded, the nurse uses a form that has been developed by the health care facility. Through the use of interviewing skills, the nursing history elicits information from the client about their current and past health problems, their lifestyle, activities of living and their psychosocial history. A nursing history centres on the client's description of their physical, psychological and emotional reactions to their illness and on the resultant changes to their lifestyle. A nursing history:

- Is the first stage of problem solving and planning for immediate and long-term client care
- Establishes an information base on which nursing diagnoses and plans for care can be built
- Helps nurses to initiate a positive relationship with the client and enables the nurse to observe the client's verbal and non-verbal communication
- Provides clients with an opportunity to discuss their feelings about themselves and their health problems
- Helps to reveal any past, present and potential problems that may require nursing intervention
- Helps clients to remember certain aspects of their illness that may have been forgotten or omitted
- Provides a written framework in which to record information about the client's physical, functional, psychological and emotional state
- Creates a reference point from which the nurse can monitor a client's progress throughout the illness (Crisp & Taylor 2005).

A nursing history should be obtained as soon as possible after the client's admission to the health care agency and should be conducted, when feasible, by the nurse with primary responsibility for planning the client's care. Before beginning the interview the nurse must explain its purpose so the client understands why certain questions will be asked. The interview setting should be quiet and private for the client to feel comfortable about discussing personal details. If a client is too ill or is unable to communicate effectively (perhaps because of language barriers), a nursing history may be obtained by talking with a family member. It is important to record on the nursing assessment form from whom the information is obtained. The nurse may need to reassure the client that the conversation will be confidential (Crisp & Taylor 2005).

It is essential that any information obtained during the interview is documented accurately and concisely, as the nursing assessment form is retained for future reference together with other documentation. The basic information, which should be obtained in a nursing history includes:

- Medical diagnosis
- Previous illnesses and admissions to hospital
- Any medications or known allergies
- The client's perception of their current state of health
- Social data; for example, type of accommodation and home conditions, interests and recreational activities, next of kin and/or significant others in their life, significant life crises, employment status, religious beliefs and practices, the name by which the client prefers to be called
- Performance of the activities of daily living; for example, degree of independence or any difficulty in maintaining a safe environment, communicating, breathing, eating and drinking, eliminating, personal hygiene and dressing, controlling body temperature, mobilising, working and playing, expressing sexuality, sleeping, concerns about dying and grieving
- Use of any prosthesis; for example, walking stick or artificial limb, and any impairments; for example, visual, auditory, or speech
- Habits; for example, use of alcohol, nicotine or non-prescription drugs (Alfaro-LeFevre 2005).

Physical examination and observation

The physical examination is conducted by a medical officer and findings are recorded in the client's notes. The medical officer uses the techniques of inspection, palpation, percussion and auscultation to detect any abnormalities that may provide information about the client's health problem. The nurse is able to refer to the medical officer's documentation for information about the client that is relevant to the planning and implementation of nursing care.

Observation of the client is performed by the nurse during the interview and requires the incorporation of a head-to-toe assessment, which relies on utilising all the senses and good communication skills. Open-ended questions will allow the client to elaborate, to tell their story and to express themself; for example: 'How would you describe the pain in your arm?' This type of question also helps the nurse to gather more information. Closed questions elicit a yes or no or more limited response and limit the development of rapport; for example: 'Do you ever get short of breath?'

The head-to-toe assessment involves assessing factors such as skin colour, general appearance, degree of mobility and independence, emotional status and the presence of obvious abnormalities, such as a rash. Information about the client's general physical status is obtained by measuring body temperature, pulse, ventilations and blood pressure. The client's weight (mass) and height are also measured and recorded. This information provides baseline data on which to assess the client's present health status and may be useful for identifying actual or potential nursing problems (Jarvis 2008).

Cultural considerations in health assessment

Values provide the foundation for beliefs, attitudes and behaviours.

Beliefs include opinions, knowledge and faith about various aspects of the world. How the individual defines illness is based on his or her belief system, for example, Chinese health beliefs in terms of yin (e.g. cold) and yang (e.g. hot). Chinese medicine treatments usually involve restoring balance by applying opposing forces, for example, application of the appropriate 'hot' remedy to treat a 'cold' illness, and vice versa.

Customs are learned behaviours that the nurse can easily assess through observation and direct questioning. Customs include dietary practices, communication patterns, religious practices and health behaviours.

Heredity is any information concerning ethnic, cultural or racial heritage and is also important for assessing the person's susceptibility to specific genetic disorders (Jarvis 2008).

Socioeconomic status is important in assessing health. Public health records show that people in lower socio-economic groups have the highest rates of death and disease resulting from virtually every health problem. For more information on cultural diversity, see Chapter 9.

Laboratory and diagnostic tests

Laboratory and diagnostic tests, which are the most objective form of assessment data, provide another source of information about the client. Both subjective and objective data are required for comprehensive assessment of the client, as they provide more information than either could provide alone. For example, during the nursing interview a client may reveal that she feels tired constantly (subjective data). The nurse observes that she looks extremely pale and the laboratory test results indicate that her haemoglobin level is below normal (objective data). Thus, the laboratory test data provide verification of the alterations from normal (tiredness and pallor) identified during the interview. (See Clinical Interest Box 19.1 for a case study of the assessment phase.)

NURSING DIAGNOSIS

The second step in the nursing process involves analysing and interpreting the information obtained to identify actual or potential problems of the client that the nurse can help to resolve or prevent through nursing intervention. The term nursing diagnosis is frequently used to describe a statement of an actual or potential problem that a client is experiencing with the activities of daily living. Most health agencies have a listing of accepted nursing diagnoses but in Australia a

CLINICAL INTEREST BOX 19.1
Case study — the assessment phase

At the start of the assessment phase for Mrs Brown, 77, admitted to hospital at 1800 hours on 20 June 2009 for surgery the following day, the nurse came to obtain a nursing history. The nurse introduced herself and explained that the purpose of the nursing history was to obtain the information necessary to develop a care plan for her.

The nurse drew the screens around the bed, sat down and began to talk with Mrs Brown. She asked the client by what name she preferred to be known and was informed that 'Mrs Brown' would be fine, as she was not enamoured with her given name of Annie. During the 20-minute discussion with Mrs Brown, the nurse obtained and recorded the following information:

- Mrs Brown's husband had died of cancer 2 years previously. She had one daughter and one son, who both lived some distance away. Her daughter came to stay with her once or twice a month, while her son visited 2–3 times a year. Neither of her children had married
- Mrs Brown lived alone in the house she had shared with her husband since their marriage. The house had all the facilities she required, but was located on a large block so that Mrs Brown was experiencing some difficulty in maintaining the garden without her husband's assistance. Mrs Brown had one cat, which she enjoyed looking after and said, 'She is good company'
- Mrs Brown had been an active member of several organisations but had given up some of her social activities over the past 18 months when her eyesight began to fail. She still enjoyed reading, watching television and working in the garden
- The client had had both her children in the same hospital and was admitted for 1 day, 5 years ago, to have an operation on her wrist. She has also spent 3 days in hospital for treatment of a fractured ankle
- Mrs Brown's past health problems included a deep vein thrombosis, a fractured wrist and a urinary tract infection
- Her current admission was so that she could have a surgery to remove a tumour from her right eye. Mrs Brown told the nurse that her vision had been deteriorating over the past 2 years and that she had difficulty in seeing many things unless they were very close. She quite frequently bumped into, or tripped over, objects in her path. She understood that she would be in hospital for about 3–4 days and would be required to instil eye drops and wear an eye pad for several days after that. She expressed some anxiety over her eyesight, as her mother had become totally blind at about the same age. Mrs Brown was also concerned as to how she would manage at home after the operation during the time her right eye was covered
- Mrs Brown had no difficulty in carrying out most of the activities of living except that she was frightened of slipping during her evening bath or shower. She enjoyed porridge for breakfast, ate a lot of fruit during the day and had experienced no problems with elimination. She usually went to bed at about 2200 hours and slept well without the use of any medication
- Mrs Brown appeared to be generally healthy, she wore glasses for reading and watching television, and she appeared to be slightly hard of hearing.

Recordings of Mrs Brown's vital signs showed that her temperature was 37°C, pulse 76/min and regular, ventilations 18/min, blood pressure 130/70 mmHg. She weighed 64 kg and her urine sample showed no evidence of any abnormalities.

After the interview with Mrs Brown the nurse looked at her medical history to see if there was any further information relevant to the delivery of nursing care. She observed that the medical officer who had examined Mrs Brown had not detected any additional pathological abnormalities. The results of her chest X-ray, electrocardiogram and full blood examination were within acceptable ranges.

complete classification of approved nursing diagnoses has not yet been compiled (Carpenito-Moyet 2005). Many health agencies use the diagnostic categories accepted by the North American Nursing Diagnosis Association (NANDA). Appendix 6 (online) contains a comprehensive list of NANDA diagnoses.

A nursing diagnosis is made after all a client's information has been obtained and compared with normal functioning for that client. The nurse then makes assessments or inferences about the significance of the information and identifies the client's problems. When formulating a nursing diagnosis the nurse should ask herself, 'Is there a problem that nursing intervention can help to resolve?'. Stating the problem (making a nursing diagnosis) can be a difficult task, as nurses sometimes become confused about problems versus needs. A problem is a difficulty the client is experiencing (actual) or may experience (potential). Another difficulty in stating a nursing diagnosis is that a nurse may state the problem as a medical diagnosis. The goal of a medical diagnosis is to identify the disease, whereas the goal of a nursing diagnosis is to identify the actual or potential health problems of the client. To illustrate the difference between a medical and nursing diagnosis, consider, for example, an elderly male admitted to hospital for investigation and treatment of his illness. He has presented with joint pain, swelling, stiffness and grating of some joints during motion and he has limited movement. The medical officer made a medical diagnosis of osteoarthritis, as opposed to a nursing diagnosis, which would state 'restricted mobility related to painful joints'.

A nursing diagnosis consists of two parts: the first part states the problem (restricted mobility), while the second part states the possible cause of the problem (painful joints). If the problem is a potential one, the words 'potential for' or 'at risk of' are written before the problem; for example, 'potential for restricted mobility related to painful joints'. Formulation of nursing diagnoses requires experience in nursing, and practice. Once the client's problems are identified, each nursing diagnosis is placed in order of importance on the nursing care plan.

PLANNING

After the client's problems have been identified and the nursing diagnoses formulated, the nurse plans the care to be implemented. Planning involves setting goals, establishing priorities and determining nursing interventions to achieve the goals (Carpenito-Moyet 2005).

Setting goals

Goals establish the framework for a nursing care plan. Goals, or objectives, are the outcomes or results expected as a consequence of nursing care activities. Therefore, for each nursing diagnosis (problem) the nurse, in conjunction with the client, sets the goals to be achieved. A goal may be short term; that is, one that is expected to be achieved in a relatively short time such as hours or days. A long-term goal is one that is to be achieved in the future, for example, within several weeks or months.

Goals are expressed specifically and in behavioural terms. By expressing a goal specifically, everyone involved in the client's care knows the expected outcome. Goals are written using verbs to express the expected behaviour and as such are observable and measurable. The expected outcomes describe the behaviour the client is expected to attain. For example, 'The client will walk the length of the ward without assistance'. It is more helpful to all concerned if a timeframe is included in the goal, for example, 'The client will walk the length of the ward without assistance by October 2'. Any goals that are set must be realistic and attainable in terms of the client's limits and the ability of the nurse to assist them.

Priorities

Priorities are established after the nursing diagnoses have been formulated and specific goals have been set, by grading them in order of importance. High priority goals are those that require immediate attention, while low priority goals are those that do not need to be attained as quickly. Basic physiological needs, such as the need for oxygen, nutrition or water, are given priority over the other needs.

Determining nursing interventions

Nursing interventions involve selecting the activities that are expected to help the client achieve the set goals (expected outcomes). To select the most appropriate nursing activities (interventions) all possible alternatives are discussed, generally in consultation with the client. Selecting appropriate nursing interventions must be based on sound nursing knowledge, using a scientific problem-solving approach, with the client's participation when possible. After a decision has been made on the measures to be implemented, statements defining the selected actions are written in the nursing care plan. For example, one selected nursing activity may be expressed as 'perform active leg and feet exercises every 2 hours while in bed'.

All proposed nursing interventions must be written specifically and in adequate detail to enable all nursing personnel to carry them out correctly. Interventions may consist of activities that the nurse will perform, or actions to be taken by the client with or without assistance from the nurse.

Nursing care plans

The nursing care plan is a document developed by the health care agency. The structure of the care plan may vary between health agencies. Some agencies may have computerised care plans. Nurses need to familiarise themselves with the nursing care plan and all other documentation used within the health care agency where they are working. While not formally a legal document, nursing care plans can be requested and have been used in legal situations. Nurses need to adhere to the legal and ethical guidelines for documenting (Chapter 20). Nursing care plans may vary in structure from one place to another but the basic principles will remain the same. The nurse should be able to clearly identify:

- The nursing diagnoses
- The goals or expected outcomes
- The specific nursing interventions for each goal
- Whether the goals are being achieved (evaluation).

Traditionally, nursing care plans are written using the headings of the nursing process and are set out in a table using columns. For teaching purposes an additional column is often used that requires new nurses and students to include their rationale for the interventions that they have chosen. This encourages new nurses to think about the reasons and the scientific rationale for implementing their interventions. Often, supporting evidence or reference to literature is required from students during the learning phase. The rationale column would not normally be included on care plans found in wards, nursing homes or other health care agencies. Figure 19.2 shows a template for a student care plan used to allow students and new nurses to practise the steps required for the delivery of nursing care.

While the structure of a nursing plan may vary between health care settings, the principles of care planning remain the same. A correctly formulated nursing care plan facilitates the coordination and continuity of care. In Clinical Interest Box 19.2, after the nurse had identified Mrs Brown's problems she was then able to plan the care to be implemented. For each nursing diagnosis the nurse set objectives (expected outcomes) and decided on the nursing actions that would help Mrs Brown to achieve those objectives, and developed a nursing care plan. Table 19.1 is an example of a fully documented (commonly used) care plan, using the case study of Mrs Brown.

IMPLEMENTATION

Implementation means putting the nursing plan into action (nursing interventions) and is the actual performance of the activities that have been selected to help the client achieve the set goals. The client's needs are reassessed

Assessment	Diagnosis	Goal	Interventions	Rationale	Evaluation
Include all data relevant to the diagnosis contained in column 2	Prioritised nursing diagnoses, in order of importance or highest need	Desired goals and outcomes Date started	Nursing actions — the 'who, what, when and how'	The scientific reason each intervention was chosen, i.e., the 'why'	Was the goal achieved? Is there a need to continue interventions, cease interventions or re-evaluate the care? Date intervention ceased

Figure 19.2 | Template for a student care plan

CLINICAL INTEREST BOX 19.2
Case study — the nursing diagnosis phase

Based on the data obtained during the assessment phase, the nurse determined that Mrs Brown's actual and potential problems were:

- Impaired vision, which caused her to be more vulnerable to accidents; for example, falls and burns
- Anxiety about her vision and how she would manage after the operation
- Some difficulty in maintaining her home garden
- Some hearing impairment
- Potential for pain and discomfort after the operation
- Potential inability to perform the activities of living independently after the operation while her right eye was covered.

She was then able to formulate the following nursing diagnoses:

- Anxiety related to impaired eyesight
- Impaired ability to communicate because of impaired vision and hearing
- Potential for accidents because of impaired vision
- Potential for pain and discomfort related to the operation
- Potential for altered independence while right eye was covered.

continuously during the implementation stage so that any new needs can be identified and so that the nursing care plan can be modified or adapted. During this stage of the nursing process the planned nursing interventions are implemented to achieve the goals, the plan is reviewed and other appropriate measures are implemented. It is important that all nursing care that is being provided for the client appears on the care plan. Therefore, nursing interventions need to be clear, concise and at the same time comprehensive (Carpenito-Moyet 2005).

As problems are solved, the nursing diagnoses are revised and deleted from the care plan if they are no longer relevant. As new nursing diagnoses are made they are added to the plan, together with specific goals and selected nursing

TABLE 19.1 | NURSING CARE PLAN FOR MRS BROWN (SEE CLINICAL INTEREST BOXES 19.1 AND 19.2)

Nursing diagnoses	Goals/expected outcomes	Nursing interventions	Rationales	Evaluation	Date ceased
Anxiety related to impaired eyesight manifested by verbalisation of concerns	To understand the implications of surgery on her vision	1. Spend time with Mrs Brown	1. Allows Mrs Brown to express her fears and concerns	1. Is able to communicate her anxieties verbally	21.6.09
		2. Explain all pre- and postoperative procedures, their purpose and possible implications	2. Explaining all expected procedures will allay anxiety by removing the 'fear of the unknown'	2. States that she understands the nursing actions	21.6.09
		3. Arrange for the surgeon to explain to Mrs Brown how her eyesight should be improved after the operation. Explain that new glasses will be prescribed after the surgery to aid her vision	3. All medical interventions are explained by a medical officer. This ensures that the client fully understands the expected positive effects as well as the potential negative effects	3. States that she has understood the surgeon's explanation and feels reassured. Understands that the new glasses will be provided soon after her discharge	21.6.09

(Continued)

actions to achieve those goals. During implementation of the nursing interventions the nurse continuously reassessed Mrs Brown to evaluate the effectiveness of the nursing care plan and to detect any new problems.

EVALUATION

After the planned nursing interventions have been implemented, the nurse must then evaluate the results to determine whether the interventions were effective. Evaluation is the process of determining the extent to which the set goals or objectives have been achieved, and enables the nurse to monitor the effectiveness of the nursing care plan. Whether the plan was a success or not is determined by comparing the client's response to the nursing interventions, with the set goals and set timeframe. Evaluation also enables the nurse to identify any new health care problems experienced by the client (Carpenito-Moyet 2005).

Evaluation is made by examining the results of the interventions, assessing the client for possible side effects and adverse reactions to the nursing interventions, and by analysing the results. Analysis involves determining whether the client is better or worse or shows no change: in other words, have the set goals been achieved? Based on the data obtained from the evaluation, a nursing judgment

TABLE 19.1 | NURSING CARE PLAN FOR MRS BROWN (SEE CLINICAL INTEREST BOXES 19.1 AND 19.2) — cont'd

Nursing diagnoses	Goals/expected outcomes	Nursing interventions	Rationales	Evaluation	Date ceased
Impaired ability to communicate due to impaired vision, manifested by client not being able to recognise non-verbal forms of communication	To communicate effectively	1. Prompt Mrs Brown to wear her current glasses 2. Face Mrs Brown when speaking and speak clearly 3. Attract her attention before starting to speak 4. Use gestures to enhance the spoken word 5. Ensure adequate lighting and reduced glare	1. When Mrs Brown wears her prescription glasses she is able to clearly visualise who is speaking to her 2. By facing Mrs Brown she will be aware that the nurse is talking to her 3. Gently touching Mrs Brown on the shoulder alerts her to your presence 4. Using non-verbal communication emphasises the verbal dialogue 5. Adequate lighting will enhance visual perception	Occasionally needs reminding Is able to participate in communication effectively	21.6.09
Potential for accidents due to impaired vision, manifested by client bumping into furniture	To provide a safe environment	1. One nurse to assist when ambulating 2. Remove obstacles from path 3. Place call bell within easy reach, place personal items within easy reach, in front of client 4. Adjust the bed to the low position 5. Assist with personal hygiene, grooming and meals where required	1. Walking alongside Mrs Brown will improve her confidence and ensure that she does not walk into any obstacles 2. Keeping the area free from excess clutter will minimise the obstacles that Mrs Brown can come into contact with 3. Keeping items within reach of Mrs Brown will ensure that she does not have to ambulate without supervision 4. This ensures that Mrs Brown will not trip or fall as she gets into or out of bed 5. This enables Mrs Brown to receive optimal care in all areas mentioned	No accidents resulted during client's stay	21.6.09

TABLE 19.1 | NURSING CARE PLAN FOR MRS BROWN (SEE CLINICAL INTEREST BOXES 19.1 AND 19.2) — cont'd

Nursing diagnoses	Goals/expected outcomes	Nursing interventions	Rationales	Evaluation	Date ceased
Potential for pain and discomfort related to the operation, manifested by eye pads	Mrs Brown will be pain free at all times	1. Assist Mrs Brown into a comfortable position 2. Assess client continually for pain, using a pain scale of 0–10, where 0 represents no pain and 10 represents maximum pain 3. Apply eye pad and shield correctly	1. Changing position can relieve discomfort and reassure client that you are there to help 2. Monitoring client can assess if pain is increasing or remaining at a constant low level. Allows methods of pain management to be used more affectively before pain becomes severe 3. When eye pad and shield are correctly positioned, the level of discomfort and irritation is decreased	1. Mrs Brown states that pain level is kept at a low scale of less than 5 2. States it is more of an uncomfortable sensation rather than a painful one	21.6.09
Potential for altered independence while right eye is covered, manifested by Mrs Brown asking staff to perform simple tasks for her	To achieve independence within client's limitations before discharge from hospital	1. Allow Mrs Brown adequate time to perform activities of daily living within her capabilities 2. Assist when Mrs Brown requests help or is unable to perform independently 3. Prepare a discharge plan 4. Contact home nursing service to organise nursing support to instil prescribed eye drops 5. Contact community agencies to arrange Home Help and Meals on Wheels on Mrs Brown's return to home	1. Promotes independence while ensuring Mrs Brown is aware that you are there to assist her if necessary 2. Avoids frustration and ensures that an accident does not occur when Mrs Brown attempts tasks beyond her current capabilities 3. A discharge plan will ensure that Mrs Brown's carers are aware of her current abilities 4. A professional health care worker will instil prescribed eye drops accurately and be able to assess for signs of improvement or infection 5. Extra home services will ensure that Mrs Brown does not have to perform tasks that she is unable to perform without supervision	1. Mrs Brown performs most activities of daily living with minimal supervision on day of discharge 2. No accidents occurred at time of report 3. Discharge plan formulated and given to Mrs Brown, who states that she understands what to expect when she is discharged 4. Community services contacted and will start from 22.6.09	21.6.09 21.6.09

is made. Evaluation therefore allows the nurse to revise and, if necessary, modify or change the plan at any stage. If the set goals have been achieved the plan is deemed to be successful and the nursing interventions can usually be terminated. If the goals have not been achieved the client's needs must be reassessed, new nursing diagnoses formulated if necessary, and the plan changed and re-implemented. (See Clinical Interest Box 19.3 for a case study of the evaluation phase.)

Evaluation is performed continuously throughout the nursing process, as it is the most important method of determining the effectiveness of a nursing care plan. Effectiveness of a nursing care plan can also be determined by another method of evaluation — a nursing audit. A nursing audit is a thorough investigation made to evaluate the overall nursing care received by a client. An audit is generally performed by an experienced nurse who does not actually work in the area where the audit is being carried out, or an external committee. Each health care agency develops its own nursing audit form, which is a checklist

CLINICAL INTEREST BOX 19.3
Case study — EVALUATION

Mrs Brown recovered well after the operation to her right eye and was required to wear an eye pad during the day. At night the soft eye pad was covered by a rigid shield to provide added protection. During the day, prescribed eye drops were instilled every 6 hours.

Mrs Brown experienced some pain in the immediate postoperative period but this was relieved when analgesic medications were administered.

She required some assistance with bathing, dressing, mobilising, and managing meals for the first 2 days. By the 3rd day she was able to perform the activities of daily living independently, with minimal supervision.

She was unable to instil the eye drops or apply the eye pad correctly, so the visiting nurse service was contacted and twice-daily home visits were arranged. As she did not feel confident in her ability to shop for or prepare food or attend to all the housework for a few days, Home Help and Meals on Wheels were arranged for her.

On the 3rd day after the operation, Mrs Brown was discharged. A discharge plan was completed and the only remaining problem was 'potential altered independence while right eye is covered'. She was pleased to be going home and expressed the belief that she would be able to manage with the assistance of the support services that had been arranged. The nurse ensured that Mrs Brown knew what times the visiting nurse would be coming to instil the drops and apply an eye pad. She was advised to wear the rigid shield over the eye pad when she retired for the night.

An appointment was made to see the surgeon the following week. Throughout the process of implementation and evaluation, the nurse constantly assessed Mrs Brown. As a problem was solved, the nursing interventions were discontinued (Table 19.1). For example, Mrs Brown was not experiencing any pain or discomfort by the second postoperative day, so analgesic medications were no longer required.

that includes specific criteria for each category of care. A nursing audit may be made during the client's hospitalisation or after discharge from hospital. Appropriately qualified professional auditors may also conduct audits on health care agencies. The purpose of an audit is to improve the quality of client care (Crisp & Taylor 2005).

SUMMARY

The nursing process forms the basis for all nursing practice. It is an ongoing process that relies on the five steps of assessment, nursing diagnosis, planning, implementation and evaluation. These steps should not be viewed in isolation — they are not mutually exclusive and are equally important to ensure quality client care. The nursing process provides nurses with a scientific method of problem solving and a methodical framework for the delivery of nursing care.

REVIEW EXERCISES

1. State five reasons why a nursing history is performed when a new client is admitted to a health care facility.
2. Information gathered from a nursing history should be accurate and precise. Give five pieces of basic information that should always be included.
3. Discuss the difference between a medical diagnosis and a nursing diagnosis.

CRITICAL THINKING EXERCISES

Mrs Allen is a 67-year-old widow who has eight children, who are all married. She has seven grandchildren, who she looks after several times a week. Her interests are gardening, reading and playing cards with her friends. She attends the local Catholic Church and is involved in community work. She smokes about 10 cigarettes a day and enjoys a social drink. She has a history of hypertension. She is being admitted on 10/10/09 for a hysterectomy.

Using the nursing process:

1. What questions would be important to ask if you were to conduct an assessment and interview your client?
2. What nursing diagnoses would you consider for this client?
3. What nursing interventions would be appropriate?
4. Develop a nursing care plan for this client (practise using the rationale column).
5. How will you evaluate the care you have prescribed?

REFERENCES AND FURTHER READING

Alfaro-LeFevre R (2005) *Applying Nursing Process: A Tool for Critical Thinking*, 6th edn. Lippincott, Philadelphia

Barkauskas V, Stoltenberg-Allen K, Baumann L, Darling-Fisher C (1994) *Health & Physical Assessment*. Mosby, St Louis

Carpenito-Moyet LJ (2005) *Nursing Diagnosis: Application to Clinical Practice*. Lippincott Williams & Wilkins, Philadelphia

Christensen B, Kockrow E (1999) *Foundations of Nursing*, 3rd edn. Mosby, Missouri

Crisp J & Taylor C (2005) *Potter & Perry's Fundamentals of Nursing*, 2nd edn. Elsevier Australia, Sydney

Game C, Anderson RE, Kidd JR (1990) *Medical-Surgical Nursing: A Core Text*. Churchill Livingstone, Melbourne

Jarvis C (2008) *Physical assessment and health examination*, 5th edn. Elsevier, Canada

Kim MJ, McFarland GK, McLane AM (1991) *Pocket Guide to Nursing Diagnoses*, 5th edn. Mosby, St Louis

North American Nursing Diagnosis Association (NANDA) International (2003–2004) *Nursing Diagnosis: Definitions and Classification*, 5th edn. NANDA

Roper N, Logan WW, Tierney AJ (1990) *The Elements of Nursing*, 3rd edn. Churchill Livingstone, Edinburgh

ONLINE RESOURCES

Sample nursing care plan: http://www.iun.edu/-libemb/nursing/careplan.htm

Chapter 20

DOCUMENTATION AND REPORTING SKILLS

OBJECTIVES

- Define the key terms/concepts
- Discuss the legal and ethical considerations associated with documentation and report writing
- Identify the purpose of documentation
- Outline the guidelines for documenting client information
- Identify the types of documentation formats in use
- Review the patient classification system associated with residential aged health care
- Review case management and critical pathway systems
- Determine the principles for reporting client information
- Develop and practise the skills of verbal and written reporting and recording in the delivery of client care

KEY TERMS/CONCEPTS

case management
charting by exception
critical pathways
flow charting
Kardex
objective data
resident
resident classification scale (RCS)
SOAP format
subjective data

CHAPTER FOCUS

Verbal reporting and documentation are two ways in which communication takes place among members of the health care team. Both are an account of what has been assessed or observed about a client and the care that has been implemented. Health care team members rely on reports and records to deliver care that is directed towards mutually agreed goals. Continuity of care and the pursuit of common objectives depend upon effective communication between members of the health care team, which involves accurate and precise verbal and written reporting and recording of information.

LIVED EXPERIENCE

After working in acute care for so long I was overwhelmed with the amount of paperwork involved with aged care. It took a while to get my head around all the jargon but I now understand why it is all so important.

Kelly, Registered Nurse

Documentation of nursing interventions and management associated with client health status serves two broad purposes: it is a means by which members of the health care team can provide appropriate care for the client, while also becoming a historical outline of the client's care for future reference if needed; and it is a contemporaneous record of events that have taken place and is therefore most likely an accurate record of those events (Crisp & Taylor 2005).

Both these purposes have legal implications for all concerned. As a means of client care, clinical records can be used in court either to prove or to refute a claim of negligence on the part of a health professional. Given the contemporaneous nature of a client's clinical records, the courts may use them to determine what care was or was not given, and the condition of the client at any particular time. Nurses therefore need to be mindful of these potential legal uses and develop their writing skills accordingly.

In addition, nurses need to meet professional and ethical responsibilities to maintain accurate records in relation to the treatment and care given to clients. For nurses, sound documenting skills are unquestionably good nursing practice and essential in facilitating effective nursing care.

PURPOSE OF DOCUMENTATION

The purpose of documentation is to facilitate optimal client outcome through communicating accurate, objective and contemporaneous descriptions of clients' health status and ongoing care. Documentation completed through professional and accurate writing, with legislative and ethical requirements in mind, helps to ensure that continuity of client care is provided. All clients require documentation, which includes records of assessment, diagnosis, planned interventions and subsequent care evaluations (Crisp & Taylor 2005).

Documentation facilitates:

- Communication of relevant clinical data between appropriate people
- Assessment of client health status, existing needs and the care provided by health professionals
- Auditing of service standards and adherence with legislative and ethical requirements
- Education and research
- Compliance with legal requirements
- Maintenance of professional standards.

Records, which promote continuity of care, are the means by which various members of the health care team communicate information about the client's condition and the type of care that has been implemented. Written records (progress notes) provide permanent and accurate assessment of clients, their health status and progress, and the data necessary to plan and implement care. As part of quality assurance programs, health care agencies perform audits in which the information contained in client records is reviewed on a regular basis. Audits are performed to determine the degree to which specified quality assurance standards have been met (Berglund & Saltman 2002).

Written records provide a great deal of information, for example, about nursing diagnoses and evaluation of care that has been implemented, which may be used for educational purposes. The information contained in records may also serve as a source of data for research. Records also become a legal document, for example, if a client takes legal action against a health care agency, client records can be used as evidence in courts of law, where they are read and interpreted by lawyers. In addition, some records are now accessible by clients under the *Freedom of Information Act* (1982). Written records assist to ensure the continuity of client care through professional, accurate and contemporary documentation.

The two most commonly used record formats are the traditional source records and the problem-oriented records. In the source method, information is grouped according to its source; for example, the record is divided into the nurse's notes, the medical officer's record, laboratory reports and the physiotherapist's report. Using this method each member of the health care team uses a separate section of the record to record data. While this method of recording enables each category of health care team member to make detailed entries, it does lead to the fragmentation of data, as the information is not written according to the client's identified problems.

The problem-oriented method groups information from all members of the health care team into sections according to a client's specific health problems, whereby each member of the team contributes to a single list of identified client problems. When this system is used it is easy to recognise and locate the client's health care problems on a single record. While each health care agency adopts its own record format, many use a problem-oriented system of total client recording that includes all the information relevant to a client's care (Berglund & Saltman 2002).

DOCUMENTATION GUIDELINES AND PRINCIPLES

Documentation must always be completed in a professional, accurate and objective manner. Factors that are to be considered when completing documentation in relation to care or treatment provided to a client include:

- Entries should be contemporaneous (as it happens) with the event and recorded in chronological order
- Even routine observations and assessments of changes of a client's condition must be recorded; if no entry has been made it may be inferred that no observation or subsequent care was provided
- Ink is used, as pencil does not provide a permanent record
- Writing is neat and legible, as illegible entries can be misinterpreted
- The client's full name, hospital number and other pertinent details are clearly stated on each sheet
- The date and time are included for each entry
- Only approved abbreviations are used, to avoid misinterpretations

- Correct spelling is used; for example, in relation to recording medications
- Any errors made are not erased or scratched out. Instead, the nurse should draw a single line through the error, write the word 'error' and initial it or sign their name. Under no circumstances should any form of white out (e.g. Liquid Paper, Tippex) be used when documenting in progress notes or assessment entries.
- No lines or spaces are left. A line should be drawn through the blank space in a partially completed line of writing to prevent others from recording in a space with someone else's signature
- Nursing actions are not recorded before they have been performed. Once performed they are recorded immediately to avoid errors or omissions
- Recording is performed in a logical and sequential manner. An organised record, for example progress notes, addresses each topic thoroughly before a new topic is introduced
- The information is accurate, concise and factual. Objectivity of entries is maintained by reflecting on what has actually been seen, heard, smelt or touched by the nurse making the entry. Subjective statements and assumptions should be avoided. Information needs to be specific and the nurse must avoid using ambiguous statements in which the meaning is unclear
- When recording subjective data the client's own words are used whenever possible, using quotation marks to indicate that the statement is a direct quote
- Each entry is signed by the person who records it. Most health care agencies require that a full signature, printed surname and designation is included; for example, Jane Smith (RN Div 2)
- The nurse adheres to the health care agency's policies regarding charting and documentation
- Confidentiality is respected; for example, avoid leaving documentation in an area where it can be read by unauthorised persons. Nurses are legally and ethically required to maintain confidentiality about any information relating to a client
- Transcription of information should be avoided whenever possible, as this practice increases the potential for error to occur (Crisp & Taylor 2005).

COMPUTERS

In major health care agencies computers are used to record client information. With computerised systems recording significant amounts of client information it is important for nurses to become familiar with any such systems being used in their workplace. An issue of concern in the use of computer technology is the potential threat to the privacy of the client. Policies and procedures in relation to client health information need to be in place and adhered to by nurses to protect individual rights to privacy and confidentiality. Further information on computers in nursing is covered in Chapter 25.

REPORTING

Health professionals must always read the clinical records, as verbal handovers at a change of shift are by their very nature only a summary of events that have taken place over the previous shift and should therefore be treated as complementary to the written report. However, reporting routinely involves the spoken or written exchange of information. A nurse has a responsibility to report verbally, as needed, details of the observations and the nursing care that has been implemented. When reporting information verbally the nurse should provide prompt, accurate and concise information to the health care professional who is involved in the delivery of client care (Crisp & Taylor 2005).

When reporting a client's symptoms, such as nausea or pain, the following details should be provided:

- Description of the event
- Severity, onset and location of the symptom
- Frequency and duration
- Any precipitating or aggravating factors
- Any associated symptoms.

For example, rather than just saying that a client has pain, it is more beneficial to provide detailed information, such as:

> Mrs Brown was lying down with her legs drawn up to her abdomen. When I asked her how she was feeling she told me she had suddenly developed severe pain in the right side of her abdomen after eating lunch. She has had the pain intermittently for 20 minutes, she is pale and is feeling nauseated. Her temperature is 37°C, pulse 90, ventilations 24, and her blood pressure is 130/70.

Detailed information such as in this example is objective rather than subjective, and enables any other subsequent nurse involved in providing care to make a better decision on what course of action to take.

When reporting about a client's behaviour (for example, manifestations of anxiety or confusion) the following details should be provided:

- The actual behaviours exhibited; for example, crying, restlessness, or a client's inability to remember their name
- Any precipitating or aggravating factors, if known
- The nursing interventions or actions taken
- The client's response to nursing interventions or actions provided.

When reporting a client's behaviour, the nurse must be objective and avoid the temptation of placing one's own interpretation on observations made. Assumptions and interpretations can be both inaccurate and misleading. For example, an objective observation would be: 'Mr Smith is crying', whereas a subjective interpretation of his behaviour might be: 'Mr Smith seems depressed'. While that may very well be the cause of his crying, he may be crying for a variety of other reasons. A more useful and accurate report would be:

> When I went into his room I noticed that Mr Smith was crying. I went to him, put my arm around his shoulder and asked him if I could help. He told me that he was very anxious about the results of his tests. I told him I would ask you to speak to him about them, and he said he would appreciate that.

When reporting about the effects of treatments, such as medications, details should be provided on the time the treatment was performed, the client's response and whether the treatment produced the desired or any adverse reactions, and the client's vital signs. For example, after administering intramuscular morphine 10 mg the nurse may report:

> Since Mrs Jones was given intramuscular morphine 10 mg at 1300 hours, she is not experiencing any pain, is resting quietly, and her vital signs are: temperature 36.8°C, pulse 82, ventilations 18, and blood pressure 120/70.

Alternatively, the report may be:

> Mrs Jones is still in pain since her injection of morphine 10 mg at 1300. She rated her pain as being 8 on a scale of 1–10, she is feeling nauseated, is sweating and pale, and her pulse rate has dropped from 80 to 58.

In addition to verbal reports, written reports are made on all aspects of a client's care and progress. To promote continuity of care, a verbal report, using written records, is given on each client at each change of shift. The nurse who is giving the report should do so in a methodical manner, beginning with basic information on the reason for the client being in hospital, followed by a detailed description of their progress. Various methods of giving change-of-shift reports may be used, such as reading from the care plan, and reports may be conducted in a nurse's office or while walking around and visiting each client. If the latter method is used, nurses must consider associated confidentiality responsibilities and avoid discussing any information in the immediate vicinity of the client that may be distressing to them (Crisp & Taylor 2005).

A report on each client in the acute setting generally includes:

- The client's name, age and sex
- The medical diagnosis
- The name of the medical officer
- Nursing diagnoses or problems — whether specific goals have been achieved, specific problems resolved, or whether any parts of the nursing care plan have been changed
- General description of the client's physical and psychological status and any recent changes in condition
- The client's degree of independence in performing the activities of daily living
- The client's response to nursing intervention and treatments
- Details of any diagnostic tests or surgical interventions that have been, or are to be, performed
- Details of any new treatments; for example, intravenous therapy, that have been prescribed
- Details of significant medications; for example, narcotic analgesics, and their effects
- Any dietary or fluid restrictions or modifications, and whether the client's fluid input and output are being measured and recorded
- Details of the condition of any wound; for example, degree of healing, amount and type of any discharge
- Details of any deviations from normal; for example, of the client's vital signs or excreta
- Pertinent information concerning the client's family or other significant people.

As a verbal report is being given, the nurse who is receiving the information should be provided with an accurate assessment of each client and their current condition. Use of the nursing process enables the nurse who is giving the report to systematically review the client's medical diagnosis, presenting associated problems, nursing diagnoses, and the nursing interventions and goals as stated on the care plan.

In addition to giving verbal reports at each change of shift, team conferences are held regularly to evaluate the progress of clients. The nursing team may hold a daily conference to review each client and their nursing care plan, or a conference may be held at which various members of the team, such as nurses, medical officer and physiotherapist meet to discuss client care and to exchange information. Team conferences are conducted in a variety of settings, including hospitals, rehabilitation and psychiatric units and community health agencies. The purpose of such a conference is to evaluate:

- A client's health problems
- Progress towards the goals that have been set
- The interventions that have been planned and implemented
- A client's progress
- Plans for discharge.

DOCUMENTATION

The various types of records that may be used by a health care agency include:

- Nursing and medical admission histories
- Client interview forms
- Nursing care plans
- Flow charts
- Progress notes/reports
- Kardex (discussed below)
- Laboratory/diagnostic test reports
- Consent forms
- Incident reports
- Preoperative anaesthetic records, and postoperative surgical reports
- Therapeutic order sheets
- Medication records
- Discharge summaries.

The nurse is most likely to be regularly involved in recording information on client interview forms, nursing care plans, various flow charts, progress notes and Kardex. Information on nursing care plans is provided in Chapter 19.

Flow charts are used to record certain assessments or

measurements, and provide an efficient method of recording information such as:

- Vital signs
- Neurological assessments
- Fluid input and output; for example, fluid-balance and intravenous therapy charts.

Sample flow charts are provided in Figures 20.1, 20.2 and 20.3.

The use of flow charts facilitates a thorough assessment by providing a framework for entries, instead of using open-ended narrative charting that involves an explanation or account of events or developments.

Progress notes involve recording information on the document that describes the client's progress. Using the problem-oriented method, all members of the health care team contribute to the progress notes by documenting information about a client's identified problems. A specific format that some health care agencies use for writing descriptive notes is referred to as the *SOAP format*. The letters SOAP stand for *subjective* statement (made by the client) that describe their perception of a problem; *objective* data, which consists of information that can be measured, obtained via observations or tests; *assessment* of the subjective and objective data available; and the *plan* that is developed in response to assessment. Clinical Interest Box 20.1 gives an example of use of the SOAP format. Some health care agencies also extend the SOAP format to include IER, making the acronym SOAPIER. The letter *I* stands for implementation of the plan, *E* stands for evaluation, and *R* stands for reassessment of the client's problems and needs.

Charting by exception progress note entries involve streamlining documentation by reducing repetitive and time-consuming charting. The assumption with charting by exception is that all standards are met with a normal or expected response unless otherwise documented. By only documenting out-of-the-ordinary developments in a client's condition, any changes are more readily identified (Crisp & Taylor 2005).

The *Kardex* system consists of flip-over cards, one for each client, which contain pertinent information about a client's ongoing plan of care. If Kardex is used, nurses are able to refer to it frequently throughout their shift and during the change-of-shift report. Each card provides a summary of information, such as medical diagnosis, medical officer's orders, nursing care plan, details related to the activities of daily living, and specific orders related to diet, current medications, scheduled tests or procedures, etc. Kardex provides a quick and easily accessible source of current information about each client (Crisp & Taylor 2005).

CLINICAL INTEREST BOX 20.1
SOAP format

24/7/08 1000 hours At risk of falling related to reduced mobility, manifested by left-sided weakness:

S. Resident states 'I don't have much feeling in my left leg and I feel dizzy'

O. Resident has an unsteady gait, holding handrails, reluctant to take any steps

A. Resident experiencing vertigo and loss of balance when walking, and associated anxiety, as was evident with previously assisted attempts to ambulate

P. Assisted to chair and requested resident not to attempt walking or transferring self without staff. Physiotherapist contacted for further review.

RESIDENT CLASSIFICATION SCALE (RCS)

The resident classification scale (RCS) questionnaire is an assessment system used to establish the care needs and level of assistance provided to residents (clients) for the purpose of allocating appropriate funding for all residential aged-care facilities funded by the Commonwealth Government. Current Commonwealth funding is based on eight categories, numbered 1–8 for each resident. Category 1 is the highest-funded category and reflects a resident with extensive care needs. Category 8 attracts no funding, indicating that the resident has minimal needs requiring professional support (Department of Health and Ageing 2005).

Each RCS questionnaire item requires considerable analysis and collectively assists in determining the resident's RCS overall category. The RCS questions that make up the assessment tool each require a rating of A, B, C or D to be made (A meaning no care need, to D meaning high care need) in relation to specified care needs and associated interventions provided to the resident. The process involves extensive documentation comprising a thorough systematic assessment, planning, implementation and evaluation process of the resident's specific needs.

Initial RCS appraisals involve three primary steps that need to be completed by the service provider before the department can classify a resident for funding purposes:

- Assessing the resident's abilities and care needs in writing with regard to aspects of care, which may include physical, emotional, psychological, social, cultural and spiritual needs
- Care planning, involving the identification of strategies to meet the resident's needs and to maximise their existing abilities. The strategies or interventions considered appropriate need to be documented in the care plan
- Submission of the completed application to the Department of Health and Ageing for classification.

Subsequent RCS re-appraisals for reclassifying existing residents in residential care involve the service provider completing a similar process. The initial assessment of all new clients is conducted over a minimum 21-day period, with the categories claimed generally valid for 12 months.

FLUID BALANCE WORKSHEET ONLY

ATTACH LABEL OR RECORD PATIENTS:

U.R. NUMBER:

SURNAME:

GIVEN NAME:

DOB:

DATE: / /

DO NOT FILE IN MEDICAL RECORDS FOLDER

	INTAKE IN ML				OUTPUT IN ML			
Time	Oral	Intra venous	Gastric Tube	NATURE OF FLUID	Urine	Vomitus or Aspiration	Bowel Fistula Blood Loss	REMARKS
TOTAL				TOTAL				

Each day transfer the TOTALS over 24 hours to SUMMARY SHEET and start a new work sheet

FLUID BALANCE

Figure 20.1 | Fluid balance chart *(reproduced with permission from Broadmeadows Health Service, Broadmeadows, Victoria)*

THE ALFRED

U.R.

Surname

GRAPHIC OBSERVATIONS CHART WITH PAIN SCALE

Given Names

PARAMETERS TO BE MONITORED AND RECORDED

	Date	Frequency of observations	Signature
Vital Signs (T°, BP, P, R, O_2 Sat)			
Surgical drain output			
Pain Score			
Sedation score (Refer to Observation guide on reverse of form) NB If patient receiving epidural/PCA, record on MR P-26			
Urinalysis			
Weight			

RISK ASSESSMENT

Norton Score (On admission and daily)

Date	Score	Date	Score

Falls Risk Assessment Score (On admission and as per care plan)

Date	Score	Date	Score

ADMISSION URINALYSIS

Date	pH	Protein	Glucose	Ketones	Bilirubin	Blood	Urobilinogen

Urinalysis

Date	pH	Protein	Glucose	Ketones	Bilirubin	Blood	Urobilinogen

WEIGHT

Date									
Weight									

HEIGHT

2050 © Alfred Hosp 4/03

GRAPHIC OBSERVATIONS CHART WITH PAIN SCALE

MR R-61

Figure 20.2 | Graphic observation chart *(reproduced with permission from The Alfred Hospital, Melbourne, Vic)*

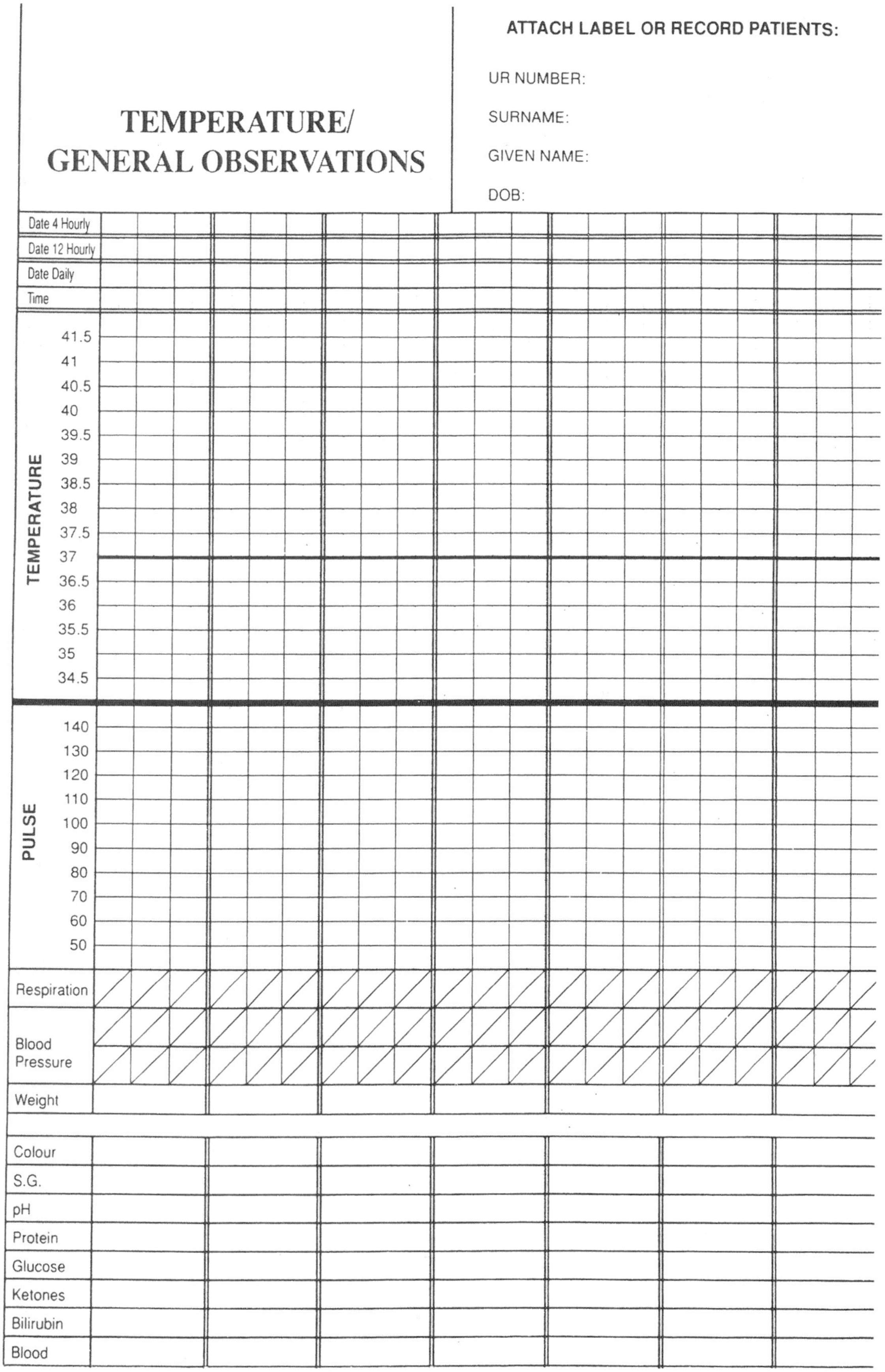

TEMPERATURE/ GENERAL OBSERVATIONS

ATTACH LABEL OR RECORD PATIENTS:

UR NUMBER:

SURNAME:

GIVEN NAME:

DOB:

Date 4 Hourly	
Date 12 Hourly	
Date Daily	
Time	
TEMPERATURE	41.5
	41
	40.5
	40
	39.5
	39
	38.5
	38
	37.5
	37
	36.5
	36
	35.5
	35
	34.5
PULSE	140
	130
	120
	110
	100
	90
	80
	70
	60
	50
Respiration	
Blood Pressure	
Weight	
Colour	
S.G.	
pH	
Protein	
Glucose	
Ketones	
Bilirubin	
Blood	

Figure 20.3 | General observations chart *(Sydney Children's Hospital, Westmead)*

The importance of accurate and extensive assessment, planning, implementation and evaluation of care needs and interventions is highlighted by manuals on residential care, documentation and accountability produced by the Department of Health and Ageing. Refer to these manuals to develop a greater understanding of the RCS system (Department of Health and Ageing 2005).

CASEMIX, CASE MANAGEMENT AND CRITICAL PATHWAYS

Casemix is a scientific approach used to describe the mix, or types of cases, for which care is provided in a care delivery setting. In the acute hospital setting, casemix classification systems provide information that can be used to help hospital management and health care funding authorities to make more informed decisions about which types of clients should be catered for, how many clients to treat, and what funding and staffing is required (Department of Health and Ageing 2005).

While casemix management systems help to classify, cost and manage overall client care, they do not help organise and coordinate the delivery of care to individual clients. Nurses have traditionally addressed this through nursing care plans; however, these are time consuming even for clients undergoing routine procedures and do not include the care provided by other health care professionals.

The case management model of delivering care uses a multidisciplinary plan of care that is summarised into critical pathways. These are usually 1–2-page formats that include key interventions and expected outcomes that allow the health care team to follow integrated care plans for the client problems specific to a medical condition or surgical procedure. The critical paths are used on each shift to direct and monitor the flow of client care. Because of the nature of human responses, there are on occasion variances in expected outcomes as the client's progress deviates from the critical path plan. A subsequent action plan in response to the client's problems will need to be developed and implemented.

A critical pathway (Figure 20.4) is a time-oriented tool used to synchronise the activities of every member of the client's health care team, thereby enhancing the provision of care on a timely basis, minimising delays, omissions and cancellations (Carpenito-Moyet 2005).

SUMMARY

Reporting and recording are the two major ways in which communication takes place among members of the health care team. Continuity of care and the pursuit of common objectives depend on effective communication, which involves accurate and precise verbal and written reporting and recording of information. A nurse has a responsibility to report verbally, to other health professionals, details of the observations made and the nursing care implemented.

A verbal report, using written records, is given for each client at each change of shift. The report must be delivered in such a way that the nurse who is receiving it obtains an accurate assessment of each client and their current condition. In addition to change-of-shift reports, team conferences are held regularly to evaluate the progress of clients.

All pertinent information is recorded in writing to provide a permanent form of communication about each client. Written records, in whatever format, are used for the purposes of communication, assessment, auditing, education and research, and legal documentation.

REVIEW EXERCISES

1. What are the two broad purposes served by the documentation of nursing interventions and management, associated with the client's health status, and needs?
2. A specific format that some health care agencies use for writing descriptive notes in medical records is referred to as the SOAP format. Identify what the letters stand for and provide an example of each.

CRITICAL THINKING EXERCISE

When reporting information verbally the nurse should provide prompt, accurate and concise information, with details being objective rather than subjective. With this in mind discuss the adequacy of information provided by the nurse in the following examples and the reasons for your conclusion.

When reporting measurements or observations of body excreta or secretions, the nurse provides the following information:

Situation 1. A nurse at the handover of shift uses expressions such as 'her pulse is normal', or 'her urine looks alright'.

Situation 2. Another nurse reporting says: 'Mrs Jones's pulse is 80, regular, and strong, urine is amber-coloured, clear, and has no offensive odour'.

REFERENCES AND FURTHER READING

Berglund CA, Saltman D (2002) *Communication for health care*. Oxford University Press, Melbourne

Carpenito-Moyet LJ (2005) *Nursing Diagnosis: Application to Clinical Practice*. Lippincott, Williams and Wilkins, Philadelphia

Crisp J, Taylor C (eds) (2005) *Potter & Perry's Fundamentals of Nursing*, 2nd edn. Elsevier Australia, Sydney

Department of Health and Ageing (2005) *The Residential Care Manual*. Commonwealth of Australia, Canberra

Forrester K, Griffiths D (2005) *Essentials of Law for Health Professionals*, 2nd edn. Elsevier Australia, Sydney

Perry AG, Potter PA (2008) *Clinical Nursing Skills & Techniques*, 6th edn. Mosby, St Louis

Richmond J (ed.) (1997) *Nursing Documentation: Writing What We Do*. AusMed Publications, Melbourne

Victorian Legislation and Parliamentary Documents (1992) *Version No. 060 Freedom of Information Act 1982*. Act No. 9859/1982 Version incorporating amendments as at 12 December 2005. Online. Available: http://www.dms.dpc.vic.gov.au/ [accessed 9 March 2008]

LIVERPOOL HEALTH SERVICE CLINICAL PATHWAY LAPAROSCOPIC STERILISATION	Affix ID Label Here MRN Surname Given Names Address - Street Suburb Postcode Date of Birth Sex AMO Hospital Name

INSTRUCTIONS

This Care Path is a guide only. Always evaluate the appropriateness of each intervention for each patient.
All staff completing this form must provide signature details on page 9 and 10.
Document all variances on the Variance sheet.

		Pre-admission Date / /	Time	Initial	Pre-admission clinic Date / /	Time	Initial
ANAESTHETIST	**Education**				☐ Pain Management		
	Consults				☐ Anaesthetist		
	Documentation & Clerking				☐ Anaesthetic Assessment complete ☐ Patient meets D.O. Admission Criteria		
	Diagnostics				Tests required ☐ Yes ☐ No Tests / Req / Ord / Res Rec ECG ☐ ☐ ☐ CXR ☐ ☐ ☐ Bloods ☐ ☐ ☐ Other ☐ ☐ ☐		
	Medications				Anxiolytic ☐ Yes ☐ No ↓ ☐ Ordered NSAID Pre Med ☐ Yes ☐ No ↓ ☐ Ordered Antiemetic ☐ Yes ☐ No ↓ ☐ Ordered Other .... ↓ ☐ Ordered		
NURSE & CLERICAL	**Discharge Planning**	Referral to discharge planner required: ☐ Yes ☐ No ↓ Referral from complete (see protocol): ☐ Yes ☐ No			Reassess if Referral to Discharge Planner required ☐ Yes ☐ No ↓ Referral form complete (see Protocol): ☐ Yes ☐ No		
	Patient Instructions Information	☐ "Patient Pathway" posted or given to non clinic patient			☐ Patient Pathway given to patient and discussed		
	Consults				☐ Nurse		
	Documentation & Clerking	☐ Request for Admission (CR5) received ☐ Consent complete. (Parts A+B) ☐ Lap Sterilisation consent complete ☐ HAQ complete ☐ HAQ screened ☐ GPSH complete ☐ GPSH screened ☐ Booked on HOSPAS ☐ OT date set Classification made per clinic criteria ☐ For Clinic ☐ No Clinic			Patient notified of clinic appointment by: ☐ Phone ☐ Mail ☐ In Person ☐ Appointment confirmed Old notes: ☐ Received ☐ Returned Test results to clinic from: ☐ Mail ☐ HOSLAB ☐ Fax ☐ Clinic attendance logged ☐ MRN & labels All results: ☐ Returned to Periop Clerk ☐ In notes		
	Diagnostics	Pregnancy test required ☐ Yes ☐ No ☐ Ordered ↓ ☐ Results received					
	Observations				☐ Weight ☐ Heart Rate ☐ BP		
	Special Needs				Interpreter required ☐ Yes ☐ No		

FILE IN MEDICAL RECORD

REORDER FROM PRINT ROOM (PHOTOCOPY)

CLINICAL PATHWAY - LAPAROSCOPIC STERILISATION

CR 122.11

Jul 98/ Rev 2

Page 1 of 10

Figure 20.4 | A sample critical pathway *(reproduced with permission from Liverpool Hospital, NSW)*

Allergies / Sensitivities

Date ______________________ Escort Arranged __________________________ Y / N

Temperature. Pulse. Resp. BP

Premedication ordered _______ Y / N Given by __________________________ Time _________

Time last food taken: ______________________ Teeth Natural/Bridged/Capped

Time last fluid taken: ______________________ Dentures Full/Partial

Time last voided: ______________________ Upper/Lower

With patient/Removed on ward

Jewellery Taped/Removed

SPECIAL ATTENTION eg. Prosthesis, diabetes, spectacles, hearing aids:

____

____

____

Identification Armband Y / N

Consent A+B signed + complete Y / N Request for Admission Y / N

Previous medical records Y / N X-Rays with patient Y / N

Ward Nurse ______________________ OR Nurse ______________________

Surgeon ______________________ **Anaesthetist** ______________________

COMPLIANCE STATEMENT

Name ____ (Print)

before coming into Hospital

- I have received instructions about being treated in Liverpool Hospital as a Perioperative Patient.
- I have followed the instructions about eating & drinking before my operation.
- I have and will give complete and accurate answers to all questions about my health and arrangements for the day of operation.
- I have arranged transport home with a responsible adult.

After my operation

- I will stay with a responsible adult on the night after my operation.
- I will not drive, drink alcohol, or operate complex machinery until the morning after my operation.
- I will follow any other instructions given to me about my care after discharge.
- I will contact the Hospital if there are any problems within 24 hours after the operation.
- I will not sign any legal or important documents within 24 hours of my operation.
- I will not travel home on Public Transport.

Signed ____ Date: / /

Witness ____ Date: / /

Page 2 of 10

Figure 20.4 | A sample critical pathway—cont'd *(reproduced with permission from Liverpool Hospital, NSW)*

Unit 7

Assessing health

Chapter 21
VITAL SIGNS

OBJECTIVES

- Define the key terms/concepts
- Describe factors that affect the vital signs
- Identify the variations in acceptable ranges for body temperature, pulse, respirations and blood pressure that occur from infancy to old age
- Describe advantages and disadvantages of using each body temperature site
- State the factors involved in the maintenance of the pulse and blood pressure
- Identify the sites commonly used to assess the pulse and state the reasons for their use
- State the factors necessary for an adequate supply of oxygen to the cells
- Identify the characteristics that should be included in a respiratory assessment
- Describe the various methods and sites to measure blood pressure

KEY TERMS/CONCEPTS

bradycardia
bradypnoea
Cheyne–Stokes breathing
cyanosis
dyspnoea
external and internal respiration
hypertension
hyperthermia
hypotension
hypothermia
hypoxia
Korotkoff sounds
Kussmaul's breathing
oxygen saturation
respiration
tachycardia
tachypnoea
vital signs

CHAPTER FOCUS

Assessment is an essential part of the nursing process, as it enables the nurse to obtain information about the client that will facilitate the identification of problems relating to their health status. When the client's actual or potential problems or concerns are identified, steps can be taken to plan appropriate care to meet their needs.

Continued assessment enables the nurse to determine the progress being made by the client, any change in the client's condition, and the effectiveness of the nursing care plan in meeting the client's needs. Accurate assessments made, recorded and reported by nurses also assist the medical officer in making a diagnosis, planning a program of treatment or altering a plan of treatment in light of reported changes in a client's condition. Information on the nursing process is provided in Chapter 19 and should be referred to in conjunction with this chapter.

Vital signs are a quick and efficient way of monitoring a client's condition or identifying problems and evaluating the client's response to interventions. The nurse has an essential role to play in assessing clients and in recording and reporting the findings. To assess a client effectively the nurse requires knowledge of the acceptable ranges in measurements of vital signs to identify any deviations or abnormalities. This chapter focuses on use of the physical senses and equipment to assess a patient's physical and mental condition and the signs and symptoms that may be indicative of change.

LIVED EXPERIENCE

The last time I was admitted into hospital I had a young student nurse look after me. The student was very meticulous and looked after all my needs. The only time that I felt uncomfortable and a little scared was the first time he took my blood pressure. He pumped up the cuff, with an intense look on his face, and deflated it. He then proceeded to do this three times and then, without telling me what was wrong, left the room with a panicked look on his face, telling me that he would have to go and get his teacher. I was so worried — I thought there was something wrong with me and that I wouldn't be able to go home. As I sat there waiting, thinking the worst, the student came back with the teacher and it turned out that he hadn't switched on the stethoscope!

Bill, age 57

GUIDELINES FOR TAKING VITAL SIGNS

The vital signs (temperature, respirations, pulse and blood pressure) indicate the body's ability to regulate body temperature, maintain blood flow, and oxygenate body tissues. Oxygen saturation is an additional vital sign obtained through pulse oximetry that reflects the ability of the cardiac and respiratory system to maintain adequate oxygenation. Pain assessment is considered a fifth vital sign (see chapter 35) (Elkin et al 2008). When checking vital signs, or 'taking an individual's observations', a nurse must be able to measure the vital signs correctly, understand and interpret the values, communicate the findings appropriately and begin interventions as required. Vital signs are taken:

- When a client is first admitted to a health care facility
- On a routine schedule according to a medical officer's order or hospital policy
- When assessing a client during home health visits
- Before and after a surgical procedure
- Before and after an invasive diagnostic procedure
- Before and after administration of certain medications that affect the cardiovascular, respiratory or temperature control function
- When a client's general physical condition changes
- Before and after nursing interventions influencing a vital sign
- When a client reports non-specific symptoms of physical distress; for example, 'feeling funny'
- Before, during and after a transfusion of blood products (Elkin et al 2008).

When taking vital signs the nurse should:

- Take the vital signs, interpret their significance and make decisions about client care
- Check that the equipment is functional and appropriate
- Know the acceptable range for all vital signs
- Know the client's usual range of vital signs
- Know the client's medical history, therapies and medications prescribed
- Control or minimise environmental factors that may affect the vital signs
- Use an organised systematic approach
- Describe the frequency of vital sign assessment on the basis of the client's condition
- Analyse the results of vital sign measurement
- Know other physical signs or symptoms and be aware of the client's ongoing health status
- Verify and communicate significant changes in vital signs to the Registered Nurse (RN) and the medical officer.

INTERPRETING OBSERVATIONS

Interpreting specific observations depends on:

- Comparison with the acceptable ranges for a given group of people
- Knowledge of the results of previous observations of a particular client
- The sum total of all observations at the time of the present observation.

For example, to interpret the significance of a client's pulse rate the nurse needs to know the acceptable pulse rate for people of that client's age group, and the client's previous pulse rate. Pulse and other observations or assessments, such as blood pressure, temperature, respirations, colour and degree of mental alertness, provide information that enables more accurate interpretation of a client's condition. Therefore, while a single observation provides some information about a client, several observations enable a more accurate assessment of their condition.

Interpreting any observation involves a decision as to its significance. The nurse has a responsibility to report observations to the nurse in charge, who makes a decision, for example, to assess the client more frequently, take immediate action or notify the medical officer.

BODY TEMPERATURE

Measuring body temperature provides the nurse with an objective assessment of the body's ability to maintain temperature regulation, identifies deviations from the acceptable range and monitors any changes.

The human body is warm blooded, with inbuilt mechanisms that maintain a balance between heat production and heat loss. As a result the internal or core temperature is stable. During ill-health the balance may be upset and considerable stress may be placed on the body's adaptive mechanisms if the temperature does not remain within the acceptable range. The temperature range of a normal adult depends on age, physical activity, status of hydration, and state of health, including the presence of infection (Elkin et al 2008).

REGULATION OF BODY TEMPERATURE

Body temperature is controlled by both voluntary actions and involuntary mechanisms. The surface temperature of the body varies with changes in the environmental temperature, and people adjust to these changes by adapting their immediate surroundings; for example, selecting appropriate clothing, moving away from or towards the source of heat or cold, and altering the temperature of heaters or coolers can help to provide a comfortable environmental temperature.

Core temperature is maintained by inbuilt mechanisms concerned with the production of heat and its dissipation.

These regulatory mechanisms, which ensure a balance between heat production and loss is achieved, are situated in the hypothalamus, where neurons respond to changes in the temperature of the blood circulating through the brain. There are also temperature receptors in the skin and some internal organs, which transmit signals to the central nervous system to help control body temperature.

HEAT PRODUCTION AND HEAT LOSS

Heat is continually being produced by the process of cellular metabolism and is constantly being lost to the environment through the following processes.

Radiation

Body heat is transferred to cooler objects in the environment. Loss of heat by radiation means loss in the form of infrared rays. If the temperature of the body is higher than the temperature of the environment, more heat is radiated from the body.

Conduction

Only small quantities of heat are lost from the body by direct conduction from the body's surface to other objects, for example, a bed or a chair. Loss of heat by conduction to the air represents a large proportion of the body's heat loss, unless the temperature of the air immediately adjacent to the skin is the same as the temperature of the skin.

Convection

Convection is the dispersion of heat by air currents. The body usually has a small amount of warm air next to it. This warm air rises and is replaced by cooler air. People always lose a small amount of heat through convection.

Evaporation

Insensible evaporation of water directly through the skin results from continual diffusion of water molecules, regardless of body temperature. When the body becomes overheated, large quantities of sweat are secreted onto the surface of the skin to provide rapid evaporative cooling of the body.

Balancing heat production and heat loss

Heat balance occurs when the rates of heat production and loss are equal. When the body temperature rises, impulses from the hypothalamus to the skin arterioles are decreased, causing vasodilation, with loss of heat occurring from radiation, conduction, convection, and evaporation of sweat. When the body temperature falls, the impulses are increased, causing vasoconstriction of the skin arterioles, reducing heat loss and increasing the flow of blood to vital internal organs. Shivering is an important source of heat, which is initiated by impulses travelling to the skeletal muscles. These impulses cause increased skeletal muscle tone, resulting in increased muscle metabolism and increased rate of heat production.

FACTORS AFFECTING BODY TEMPERATURE

In health, a range of processes and activities affect body temperature. These include age, diurnal variations, exercise, hormones, stress and environment. Factors that lower the body temperature include exposure to a cold damp environment, insufficient warm clothing, and an under-secretion of the hormone thyroxine. Factors that raise the body temperature include:

- Exposure to a hot humid environment
- Strenuous muscular activity
- Intake of foods high in fat or carbohydrates
- Strong emotions such as anger
- An over-secretion of the hormone thyroxine
- Insufficient fluid intake.

Actions to assist the physiological processes of body temperature control include:

- Maintaining immediate surroundings at a comfortable temperature
- Adapting clothing to suit the climate
- Adjusting intake of food and fluids to suit the climate
- Adjusting the level of physical exercise.

ASSESSING BODY TEMPERATURE

To assess a client's temperature the nurse uses both observational skills and a clinical thermometer. Using the senses of sight and touch the nurse can observe the client's skin colour and temperature. Correct use of the thermometer will provide an accurate measurement of body temperature. As a result, the nurse is able to plan and implement appropriate nursing actions to assist the client in maintaining body temperature.

The frequency with which a client's temperature is measured depends on continued assessment of their individual needs, and the nursing policies of the institution (Clinical Interest Box 21.1). Residents of long-term care facilities generally do not have their temperature measured as often as acutely ill people who require more frequent monitoring of their condition. Measuring the individual's temperature together with assessment of the other vital signs is an important method of determining their general condition. Assessment of these vital signs enables the nurse to establish baseline measurements that can be compared with future readings, and to monitor the individual's response to treatment.

CLINICAL INTEREST BOX 21.1
Measuring temperature in older adults

- The temperature of older adults is at the lower end of normal temperature range: 36°C
- Temperatures considered within acceptable range may reflect a fever in an older adult
- Older adults are sensitive to slight changes in temperature

MEASURING BODY TEMPERATURE

Several types of clinical thermometers are used to measure body temperature. The most commonly used types are electronic, tympanic electronic and chemical dot single use or reusable. Electronic thermometers (Figure 21.1) are most commonly used in health care facilities. The electronic thermometer is battery operated and a cover is placed over the probe before use and disposed of after the temperature has been measured. An electronic thermometer enables an accurate temperature reading to be obtained within a few seconds and may also be used when it is necessary to monitor a client's temperature continuously. A signal device indicates when the temperature has registered, and the reading may be obtained from either a digital display or a printout. All types of thermometer are calibrated in the Centigrade scale.

BODY TEMPERATURE SITES

Body temperature may be measured using the oral, tympanic membrane or axillary sites, on the skin or in the groin. The taking of rectal temperature with a rectal thermometer is rarely performed because of the trauma and pain it causes individuals and because of the risk of cross-contamination. It is no longer performed on neonates.

Tympanic site

The tympanic membrane is now the most commonly used site for taking temperature. An otoscope-like speculum with an infrared sensor tip detects heat radiated from the tympanic membrane. Within 2–5 seconds of placement in the auditory canal, a reading appears on the display unit. A sound signals when the peak temperature reading has been measured (Figure 21.2). The advantages of using this site is that it is easily accessible; minimal client repositioning; unaffected by oral intake of food, fluids or smoking and can be used with clients with tachypnoea without affecting breathing. Disadvantages of using this site are that: it can be uncomfortable and involves the risk of injuring the tympanic membrane if the probe is inserted too far; repeated measurements can vary and the presence of cerumen (wax) and purulent discharge can affect the reading; it requires removal of hearing aid before measurement; it requires disposable sensor cover available only in one size; it does not obtain continuous measurement and can be affected by ambient temperature devices; for example, heaters (Elkin et al 2008).

The oral site

The thermometer is placed under the person's tongue, to one side of the frenulum, to ensure that it is in contact with a heat pocket, and the person closes their lips. The advantages of this site are: it is easily accessible; comfortable for the client; reflects rapid change in core temperature and provides accurate surface temperature reading. Some disadvantages of this site are: causes in delay in measurement if client has recently ingested hot/cold fluids or foods, smoked, or received oxygen by mask or nasal cannula (Elkin et al 2008). So that an accurate measurement can be obtained safely, the person must be:

- Able to close their lips completely and retain the thermometer in the correct position
- Able to breathe comfortably through their nose for the length of time the thermometer is in their mouth
- Rested and not have consumed cold or hot fluids in the previous 15–30 minutes.

The oral site is unsuitable for people who:

- Have an oral infection or painful mouth
- Have recently had oral surgery

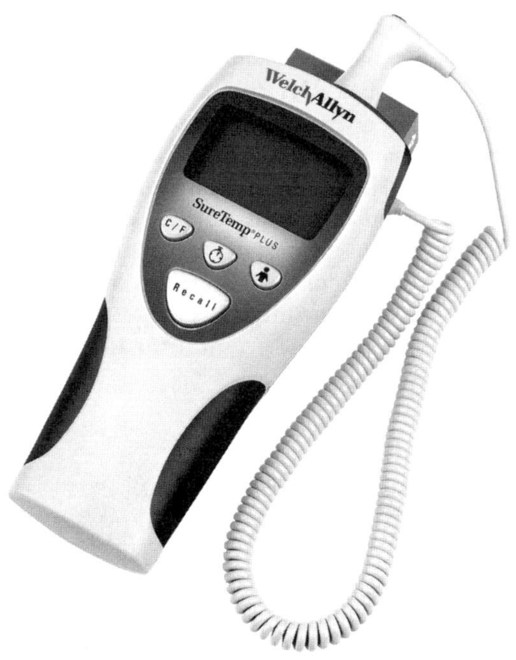

Figure 21.1 | An electronic thermometer *(photo courtesy of Welch Allyn Australia Pty Ltd)*

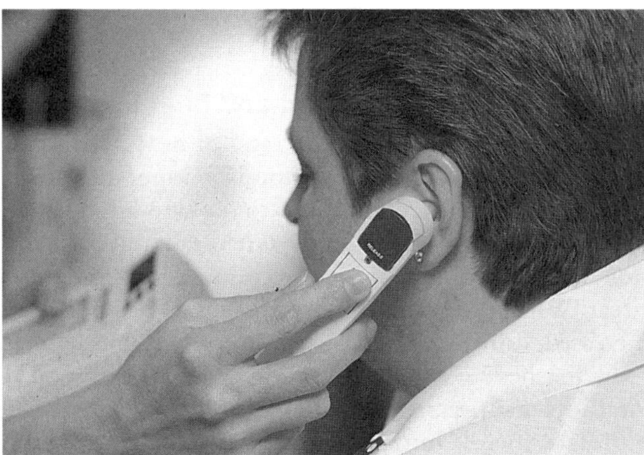

Figure 21.2 | Measuring temperature with tympanic thermometer *(Potter & Perry 2008: 514)*

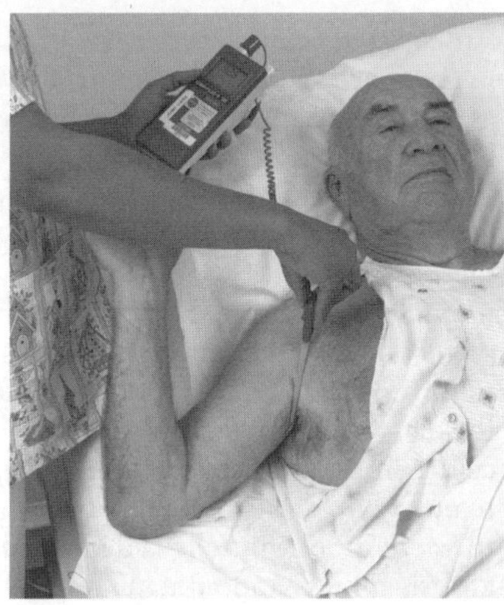

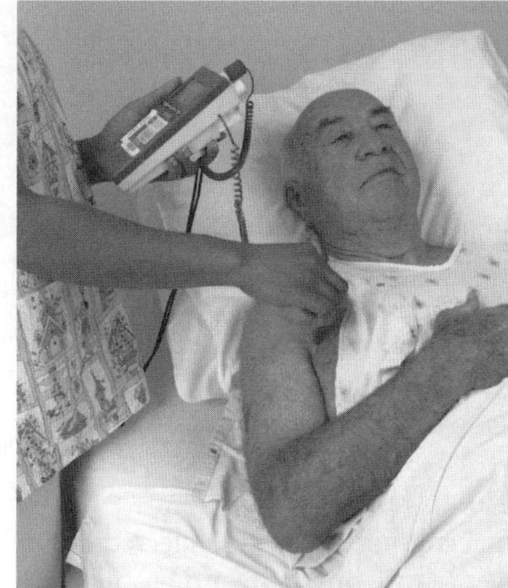

Figure 21.3 | Taking temperature from the axilla *(Elkin et al 2008)*

- Experience any impairment of breathing or obstruction of the nasal passages
- Are unconscious.

The axilla

Using the axilla (Figure 21.3) provides a less accurate measurement of body temperature, but may be used when it is not possible to measure the temperature orally (Clinical Interest Box 21.2). It is safe and non-invasive and can be used with newborns and unconscious clients. The thermometer is placed in the axilla in contact with two dry skin surfaces and is kept in place in the axilla by bringing the person's arm over their chest. A disadvantage of using this site is that the thermometer must be left in place for a long time to obtain an accurate measurement; it can be affected by exposure to the environment and requires continuous positioning by the nurse (Elkin et al 2008).

The skin

Various types of single-use disposable thermometers are available. A temperature-sensitive strip of tape is placed on the forehead or abdomen to record the heat of the body (Figure 21.4). These are often used in newborn nurseries. Directions on the package explain how to use these thermometers. Most disposable thermometers will register the temperature within 60 seconds. The advantages of this site is that it is inexpensive; provides continuous reading and is safe and non-invasive. The disadvantages are that measurement lags behind other sites during temperature changes; sometimes affected by environmental temperature and diaphoresis or sweat can impair adhesion (Elkin et al 2008).

CLINICAL INTEREST BOX 21.2
Axillary temperature in paediatrics

- Axillary temperature cannot be relied on to detect fevers in infants and young children
- Axillary or skin temperature is safest for newborns. The thermometer must be kept in place for 5 minutes
- Infants are sensitive to slight changes in environmental temperatures

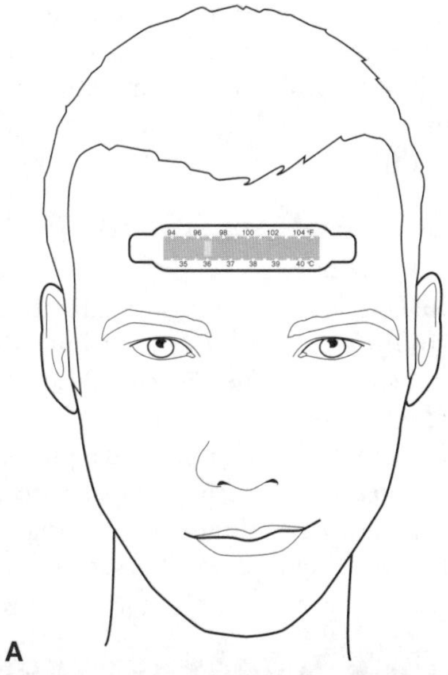

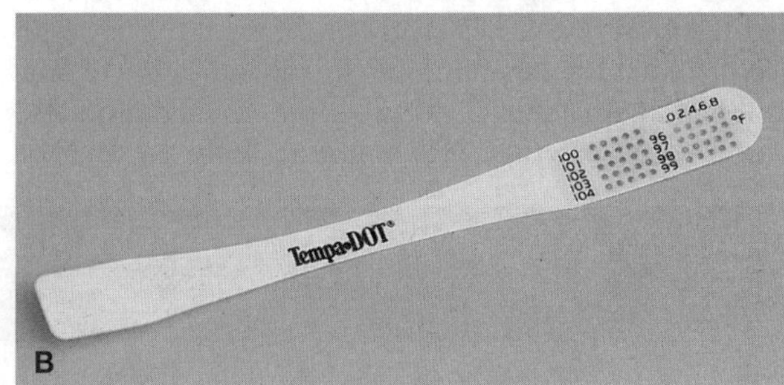

Figure 21.4 | Disposable thermometers
A: A temperature-sensitive skin tape.
B: Disposable, single-use thermometer strip *(photo B: Potter & Perry 2008)*

STEPS IN OBTAINING AN ACCURATE MEASUREMENT OF BODY TEMPERATURE

To obtain an accurate measurement of body temperature and to promote the client's comfort and safety, the nurse should:

- Select the appropriate site
- Check that the thermometer is undamaged, not contaminated and is working properly
- Ensure that the person is informed of the procedure
- Ensure that the person is rested
- Position the person according to the site selected
- Wash hands to prevent cross-infection and ensure that the thermometer has been disinfected before the procedure
- Use the correct probe for the site selected when using an electronic thermometer.

Depending on the site being used, some variations occur in the time that the thermometer is left in position, the normal range of temperature, and the position in which the person is placed (Table 21.1). Because of variations between sites it is important to note on the observation or vital sign charts what method was used to take the temperature. For example, if the temperature was taken orally, the temperature would be recorded: 36.7 PO (Latin: *per os* [by mouth]).

PROCEDURE FOR MEASURING BODY TEMPERATURE

While the actual procedure for measuring temperature may vary slightly in different health care settings, the general principles remain the same. The nurse should assess the needs of each individual and refer to the institution's policy manual for information about the technique and equipment. Table 21.2 lists guidelines for measuring temperature using each body site. Temperature measurements are usually recorded on graph-style charts (Figure 21.5). These enable the pattern of temperature variations to be observed readily.

ALTERATIONS IN BODY TEMPERATURE

Body temperature reflects body function, and a deviation from acceptable temperature range is an indication of body dysfunction. An imbalance between the production and loss of heat results in a rise or fall in normal body temperature. An elevated temperature is referred to as hyperthermia, pyrexia or fever. A temperature above 41°C is referred to as hyperpyrexia. A temperature below the acceptable range is referred to as hypothermia.

Hyperthermia occurs when cells are injured, or invaded by pathogens that release chemical substances called pyrogens, which act on the hypothalamus and cause a rise in body temperature. Hyperthermia is a manifestation of metabolic disorder, infection, neurological disease, severe trauma or neoplasm. Hypothermia refers to a lowering of the temperature of the entire body. The thermal regulating centre in the hypothalamus is greatly impaired when the temperature of the body falls below 34.4°C. At this level, the activity of the cells is decreased, less heat produced and sleepiness and coma can develop. Those at risk of hypothermia include postoperative clients, who have been cooled during surgery, newborn infants, elderly or debilitated clients, and any person who is subjected to prolonged exposure to a cold environment (de Wit 2005). Alterations in body temperature produce certain physiological effects, as shown in Table 21.3.

NURSING CARE OF A CLIENT WITH ALTERED BODY TEMPERATURE

Hyperthermia

The aims of nursing a client with hyperthermia include:

- Reducing body temperature to an acceptable range
- Relieving any associated discomfort
- Encouraging rest to decrease the production of body heat
- Maintaining nutritional and fluid status.

These aims can be achieved by implementing certain nursing actions, which include:

- Assessing the client's temperature after the administration of any prescribed medication such as antipyretics and antibiotics
- Sponging the client with tepid water. This procedure causes the superficial blood vessels to dilate and release heat, thereby reducing body temperature. The client is undressed and covered with a bath blanket. Using water at a temperature of 27–30°C each part of the client's body is sponged. Long slow strokes should be used, leaving beads of water on the skin to encourage loss of heat by evaporation. The skin may be gently patted dry, but rubbing should be avoided,

TABLE 21.1 | MEASURING BODY TEMPERATURE

	Oral	Axilla	Skin	Tympanic
Time thermometer is left in position for	1 minute	3 minutes	60 seconds	2–5 seconds
Normal range of temperature	36–37.2°C	36–37°C	36–37°C	35.5–37.6°C
Position of client	Lying or sitting	Lying or sitting with arm across the chest	Lying or sitting	Lying or sitting

S.M.O ____________________

WARD ____________________

____

IDENTIFICATION

PATIENT'S NAME ____________________

DATE									
DAYS AFTER	ADMISSION								
	OPERATION								
HOUR		2 6 10 14 18 22	2 6 10 14 18 22	2 6 10 14 18 22	2 6 10 14 18 22	2 6 10 14 18 22	2 6 10 14 18 22	2 6 10 14 18 22	
BLOOD PRESSURE	TEMPERATURE								
260	41.5								
250	41								
240	40.5								
230	40								
220	39.5								
210	39								
200	38.5								
190	38								
180	37.5								
170	37								
160	36.5								
150	36								
140	140								
	PULSE								
130	130								
120	120								
110	110								
100	100								
90	90								
80	80								
70	70								
60	60								
50	50								
40	40								

	GIRTH								
	HEIGHT								
	WEIGHT								
INTAKE	ORAL								
	N/G								
	IV								
	TOTAL								
OUTPUT	URINE								
	N/G								
	VOMITUS								
	DT								
	TOTAL								
	STOOLS								
	APERIENT								

URINALYSIS	AMOUNT								
	SP GRAVITY								
	ALBUMIN								
	SUGAR								
	BLOOD								
	BILE								

Figure 21.5 | A vital signs graph-style chart

TABLE 21.2 | GUIDELINES FOR MEASURING BODY TEMPERATURE

Action	Rationale
Review and carry out the standard steps in Appendix 1	
Measuring body temperature with a tympanic membrane electronic thermometer	
Assist client in assuming a comfortable position, with head turned away from the nurse	Ensures comfort and exposes auditory canal for accurate temperature measurement
Observe for ear wax (cerumen) in client's ear canal	Lens cover of speculum must not be impeded by earwax (will not obtain an accurate measurement). Switch to other ear or select an alternative measurement site
Remove thermometer from charging base and slide disposable speculum cover over otoscope-like tip until it locks into place	Base provides a battery power. Soft plastic probe cover prevents transmission of microorganisms
If holding handheld unit with right hand, obtain temperature from client's right ear; left handed persons should obtain temperature from client's left ear	The less acute angle of approach the better the probe will seal inside the auditory canal
Insert speculum into ear canal, following manufacturer's instructions for tympanic probe positioning. Pull pinna backward, up and out for an adult, move thermometer in a figure-eight pattern, fit probe snug in canal and do not move point towards the nose	Correct positioning of probe will ensure accurate readings
As soon as probe is in place, depress scan button. Leave thermometer probe in place until an audible signal is given and client's temperature appears on the digital display	Depression of scan button causes infrared energy to be detected
Carefully remove speculum from auditory meatus. Push ejection button on unit to discard plastic probe cover into an appropriate receptacle	Reduces transmission of microorganisms
Return handheld unit to charging base	Protects sensor tip from damage and keeps unit charged ready for next use
Assist client in reassuming a comfortable position	Restores comfort and sense of wellbeing
Wash hands	Reduces risk of transmission of microorganisms
Discuss findings with client as needed	Promotes participation in care and understanding of health status
Record the time and temperature on the vital signs chart. Record measurements in the nurse's notes if the temperature was elevated	Verifies that temperature was taken and makes measurement data available
Measurement of body temperature with electronic thermometer	
Oral temperature	
Remove thermometer from charging unit. Slide disposable plastic probe cover over thermometer probe until cover locks in place	Charging provides battery power. Soft plastic cover prevents transmission of microorganisms
Gently place thermometer probe under the tongue in posterior sublingual pocket lateral to centre of jaw	Heat from superficial blood vessels in sublingual pocket produces temperature reading
Ask client to hold thermometer probe with lips closed	Maintains proper position of thermometer during recording
Leave thermometer probe in place until audible signal occurs and client's temperature appears on digital display	To ensure accurate reading, probe must stay in place until signal occurs
Remove thermometer probe from under client's tongue, push ejection button and discard plastic probe cover into an appropriate receptacle	Reduces risk of transmission of microorganisms
Return thermometer to storage position of thermometer unit and return to charger	Maintains battery charge
Discuss findings with client as needed	Promotes participation in care and understanding of health status
Record the time and temperature on the vital signs chart. Record measurements in the nurse's notes if temperature was elevated	Verifies that temperature was taken and makes measurement data available

TABLE 21.2 | GUIDELINES FOR MEASURING BODY TEMPERATURE—cont'd

Action	Rationale
Axillary temperature	
Remove thermometer from charging unit. Slide disposable plastic probe cover over thermometer probe until cover locks in place	Charging provides battery power. Soft plastic cover prevents transmission of microorganisms
Raise client's arm away from torso and make sure the axilla is dry	Moisture may interfere with accurate reading
Place thermometer into centre of axilla, lower arm over probe and place arm across client's chest	Maintains position of thermometer against blood vessels in axilla
Hold thermometer in place until audible signal occurs and client's temperature appears on digital display, remove probe from axilla	To ensure an accurate reading
Push ejection button on thermometer probe stem to discard plastic probe cover into an appropriate receptacle.	Reduces risk of transmission of microorganisms
Return thermometer to storage position of thermometer unit and return to charger	Maintains battery charge
Discuss findings with client as needed	Promotes participation in care and understanding of health status
Record the time and temperature on the vital signs chart. Record measurements in the nurse's notes if temperature was elevated	Verifies that temperature was taken and makes measurement data available

Special note:
- In an infant or young child it may be necessary to hold the arm against the child's side when using axillary method. If infant is in a side-lying position, the lower axilla will record the higher temperature
- Do not use axilla if skin lesions are present because local temperature may be altered and area may be painful to touch

TABLE 21.3 | EFFECTS OF ALTERED BODY TEMPERATURE

Hyperthermia	Hypothermia
Elevated temperature, pulse and ventilation rates (rigor may occur)	Subnormal temperature, decreased pulse and ventilation rates
Warm flushed skin and sweating may be present	Cool, pale or mottled dry skin
Restlessness, drowsiness or confusion	Drowsiness, shivering
Aching muscles and joints	Muscle weakness
Headache	Mental confusion
Photophobia	Unconsciousness (if prolonged)
Loss of appetite	
Increased thirst	
Dehydration (if prolonged)	

as this increases cell metabolism and heat production. During the sponge the client must be observed for shivering, pallor, mottling or cyanosis, or a rapid, weak or irregular pulse. If any adverse reactions occur, the sponge must be discontinued immediately. During, and on completion of, the sponge the client should be advised to avoid unnecessary movement, as muscular activity increases heat production. The client's temperature, pulse and respirations should be measured 30 minutes after the sponge to assess the effectiveness of the procedure

- Promoting the client's general comfort by providing loose, light, clean and dry nightwear and bed linen. To maintain clean and dry skin, the client's hygiene needs must be attended to
- Regular mouth care, including mouth rinses and the application of a lip cream, which will help reduce any oral dryness associated with hyperthermia
- Ensuring that the room is quiet and free from harsh light and ventilated adequately
- Encouraging the client to rest or sleep as much as possible, as reducing the level of physical activity will decrease the production of body heat
- Continually checking the client's skin colour,

temperature and general condition to assess the effectiveness of nursing interventions
- Maintaining optimal nutritional status to cater for the increased metabolic demand associated with hyperthermia. The client should be provided with light appetising meals that provide essential nutrients. If appetite is poor, extra kilojoules may be provided by adding glucose to oral fluids
- Providing adequate fluids, which are necessary to prevent dehydration. The client should be encouraged to drink large amounts of cool or iced fluids. If the person is unable to tolerate fluids orally, intravenous administration of fluids may be necessary. The input and output of all fluids should be closely monitored and the person observed for any signs of dehydration.

Information on the signs and symptoms of dehydration is provided in Chapter 30.

A rigor sometimes occurs in response to the physiological processes associated with hyperthermia. The nurse should assess the client's condition throughout the three typical stages of a rigor, and implement nursing actions necessary to promote client comfort:
- Stage 1: As the body temperature begins to rise the client feels cold and may shiver violently. Comfort should be promoted by keeping the client warm but avoiding overheating. The intake of fluids should be encouraged
- Stage 2: The temperature rises to approximately 40°C and the client feels very hot and uncomfortable. Minimal clothing and bed linen should be used and other actions to reduce the body temperature should be implemented; for example, encouraging the client to drink large amounts of cool fluid
- Stage 3: Profuse sweating occurs and as a result body temperature begins to fall. Actions to reduce temperature should be stopped and any damp clothing or bed linen should be changed to maintain a dry environment. The client should be encouraged to rest quietly in an attempt to reduce the production of body heat.

Chapter 48 covers emergency care of an individual with hyperthermia.

Hypothermia

The aims of nursing a client with hypothermia include:
- Restoring body temperature to an acceptable range
- Relieving any discomfort associated with hypothermia
- Encouraging mobilisation to increase the production of body heat
- Maintaining nutritional and fluid status.

These aims can be achieved by implementing certain nursing actions which include:
- Helping to increase the client's temperature by gradually rewarming them. Rapid rewarming and the direct application of heat to the body surface should be avoided, as these actions cause peripheral vasodilation and diversion of blood away from vital internal organs. The environmental temperature should be kept between 26°C and 29°C
- Providing lightweight warm clothing and bed linen. A hypothermia or 'space' blanket may be used in an effort to restore normal body temperature
- Promoting general comfort by attending to the client's position and hygiene needs
- Encouraging mobilisation as the temperature begins to rise, in an effort to increase production of body heat.
- Encouraging the client to consume warm food and fluids, particularly those containing carbohydrate, to assist the production of body heat
- Continually checking the client's temperature and general condition to assess the effectiveness of nursing interventions.

Chapter 48 covers the emergency care of a person with hypothermia. Clinical Interest Box 21.3 outlines the possible nursing diagnoses for a client with body temperature alteration.

CLINICAL INTEREST BOX 21.3
Nursing diagnoses for clients with body temperature alterations

Altered body temperature is a risk for:
- Hyperthermia
- Hypothermia
- Ineffective thermoregulation

PULSE

Measuring the pulse and blood pressure provides the nurse with an objective assessment of a client's cardiovascular and fluid status. By monitoring the pulse and blood pressure the nurse can identify deviations from acceptable ranges and detect any changes.

As described in Chapter 38, the cardiovascular system transports essential substances to the tissue cells, and waste substances from the tissue cells to various organs for excretion. An adequate supply of blood is necessary for the cells to function effectively, and any disruption to the blood supply may have serious consequences. An adequate flow of blood throughout the body is dependent on the ability of the heart to pump, the ability of the blood vessels to transport the blood, and the quantity and quality of the blood.

The most important factor responsible for the transport of substances to the tissues is cardiac output. Cardiac output is the volume of blood pumped by each ventricle during each minute, and is the product of the volume of blood pumped at each beat (stroke volume) and the number of beats during one minute (heart rate). A healthy heart in a healthy adult ejects 5–6 litres of blood per minute. This amount can be increased by an increase in either heart rate and/or stroke volume and can also vary with:

- Body size, as cardiac output increases in proportion to the surface area of the body
- Age, as with increasing age the cardiac output decreases
- Posture, as cardiac output is greater when a person is standing
- Exercise, as the greater the degree of physical activity the greater the cardiac output needs to be. Strenuous physical activity can result in an increased heart rate and a cardiac output of 30 L/min
- A sudden increase in total blood volume; for example, the infusion of fluid intravenously
- Certain disease states — cardiac output is increased in conditions such as pulmonary disease and anaemia, and is decreased in conditions such as shock or myocardial infarction.

The rate at which the heart beats is controlled by the conducting system of the heart and the autonomic nervous system. The sinoatrial node initiates impulses that spread throughout the conducting system and to all areas of the cardiac muscle, resulting in atrial then ventricular contraction. Stimulation of the parasympathetic nerve fibres, primarily the vagus nerves, reduces the heart rate, while stimulation of the sympathetic nerve fibres increases the heart rate. Various chemicals and ions can also affect heart activity; for example, adrenaline inhibits the parasympathetic nerves, resulting in increased heart rate. An excess of potassium ions in the blood decreases the ability of the heart to contract. Heart, and therefore pulse, rate varies according to age, sex, body build, level of physical activity and emotions.

Assessing the pulse

Cardiovascular function is assessed by observing the general appearance of the client and detecting the signs and symptoms of dysfunction, such as cyanosis, pallor, cool skin temperature, oedema and dyspnoea. Cardiovascular status is also assessed by monitoring the pulse and blood pressure. The frequency with which the pulse and blood pressure are assessed depends on the person's condition and how closely it needs to be monitored. Residents in long-term care facilities will generally require pulse and blood pressure measurement infrequently, whereas people who are acutely ill may have the measurements performed at intervals ranging from every 30 minutes to six times a day.

Assessing the arterial pulse provides significant information about a person's cardiac function and peripheral perfusion. As the heart beats it ejects blood from the left ventricle into the aorta. Each beat of the heart produces a wave of blood through the arteries so that there is regular recurrent expansion and contraction of the arteries. The waves of blood that cause pulsation through the arteries are palpable as a pulse, which can be felt when a superficial artery is partially compressed by the fingers, and is most easily felt over a large artery that lies close to the skin and crosses over a bone or firm tissue. Table 21.4 gives guidelines for taking a pulse.

PULSE SITES

The pulse sites (Figure 21.6), where the pulse may be palpated are:

- Temporal: the temporal artery is palpated immediately in front of the ear
- Carotid: the carotid artery is palpated at the front of the neck, to the side of the thyroid cartilage
- Apical: the apical pulse is the beat heard at the apex of the heart, and is assessed using a stethoscope. The stethoscope is placed over the apex of the heart, in the left centre of the chest just below nipple level
- Brachial: the brachial artery is palpated in the antecubital fossa at the elbow joint
- Radial: the radial artery is palpated in the wrist just above the thumb
- Femoral: the femoral artery is palpated in the inguinal area
- Popliteal: the popliteal artery is palpated at the back of the knee (Figure 21.7)
- Posterior tibial: the posterior tibial artery is palpated just behind the medial malleolus of the ankle (Figure 21.8)
- Pedal: the dorsalis pedis artery is palpated on the anterior surface of the foot (Figure 21.9).

The radial artery is the most commonly used site, as it is conveniently located and readily accessible (Figure 21.10). The temporal or carotid sites may be used if it is difficult to palpate the radial artery easily, for example, if a client

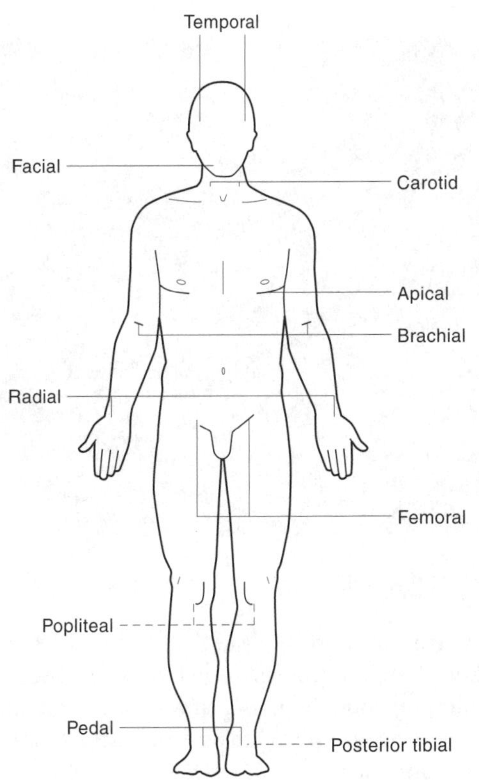

Figure 21.6 | Location of the pulse sites

TABLE 21.4 | GUIDELINES FOR PULSE MEASUREMENT

Action	Rationale
Review and carry out the standard steps in Appendix 1	
If client is supine, place client's forearm straight alongside or across lower chest or upper abdomen with wrist extended straight. If sitting, bend client's elbow 90 degrees and support lower arm on chair or on nurse's arm.	Relaxed position of lower arm permits full exposure of artery to palpation
Place the index and middle fingers over the site and press gently until pulsation can be felt	The assessor's thumb is not used, as it has a strong pulse and may be felt instead of the client's pulse. Pressure that is too light will fail to detect the pulse, and firm pressure may obliterate the pulse
Using a watch with a second hand, count the pulse for one minute. While the rate is being counted, the rhythm and volume are also assessed. If pulse is regular count rate for 30 seconds and multiply total by 2. If pulse is irregular, count rate for 60 seconds. Assess frequency and pattern of irregularity and compare radial pulses bilaterally.	Allows sufficient time to detect the rate and any abnormalities. It requires 30 seconds to determine if the pulse is regular in rhythm. Inefficient contraction of heart fails to transmit pulse wave, interfering with cardiac output, resulting in irregular pulse. Longer time period ensures more accurate count. A marked difference between radial pulses may indicate arterial flow is compromised in one extremity and action should be taken immediately.
Document the time of assessment and the rate and characteristics of the pulse. Record the pulse measurement	A record provides information about the client's condition
Any abnormalities must be reported immediately, as an apical measurement may be indicated	An apical measurement provides a more accurate assessment of the pulse
Wash and dry hands	Prevents risk of transmission of microorganisms
Special note: If pulse is irregular, assess for a pulse deficit. Count apical pulse while colleague counts radial pulse. Begin apical pulse, initiating counting by a signal to simultaneously assess pulses for a full minute. If pulse count differs by more than 2 beats per minute, a pulse deficit exists, which may indicate alteration in cardiac output	
(deWit 2005; Elkin et al 2008)	

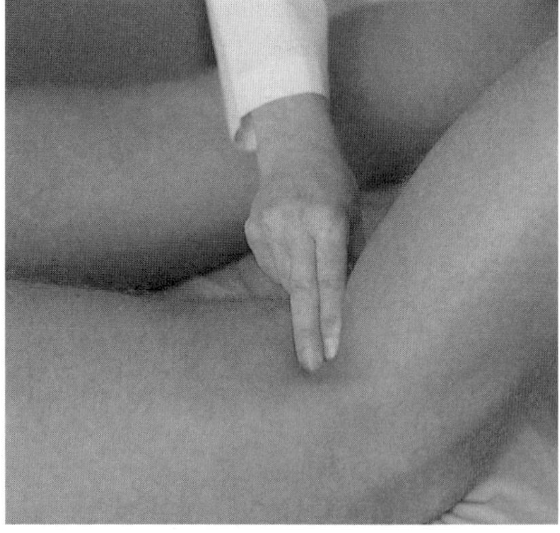

Figure 21.7 | Measuring the popliteal pulse *(Elkin et al 2008)*

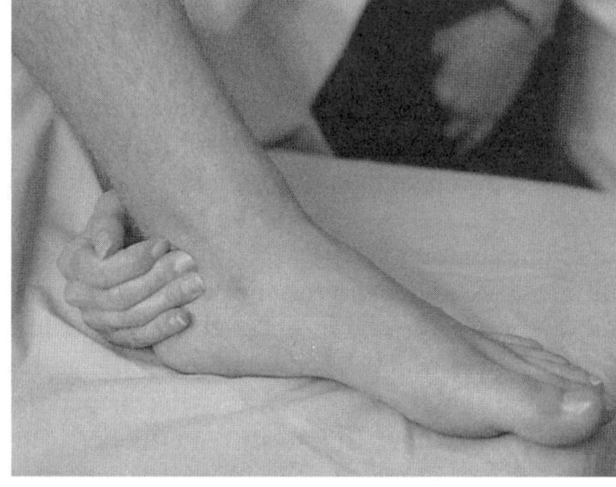

Figure 21.8 | Measuring the posterior tibial pulse *(Elkin et al 2008)*

has both arms encased in plaster. The remaining sites are used when there are specific indications for assessing the flow of blood through a particular artery; for example, the popliteal and pedal pulses are assessed after certain types of surgery to the leg.

The apical pulse is assessed when a more accurate estimation of heart rate or rhythm is required or when there is any doubt about the rate or rhythm of a peripheral pulse (Figure 21.11). It is routinely used for infants and children up to 3 years of age. Apical–radial pulse assessment may be indicated for clients with certain cardiovascular disorders. The apical and radial rates should be identical, and are usually measured by two different people. One person palpates and assesses the radial pulse while a second person assesses the apical pulses at the same time. Some heart beats that can be detected at the apex are not strong enough to

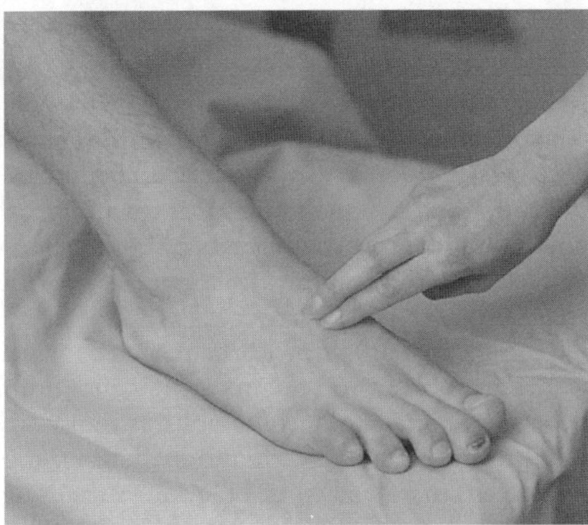

Figure 21.9 | Measuring the pedal pulse *(Elkin et al 2008)*

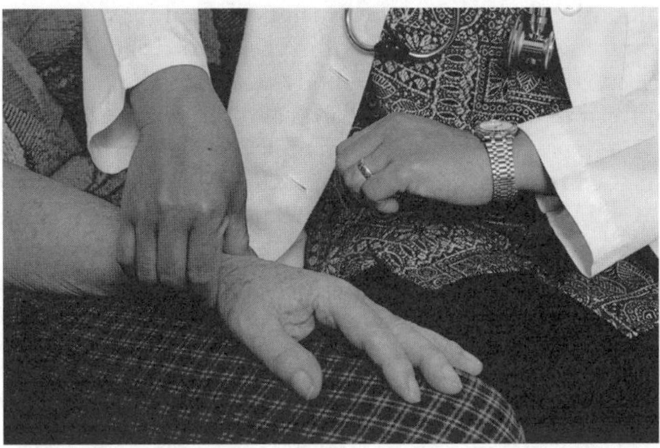

Figure 21.10 | Measuring the radial pulse *(deWit 2005)*

be palpated at peripheral sites. Any difference between the two measurements is called the pulse deficit, and should be reported immediately.

CHARACTER OF THE PULSE

The pulse is assessed for rate, rhythm and volume:

- **Rate** — the pulse rate is the number of beats per minute, and the acceptable rate varies according to age: 120–140 beats/min for an infant, 90–120 beats/min for a child, 60–100 beats/min for an adult. It should be noted that athletes and other physically fit individuals commonly have a pulse rate below 60 beats/min. A large proportion of elderly people also have a pulse rate below 60 beats/min
- **Rhythm** — the rhythm of the pulse is the regularity with which the beats occur. A normal pulse has a regular rhythm, with the same intervals between each beat
- **Volume** — the volume refers to the strength of the beat, and an acceptable pulse is strong and easily palpated.

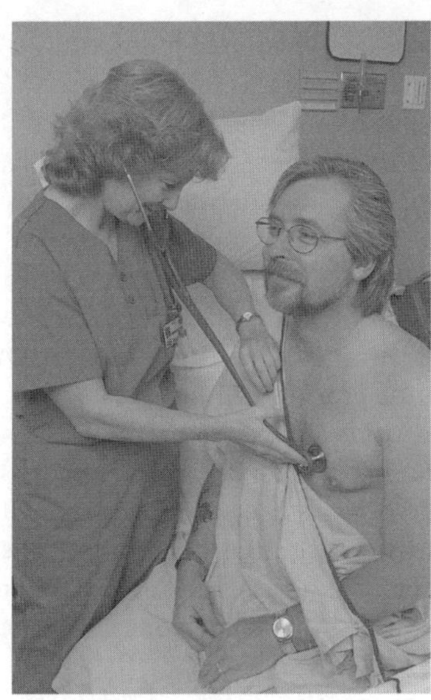

Figure 21.11 | Counting the apical pulse *(deWit 2005)*

FACTORS AFFECTING PULSE RATE

The pulse rate varies according to age (Clinical Interest Box 21.4), sex, body build, level of physical activity, fever, medications, haemorrhage, position changes, stress and emotions. The pulse may also be affected during various disease states, which result in alterations to its character.

Rate

An increase in the pulse rate above 100 beats/min is called *tachycardia* and may result from fear, anxiety, excitement, anger or pain. Tachycardia may also occur in conditions such as haemorrhage, shock, fever, thyrotoxicosis or congestive cardiac failure. A decrease in the pulse rate below 60 beats/min is called *bradycardia* and may occur during absolute relaxation or sleep. Bradycardia may also occur in conditions such as cerebral haemorrhage, heart block, myxoedema or drug toxicity, such as with digitalis.

Rhythm

An irregular rhythm, when the intervals between each beat vary, is called arrhythmia, or dysrhythmia, and may occur in conditions such as electrolyte imbalance or cardiac tissue damage. Examples of irregular rhythm include:

- Ectopic beats, which are premature heartbeats and may be occasional or frequent
- Coupled beats (or bigeminal pulse), in which two

CLINICAL INTEREST BOX 21.4
The pulse in older adults

It is often difficult to palpate the pulse of an older adult or obese client. A stethoscope provides a more accurate reading.

Once elevated, the pulse rate of an older adult takes longer to return to a normal resting rate.

beats in close succession are followed by a pause during which no pulse is felt
- Atrial fibrillation, in which fibrillation of the atria results in random, rapid contractions and, consequently, an irregular pulse.

Volume

An increased volume, when the pulse is referred to as being full and bounding, can result from strenuous physical exercise or strong emotions. An increased volume can also occur in conditions such as hypertension, thyrotoxicosis or aortic valve incompetence. A decreased volume, when the pulse is referred to as being weak and thready, can occur in conditions such as haemorrhage, shock, acute myocardial infarction or cardiac failure. When the pulse is so weak that it cannot be palpated it is referred to as being imperceptible.

When assessing the pulse, any deviations from the client's acceptable range should be reported immediately and documented. Pulse measurements are recorded on a chart (Figure 21.5). Each health care institution adopts its own printed form of graph and method for recording pulse measurements, together with the other vital signs. Commonly, the chart also provides space for recording other information, such as the client's weight. Clinical Interest Box 21.5 outlines the possible nursing diagnoses for alterations in pulse assessment.

RESPIRATION

Oxygen, a colourless and odourless gas, makes up about 20% of the atmosphere, and is essential for sustaining most forms of life. Every cell in the human body requires oxygen for metabolism and must get rid of the metabolic waste product, carbon dioxide. The intake of oxygen and the elimination of carbon dioxide is achieved through the respiratory system. The respiratory system delivers oxygen from the atmosphere to the bloodstream, and carbon dioxide from the bloodstream to the atmosphere, through the act of breathing or ventilation. During breathing the lungs inflate and deflate about 20 times every minute.

CLINICAL INTEREST BOX 21.5
Nursing diagnoses using pulse assessment data as defining characteristics

- Activity intolerance
- Anxiety
- Cardiac output, decreased
- Fear
- Fluid volume deficit
- Fluid volume excess
- Impaired gas exchange
- Hyperthermia
- Hypothermia
- Tissue perfusion, altered
- Pain

Inspiration of air occurs as the diaphragm contracts and flattens, thus enlarging the thoracic cavity. At the same time the ribs are pulled up and outwards by the action of the intercostal muscles. As the chest expands, air enters the lungs. Exhalation occurs as the ventilatory muscles relax and the chest returns to its minimum size, thus expelling air from the lungs. (Further information about the structure and function of the respiratory system is provided in Chapter 38.)

The cardiovascular system is the means by which the gases are transported to and from the cells. From the lungs, oxygen, bound to haemoglobin, is transported in the blood to the cells, and carbon dioxide from the cells is transported, dissolved in the blood, to the lungs for excretion. Respiration is the exchange of oxygen and carbon dioxide. *External respiration* is the exchange of oxygen and carbon dioxide between the external environment and the blood by the process of diffusion in the lungs. *Internal respiration* is the exchange of oxygen and carbon dioxide between the blood and the body tissues by the process of diffusion between the capillaries and the cell membrane.

The passage of oxygen from the atmosphere to the alveoli in the lungs and the passage of carbon dioxide from the alveoli to the atmosphere require an unobstructed airway. In addition, the entire process of respiration requires:

- Adequate oxygen in the atmosphere
- A functioning respiratory tract
- Functioning thoracic muscles and nerves to control the thoracic cage
- Blood to transport the gases
- Capillaries in close proximity to the cells to allow the exchange of gases.

Regulation of breathing and respiration

The automatic control of breathing stems from the respiratory centres located in the brainstem. From these sites, impulses travel along the spinal cord to the nerves that control the diaphragm and intercostal muscles. Reflex responses and chemical signals control these nerve centres and thus the rate of breathing. During actions such as speaking and swallowing, impulses from the throat are conveyed to the respiratory centre and breathing stops temporarily. The chemical control of breathing mainly depends on the level of carbon dioxide in the blood. The presence of excess carbon dioxide causes the respiratory rate to increase until the excess carbon dioxide is eliminated. Conversely, a decreased carbon dioxide level slows the respiratory rate.

Factors affecting respiratory function

Factors that affect the process of respiration include:

- **Availability of oxygen**. Oxygen makes up 20% of the air and normally this is sufficient to meet the needs of the body, but a decrease in this amount of oxygen can cause problems. Two instances where the available oxygen may be deficient are:

- High altitude. The total pressure of all gases in the air decreases at high altitude. As the total pressure decreases, the oxygen pressure decreases proportionately, and people experience difficulty in obtaining adequate oxygen until they become acclimatised. As a result, the respiratory rate is increased in an attempt to supply the body with sufficient oxygen
- The presence of noxious gases. Noxious gases in the air displace the oxygen and reduce the amount normally available for inspiration.

- **Regulating mechanisms**. Any factor that interferes with the control mechanisms for breathing may cause respiratory difficulties. Respirations may be depressed by factors that reduce the activity of the respiratory centre; for example, cerebral oedema or medications such as morphine. Respirations increase when the pH of the blood is lowered, as a respiratory response to rid the body of the excess acid.
- **Passage of oxygen and carbon dioxide**. The efficiency of respiration can be affected by any factor that obstructs the patency of the respiratory tract or the actions of the respiratory muscles. For example, an accumulation of secretions resulting from a reduced cough reflex. Respirations may be reduced by factors that affect the actions of the respiratory muscles, for example, injury or disease that restricts the movements of the diaphragm.
- **Diffusion of oxygen and carbon dioxide**. Any dysfunction of the lungs (e.g. pulmonary oedema, asthma or chronic obstructive airways disease) may impede the transfer of oxygen and carbon dioxide. (Information on these and other respiratory disorders is provided in Chapter 38.)
- **Transport of oxygen and carbon dioxide to and from the cells**. Any condition affecting the efficiency of the heart, the blood vessels or the blood can interfere with the transportation of oxygen to the cells and carbon dioxide away from the cells. Such conditions include congestive cardiac failure, atherosclerosis and anaemia. (Information on these and other cardiovascular disorders is provided in Chapter 38.)
- **Influences on the rate, depth and rhythm of breathing**. Several factors influence the characteristics of breathing; for example, the degree of physical activity. Oxygen requirements are greatest during exertion and least during sleep. The respiratory rate and depth vary in response to the body's demand for oxygen; for example, during strenuous exercise the volume of air drawn into the lungs with each breath may be increased from the usual 500 mL to as much as 4000 mL. Changes in mood or emotion may also affect the rate, depth and rhythm of ventilation. For example, the respiration rate is commonly increased during anxiety, pain or anger. Smoking also affects breathing and often causes short-term effects such as coughing and shortness of breath, or long-term effects such as severe dyspnoea, resulting from emphysema.

ASSESSING RESPIRATIONS

A client's respiratory status is assessed to ascertain whether they are receiving an adequate supply of oxygen to meet their body's needs. Assessment is made by observing them for signs and symptoms of an inadequate oxygen supply, identifying any deviations from normal and by assessing their respirations. Assessing respiratory status and identifying any actual or potential problems are assisted by obtaining information from the client regarding:

- Allergic reactions, such as coughing, sneezing or shortness of breath that occur as a result of exposure to allergens such as dust, pet hairs or pollen
- Exposure to environmental air pollutants such as chemical wastes
- Smoking habits
- Presence of a cough and/or the production of sputum
- Chest pain.

It is important to observe the skin colour for signs of cyanosis. *Cyanosis* is a bluish discolouration of the skin and mucous membranes due to inadequate oxygenation and can be either peripheral or central. Peripheral cyanosis is caused by local vasoconstriction and is usually visible only in the nail beds and sometimes the lips. Central cyanosis is the result of prolonged hypoxia (diminished availability of oxygen to the body tissues) and affects all body organs. It is most visible in highly vascular areas such as the lips, nail beds, tip of the nose, the external ear and the underside of the tongue. In people with naturally dark brown or black skin, cyanosis can be most readily detected by inspecting the mucosa inside the lips.

The client should be observed for signs and symptoms of hypoxia. Hypoxia may result from disorders that limit the volume of air entering the lungs or from obstructive lung diseases such as asthma and emphysema. The signs and symptoms of hypoxia and respiratory distress include:

- Elevated blood pressure and pulse rate
- Shortness of breath and fatigue
- Cyanosis
- Abnormal ventilations
- Use of accessory muscles during breathing and flaring of the nares
- Retraction of the sternum and intercostal muscles
- Apprehension or agitation
- Confusion or reduced level of consciousness
- Visible perspiration.

A person who has a chronic respiratory disorder should also be observed for a barrel-shaped chest, which is a thoracic deformity commonly associated with chronic obstructive airways disease. When chronic hypoxia exists, a person experiences general fatigue and intolerance to exercise and may have clubbing of the fingers.

Assessing respirations provides information about the

client's respiratory status and aids in evaluating airway patency, the status of the respiratory muscles and the client's metabolic state. Clients have their respirations assessed, together with their other vital signs, when they are admitted to hospital. The frequency with which respirations are subsequently assessed depends on how closely the client's condition needs to be monitored. Residents in long-term care facilities commonly have their respirations assessed less often than acutely ill clients, whose condition may need to be monitored at intervals ranging from every 30 minutes to six times a day.

Respirations are assessed without the client's knowledge by noting the rise and fall of the chest. If a person is aware that their respirations are being assessed they may become conscious of them and may unintentionally change their character. The nurse may assess the respirations by observing the person or by placing a hand on the client's chest to feel the rise and fall. To avoid making the client aware that their respirations are being assessed, the nurse may place fingers on the person's radial pulse site and continue as if counting the pulse.

Respirations are assessed for rate, rhythm, depth and sound:

- **Rate**. The respiratory rate is the number of respirations per minute. One inhalation and one exhalation equals one respiration (Figure 21.12). The rate of respiration varies according to age, level of activity and emotions. The normal respiratory rates according to age are about 30–60/min for a newborn, 28–40/min for an infant, 20–28/min for a child, 12–20/min for an adult
- **Rhythm**. The rhythm of respiration is the pattern or regularity of breathing. Normal respirations are evenly spaced, with little variation from one breath to another
- **Depth**. Depth of respirations depends on the volume of air being inhaled and exhaled with each respiration. The depth should be constant with each breath and is assessed by observing the client's chest movement for adequate expansion. Respirations are described as being normal, shallow or deep
- **Sound**. Normal respirations are inaudible.

Table 21.5 gives guidelines for measuring respirations.

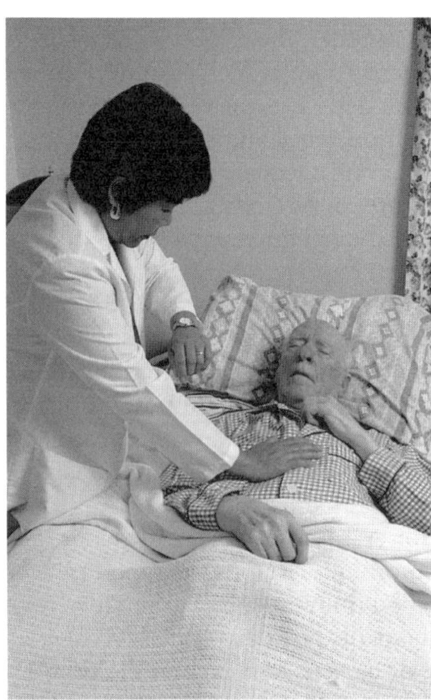

Figure 21.12 | Measuring respirations *(deWit 2005)*

> **CLINICAL INTEREST BOX 21.6**
> **Respiration in older adults**
>
> - Ageing causes ossification of costal cartilage and downward slanting of ribs, resulting in a more rigid rib cage, which reduces chest wall expansion
> - Depth of respirations tend to decrease with ageing

ALTERATIONS IN RESPIRATIONS

Many factors may cause alterations to the rate, rhythm, depth or sound of respirations and deviation from the acceptable range and pattern.

Rate

An increase in the rate above the acceptable range is called *tachypnoea* and may occur as a result of physical exercise; states such as fear, pain, anxiety, excitement or anger; disease states such as fever, infection, respiratory disorders, thyrotoxicosis and congestive cardiac failure. A decrease in the rate below the acceptable range is called *bradypnoea* and may occur as a result of absolute rest or sleep, trauma to the brain, uraemia, diabetic coma, or medications that depress the respiratory centre, such as morphine.

Rhythm

The normal regular pattern of breathing may be altered by a variety of disease states. In obstructive airways disease, such as asthma, chronic bronchitis or emphysema, there is a prolonged expiratory phase. In heart failure or increased intracranial pressure, *Cheyne–Stokes breathing* may occur. This is an abnormal pattern characterised by periods of apnoea. The cycle of Cheyne–Stokes breathing begins with slow shallow breaths that gradually increase in depth and rate. Breathing then gradually becomes slower and more shallow, culminating in a 10–60 second period without ventilation (apnoea), before the cycle is repeated.

Depth

If a person inhales and exhales only small amounts of air, the respirations are described as shallow. *Hypoventilation* is the term used to describe a reduced rate and depth of ventilation, and may occur as a result of a decreased response of the respiratory centre to carbon dioxide, or in respiratory disorders such as bronchitis or atelectasis. Unresolved

TABLE 21.5 | GUIDELINES FOR MEASURING RESPIRATIONS

Action	Rationale
Review and carry out the standard steps in Appendix 1	
Ensure that the individual is resting in a position of comfort	Exercise or discomfort alters the nature of respirations
Check client's previous baseline respirations	It is important to know the client's usual respiration rate to compare changes with that measurement
Using a watch with a second hand, without changing the position of your hand on the pulse and without the client's knowledge, count the respirations for 1 minute	Maintaining the same position keeps client from being aware that you are counting respirations. Inconspicuous assessment prevents client from consciously or unintentionally altering rate and depth of breathing. The intervals between respirations may be inconsistent, and counting for a full minute enables an accurate measurement of rate
Place client's arm (or your hand) in relaxed position across the abdomen or lower chest, directly over client's upper abdomen	Client's or nurse's hand rises and falls during the respiratory cycle, which makes it easier to count the respirations
While measuring the rate, also observe the rhythm, depth and sound of respirations	A complete assessment of respirations is necessary
If rhythm is regular, count number of respirations in 30 seconds and multiply by 2. If rhythm is greater than 16 respirations per minute, count for a full minute	Respiratory rate is equivalent to number of respirations per minute. Suspected irregularities require assessment for at least 1 minute
Document the time of measurement and the rate and character of the respirations on the appropriate chart using numbers or dots	A record of the respirations provides information about the client's condition to members of the health team
Report any deviations from usual acceptable ranges	Appropriate care may be planned and implemented
Special note: Occasional periods of apnoea are a symptom of underlying disease in the adult and must be reported to the medical officer or nurse in charge. Irregular respirations and short episodes of apnoea are normal in a newborn.	
(deWit 2005; Elkin et al 2008)	

hypoventilation results in hypoxia and increased amounts of carbon dioxide in the blood.

When large amounts of air are inhaled and exhaled the respirations are described as deep. *Kussmaul's breathing* is the term used to describe abnormally deep, very rapid, sighing respirations. This pattern of breathing may occur as a result of disorders such as renal failure or metabolic acidosis.

Dyspnoea is the term used to describe shortness of breath or difficulty in breathing and may occur after strenuous exercise (temporarily) or as a result of certain respiratory or cardiac disorders. Dyspnoea is commonly accompanied by hypoventilation or hyperventilation.

Hyperventilation is the term used to describe rapid deep breathing. Sustained hyperventilation, which is sometimes a consequence of extreme anxiety, causes loss of carbon dioxide and a decrease in carbonic acid concentration in the blood. This can cause alkalosis to occur.

Orthopnoea is the term used to describe the condition in which an individual must sit up or stand to breathe deeply or comfortably. This condition occurs in various respiratory or cardiac disorders, such as emphysema, pulmonary oedema and asthma.

Pursed-lip breathing is a technique commonly employed by people with severe dyspnoea or orthopnoea, for example, as a consequence of emphysema. This technique of breathing funnels expired air through a narrow opening, thus creating a positive back pressure on the airways to keep them open.

Sound

Abnormal breath sounds can occur when air passes through narrowed airways or moisture or when there is inflammation of the lungs or pleura.

Stertorous breathing is the term used to describe laboured respirations that have a snoring sound, which commonly result from an obstructed airway.

Wheezing results from narrowed airways, such as in asthma, and respirations sound high pitched and squeaking.

Bubbling refers to gurgling sounds heard as air passes through moist secretions in the respiratory tract.

Crackles refers to an abnormal non-musical sound heard on auscultation of the lungs during inspiration. Sounds like hair rubbed between the fingers next to the ear (deWit 2005).

Stridor results from an obstruction or spasm in the trachea or larynx, as in laryngotracheobronchitis (croup), in which the respirations have a high-pitched musical sound, particularly on inspiration.

CLINICAL INTEREST BOX 21.7
Nursing diagnoses using respiratory assessment data as defining characteristics

- Activity intolerance
- Airway clearance, ineffective
- Anxiety
- Breathing pattern, ineffective
- Gas exchange, impaired
- Pain
- Tissue perfusion, altered

When the nurse is assessing a client's breathing, any deviations from the acceptable range and sound should be reported immediately so that appropriate actions can be planned and implemented. Respiration rates are documented using numbers or dots on a chart similar to the one illustrated in Figure 21.6.

In certain circumstances an instrument called a spirometer is used to assess pulmonary function by measuring and recording the volume of inhaled and exhaled air. Clinical Interest Box 21.7 outlines the possible nursing diagnoses for alterations in respirations.

PULSE OXIMETRY — MEASURING OXYGEN SATURATION

Pulse oximetry is the non-invasive measurement of arterial blood oxygen saturation; that is, the extent to which haemoglobin is loaded with oxygen and is expressed as a percentage; for example an SaO_2 indicates that 96% of the haemoglobin molecules are carrying oxygen molecules. A pulse oximeter is a probe with a light-emitting diode (LED) connected by cable to an oximeter. Light waves emitted by the LED are absorbed then reflected back by oxygenated and deoxygenated haemoglobin molecules. The reflected light is processed by the oximeter, which calculates pulse oxygen saturation (SpO_2).

SpO_2 is a reliable estimate of arterial oxygen saturation and is a simple painless measurement (Figure 21.13). The nurse usually attaches a non-invasive sensor to the client's finger, toe or bridge of nose. In addition, sensors for infants and children can be applied to the palm or the sole of the foot. Spot check oximetry readings have little clinical value. Trends over time provide the best information about the client's oxygenation. The measurement though can be affected by factors that affect light transmission, such as outside light sources or client motion. Avoid direct sunlight or fluorescent lighting when using an oximeter. Conditions that decrease arterial blood flow such as peripheral vascular disease, hypothermia, medications, hypotension or peripheral oedema affect accurate determination of SpO_2 (see Clinical Interest Boxes 21.8 and 21.9). Guidelines for measuring oxygen saturation are outlined in Table 21.6.

CLINICAL INTEREST BOX 21.8
Pulse oximetry in older adults

Identifying an acceptable pulse oximeter probe site may be difficult with older adults because of the likelihood of peripheral vascular disease, decreased carbon dioxide level, cold-induced vasoconstriction and anaemia.

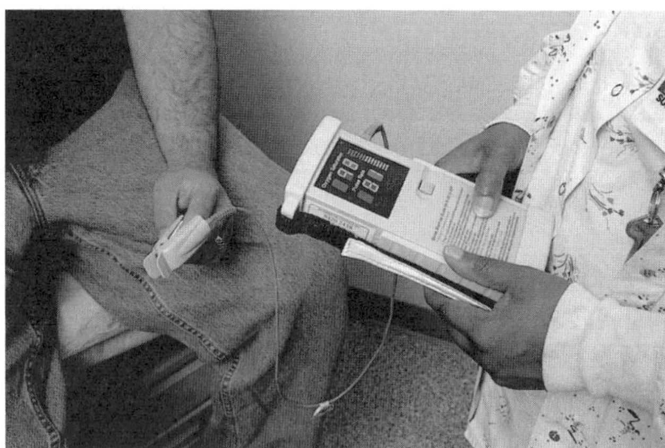

Figure 21.13 | Pulse oximetry *(deWit 2005)*

BLOOD PRESSURE

Measuring blood pressure provides significant information about the individual's cardiovascular function. A series of blood pressure measurements may show the development of a trend and is therefore more significant than a single measurement. Blood pressure is the force exerted by the blood on the walls of the blood vessels as the heart contracts

CLINICAL INTEREST BOX 21.9
Factors affecting determination of pulse oxygen saturation

Interference with Light Transmission

- Outside light sources can interfere with the oximeter's ability to process reflected light.
- Carbon monoxide (caused by smoke inhalation or poisoning) artificially elevates SpO_2 by absorbing light similar to oxygen.
- Client motion can interfere with the oximeter's ability to process reflected light.
- Jaundice may interfere with the oximeter's ability to process reflected light.
- Intravascular dyes (methylene blue) absorb light similar to deoxyhaemoglobin and artificially lower saturation.

Reduction of Arterial Pulsations

- Peripheral vascular disease (Raynaud's disease, atherosclerosis) can reduce pulse volume.
- Hypothermia at assessment site decreases peripheral blood flow.
- Pharmacological vasoconstrictors (epinephrine, phenylnephrine, dopamine) will decrease peripheral pulse volume.
- Low cardiac output and hypotension decrease blood flow to peripheral arteries.
- Peripheral oedema can obscure arterial pulsation.

(Elkin et al 2008)

TABLE 21.6 | GUIDELINES FOR MEASURING OXYGEN SATURATION

Action	Rationale
Review and carry out the standard steps in Appendix 1	
Instruct client to breathe normally	Prevents large fluctuations in respiration and possible error in reading
If finger is to be used, remove nail polish	Opaque coatings decrease light transmission
Determine capillary refill at site. If less than 3 seconds, select alternative site	Cool temperature with vasoconstriction or vascular disease may decrease circulation, impede refill, and prevent sensor from measuring SpO_2
Position client comfortably. If finger is chosen as monitoring site, support lower arm. Instruct client to keep sensor probe site still	Movement interferes with SpO_2 determination. Pressure of sensor probe's spring tension on finger or earlobe may be uncomfortable
Attach sensor probe to monitoring site	Select sensor site based on peripheral circulation and extremity temperature
Turn on oximeter by activating power and observe pulse waveform. Correlate oximeter pulse rate with client's radial pulse	Enables detection of valid pulse
Read SpO_2 on digital display	Reading may take from 10 to 30 seconds
If continuous SpO_2 monitoring is planned, verify SpO_2 alarm limits, which are preset by the manufacturer at a low of 85% and a high of 100%. Limits for SpO_2 and pulse rate should be determined as indicated by client's condition. Verify that alarms are on, assess skin integrity under sensor every 2 hours. Relocate sensor at least every 4 hours, and more frequently if skin integrity is altered	Spring tension of sensor of sensitivity to disposable sensor adhesive can cause skin irritation and lead to disruption of skin integrity
If intermittent or spot-checking SpO_2 measurements are planned, remove sensor probe and turn oximeter power off. Store sensor probe in appropriate location	Sensor probes are expensive and vulnerable to damage
Discuss findings with client as needed	Promotes participation in care and understanding of health status
Remove probe and turn oximeter power off	Maintains battery charge
Assist client in returning to comfortable position	Restores comfort and promotes sense of wellbeing
Wash hands	Reduces risk of transmission of microorganisms

Special Note:

- Do not attach probe to finger, ear or bridge of nose if area is oedematous or skin integrity is compromised. Do not attach sensor to fingers that are hypothermic. Do not place sensor on same extremity as electronic blood pressure cuff. Blood flow to finger will be temporarily interrupted when cuff inflates and cause inaccurate blood pressure reading that triggers alarm.
- If oximeter pulse rate, client's radial pulse rate and apical pulse rate are different, re-evaluate oximeter sensor placement and reassess pulse rates

(deWit 2005; Elkin et al 2008)

and relaxes. The pressure that the blood exerts against arterial walls during contraction of the left ventricle is called the systolic pressure. Diastolic pressure is the arterial pressure during left ventricular relaxation, and is a measurement of the minimum pressure being exerted on the arterial walls.

Blood pressure is maintained by the complex interaction of the body's homeostatic mechanisms and is related to:

- Cardiac output
- The force of ventricular contractions
- The viscosity (thickness) of the blood
- Peripheral vascular resistance
- Elasticity of blood vessel walls.

Blood pressure exerts force on the walls of arteries, veins and on the chambers of the heart. Usually arterial blood pressure is measured and involves measuring the systolic and diastolic pressures. It is generally measured by a non-invasive or indirect method, using a manometer and a stethoscope. It may also be measured directly by the insertion of a probe or catheter into a blood vessel. Blood pressure varies according to age, time of day, body posture and emotions.

ASSESSING BLOOD PRESSURE

Indirect blood pressure measurement is made using one of several devices (Figure 21.14), which include:

- The sphygmomanometer, which includes a pressure

manometer, an occlusive cloth or vinyl cuff that encloses an inflatable rubber bladder, and a pressure bulb with a release valve that inflates the bladder.
- An electronic device, where the measurement is displayed on a screen.

The sphygmomanometer consists of a cloth-covered rubber bag (the cuff) from which two rubber tubes extend. One of the tubes is connected to a hand-operated bulb that has a valve which can be tightened and released. The second tube is connected to the manometer, that registers millimetre calibrations. Thus, blood pressure is measured in millimetres of mercury (mmHg). Blood pressure cuffs come in various sizes because the bladder must be the correct width and length for the client's arm (Figure 21.15). If the bladder is too narrow, the blood pressure reading will be erroneously elevated; if it is too wide, the reading will be erroneously low (Berman et al 2007). Blood pressure is not a routine part of assessment in children under age 3.

Avoid speaking to the client for at least 1 minute before initiating a blood pressure recording. Talking to a client when the blood pressure is being assessed can increase readings 10–40%.

ELECTRONIC BLOOD-PRESSURE DEVICES

These devices are sometimes applied when frequent blood pressure assessment is required, such as in the critically ill or potentially unstable client. The system includes either a microphone or a pressure sensor built into the inflatable cuff. The microphone or acoustic system hears Korotkoff sounds and registers diastolic and systolic readings. The pressure sensor or ultrasonic system responds to the pressure waves generated by the movement of blood through the artery.

Korotkoff sounds are sounds heard during the taking of blood pressure using a sphygmomanometer and stethoscope. In some clients, the sounds are clear and distinct, whereas in others, only the beginning and ending sounds are heard.

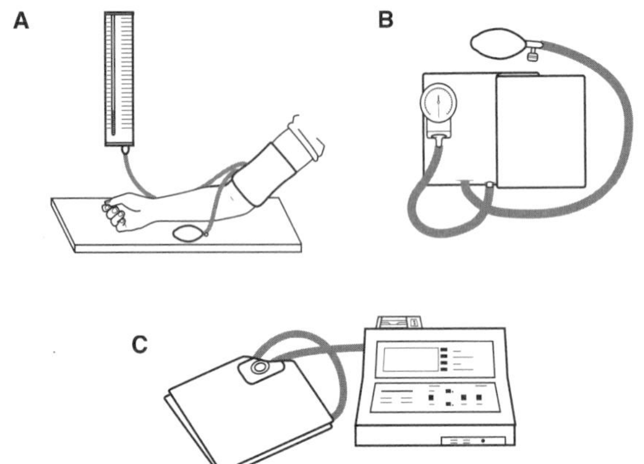

Figure 21.14 | Devices for measuring blood pressure
A: Mercury manometer and cuff
B: Aneroid manometer and cuff
C: Electronic sphygmomanometer

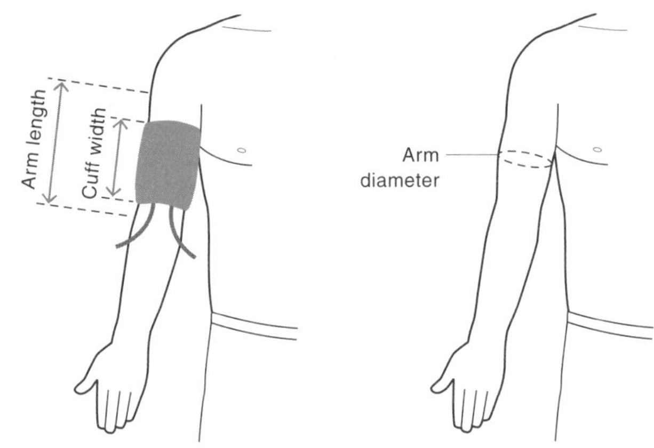

Figure 21.15 | Guidelines for proper blood pressure cuff size Cuff width = 20% more than upper arm diameter, or 40% of circumference and two-thirds of arm length *(adapted from Perry & Potter 2008)*

As air is released from the cuff, pressure on the brachial artery is decreased and the blood is heard pulsing through the vessel. These sounds are described in phases:
- **Phase I:** — systolic pressure indicated by a sharp thump
- **Phase II:** — A blowing or whooshing sound that increases as the cuff is deflated
- **Phase III:** — crisp intense tapping that occurs with each heartbeat
- **Phase IV:**— a softer blowing sound that fades
- **Phase V:** — silence (deWit 2005; Elkin et al 2008).

A baseline blood pressure should be obtained using the auscultatory method before applying automatic devices. A comparison assists in evaluating a client's status and allows proper programming of the device. The advantages of automatic devices are the ease of use and efficiency when repeated or frequent measurements are indicated. No stethoscope is required. The microphone or pressure sensor must be positioned directly over the artery for proper function.

PALPATION

The indirect palpation technique is useful for clients whose atrial pulsations are too weak to create Korotkoff sounds, such as with severe blood loss and decreased heart contractility. The diastolic pressure is difficult to determine by palpation. When the palpation technique is used, the systolic value and the manner in which it was measured are recorded, for example, RA 90/–, palpated, supine. Clinical Interest Box 21.10 outlines the method for palpating the systolic blood pressure.

ASSESSING BLOOD PRESSURE IN LOWER EXTREMITIES

Dressings, casts, IV catheters, arteriovenous fistulas or shunts and axillary lymph-node dissection can make the upper extremities inaccessible. Blood pressure must then

CLINICAL INTEREST BOX 21.10
Palpating the systolic blood pressure

- Apply blood pressure cuff to the upper arm in the same method as the auscultation method
- Continually palpate the radial artery
- Inflate blood pressure cuff 30 mmHg above the point at which the radial pulse can no longer be palpated
- Release valve and allow mercury to fall 2 mmHg/s
- As soon as the radial pulse is palpable, note the manometer reading, which is the systolic blood pressure

(Perry & Potter 2001)

be measured in the lower extremities. The popliteal artery, palpable behind the knee in the popliteal fossa, is the site for auscultation. The cuff must be wide enough and long enough. Placing the client in a prone position is best, or with the knee flexed slightly for easier access to the artery. The cuff is positioned 2.5 cm above the popliteal artery, with the bladder over the posterior aspect of the mid-thigh (Figure 21.16). Systolic pressure in the legs is usually higher by 10–40 mmHg than in the brachial artery, but the diastolic pressure is the same.

BLOOD PRESSURE SITES

The site commonly used to measure arterial blood pressure indirectly is the brachial artery in the antecubital fossa at the elbow joint (Figure 21.17). Less commonly, it may be measured at the popliteal artery behind the knee. Guidelines for measuring blood pressure are outlined in Table 21.7.

Blood pressure measurements may be recorded using dots on a graph similar to the one illustrated in Figure 21.5, or in longhand. If the longhand method of recording is used, the systolic pressure is recorded above the diastolic pressure, for example, 120/70 mmHg. If taking a client's blood pressure for the first time during the current admission, it should be taken in both arms. There should be a difference of no more than 5–10 mmHg between the arms. The arm found to have the higher pressure should be used for subsequent examinations. Document and record where appropriate which arm to use. Figure 21.18 provides the usual site for measuring blood pressure and placement of the stethoscope diaphragm.

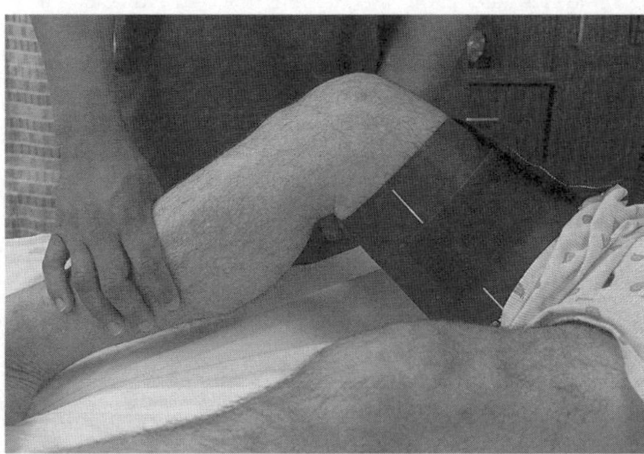

Figure 21.16 | Lower extremity blood pressure cuff positioning *(Potter & Perry 2008)*

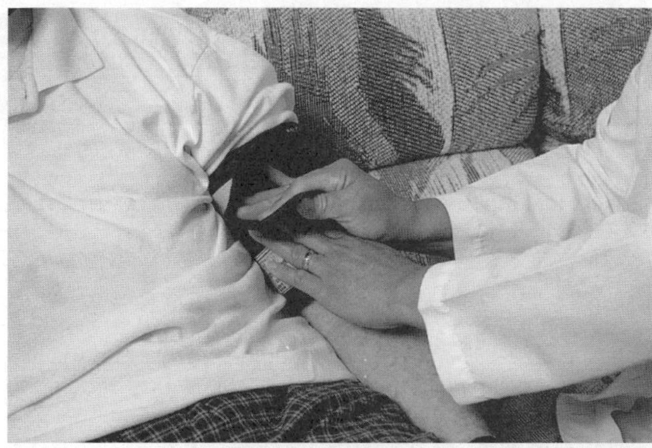

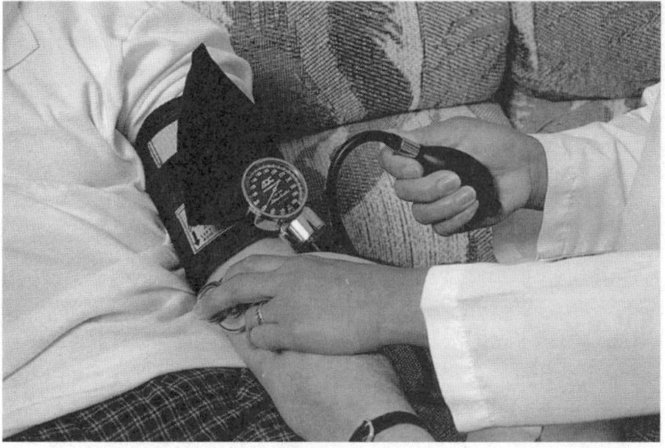

Figure 21.17 | Upper extremity blood pressure cuff positioning *(deWit 2005)*

ALTERATIONS IN BLOOD PRESSURE

It is generally considered that an acceptable systolic blood pressure for an adult is 100–120 mmHg, and acceptable diastolic blood pressure ranges from 60–80 mmHg.

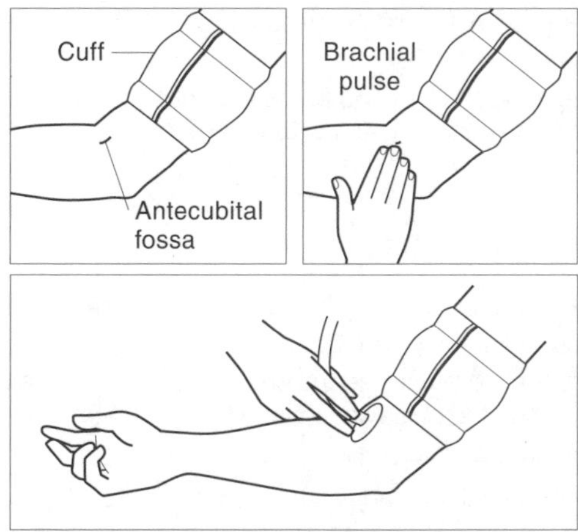

Figure 21.18 | The usual site for measuring blood pressure
The diaphragm of the stethoscope is placed over the brachial artery

TABLE 21.7 | GUIDELINES FOR MEASURING BLOOD PRESSURE

Action	Rationale
Review and carry out the standard steps in Appendix 1	
Ensure that the client is rested and in a position of comfort. Provide privacy and reduce environmental noise	Activity or discomfort may increase blood pressure. Allows you to hear the blood pressure sounds more accurately and puts the client at ease
Remove any constricting clothing from the client's arm. Support the arm in an extended position with the palm facing up. Position the arm so that the brachial artery is at the level of the heart. If sitting, client should be instructed to keep feet flat on floor without legs crossed	Tight clothing may reduce blood flow or create venous congestion in the arm. Correct arm placement enables accurate blood pressure measurement. If arm is extended and not supported, client may perform isometric exercise that can increase diastolic pressure 10%. Placement of arm above the level of the heart causes false-low readings. Placement of arm lower than the level of the heart causes false-high readings. Even in the supine position a diastolic increase of as much as 3 to 4 mmHg can occur for each 5 cm the arm is below the level of the heart
Select an appropriate cuff size	A cuff that is too small may result in a false high reading, while a cuff that is too large may result in a false low reading
Check for air leaks in the cuff, tubing and valves of the sphygmomanometer	Leakage of air may result in an inaccurate measurement
Squeeze the cuff to expel any air, then tighten the valve	Prepares the cuff for use
Two-step method	**Rationale**
Palpate the brachial artery. Position the cuff so that the rubber bag is centred over the brachial artery, with the lower edge of the cuff 2.5–5 cm above the antecubital fossa. Wrap the cuff smoothly and firmly around the upper arm, and secure it in position	Inform the client of the blood pressure. If possible, discuss risk factors for high blood pressure. If blood pressure is elevated, inquire as to any factors that may have affected blood pressure, including general health, life stress, or diet changes. If client takes blood pressure medication, determine if anything has interfered with prescribed regimen.
Position the sphygmomanometer on a level surface, at eye level	An incorrectly placed, or loosely applied, cuff may result in an inaccurate measurement
Palpate the radial pulse and, with the fingers on the pulse, inflate the cuff until the palpated pulse can no longer be felt. Read the pressure reading	Errors in measurement can occur if the manometer is not vertical This measurement provides an approximation of the systolic pressure, and prevents the cuff from subsequently being overinflated
Deflate the cuff	Restores circulation to the arm
Place the disc of the stethoscope over the brachial artery in the antecubital fossa. Reinflate the cuff 30 mmHg above the approximate systolic pressure read during the previous inflation	Pulse beat can be heard when the disc is placed directly over the artery, allowing for precise measurement of the systolic pressure
Use the valve on the hand pump to release air, and slowly deflate the cuff — no faster than 5 mmHg per second	If the cuff is deflated too rapidly, there will be insufficient time to assess the pressure accurately. Deflating too rapidly or too slowly gives false readings. Avoid contact of the stethoscope tubing with the clothing, cuff or tubing of the sphygmomanometer to decrease the possibility of extraneous noise
Note the pressure reading as soon as the pulse beat is heard through the stethoscope	This measurement indicates the systolic pressure
Continue to slowly deflate the cuff. Note the pressure reading as soon as the pulse sounds muffled or disappears	This measurement indicates the diastolic pressure
Deflate the cuff completely	Releases remaining air
Remove the cuff and adjust the individual's clothing	Promotes comfort
Record the measurement immediately	Prevents errors or omissions
Wash and dry hands. Clean earpieces and diaphragm of stethoscope and cuff with alcohol swab	Reduces risk of transmission of microorganisms
Report any deviations from normal	Appropriate care can be planned and implemented

TABLE 21.7 | GUIDELINES FOR MEASURING BLOOD PRESSURE—cont'd

One-step method	Rationale
Place stethoscope earpieces in ears and be sure sounds are clear and not muffled	Ensures each earpiece follows angle of ear canal to facilitate hearing
Relocate brachial artery, and place diaphragm of stethoscope over it. Do not allow chest-piece to touch cuff or clothing	Proper stethoscope placement ensures optimal reception
Close valve of pressure bulb clockwise until tight	Tightening of valve prevents air leak during inflation
Quickly inflate cuff to 30 mmHg above client's usual systolic pressure	Inflation above systolic level ensures accurate measure of systolic pressure
Slowly release pressure bulb valve, and allow manometer needle to fall at a rate of 2–3 mmHg/sec. Note point on manometer when you hear the first sound. The sound will slowly increase in intensity	Too rapid or slow a decline in pressure release causes inaccurate readings. The first Korotkoff sounds reflect systolic pressure
Continue to deflate cuff gradually, noting point at which sound disappears in adults. Note pressure to nearest 2 mmHg. Listen for 20 to 30 mmHg after the last sound, and then allow remaining air to escape quickly	Beginning of the fifth Korotkoff sound is an indicator of diastolic pressure in adults. Fourth Korotkoff sound involves distinct muffling of sounds and is an indication of diastolic pressure in children
Remove the cuff and adjust the individual's clothing	Promotes comfort
Record the measurement immediately	Prevents errors or omissions
Wash and dry hands. Clean earpieces and diaphragm of stethoscope and cuff with alcohol swab	Reduces risk of transmission of microorganisms
Report any deviations from normal	Appropriate care can be planned and implemented
Special note: Inform the client of the blood pressure. If possible, discuss risk factors for high blood pressure. If blood pressure is elevated, inquire as to any factors that may have affected blood pressure, including general health, life stress, or diet changes. If client takes blood pressure medication, determine if anything has interfered with prescribed regimen.	
(deWit 2005; Elkin et al 2008)	

Commonly, systolic pressure is regarded as being elevated when it is higher than 120 mmHg, and diastolic pressure elevated when it is above 80 mmHg (Clinical Interest Box 21.11).

The significance of a recorded blood pressure level can only be reliably assessed in the knowledge of previous levels, and in relation to the client's current health state. For example, a person with a blood pressure of 95/60 mmHg may be perfectly healthy. Conversely, a person displaying signs of clinical shock but with a blood pressure of 135/90 mmHg may normally have a blood pressure exceeding this level.

At times it may be necessary to measure the blood pressure with the client assuming first a lying then a standing position, particularly if the client is on certain medications and/or has certain cardiovascular problems. It is important to report and document any differences observed between the two measurements.

If the blood pressure is to be measured frequently, for example, every half hour, the cuff may be left on the person's arm but, after each measurement, the nurse must ensure that the cuff is deflated completely. Care must be taken to avoid inflating the cuff repeatedly within a short time, as this action may result in venous congestion and cause the client pain.

Hypertension is the term used to describe an elevated arterial blood pressure. Hypertension is a feature of many disease states but frequently its cause is unclear. When no cause can be detected, hypertension is described as 'essential'. The potential for onset of hypertension increases with obesity, smoking, a family history of high blood pressure, or high serum sodium or cholesterol levels. Hypertension is associated with cardiac enlargement, heart failure, coronary artery disease and cerebrovascular accidents. Sustained hypertension is associated with a high mortality rate, so the importance of preventing and controlling hypertension is considerable.

Hypotension is the term used to describe a low blood pressure in relation to the client's usual pressure. Hypotension is associated with low cardiac output states,

CLINICAL INTEREST BOX 21.11
Hypertension in older adults

Hypertension is common in older adults. An older adult's blood pressure range is usually 140–160/80–90 mmHg. Systolic blood pressure is a better predictor of coronary heart disease, heart failure and stroke than is diastolic blood pressure.

Older adults are instructed to change position slowly and pause after each change to avoid postural hypotension and to prevent injuries.

CLINICAL INTEREST BOX 21.12
Nursing diagnoses using blood pressure data as defining characteristics

- Activity intolerance
- Anxiety
- Cardiac output, decreased
- Fluid volume deficit
- Injury, risk for
- Pain
- Tissue perfusion, altered

for example, left ventricular failure, and with hypovolaemic and cardiogenic shock. With sustained hypotension the blood pressure is not adequate for normal tissue perfusion and oxygenation and may result in renal failure. Clinical Interest Box 21.12 outlines the possible nursing diagnoses for alterations in blood pressure.

SUMMARY

Vital signs reflect changes in body function that otherwise might not be observed. Various sites and methods can be used to assess vital signs, and the nurse selects the site and method that is safest for the client and that will provide the most accurate measurement possible. It is important to note that changes in one vital sign can trigger changes in other vital signs.

Vital signs are generally assessed when a client is admitted to a health care agency, to establish baseline data, and when there is a change or possibility of change in the client's condition. Data obtained from measurements of vital signs are then used to plan and implement appropriate nursing interventions. Measurements of vital signs are also used to evaluate a client's response to nursing interventions or prescribed medical therapy. It is important for the nurse to have knowledge of the normal ranges of vital signs and of the factors that regulate and influence vital signs, as this helps the nurse interpret the measurements that deviate from normal (Berman et al 2007).

REVIEW EXERCISES

1. What are the factors that can affect vital signs?
2. What are the advantages and disadvantages of using each body-temperature site?
3. What factors are involved in the maintenance of the pulse and blood pressure?
4. What characteristics should be included in a respiratory assessment?
5. What are the normal ranges for all the vital signs across the life span?

CRITICAL THINKING EXERCISES

1. Ms Hill has just given birth to a healthy baby boy. After the delivery she has a postpartum haemorrhage and loses 1200 mL of blood. Would you expect Ms Hill's blood pressure to increase or decrease? State the reason for your choice.
2. Give two reasons for taking a person's lying and standing blood pressure.
3. Mr Russell has just had a cigarette. The medical officer has just asked you to take Mr Russell's vital signs. What would you do? State the reason for your answer.
4. Mrs Seagal, 56, was admitted to your ward for repair of a hip fracture.

In the observation chart below, identify the information described in the following questions, then answer the questions:

Admission obs	T – 36.7,	P – 100,	R – 22,	B/P – 140/90:1600 hrs
Preoperative obs	T – 36.4,	P – 80,	R – 18,	B/P – 130/70:0800 hrs
Postoperative obs	T – 35.8,	P – 60,	R – 16,	B/P – 120/70:1400 hrs
	T – 36.4,	P – 80,	R – 18,	B/P – 130/70:1800 hrs
	T – 36.4,	P – 76,	R – 18,	B/P – 120/70:2000 hrs
Day 1 Post op	T – 36.4,	P – 80,	R – 20,	B/P – 130/70:1000 hrs
	T – 36.4,	P – 80,	R – 20,	B/P – 130/70:1800 hrs
	T – 36.8,	P – 88,	R – 20,	B/P – 130/70:2200 hrs
Day 2 Post op	T – 37.0,	P – 88,	R – 20,	B/P – 130/70:0100 hrs
	T – 37.8,	P – 90,	R – 22,	B/P – 135/80:1400 hrs
	T – 38.5,	P – 90,	R – 22,	B/P – 135/90:2000 hrs
Day 3 Post op	T – 37.4,	P – 88,	R – 22,	B/P – 135/70:0700 hrs

a) Suggest a reason why, on the day of her admission, Mrs Seagal's vital signs were slightly elevated.
b) Suggest a reason why Mrs Seagal's vital signs had decreased on the preoperative assessment.
c) What could you infer from the overall change in vital signs in the postoperative period?
d) What further objective and subjective data would you need to collect to confirm your assumptions?

REFERENCES AND FURTHER READING

Berman AJ, Kozier B, Snyder S (2007) *Kozier and Erbs Fundamentals of Nursing: Concepts, Process, and Practice*, 8th edn. Prentice-Hall, Upper Saddle River, NJ

Crisp J, Taylor C (eds) (2005) *Potter & Perry's Fundamentals of Nursing*, 2nd edn. Elsevier Australia, Sydney

deWit SC (2005) *Fundamental Concepts and Skills for Nursing*, 2nd edn. WB Saunders, Philadelphia

Elkin M, Perry A, Potter P (2008) *Nursing Interventions and Clinical Skills*, 4th edn. Mosby Elsevier, Canada

Perry AG, Potter PA (2001) *Clinical Nursing Skills and Techniques*, 5th edn. Mosby, St Louis

Potter PA, Perry AG (2008) *Fundamentals of Nursing*, 7th edn. Elsevier Mosby, St Louis

ONLINE RESOURCE

Changes in vital signs with ageing: www.nlm.nih.gov/medlineplus/ency/article/004019.htm

Chapter 22

ADDITIONAL CLINICAL MEASUREMENTS

OBJECTIVES

- Define the key terms/concepts
- Understand the factors that affect urinary elimination
- Demonstrate the ability to measure urine output, perform urinalysis, report and record results of urine tests accurately
- Explain factors that affect blood glucose levels and note the significance of deviations from normal
- Demonstrate the ability to perform and record blood glucose levels safely and accurately
- Identify deviations from usual body weight and their possible causes
- Demonstrate the ability to measure, report and record body weight accurately

KEY TERMS/CONCEPTS

bilirubinuria
blood glucose levels
glycosuria
haematuria
hyperglycaemia
hypoglycaemia
ketones
ketonuria
protein
proteinuria
urinalysis

CHAPTER FOCUS

Clinical measurement procedures provide important information about complex chemical reactions that affect the physiological functioning of the body. Laboratory examinations of blood, urine and other body fluids provide accurate information about the function of various organs and physiological mechanisms. This information is helpful in making or confirming a diagnosis or in evaluating the effectiveness of a treatment. This chapter introduces basic information about common clinical measurements and procedures (additional to vital signs) that help in the assessment of a client who enters a health care facility.

LIVED EXPERIENCE

My grandfather, James, is 88 years old and sometimes we have to test his blood glucose 2–4 times a day. He was starting to lose sensitivity in his fingertips from the frequent finger-sticks and was becoming very distressed. The nurse told us about a glucometer that allows testing from alternative sites. We have bought one and it is so much better.

Rebecca, James's granddaughter

URINALYSIS

ELIMINATION OF URINE

The elimination of urine, or voiding, should be voluntary and painless. The frequency with which urine is passed varies with each individual. Factors that affect the frequency of voiding and the volume of urine include fluid input, bladder capacity, response to the need to void and the availability of toilet facilities. The frequency of voiding, and often the amount of urine voided, can be increased by a large fluid input, fear or anxiety, exposure to a cold environment, and some disease states, and decreased by a low fluid input, exposure to a hot environment, and some disease states.

Urine is composed of 96% water, 2% urea and 2% mineral salts. Normal urine has the following characteristics:

- It is voided without pain or discomfort
- It is clear and light-amber in colour
- It has a slight aromatic odour that increases when left to stand
- It has a pH of between 4.5 and 8.0; that is, slightly acidic (average is 6.0). pH is a scale representing the relative acidity or alkalinity of a solution, with the numerical value indicating the concentration of hydrogen ions. A value of 7.0 is neutral, below 7.0 is acid, and above 7.0 is alkaline
- It has a specific gravity of between 1.005 and 1.030. Specific gravity is a measure of the concentration of particles in the urine and reflects the ability of the kidneys to concentrate or dilute urine
- It is excreted in amounts of between 1000 mL and 2000 mL in 24 hours.

COLLECTION OF A URINE SAMPLE

The nurse may be required to collect urine for observation or testing in the ward, or so that a specimen can be sent to the laboratory for analysis. Key aspects related to the collection of urine include:

- Thorough washing and drying of the hands before and after collection to prevent cross-infection
- The container in which the urine is collected must be clean, and in some instances sterile, to ensure collection of a specimen free from external contamination
- If testing or laboratory analysis is required, contamination of the container and urine must be prevented throughout the procedure
- Adequate information about the client and the specimen must be provided. The label on the specimen container must contain the client's name, registration number, the date and time of collection and the method used to collect the specimen; for example, catheter specimen of urine. When a specimen is despatched for laboratory analysis it must be accompanied by the medical officer's request form. The medical officer requests the collection of a specimen and indicates on the form the specific laboratory tests to be performed
- Specimens must be sent to the laboratory as soon as possible after collection; if there is a delay in despatch, the specimen may require refrigeration
- If the client is responsible for collecting the urine specimen, the nurse should provide the client with information necessary to ensure that the collection is performed correctly.

Avoiding contamination

If urine is to be collected for observation or testing in the ward, the individual is requested to void into a clean bedpan or urinal. The urine should not be contaminated, for example, by faeces or menstrual blood, as a false assessment may result. The urine is transferred from the toilet utensil into a clean container in preparation for observation or testing.

Timed urine collection

Some tests require urine to be collected over 2–72 hours. The 24-hour timed collection is the most common. All urine excreted during the timed period is collected and sent for laboratory analysis to measure the quantity of various substances present, such as specific hormones. The required equipment consists of: a large-volume, screw-topped labelled container and a jug to transfer urine into the container. A suggested method of collecting a timed urine specimen is outlined in Table 22.1.

Mid-stream urine specimen

The aim of this method of collection is to collect the middle portion of the stream of urine to obtain a sample of urine that is not contaminated by microorganisms from outside the urinary tract. The urine is sent to the laboratory to be tested for the presence of microorganisms and their sensitivity to antimicrobial drugs. The required equipment consists of:

- A sterile container, such as a kidney dish
- Disposable gloves (for the nurse)
- A labelled sterile specimen container
- A completed laboratory request form
- Warm water and cotton wool balls for a perineal wash
- A towel, soap and washcloth
- Provision of appropriate toilet facilities.

A suggested method of collection is outlined in Table 22.2.

It is easiest for a client to obtain a mid-stream voided specimen while using toilet facilities rather than a bedpan or urinal. As most clients will be capable of performing this procedure independently, it is important that they are provided with adequate information about the technique. The nurse performs the procedure if the person is dependent.

Using a collection bag

A urine collection bag may be used to obtain a specimen from a client who is unable to control the flow of urine, for example, a person who is incontinent, unconscious or confused. It is not possible to obtain mid-stream urine

TABLE 22.1 | GUIDELINES FOR TIMED URINE COLLECTION

Action	Rationale
Review and carry out the standard steps in Appendix 1	
The bladder is emptied completely and the urine discarded. Note the time of collection	Collection begins with the bladder empty. Only urine secreted during the time allocated is collected
From the starting time of collection onwards, each specimen of urine voided in the time requested is added to the container	All urine voided in that period is collected to ensure an accurate test result
The container of urine is refrigerated until the collection is complete	Keeping the urine cold helps prevent decomposition
At the end of 24 hours the bladder is emptied and the urine added to the container	The last voiding empties the bladder and completes the 24-hour collection
Encourage client to drink two glasses of water an hour before timed urine collection ends. Ensure that the client is not on restricted fluids	Facilitates client's ability to void at the end of the period
Ensure that the label on the container has all the relevant information. Despatch specimen to the laboratory as soon as possible with the request form, or store specimen in refrigerator	Accurate documentation is necessary to avoid errors
If any of the urine is inadvertently discarded, the collection may need to be abandoned and the procedure restarted	Inaccurate results will be obtained if all urine excreted over the 24-hour period is not acquired
(deWit 2005)	

TABLE 22.2 | GUIDELINES FOR MID-STREAM URINE COLLECTION

Action	Rationale
Review and carry out the standard steps in Appendix 1	
Explain to client and/or family member reason specimen is needed, how client can assist (when applicable), and how to obtain a specimen that is free of tissue and stool	Promotes cooperation and client participation. In some cases client can collect clean-voided specimen independently
Give client or family member towel, wash-cloth and soap to cleanse perineum, or assist client (after application of clean gloves) with cleansing perineum	Clients usually prefer to wash their own perineal area when possible. Prevents external microorganisms from contaminating the specimen
Using surgical asepsis, open outer package of commercial specimen kit	Maintains sterility of specimen container
Apply sterile gloves	Prevents introduction of microorganisms into urine specimen from nurse's hands
Client voids 30–60 mL of urine into the toilet or toilet utensil	Flushes any residual microorganisms out of the urethra
Collect the next 20–30 mL of urine in a sterile container, e.g. sterile kidney dish	This is the middle stream of urine and is the portion sent for analysis
The person completes voiding into the toilet or toilet utensil	The remainder of the urine is not required for collection
Pour collected urine specimen into labelled sterile specimen container and remove gloves	Prevents cross-infection
Despatch specimen to the laboratory as soon as possible with the request form, or store specimen in refrigerator	Decomposition and cell growth occur if urine is left standing, and may provide a false result
The procedure should be documented	Appropriate care can be planned and implemented
Special note: Indicate on laboratory slip if client is menstruating	
(deWit 2005; Elkin et al 2008)	

collection from a child who is not toilet trained; in this case, urine for culture should be obtained by using a sterile plastic urine-collecting bag that adheres to the perineum. The required equipment consists of:

- A collection bag of suitable size (i.e. paediatric or adult)
- A sterile labelled specimen container
- A completed laboratory request form

- Clean disposable gloves and items for cleansing the genital area, such as soap, water, washcloth and towel.

A suggested method of collecting a sample of urine using a collection bag is outlined in Table 22.3.

Collecting a sterile urine specimen from a client with an indwelling urinary catheter

A catheter specimen of urine is obtained from a client who has an indwelling catheter (Figure 22.1). The insertion of a catheter for the sole purpose of obtaining a urine specimen is generally avoided because of the risk of introducing microorganisms into the urinary tract. To reduce this risk when obtaining a specimen of urine from an indwelling catheter, it is important to maintain a closed urinary drainage system. For this reason, collecting a specimen from the end of the catheter connected to the drainage tubing should be avoided. Instead, the urine should be aspirated through the sampling port using a sterile syringe and needle. A urine specimen for culture tests should not be collected from a urinary drainage bag unless it is the first urine to drain into a new sterile bag. Bacteria can ascend up into the drainage bag from surfaces it makes contact with, and grow rapidly. This can give a false measurement of bacteria in the urine.

The equipment necessary consists of a sterile syringe and needle, alcohol swabs or disinfectant swabs, sterile labelled specimen container, completed laboratory request form, clean disposable gloves and a clamp. The recommended method for obtaining a urine specimen from a catheter is outlined in Table 22.4.

If it is not possible to aspirate the urine with a syringe and needle, the catheter may be clamped to allow urine to accumulate in the bladder. The clamp is then released, and the catheter disconnected from the drainage tubing. This must be done using aseptic technique to avoid introducing microorganisms. The area where the catheter joins the drainage tube should be wiped with an alcohol swab. The catheter is disconnected and the urine allowed to drain from it into the sterile specimen container. Avoid touching the inside of the sterile container with the catheter, and do not allow the open ends of the drainage tube or catheter to become contaminated. Both connection sites should be wiped with an alcohol swab before being rejoined. The nurse must thoroughly wash and dry their hands before and after the procedure.

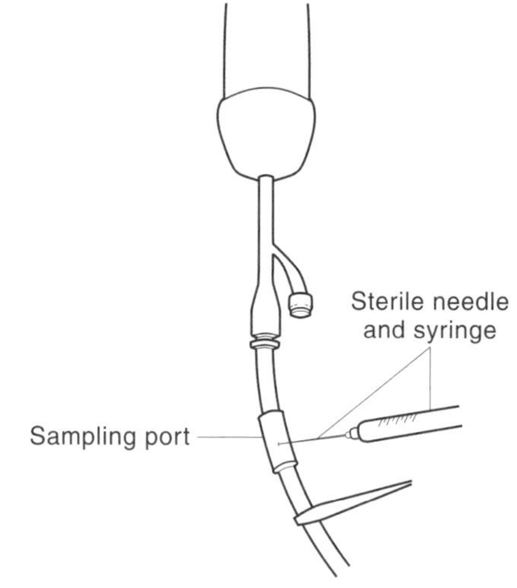

Figure 22.1 | Obtaining a sample of urine from a catheter

TABLE 22.3 | GUIDELINES FOR BAG COLLECTION OF URINE

Action	Rationale
Review and carry out the standard steps in Appendix 1	
Place the person in a supine position if possible	Facilitates application of the bag
Cleanse the perineal area, swabbing towards the anus. Ensure that the urethral meatus is clean and dry	Prevents contamination of the urine by microorganisms from the surrounding skin
Remove the covering from the bag's adhesive surfaces and apply the bag. The bag should enclose the urethral meatus, but not the anus	The bag must be correctly positioned and firmly secured to avoid leakage
Press the adhesive surfaces onto the skin (if necessary, the surrounding skin is shaved before applying the bag)	Promotes adherence of the bag to the skin
Check frequently and gently remove the bag when sufficient urine has been collected	Avoids damage to the skin
Transfer the urine into the specimen container	Prepares specimen for testing or despatch to the laboratory
Reposition the client and adjust the bedclothes to meet needs	Promotes comfort
Despatch specimen to the laboratory as soon as possible with the request form, or store specimen in refrigerator	Decomposition and cell growth occur if urine is left standing
Wash and dry hands	Prevents cross-infection
(deWit 2005)	

TABLE 22.4 | COLLECTING URINE FROM AN INDWELLING URINARY CATHETER

Action	Rationale
Review and carry out the standard steps in Appendix 1	
Explain procedure to client	Minimises anxiety when nurse manipulates catheter and aspirates urine with needle and syringe
Clamp the catheter about 30 minutes before the specimen is to be collected	Allows urine to accumulate in the bladder so that a specimen can be obtained
Wash and dry hands and put on disposable gloves and goggles	Prevents risk of transferring microorganisms
Position client so catheter port is easily accessible. Wipe the sampling port with an alcohol swab	Prevents entry of microorganisms into catheter
Attach the needle to the syringe and insert the needle at 45 degree angle just above where catheter is attached to drainage tube at built-in sampling port in silastic, silicone or plastic catheter into the port. Aspirate the specimen of urine into the syringe and transfer it into the specimen container	The needle should not be inserted into the shaft of the catheter, as this may result in subsequent leakage of urine
Wipe the puncture area on the catheter with an alcohol swab	Prevents entry of microorganisms into catheter
Unclamp the catheter	Allows urine to flow again
Dispose of the used swabs, gloves, syringe and needle safely	Prevents risk of transferring microorganisms and injury
Wash and dry hands	Prevents cross-infection
Despatch specimen to the laboratory as soon as possible with the request form, or store specimen in refrigerator	Prevents decomposition of urine or cell growth

(deWit 2005; Elkin et al 2008)

Suprapubic bladder aspiration

This procedure is not commonly performed but, when necessary, it is performed by a medical officer using sterile equipment and aseptic technique. It involves insertion of a needle through the skin over the suprapubic area into the bladder. A quantity of urine is aspirated, placed in a sterile container and despatched to the laboratory. After this procedure the nurse should observe the puncture site for bleeding, and the urine for the presence of blood.

EXAMINATION OF URINE

To detect and identify abnormalities, urine is examined by observation, by chemical testing in the ward or by analysis in the laboratory. Abnormalities that can be detected by observation are listed in Table 22.5.

URINALYSIS

Testing the urine for abnormalities is referred to as urinalysis and is commonly performed when a person is admitted to a health care facility. The frequency with which it is subsequently performed depends on the client's condition and prescribed management. Chemical reagent strips are used to test urine for several substances at the one time or for one specific substance (Figure 22.2). Urinalysis provides information about:

- The condition and function of the urinary system
- The presence of pathogenic microorganisms in the urinary tract or urine
- The presence of nutrient materials that are normally transported to the body cells but may have been excreted in the urine, e.g. glucose
- The presence of a systemic disease unrelated to disorders of the urinary system
- The acid–base balance of the body.

As urinalysis is an important diagnostic aid and a measure of the effectiveness of certain treatments, accuracy of performance is essential. Key aspects of performing urinalysis are outlined in Table 22.6. The required equipment consists of:

- A clean container of urine
- Paper and pen
- Watch with a second hand
- Clean disposable gloves
- Goggles
- Biochemical testing agents and the manufacturer's colour comparison charts.

A variety of different chemical strips are used to test urine for abnormalities, and the nurse should become familiar with their use. These abnormalities, which can be detected by various tests, and their possible causes are listed in Table 22.7. Urinalysis may also be done with an automated urine chemistry analyser (see Clinical Interest Box 22.1).

STRAINING URINE

Stones, or calculi, are insoluble substances formed from mineral salts that may develop in the kidneys. They can range in size from microscopic, through resembling grains of sand or gravel, to several centimetres in diameter. If it is known or suspected that a client has developed renal

TABLE 22.5 | ABNORMALITIES OF URINE DETECTED BY OBSERVATION

Observation	Deviation from normal	Possible cause
Colour	Pale	High fluid intake, other factors that dilute the urine, such as diuretic medication or disease, e.g. diabetes mellitus
	Dark or brown	Concentrated urine due to dehydration or presence of bile pigment, e.g. in liver or gall bladder disease
	Smokey	Presence of occult blood
	Red	Presence of frank blood
	Bright yellow, blue or green	Specific medications
	Mucus plugs, viscous, thick	White blood cells, bacteria, pus, or contaminants such as prostatic fluid or vaginal discharge may cause cloudy urine
Odour	Ammonia	Decomposing urine
	Foul-smelling 'fishy' odour	Infected urine
	Sweet smelling	Presence of glucose, e.g. in diabetes mellitus
Foreign substances	Pus	Urinary tract infection
	Stones, gravel	Calculi in urinary tract
Amount	Higher than normal in 24 hours	High fluid intake, diuretic medications, diseases, e.g. diabetes mellitus
	Lower than normal in 24 hours	Obstruction to the flow of urine Diseases that reduce the normal production of urine, e.g. renal failure

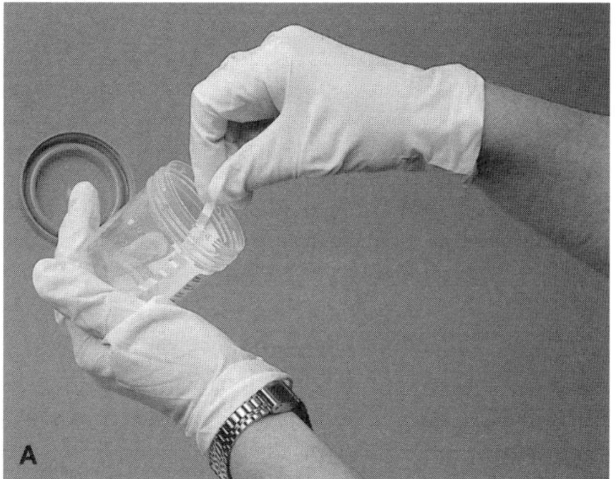

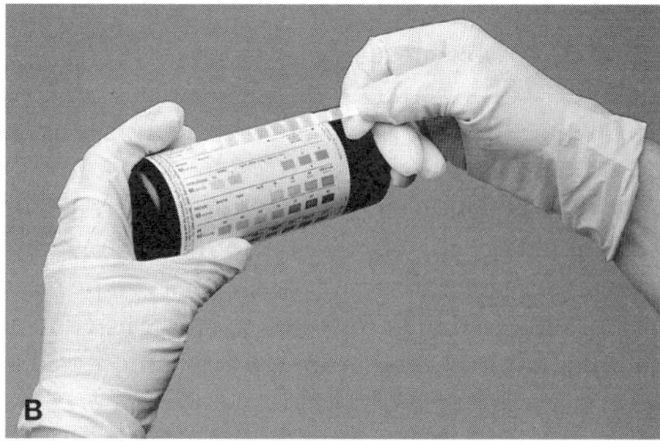

Figure 22.2 | Performing a urinalysis
A: Wet the dipstick with the urine sample, ensuring that each coloured square is moistened
B: Compare the colour on the bottle with the colour of the strip at the correct time interval *(deWit 2005)*

CLINICAL INTEREST BOX 22.1
Automated urinalysis

Automated urine chemistry analysers are becoming prevalent in acute-care facilities. These automated analysers are able to perform urinalysis, hCG (human chorionic gonadotrophin) testing (pregnancy testing) and an albumin-creatinine ratio (ACR), which signifies renal or chronic disease. Samples are analysed automatically and results are usually printed out within 1 minute and can be used to rapidly identify urines that do not need further processing.

The technique involves blotting the reagent strip by dipping it into the urine sample, placing the strip on the test strip table then pressing the start button. The instrument then analyses, displays and prints test results.

calculi, the urine is observed carefully by straining it to detect the passage of stones. Any stones collected are sent for laboratory examination, which reveals their exact composition and helps to identify their cause. The urine is strained by pouring it through a fine substance such as gauze or filter paper.

MONITORING BLOOD GLUCOSE LEVELS

Blood glucose monitoring is an accurate method of assessing the effectiveness of diet, exercise levels and medication therapy and to gain information regarding a client's current blood glucose level. Blood glucose monitoring is performed by obtaining a drop of capillary blood, which is applied to a reagent strip. The colour of the strip is then compared with a standard, either visually or with a reflectance meter. A variety of blood glucose monitoring machines are available,

TABLE 22.6 | GUIDELINES FOR URINALYSIS*

Action	Rationale
Review and carry out the standard steps in Appendix 1	
Wash hands and put on disposable gloves and goggles	Prevents risk of transferring microorganisms and is a standard precaution for handling body fluids
Obtain urine that is free from contamination by faeces, menstrual blood or body secretions and test within 30 minutes	Test results can be affected by the presence of contaminants or changes that occur when urine is left standing
A clean dry container should be used to hold the urine	Contaminants, e.g. disinfectant, can affect test results
Assemble all the required equipment before beginning the test	The procedure should not be interrupted after testing has begun
Immerse chemical reagent strip into urine specimen	Immersion exposes reagent to the urine constituents
Remove strip immediately from container and tap it gently against the container's side. Hold strip in horizontal position	Excess urine can dilute chemical reagent. Prevents mixing of chemical reagents
Follow the manufacturer's instructions regarding the use of biochemical reagents:	
• Check expiry date	Out-of-date chemicals lose their efficiency
• Avoid unnecessary exposure to air, light or moisture	Prevents loss of reactivity
• Avoid contact with the chemical agents by the fingers	Prevents contamination
• Do not transfer reagents from their original bottles into others	Prevents deterioration and loss of reactivity
• Time for number of seconds specified on the container, and compare colour of strip with colour chart	Accurate timing is essential to provide quantitative results
If abnormalities are detected, do not discard the urine until the results have been reported	Further testing may be indicated
Report and document test results immediately	Avoids errors or omissions
Dispose of used chemical tablets or strips. Rinse and clean any containers. Wash and dry hands	Prevents cross-infection

* In older adults, urine testing is considered unreliable because of age-related renal function changes. Also, certain medications, foods and vitamins may discolour the urine and interfere with accurate reading of test results.
(deWit 2005; Elkin et al 2008)

including ones with automatic finger-pricking, which run either on batteries or from mains power (Figure 22.3).

The aim of self blood glucose monitoring is to assist clients with diabetes to assume more independence in managing their condition. Each person using blood glucose monitoring receives individual instruction in the technique, from a diabetes health educator, for example. People with diabetes are advised on the appropriate times at which to perform the test and are shown how to make suitable adjustments to their insulin dose if the blood glucose levels are above or below those recommended. If the nurse is required to perform blood glucose monitoring they should also receive instruction in the technique and should become familiar with the manufacturer's instructions accompanying each monitoring device. Table 22.8 provides guidelines for blood glucose monitoring. Clinical Interest Box 22.2 discusses non-invasive blood glucose monitoring.

CLINICAL INTEREST BOX 22.2
Non-invasive blood glucose monitoring

In March 2001 the US Food and Drug Administration approved a non-invasive blood glucose monitoring device for adults with diabetes. This means that blood glucose levels can be checked without puncturing the skin for a blood sample. The GlucoWatch Biographer was approved to detect glucose level trends and patterns in adults aged 18 and older with diabetes. It must be used along with conventional blood glucose monitoring of blood samples. The device, which looks like a wristwatch, pulls body fluid from the skin using small electric currents. It checks blood glucose levels every 20 minutes.

(National Diabetes Information Clearinghouse 2003)

COLLECTING BLOOD SPECIMENS — VENIPUNCTURE WITH SYRINGE, VENIPUNCTURE WITH VACUTAINER AND BLOOD CULTURES

Blood tests, one of the most commonly used diagnostic measures, yield valuable information about a client's nutritional, haematological, metabolic, immune and biochemical status. These tests allow health care providers to screen clients for early signs of physical illness, monitor changes in acute or chronic diseases, and evaluate responses to therapies. As veins are major sources of blood for both laboratory tests and routes for intravenous (IV) fluid or blood administration, maintaining their integrity is essential. It is

TABLE 22.7 | RESULTS OF URINALYSIS

Test	Normal values	Deviation	Possible causes
pH	4.5–8.0	Elevated (alkaline [above 8.0])	Urinary tract infection, chronic cystitis, metabolic or respiratory alkalosis, acute and chronic renal failure, low-protein diet
		Lowered (acidic [below 4.5])	Diabetic acidosis, fever, pulmonary emphysema, diarrhoea and dehydration, high-protein diet
Specific gravity	1.010–1.030	Elevated (above 1.030)	Low fluid input, vomiting, diarrhoea, hepatic disease, congestive cardiac failure, presence of abnormal substances in the urine, e.g. protein
		Lowered (below 1.010)	High fluid input, diabetes insipidus, certain kidney diseases
Protein (proteinuria)	Nil	Present	Kidney infections
			Acute glomerulonephritis, pyelonephritis, diabetes mellitus (types 1 and 2), acute febrile states, hypertension, congestive cardiac failure
Glucose (glycosuria)	Nil	Present	Diabetes mellitus (types 1 and 2), pancreatitis, pain, Cushing's syndrome, hyperthyroidism, administration of corticosteroids, stress
Ketones (ketonuria)	Nil	Present	Diabetes mellitus (type 1), fever, starvation, pregnancy, trauma, vomiting and diarrhoea
Bilirubin (bilirubinuria)	Nil	Present	Liver disease (hepatitis, cirrhosis), biliary obstruction
Blood (haematuria)	Nil	Present	Urinary tract disease or trauma, acute nephritis, renal calculi, renal carcinoma, use of anticoagulants, chronic kidney infection
Nitrite	Nil	Present	Urinary tract infections, pyelonephritis, cystitis, urethritis
Urobilinogen	0.1–1.0	Elevated (above 1.0)	Liver disorders (cirrhosis, hepatitis), congestive cardiac failure, blood disorders, e.g. haemolytic anaemia, pernicious anaemia, thalassaemia
		Lowered (below 0.1)	Obstruction of the bile duct, antibiotic therapy, cancer of head of pancreas
Leukocytes	Very few	Increased	Urinary tract infection, bacteriuria

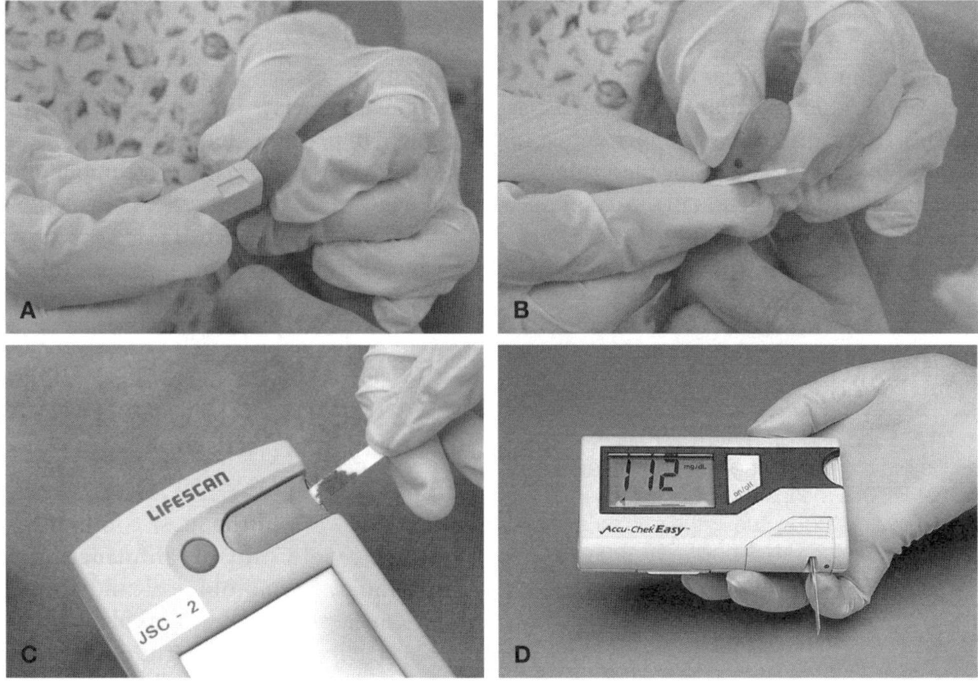

Figure 22.3 | Performing a blood glucose level test

A: Piercing the fingertip **B**: Transferring blood droplet to test pad **C**: Placing reagent strip into meter **D**: Reading meter

(Perry & Potter 2001)

TABLE 22.8 | GUIDELINES FOR MEASURING BLOOD GLUCOSE LEVELS*

Action	Rationale
Review and carry out the standard steps in Appendix 1	
Explain to client what is happening throughout procedure	Promotes participation in care and understanding of health status
Gather all necessary equipment before starting procedure (glucometer, reagent strips, warm washcloth, paper towel, sharps container, disposable gloves, goggles)	Prevents hunting for supplies when ready to perform test
Provide privacy for client if possible and appropriate	Promotes client comfort
Select appropriate puncture site in consultation with client	Ensures free flow of blood after puncture
Dilate the capillaries by applying a warm compress	Promotes vasodilation
Assist client to wash hands with soap and water then dry them	Promotes skin cleansing
Ensure that reagent strip and glucometer are calibrated — check the code on the test strip vial	Some machines must be calibrated so that an accurate reading is obtained. Code on test strip must match code entered into the glucose meter
Check expiry date for reagent strip	Ensures accurate reading is obtained
Choose a vascular area for puncture site. In stable adults, select lateral side of finger; be sure to avoid central tip of finger, which has more dense nerve supply. Hold area to be punctured in a dependent position while gently massaging finger towards puncture site	Increases blood flow to area before puncture
Position lancet correctly (to the side of the finger) and pierce the skin sharply and quickly**	Ensures proper skin penetration
Correctly apply the blood to the reagent patch on the strip	Ensures proper coverage of test pad on reagent strip
Apply correct pressure to the puncture site	Promotes haemostasis
Remove excess blood from the strip according to the manufacturer's instructions	For meter to read glucose levels, some strips must be dry
Place the strip in the glucometer, according to the manufacturer's instructions	Strip must be inserted correctly to obtain an accurate reading
Read the result from the glucometer and compare colour change on the strip with the standardised colour chart on the container	Each meter has a specified time for reading glucose level
Check puncture site for any bleeding before leaving client and apply a band aid to the puncture wound if required	Can be a source of discomfort for the client. Prevents further bleeding and protects wound
Wash hands after procedure and dispose of contaminated equipment, sharps and gloves appropriately	Reduces risk of transmission of infection
Record results accurately on chart and in correct location in client's history. Share the result with the client and then report the observation to the Registered Nurse	Keeps client informed. Documentation provides a record of the reading

* Normal blood glucose reading should read between 3.5 and 8.0 mmol/L.

** The puncture depth of the lancet needle can be adjusted by pushing the lancet further in or pulling it out a little from the holder. This procedure should never be performed without the use of gloves because of the risk of contamination with blood. Small children will need to be held by the parent or another nurse. Children should be told there will be a tiny sting and that they will see a little drop of blood. (Children should always be told the truth.) Having children use a finger puppet on the other hand will sometimes distract them from the procedure sufficiently for them to stay still.

(deWit 2005; Elkin et al 2008)

important to use the most distal sites first, and retain one or more appropriate sites for IV access. Do not draw blood from a site proximal to an IV insertion site. After obtaining a specimen, place it directly into the appropriate blood tube. A colour-coding system for the tops of the collection tubes is used to indicate the type of specimen that can be collected within that tube. Special blood tubes are available, containing anti-coagulants, because some tests cannot be performed on clotted or haemolysed specimens.

Blood cultures aid in the detection of bacteria in the blood. It is important that at least two culture specimens be drawn from two different sites. If only one culture produces bacteria, the assumption is that the bacteria were skin contaminants rather than the infecting agent. Bacteraemia exists when both cultures grow the infectious agent (Elkin et al 2008). Table 22.9 provides guidelines for collecting blood specimens.

TABLE 22.9 | GUIDELINES FOR COLLECTING BLOOD SPECIMENS — VENIPUNCTURE WITH SYRINGE, VENIPUNCTURE WITH VACUTAINER, AND BLOOD CULTURES

Action	
Review and carry out the standard steps in Appendix 1	
Explain to client what is happening throughout procedure Gather all necessary equipment before starting procedure (alcohol or antiseptic swab; clean gloves; sterile gauze pad; tourniquet; adhesive bandage or adhesive tape; appropriate blood tubes; completed identification labels; completed laboratory request; small plastic bag for delivery of specimen to laboratory) Provide privacy for client if possible and appropriate	
Steps	**Rationale**
1 . . .	
2 Assist client with lying supine or sitting in semi-Fowler's position or in a chair with arm supported and elbow extended. Place small pillow or towel under upper arm. (Option: lower arm briefly so it fills hand and lower arm with blood.)	Helps to stabilise extremity. Supported position in bed reduces chance of injury to client if fainting occurs.
3 Apply tourniquet so that it can be removed by pulling end with single motion.	Tourniquet blocks venous return to heart from extremity, causing veins to dilate for easier visibility.
a. Position the tourniquet 5 to 10 cm (2 to 4 inches) above venipuncture site selected.	
b. Cross the tourniquet over the client's arm, holding the tourniquet between your fingers close to the arm (see illustration). Tourniquet may be placed over gown sleeve to protect skin.	
c. Tuck a loop between the client's arm and the tourniquet so that the free end can be easily grasped (see illustration).	Free end can be pulled to release tourniquet after venipuncture.
Special note: Palpate distal pulse (e.g. radial) below tourniquet. If pulse is not palpable, the tourniquet is too tight and is impeding arterial blood flow. If this happens, remove and wait 60 seconds before reapplying tourniquet more loosely or assessing other extremity. Keep tourniquet in place no longer than 1 minute. Minimises effects of haemoconcentration and haemolysis. Prolonged time may alter test results and cause pain and venous stasis (e.g. falsely elevated serum potassium level) (Malarkey and McMorrow 2005).	
4 Ask the client to gently open and close fist several times, finally leaving fist clenched.	
5 Quickly inspect extremity for best venipuncture site, looking for straight, prominent vein without swelling or haematoma. Of the three veins located in the antecubital area, the median cubital vein is preferred (see illustration).	This vein is large, well anchored (does not easily move), closer to the surface of the skin, and less painful to puncture. Straight and intact veins are easiest to puncture. The veins of the lower arm and hand are preferred for administering IV fluids.
6 Palpate selected vein with finger (see illustration). Note if vein is firm and rebounds when palpated or if vein feels rigid and cordlike and rolls when palpated.	A healthy vein is elastic and rebounds on palpation. Thrombosed vein is rigid, rolls easily and is difficult to puncture.

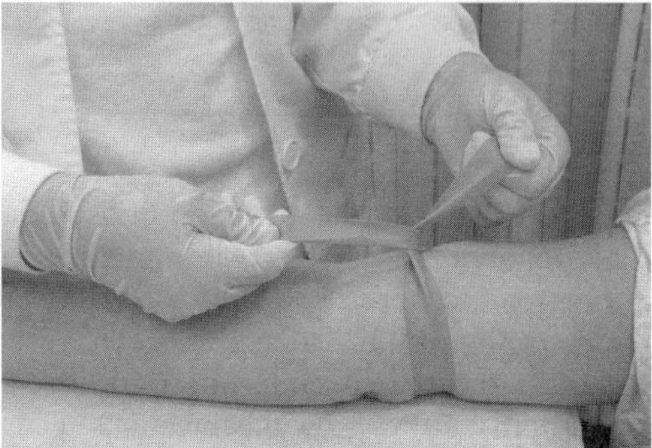

STEP 3b. Cross tourniquet over the arm.

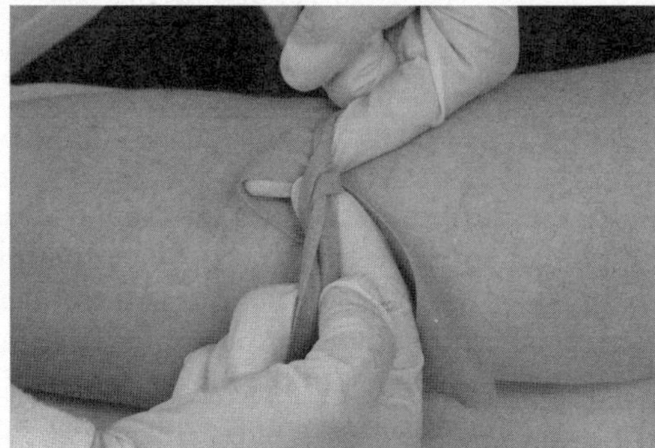

STEP 3c. Tuck a loop between the client's arm and tourniquet.

TABLE 22.9 | GUIDELINES FOR COLLECTING BLOOD SPECIMENS — VENIPUNCTURE WITH SYRINGE, VENIPUNCTURE WITH VACUTAINER, AND BLOOD CULTURES — cont'd

Steps	Rationale
Special note: Avoid vigorously slapping veins because this can cause vasospasm.	
7 Obtain blood specimen.	
a. Syringe Method:	
(1) Have syringe with appropriate needle attached.	
(2) Cleanse venipuncture site with antiseptic swabs, moving in a circular motion from site outwards for about 5 cm (2 inches) (see illustration). Allow to dry.	Antimicrobial agent cleans skin surface of resident bacteria so organisms do not enter puncture site. Allowing antiseptic to dry completes its antimicrobial task and reduces 'sting' of venipuncture. Alcohol left on skin can cause haemolysis of sample.
(a) If drawing sample for blood alcohol level or blood cultures, use only antiseptic swab rather than alcohol swab.	Ensures accurate test results.
(3) Remove needle cover and inform client of 'stick' lasting only a few seconds.	Prepares client and prevents sudden movement from the needle.
(4) Place thumb or forefinger of nondominant hand 2.5 cm (1 inch) below site, and gently pull skin taut. Stretch skin steadily until vein is stabilised.	Stabilises vein and minimises rolling during needle insertion.
(5) Hold syringe and needle at a 15- to 30-degree angle from client's arm with the bevel up.	Angle and bevel up position facilitate entry of the needle into the vein.
(6) Slowly insert needle into vein (see illustration), stopping when a 'pop' is felt as the needle enters vein.	Prevents puncture through the opposite side of the vein.

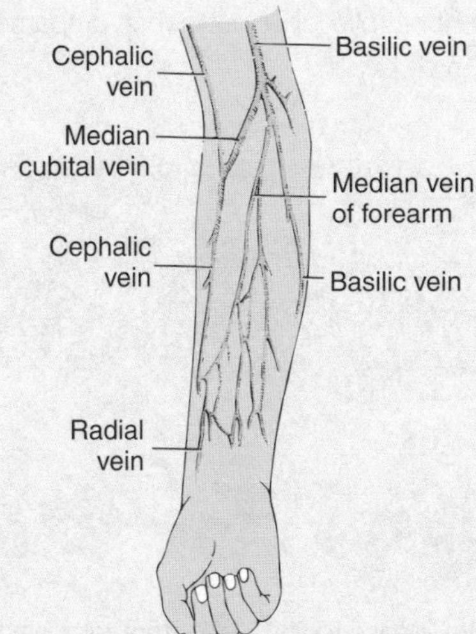

STEP 5 Location of antecubital veins.

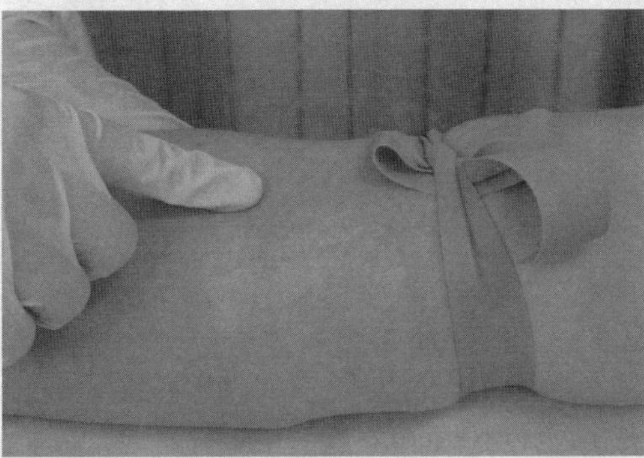

STEP 6 Palpate vein.

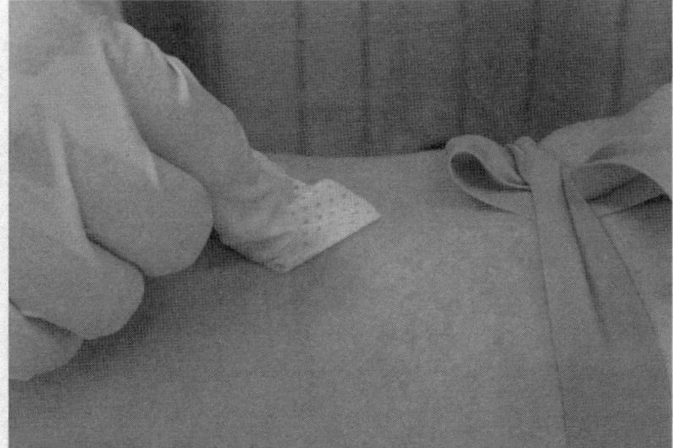

STEP 7a(2). Cleanse venipuncture site with antiseptic solution.

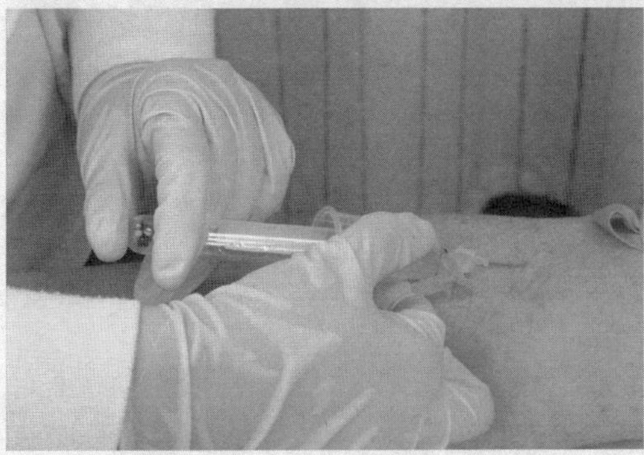

STEP 7a(6). Perform venipuncture.

(Continued)

TABLE 22.9 | GUIDELINES FOR COLLECTING BLOOD SPECIMENS — VENIPUNCTURE WITH SYRINGE, VENIPUNCTURE WITH VACUTAINER, AND BLOOD CULTURES — cont'd

Steps	Rationale
(7) Hold syringe securely, and pull back gently on plunger (see illustration).	Creates a vacuum for withdrawal of blood specimen.
(8) Observe for blood return and withdraw until desired amount of blood is obtained.	Verifies placement in the vein.
(9) Release tourniquet before removing needle (see illustration).	Reduces bleeding at site.
(10) Apply 2 × 2 gauze pad or alcohol swab over puncture site without pressure. Quickly, but carefully, withdraw needle and apply pressure after removal of needle (see illustration).	Minimises discomfort and trauma to vein.
(11) Activate needle safety cover and immediately discard needle in proper receptacle.	Phlebotomy equipment must include needle safety devices. Reduces risk of needlestick injury (OSHA 2001).
b. Vacutainer System Method:	
(1) Attach double-ended needle to Vacutainer tube (see illustration).	
(2) Have proper blood specimen tubes resting inside Vacutainer, but do not puncture rubber stopper.	Tubes are usually colour coded to indicate intended use based on size of tube and presence or absence of a chemical additive. Puncture of stopper results in loss of vacuum.
(3) Cleanse venipuncture site with alcohol swab (70% isopropyl alcohol) using a circular motion out from site for approximately 5 cm (2 inches). Allow to dry.	Antimicrobial agent cleans skin surface of resident bacteria so organisms do not enter puncture site. Allowing alcohol to dry reduces 'sting' of venipuncture. Alcohol left on skin can cause haemolysis of sample.
(4) Remove needle cover, and inform client that 'stick' lasting only a few seconds will be felt.	Client has better control over anxiety when prepared about what to expect.

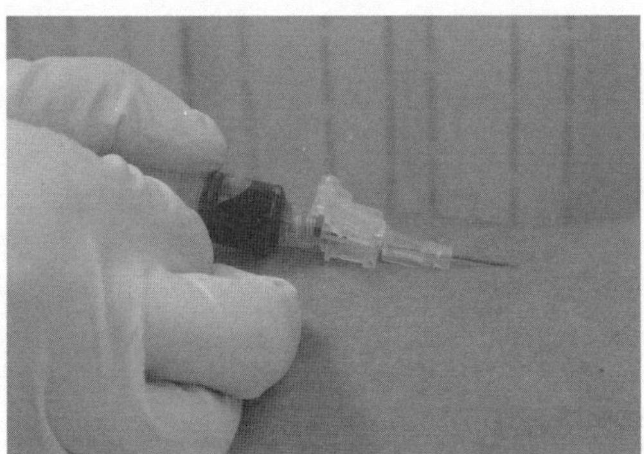

STEP 7a(7). Pull back on plunger.

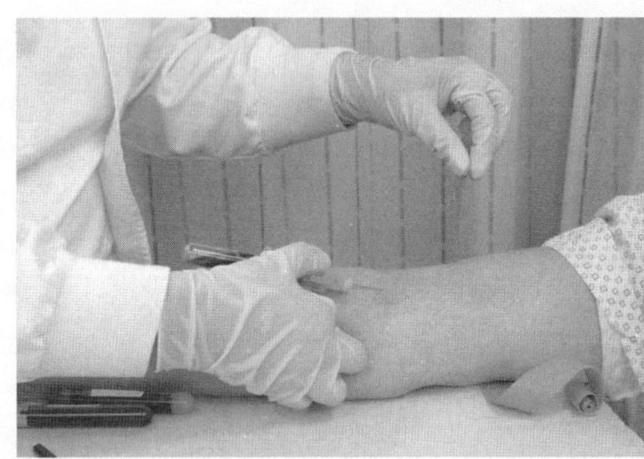

STEP 7a(9). Release tourniquet before removing needle.

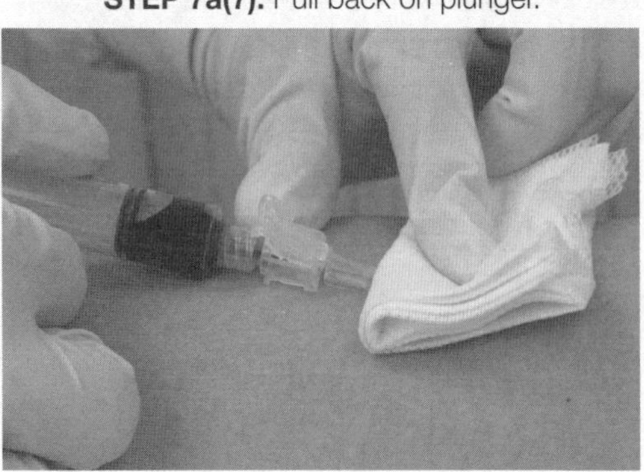

STEP 7a(10). Apply gauze over puncture site.

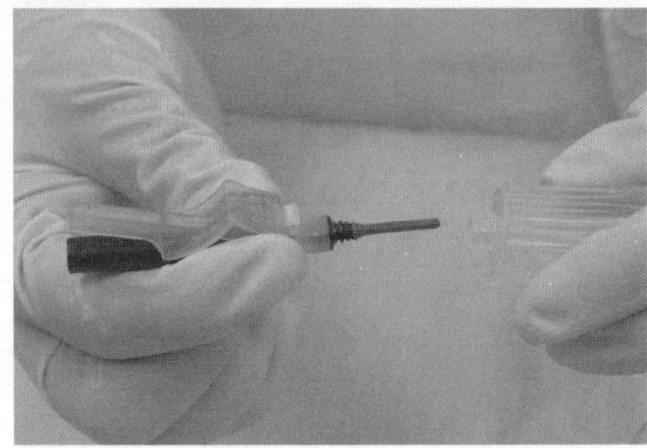

STEP 7b(1). Attach double-ended needle.

TABLE 22.9 | GUIDELINES FOR COLLECTING BLOOD SPECIMENS — VENIPUNCTURE WITH SYRINGE, VENIPUNCTURE WITH VACUTAINER, AND BLOOD CULTURES — cont'd

Steps	Rationale
(5) Place thumb or forefinger of nondominant hand 2.5 cm (1 inch) *below* site, and pull skin taut. Stretch skin down until vein is stabilised.	Position of finger below site prevents accidental needle stick. Stretching helps to stabilise vein and prevent rolling during needle insertion.
(6) Hold Vacutainer needle at 15- to 30-degree angle from arm with bevel of needle up.	Reduces chance of penetrating both sides of vein during insertion and is less traumatic to the vein.
(7) Slowly insert needle into vein (see illustration).	Prevents puncture on opposite side.
(8) Grasp Vacutainer securely, and advance specimen tube into needle of holder (do not advance needle in vein).	Pushing needle through stopper breaks vacuum and causes flow of blood into tube. If needle in vein advances, vein may become punctured on other side.
(9) Note flow of blood into tube, which should be fairly rapid (see illustration).	Failure of blood to appear indicates that vacuum in tube is lost or needle is not in vein.
(10) After specimen tube is filled, grasp Vacutainer firmly and remove tube. Insert additional specimen tubes as needed.	Prevents needle from advancing or dislodging. Tubes with additives should be inverted as soon as possible.
Special note: When filling tubes with an anticoagulant additive, let tube fill until the vacuum is exhausted. Ratio of blood to additive is important. Gently rotate the tube back and forth 8 to 10 times. Prevents clotting as additives are mixed with blood. Shaking can cause haemolysis of red blood cells (RBCs), producing inaccurate test results.	
(11) Release tourniquet and apply gauze; see Steps 7a(9) and 7a(10).	Reduces bleeding at site when needle is withdrawn.
c. Blood Culture:	
(1) Cleanse venipuncture site with antiseptic swab (check agency policy). Allow to dry.	Antimicrobial agent cleans skin surface so organisms do not enter puncture site or contaminate culture. Drying ensures complete antimicrobial action.
(2) Clean bottle tops of Vacutainer tubes or culture bottles. Check agency policy regarding cleaning with 70% alcohol after cleaning with antiseptic solution and air-drying.	Ensures specimen is sterile.
(3) Collect 10 to 15 mL of venous blood by venipuncture from each venipuncture site.	Cultures must be obtained from two sites to confirm culture growth.
(4) Discard needle on syringe; replace with new sterile needle before injecting blood sample into culture bottles.	Maintains sterile technique and prevents contamination of specimen.
(5) If both aerobic and anaerobic cultures are needed, fill the anaerobic container first (Pagana and Pagana 2005).	Anaerobic organisms may take longer to grow.
(6) Gently mix blood in the culture bottle.	Mixes medium and blood.
(7) Release tourniquet and apply gauze; see Steps 7a(9) and 7a(10).	

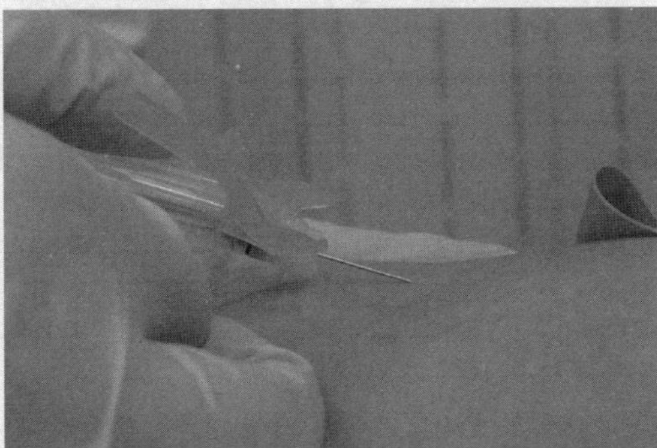

STEP 7b(7). Insert Vacutainer needle into vein.

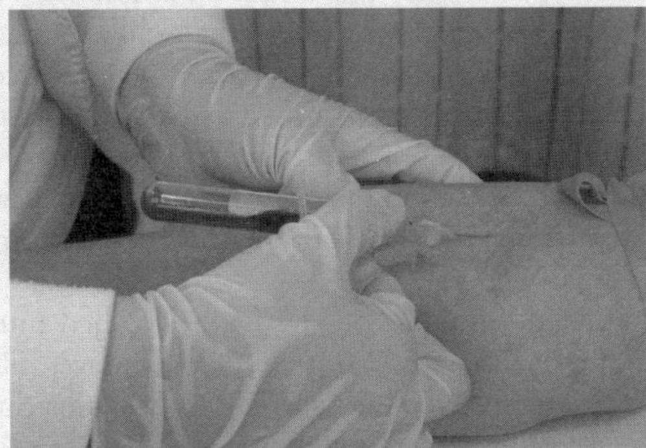

STEP 7b(9). Note rapid flow of blood into tube.

(Continued)

TABLE 22.9 | GUIDELINES FOR COLLECTING BLOOD SPECIMENS — VENIPUNCTURE WITH SYRINGE, VENIPUNCTURE WITH VACUTAINER, AND BLOOD CULTURES — cont'd

Steps	Rationale
8 For blood obtained by syringe, transfer specimens to appropriate specimen tubes. Insert needle through stopper of blood collection tube and allow vacuum to fill the tube. Do not force blood into tube.	Forcing blood into tube may cause haemolysis of RBCs.
9 Take blood tubes containing additives; gently rotate back and forth 8 to 10 times.	Additives should be mixed with blood to prevent clotting. Shaking can cause haemolysis of blood cells, producing inaccurate results.
10 Observe for any sign of blood on outside of tube; wipe with 70% alcohol.	
11 Carefully discard uncapped sharps into appropriate container. If needle has built-in safety device, activate (see illustration) and then discard.	One-handed technique helps to avoid needlestick injury (OSHA 2001).
12 Label the specimen with the client identifiers, date and time. Affix proper requisition.	Ensures diagnostic information reported on correct client.
13 Place all specimens in appropriate bag for transfer. Transport cultures immediately to laboratory (or at least within 30 minutes).	

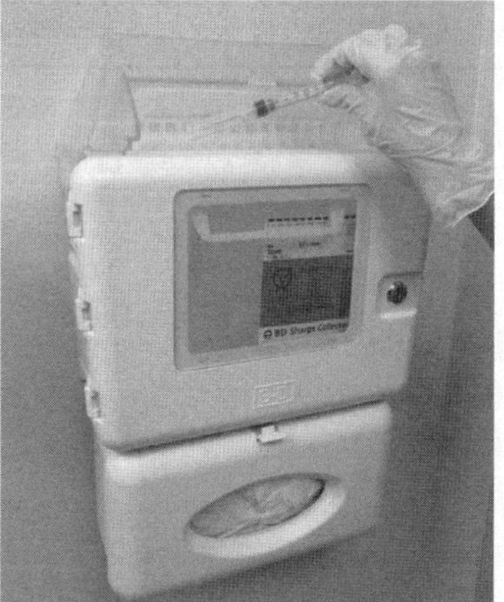

STEP 11 Needle with safety cover.

(Elkin et al 2008)

ASSISTING WITH ELECTROCARDIOGRAM

An electrocardiogram (ECG) is a graphical representation of the heart's electrical activities, or conduction system. The electrical impulse of each heartbeat originates within the sinoatrial (SA) node, which is in the right atrium. The electrical activity of the conduction system is recorded on an ECG. An ECG may be performed to determine baseline cardiac function, to help evaluate response to cardiac medications, to help monitor recovery after a myocardial infarction, or when the client experiences chest discomfort (Elkin et al 2008).

The normal sequence on the ECG is called normal sinus rhythm (NSR), which contains PQRST waves (Figure 22.4). The PR interval represents atrial depolarisation during which the atria empty their blood supply into the ventricles. The QRS interval represents ventricular depolarisation, during which ventricular contraction occurs. The remainder of the wave-form through the end of the T-wave signifies ventricular repolarisation. Disturbances in conduction may occur when impulses cannot travel through the normal pathways, called an arrhythmia. Arrhythmias may occur as a response to ischaemia, valvular abnormality, anxiety, drug toxicity, or acid–base or electrolyte imbalance. Table 22.10 provides guidelines for assisting with electrocardiogram (Elkin et al 2008).

A holter monitor is a small, portable device that records electrical activity of the heart for as long as 24 hours. This makes it possible to monitor the cardiac rhythm for ambulatory clients during activity, rest and sleep. Clients keep a diary of activity, noting when they experience rapid heart beats or periods of dizziness. Correlation between activities and abnormal electrical activity can then be determined (Elkin et al 2008).

WEIGHT AND HEIGHT MEASUREMENTS

A person's general level of health can be reflected in the ratio of height to weight. Obtaining an accurate body weight is important because it is one parameter used to evaluate

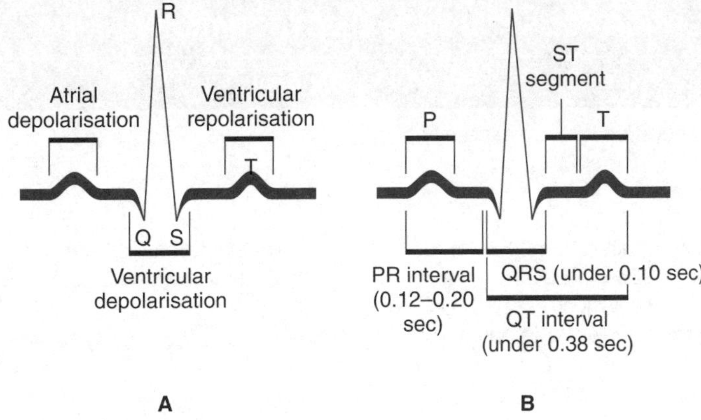

Figure 22.4 | Normal ECG waves and intervals *(Pagana & Pagana 2002)*

and treat many diseases, including congestive heart failure (CHF), fluid overload and renal failure (Elkin et al 2008). Weight is a routine measure taken during health screenings and health care visits. Both are routine when clients are admitted to a health care facility. A nurse measures the height and weight of infants and children to assess growth and development. In older adults, height and weight coupled with a nutritional assessment are important in determining the cause and treatment for chronic disease and in assessing the older adult who has difficulty in eating. The nurse should look for overall trends in height and weight changes. The assessment process screens for abnormal weight changes. The nursing history can help to focus on possible causes for a change in weight (Table 22.11).

Before taking measurements the nurse asks the client what their current height and weight are. Standardised tables can help reveal the normal expected weight for a client at a given height (Figure 22.5).

Clients should be weighed at the same time of day, on the same scale and in the same clothes to allow an objective comparison of subsequent weights. Medical and nursing decisions in relation to drug calculations, lifting and positioning may be based on weight changes. Clients capable of weight bearing would use a standing scale. The nurse needs to make sure that this is calibrated to zero. The client stands and remains still on the scales. The electronic scales calibrate automatically and then display the weight within seconds (Figure 22.6). Stretcher and chair scales are available for clients unable to bear weight. After being transferred to the scale the client is lifted above the bed by a hydraulic device and the weight is measured on a balance beam or digital display. If a client has lost more than 5% of body weight in a month or 10% in 6 months, the loss is significant.

Infants can be weighed in baskets or on platform scales. The nurse removes the infant's clothing and weighs them

TABLE 22.10 | GUIDELINES FOR ASSISTING WITH ELECTROCARDIOGRAM

Review and carry out the standard steps in Appendix 1

Steps	Rationale
1 . . .	
2 Expose client's chest and arms, and cleanse and prepare skin using alcohol wipes.	Alcohol removes oil and fat from the skin and minimises artifact caused by inadequate contact with the skin (Chernecky and Berger 2004).
3 If large amounts of hair are present, it may be necessary to clip hair at the placement sites.	Promotes adherence of leads (electrodes) to chest or extremity.
4 Apply self-sticking electrodes, or apply electrode paste and attach leads. For 12-lead ECG (see illustration): a. Chest (precordial leads) V_1—Fourth intercostal space (ICS) at right sternal border V_2—Fourth ICS at left sternal border V_3—Midway between V2 and V4 V_4—Fifth ICS at midclavicular line V_5—Left anterior axillary line at level of V4 horizontally V_6—Left midaxillary line at level of V4 horizontally	Position of leads promotes proper display of ECG on paper.

(Continued)

TABLE 22.10 | GUIDELINES FOR ASSISTING WITH ELECTROCARDIOGRAM — cont'd

Steps	Rationale
b. Extremities: one on lower portion of each extremity aVr—Right wrist aVl—Left wrist aVf—Left ankle	
5 Turn on machine, enter in any required demographical information and obtain tracing; 12-lead ECG may be obtained without removing precordial leads.	Transfers electrocardiac conduction on ECG tracing paper for subsequent analysis by cardiologist.
6 Disconnect leads and wipe excess electrode paste from chest.	Promotes comfort and hygiene.

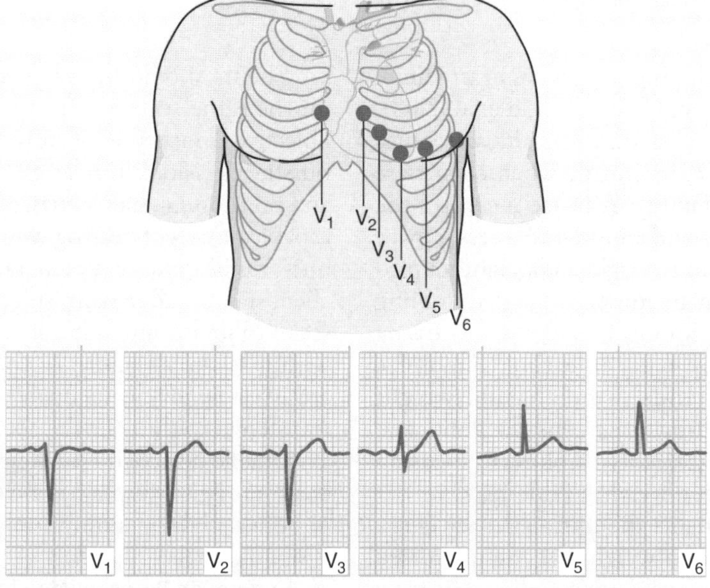

STEP 4 Placement of ECG leads and corresponding ECG waves. (From Phipps WJ and others: *Medical-surgical nursing: health and illness perspectives*, 7th edn, St Louis, 2003, Mosby.)

(Elkin et al 2008)

TABLE 22.11 | NURSING HISTORY FOR WEIGHT ASSESSMENT

Assessment category	Rationale
Ask about total weight lost or gained; compare with usual weight; note time period for loss (e.g. gradual, sudden, desired or undesired)	Determines severity of problem and may reveal if related to disease process, change in eating pattern, or pregnancy
If weight loss desired, ask about eating pattern, diet plan followed, usual daily calorie intake and appetite	Helps to determine appropriateness if diet plan followed
If weight loss undesired, ask about anorexia, vomiting, diarrhoea, thirst, frequent urination and change in lifestyle or activity	Focuses on problem that may cause weight loss (e.g. gastrointestinal problems)
Assess if client has noted changes in social aspects of eating: more meals in restaurants, rushing to eat meals, stress at work or skipping meals	Lifestyle changes can contribute to weight changes
Assess if client takes chemotherapy, diuretics, insulin, psychotropics, steroids, non-prescription diet pills or laxatives	Weight gain or loss can be side effects of these medications

(deWit 2005; Elkin et al 2008)

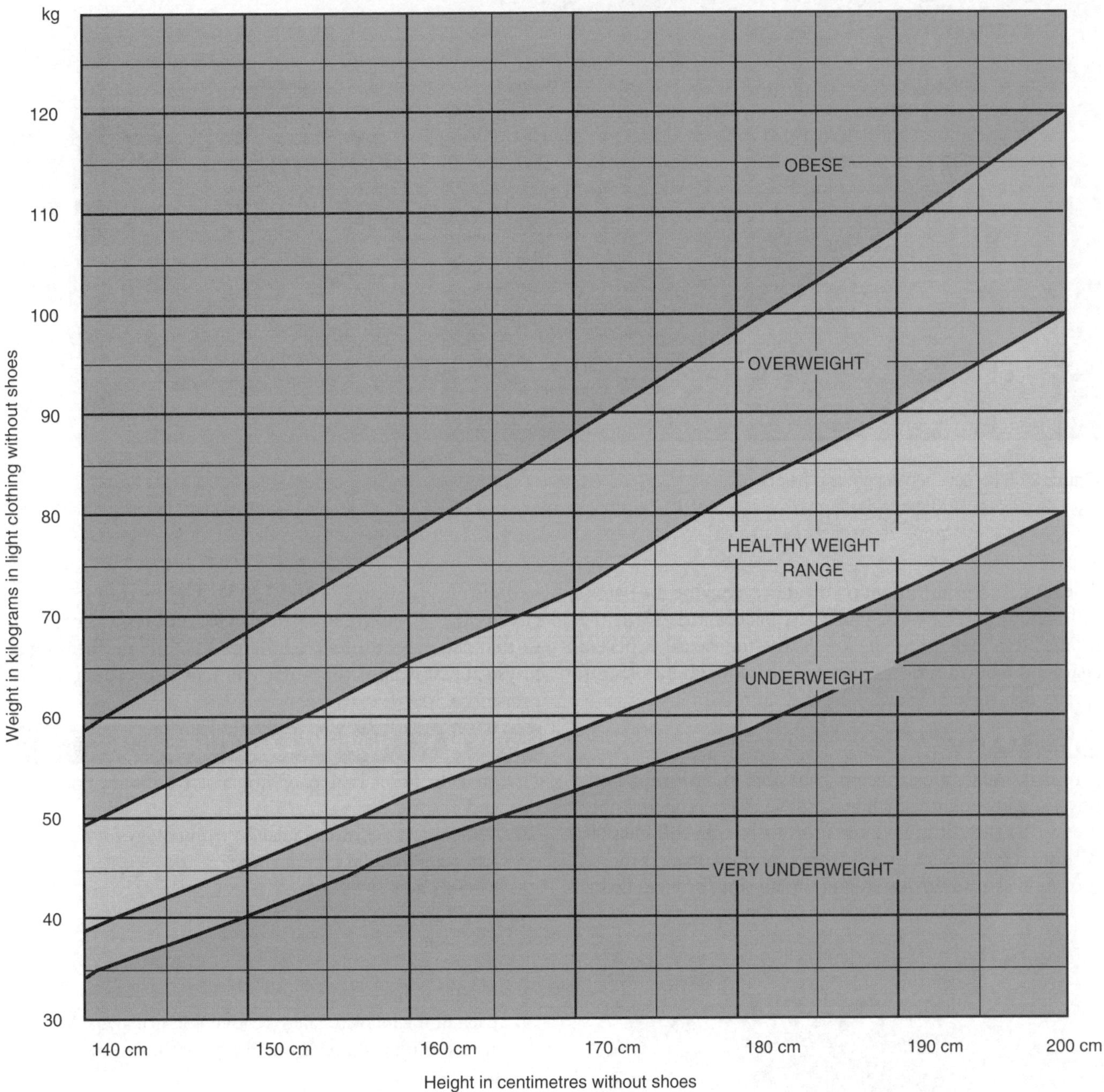

Figure 22.5 | The Australian Nutrition Foundation weight-for-height chart *(reproduced with permission from Nutrition Australia)*

in dry disposable nappies to ensure accurate readings. The weight can be adjusted later for the weight of the nappy. The room should be warm and a light cloth or paper placed on the scale's surface prevents cross-infection from urine and faeces. Infant weight is measured in grams.

Different techniques are used for measuring the height of weight-bearing clients. Clients able to stand remove their shoes. A paper towel can be placed on the scale platform or floor so that the client's feet remain clean. A measuring stick or tape is attached vertically to the weight scales or wall. The nurse asks the client to stand erect. On a standing scale, a metal rod attached to the back of the scale swings out and over the crown of the head.

Portable devices are available that provide a reliable means to measure height. A non-weight-bearing client, such as an infant, is positioned supine on a firm surface.

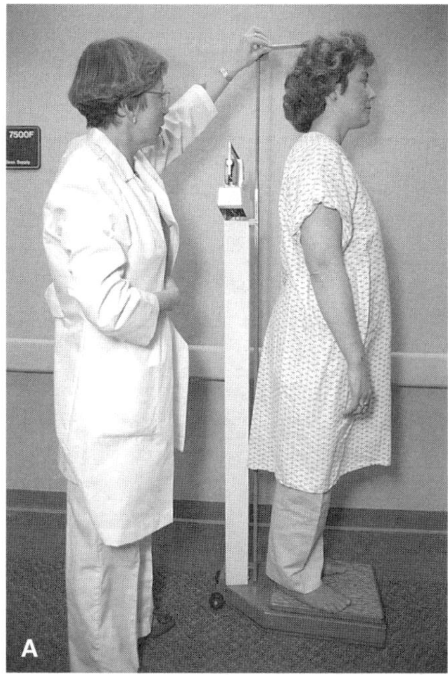

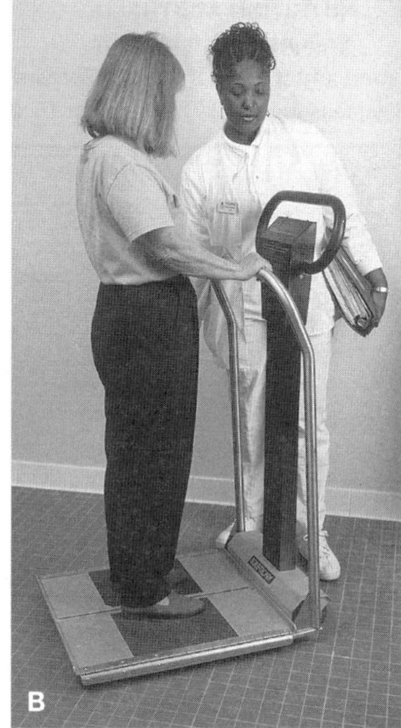

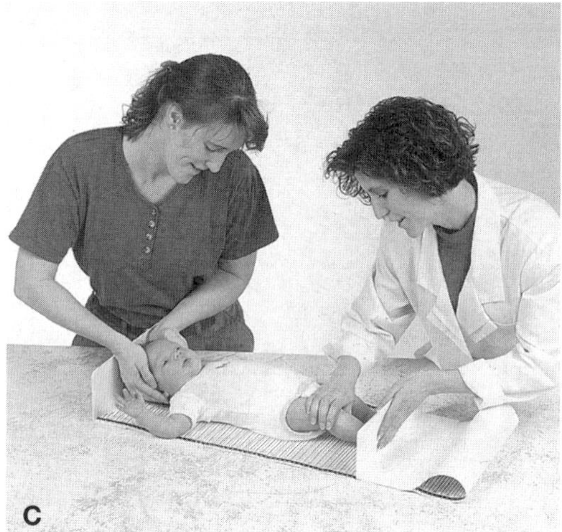

Figure 22.6 | Measuring weight and height

A: Adjustable scales *(Potter & Perry 2001)* **B**: Electronic scales *(Potter & Perry 2001)* **C**: Measurement of infant length *(Courtesy Seca Corporation, Hanover, MD)*

The nurse places the infant on the device, having the parent hold the infant's head against the headboard. With the infant's legs straight at the knees, the footboard is placed against the bottom of the infant's feet. The infant's length is recorded to the nearest 0.5 cm (Figure 22.7).

SUMMARY

Enrolled Nurses are expected to be able to perform a basic physical assessment, which includes vital signs and, possibly, measuring the clinical parameters outlined in this chapter. Although assessment is the first step of the nursing process, thorough assessment also requires planning, implementing and also evaluation (deWit 2005). The nurse must also ensure that all specimens are collected and tested correctly so that accurate results are obtained. While performing a physical assessment the nurse can teach the client about preventive health care.

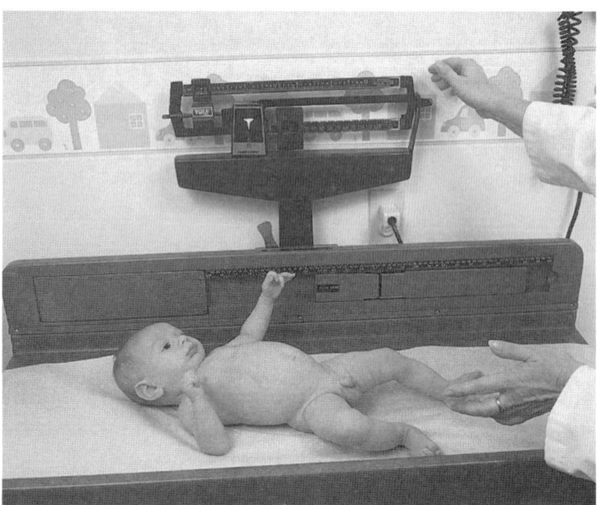

Figure 22.7 | Weighing an infant *(Jarvis 2008)*

REVIEW EXERCISES

1. State the normal values on urinalysis for specific gravity and pH.
2. Write down the correct medical terminology for the following if found on urinalysis:
   - Ketones
   - Glucose
   - Blood
   - Protein
   - Bilirubin.
3. Each of the following may be found on urinalysis. Write at least three conditions that may be indicated by the presence of each:
   - Glucose
   - Bilirubin
   - Leukocytes
   - Blood
   - Ketones
   - Nitrites
   - Protein.
4. For a person who does not have diabetes mellitus, state what the normal range for blood glucose level should be.
5. Define hyperglycaemia and hypoglycaemia.
6. The preferred vein for venipuncture for phlebotomy is:
   a. The antecubital vein, which is less painful

b. The basilic vein, which is straight
c. The cephalic vein, which is in the hand and well anchored
d. The median cubital vein, which is larger, well anchored and closer to the surface.

CRITICAL THINKING EXERCISES

1. Mrs Ngu presented to the clinic complaining of symptoms of urgency, frequency and pain on urination. The Registered Nurse asks you, the Enrolled Nurse, to perform a urinalysis. What would you expect to find on urinalysis and why?
2. Describe the significance of finding a high level of ketones in the urine of an individual with type 1 diabetes mellitus.
3. Where is the best location on a person's finger to perform a blood glucose test and why?
4. Mr Midler has congestive cardiac failure and manifests the following signs and symptoms: breathlessness, anorexia, peripheral oedema and mouth ulcers. The doctor has asked that Mr Midler be weighed daily.
   a) What could be the reason for this request?
   b) A fluid balance chart (FBC) has been ordered for Mr Midler. The following information is recorded on the FBC:
      1200 hrs — orange juice 150 mL, soup 200 mL
      1400 hrs — cup of tea 180 mL
      1600 hrs — water 120 mL
      1630 hrs — cup of tea 120 mL
      2130 hrs — voided 150 mL urine
      0800 hrs — cup of tea 250 mL, water 100 mL
      1030 hrs — cup of tea 100 mL
      1100 hrs — voided 250 mL
      i) What is Mr Midler's total fluid intake over the 24 hours?
      ii) What is his total fluid output over the 24 hours?
      iii) Is the FBC in a positive or negative balance?
      iv) When you weigh Mr Midler the next morning, would you expect him to have lost weight or to have gained weight?
      v) State in kilograms how much weight he would have either gained or lost.

REFERENCES AND FURTHER READING

Berman AJ, Kozier B, Snyder S (2008) *Kozier and Erbs Fundamentals of Nursing: Concepts, Process, and Practice*, 8th edn. Prentice-Hall, Upper Saddle River, New Jersey

Clinitek 50: Urine Chemistry Analyzer [booklet]. Clin 2708 Medicus PDA. Bayer Australia Limited, Health Care Business Group, Sydney

Crisp J, Taylor C (eds) (2005) *Potter & Perry's Fundamentals of Nursing*, 2nd edn. Elsevier Australia, Sydney

deWit SC (2005) *Fundamental Concepts and Skills for Nursing*, 2nd edn. WB Saunders, Philadelphia

Elkin M, Perry A, Potter P (2008) *Nursing Interventions and Clinical Skills*, 4th edn. Mosby Elsevier, Canada

Jarvis C (2008) *Physical Examination and Health Assessment*, 4th edn. WB Saunders, Philadelphia

Kozier B, Erb G, Berman AJ, Snyder S (2007) *Fundamentals of Nursing: Concepts, Process and Practice*, 8th edn. Prentice-Hall, Upper Saddle River, NJ

Pagana KD, Pagana TJ (2002) *Mosby's manual of diagnostic and laboratory tests*, 2nd edn. Mosby, St Louis

Perry AG, Potter PA (2001) *Clinical Nursing Skills and Techniques*, 5th edn. Mosby, St Louis

Potter PA, Perry AG (2004) *Fundamentals of Nursing*, 6th edn. Elsevier Mosby, St Louis

Seidel HM et al (2006) *Mosby's Guide to Physical Examination*, 6th edn. Elsevier Mosby, St Louis

ONLINE RESOURCES

National Diabetes Information Clearinghouse: http://diabetes.niddk.nih.gov

Chapter 23

GENERAL HEALTH ASSESSMENT

OBJECTIVES

- Define the key terms/concepts
- Describe the techniques used with each assessment skill
- Discuss the importance of understanding cultural diversity when assessing clients
- Identify information from the nursing history before a physical assessment
- Discuss normal physical findings for clients across the lifespan
- Document assessment findings on appropriate forms

KEY TERMS/CONCEPTS

auscultation
inspection
olfaction
palpation
percussion

CHAPTER FOCUS

A comprehensive assessment is performed on admission to a health care facility. This assessment involves a detailed review of the client's condition, with the nurse collecting a nursing history and performing a behavioural and physical examination. Periodic assessments are performed on a regular basis in nearly every health care setting. In acute-care settings a brief assessment is performed at the beginning of each shift to identify changes in the client's status compared with the previous assessment. Effective assessment skills can quickly identify new signs and symptoms that indicate complications of an illness or adverse side effects of medical therapy. In aged care facilities, nurses complete similar assessments weekly, monthly or more frequently when a resident's health status changes (Elkin et al 2008). This chapter outlines how to undertake a general health assessment of clients across the lifespan.

LIVED EXPERIENCE

Over the years working as a nurse I have learnt that when admitting clients and obtaining a nursing history, the questions asked need to be specific. I once had a client tell me that her bowel habits were 'regular'. I later found out that regular for this client was once a week! Another client told me that he only drank alcohol socially. It turned out that he went out every night of the week with friends and had two or three alcoholic drinks after work.

Stephanie, Registered Nurse for 15 years

PHYSICAL ASSESSMENT

A physical assessment of clients in a health care facility is obtained to:

- Gather baseline data about the client's health
- Supplement, confirm or refute data obtained in the nursing history
- Confirm and identify nursing diagnoses
- Make clinical judgments about a client's changing health status and management.

A nurse must learn how to really discern a client's condition so that, even in passing or without conscious effort, clues to client health or ill-health are not missed. This includes being aware of clients and their general appearance, colour, expression and body posture. During closer contact with the client, no significant external feature should escape the nurse's notice. The nurse must be able to recognise deviations from what is acceptable and usual for the client. To do this the nurse must know what to look for and what constitutes the acceptable and usual for each client.

Clients are assessed when they are first admitted to a health care institution or when community or home nursing care is initiated. Thereafter, assessment is performed continuously to evaluate client progress and to identify changing needs. Table 23.1 lists the observations to be made during the admission assessment, the acceptable findings and various deviations from the norm. In addition to the observations listed in this table, the nurse must assess the client's:

- Degree of independence
- Ability to perform the activities of daily living
- Ability to interact with others
- Reactions and responses to treatment; for example, medications
- Basic needs; for example, for food, water, oxygen, safety, exercise and comfort
- Specific needs; for example, for wound care or pain relief
- Excretions and secretions; for example, urine, faeces, vomitus, wound drainage.

Information on these topics is provided in the relevant chapters; for example, Chapter 27 addresses comfort needs and Chapter 35 addresses the need for freedom from pain.

Subjective and objective data are included in the assessment of the client. Subjective data are collected by interviewing the client during the nursing history. This includes information that can only be described or verified by the client. Family members and caregivers can also contribute to subjective data about the client. Subjective data are also referred to as symptoms. Objective data are data that can be observed and measured. These types of data are obtained using inspection, palpation, percussion, auscultation and olfaction during the physical examination. Objective data are also called signs. Although subjective data are usually obtained by interview and objective data are obtained by physical examination, it is common for the client to provide subjective data while the nurse is performing the physical examination, and it is also common for the nurse to observe objective signs while interviewing the client during the history (Brown et al 2008).

ASSESSMENT TECHNIQUES

Inspection, palpation, percussion, auscultation and olfaction are the five basic assessment techniques. Each skill enables the nurse to collect a broad range of physical data about clients (Brown et al 2008).

Assessment through inspection

While observation of all the aspects mentioned in this chapter is essential, one of the most important skills a nurse develops is the ability to look at a client and determine whether they are comfortable. A client's comfort depends on many things, the most basic of which are that needs for hygiene, posture, maintenance of body temperature and freedom from pain are met. deWit (2005) lists the following items that the nurse observes and assesses when looking at a client:

- Rest and activity needs:
  — body proportion and appearance
  — range of motion in joints
  — muscular strength
  — balance
  — ability to perform activities of daily living
  — sleep pattern
  — pain
- Nutritional, fluid and electrolyte needs:
  — height and usual weight
  — unusual gain or loss of weight
  — amount and types of foods eaten
  — compliance with prescribed diet
  — fluid intake and output
  — abnormal loss of body fluid
  — skin turgor and moistness of mucous membranes
- Safety and security:
  — potential risks for injury
  — sensory deficits
  — ability to speak and understand English
  — need for side rails or safety devices
- Hygiene and grooming:
  — ability to bathe, dress and groom self
  — amount of assistance needed
- Oxygenation and circulation needs:
  — rate and depth of breathing; breath sounds; cough or sputum production
  — level of consciousness
  — blood pressure
  — pulse rate and characteristics
  — peripheral pulses
  — skin colour and temperature
- Psychosocial needs:
  — desire for spiritual assistance
  — supports

TABLE 23.1 | ADMISSION ASSESSMENT

Aspect	Normal	Deviations from normal
General physical appearance	Normal weight for age, sex, height, body build	Overweight, underweight
	Personal hygiene and grooming satisfactory	Appears to be neglected
Skin	Normal colour for race	Pallor, cyanosis, jaundice
	Neither dry nor moist	Excessively dry or moist
	Normal temperature	Elevated temperature, localised warmth or coldness
	Smooth	Rough, or localised changes or irregularities
	Elastic	Diminished by dehydration or oedema
	No lesions	Rashes, bruises, scars, abrasions, ulcers, nodules
Hair	Normal texture for age, race	Brittle, dry, coarse
	Normal distribution	Areas of hair loss
	Scalp clean and healthy	Dandruff, lesions, lice
	Shiny and clean	Dull, neglected
Nails	Transparent	Streaks (red or white)
	Smooth	Ridged
	Convex	Concave curves
	Pink nail beds	Cyanosed, pale
Eyes	Sclerae and corneas clear	Pale, inflamed, jaundiced
	Eyelashes turn out and away	Rubbing on eyeball
	Open eyelids do not fall over pupils	Ptosis (drooping)
	Pupils equal and reacting to light	Dilated, pinpoint, unequal, non-reactive
	No discharge	Watery or purulent discharge
	Tolerance to light	Photophobia (intolerance to light)
	Normal visual acuity	Visual impairment
Ears	Normal hearing acuity	Hearing impairment
	Ear canal clean	Inflamed, presence of excessive wax
	No discharge	Watery or purulent discharge
		Itching, pain, tinnitus
Mouth	Lips pink, moist, smooth	Pale, cyanosed, dry, cracked
	Mucosa pink, moist, glistening	Pale, cyanosed, dry, ulcers, cracks
	Gums pink, moist, smooth	Inflamed, swollen, bleeding, lesions
	Teeth white, straight, smooth	Discoloured, chalky, decayed
	Tongue pinky red, moist	Coated, cracked
	Breath fresh	Halitosis (bad breath), ketone odour
Thorax and lungs	Normal-shaped chest	Barrel-shaped chest
	Normal breath sounds	Wheezing, rales, gurgles, dry or moist cough
Abdomen	Slightly convex, symmetrical	Excessively concave, asymmetrical, distended
Posture and gait	Able to sit, stand and walk normally	Postural abnormalities, e.g. kyphosis, scoliosis; abnormal gait
Mobility	Full range of joint motion	Stiffness or instability of a joint, unusual joint movement, swelling of a joint, pain on movement
Muscle tone and strength	Normal tone and strength	Increased or decreased tone, decreased strength
Speech	Ability to speak clearly	Speech impairment, e.g. lisp or stammer
Mental and emotional status	Appropriate emotional responses	Responses inappropriate, apprehension, anxiety, depression, hostility
Level of consciousness and orientation	Alert, responsive, oriented to time, place, person	Disoriented, unresponsive to stimuli, shortened attention span
Presence of prosthesis or aids	None, although aids to sight and hearing are common	Spectacles, contact lenses, artificial eye, hearing aids, walking sticks, frames, wheelchairs, artificial limb, dentures

— usual coping mechanisms
— financial concerns
— fears and concerns

- Elimination:
  — characteristics and amount of urinary output
  — characteristics and regularity of bowel movements
  — alterations in elimination
  — presence of pain, burning or other discomfort.

As well as observing and assessing the client and their needs, the nurse must also use the sense of sight to assess the functioning of equipment used in client care. Nurses assess various items of equipment to determine whether they are functioning correctly when they are in use, for example:

- Intravenous fluid apparatus
- Oxygen apparatus
- Urinary drainage systems
- Wound drainage systems
- Traction apparatus.

While Enrolled Nurses (ENs) may not be directly responsible for the management of specific items of equipment, they have a responsibility to observe their functioning and report immediately to the Registered Nurse (RN) if any malfunction is suspected.

Assessment through palpation

Palpation uses the sense of touch. Through palpation the hands make delicate and sensitive measurements of specific physical signs. Palpation detects resistance, resilience, roughness, texture, temperature and mobility. The nurse uses different parts of the hand to detect specific characteristics. For example, the back of the hand is sensitive to temperature variations. The pads of the fingertips detect subtle changes in texture, shape, size, consistency and pulsation of body parts. The palm of the hand is sensitive to vibration. The nurse measures position, consistency and turgor by lightly grasping the body part with fingertips. Assist the client to relax and position comfortably as muscle tension during palpation impairs the ability to palpate correctly. Asking the client to take slow, deep breaths enhances muscle relaxation. Palpate tender areas and ask client to point out areas that are more sensitive and note any nonverbal signs of discomfort (Elkin et al 2008).

The sense of touch should be developed so that a nurse is able to detect abnormalities such as:

- Abnormally hot, cool, moist, dry, inelastic or roughened skin
- An excessively hard or soft peripheral vein
- A rapid, slow, weak or irregular pulse
- Rigid or flaccid muscles
- Swelling of part of the body; for example, a joint.

Touch is also used when examining a client by palpation or percussion. Palpation, usually performed by a medical officer or a RN, is a technique whereby the examiner feels the texture, size, consistency and location of certain parts of the body with the hands. For example, the examiner may palpate the upper abdomen to determine the size of the liver.

Assessment through percussion

Percussion, usually performed by a medical officer or a RN, is a technique in which the examiner strikes the body surface with a finger, producing vibration and sound. An abnormal sound suggests the presence of a mass or accumulation of fluid within an organ or cavity. For example, the examiner may percuss the posterior chest wall to determine the presence of fluid in the lungs.

Assessment using the sense of hearing (auscultation)

It is important that a nurse learns to listen effectively, so that not only what a client says is registered but also the tone of voice, which often conveys a great deal. A nurse must also learn how to recognise abnormal sounds. Information on the art of effective listening in communication is provided in Chapter 29 and emphasises the importance of recognising that listening is an active process that involves much more than just hearing the spoken word. In client care, recognising abnormal sounds involves the ability to detect:

- Abnormalities of breathing; for example, respirations that are wheezing, noisy or distressed
- Abnormalities of heart sounds, blood pressure, bowel sounds or fetal heart sounds, when using a stethoscope
- Manifestations of a client's distress; for example, coughing, expectorating sputum, vomiting, crying or moaning
- Changes in the sound or rhythm of technical equipment such as suction or artificial ventilation apparatus.

Auscultation is listening with a stethoscope to sounds produced by the body. To auscultate correctly, listen in a quiet environment. To be successful, the nurse must first be able to recognise normal sounds from each body structure, including the passage of blood through an artery, heart sounds and movement of air through the lungs (Elkin et al 2008).

Assessment using the sense of smell (olfaction)

A well-developed sense of smell enables a nurse to detect odours that are characteristic of certain conditions. Some alterations in body function and certain bacteria create characteristic odours, for example:

- The 'fishy' smell of infected urine
- The ammonia odour associated with concentrated or decomposed urine
- The musty or offensive odour of an infected wound
- The offensive rotting odour associated with gangrene (tissue necrosis)
- The smell of ketones on the breath in ketoacidosis (accumulation of ketones in the body)
- The smell of alcohol on the breath — due to ingestion of alcohol
- Halitosis (offensive breath) accompanying mouth infections; for example, gingivitis or certain disorders of the digestive system; for example, appendicitis
- The foul odour associated with steatorrhoea (abnormal amount of fat in the faeces)
- The characteristic odour associated with melaena (abnormal black tarry stool containing blood)

- The faecal odour of vomitus associated with a bowel obstruction
- Bromhidrosis (offensive smelling perspiration) caused by bacterial decomposition of perspiration on the skin.

Assessment using equipment

A nurse should acquire proficiency in the correct operation of equipment used to provide information about a client; for example:

- Clinical thermometer
- Sphygmomanometer
- Stethoscope
- Weighing scales
- Urine-testing equipment
- Tape-measure; for example, to measure head, limb or abdominal circumference
- Auriscope, to visualise the ear canal
- Pen-light torch.

GUIDELINES FOR CONDUCTING A GENERAL HEALTH ASSESSMENT

When starting a general health assessment the nurse should:

- Set priorities for assessment based on a client's presenting signs and symptoms
- Use a head-to-toe approach, as this facilitates an effective assessment
- Encourage the client to be an active participant — the client can often let the nurse know when actual changes have occurred
- Respect the client's race, gender, age and cultural beliefs
- Follow standard precautions for infection control
- Consider the possibility of latex allergy
- Record quick notes to facilitate accurate documentation
- Integrate health promotion and education into physical assessment activities.

GENERAL SURVEY

If a client has any acute distress, such as difficulty in breathing, pain or anxiety, defer the general survey until later. A general survey includes the following steps:

- Review baseline vital signs
- Determine the client's need for an interpreter to be available (if an older adult has difficulty with memory, gather data from a family member or other person of significance to the client)
- Identify the client's normal height and weight
- Review the client's past fluid intake and output
- Identify the client's general perceptions about their personal health
- Assess the client's responses (may need to assess the client's orientation to person, place and time) (Clinical Interest Box 23.1)

CLINICAL INTEREST BOX 23.1
Symptoms that may indicate dementia

Learning and retaining new information
Trouble remembering recent conversations, events and appointments
Frequently misplaces objects

Handling complex tasks
Difficulty following a complex train of thought
Difficulty performing tasks that require many steps

Reasoning ability
Unable to develop a plan to address problems at work or home
Displays uncharacteristic disregard for rules of social conduct

Spatial ability and orientation
Difficulty driving
Difficulty in organising objects around the house
Difficulty finding way around familiar places

Language
Increasing difficulty with expressing self
Difficulty following conversations

Behaviour
Appears more passive and less responsive
More irritable and suspicious than usual
Misinterprets visual and auditory stimuli

(Perry & Potter 2002: 263. Data from Agency for Health Care Policy and Research 1996)

- Assess posture and position and body movements
- Assess speech
- Observe hygiene and grooming:
  - — observe the colour, distribution, quantity, thickness, texture and lubrication of hair
  - — inspect the condition of the nails
  - — assess the presence or absence of body odour
- Assess the eyes:
  - — inspect pupils for size, shape and equality
  - — note the condition of the client's vision
- Assess hearing
- Inspect the nose externally for shape, skin colour, alignment and presence of deformity or inflammation. Note the colour of the mucosa and any lesions, discharge, swelling or presence of bleeding
- In clients with nasogastric tubes, inspect the nares for excoriation or inflammation
- Assess the mouth, inspect the oral mucosa, tongue, teeth and gums for hydration; determine whether the client wears dentures
- Ask the client if they have noticed any changes in the skin
- Inspect the skin surfaces, comparing the skin colour of symmetrical body parts
- Use non-gloved fingertips to palpate skin surfaces to feel moisture of intact skin
- Inspect the character of any secretions: note colour, odour, amount and consistency
- Assess skin turgor. (In an older adult the skin is less elastic and drier than the skin of a younger person.

Skin turgor is not an accurate measure of hydration in the older adult. Checking the mucous membranes is a better assessment technique.)
- Assess the condition of the skin for pressure areas
- Assess the client's affect and mood, as this reflects the client's mental status, consciousness, feelings and emotional status
- Observe the client's interaction with their spouse or partner, older adult child or carer
- Observe for signs of abuse:
  — for a child, blood on underclothing, pain in the genital area or difficulty in sitting or walking may be indicative of child sexual abuse
  — for a female client, injury or trauma inconsistent with a reported cause, or obvious injuries to face or neck, could indicate domestic violence
  — for an older adult, injury or trauma inconsistent with a reported cause, injuries in unusual locations (neck or genitalia), pattern injuries (left when an object is used to strike a person and leaves an imprint), parallel injuries (bilateral bruising in upper arms, suggesting client was shaken) and burns may suggest abuse.

A nursing care plan is prepared from the information gathered from this assessment.

ROUTINE SHIFT ASSESSMENT

Each client should also be assessed at the beginning of each shift, as this helps the nurse to establish priorities of care and organise the work for the shift. The nurse introduces themself to each client at the start of the shift and observes:
- Skin colour
- Appearance
- Ease of respiration
- How the client is feeling
- Ability to respond to questions
- Ability to communicate
- Level of consciousness
- Vital signs
- Voiding status
- Ability to move easily
- Skin lesions or pressure areas
- Presence of oedema.

It is important to note that a client should be assessed whenever you first have contact with that client. Nurses also need to:
- Ascertain the time of the last bowel movement
- Check tubes and equipment (IV lines, nasogastric tubes, urinary catheters, dressings, wound suction devices, oxygen rates, traction)
- Ensure that call bell, TV control, water and tissues are in reach
- Check that room temperature is suitable
- Determine which supplies will be needed in the room for the remainder of the shift.

Table 23.2 outlines the routine shift assessment.

DIAGNOSTIC PROCEDURES

Shortly after admission, or at any time during a stay in a health care facility, the client may be required to have one or various diagnostic tests or examinations performed. For most people, any test or examination is a cause for anxiety and apprehension. The client may experience discomfort, pain or embarrassment during a procedure and may be apprehensive about the results. The nurse is in a key position to reduce or minimise anxiety, embarrassment and discomfort.

EXAMINING THE CLIENT

When admitted to a health care facility, a medical officer or RN gives each client a comprehensive physical examination. The person is assessed by various techniques, such as auscultation, percussion and palpation, which were described earlier in the chapter. Further examinations may be performed during the client's stay.

Before the examination

Preparing the client before the examination involves:
- A full explanation of the type of examination to be performed
- An opportunity to empty the bladder and/or bowel. The client will feel more comfortable and the examination will be performed more effectively if the bladder and rectum are empty
- Providing privacy by closing any doors or windows or by drawing the screens around the bed
- Providing a drape for warmth and privacy. The upper bedclothes should be folded to the bottom of the bed
- Assistance to the required position (information on various positions is provided in Chapter 33). The pillows should be arranged to provide comfort and support. The positions normally used are:
  — for examining the chest and back the client is assisted into a sitting position. The nightgown or pyjama top is undone or removed if necessary and a drape positioned to provide privacy
  — for examining the abdomen the client is assisted into the recumbent position. The clothing is adjusted to expose the abdomen and a drape is positioned to provide privacy
  — for a rectal examination the client is assisted to assume the left lateral position. A drape is positioned so that only the anal area is exposed
  — for a vaginal examination the client is assisted to assume either the dorsal or Simm's position, according to the medical officer's instructions. Adequate draping is necessary to ensure that only the vaginal area is exposed.

Before the examination the nurse may need to assist the medical officer in collecting the equipment required. Check each health facility's protocol for the list of equipment and procedure outline.

TABLE 23.2 | CHECKLIST FOR ROUTINE SHIFT ASSESSMENT

1 Mental and Neurological Status **a.** Level of consciousness (LOC)/responsiveness **b.** Alertness/orientation **c.** Pupils equal, round, and reactive to light and accommodation (PERRLA) **d.** Mood **e.** Behaviour **2** Vital Signs **a.** Blood pressure **b.** Pulse **c.** Respiration **d.** Temperature **e.** Pain and comfort level **3** Motor Sensory Function **a.** Range of motion (ROM) **b.** Movement **c.** Strength **d.** Presence of numbness or tingling **4** Integument (Skin/Mucous Membranes) **a.** Colour **b.** Temperature **c.** Turgor **d.** Moisture **e.** Oedema **f.** Integrity	**5** Cardiopulmonary System **a.** Heart sounds **b.** Apical rate and rhythm **c.** Lung sounds **d.** Breathing pattern **e.** Peripheral pulses **f.** Capillary refill **6** Gastrointestinal (GI) System **a.** Bowel sounds **b.** Abdominal palpation **c.** Degree of abdominal distention **d.** Bowel elimination problems (e.g. diarrhoea, constipation, flatulence) **7** Wounds **a.** Cleanliness **b.** Presence of swelling, redness, infection, or drainage **c.** Bandage/dressing **8** Invasive Tubes (e.g. Intravenous [IV] Lines, Nasogastric [NG] Tubes, Wound Drains, Catheters) **a.** Device and location **b.** IV line: Correct fluid/medicine infusing **c.** Patency and position **d.** Presence of redness, swelling or tenderness at site **e.** Drainage rate or infusion rate **f.** Date of last tubing change

(Elkin et al 2008)

During the examination

During the examination the nurse should remain with the client to provide physical and emotional support and assist when a change of position is required, remembering to provide adequate physical support and privacy. Emotional support is partially provided by the nurse's presence, and further support may be given in the form of encouragement and explanations of what is to happen. The nurse may also be required to assist the medical officer or receive any specimen obtained.

After the examination

The client is assisted into a position of comfort, clothing is readjusted and the bedclothes are arranged to meet needs. If a rectal or vaginal examination was performed, the person should be provided with tissues to wipe off any excess lubricant. The equipment is removed and attended to in the appropriate manner. Any specimens are despatched to the laboratory as soon as possible. The examination and the person's response to it is reported to the nurse in charge and documented.

DIAGNOSTIC INVESTIGATIONS

Apart from the physical examination, specific tests may be performed to assist diagnosis or aid in evaluating the client's condition. Diagnostic procedures include:

- Radiological examination
- Ultrasonography
- Blood tests
- Urine tests
- Histological tests
- Microbiological tests
- Endoscopy
- Recording electrical activity
- CT scanning.

The nurse may be involved in preparing the client before a diagnostic procedure, assisting throughout the procedure and providing care after the procedure. To determine the specific preparation and post-test care required for each procedure, the nurse should refer to the health care facility's policy manual.

Preparing the client before any diagnostic procedure involves both physical and psychological preparation. The nurse should explain the purpose of the test and the procedure. If the client understands what is to happen and why, they may be less anxious about the test. The nurse should ensure that the client is informed of when, where and who will perform the test, and that the client's informed consent has been obtained. Many tests, especially those of an invasive nature, require that the client gives informed consent for the test to be performed. Clinical Interest Box 23.2 lists examples of possible nursing diagnosis.

ASSESSING INFANTS AND CHILDREN

A nursing history is obtained from the parents and from the child if they are old enough. As much information as possible should be obtained to enable the nurse to

CLINICAL INTEREST BOX 23.2
Examples of nursing diagnoses made after nursing assessment

- Imbalanced nutrition: less than body requirements or more than body requirements
- Deficient fluid volume or excess fluid volume
- Anxiety or fear
- Bathing/hygiene self-care deficit
- Impaired physical mobility
- Impaired wheelchair mobility
- Impaired bed mobility
- Impaired skin integrity
- Ineffective breathing pattern
- Ineffective peripheral tissue perfusion
- Pain
- Dysfunctional family processes
- Carer strain

understand habits and to establish a greater similarity between the home and hospital environments. Information obtained should include:

- Family data; for example, the child's name or nickname, date of birth and age, names of other family members, parents' occupations
- Medical history; for example, details of any infectious diseases suffered by the child, any known exposure to infectious diseases within recent weeks, details of immunisation against infectious diseases, any known allergies, current medications, and details about any current illness or disability other than that for which the child is being admitted. Table 23.3 outlines the common disorders of infancy, childhood and adolescence to be aware of
- Whether the child has ever been admitted to hospital before and, if so, how they reacted to the experience
- Activities of daily living; that is, information about eating, sleeping, elimination, hygiene and play. Table 23.4 lists the information that should be obtained about the child's activities of daily living.

As nurses are with hospitalised children constantly, they have a vital role to play in assessment and accurate reporting. Changes in a child's condition can occur with alarming rapidity, and a child's reactions to illness and to treatment can be dramatic, so constant vigilance by the nurse is essential. Because infants and young children are unable to communicate their feelings they need to be closely observed for indications of pain, a change in condition or the onset of complications. Nurses must have a sound knowledge of what is considered normal so that they are able to recognise an abnormal situation.

Assessing an infant or child (Table 23.5) also involves measuring the vital signs, weight and height. Information on assessing vital signs is provided in Chapters 21 and 22.

When measuring temperature, the route selected depends on the age and condition of the child. The axillary route is generally selected for infants and young children whereas the oral route may be more suitable for an older child. It may be easier to assess the pulse of infants or young children while they are asleep, or by selecting the temporal pulse site in preference to the radial site. An infant's pulse may be assessed apically by placing the diaphragm of a stethoscope over the apex of the heart.

To obtain an accurate measurement, respirations are best measured when the child is asleep or resting quietly. In general, particularly with infants and young children, the pulse and respirations are measured before the temperature.

Blood pressure measurements are performed using the same techniques as those used for adults, but with equipment that is designed for paediatric use, for example, a small cuff.

Weight (mass) is measured using a type of scale appropriate for the child; for example, infants are weighed on infant scales, while older children are weighed on a chair or standing scale.

Height is measured with the older child in a standing position, while recumbent length is a more reliable form of height measurement in infants and young children.

Head circumference is generally measured in children up to 3 years of age, and in any child whose head size is questionable. The head is measured at its greatest circumference by placing a tape measure around the head, slightly above the eyebrows and around the occipital prominence at the back of the skull.

CHILD ABUSE

Child abuse, or maltreatment, can be identified as any situation in which a child is non-accidentally harmed physically, mentally or emotionally. Child abuse results from psychological, sociological, cultural and environmental factors. Studies have shown that child abuse is due to these and other factors, often in combination, and that there is no reliably identifiable single cause. Because nurses may come into contact with a child who has been abused, it is important that they have some knowledge and understanding about child abuse.

Many health care facilities, especially those with paediatric facilities, have clearly defined protocols for managing abused children and their families, and nurses who are working with children should make certain they understand the procedures to be followed when child abuse is suspected. Many health care facilities also have multidisciplinary teams to assist in diagnosis, assessment and treatment.

Preventing child abuse and neglect is very important and involves:

- Identifying families at risk for potential abuse
- Providing supportive services; for example, parents anonymous groups, day care facilities, foster care, volunteer coordinators, family aides, individual counselling

TABLE 23.3 | COMMON DISORDERS OF INFANCY, CHILDHOOD AND ADOLESCENCE

Disorder	Age most likely to occur
Communicable diseases	
Pertussis (whooping cough)	Under 10 years
Infectious parotitis (mumps)	Between 2 years and adulthood
Rubeola (measles)	Early childhood
Rubella (German measles)	Childhood
Varicella (chicken pox)	Early childhood
Hepatitis A	Childhood
Enteritis	Infancy, childhood
Meningitis (viral, bacterial)	Infancy, early childhood
Sexually transmitted infections	Adolescence (or during childhood in cases of child sexual abuse)
Impetigo	Early childhood
Respiratory system disorders	
Laryngotracheobronchitis (croup)	3 months to 3 years
Acute epiglottitis	3–4 years
Tonsillitis	Childhood to adulthood
Pneumonia	Infancy, childhood
Asthma	5–6 years and onwards
Allergic rhinitis	Childhood
Otitis media (as part of viral upper respiratory tract illnesses)	Childhood
Acute bronchiolitis	Infancy
Gastrointestinal disorders	
Acute gastroenteritis	Infancy
Pyloric stenosis	Manifests 2–4 weeks postpartum
Acute appendicitis	Childhood, adolescence
Umbilical hernia	Infancy to 3–4 years
Intussusception	Infancy
Helminth infestations (worms)	Childhood
Diarrhoea	Infancy, childhood
Constipation	Childhood, adolescence
Skin disorders	
Nappy dermatitis (rash)	Infancy
Eczema	Infancy, early childhood
Seborrhoeic dermatitis	Infancy
Scabies	Childhood
Miliaria (prickly heat)	Infancy
Acne	Adolescence
Genitourinary disorders	
Urinary tract infection	Childhood
Enuresis (bed-wetting)	Childhood (4–8 years)
Acute glomerulonephritis	5–10 years
Menstrual problems	Pre-teen and teenage years
Circulatory system disorders	
Anaemia	Infancy, childhood, adolescence
Leukaemia	Childhood
Haemophilia	Manifests in early childhood
Atrial/septal heart defects	Congenital — manifests in infancy or early childhood
Idiopathic thrombocytopenic purpura	3–7 years
Neurological conditions	
Convulsions	6 months to 6 years
Epilepsy	Generally appears between 4 and 8 years
Cerebral palsy	Infancy

TABLE 23.3 | COMMON DISORDERS OF INFANCY, CHILDHOOD AND ADOLESCENCE — cont'd

Disorder	Age most likely to occur
Metabolic and nutritional disorders	
Coeliac disease	Manifests within 6 months after birth
Cystic fibrosis	Manifests in infancy
Obesity	Childhood or adolescence
Protein-kilojoule malnutrition	Infancy
Rickets	Infancy
Musculoskeletal disorders	
Congenital hip dysplasia	Manifests in infancy
Osteogenesis imperfecta	Manifests at birth or soon afterwards
Scoliosis	Childhood, adolescence
Traumatic disorders	
Choking, suffocation	Infancy, early childhood
Poisoning	Early childhood
Burns	Infancy, early childhood
Foreign objects lodged in a body orifice	Early childhood
Bites, lacerations, stings, abrasions	Childhood
Fractures, dislocations	Childhood, adolescence
Sudden infant death syndrome (SIDS)	Before 2 years
Abuse (physical, sexual, emotional)	Any age from infancy to adolescence
Behavioural or psychological disorders	
Hyperactivity, temper tantrums, concentration problems	Childhood
Autism	Manifests in infancy or early childhood
Eating disorders; anorexia nervosa, bulimia nervosa	Late childhood, adolescence
Substance abuse	Late childhood, adolescence

TABLE 23.4 | PAEDIATRIC NURSING HISTORY (ACTIVITIES OF DAILY LIVING)

Activity	Information obtained
Eating and drinking	Food and beverage likes and dislikes Any foods the child is not allowed to eat or is allergic to Usual appetite Feeding habits: cup, spoon, bottle, eats by self, needs assistance Special cultural requirements or habits If bottle fed, the formula and frequency of feeds
Sleeping	Usual time of sleep and waking Routine before sleep: drink, bedtime story, favourite toy or blanket, night-light Bed or cot Sleeps alone or with others Any problems, e.g. nightmares or sleepwalking
Elimination	Toilet trained or not Use of toilet, pot or nappies Use of words to communicate need to urinate and defecate Any problems, e.g. bed-wetting, constipation
Hygiene	Usual habits: bath or shower, hair and dental care Any problems/dislikes, e.g. having teeth cleaned Degree of assistance required Care of any prosthesis, e.g. glasses, contact lenses, orthodontic appliances, hearing aid
Play	Favourite toys and activities Attends crèche, playgroup, pre-school, school Favourite television programs, any restrictions Prefers to play with others or by self Any imaginary playmate

TABLE 23.5 | ASSESSING INFANTS AND CHILDREN

Item assessed	Observations
General appearance	Facial expression: alert, anxious, placid, pained, apathetic Posture: favouring a body part, e.g. knees drawn up to relax the abdominal muscles may indicate abdominal pain, or sitting up to relieve breathing difficulties; unusual gait, curvatures in posture, e.g. lateral curvature of the spine Range of joint motion Hygiene: cleanliness, unusual odour; condition of the hair, nails and teeth Nutritional status: overweight, underweight Behaviour: personality, level of activity, reactions to stress, interactions with others, listless, overactive; aggressive or regressive behaviour (a child's interaction with parents may provide valuable information about the child's behaviour) Development: speech, motor skills, degree of coordination
Skin	Colour, texture, temperature, moisture, turgor Lesions, scratches, bruises, scaliness, evidence of infestation, scars, bite marks, inflammation, rashes, oedema
Hair	Quality, texture, distribution, elasticity, evidence of infestation
Nails	Colour, shape, texture, quality
Mouth	Condition of lips, tongue, teeth and gums Presence of sores, coating, bad breath, ulcers, bleeding
Eyes	Pupils: size, equality, reaction to light Colour of sclera Presence of any inflammation, discharge, excessive watering, puffiness of the lids, squint, ptosis Any defects of vision
Ears	Accumulation of wax, discharge, presence of pain Any hearing defects
Chest and lungs	Shape, symmetry, movement of the chest Respirations are assessed for rate, rhythm, depth and quality. The character of breath sounds is noted, e.g. noisy, wheezing, grunting
Abdomen	Contour of the abdomen, e.g. distension or rigidity Condition of the skin covering the abdomen Movement, e.g. visible peristalsis Presence of hernias
Infant cries (the only way an infant can express feelings)	Characteristic for each infant, but common features include: • An angry cry with fist in the mouth (indicates hunger) • An angry cry with excessive movement of the arms and legs (indicates frustration) • A shrill, spasmodic cry (indicates pain) • A weak whimpering cry (indicates general weakness) • A fretful cry (may indicate loneliness, hunger, discomfort or boredom) • A hoarse cry (indicates an infection or obstruction of the respiratory tract) • A shrill cry (may indicate cerebral irritation)
Faeces	Colour, quantity, consistency, odour, frequency A breastfed infant's stools are yellow and paste-like A bottle-fed infant's stools are pale yellow to brown, firmer in consistency and have a more offensive odour Abnormalities include: • Green frothy stools • Pale offensive bulky stools • Watery stools • Presence of blood, mucus, parasites
Urine	Colour, quantity, odour, frequency

- Promoting parenting skills and parental attachment
- Alleviating stresses in particular families
- Removing a child from an abusive or potentially abusive situation.

Child abuse may be classed as:

- Physical abuse
- Neglect
- Failure to thrive
- Emotional deprivation and abuse
- Sexual abuse.

Signs of physical abuse may be readily identified or they may be less obvious and difficult to recognise. Some of the signs that should alert medical officers, nurses and others who work with children, include:

- Delay in seeking treatment for an injury
- Inadequate explanation of the cause of injuries
- Multiple injuries; for example, bruises, scratches, burns and bite marks
- The site of injuries; for example, localised burns on the buttocks or soles of the feet
- Presentation of the parents; for example, showing a lack of concern for the child or inability to comfort a distressed child
- Manifestations of developmental delay in a child; for example, delay in development of language skills.

Signs of emotional deprivation or abuse are generally more difficult to recognise. Emotional deprivation may be evident when signs of *failure to thrive* are present. Failure to thrive is generally defined as an underweight malnourished infant with a height and head circumference below normal. Although failure to thrive may be caused by emotional deprivation, other causes are organic ones or accidental underfeeding. Emotional abuse occurs when the child is not provided with the type of environment that is required for their optimal growth and development. The child may be subjected to continual verbal abuse, hostility and rejection.

Sexual abuse in children may present in a variety of ways:

- A history of sexual abuse from the child or a family member
- Vague abdominal pains or persistent or unexplained vaginal discharge
- Sexually transmitted infection
- Unexplained genital trauma
- Running away from home
- Sexually provocative behaviour.

RECORDING AND REPORTING

After conducting a general health assessment the nurse should document the collected data as follows:

- Record the client's vital signs on the vital signs chart
- Record the description of alterations in the client's general appearance
- Describe the client's behaviours using appropriate terminology. Include the client's description of their own signs and symptoms
- Report abnormalities and acute symptoms to the RN or medical officer.

TEACHING CONSIDERATIONS

While conducting the general survey, the nurse should use this as an opportunity to undertake health education with the client. The following could be incorporated:

- During the general survey, inform the client of the acceptable ranges for vital signs and normal weight for height
- Discuss the client's dietary intake and discuss any problems the client has in terms of food preparation or food selection
- If the client has been undertaking any high-risk behaviour activity such as smoking, overexposure to the sun, drinking alcohol, etc, discuss the health issues of these.

SUMMARY

The general health assessment is conducted to assess the function and integrity of the client's body. The health assessment is conducted in a systematic manner that requires the fewest position changes for the client. The data obtained in the physical health examination supplement, confirm or refute data obtained during the nursing history. These data can also help the nurse to establish nursing diagnoses, plan the client's care and evaluate the outcomes of nursing care (Berman et al 2007). Data collection is a vital part of a physical assessment and requires a comprehensive interview. A holistic assessment requires psychosocial and cultural data (deWit 2005).

REVIEW EXERCISES

1. What are the reasons that a physical assessment is performed on a client when admitted to a health care facility?
2. What are the three methods of assessment that a medical officer or RN would use when examining a client?
3. If you were admitting a child to the ward, what extra assessments would you perform?

CRITICAL THINKING EXERCISES

1. What assessment techniques should an EN use for the following clients:
   a) A client suspected of having a head injury?
   b) A client with a cast on the lower leg?
   c) A client reporting abdominal pain?
   d) A client being admitted for a surgical procedure?
2. What would you do if you were required to assess a client of the opposite sex and the person says he or she doesn't want you to do the assessment?
3. Mr Leonard enters the hospital with a history of weight loss and general fatigue. Describe three body systems that might be involved. What questions might you ask Mr Leonard to discover what primary system is involved?
4. Mrs Weigard, 76, is married and comes to outpatients with the complaint of 'severe burning in my hands and wrists'. She was diagnosed with arthritis more than a year ago. What type of questions might you ask of Mrs Weigard to assess how this has affected her lifestyle?

REFERENCES AND FURTHER READING

Agency for Health Care Policy and Research (1996) *Recognition and Initial Assessment of Alzheimer's Disease and Related Dementias*. Agency for Health Care Policy and Research, Rockville, MD

Berman AJ, Kozier B, Snyder S (2008) *Kozier and Erbs Fundamentals of Nursing: Concepts, Process, and*

Practice, 8th edn. Prentice-Hall, Upper Saddle River, NJ
Brown D, Edwards H (2008) *Lewis's Medical-Surgical Nursing: Assessment and Management of Clinical Problems*, 2nd edn. Mosby Elsevier Australia, Sydney
Crisp J, Taylor C (eds) (2005) *Potter & Perry's Fundamentals of Nursing*, 2nd edn. Elsevier Australia, Sydney: 739–42, 1348, 1351
deWit SC (2001) *Fundamental Concepts and Skills for Nursing*. WB Saunders, Philadelphia
Elkin M, Perry A, Potter P (2008) *Nursing Interventions and Clinical Skills*, 4th edn. Mosby Elsevier, Canada
Perry AG, Potter PA (2002) *Clinical Nursing Skills and Techniques*, 5th edn. Mosby, St Louis

Chapter 24

ADMISSION, TRANSFER AND DISCHARGE PROCESS

OBJECTIVES

- Define the key terms/concepts
- Describe the planning and implementation of care for the client who requires admission, transfer or discharge
- Describe the planning and implementation of care for the client who requires a diagnostic procedure
- Describe the means by which a child may be prepared for admission to hospital
- Outline the special aspects related to admission of a child
- State the responsibilities of the nurse in relation to assessment and observation of children

KEY TERMS/CONCEPTS

admission process
discharge process
stress
stressors
transfer process

CHAPTER FOCUS

Admission to a health care facility such as a hospital is a major event for clients and for their significant others, as they are often anxious about the admission, the illness and its implications. It is therefore most important that the nurse is familiar with the admission protocol so they can carry out the necessary activities in a manner which will help to reduce anxiety. This chapter outlines the admission process, transferring and discharge of children, adolescents and adults.

LIVED EXPERIENCE

My great-aunt had been developing memory loss over a year. She developed a urinary tract infection and became very confused, and was admitted into hospital for treatment. It was decided that she was too confused to ever go back home to her unit. She was transferred directly from hospital into an aged-care facility, never to return home to her own space and possessions. I remember feeling sad for my great-aunt who had been a single independent woman all her life. I never thought that for some people being admitted into hospital could mean that they may never resume their lifestyle again and how stressful and depressing this can be for the individual and their family.

Beth, age 36, great-niece

TYPES OF ADMISSION

Admissions are classified as either elective or non-elective. An elective admission is a planned admission, when individuals know in advance that they will be entering a health care facility. In many instances a person's name will have been placed on a waiting list until a bed becomes available. A non-elective or emergency admission is one in which admission to a health care facility has suddenly become necessary. The person may be acutely ill or severely injured. Admission may be arranged by a medical officer (local general practitioner) or may be via the emergency department of a hospital, without the person having been seen by a medical officer.

Health care facilities adopt admissions and discharge policy whereby people for elective admission report to the admitting department on a specified date at a specified time. Implementing this policy promotes efficient admission procedures and subsequent care of the individual. Before an elective admission the person visits the admitting department to arrange the date and time. At this visit the individual is given a printed information leaflet providing details about the admission. Information on the leaflet includes a list of items the person should bring with them; details about visiting hours; the facilities available (such as the kiosk and telephone service); and any instructions regarding pre-admission investigations or procedures that have been prescribed. Alternatively, this may be conducted over the phone or by mail.

REACTIONS TO ADMISSION

Most people face admission to a health care facility with reluctance, while others may experience relief that something is being done to deal with their illness. Whether a person is to be admitted for a brief or an extended period, any admission is associated with various potential stressors. Previous admissions can affect a person's reactions and expectations, while an individual being admitted for the first time faces the unknown. Elective admission for a relatively minor condition generally causes less stress than does an emergency admission. The nurse must remember that although many anxieties about, and reactions to, admission are common to most people, each person is an individual.

Stress is a phenomenon in which the individual perceives environmental stimuli as taxing their physiological, psychological or sociological systems. Stressors, which may be classified as either physical or psychological, are factors that require a response or change. Apart from the implications of the reason for admission, admission to hospital is a major stressor for most people. Features of admission that produce stress and pose a threat to self-concept, self-esteem and body image include:

- Loss of independence and control over events
- Disruption to relationships
- Unfamiliar environment, equipment and personnel
- Possible loss of income
- Possible effects on employment prospects
- The nature and implications of the illness
- Painful and/or embarrassing tests or procedures
- Worry to others of significance to the client (often referred to as 'significant others')
- Restrictions on the activities of living
- Loss of privacy and dignity
- Loss of emotional or moral support
- Fear of dying and death.

Reactions to stress and coping mechanisms are described in Chapter 13 and include:

- Nervousness
- Anxiety
- Irritability
- Emotional lability
- Anger or hostility
- Decreased tolerance towards other people
- Forgetfulness
- Confusion
- Indifference
- Withdrawal
- Depression
- Difficulty in sleeping
- Physical manifestations; for example, palpitations, headaches, loss of appetite or gastrointestinal disturbances.

The nurse should therefore attempt to reduce the stressors related to admission to a health care facility. The nurse should approach the client in a warm and empathetic manner and provide information about the admission procedures and subsequent activities. The nurse should implement ways of maintaining the client's independence, self-esteem and dignity. One of the most important ways in which this can be achieved is to involve the individual in planning and evaluating care.

THE ADMISSION PROCESS

ADMITTING AN ADULT TO A HEALTH CARE FACILITY

The process of admission prepares the individual for their stay in the health care facility. Admission procedures that are efficient and demonstrate appropriate concern for the individual will help to ease anxiety. Effective admission procedures are directed towards:

- Verifying the client's identity
- Assessing the client's physical and psychological status
- Promoting the client's comfort in an unfamiliar environment
- Providing items needed for care
- Providing the client with information about various practices and protocol.

Room preparation

Before the client is admitted to the unit, the nursing team will determine the location of their bed. Depending on need and availability, the client may be admitted into a single or shared room. Before the client arrives the nurse should check to see that the room is in order and that all the necessary items are available. The room should contain a bed, bedside locker, over-bed table, chair and wardrobe. The bed may need to be adapted to meet specific needs; for example, by providing extra pillows, a bed-cradle, a sheepskin blanket, or a fracture board under the mattress.

Although the items placed in the room may vary slightly in different health care facilities, the basic items provided for each individual are two bath towels, two face washers and an information booklet. Extra items, such as oxygen equipment, suction apparatus, side rails for the bed or an intravenous pole are placed in the room if required. The top of the bedclothes may be turned back or they may be folded down to receive a client who arrives on a trolley.

Reception of the client

Chapter 23 provides details of the admission assessment. Before arrival in the unit (unless it is an emergency admission) the client reports to the admitting department. Here a member of the clerical staff obtains and records information including the person's full name; age; sex; marital status; religion; address; the name, address and telephone number of next of kin; and details about any hospital insurance. An identification band (Figure 24.1) is placed on the client's wrist as a basic safety precaution against mistaken identity and treatment. Some facilities require clients to wear two identification bands, one on the wrist and one on the ankle. The person is advised whether to attend the X-ray or pathology department before admission to the unit. The individual is then escorted to the unit, where a nurse receives them.

The nurse who is responsible for admission to the unit should greet the client, and any accompanying relative or friend, in a warm and friendly manner. The nurse should address the person by name and introduce themselves, then escort the person to the room and begin the process of admission. Depending on the circumstances, a relative or friend may be present and may be offered a seat in a waiting area.

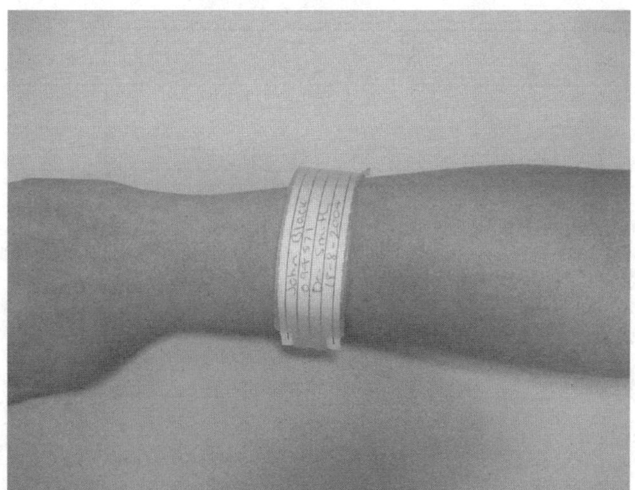

Figure 24.1 | Identification band

The admission procedure is basically the same in most health care facilities but will vary in detail in different settings, and in sequence, according to circumstances. The client is taken to the room and introduced to any other person in the room. If sharing a room, privacy must be ensured. The client is shown the general layout of the room and where to put personal belongings. It is important that the client is shown how to use the signal device, any fitted television or radio controls, and lights. The client's identification band should be checked and compared with the card on the bed to see that they are correct. The client is shown the location of the bathroom, toilet, sitting room and telephones. Depending on circumstances, the client may remain in day clothes and be able to walk about the ward, or may be required to change into night clothes and get into bed.

Although the client will have been advised not to bring valuable items, documentation is made of any personal effects. It is not generally necessary to itemise clothing, but a list is compiled of any items of value, such as a wristwatch, jewellery, television set, radio and money. Some health care facilities also require that documentation is made of any prosthesis, such as dentures, a hearing aid or artificial limb. If the client has a large sum of money they are advised to either send it home or to place it in the health care facility's safe. A 'valuables' envelope is provided for the safe-keeping of money or valuable items. It is very important to inform the client that the health care facility does not accept responsibility for valuable items unless they are deposited in the safe. The nurse should refer to the facility's policy regarding the procedure to be followed when the person's valuables are to be stored.

Many health care facilities have a booklet that contains information about various aspects of the organisation. The booklet contains details such as visiting times; meal times; how to identify the various personnel; kiosk, telephone, television and laundry facilities available; regulations regarding smoking, and the time the individual is expected to vacate the room on discharge.

As soon as practicable, assessment is made of vital signs and weight, and the information documented. A sample of urine is obtained and urinalysis performed. (Information on vital signs and urinalysis are provided in Chapters 21 and 22.) The client's height may also be measured and documented.

Throughout the admission procedure, the nurse should discreetly observe the client to gain information that will assist in planning care. Assessment is made, and documented (Figure 24.2), of the client's:

- General physical appearance
- Degree of mobility
- Level of independence
- Psychological status

BROADMEADOWS HEALTH SERVICE

NURSING ADMISSION ASSESSMENT

AFFIX PATIENT IDENTIFICATION LABEL HERE

U.R. NUMBER: ______________________

SURNAME: ______________________

GIVEN NAME: ______________________

DATE OF BIRTH: ____/____/____

Date of Admission: ____/____/____ Time: __________ Admitted From: ______________________

Reason for Admission: ______________________

____

____

1) CLINICAL ASSESSEMENT ON ADMISSION:

T __________ P __________ R __________ BP Lying __________ BP Standing __________

Weight __________ O_2 Saturation __________ BSL __________ ECG __________

Urine colour __________ Odour __________ U/A __________ SG __________ PH __________

Pupils: ● ● ● ● ● ● ● ●

1 2 3 4 5 6 7 8

Pupil Size: left right

Pupil Reaction: left right

2) BEHAVIOUR / MOOD: (Circle appropriate response)

Alert Confused Drowsy Disoriented Agitated Non-Responsive

General Comments: ______________________

Memory (past and present): ______________________

Mood (Please circle): Depressed Normal Elevated

Dysfunctional Behaviour (note any specific concerns): ______________________

3) COMMUNICATION

Preferred language spoken: ______________________

Interpreter Required: Yes / No Interpreter Sticker: Yes

SPEECH: Impairment Yes / No Refer to Speech Pathologist: Yes / No

HEARING: Impairment Yes / No Aid: Left Ear / Right Ear

VISION: Impairment Yes / No (L) Eye: ______ (R): ______ Prosthesis: ______

Glasses Lens

Date Revised 26/6/03

NURSING ADMISSION ASSESSMENT

ON TRIAL

Figure 24.2 | Admission chart *(reproduced with permission from Broadmeadows Health Service)*

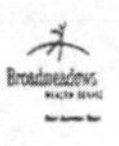

NURSING ADMISSION ASSESSMENT

4) SKIN INTEGRITY

HEAD

TRUNK

EXTREMITIES

1. Oedema
2. Rash
3. Bruised
4. Colour Change
5. Nails
6. Skin Integrity
7. Pain
8. Wound (refer to wound assessment tool)

5) PRESSURE INJURY RISK ASSESSMENT: (Waterlow Score)
Refer to the Waterlow Risk Assessment at the back of the Nursing Care Plan.

6) FALLS RISK ASSESSMENT:
Refer to the Falls Risk Assessment at the back of the Nursing Care Plan.

7) FUNCTIONAL DECLINE

Has there been a recent change in ability to maintain independence with any ADLs? Yes [ ] No [ ]

Please comment: ______________________________

____

5) NUTRITIONAL RISK SCREEN

Underweight	Yes [ ]	No [ ]
Overweight	Yes [ ]	No [ ]
Unintentional Weight Loss	Yes [ ]	No [ ]
Reduced Appetite	Yes [ ]	No [ ]
Chewing / Swallowing Problems	Yes [ ]	No [ ]
Mouth / Teeth Problems	Yes [ ]	No [ ]

6) CONTINENCE

Bladder	Yes [ ]	No [ ]
Bowel	Yes [ ]	No [ ]
Assessment commenced as per protocol		[ ]

7) ORIENTATION TO THE WARD:

[ ] Call Bell	[ ] Meal Times	[ ] Personal Clothing	[ ] Telephone
[ ] Bathroom / Toilet	[ ] Valuables	[ ] Television	[ ] Lights
[ ] Visiting Hours	[ ] Smoking Regulations	[ ] Dining / Sitting Rooms	

PCU / ECU2 / REHAB Specialty routine explained: Yes [ ] No [ ]

8) RELIGIOUS BELIEFS: Religion: ______________________________

Is there anything we can do to accommodate your cultural or religious beliefs? ______________________________

____

____

ON TRIAL

Date Revised 26/6/03

______________________________ ______________________________ ______/______/______

Figure 24.2 | Admission chart — cont'd

- Skin
- Hearing and visual acuity
- Ability to communicate
- Level of consciousness and orientation
- Gait and posture
- Use of any prostheses or aids.

At the time of admission or as soon as possible afterwards, a nursing history is compiled and a nursing care plan developed. (Information on these and other aspects of the nursing process are provided in Chapters 19 and 20.)

The client should be provided with a flask of fluid and offered a cup of tea or coffee, unless oral fluids are contraindicated. Anybody accompanying the client may also be offered a drink or shown where to find the kiosk. This is of particular importance if it is an emergency admission. The client's significant others may be very distressed, and may appreciate being shown to an area where they can sit and rest for a while. The health care facility may also provide accommodation for the relatives if the client is very ill.

Before leaving the room the nurse should ensure that the client and significant others have been given all the information they require. The nurse should answer any questions or, if not able to, refer them to the nurse in charge. The nurse should also bear in mind that a person who is stressed tends not to hear or remember all the information given; therefore, ensure that the information is repeated whenever necessary.

ADMITTING A CHILD TO A HEALTH CARE FACILITY

When a child has a condition that requires hospitalisation the nurse should understand the effects of admission on the child and parents. Admission to hospital may be planned or unexpected and the nurse should realise that an emergency admission is a time of crisis for the child and family, as there is no time to prepare them for the event. Children must never be threatened with hospitalisation as a form of punishment, nor should they be told they will be going on a holiday rather than telling them they are to be admitted to hospital.

A range of factors influence the way in which a child and the child's family react when illness or an injury make it necessary for the child to be admitted to hospital. These include:

- The age of the child and ability to comprehend the situation
- The amount of preparation of the child by the parents before admission. An emotionally secure child usually adapts well if given a realistic explanation of hospital life, is told the reason for admission and what will happen and has an assurance that one or both parents will spend as much time as possible with the child. Many parents fail to prepare a child for hospitalisation and in some cases may transmit their own fears and misconceptions, with the result that admission to hospital is a very frightening and traumatic experience for the child
- The condition of the child. An acutely ill or severely injured child may not be totally aware of the situation but the parents will be distressed and apprehensive
- The cultural background of the child. In some cultures there is an extended and very closely knit family pattern and the child who is accustomed to the loving protection and guidance from parents, grandparents, aunts and uncles can be quite devastated when separated from such an environment. In other situations, in which a child leads a lonely existence with little companionship or family support, the company of other children and the attention received in hospital may be very welcome
- The reaction shown by the parents can markedly influence a child's reaction to illness and hospitalisation. Anxiety, tension, worry or emotional outbursts on the parents' part are likely to increase the child's feelings of fear and insecurity, whereas serene, calm, confident and supportive parent's can allay the child's fears and promote a feeling of security
- The relationship between the hospital staff and the child's parents is a very important factor, particularly in the case of an older child, who will relate more readily to nurses who have established rapport with the parents.

The role of the parents during a child's illness is now acknowledged as being of the utmost importance and most hospitals allow unrestricted visiting, while many provide accommodation facilities for the parents of children who are very sick. The parent should be encouraged to participate in the care of the child, with guidance and help from the nurse assigned to the particular child. When a parent is prevented from spending much time with the sick child because of home commitments or for economic reasons, a social worker may be consulted with a view to discussing and arranging help for the parent.

Preparation for admission

Children accept admission to hospital much better if they have been adequately prepared beforehand. While it is not possible to explain hospitalisation to infants, children from about age 2 can be helped to adjust to this significant event by adequate preparation. Preparation is directed towards overcoming fears and anxieties, such as the fear of:

- Separation
- Bodily injury and pain
- Loss of routine and rituals
- Physical restrictions
- Enforced dependency and loss of independence
- Strangers
- Loss of body image.

Preparation for admission involves explaining what will happen in language appropriate for the child's level of comprehension. Many excellent publications are available, some in picture form, which may be used to reinforce explanations. Parents should encourage their child to discuss all aspects of hospitalisation to help overcome any fears and anxieties. Many hospitals encourage visits to the ward before admission so that the child can see the area and meet some of the personnel who will be involved in their care. Another way of preparing children is to allow them to decide the items they want to take to hospital and allowing them to pack their own case in readiness for the trip.

Parents may also experience many fears and anxieties when their child is to be admitted to hospital. They can be helped to overcome anxiety if they are provided with information about the child's condition and aspects of their hospitalisation. They must be given opportunities to ask any questions and discuss their anxieties. The emphasis on parental involvement and family-centred care can do much to relieve anxiety. The parents should be informed of the facilities available if they wish to stay with their child, and they are encouraged to participate in the child's care.

In an emergency admission there is no time to prepare the child or parents and the event can therefore be very traumatic for both. Encouraging one or both parents to stay as long as possible can reduce some of the child's fears and anxieties.

Many children go through various phases of disturbance when they are hospitalised, particularly if they are separated from the parents. During the initial phase, that of protest, the child may cry or scream for their parents and refuse the attention of anyone else. It is not unusual for the child to stop protesting only when physically exhausted. During the second stage, that of despair, the crying generally subsides and the child may become withdrawn and apathetic. The child may feel abandoned and experience feelings of hopelessness and grief. During the third stage, that of detachment, the child appears to have adjusted to the separation but in reality the child is detaching from the parents in an attempt to escape the pain and wishing they were there. When the parents do visit, the child may react with disinterest and, unless the parents understand these reactions, they may become very distressed. To respond appropriately, nurses need to be aware of the phases and signs of separation anxiety. Much paediatric nursing care is directed towards helping the child and the parents adjust to the reality of hospitalisation.

Admission

Admission to hospital can be frightening for a child and distressing for the family. As most children respond to their parents' reactions, it is important that the nurse gains the parents' confidence from the time of admission. This is reassuring to the child, who is quick to sense the parents' reactions.

Before admission, the nurse in charge of the ward assigns a room based on the child's age and diagnosis. Whenever possible, children of the same age group with similar types of illnesses are placed in the same room. Other children in the room should be informed of the pending arrival of a new patient so that they can be welcomed. The room should be prepared and all the necessary documents and items of equipment placed nearby so that the admitting nurse will not have to leave the child.

The admission procedure may vary slightly between hospitals, depending on hospital policy and the prevailing circumstances. Admitting a child involves assessing vital signs, measuring height and weight, placing an identity band on the child's wrist and/or ankle, obtaining a sample of urine for urinalysis, introductions to other children in the room, and orienting the family to the available facilities, such as signal devices, television controls, telephone, bathroom and toilet. The child and parents should be shown the playroom and dining areas and the parents should be provided with details about the rooming-in facilities.

During admission, the parents are encouraged to remain with the child and to assist with activities such as undressing and settling at night. The use of each piece of equipment should be explained, and the child may be encouraged to handle some of the items to allay fears. Most children and parents will react and adapt better if they are informed in advance of the possibility of treatments involving the use of intravenous therapy equipment, drainage tubes, dressings, plasters or oxygen apparatus.

GENERAL ASPECTS OF PAEDIATRIC NURSING

Care of children differs from the care of adults in many ways; for example, the inability of very young children to communicate necessitates special skills of observation and interpretation. Each child must be treated as an individual but there are certain aspects of care which apply to all children:

- Complete honesty is important. Simple explanations before any procedure is performed should be given in language appropriate for the child's level of development and comprehension. A child should not be told that a technique or procedure will not hurt if in fact it is likely to do so. The nurse should be patient and be prepared to take the time necessary to help the child understand, and to allay anxiety
- The nurse should recognise the child's need for love and a feeling of security. Parents should be encouraged to room-in or to spend as much time as possible with their child. If the parent(s) cannot be with the child all the time, the nurse should give extra attention and demonstrate affection towards the child
- Whenever possible the same nurse(s) should care for the child during hospitalisation. An attempt should be made to maintain a routine similar to the one the child is accustomed to at home. A similar routine makes hospital life less bewildering for a child and promotes a feeling of security

- Efforts should be made to minimise a hospital-type environment, for example, by encouraging the child to wear their own clothes, to sit at a table for meals, and by allowing the child to keep as many attachments to home as possible, such as family photographs and their own toys
- Lessen the feeling of separation from home by encouraging the child to talk about home, family, pets, friends and school. If the parent(s) cannot be with the child all the time, it is sometimes helpful if they leave small parcels for the child to open each day. Visits by siblings, other relatives and friends should be encouraged
- Show respect for the dignity of the child and their right to privacy. Undue exposure, for example when dressing, can cause embarrassment, especially for an older child
- Maintain the degree of independence and the behaviour patterns established by the parents. It can be distressing for the parents, and detrimental to the child, if a child's development is retarded as a result of a period spent in hospital
- Allow for periods of regression during hospitalisation and recognise that regressive behaviour is a feature of illness. For example, a child who was previously toilet-trained may regress to bed-wetting
- Provide opportunities for play. Play is an activity by which a child can practise and perfect skills, give expression to thoughts and feelings, be creative, perfect language and be prepared for adult behaviour and roles. Play within a hospital environment is a valuable means of teaching and of reducing anxiety. A range of play materials should be provided that are suitable for the child's level of development, condition and capabilities. Some paediatric facilities provide play therapists, whose function is to ensure that a child is occupied, has the opportunity to play and be creative, and is provided with an outlet to release pent-up feelings
- Provide an atmosphere and opportunities that encourage free expression of feelings by the child and parents
- Preparation for discharge from hospital involves providing the parents, and child if able to understand, with information about medications or other forms of treatment or care required, arranging appointments and/or contact with the visiting nurse service, and ensuring that the parents understand that the child may experience some behavioural problems after returning home; for example, sleep disturbances, difficulties at school, or regressive behaviours.

ADMITTING AN ADOLESCENT TO A HEALTH CARE FACILITY

Adolescence is a stage of development characterised by sudden physical changes and social and emotional maturing. It is frequently described as a transition period between childhood and adulthood, which begins with the gradual appearance of secondary sex characteristics and ends with cessation of body growth. (Further information on growth and development during adolescence is provided in Chapter 17.)

When an adolescent requires admission to hospital, the most appropriate environment is a ward or unit that has been specially designed to cater for the needs of adolescents. It is not usually appropriate for an adolescent to be nursed in a paediatric ward or in a ward where the patients are middle aged or elderly. When a special ward is not available the adolescent should be placed in a room where the other occupants are about the same age and the same gender.

Because the adolescent is seeking independence, the nurse should try to involve them in their own care as much as possible. The adolescent should be encouraged to participate in decision making and care planning and should be allowed the maximum amount of independence appropriate to the situation.

Accidents are the greatest cause of deaths in the adolescent age group, as their tendency for risk-taking behaviour together with feelings of indestructibility make them particularly prone to accidents, especially those involving motor vehicles and sports.

DISCHARGE PLANNING

Effective discharge from a health care facility requires careful planning and continuing assessment of the client's needs during their stay. Ideally, discharge planning begins soon after the client's admission. The purpose of discharge planning is to assist the client to make a smooth transition from one setting or level of care to another without impending the progress already achieved, and to provide for other health needs that are still not met. Discharge planning is directed towards teaching the client and significant others about the condition and its effects on lifestyle, providing instructions for performing self-care activities, informing the client of any dietary or activity restrictions, and arranging for any follow-up care that may be necessary.

The concept of continuity of care recognises that the client's needs change and that the type of services necessary to support these needs also change. Health services that may be required after the client's discharge include long-term and rehabilitation settings, nursing home or day care centres. Services outside the health care facility setting include community nursing, home nursing resources and community facilities such as 'meals on wheels'. Because of shortened hospital stays it is often unrealistic to teach clients everything they need to know. Referral to a home health agency for follow-up teaching may be necessary. In such situations the hospital nurse needs to prepare clients with sufficient information and supplies to manage at home for at least a few days until the home health nurse arrives.

Discharge planning is a team approach involving the client and significant others, the medical officer, nurses and other health care team members, such as the occupational therapist, physiotherapist and dietician. The steps involved in discharge planning are:

- Assessing the client and their significant others
- Analysing data to identify specific needs
- Planning to meet those needs
- Implementing the plan
- Evaluating the discharge planning process and the results (Figure 24.3).

PREPARING CLIENTS TO GO HOME

Nurses preparing the client to go home need to assess:

- The client's personal and health data
- The client's ability to perform the activities of daily living
- Any physical, cognitive or other functional limitations that the client may have
- Carers' responses and abilities
- Adequacy of the client's financial resources
- Community supports
- Hazards or barriers that the home environment presents
- Need for health care assistance in the home (Clinical Interest Box 24.1).

The following outcomes must be evaluated for a client's discharge plan (Figure 24.4):

- Can the client and family, if appropriate, explain the diagnosis and the safe and effective use of discharge medications?
- What specialised instruction or training is required for the client and family to be able to provide proper care after discharge?
- What community support systems need to be coordinated to enable the client to return home safely?
- Are the client and family able to cope with the client's health status?
- Is relocation of the client, coordination of support systems, or transfer to another health care facility needed (Figure 24.5)?

CLINICAL INTEREST BOX 24.1
Discharge planning — home assessment parameters

Personal and health data
Age, sex, height and weight, cultural data, a medical history, current health status, surgery

Abilities to perform activities of daily living (ADLs)
Abilities for dressing, eating, toileting, bathing (bath, shower, sponge), ambulating (with or without aids such as a cane, crutches, walker, wheelchair), transferring (from bed to chair, in and out of bath, in and out of car), meal preparation, transportation and shopping.

Disabilities/limitations
Sensory losses (auditory, visual), motor losses (paralysis, amputation), communication disorder, mental confusion or depression, incontinence, etc.

Caregivers' responses/abilities
Principal caregiver's relationship to client, thoughts and feelings about client's discharge, expectations for recovery, health and coping abilities, comfort with performing required care.

Financial resources
Financial resources and needs (note equipment, supplies, medications, special foods required).

Community supports
Family members, friends, neighbours, volunteers, resources such as nutrition services, health centres, community health nurses, day programs, legal assistance, home care, respite care.

Home hazard appraisal
Safety precautions (stairs with or without handrails; lighting in rooms, hallways and stairways; night-lights in hallways or bathroom; grab bars near toilet and tub; firmly attached carpets and rugs), self-care barriers (lack of running water, lack of wheelchair access to bathroom or home, lack of space for required equipment, lack of elevator).

Need for health care assistance
Home-delivered meals; special dietary needs; volunteers for telephone reassurance, friendly visiting, transportation, shopping; assistance with bathing; assistance with housekeeping; assistance with wound care, ostomies, tubes, intravenous medications, etc.

(Berman et al 2008)

TEACHING AS PART OF DISCHARGE PLANNING

The goal is to provide clients and families with the knowledge and skills required to meet ongoing health needs. It is difficult to provide clients with information they need the evening before or the morning of discharge. Before beginning to teach, you must determine what information has already been given by the medical officer or other carers. Get the client to describe what they believe they are to do when they go home — inconsistencies can then be identified and clarification given. Be aware of possible learning barriers that affect all clients. Learning will be enhanced if spoken instructions are reinforced with written materials. A variety of modes of presentation are used, such as videotapes, booklets and discussions. The nurse should document any instruction that is given to a client.

After a family has learned how to perform any necessary carer skills, have them assume care before the client returns home. Many hospitals require family members to manage care before the client is discharged home (Perry & Potter 2002).

DAY OF DISCHARGE

When the date and time of discharge have been determined, the client and significant others are informed. Transport is arranged for the client if necessary. Before the client leaves the health care facility the nurse should check that:

- The medical officer's discharge orders for prescriptions, changes in treatment or the need for special equipment have been organised

THE ALFRED Discharge Plan

U.R. ______

Surname ______

Given Names ______

Facsimile From: ______ Phone: (03) 9276 ______

Hospital Doctor: ______ Phone: (03) 9276 ______
Primary Nurse: ______ Phone: (03) 9276 ______
Allied Health: ______ Phone: (03) 9276 ______
GP Name: ______ Phone: ______
Case Manager: Yes ❐ No ❐ Name: ______ Phone: ______
Interpreter required: Yes ❐ No ❐ Language: ______
Discharge Date: ______ Discharging Ward: ______ Discharge Destination: ______ Discharge Time: ______

Community Services Needed: Yes ❐ No ❐ Patient declined services offered ❐ (please indicate services declined in table below)
Please complete for all new and existing community services

Service	✔ if service involved	Name & title of Community Service staff member spoken to	Date service to commence	Contact phone number	Fax number
Alfred @ Home					Not Applicable
RDNS/ Community Nursing					★
Post Acute Care/ InterPAC					★
Council Services: MOW ❐ Home Help ❐ Personal Care ❐					★
Palliative Care Services					★
Mental Health Services					★
Community Health/ Rehabilitation Centre ______ ______					★
Other (specify) ______					★
Other (specify) ______					★

★ please complete the continuation of this table over the page

Follow up phone call appointment	Yes ❐ No/Refused ❐ N/A ❐	Date:	Time:

Outpatients Appointments:

Doctor/Clinic	Place/Floor	Date	Time

General Instructions:

The above material has been reviewed with me. My questions have been answered and I understand the contents. I am aware that this information will be sent to my GP and the Community Services involved in my ongoing care.

Patient's/Carer's Signature: ______ **Nurse's Signature:** ______

This message is confidential and intended only for the person to whom it is addressed. If you have received it in error please notify the sender and destroy the document. Any unauthorised disclosure, copying or distribution or taking action in reliance on its contents is prohibited and may be unlawful. Bayside Health is not liable for the proper and complete transmission of the information contained in this communication or for any delay in its receipt.

Page 1 of 2

ORIGINAL TO REMAIN IN MEDICAL RECORD Copy of front page to be given to patient on discharge and copy to be attached to call back data sheet (MR E-57)

DISCHARGE PLAN

MR E-66

1635 03/02

Figure 24.3 | Discharge sheet *(reproduced with permission of The Alfred Hospital, Melbourne)*

Table to be completed by the Alfred hospital staff member notifying/contacting the Community Service Provider.

For example: if the Palliative Care Nurse Co-ordinator contacts a Palliative Care Community Service to notify them of a patient who will be needing their service, then he/she completes the relevant line in the table (palliative care services). If however, Nursing staff or another staff member (Allied Health etc) make this initial contact with the Community Service Provider, they are responsible for completing this line in the table.

Service	Notification method	Date * notified __/__/__	EDD ** provided __/__/__	Date confirmed if appropriate	Name and Title of Alfred staff member ***	Pager number if appropriate
RDNS/ Community Nursing	ph ❐ fax ❐ in person ❐					
Post Acute Care/ InterPAC	ph ❐ fax ❐ in person ❐					
Council Services: MOW ❐ Home Help ❐ Personal Care ❐	ph ❐ fax ❐ in person ❐					
Palliative Care Services	ph ❐ fax ❐ in person ❐					
Mental Health Services	ph ❐ fax ❐ in person ❐					
Community Health/ Rehabilitation Centre	ph ❐ fax ❐ in person ❐ ph ❐ fax ❐ in person ❐					
Other (specify) ________	ph ❐ fax ❐ in person ❐					
Other (specify) ________	ph ❐ fax ❐ in person ❐					

* Date notified – date external Community Service Provider notified. This should be **at least 2 days prior to discharge** (or day prior to discharge if LOS ≤ 3 days).

** EDD provided – please indicate the estimated discharge date provided to the Community Service Provider on notification.

*** Contact details of the Alfred staff member notifying the Community Service Provider and which have been provided to the Community Service Provider if they require any additional information regarding the patient.

Discharge Checklist:

Routine requirements	Yes	No	N/A	Provided and explained by:
Discharge Medications				
Medication Education - verbal ❐ - written ❐				
Medical Certificate/Other paperwork (Centrelink, WorkCover, TAC)				
Wound Care/Other Education Information				
Dressing Materials				
Clothing/Valuables returned				
Private X-rays returned				
Aids/Equipment required				
Transport type:			By Whom:	

1635 03/02

Page 2 of 2

ORIGINAL TO REMAIN IN MEDICAL RECORD

Figure 24.3 | Discharge sheet — cont'd

DISCHARGE PLANNING ASSESSMENT PART B

TO BE COMMENCED ON ADMISSION AND COMPLETED PRIOR TO DISCHARGE

ACCOMMODATION

☐ NURSING HOME ☐ HOSTEL ☐ RETIREMENT VILLAGE
☐ BOARDING HOUSE ☐ OWN HOUSE/UNIT ☐ RENTED HOUSE/FLAT

NUMBER OF STAIRS: FRONT/BACK ______ INTERNAL ______

COMMUNITY ASSISTANCE BEFORE ADMISSION

☐ DOMICILIARY NURSES ☐ MEALS ON WHEELS ☐ HOME HELP ______
☐ COMMUNITY NURSES ☐ Q.A.S. ☐ OTHER ______
☐ NIL ☐ HOME MEDICAL AIDS ______

DOMESTIC ARRANGEMENTS

☐ LIVES ALONE ☐ WITH FAMILY ☐ OTHER ______

CONCERNS RE MANAGEMENT AT HOME

PATIENT ______

CARER ______

LEVEL OF A.D.Ls.

RequiresAssistanceWith:	***Before Admission***		***At Discharge***	
HYGIENE/GROOMING:	☐ NO	☐ YES	☐ NO	☐ YES
TOILETING:	☐ NO	☐ YES	☐ NO	☐ YES
MOBILISING (Incl. Transfers)	☐ NO	☐ YES	☐ NO	☐ YES
MEALS:	☐ NO	☐ YES	☐ NO	☐ YES
CLEANING/LAUNDRY:	☐ NO	☐ YES	☐ NO	☐ YES
SHOPPING:	☐ NO	☐ YES	☐ NO	☐ YES
WOUND/ULCER/STOMA CARE:	☐ NO	☐ YES	☐ NO	☐ YES
MEDICATIONS:	☐ NO	☐ YES	☐ NO	☐ YES
TRANSPORT:	☐ NO	☐ YES	☐ NO	☐ YES
FINANCES:	☐ NO	☐ YES	☐ NO	☐ YES
COMMUNICATION:	☐ NO	☐ YES	☐ NO	☐ YES

DISCHARGE PROBLEMS IDENTIFIED

1 ______
2 ______
3 ______
4 ______

REFERRED TO: ☐ C.L.N. ☐ S.W. ☐ O.T. ☐ O.P.D. ☐ L.M.O. ☐ PHYSIO. ☐ GARU.

SIGNATURE ______ **STATUS:** ______ **TIME:** ______

PRINT NAME ______ **UNIT:** ______ **DATE:** ______

IP C:\DESIGN41\RCJ96NOV\RC1970FX.DS4 CMIU

Figure 24.4 | Discharge risk assessment form *(reproduced with permission of Royal Brisbane Hospital, Brisbane, Qld)*

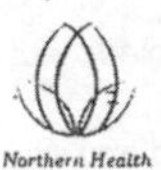

INTERHOSPITAL NURSING TRANSFER

U.R. NUMBER: ____________________

SURNAME: ____________________

GIVEN NAME: ____________________

DATE OF BIRTH: ____/____/____ SEX: ________

NORTHERN HEALTH

Transferred from:

☐ **NORTHERN HEALTH**
185 Cooper Street, Epping Victoria 3076
Phone: 8405 8000 Fax. 8405 8344

☐ **BUNDOORA EXTENDED CARE CENTRE**
1231 Plenty Road, Bundoora, Victoria, 3083
Phone: 9495 3100 Fax: 9467 4365

☐ **BROADMEADOWS HEALTH SERVICE**
35 Johnstone Street, Broadmeadows, Victoria 3047
Phone: 8345 5127 Fax: 8345 5353

Transferred to: ____________________

Northern Health Consultant Doctor: ____________________

Local Doctor: ____________________ Phone: ____________ Fax: ____________

Admission Date: ____/____/____ Transfer Date: ____/____/____

PERSONAL DETAILS:

Next of kin (1): Name: ____________ Relationship: ____________ Phone: ____________

Next of kin (2): Name: ____________ Relationship: ____________ Phone: ____________

N.O.K aware of patient's condition?: YES / NO N.O.K. aware of transfer?: YES / NO

Clothing sent with patient?: YES / NO Valuables sent with patient?: YES / NO

Details of belongings: ____________________

____

Dentures with patient: Upper / Lower / None Spectacles with patient?: YES / NO

Other aids / prostheses sent with patient: ____________________

RELEVANT MEDICAL DETAILS:

DIAGNOSIS: ____________________

REASON FOR TRANSFER: ____________________

METHOD OF TRANSPORT FOR TRANSFER (e.g. ambulance): ____________________

DOES THIS PATIENT NEED AN ESCORT? YES / NO If Yes, escorted by: ____________________

PROCEDURES / OPERATIONS: ____________________

COMPLICATIONS: ____________________

PAST MEDICAL HISTORY: ____________________

____

____

SOCIAL CIRCUMSTANCES: ____________________

____

CONSCIOUS STATE (eg confused?): ____________________

BEHAVIOUR: ____________________

LANGUAGE SPOKEN: ____________________ Interpreter Required? YES/NO

SPEECH IMPAIRMENT: ____________________

HEARING IMPAIRMENT: ____________________ Hearing Aid with patient? Right / Left / None

THE NORTHERN HOSPITAL

FORM 11404 MAY '02D

Figure 24.5 | Transfer form *(reproduced with permission from Northern Health, Victoria)*

MOBILITY: **On Bed:** Independent / Supervision / Able to Assist - 1 staff / Able to Assist - 2 staff / Not Able to Assist

Off Bed: Independent / Supervision / Able to Assist - 1 staff / Able to Assist - 2 staff / Not Able to Assist

Manual Handling Aids: ______

Gait Aids: ______

FALLS: High risk / Low risk ______

Falls in last 12-months? YES / NO Fall during current admission: YES / NO

Preventative Strategies: ______

PERSONAL HYGIENE: Independent / Supervision / Able to Assist - 1 staff / Able to Assist - 2 staff / Not Able to Assist

PRESSURE AREAS: Nil / Present Details: ______

Preventative Strategies ______

WOUND / DRESSINGS: ______

______

INTAKE: Oral / Intravenous / Naso - gastric / P.E.G.

DETAILS (include diet): ______

OUTPUT: **Urine:** Continent / Incontinent

Urinary Catheter: YES / NO Insertion Date: ____/____/____ Size: ______

DETAILS: ______

Faeces: Continent / Incontinent

Bowels last opened: ______

DETAILS (include aperients required): ______

Stoma: YES / NO DETAILS: ______

OTHER GENERAL COMMENTS: ______

______

______

MOST RECENT (relevant) VITAL SIGNS PRIOR TO TRANSFER: Temp: ______ Pulse: ______ Resp: ______ BP: ______

O_2 Sat: ______ BSL: ______ Other: ______

CURRENT MEDICATIONS: See attached photocopy of Medication Chart

ALLERGIES (Drug, Food etc): ______

OTHER ALERTS (eg MRSA): ______

Doctor's letter sent: YES / NO R.N.'s SIGNATURE: ______

X - rays sent: YES / NO PRINT NAME: ______

Photocopy Medication Chart: YES / NO WARD: ______

Medications sent: YES / NO CONTACT PHONE NUMBER: ______

Allied Health letter sent: YES / NO

File original copy in medical record **Duplicate copy to be sent to transferring hospital with patient**

Figure 24.5 | Transfer form — cont'd

- All personal possessions have been collected and packed, including any articles of value being held in the health care facility's safe
- The client is assisted to dress, if necessary
- Any dressings or bandages have been applied as necessary
- The client is provided with any prescribed medications together with instructions for their administration. The health care facility generally provides an instruction/information sheet that includes this
- The client is aware of, and understands, any dietary or activity restrictions
- The visiting nurse service has been notified if the client requires this service
- The medical officer has informed the client of any future appointments at a medical centre or at a health care facility
- The client is confident about performing any self-care activities that have been taught, such as administering insulin, dressing a wound or caring for a colostomy
- The client and significant others are aware of whom to contact should there be any problems after discharge.

When the client is ready to leave the unit or ward, they are escorted to the discharge department and any documentation completed. The client is then escorted to the exit. In the unit, the nurse reports to the nurse in charge and documents that the discharge has been completed (Clinical Interest Boxes 24.2 and 24.3).

Research has demonstrated that older adults are vulnerable to poor outcomes during the first few weeks after discharge. This reinforces the importance of either telephone or home health care follow-up for older adults after discharge to address needs associated with functional decline and, by doing so, preventing readmission (Perry & Potter 2002).

CLINICAL INTEREST BOX 24.2
Client risk factors for discharge planning

- Lack of knowledge of treatment plan
- Altered cognition
- Newly diagnosed chronic disease
- Major or radical surgery
- More than three active medical problems
- Social isolation
- Emotional or mental instability
- Visual and hearing deficits
- Takes more than five drugs
- Lack of financial resources
- Lack of available or approximate referral sources
- Terminal illness
- Lack of in-home care provider

(Burgess & Ragland 1983 in Potter & Perry 2002; Blaylock & Cason 1992)

CLINICAL INTEREST BOX 24.3
Elements of a written discharge summary form

- Mode of discharge: ambulatory, wheelchair, stretcher
- Instructions for self-care activities: activity, diet, medications, special treatments such as wound care, self-catheterisation, tracheotomy care
- Signs and symptoms of complications or drug reactions to be observant for
- Signs and symptoms that are normal for the person
- Correct settings for any equipment required
- Planned follow-up appointment at the doctor's office or clinic
- Explanation of pertinent emergency procedures
- Client's signature, showing understanding of instructions

(Perry & Potter 2002)

Discharge against medical advice

A person may at any time decide to leave a health care facility against the advice of the medical officer. If this occurs the nurse must immediately report the incident to the nurse in charge, and notify the individual's medical officer. If the individual cannot be dissuaded from leaving, they are asked to sign a statement to the effect that they are leaving at their own risk and that they are responsible for the consequences. If the client refuses to sign, this must be documented. The document is signed by at least one witness; this may be the medical officer or the nurse in charge. The incident is fully reported in the individual's notes.

Transfer

Sometimes it is necessary to transfer a client from one unit or ward at a health care facility to another, or to another facility. Transfer of a client may be necessary for a variety of reasons, such as a change in condition, demand for available beds, or the requirement to be isolated from others. Whatever the reason, a transfer may be a distressing experience for the client, who is likely to feel apprehensive about the need to adapt to new surroundings and personnel. Conversely, the transfer may be welcomed as an indication of an improvement in the client's condition, for example, being transferred from an intensive care unit to a general ward. Keep in mind that being transferred from the hospital to a rehabilitation or long-term facility can be confusing and frightening for older adults. Whenever possible, have family or a close friend either travel with the client or meet them when they arrive at the new facility.

When a client is to be transferred it is essential that both the client and significant others are informed as soon as possible. A full explanation of the reasons for the transfer provides the person with time to adjust and provides their significant others time to make any changes necessary. In addition to preparing the client for the transfer, it is necessary to inform the staff in the receiving unit or facility of the client's condition and care plan. Arrangements for

CLINICAL INTEREST BOX 24.4
Nursing diagnoses — planning for discharge

- Altered health maintenance
- Altered protection
- Ineffective management of therapeutic regimen
- Knowledge deficit
- Non-compliance
- High risk for infection
- High risk for injury
- Health-seeking behaviours
- Self-care deficit

transportation are made if necessary. Key aspects involved in the transfer are:

- Informing the client of the date and time the transfer is to occur
- Assessing whether the client is able to walk or if a wheelchair or trolley is required
- Arranging transportation, e.g. an ambulance, if being transferred to another facility
- Notifying the receiving unit or facility of the date and time of the transfer
- Notifying the admissions department of the transfer
- Assisting the person to pack all personal possessions. The nurse should check the entire room to ensure that nothing is left behind
- Assembling the documents that are to accompany the client
- The medications are either sent with the client or returned to the facility's pharmacy department
- Accompanying the client to the receiving unit, the ambulance or private car
- Introducing the client to the nursing staff in the receiving unit and remaining with them until the staff have received the client into their care
- Reporting to the nurse in charge and documenting that the transfer has been accomplished (Figure 24.5).

Possible nursing diagnoses related to discharge planning are listed in Clinical Interest Box 24.4.

SUMMARY

Admission to a health care facility, whether elective or emergency, is a major event for an individual. Both the person and their significant others are generally anxious about the admission and its implications. The individual may react to admission in one or more ways; for example, with apprehension, irritability, anger, depression or relief. The nurse should perform the process of admission in a warm, efficient and empathetic manner to minimise any anxiety.

Before admission, the unit is prepared to receive the individual. Reception of the individual is directed towards verifying the client's identity, assessing the physical and psychological status, promoting the client's comfort in an unfamiliar environment, providing items needed for care and providing the client with information.

The client may be transferred to another ward, unit or health care facility. A full explanation of the reason for the transfer should be provided to the person and to significant others. Discharge planning, which begins soon after admission, is directed towards assisting the individual to make a smooth transition from one setting to another. Discharge planning involves assessment, analysis of data, planning, implementation and evaluation.

REVIEW EXERCISES

1. How would you plan and implement the care for the client who requires admission, transfer or discharge?
2. What information would you give to parents or carers of a child to help them prepare the child for admission to hospital?
3. What are the responsibilities of the nurse in relation to assessment and observation of children?

CRITICAL THINKING EXERCISES

1. Two-year-old Thomas has been admitted to the hospital with gastroenteritis. His parents wish to participate in his care but will not be able to stay with him continuously. His father works night duty and his mother needs to care for his older siblings at home. Identify nursing measures that will minimise separation anxiety for Thomas.
2. What might you say to make a nervous client and family feel more relaxed during admission?
3. Mr D'Arcy, aged 66, has emphysema and is admitted to your health care facility often. On assessment you discover he is homeless and spends nights in a refuge in the city. What do you need to consider before discharging Mr D'Arcy?

REFERENCES AND FURTHER READING

Berman AJ, Kozier B, Snyder S (2008) *Kozier and Erbs Fundamentals of Nursing: Concepts, Process, and Practice*, 8th edn. Prentice-Hall, Upper Saddle River, NJ

Blaylock A, Cason CL (1992) Discharge planning: predicting patients' needs. *Journal of Gerontological Nursing* 18(7): 8

Burgess W, Ragland EC (1983) *Community Health Nursing: Philosophy, Process, Practice.* Appleton-Century-Crofts, Norwalk CT

Crisp J, Taylor C (eds) (2005) *Potter & Perry's Fundamentals of Nursing*, 2nd edn. Elsevier Australia, Sydney

deWit SC (2005) *Fundamental Concepts and Skills for Nursing*, 2nd edn. WB Saunders, Philadelphia

Kozier B, Erb G, Berman AJ, Snyder S (2004) *Fundamentals of Nursing: Concepts, Process and Practice*, 7th edn. Prentice-Hall, Upper Saddle River, NJ

Perry AG, Potter PA (2002) *Clinical Nursing Skills and Techniques*, 5th edn. Mosby, St Louis

Unit 8

Important components of nursing care

Chapter 25

INFECTION PREVENTION AND CONTROL

OBJECTIVES

- Define the key terms/concepts
- Name the major groups of microorganisms and state the characteristics of each group
- Explain the links in the chain of infection
- Describe the body's normal defences against infection
- Explain the differences between innate immunity and acquired immunity
- Identify factors that increase susceptibility to infection
- Differentiate between standard and additional precautions
- Explain nursing responsibilities in relation to preventing transmission of infection
- Define the concepts of medical and surgical asepsis
- Demonstrate recommended and approved infection control techniques when carrying out nursing activities
- Describe the role of the infection control nurse

KEY TERMS/CONCEPTS

aerobes
anaerobes
antibiotic
antigen
antimicrobial
asepsis
asymptomatic
autoclave
bacteria
carrier
chain of infection
communicable disease
disinfection
fomites
immunity
immunocompromised host
immunosuppression
incubation
infection
microorganism
normal flora
nosocomial infection
pathogen
phagocytosis
sterile
vector
virulence
virus

CHAPTER FOCUS

Infection prevention and control is a priority in nursing. Infectious diseases have not disappeared with advances in drug and medical therapy, and in some cases microorganisms have developed drug-resistant strains. Control and prevention of infection is an essential component of every nursing activity. Nurses require knowledge about microorganisms, the infectious process and the application of infection control principles to prevent the spread of microorganisms. This knowledge helps nurses to minimise the incidence of infection and the spread of infection between clients, and to protect themselves and other health care workers from contact with infectious material or exposure to communicable diseases. Nurses are also in a prime position to educate their clients about activities that increase personal resistance to infection and control the spread of infection in the home.

LIVED EXPERIENCE

Early in my first year at college when I was a student nurse, we learned about hand washing. I've never forgotten because we did this thing that surprised us all. We all washed our hands and then rubbed on gel that would glitter in the dark to show up any areas where microorganisms were still present. Well, I thought I had washed my hands thoroughly but when the lights went out there was glitter around my nails, between my fingers and on the backs of my hands. I understood then the importance of an effective hand wash.

Anne-Marie Roberts, Enrolled Nurse

Nurses, together with all health care workers, share the responsibility of preventing the spread of infection between themselves and clients and between one client and another. Clients in health care settings are at risk of acquiring infections because of lowered resistance and increased exposure to microorganisms. Sources of infecting microorganisms can be people or environmental objects, such as medical or nursing equipment that has become contaminated.

MICROORGANISMS AND INFECTION

Microorganisms are forms of animal or plant life too small to be seen without the aid of a microscope. One of three events occurs when microorganisms invade the body. They are destroyed by the body's immune defence mechanisms, they stay within the body without causing disease, or they cause infection or an infectious disease.

DISTRIBUTION OF MICROORGANISMS

Millions of microorganisms are found in every situation where it is possible for life to exist. Microorganisms are present in air, water, soil, dust, in and on food, on every surface and in and on the bodies of living organisms, including human beings.

Microorganisms may be pathogenic or non-pathogenic. Only a small proportion of the microorganisms that abound in nature are pathogenic, meaning that they are capable of causing disease. Non-pathogenic microorganisms do not cause disease under normal circumstances and when in their normal environment. Those that normally reside on or in the human body and cause no harm are termed the body's normal flora. Normal flora defends the body by curbing invasion by pathogenic microorganisms. They achieve this by occupying receptor sites on host cells, consuming the available nutrients and by secreting substances toxic to invading microorganisms. However, these protective non-pathogenic microorganisms can become pathogenic if they are moved from their normal environment to another. For example, *Escherichia coli* bacteria are microorganisms that normally reside in the small bowel and colon of the human intestinal tract and under normal circumstances cause no ill effects. If transferred somewhere else, to the renal system for example, they will cause a urinary tract or kidney infection.

Normal flora are resident on the skin, on the mucous membranes of the upper respiratory tract, in the intestines and in the vagina. These are the helpful bacteria necessary for a number of functions, including the production of some vitamins, breaking down the cellulose content of the diet for excretion in faeces and preventing the overgrowth of other organisms.

Infective pathogens are the organisms that are able to overcome the normal defences of the body, invade the tissues, multiply and produce poisonous substances such as toxins that damage the tissues and cause disease. Bacteria of the genus *Streptococcus*, for example, are commonly responsible for causing throat infections and more serious conditions such as rheumatic fever and scarlet fever.

ORGANISMS THAT CAUSE INFECTION

An infection is the entry and multiplication of an infectious agent (pathogen) in the tissues of a host. If the infectious agent fails to cause injury to cells or tissues and the client has no signs and symptoms of infection the infection is said to be asymptomatic. If the pathogens multiply and cause clinical signs and symptoms, such as pain, high temperature or lethargy, the infection is said to be symptomatic. Infective diseases that are readily communicable from person to person are called infectious or contagious. Virulence is a term used to describe the pathogenicity of an organism or, in other words, the extent to which it is capable of causing disease. The potential for microorganisms to cause disease depends on virulence, a sufficient number of organisms being present, and their ability to enter and survive in the host.

TYPES OF MICROORGANISMS

The major groups of microorganisms are classified according to size, structure and method of reproduction. Microorganisms include bacteria, viruses, fungi, protozoa and helminths.

Bacteria

Bacteria are single-celled microscopic organisms without a nucleus that have the capacity to reproduce rapidly. Bacteria may be classified by reactions to laboratory techniques and by their appearance. Gram-staining, growing bacteria by culture and sensitivity testing are some of the laboratory techniques that identify bacteria and determine which antibiotic will be effective against them. Gram-staining involves placing live bacteria onto a microscope slide then applying methyl violet followed by iodine solution. The cells are stained blue at this stage. They are then treated briefly with acetone. Bacteria that retain the original blue stain are Gram-positive. Gram-negative cells are de-colourised by the acetone and appear red (Wilson 2000). Gram-negative bacteria are the more dangerous because they produce an endotoxin that can cause haemorrhagic shock and severe gastrointestinal disturbance, such as acute diarrhoea. They also lower the client's resistance to other pathogens, making them susceptible to other different infections.

To culture (grow a sample of) bacteria, a sample from the client is transferred to growth medium, such as nutrient agar, that promotes multiplication and growth. When bacteria are present in sufficient quantity, sensitivity tests are carried out to determine the appropriate antibiotic to prescribe (deWit 2005).

Some species of bacteria have the ability to develop highly resistant round or oval structures, called spores, when they are exposed to adverse conditions such as lack of nutrients and/or water. Spores are resistant to disinfectants

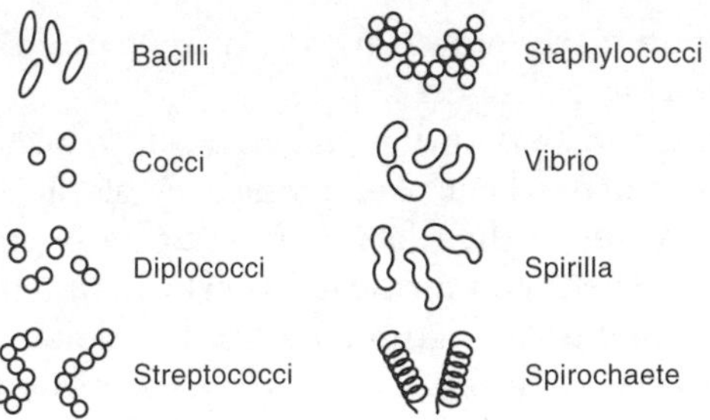

Figure 25.1 | Bacterial shapes

and to high or low temperatures, so they are difficult to destroy. They are resistant to sunlight and even freezing conditions so may remain viable in adverse environments for many years. They germinate when the environmental conditions become favourable, and this allows the bacterial cell within to begin multiplying (Wilson 2000).

Bacteria appear in a variety of sizes, shapes and arrangements. There are three main shapes — rod shaped (bacilli), round (cocci) and spiral shaped (spirilla, vibrios and spirochaetes). Figure 25.1 provides examples of bacterial shapes.

Diseases caused by cocci include meningitis, gonorrhoea, pneumonia and skin infections such as boils and impetigo; diseases caused by bacilli include tetanus, diphtheria, tuberculosis (TB) and Legionnaires' disease; the disease most commonly caused by spirochaete infection is syphilis. Different kinds of bacteria tend to affect different organs and systems of the body, producing a range of infectious diseases, each with its own group of symptoms. Bacteria make up the largest group of pathogens and are usually treated with antibiotics. The advent of antibiotics in the 1940s provided a powerful weapon to treat bacterial infections; however, because bacteria continually mutate as they divide, some had natural resistance to the effects of antibiotics and have developed into resistant strains. These pathogens include methicillin-resistant *Staphylococcus aureus* (MRSA), vancomycin-resistant *Enterococcus* (VRE) and penicillin-resistant *Pneumococcus*. These multi-drug-resistant organisms are dangerous threats, and emphasise the need for nurses and all health care workers to practise effective infection prevention and control measures (Wilson 2005).

Rickettsiae and *Chlamydiae* are microorganisms classified as specialised bacteria but they are smaller than most other bacteria and can only reproduce within the living cells of a host. Organisms that can only multiply within living cells are called parasites. *Rickettsiae* are often carried by arthropod vectors such as fleas, ticks and lice. A vector is the term used for a carrier that transfers an infective agent from one host to another. Body lice, for example, are arthropod vectors that carry the *Rickettsiae* responsible for epidemic typhus. Arthropods are creatures with jointed legs and include insects and ticks. Arthropods that live on the body's surface (skin and mucous membranes) are called ectoparasites. Ectoparasites are responsible for conditions such as scabies and head or pubic lice (see Chapters 27 and 37 concerning nursing care for these conditions).

Chlamydial organisms are the cause of several significant human illnesses, including trachoma, the leading cause of blindness in the world today. *Chlamydiae trachomatis* is the cause of a prevalent sexually transmitted disease that can result in problems ranging from urethritis to serious inflammation of the reproductive system. Infection with *Chlamydiae trachomatis* can lead to pelvic inflammatory disease in women, with consequences such as infertility, ectopic pregnancy or miscarriage.

Mycoplasmas are a type of ultramicroscopic bacteria that lack a cell wall. They are responsible for some respiratory and genital-tract infections in humans. *Mycoplasma pneumoniae* causes a virulent type of pneumonia that spreads via respiratory secretions and is transmitted slowly but easily between humans (Wilson 2005; Wilson 2000).

Viruses

Viruses are specialised microorganisms with a number of distinctive characteristics:

- Most are ultramicroscopic, meaning that they are too small to be seen with a light microscope and can be viewed only with an electron microscope
- They have no cell structure and they lack a rigid cell wall
- They are intracellular parasites, meaning that they can grow and reproduce only when resident within a host cell, and cannot be cultured on dead or artificial media.

The major viral diseases of concern within the health care setting are infectious mononucleosis (glandular fever [Epstein–Barr virus infection]), cytomegalovirus infection, herpes simplex virus infection, viral hepatitis (hepatitis A, B and C viruses), influenza, measles, human immunodeficiency virus (HIV) infection, respiratory syncytial virus infection, rotaviral enteritis, chickenpox (varicella virus), shingles (herpes zoster virus), rubella (German measles), viral haemorrhagic fevers and, most recently, severe acute respiratory syndrome (SARS, caused by a novel coronavirus) (Lashley & Durham 2007; Wilson 2005; Wilson 2000).

Fungi

Fungi are tiny organisms such as moulds and yeasts that belong to the world of plants but contain no chlorophyll. Fungi are present in the soil, air and water and they multiply by producing various kinds of spores. Most species of fungi are non-pathogenic, but a few cause disease. There are three types of fungal (mycotic) infections: superficial, which affect the skin, mucous membranes, hair and nails; intermediate, which affect subcutaneous tissues; and systemic, which infect deep tissues and organs. Tinea (ringworm) is one genus of the fungal group of organisms called dermatophytes. Tinea species cause superficial infections of the keratin found in skin, scalp and nails. Sometimes antibiotic medications alter the body's normal flora, providing an environment that allows fungal infections such as vaginal candidiasis (vaginal thrush) and tinea pedis (athlete's foot) to develop (Wilson 2000).

Protozoa

Protozoa are single-cell organisms of the animal kingdom. All protozoa require large amounts of water and are abundant in soil and water, and in and on plants and animals. They are classified according to their ability to move. Amoebic dysentery and giardiasis are serious conditions caused by protozoan parasites. The route of entry is usually by ingestion of contaminated water or food, which commonly results in severe diarrhoea.

Some protozoans are transmitted by insects (vectors) to man. Pathogenic protozoa include the plasmodium species, which is carried by mosquitoes and causes malaria. Malaria still causes over three million deaths each year in the more tropical regions of the world (Herlihy & Maebius 2000). Certain strains of protozoa are a major cause of opportunistic infections, meaning that they take the opportunity to establish themselves in a host whose resistance is lowered. For example, *Pneumocystis carinii* is commonly the cause of pneumonia in people with acquired immune deficiency syndrome (AIDS), whose immune systems are weakened by the presence of the AIDS virus (HIV) (Lashley & Durham 2007).

Helminths

Helminths are parasitic worms, or flukes — multicellular animals that are pathogenic to humans. They are classified according to external appearance: flatworms (platyhelminths) or roundworms (nematodes). Parasitic worms often live in relative balance with human hosts, taking only enough nutrients to survive without destroying the health of the host. Most worm infections are transmitted from person to person via faeces that contaminate food and water. Flatworms include tapeworms and flukes that reside in the intestine of the host. Tapeworms commonly enter the human body via contaminated or insufficiently cooked pork and may grow 1–12 metres in length. Flukes are not common in Australia or New Zealand but are a serious problem in many Asian, tropical and subtropical countries. They enter the body via improperly cooked fish and invade the blood and organs such as the liver, lungs and intestines. Infestation by large flatworms causes anaemia, fatigue, abdominal pain and weight loss.

Roundworms include ascarides, hookworms, trichinae, pinworms and a minute worm that causes filariasis (elephantitis). Pinworm is one of the most common parasitic worms. It affects children more often than adults. This nematode is less than a centimetre long and inhabits the upper part of the large intestine, but lays its eggs on the outer perianal area of the host. The deposition of the eggs causes irritation, the child scratches, hands are contaminated and eggs are transferred from hand to mouth and sometimes to friends. This circular pattern of reinfestation makes pinworm particularly hard to control (King, Belman & Kramer 2001).

The diagnosis of worm infestation is made by microscopic examination of the client's faeces, which reveals the presence of adult worms or their larvae. Infestation by parasitic worms is treated with medications called anthelmintics (Bryant, Knights & Salerno 2006). Education of clients regarding prevention of spread and reinfestation is essential. Table 25.1 provides a list of common infection-causing organisms.

CHAIN OF INFECTION

Infection is a state that exists when pathogenic microorganisms have invaded and multiplied in the tissues and there are manifestations of damage to the tissues. The process of the spread of infection can be conceived as a chain of events. Each event is a link in the chain and must occur sequentially for an infection to develop. For the chain of events to continue, the following elements must be present:

- Reservoir where pathogens can reside
- Pathogenic organisms in sufficient numbers (causative agent)
- Portal of exit from the reservoir (an escape route)
- Mode of transmission (vehicle to transport to new destination)
- Portal of entry to the new host
- Susceptible new host.

Figure 25.2 illustrates the chain of infection. Infection prevention and control is directed towards breaking the links in the chain of infection.

RESERVOIRS (SOURCES) OF INFECTION

The reservoirs of pathogenic microorganisms are human, animal or inanimate sources. A reservoir is a place where a pathogen can survive but may or may not multiply. The presence of microorganisms does not always cause a person to be ill. In humans, microorganisms can thrive in reservoirs

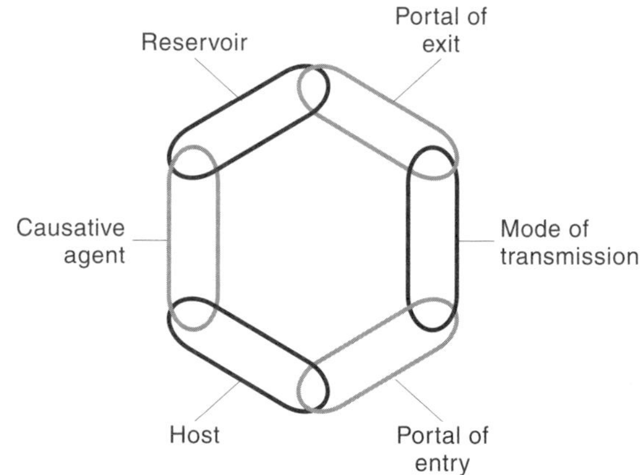

Figure 25.2 | Chain of infection

TABLE 25.1 | COMMON PATHOGENS AND THE INFECTIONS/CONDITIONS THEY CAUSE

Organism class and examples	Main location (reservoir)	Resulting infection/condition
Bacteria		
Escherichia coli, Neisseria meningitides, Neisseria gonorrhoeae	Colon, upper respiratory tract, genitourinary tract, rectum	Gastroenteritis, urinary tract infections, meningitis, gonorrhoea, pelvic inflammatory disease, infectious arthritis
Pseudomonas aeruginosa, Staphylococcus aureus	Gastrointestinal tract, nose, skin (especially axillae, perineum and groin)	Skin, ear and urinary tract infections; wound infection; cellulitis; pneumonia; impetigo; carbuncle
Streptococcus A group	Nose, mouth and throat	Throat infection, wound infection
B group	Vagina	Urinary tract infection
C and G groups	Skin and mucous membranes	Wound infection and a range of nosocomial infections
***Rickettsiae* & *Chlamydiae* (specialised bacteria — intracellular parasites mostly transmitted via animal, bird or insect vectors)**		
Rickettsiae prowazekii *Chlamydiae trachomatis*	Body lice, areas containing columnar epithelial cells (e.g. conjunctiva, cervix, urethra, respiratory tract and gastrointestinal tract)	Typhus, trachoma, conjunctivitis, genital-tract infections
Mycoplasmas (atypical, very small bacteria found in soil and the general environment)		
Mycoplasma pneumonia	Respiratory tract	Respiratory infection, pneumonia
Mycoplasma hominis	Genitourinary tract	Pyelonephritis, pelvic inflammatory disease
Ureaplasma urealyticum	Genitourinary tract	Urethritis
Viruses		
Hepatitis A	Faeces	Hepatitis A
Hepatitis B and C	Blood and body fluids	Hepatitis B and C
Herpes simplex virus (HSV)	Lesions on skin or mucous membranes; saliva	Cold sores (HSV type 1) and sexually transmitted infection (HSV type 2), aseptic meningitis
Human immunodeficiency virus (HIV)	Blood, all body secretions	Acquired immune deficiency syndrome (AIDS)
Fungi		
Candida albicans	Mouth, skin, colon, genital tract	Thrush, vaginitis, pneumonia, sepsis
Aspergillus organisms	Soil, dust, mouth, skin, colon, genital tract	Aspergillosis, pneumonia, sepsis
Protozoa		
Plasmodium falciparum	Blood	Malaria
Helminths		
Enterobius vermicularis (pinworm)	Large colon	Perianal itching

(in Potter & Perry 2008, modified from Ritter 2005)

such as open wounds, nasal passages, skin crevices and in the blood.

Human sources

Most organisms that infect humans are acquired from human sources. A variety of organisms, normal flora, reside on the surface of the skin and within body cavities, fluids and discharges. Some areas of the body contain larger populations of normal flora than others, for example, the skin, respiratory tract, colon, mouth and vagina. Areas of the body that are usually considered sterile (without normal flora) include the spinal fluid and blood, the urinary system and the peritoneal cavity. The entrance of a foreign object or organism into a sterile site leads to a high risk of infection. Auto-infection occurs when normal flora cause infection by being transferred from their normal place of residence to a different site in the same host. Crossinfection may occur when organisms from one person are transferred to another person, for example, when organisms on a nurse's hands are transferred to a client's wound.

A person incubating a disease is another source of infection. An incubation period is the time between the entrance of the pathogen into the host and the appearance of the clinical symptoms of the disease. During the incubation period the organisms multiply and can be transmitted and infect others before the host or anyone else knows the disease is present. Nurses therefore should treat every client as if they were a potential source of infection.

A person with an infection can liberate large numbers of pathogens into the environment. In some diseases the risk of infecting others may last only a short time; in others, pathogens continue to be released by the infected person over a long period; for example, the tuberculosis *Mycobacterium* may be present in the host for many years (Wilson 2000; Wilson 2005).

A carrier is an individual who is the host for pathogenic microorganisms. An individual may be a carrier during the incubation period of a disease, after an attack of the disease, or without ever experiencing symptoms of the disease that the organism causes.

Animal sources

Animals, birds and insects (vectors) can also be reservoirs for infectious organisms; for example, Q fever is caused by a parasite found in cattle, psittacosis is transmitted from birds and malaria from mosquitoes.

Inanimate sources

Soil, seawater, food, water and milk are additional reservoirs for pathogens. Many organisms live in the soil and obtain their nourishment from decaying vegetable and animal matter. Some anaerobic spore-forming bacteria cause disease if they gain entry to human tissue; for example, *Clostridium tetani* lives in the soil and, if it enters the body, can cause the illness known as tetanus, which results in serious damage to the nervous system. Route of entry to a human host is via puncture wounds, cuts or other lesions. Because anaerobic bacteria can only survive and multiply in the absence of oxygen, they can survive if they are present in canned or vacuum-packed foods. If the toxin they produce is ingested the result may be extremely serious or even lethal.

To grow and reproduce, organisms require a suitable environment. Environment relates to the availability of food and water, the level of light, oxygen and heat and the pH range. Microorganisms thrive most effectively in warm dark environments such as those within body cavities and under wound dressings. The need for oxygen varies with different groups of bacteria. Some can survive with or without oxygen (facultative anaerobes), some need oxygen (obligate aerobes), while others survive only in the absence of oxygen (anaerobes). Large numbers of anaerobes are present in the human intestine. Most microorganisms grow only in certain temperature ranges. The ideal temperature for most human pathogens is about 37°C but it is possible for some to multiply in temperatures ranging from10–60°C. Most microorganisms survive most efficiently in an environment within a pH range of 5–8.

PORTALS OF EXIT FROM THE RESERVOIR

If microorganisms are to enter another host and cause disease, they must first find a portal of exit, then a new site in which to reside. When the human body provides the reservoir, microorganisms can exit through a variety of sites, discussed below.

Skin and mucous membranes

Any break in the skin or mucous membranes can lead to infection. A surgical wound, for example, can be an entry point, a portal of exit and a reservoir for a pathogen.

Gastrointestinal tract

Although most organisms of the mouth are normal flora, the mouth is one of the most bacterially contaminated sites of the body; therefore, saliva (including kissing) is a portal of exit for pathogens. Other portals of exit include expectorated sputum, faeces, vomitus, bile or discharge from wounds. Any drainage tube or opening from the gastrointestinal tract is a potential portal of exit.

Urinary tract

When there is an infection of the genitourinary tract, microorganisms can exit via the urine.

Respiratory tract

Pathogens that infect the respiratory tract can be released through sneezing, coughing, talking or even breathing. The nose or mouth should be covered when sneezing or coughing, and disposable tissues should be used to control the exit of microorganisms. In some health care institutions, routine investigations are performed, such as nose and throat swabbing, to ensure that team members are not harbouring pathogenic microorganisms that can be transmitted to others via respiratory secretions. Such precautions are particularly important in promoting the safety of more vulnerable clients in areas such as operating rooms, burns units or neonatal units. For example, nurses whose swabs test positive for staphylococcal organisms would not be allocated to work with vulnerable clients.

Blood

Blood is normally sterile but, when a client has a blood-borne infectious disease such as hepatitis B or C or AIDS, it becomes a reservoir for the causative pathogens. Any break in the skin that allows blood to escape, and menstrual blood from the vagina, are portals of exit for blood-borne pathogens.

Reproductive tract

A male's urethral meatus or a female's vaginal canal can provide the means of exit for pathogens that are transferred from the body via semen or vaginal discharge. Chlamydia, herpes simplex, gonorrhoea and syphilis are examples of infectious diseases transmitted in this way.

MODES OF TRANSMISSION

Microorganisms move from a reservoir to a new host in a variety of ways. Diseases may be transmitted via the airborne (inhalation), contact (touching) or alimentary (ingestion) routes and the same microorganism may be spread by more than one route. For example, the varicella zoster virus, which causes chicken pox, can be acquired through inhalation of infected respiratory droplets as well as through contact with infected fluid leaking from skin lesions. Any substance that carries pathogens is known as the vehicle of transmission. Food, water, blood, urine, saliva or vomitus may provide a vehicle for transmission.

Airborne transmission

Airborne dissemination may occur via either airborne droplet (droplet nuclei) or dust particle. Tiny pathogens can be carried on airborne particles such as dust, water and respiratory droplets and, if inhaled by a susceptible host, cause infection. Pathogens expelled from the respiratory tract during coughing, sneezing or talking can be transmitted to a susceptible host by this route. The distance and extent of distribution depends on the force of the expulsion and gravity. Droplet transmission can also occur during medical procedures such as suctioning and bronchoscopy. Examples of illnesses spread by droplet nuclei are measles, rubella, influenza, pneumonia, meningitis, meningococcal disease and TB.

Droplets of moisture that contain organisms do not have to be inhaled to spread infection. They contaminate all surfaces on which they fall, so transmission can occur via indirect contact. Dust consists of environmental dust particles, dead skin, flakes, fluff from clothing, dried secretions and microorganisms. It is liberated from humans by means of normal body movements and from clothing during normal activity and dispersed by sweeping, dusting, bed making and other physical activities. It then settles on all surfaces in the environment. Microorganisms can therefore settle on and contaminate items such as clothing and bedclothes, books, papers, crockery, cutlery, toys, toilet utensils, furniture and fittings, dressing materials, needles, tubing, instruments and stethoscopes. Non-living, inanimate objects that can transmit microorganisms are called fomites. Indirect contact occurs when there is personal contact of the host with fomites in the environment.

Airborne transmission includes the spread of pathogens that may happen during procedures such as bed-making or manual washing of instruments or equipment. Microorganisms that are displaced into the atmosphere are carried and distributed by air currents. Ventilation and air-conditioning systems can rapidly distribute microorganisms.

Contact transmission

This is the most significant route of transmission in health care settings (Wilson 2000). Microorganisms can be transferred directly from one individual to another by physical contact between an infected person and a new host. Contact transmission can occur by touching the skin or body fluids of a client with an infection, or through the use of contaminated nursing or medical equipment. The hands can be the means of transfer if, after contact with an infectious client, they are not washed adequately before tending another client. Effective hand washing is the single most important way to limit cross-contamination and the spread of infection. Cross-contamination is said to have occurred when pathogens have been transmitted from one person or object to another. Contact transmission can also occur as a result of sexual activity or from a mother to an unborn baby via the placenta (transplacentally).

Many diseases are spread by direct contact, including glandular fever, caused by the Epstein–Barr virus. Some disorders can be transmitted by airborne droplet or by direct contact. The common cold or influenza, for example, can be transmitted as a result of pathogens released when sneezing, coughing or talking being carried on airborne droplets and inhaled by another person, while directly touching nasal or oral secretions can result in direct contact transmission.

Transmission by ingestion

Microorganisms can enter the gastrointestinal tract in a variety of ways, including via infected food or water, contaminated eating or drinking utensils or hands or, more often in children than adults, via contaminated objects being placed in the mouth. A person with a gastrointestinal infection can transfer infection via their hands if they are not washed effectively after defecation.

Contaminated food and water are responsible for the spread of diseases such as Creutzfeldt-Jakob disease (CJD) and cholera. Food poisoning results from ingesting food contaminated with toxic substances or bacteria that contain toxins; for example, *Salmonella enteritidis* is a bacteria that produces toxins resulting in food poisoning. Food or water may become contaminated:

- When handled by someone who has an infection or who is a carrier
- By rats, mice or insects (vectors) gaining access to food
- When food is stored at warm temperatures, which encourages the growth of bacteria
- By cooking methods that use temperatures low enough to promote bacterial growth but not high enough to destroy bacteria
- If there are unhygienic conditions where food is prepared or processed (e.g. dirty utensils, dirty

Box 25.1 | Modes of transmission of microorganisms

AIRBORNE

Droplet nuclei or residue or evaporated droplets suspended in air (e.g. sneezing, coughing)

Carried on dust particles inhaled by susceptible host

CONTACT

Direct

Contact with infectious person's body excreta

Person-to-person physical contact (e.g. sexual intercourse)

Indirect

Contact of susceptible host with contaminated article (e.g. used needles, dressings)

Ingestion

Contaminated vehicle consumed by susceptible host (e.g. water, food, drugs or other substance)

Pathogen enters gastrointestinal tract via contaminated eating utensils, cups or crockery

VECTOR

External mechanical transfer (e.g. flies)

Internal transmission (e.g. bites/stings of disease-carrying vectors)

kitchens, inadequate hand-washing facilities, inadequate refrigeration) or infestations of rats, mice, flies, ants or cockroaches.

Vector transmission

Vector-borne transmission (via mosquitoes, flies, rats and other animals) as a health concern is not as significant in Australia and New Zealand as it is in other parts of the world. Examples of microorganisms spread by this mode are *Plasmodium falciparum* (malaria) and *Yersinia pestis* (plague).

Box 25.1 summarises the modes of transmission of microorganisms.

PORTALS OF ENTRY

Microorganisms can enter the body through the same routes they use for exiting:

- Inhalation into the respiratory tract
- Ingestion through the mouth into the alimentary canal
- Inoculation through the skin or mucous membrane, which can occur when the skin becomes cracked or when tissue integrity is disturbed during injury, surgical procedures, injections, bites or stings
- Transplacental entry occurs when organisms from a pregnant woman cross the placenta to enter the fetal circulation (e.g. toxoplasmosis).

Measures that control the exit of microorganisms also control the entrance of pathogens, and include:

- Maintaining skin and mucous-membrane integrity
- Correct handling of urinary catheters and drainage sets
- Cleansing the genital area in a direction away from the urinary meatus to the rectum
- Implementing aseptic techniques, using sterile equipment during invasive procedures
- Cleansing wounds outwards from the wound site, to prevent the entrance of microorganisms.

SUSCEPTIBLE HOST

Susceptibility is the degree of resistance an individual has to pathogens. Whether a person acquires an infection depends on their susceptibility to the infectious agent. A susceptible host is the last link in the chain of infection. Susceptibility can be reduced by lifestyle practices that boost resistance, such as healthy nutrition, adequate exercise, rest and sleep, stress-management activities and effective hygiene practices. The body has certain natural resources that confer a degree of resistance against infection by invading pathogens.

RESISTANCE TO INFECTION

The body has two main lines of resistance to infection: non-specific defences and a specific immune response. Non-specific defences are those that defend naturally against any invading organism or foreign matter. The specific immune response defends against specific foreign agents, such as a specific bacteria, virus, pollen or toxin.

NON-SPECIFIC DEFENCE AGAINST INFECTION

Non-specific defences can be divided into two categories, external and internal. External defences are the mechanical and chemical barriers that protect the potential entry points for invasion by microorganisms. Internal defences are the automatic protective actions of the inflammatory process, phagocytic cells, 'natural killer' cells and protective proteins.

External mechanical and chemical barriers

These are the natural physical barriers that prevent micro-organisms from entering the body or expel them before they proliferate. Physical barriers include the skin, mucous membranes, normal body flora and some body secretions (Figure 25.3).

The body as a whole is protected by the skin, which forms an intact waterproof barrier against microorganisms. Sweat and sebum secreted through the skin are bactericidal for some organisms.

The gastrointestinal tract is protected by mucous membrane and the normal flora of the bowel. In addition, saliva produced by glands in the mouth contains the enzyme lysozyme, which inhibits the growth of bacteria. Acids secreted in the stomach create a low pH environment unfavourable to the survival of most pathogens. The high pH of alkaline bile secreted into the duodenum is also unfavourable to survival and is antibacterial.

The respiratory tract is protected by mucous membrane. The membrane of the upper airway is lined with hair-like

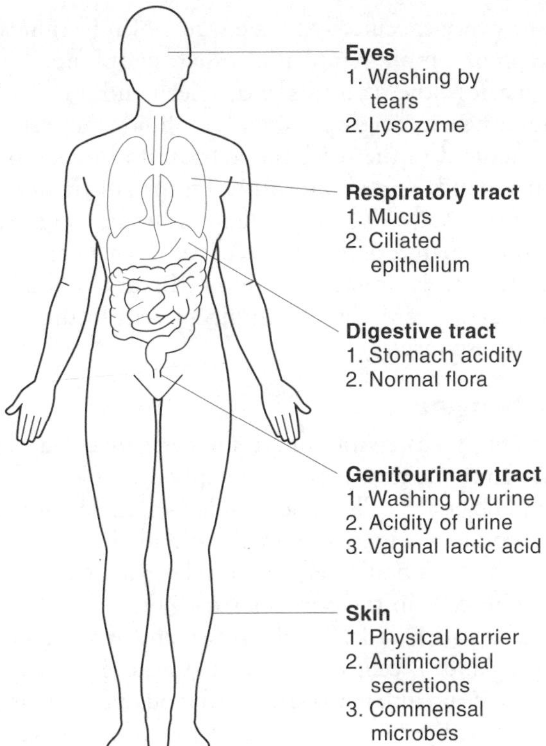

Figure 25.3 | Natural external non-specific defences against infection *(adapted from Wilson 2000)*

structures called cilia, that waft inhaled microorganisms away from the lungs and into the oropharynx to be expectorated or swallowed. Nasal secretions, like saliva, also contain lysozyme.

The eyes are protected by tears that, like saliva and nasal secretions, also contain lysozyme. The fluid secreted protects the surface of the eyes by washing them.

The vagina is protected by normal flora called lactobacilli, which cause vaginal secretions to have a local pH of 4–5, which is low enough to inhibit invasion by other microorganisms.

The urinary tract is protected by the flushing action of urine as it flows from the bladder, and the natural acidity of urine is not conducive to the survival of microorganisms.

Inflammation

Microorganisms that manage to foil the body's mechanical and chemical barriers and so gain entry to the tissues trigger an internal inflammatory response. The inflammatory response is the body's attempt to destroy as many invading organisms as possible and to confine them to the point of entry. Although often associated with infection, inflammation is the body's physical response to any form of injury or damage. It is usually characterised by four basic physical symptoms: redness, pain, heat and swelling. Histamine and other substances are released from tissues irritated by invading organisms, causing blood vessels to dilate. This increases blood flow through the damaged tissues, resulting in redness and heat. The histamine and other substances also increase the permeability of the blood vessels, resulting in fluid seeping from the blood into the tissues, which accounts for the swelling. The pressure caused by this accumulation of extracellular fluid in the tissues can also cause pain. Pain can also be caused by damage to nerve fibres or by the release of toxic chemicals from microorganisms.

Phagocytic cells

White blood cells called neutrophils and macrophages are attracted to an infection site by chemicals released from damaged cells. These white cells are phagocytes, which means that they attack the pathogens by enveloping, ingesting and then digesting them with enzymes, a process called phagocytosis.

Neutrophils have a shorter life span than macrophages. During a period of about 6–8 hours they circulate and attach onto microorganisms and digest them. Macrophages are able to engulf and ingest microorganisms over a much longer period of time. As these phagocytes carry out the destruction of microorganisms, many of them die in the process. The debris from the white cells, pathogens, damaged tissue cells and fluid in the area of inflammation accumulates to become a thick yellowish substance called pus. If the pus cannot drain to the outside of the body, cells build a wall of tissue to surround this infected debris. This contained walled-off area is an abscess. An abscess can be protective because it restricts the spread of the infection to other areas of the body. If antibiotic therapy does not effectively destroy the pathogens causing the infection and the accumulation of pus, an abscess may require surgical intervention to lance the wall to release and drain the pus from the area.

As phagocytes act they release pyrogens. Pyrogens stimulate the hypothalamus to reset the body's temperature at a higher level. This is what causes the fever associated with infection. Fever is also a defence in that many microorganisms do not thrive above certain temperatures. The higher body temperature therefore reduces the ability of certain pathogens to multiply. For this reason it is best not to reduce a fever unless it is of such intensity that there is a risk of seizures or damage to the brain.

Natural killer cells

Natural killer (NK) cells are a specialised type of lymphocyte capable of binding to and killing pathogens by breaking holes in cell membrane and releasing destructive enzymes. They are particularly effective against parasites, some virus-infected cells and some malignant tumour cells. NK cells are manufactured predominantly in the bone marrow and in the spleen.

Protective proteins

There are two groups of protective proteins — complement proteins and interferons. Complement comprises a set of about 20 proteins that help phagocytic cells identify pathogens. They do this by a series of reactions that eventuate in a protein substance, called C3b, coating the surface of the pathogens. Phagocytic cell receptors are able to recognise this substance, bind to it then ingest the pathogen. They are also involved in destroying foreign bacteria by a process called cytolysis. The complement achieves this by first changing the shape of the bacteria to a doughnut shape, then making a hole through the cell membrane. This permits ions and water to enter and swell the cell until it ruptures (Crisp & Taylor 2005).

Interferons are a group of proteins secreted by cells infected with a virus. They are capable of binding onto other surrounding cells and protecting them from viral replication. They are also able to enhance the destructive abilities of NK cells against malignant tumour cells. All cells can produce alpha and beta interferons, which interfere with the replication of viruses. T lymphocytes and NK cells can produce gamma-interferon, which coordinates and enhances the activities of other parts of the immune system (Wilson 2000).

If invading pathogens survive the external barrier defences and the other non-specific responses and continue to proliferate without effective treatment, infection may spread to other parts of the body, primarily via the circulatory and lymphatic systems.

SPECIFIC DEFENCES AGAINST INFECTION: IMMUNITY

Having immunity is the situation of being resistant to, or being unaffected by, a particular infectious disease. It means that a specific antibody has been produced to defend the body against a specific pathogen or the toxin it produces. An antigen is the term used for any foreign material, including bacteria, viruses or toxins, that stimulates an immune response in the body (Wilson 2000). Antibodies are proteins synthesised by the host that inactivate antigens. Tissues from another person, such as incorrectly matched blood or a donor organ, can also be antigens, causing an antigen–antibody response in a recipient host. The antigen–antibody response is a very specific defence because it always involves one specific antibody striving to combat one specific type of antigen. When antibodies directly react against, interact with or bind to antigens, an antigen–antibody reaction is said to have occurred. Mostly the antigen–antibody response is an important mechanism that promotes human survival. On some occasions it can cause problems; for example, an overreaction to an antigen can cause hypersensitivity and an allergic reaction such as is seen in hay fever, in people particularly allergic to bee stings, and sometimes in people who are allergic to particular medications.

The lymphatic system

The body's immune responses are under the control of the lymphatic system. It is a highly efficient system that responds very specifically to the threat of infection. It is made up of lymph, lymphatic vessels, lymph nodes, red bone marrow, the thymus gland, spleen and tonsils. The immune system develops when lymphoid stem cells are manufactured in the red bone marrow and travel to the thymus gland, spleen and other lymphoid tissues and organs in the body. These organs and tissues are coordinated to produce, mature and activate cells effective in providing the body with its immune response (Bryant et al 2006). Lymphocytes are the most significant cells in the body's immune responses.

Lymphocytes

There are two categories of lymphocytes involved in the specific immune response — T lymphocytes (T cells) and B lymphocytes (B cells). They reside in areas of lymphoid tissue around the body (Figure 25.4) and circulate in the blood. It is the job of T cells and B cells to attack antigens. Fetal stem cells in the bone marrow initiate production of T cells and B cells. T cells travel and mature in the thymus gland. B cells do not travel to the thymus gland and mature and differentiate in fetal blood or bone marrow. After maturing, both types reside in various lymphoid tissue around the body and also circulate in the blood. T cells comprise 70–80% of circulating lymphocytes, B cells comprise the other 20–30%.

Both T and B cells attack antigens. T cells are predominant in cell-mediated (cellular) immunity, which occurs through direct cell-to-cell contact of T cells with foreign cells. B cells are predominant in antibody-mediated (humoral) immunity, which involves indirect interaction with antigens through the secretion of antibodies.

Recognising 'self' cells

To function effectively at defending the body from invading organisms, these defence responses must be able to

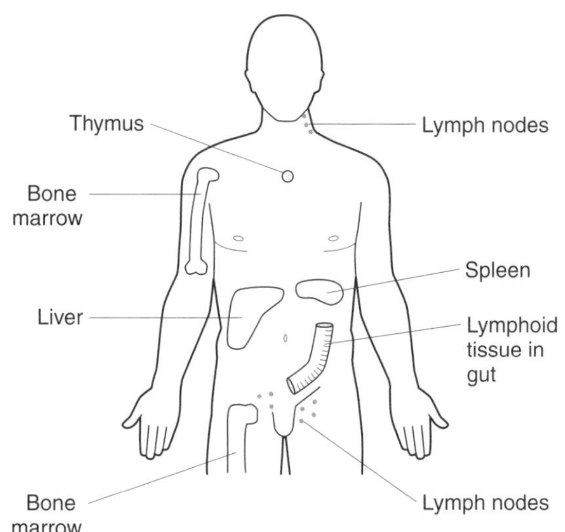

Figure 25.4 | Location of organs and tissues of the immune system *(adapted from Wilson 2000)*

distinguish between the body's own cells and foreign agents. During the period between life as a fetus and several years after birth, the thymus gland is busy setting up the antibody response system. During this process T cells are maturing. To enable the process of identifying cells that belong to the 'self' and should not be attacked, markers are placed on the outer surfaces of the body's own cells. The marker is a group of molecules called the major histocompatibility complex (MHC). Each person has their own unique MHC. This accounts for why the body recognises and attacks tissue or organs donated from others. Any T cells that recognise and respond to 'self' cells are discarded.

Malfunction of a person's immune system can cause a failure to recognise cells that belong to the self. This results in damage or destruction of 'self' cells. An attack on the body's own cells is the basis of autoimmune disorders such as rheumatoid arthritis, juvenile-onset (type 1) diabetes mellitus, pernicious anaemia, multiple sclerosis and systemic lupus erythematosus. In juvenile-onset diabetes the body attacks the islet cells of the pancreas, interfering with the production and secretion of the insulin they normally produce. It is thought that the mechanisms that cause autoimmune disorders are of genetic origin.

Cell-mediated immunity

Two types of T cells are involved in cell-mediated immunity: T-helper (CD4) cells, and cytotoxic T cells. Cell-mediated immunity is particularly effective against fungi, protozoan parasites, malignant cells and foreign tissue that is alien to the body, for example, transplanted organs (Herlihy & Maebius 2000). The following steps are involved in cellular immunity:

- Macrophages recognise antigens on the surface of pathogens and attack, using the process of phagocytosis. During digestion of the pathogen the antigen is pushed to the surface of the macrophage. The macrophage is then an antigen-presenting cell
- There are antigen receptors on the surface membranes of T-helper (CD4) cells. When an antigen-presenting macrophage meets a T cell with surface receptors that fit the antigen, binding occurs, which activates the T-helper cells
- Cytotoxic T cells also bind to specific antigens on macrophages that have digested infected foreign or malignant cells. They are triggered to release lysosomal enzymes, which destroy the cells
- Each T-helper cell carries a different surface receptor, which is able to recognise a specific antigen on another cell. T-helper cells bind to specific antigens and then proliferate by cell division (clonal replication) until there are large numbers forming a cloned group. Subgroups develop within the cloned group so that, besides the T-helper cells, there are natural killer T cells, suppressor T cells and memory T cells for that specific antigen
- The T-helper cells that are bound to antigens secrete messenger proteins called interleukins
- Interleukins activate B lymphocytes, other T lymphocytes and gamma-interferon
- Gamma-interferon promotes increased macrophage activity that increases the number of pathogens that are destroyed
- Gamma-interferon also activates T-suppressor cells that inhibit or switch off the immune response when the antigen has been eliminated. The suppressor T cells control B- and T-cell activity.
- Memory cells: some B and T cells produced in response to exposure to an antigen become memory cells. They have the ability to retain information about the initial encounter with an antigen. They are then ready to respond quickly to any future contact with the same antigen. This allows a faster immune response to a second and all future exposures to the same infecting organism.

Antibody-mediated (humoral) immunity

It is mostly B lymphocytes that are involved in the antibody-mediated response. Each B cell is programmed to produce a unique antibody. Each B cell displays its own specific antibody on its outer surface. This acts as a receptor for passing antigens. Antibodies only bind with antigens that specifically fit their unique receptor — the antigen must have a shape that precisely fits the antibody, rather like the way two pieces of a jigsaw puzzle fit together. B cells produce vast quantities of specific antibodies to lock with, then generate a reaction against, specific antigens. Antibodies are gamma globulins, one subtype of a class of proteins called immunoglobulins. Immunoglobulins are classified into five identifiable groups: IgG, IgM, IgA, IgE and IgD. Table 25.2 describes some specific properties of each class of immunoglobulin. Between them they perform these general tasks:

- Cause agglutination (clumping together) of microorganisms, which makes it easier for phagocytes to destroy antigens
- Activate complement proteins, which are important in making it easier for phagocytic cells to ingest microorganisms
- Destroy antigens on cells by the process of cytolysis
- Render microorganisms more susceptible to phagocytosis
- Neutralise toxins produced by microorganisms.

The following steps are involved in antibody-mediated immunity:

- Macrophages become antigen-presenting cells, as in cell-mediated immunity (above)
- B and T cells with appropriate receptor sites bind to antigen-presenting cells and become activated
- T-helper cells secrete a substance called lymphokine, which stimulates the bound (i.e. antigen specific) B cells to proliferate. They replicate as a clonal group.

TABLE 25.2 | FUNCTIONS OF THE FIVE CLASSES OF IMMUNOGLOBULINS

Class	Functions
IgG	Most abundant type of immunoglobulin Diffuses from blood vessels into tissue fluids Crosses the placenta in the last trimester of pregnancy (the only immunoglobulin that crosses the placental barrier) to provide infants with passive immunity Coats pathogens to make phagocytosis easier and neutralises toxins
IgM	Large immunoglobulin molecule First one produced during an immune response Confined to the blood Triggers the increased production of IgG Binds efficiently with complement proteins to activate them
IgA	Principal immunoglobulin of saliva, tears, and respiratory-, reproductive- and intestinal-tract secretions. Also found in respiratory-tract mucosa and plasma Protects exposed surfaces from antigens that enter the respiratory and gastrointestinal tracts Coats microorganisms, preventing them from adhering to epithelial cells
IgE	Provides the primary defence against environmental antigens by releasing histamine Involved in allergic responses There are some indications that IgE is involved in attacking and destroying parasitic organisms such as helminths
IgD	Maximum levels during childhood Increased levels during chronic infections Found in blood and on surfaces of lymphocytes Involved in activating B cells

The clonal group includes subgroups of plasma cells and memory cells

- Plasma cells produce large quantities of antibodies, which are carried by the circulatory system and bind with antigens on the surface of microorganisms, forming antigen–antibody complexes that are recognised by phagocytic cells, which ingest the microorganisms (Wilson 2000)
- Memory B cells retain information about the initial contact with the specific antigen and remain ready to respond quickly to future encounters with the same antigen.

On first exposure to an antigen, B cells produce quantities of plasma cells that secrete antibodies. The B cells also produce quantities of memory cells. This first exposure, the first time B cells are activated by a specific antigen, is termed the primary response. This would occur on the first exposure to the measles virus, for example. During the primary response the antibodies develop relatively slowly, with a relatively low amount in the blood plasma. This allows symptoms of the illness, such as the measles, to manifest. When the immune system is confronted with the same antigen on subsequent occasions, the body mounts a much speedier response and is able to produce antibodies in much larger numbers because the memory cells already reside in the plasma. This is termed the secondary response and is usually quick enough and strong enough to prevent the associated pathogen from becoming established and symptoms of the illness developing. This demonstrates that the body has developed immunity to the specific infectious microorganism, such as the measles virus. The antibodies to a specific disorder can be measured to determine the level of immunity a person has to a specific disorder. This measurement is called an antibody titre.

Innate immunity

Innate immunity is sometimes referred to as genetic or inborn immunity. Effective defences against potentially harmful microorganisms are present from birth and do not depend upon having previous experience with any particular microorganism. This is known as the innate immune mechanism, which is effective against a range of potentially infective agents and is, therefore, non-specific. Humans are born with inborn immunity to certain diseases that affect animals or plants, and animals and plants are not usually susceptible to the infectious diseases that afflict humans. For example, humans cannot get Dutch Elm disease and dogs and cats do not get measles or chicken pox.

Naturally acquired immunity

Acquired immunity is not present at birth but is developed during life; it may be naturally or artificially acquired. Naturally acquired immunity is gained in two ways, either passively or actively. Passive natural immunity is acquired before birth when immunoglobulins in the mother's blood are transferred across the placenta and enter the fetal blood. It is acquired after birth when a breastfed baby receives small amounts of immunoglobulins from its mother's breast milk. These are most abundant in colostrum, the milk produced very soon after delivery of the baby. Passively acquired immunity is not permanent and does not last as long as actively acquired immunity — the immunoglobulins passed from mother to baby may remain in circulation and provide immunity for only up to a few months.

Active natural immunity occurs after being exposed to an infectious organism and developing specific antibodies and many memory cells to ward off future encounters with the same pathogen. Active immunity is acquired as a result of the stimulation of an individual's immune system, with active involvement of the body in the production of its own immunoglobulins. For example, if measles, mumps or chicken pox is experienced as a child, active natural immunity to these illnesses is established.

Artificially acquired immunity

Artificial immunity is acquired in two ways: either by means of a vaccine or by injection of immunoglobulin. Vaccines are antigenic materials that induce a specific active artificial immunity to infection by a specific microorganism. Vaccines are suspensions of live, dead or attenuated (weakened) pathogens introduced into the body to stimulate the production of specific immunoglobulins. For example, the measles vaccine is developed by weakening the live measles virus that causes the illness. When injected into the recipient, the weakened virus stimulates the immune system to produce antibodies to protect against the illness. Vaccine can also be made using the toxin secreted by a pathogen. The toxin is modified to limit its ability to cause harm, while keeping it strong enough to induce immunity. The modified toxin is called a toxoid.

Specific vaccines provide protection against some infectious diseases for months or years. It is recommended that vaccination against many diseases be provided at a very young age; for example, Sabin vaccine, which is ingested orally, provides protection against poliomyelitis, and the first dose should be given when a child is only 2 months old. (For further information about vaccination, refer to the Immunise Australia website www.immunise.health.gov.au.)

Bacille Calmette–Guérin (BCG) is a freeze-dried, live attenuated vaccine available for people who are not immune to TB. A 'Mantoux test' (named after the French physician Charles Mantoux) is performed first by injecting tuberculin (a protein derivative from the tuberculosis bacillus) into the skin on the forearm. Immunity to TB is demonstrated by a positive skin reaction at 72 hours, indicated by an area of oedema 5 mm or more in diameter. (A positive reaction may be due to a current infection, a previous infection, or previous vaccination with BCG vaccine.) If the reaction to the Mantoux test is negative, BCG vaccine may be given by intradermal injection (inoculation). Other vaccines are given to provide immunity against cholera, meningococcus, diphtheria, whooping cough (pertussis vaccine), typhoid fever, typhus and influenza.

Immunoglobulin is different to vaccine. It provides artificial passive immunity because it contains antibodies (immunoglobulins) which have already been developed within a human or animal donor. The antibodies have developed in response to a specific infection that the donor has been exposed to. These 'ready prepared' antibodies are injected into a recipient with the aim of providing them with immediate antibody protection. For example, a nurse who has accidentally suffered exposure to the hepatitis B virus via a needle-stick injury and who does not have immunity may receive hepatitis B immunoglobulin in an attempt to provide instant protection from the virus. As this is passive immunity, protection is short lived.

Immunoglobulins are also available for diseases such as rubella, hepatitis A, rabies and tetanus. Tetanus immunoglobulin may be injected to treat a client with tetanus but may also be used in the management of a tetanus-prone wound. Tetanus immunoglobulin contains antibodies that counteract toxins secreted by the anaerobic *Clostridium tetanus* bacillus; it is therefore called tetanus antitoxin (TAT). Antitoxins contain antibodies that neutralise the toxins secreted by pathogens, although they do not affect the pathogens themselves. Botulism and diphtheria are other examples of conditions treated with antitoxins. Antivenoms contain antibodies that combat the ill effects of bites or stings sustained from venomous creatures such as snakes, spiders, box jellyfish and stone fish.

Worldwide immunisation programs have eradicated or substantially reduced the incidence of smallpox, diphtheria, tetanus, whooping cough and poliomyelitis. Nurses can promote the health of the community by providing education about immunisation programs. It is strongly recommended that nurses access all available immunisation protection from diseases they may themselves be exposed to, in particular TB and hepatitis A and B. Figure 25.5 indicates the different types of immunity.

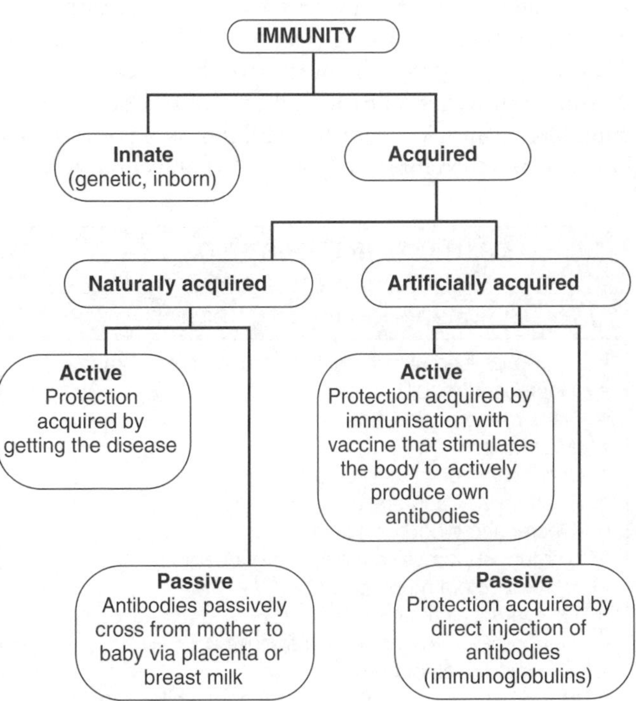

Figure 25.5 | Types of immunity *(adapted from Herlihy 2007: 221)*

FACTORS THAT INCREASE SUSCEPTIBILITY TO INFECTION

By knowing the factors that increase susceptibility to infection and by recognising the early signs and symptoms of infection, the nurse is better able to assess the client's needs, plan preventive therapy and initiate supportive nursing measures. Any reduction in the body's defences against infection places a client at risk.

CLIENT SUSCEPTIBILITY

Many general factors increase susceptibility to infection (Clinical Interest Box 25.1) and an important component of nursing practice is assessing every client for existing infection or the potential for contracting an infection. Assessment includes determining the client's:

- Health history
- Status of normal defences against infection
- Risk factors
- Knowledge about infections, prevention and control
- Age
- Nutritional status
- Level of stress and coping strategies.

Health history

Knowledge of the client's past health and illness experiences can provide information about previous exposure to communicable diseases and the status of current immunity.

Status of normal defence mechanisms

A thorough objective nursing assessment enables the nurse to determine the condition of the client's normal defences against infection. Alteration to any of the normal external or mechanical barriers provides the potential for pathogens to enter the body and thrive. A laceration, burn or abrasion, for example, destroys the protective shield that the skin normally provides, allowing an easy portal of entry for microorganisms. A client with frail, thin skin is at risk of a skin tear and therefore has a potential for infection. A client who is a chronic heavy smoker almost certainly has reduced defences against respiratory pathogens; the ability of the lungs to expand is reduced and the wafting movement of the protective cilia is impaired, leaving the client less able to propel mucus from the respiratory tract. After general surgery or any illness or procedure that further reduces mobility and lung expansion there is a high risk of the client contracting an infection such as pneumonia. A client who is dehydrated and voiding very small amounts is at risk of urinary tract infection because the normal flow of the urine is not effectively washing out microorganisms that might be entering the body via the urethra. Any reduction in the effectiveness of the body's natural defences creates a risk of infection for clients.

Any illness or disease process can affect the body's defence mechanisms and lower the client's resistance to infection. In particular, clients with disorders of the immune system are often at serious risk. Disorders of the immune system are categorised as primary or secondary disorders. Primary immunodeficiency disorders are rare disorders with genetic origins. Secondary immunodeficiency disorders are more common and frequently result from underlying disease processes or from the treatment of those diseases. Common causes include malnutrition, chronic stress, burns, diabetes mellitus and self-administration of recreational drugs and alcohol. AIDS is the most common secondary immunodeficiency disorder. Leukaemia, lymphoma and aplastic anaemia are other disorders that weaken immune defences. People with secondary immunodeficiencies experience immunosuppression and are often referred to as immunocompromised hosts. Nursing interventions for clients who are immunocompromised include eliminating contributing factors such as poor nutrition, treating the underlying condition and using sound principles of infection control.

Some medical and drug therapies, such as corticosteroid medications or chemotherapy, compromise immunity to infection. The nurse needs to assess the client's history to determine if there is an increased susceptibility to infection related to any medications or treatments.

Accurate assessment of the client's clinical condition and risk factors for infection enables the nurse to plan and implement appropriate treatment and preventive care. Nursing assessment should also determine the client's knowledge about, and ability to perform, infection prevention and control measures, such as personal hygiene care.

CLINICAL INTEREST BOX 25.1
General factors increasing susceptibility to infection

- Compromised skin integrity or mucous membranes
- Decreased mobility
- Very young or advanced age
- Malnutrition
- Alcoholism or other drug addiction
- Decreased cough reflex
- Decreased blood circulation
- Immunosuppressive therapy (e.g. chemotherapy, corticosteroid medication)
- Prematurity in infants
- Suppressed inflammatory response
- Chronic illness or chronic stress
- Suppression or insufficient number of white blood cells
- Indwelling tubes (urinary catheter, IV line)

Age

Very young and very old clients are particularly susceptible to infection. The immune systems of the very young may not be fully developed, and older age brings with it a decrease in the strength of the immune response. In particular, there is a loss of functional capacity of the cell-mediated system. This means that older clients are susceptible not only to invasion by new pathogens but also to reactivation of latent viruses and bacteria, for example, herpes zoster virus and

CLINICAL INTEREST BOX 25.2
Older adults and infection

- Older adults should be immunised annually against influenza
- Circulatory changes related to congestive heart failure and calcified mitral and aortic valves mean that older adults with these conditions are prone to pneumonia and bacterial endocarditis
- Older adults or other clients who are cognitively impaired often need special help with infection control measures (e.g. prompting to wash their hands at appropriate times)
- Symptoms of infections in older adults with dementia are often manifested as increased confusion or other changes in behaviour such as tearfulness or irritability. They may no longer have the ability to communicate their discomfort or to tell you about their symptoms verbally

Mycobacterium (Ebersole & Hess 2001). Clinical Interest Box 25.2 identifies issues concerning older adults and infection.

Normal ageing results in changes to the body's natural defences; for example the skin loses elasticity and becomes thinner. It is more easily torn and takes longer to heal, thus providing microorganisms with a portal of entry. The structure and function of all areas of the body are affected by age. For example, the cellular changes that occur in areas such as the lungs, the respiratory tract, the reproductive tract and the urinary system mean that advancing years increase susceptibility to infection. Table 25.3 identifies factors that increase susceptibility to infection in older adults.

Nutrition

Nursing assessment includes identifying clients who are at risk of inadequate dietary intake. Clients who have a debilitating illness, are confused, unable to eat without assistance, have an eating disorder, have difficulty swallowing or have any changes in the gastrointestinal tract that interfere with processing nutrients are all at risk. Any health problem that causes an inadequate intake of carbohydrates, fats, proteins and other nutrients weakens the body's defence mechanisms and healing ability. Whenever body tissues need to heal, there is an increased demand for nutrients, particularly additional protein, to aid the healing process. This means that clients with extensive tissue damage, such as might be caused by burns or other trauma, are at particular risk. High-risk clients may be assessed by a dietitian, whose role is to ensure that nutritional intake is sufficient to meet needs. This may necessitate the use of liquid nutritional supplements or parenteral nutrition. Parenteral nutrition is the administration of nutrients by a route other than the alimentary canal. All clients who have surgery also have increased demands for protein to aid healing. Nursing assessment involves monitoring the client's abilities to eat and digest food, intake and output of fluids, and bowel movements. Before discharge the nurse undertakes an evaluation of the client's abilities to maintain a healthy nutritious diet at home (see Chapter 31 for more information concerning nutrition).

Stress and coping strategies

Physical or emotional stress creates a specific response in the human body. This is the general adaptation syndrome (see Chapter 13). It causes an increase in metabolism that rapidly uses up the body's reserves of energy. Prolonged stress causes the body to continuously release excessive amounts of the steroid cortisol, which over an extended period of time leads to suppression of the immune response. Reduced immunity makes the body more susceptible to a wide range of infections (Herlihy & Maebius 2000). The nurse can assist the client to minimise the effects of stress in a variety of ways (see Chapter 13). Hospitalised clients who are susceptible to infection are at particular risk of nosocomial infections.

Nosocomial infection

A nosocomial infection is one that is acquired by a previously uninfected individual as a result of being in a health care facility. Such infections are sometimes referred to as iatrogenic or hospital-acquired infections (HAIs). A hospital is a likely place for acquiring an infection because it harbours a high population of microorganisms, including virulent strains that may be resistant to antibiotics. An infection is deemed nosocomial only if it is acquired more than 72 hours after hospitalisation. Commonly nosocomial infections are caused by organisms such as *Candida albicans*, *Escherichia coli*, *Pseudomonas* or *Staphylococcus*, hepatitis viruses or herpes zoster virus. A nosocomial infection is caused by exposure to the environment, through medical procedures or via medical officers or nurses failing to comply with infection prevention and control standards, in particular, hand washing (Lucet et al 2002).

Factors that increase a client's susceptibility to nosocomial infection include:

- Use of invasive techniques such as insertion of a urinary catheter or intravenous line and the use of endotracheal and nasogastric tubes
- Presence of a condition that alters the body's ability to combat microorganisms
- An impaired immune system.

The major types of nosocomial infections acquired by clients occur in the urinary tract, lower respiratory tract, in a surgical wound or in the blood. Infections in the blood are less common than others but lead to more serious consequences for the client. Other sites for nosocomial infections include non-surgical wounds such as decubitus ulcers, IV insertion points and the gastrointestinal tract. Nurses and all other health care workers play a vital role in preventing nosocomial infections by adhering to all

TABLE 25.3 | FACTORS THAT INCREASE SUSCEPTIBILITY TO INFECTION IN OLDER ADULTS

The normal changes of ageing means that older adults are at higher risk of infection than younger adults. Any illness experienced by an older adult increases the risk because it places increased demands on the body and a strain on its natural defence mechanisms. Nursing interventions aim to decrease this risk.

Body area	Effect of ageing process	Nursing interventions
Skin	Loses resilience because of reduced tissue elasticity and increased dryness, making the skin more susceptible to damage and slower to repair. Any opening in the skin provides a portal of entry for microorganisms	Gentle handling during bathing, moving, lifting and other procedures Careful observation of skin for signs of pressure or tears at least once each shift Use of protective aids such as sheepskins Use of skin moisturiser
Respiratory system	Decreased number of cilia lining the trachea reduces ability to move mucus, debris and dust into the pharynx Lung elasticity declines and thoracic muscle strength diminishes, making it more difficult to cough effectively so as to expel accumulated material from the airway	Increase fluid intake to thin mucous secretions Deep breathing and coughing exercises to expand the lungs and aid movement of material towards the pharynx to be expelled Effective oral hygiene to reduce potential for microorganism to invade the trachea/lungs Mobilise as soon as possible Maintain postsurgical clients (unless contraindicated) in a semi-Fowler's (semi-upright) position to promote lung expansion Motivate/support a client who smokes to reduce/break the habit
Immune system	Strength of immune responses decreases. Decreased T-cell function due to decreases in cell-mediated and humoral immunity	Recommend annual immunisation against influenza Implement all standard precautions to minimise risk of exposure to pathogens Promote exercise and healthy diet and facilitate regular rest and sleep to strengthen natural defences
Gastrointestinal system	Loss of smooth muscle in stomach and decreased peristalsis in intestine leads to slower emptying of content and any ingested microorganisms, increasing potential for colonisation Alteration to secretions of stomach acid and pepsin lead to a change in pH that interferes with ability to protect against ingested pathogens	Educate about hygienic preparation, storage and cooking of food for consumption Educate regarding hand washing and other hygiene measures to reduce potential for transference of microorganisms into the gastrointestinal tract Promote effective oral hygiene to minimise potential for microorganisms to enter the gastrointestinal tract
Urinary/renal system	Structural changes in kidney and renal vessels reduces renal blood flow. Together with general loss of functioning of body cells this results in the body, under the stress of infection, being less able to maintain adequate fluid homeostasis Hypertrophy of prostate gland in males, cystocele or rectocele and degeneration of nerves to bladder causes inadequate emptying of bladder and urine stasis. Stasis predisposes to urinary-tract infection	Monitor fluid intake/output Observe and report signs of dehydration/fluid overload Implement all standard precautions to minimise exposure to pathogens Promote intake of sufficient fluid to flush urinary system with dilute urine Encourage client to take sufficient time to empty bladder fully

(adapted from deWit 2005)

recommended infection prevention and control measures outlined in policy guidelines.

ASEPSIS AND INFECTION PREVENTION AND CONTROL

Asepsis means the absence of microorganisms. The term covers the processes of infection control that may involve exclusion of microorganisms by the physical isolation of a client with an infection, removal of microorganisms by cleansing the hands or equipment, or destruction of microorganisms by sterilisation or disinfection. Aseptic technique refers to any health care procedure in which precautions such as the use of sterile gloves and instruments are used to prevent contamination of a person, object or area by microorganisms. Techniques used to maintain asepsis can be categorised into clean (medical asepsis) and sterile techniques (surgical asepsis).

Medical asepsis refers to the use of a clean technique

that involves interfering with the chain of infection. Routine practices are aimed at reducing the number of microorganisms or containing them within a specific area. Medical asepsis does not destroy all microorganisms but reduces the risk of transmission. It prevents cross-infection or reinfection of the same client. It is the process of using cleanliness to protect items in the environment from being contaminated and by using disinfection as a method of dealing with items that have become contaminated. It involves the use of gowns, masks and gloves to protect the nurse, and use of the 'no-touch' technique when undertaking procedures such as wound dressings (see Chapter 37).

Surgical asepsis (sterile technique) involves measures that render supplies and equipment totally free of microorganisms, and practices that avoid contamination during their use. Surgical asepsis involves surgical hand washing and the use of sterile barrier clothing by those working in areas such as operating theatres. It also involves sterilisation of equipment, the use of sterile fields and special air filtration systems. Sterile techniques and surgical asepsis are discussed in more depth towards the end of this chapter.

The basic principles employed in preventing the spread of infection are the same in all situations, regardless of whether clients are cared for in the community, in aged-care facilities, in day clinics or in hospitals. Medical and surgical aseptic techniques and all infection prevention and control activities are directed towards breaking the chain of infection. Specific guidelines in Australia and New Zealand have been developed to help health care workers in this process. In Australia these are termed standard precautions and additional precautions. The principles of infection control that frame these precautions are in close alignment with infection control guidelines developed by the Ministry of Health in New Zealand.

STANDARD PRECAUTIONS AND ADDITIONAL PRECAUTIONS

Standard and additional precautions are the guidelines that relate to infection prevention and control in the workplace. The Australian Government Department of Health and Ageing (2004) provides the national guidelines for infection control in health care settings. Hard copies of these *Infection Control Guidelines* are readily available. Copies have been distributed nationally to public and private hospitals, aged care facilities, peak health organisations, state and territory health departments, health libraries and universities.

Standard precautions are the basic recommended work practices to be implemented in the treatment and care of all clients regardless of diagnosis or perceived infectious risk. Standard precautions are the first tier in a two-tiered approach to infection control. Additional precautions form the second tier and are used in situations in which clients are known or are suspected as being infected with epidemiologically significant or highly transmissible pathogens that may not be contained by the use of standard precautions alone.

Standard precautions relate to:

- Aseptic technique
- Effective hand hygiene
- Use of personal protective equipment such as gloves, gowns, masks or eye protection when appropriate
- Appropriate reprocessing of instruments and equipment
- Implementation of environmental controls
- Safe systems for the handling of blood (including dried blood) and all other body fluids, secretions and excretions (excluding sweat) regardless of whether or not they contain visible blood
- The safe handling of non-intact skin and mucous membranes.

The additional precautions are focused on three modes of transmission. Extra precautions are implemented to interrupt transmission of highly contagious or epidemiologically important pathogens that are transmitted via the respiratory droplet or airborne route, direct or indirect contact with dry skin or with contaminated surfaces, or via any combination of these routes. For example, a client with influenza, active pulmonary TB, measles, Creutzfeldt-Jakob disease or SARS would be in this category. Additional precautions are tailored to the specific infectious agent concerned and may include:

- Nursing the client in a single room (isolation) or cohort placement in cases of outbreaks, particularly for children or elderly clients
- Protection with personal respiratory filtering devices for anyone entering the client's room
- Special room ventilation systems to maintain the room air at negative pressure
- Room door opened only for staff to enter or leave
- Care only by nurses who are immune to the infection carried by the client
- Dedicated equipment
- Restricted movement of nurses and clients.

Additional precautions are not required for clients with blood-borne viruses such as HIV, hepatitis B or hepatitis C unless other factors indicate it necessary, such as the presence of an additional highly transmissible disorder such as pulmonary TB (Australian Government Department of Health and Ageing 2004).

Table 25.4 identifies the main points relating to standard and additional precautions and infection control.

IMPLEMENTING STANDARD PRECAUTIONS

Standard precautions involve activities aimed to interrupt the chain of infection. These include hand hygiene measures and use of a range of protective devices. Table 25.5 identifies nursing interventions that interrupt the chain of infection.

TABLE 25.4 | STANDARD AND ADDITIONAL PRECAUTIONS FOR INFECTION CONTROL: MAIN POINTS

Standard precautions

- Routine personal hygiene practices to be observed
- Hands to be washed before and after all significant client contacts, after contact with blood, all body fluids, secretions and excretions, non-intact skin and mucous membranes
- Gloves to be worn when touching blood, all body fluids, secretions and excretions, non-intact skin and mucous membranes. Hands to be washed before putting gloves on and after gloves are removed
- Personal protective equipment such as masks or face shields and eye protection to be worn when client care activities may generate splashes or sprays of blood, body fluids, secretions or excretions
- Impermeable gowns to be worn if clothes are likely to be soiled with blood or body fluid. Hands to be washed immediately gown is removed
- Protocols for handling and disposal of sharps and other clinical wastes to be followed at all times
- Environmental control policies to be adhered to (e.g. cleaning, disposal of linen and rubbish, disinfection, sterilisation and spills management)
- Client care equipment to be cleaned and reprocessed according to protocols or policies
- Private room unnecessary unless client unable to maintain hygiene practices in accordance with prevention and control strategies

Additional precautions

Type of transmission	Protection	Example
Airborne	Private room or cohort; use of surgical mask or respiratory protection device for TB or SARS; mask for client if transported	Varicella zoster (chicken pox), measles, TB, SARS
Droplet	Private room or cohort; use of surgical mask; mask for client if transported	Influenza, pneumonia, rubella, pertussis, mumps
Contact	Private room or cohort; gloves for direct client or environmental contact; gowns for direct contact or splashing	Respiratory syncytial virus, shigella, acute diarrhoea, scabies

HAND HYGIENE

Hand hygiene is the term that applies to routine and aseptic hand washing, the use of an antiseptic hand rub or the combined use of hand washing and antimicrobial skin cleansers to rid the hands of microorganisms. Because hands are easily contaminated, thorough hand washing is a basic and essential precaution in preventing the spread of microorganisms. Hand washing does not sterilise the skin but it does remove resident microorganisms (non-pathogenic organisms that are constantly present on the skin) and transient microorganisms (pathogens collected after contact with contaminated reservoirs).

Health professionals use three different types of hand-washing procedure, according to different situations. A routine hand wash is performed before or after direct or indirect contact with clients or equipment, for example, before handling food or food utensils. An aseptic hand wash is conducted before undertaking aseptic non-surgical procedures. A surgical hand wash (surgical scrub) is undertaken before any invasive surgical procedure such as operating-room procedures. A surgical scrub involves applying antimicrobial skin cleanser to the hands after washing them and before putting on sterile gloves. Surgical hand asepsis reduces the resident microbial count on the hands to the minimum (Boyce & Pittett 2002). Further information on surgical asepsis is provided later in this chapter. The Australian Government Department of Health and Ageing (2004) provides guidelines that outline the way each of these hand-washing procedures should be conducted to most effectively reduce transmission of microorganisms (Table 25.6).

The Australian Government Department of Health and Ageing (2004) guidelines correspond closely to those of the US Centers for Disease Control and Prevention (CDC). In response to worrying outbreaks of infection in health care facilities and in particular those involving antimicrobial-resistant microorganisms such as MRSA, the CDC advocates adherence to correct hand-washing procedures and the use of alcohol-based hand rubs (Boyce & Pittett 2002). When using an alcohol-based hand rub the manufacturer's recommendations for the quantity to use must be followed. Generally an alcohol-based hand rub is applied to the palm of one hand then the hands are rubbed together, allowing the solution to cover all surfaces of the hands and fingers until the hands are dry. The Australian Government Department of Health and Ageing (2004) infection control guidelines indicate that hand washing is the most effective measure in preventing the spread of infection and suggest that alcohol-based preparations designed for use without water should be used as an adjunct to hand washing. The use of an alcohol-based hand rub alone (without prior hand washing) should only occur in exceptional circumstances; for example, in emergency situations when there is insufficient time for hand washing.

TABLE 25.5 | INTERRUPTING THE CHAIN OF INFECTION

Link in the chain	Objective	Nursing interventions
Reservoir: • Infected person • Vector • Contaminated object	Eliminate conditions that favour growth of microorganisms Prevent transmission of microorganisms	Correct hand-washing technique Use of disposable gloves Standard precautions: handling, disinfecting/sterilising/disposing of contaminated articles Additional barrier/isolation precautions as indicated
Portal of exit — body fluids, excreta or other secretions	Prevent contamination	Correct hand-washing technique Use of disposable gloves Use of standard precautions Never recap needles; correct handling of all body fluids/sharps/other equipment Correct aseptic technique Educate clients/others regarding measures to prevent transmission
Route of transmission: • Hands • Mouth/nose • Infected lesions/body fluids • Contaminated food/water • Contaminated objects	Prevent cross-contamination; eliminate vectors	Correct hand-washing technique Use of disposable gloves Use of standard/additional precautions Correct storage/preparation of consumables Correct medical or surgical aseptic technique Isolation precautions Effective pest control
Portal of entry: • Mouth/nose • Body orifices • Openings in skin/mucous membranes	Prevent entry of microorganisms into a host	Use of standard/additional precautions Use of mask, face shield, goggles, gloves, gown Avoid putting contaminated hands/objects near mouth Waterproof occlusive covering to protect skin breaks Effective skin and oral hygiene
Susceptible host	Improve client resistance to infection; prevent infection	Assess potential for infection All above precautions Protective isolation if indicated Provide healthy nutrition/sound rest and sleep. Encourage exercise as able Protective skin care, aids as needed (e.g. sheepskin elbow/knee pads) Positioning to promote lung expansion Correct aseptic technique

(adapted from deWit 2005)

It is recommended that nurses wash their hands before and after significant contact with any client and after activities likely to cause contamination. Significant client contact includes:

- contact with, or physical examination of, a client
- emptying a drainage reservoir (e.g. catheter bag)
- delivering an injection or undertaking venipuncture.

Nursing activities that have the potential to cause contamination include:

- changing bedding or clothing soiled with urine, blood or other body secretions
- handling equipment or instruments soiled with blood or other body secretions
- undertaking invasive procedures such as inserting a urinary catheter or performing nasotracheal suctioning.

Hand washing reduces the number of microorganisms present on the hands and inhibits their growth and reproduction. Before aseptic non-sterile procedures, nurses should wash their hands for a full minute with antibacterial soap. Before surgical procedures nurses should wash their hands for 5 minutes on the first occasion for the day and for 3 minutes before each sterile procedure after that (Australian Government Department of Health and Ageing 2004). It is never acceptable to take short-cuts when washing the hands, and hand washing should always be conducted according to policy of the employing agency. The length of time recommended for hand washing sometimes varies between agencies and may depend on the products used, but it should not be less than recommended in the Australian Government Department of Health and Ageing guidelines outlined in Table 25.6. Despite good intentions, nurses frequently fail to employ an effective hand-washing technique (Lucet et al 2002), often neglecting to thoroughly wash some areas of the hands. Figure 25.6 identifies the areas of the hands most often neglected during washing.

In addition to washing, care of the hands involves:

TABLE 25.6 | HAND-WASHING TECHNIQUES

Type	Technique (How)	Duration	Drying	Example (When)
Routine hand wash	Remove jewellery. Wet hands thoroughly and lather vigorously using neutral pH liquid hand-wash solution. Rinse under running water Do not touch taps with clean hands — if elbow or foot controls are not available, use paper towel to turn taps off	10–15 seconds	Pat dry using paper towel	Prior to eating or smoking After going to the toilet Prior to significant contact with patients (e.g. physical examination, emptying a drainage reservoir [catheter bag]) Prior to administering injection or performing venipuncture Prior to and after routine use of gloves After handling any instruments or equipment soiled with blood or other body substances
Hand wash before aseptic procedures (non-surgical)	Remove jewellery. Wash hands thoroughly using an antimicrobial skin cleanser. Rinse carefully Do not touch taps with clean hands — if elbow or foot controls are not available, use paper towel to turn taps off	1 minute	Pat dry using paper towel	Prior to any non-surgical procedures that require aseptic techniques (such as inserting urinary or intravenous catheters)
Surgical hand wash	Remove jewellery. Wash hands, nails and forearms thoroughly and apply an antimicrobial skin cleanser (containing 4% w/v chlorhexidine or detergent-based povidone iodine containing 0.75 per cent available iodine or an aqueous povidone-iodine solution containing 1% available iodine). Rinse carefully, keeping hands above the elbows No-touch techniques apply	First wash for the day: 5 minutes. Subsequent washes: 3 minutes	Dry with sterile towels	Prior to any invasive surgical procedures (operating-room procedures)

(adapted from Australian Government Department of Health and Ageing 2004)

- Covering any broken or infected areas of the skin with a waterproof dressing
- Wearing disposable gloves to protect larger skin lesions
- Keeping fingernails clean and short (less than one quarter of an inch long) and not wearing artificial nails
- Removing any rings before starting any client care activity
- Keeping the skin free from cracks. If frequent immersion in water results in skin dryness, a good quality hand cream should be used
- Wearing disposable gloves (and forceps if indicated) when dealing with infective or potentially infective material (e.g. soiled dressings or blood).

RINGS, JEWELLERY AND ARTIFICIAL NAILS

There has been debate about the requirement for nurses to remove rings and other jewellery when working with clients in health care settings. There is little hard evidence that the wearing of jewellery constitutes an infection risk to staff or patients. However, it seems likely that uncleaned rings, artificial nails and other adornments harbour microorganisms that might contaminate sterile fields. The Australian Government *Infection Control Guidelines* suggest that each health care establishment should develop policies about the wearing of jewellery (including body piercings), artificial nails or nail polish by employees. It is recommended that the policies take into account the risks of transmission of infection to clients and health care workers, rather than cultural preferences (Australian Government Department of Health and Ageing 2004).

USE OF PERSONAL PROTECTIVE EQUIPMENT (PPE)

In accordance with standard precautions, personal protective equipment (PPE) is used with all clients when there is potential to come in contact with body substances or airborne microorganisms. This is because every client has the potential to transmit infection via body substances, and the risk for transmission may be unknown, even by the client. PPE includes gloves, gowns, masks or face shields and, in some circumstances, foot and hair coverings.

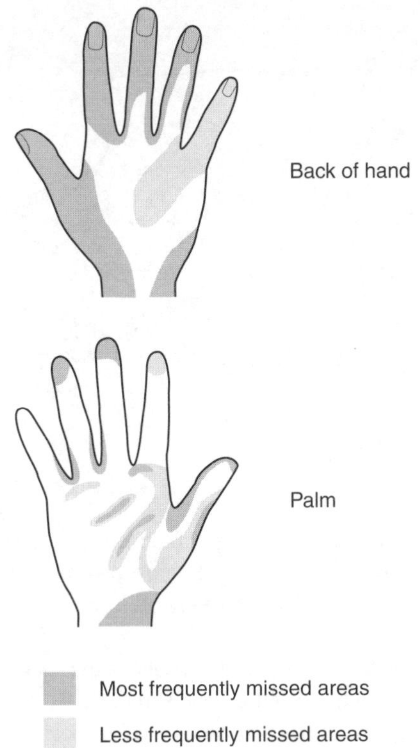

Figure 25.6 | Areas most neglected when hand washing

In determining the type of PPE to use, the nurse should consider the probability of exposure to blood and body substances, the amount and type of exposure and the route of transmission. Full protective wear is recommended for operating-room procedures, and appropriate respiratory protection should be worn by health care workers exposed to virulent microorganisms such as those causing *Mycobacterium* tuberculosis or SARS.

Gloves

The nurse should put on clean, non-sterile disposable gloves in any situation in which there is a risk of touching blood, body fluids or excretions, or any items contaminated by them. Clean gloves should also be put on just before the nurse touches mucous membranes or non-intact skin. Non-sterile gloves are adequate in these situations. Sterile gloves are needed only when a surgical or sterile procedure is to be conducted. Disposable gloves should be used as an adjunct to hand washing when there is a risk that hands might be contaminated by blood or body fluid. Hands should be washed or an alcohol-based rub applied before and after putting on gloves. Gloves should be changed before and after each client procedure and also during multiple procedures on the same client when there is a possibility of cross-contamination (Australian Government Department of Health and Ageing 2004).

Contaminated gloves should always be removed immediately after the task is completed and in such a way that the contaminated outside surfaces are enveloped within the inside surfaces, as this helps to limit the risk of transmission. Figure 25.7 illustrates the correct method of removing contaminated gloves. Once removed, gloves should be placed immediately into the appropriate waste receptacle and the hands washed. Hand washing is essential before and after gloving because gloves do not provide complete 100% protection. With the increased use of latex gloves in the workplace, allergies to latex have increased. Nurses are therefore advised not to use latex gloves unnecessarily for routine tasks when the risk of exposure to body fluids is unlikely. Nurses are also advised not to use petroleum-based hand lotions because these attract latex proteins from the gloves, increasing the risk of developing a latex allergy. Employers are obliged to supply latex-free gloves to nurses who develop sensitivity to latex (deWit 2005).

Barrier/isolation gowns

An impermeable gown is worn to prevent contamination of the clothing by pathogenic microorganisms, thus preventing cross-infection. Gowns are worn when there is a chance that the nurse's body or personal clothing might become contaminated with airborne microorganisms or a client's infected body substances. Vulnerable individuals, who for their own protection are being nursed using isolation precautions, may also wear gowns to protect from microorganisms that may be on the clothing of persons entering the room. This, for example, would apply to a client who is immunosuppressed as a result of chemotherapy, or for a client in a burns unit who has large areas of non-intact skin and is therefore at high risk of becoming infected.

A gown may be made of non-porous paper and be disposable, or may be made from cotton and be reusable. A gown should be long and large enough to cover the clothing completely, and open down the back where it is tied at the neck and waist. To put on a gown, the hands are first washed and dried. A clean gown is picked up, and held out to allow it to unfold. The arms are slipped inside the sleeves and, if it is necessary to adjust any part of the gown, this is achieved by handling the inside only. The neck tapes are tied, then the waist tapes are tied at the back. To remove a gown, the waist and neck tapes are untied, the gown is allowed to fall from the shoulders. Holding the gown by the shoulder seams, it is slipped off and turned inside out as it is being removed. The hands should be removed from the sleeves, ensuring that they do not touch the outside of the gown. The gown is placed in the soiled linen container or, if it is disposable, in the rubbish container. The hands are washed and dried before leaving the room.

Face protection devices

Depending on the mode of transmission, health care workers may wear a mask, goggles or face shield. These items are applied before entering the room. Face masks are worn to prevent the spread of microorganisms from the respiratory tract of a client to the nurse or from the nurse's respiratory tract to a client. If there is a risk of splash contamination by blood or other body fluids, a more substantial face shield

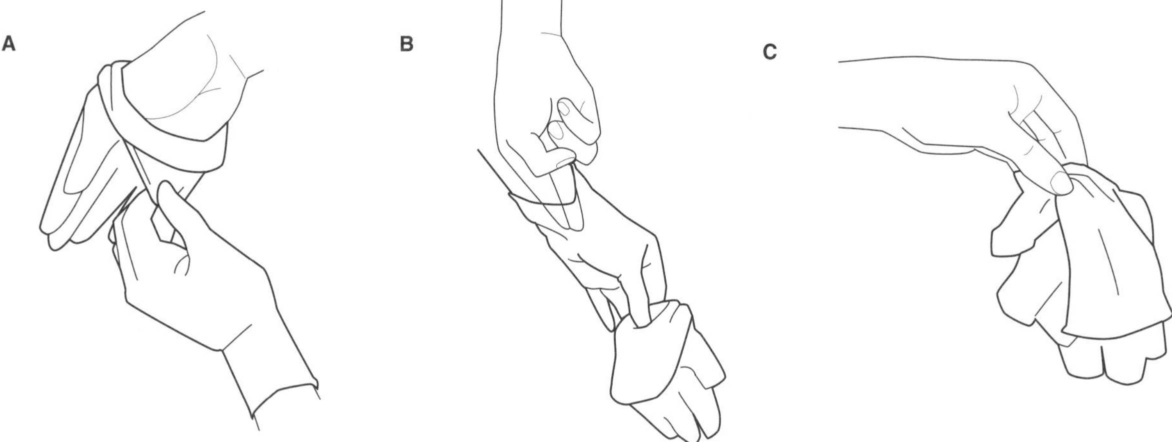

Figure 25.7 | Removing contaminated gloves

A: Removing the right glove. Take hold of the cuff on the glove on the right hand and slide it from the hand, folding the inside of the glove over the outside. This encloses the contaminated outside area. Avoid touching the skin of the right wrist or hand with the fingers of the contaminated glove on the left hand, as to do so would enable microorganisms to be transferred.

B: Removing the left glove. Grasp the glove that has been removed from the right hand in the palm of the left gloved hand. Slip two fingers from the ungloved right hand under the band of the second glove at the wrist. Roll the glove off, turning it inside out, over the first glove. This action ensures that exposure of the contaminated surfaces on both gloves is minimal, reducing the risk of transferring microorganisms.

C: Safe method of holding contaminated gloves. Ensuring that you hold and touch only the inside surface of the left-hand glove, drop the rolled up gloves into the appropriate receptacle for rubbish. The gloves should be disposed of in this way immediately after removal. This reduces the risk of spreading infection. Wash your hands promptly because there is no guarantee that gloves provide 100% protection. This also reduces the risk of developing an allergy to the latex in the gloves. Nurses who are left-handed may prefer to reverse this process.

and/or eye goggles should be worn. Disposable masks are worn and discarded immediately after use. The hands are washed and dried after the mask is removed. When a mask is used it must:

- Be handled only by the tapes or loops at either end
- Cover the nose and mouth completely
- Not be allowed to hang around the neck, as this practice results in contamination
- Be changed as soon as it becomes damp, as moisture allows microorganisms to pass through the mask.

Various types of mask and protective devices are required when the nurse is caring for clients with highly infective respiratory disorders such as TB or SARS. It is the nurse's responsibility to be aware of agency policy in relation to the type of protective device to use in particular circumstances. It is the responsibility of the agency to ensure that employees are provided with the knowledge and skills to use any specialised equipment efficiently.

Hair covers

An elasticised paper cap is the most common hair covering. It is used whenever there is a risk of the hair becoming contaminated or if microorganisms from the hair might endanger the client. Nurses wear caps in the surgical operating room environment.

Shoe covers

Disposable paper covers are worn over shoes whenever there is a risk of body substances splashing onto shoes during nursing procedures. The covers are removed before leaving the room, to prevent pathogens being carried away from the area. Over-shoe cloth or paper covers are used in the operating room environment to contain any microorganisms that might be on the shoes of operating room staff.

REPROCESSING OF INSTRUMENTS AND EQUIPMENT

Disposable equipment must be disposed of immediately after use. Non-disposable instruments and equipment must be reprocessed according to formal infection prevention and control protocols. Reprocessing protocols relate to the correct safe handling, cleaning, disinfecting and sterilising of equipment in order to reduce or eliminate microorganisms. Reprocessing of instruments and equipment includes general cleaning, disinfection (by heat and water, or chemical disinfectants) and/or sterilisation. The level of reprocessing that is necessary depends on the body site where specific items are used, and therefore the level of contamination risk involved. The levels of risk are: critical, semi-critical and non-critical. Items involved with penetration into sterile tissue, body cavities or the bloodstream (e.g. surgical instruments such as laparoscopes and arthroscopes) present a critical risk. Items that are in contact with intact non-sterile mucosa (e.g. vaginal specula, sigmoidoscopes) present a semi-critical risk. Items in contact only with intact skin (e.g. stethoscopes, non-invasive ultrasound probes) present a non-critical risk. When a critical risk is present items must be sterilised. It is also preferable to sterilise items when a semi-critical risk is present. However, chemical disinfection may be used when a semi-critical risk is present but the item will not tolerate heat. This is the case for flexible fibreoptic equipment such as endoscopes, sigmoidoscopes, gastroscopes, colonoscopes and invasive ultrasound probes. When a non-critical risk is present a minimum level of reprocessing is adequate. Minimal reprocessing involves routine cleaning and decontamination with disinfectant after cleaning as necessary.

ROUTINE CLEANING

Cleaning is an essential factor in preventing cross-infection. Cleaning is the removal from items of all foreign material, such as soil and organic material. Detergent and water is generally sufficient for routine cleaning (Australian Government Department of Health and Ageing 2004). All reusable instruments and equipment should be cleaned as soon as possible after use regardless of risk level and any other infection control measures required. If items are not thoroughly cleaned they cannot later be effectively disinfected or sterilised (Australian Government Department of Health and Ageing 2004). A plastic apron, general purpose utility gloves, and protective face and eyewear should be worn when cleaning equipment that may be contaminated with material such as blood, mucus, pus, sputum or faeces. The following steps provide a general guide to manual cleaning of instruments and equipment:

- Remove gross soiling immediately after use by rinsing in warm water (15–18°C)
- Fully disassemble instruments and immerse in warm water and detergent (enzymatic cleansers are hazardous and should only be used if indicated, e.g. for fibreoptic and other instruments where design characteristics make routine cleaning difficult)
- Remove all visible soiling with a small clean brush, working low in the sink
- Rinse thoroughly in hot water (unless contraindicated by manufacturer)
- Dry mechanically in a drying cabinet or hand dry with a clean, lint-free cloth (items must not be left to dry in ambient air)
- Inspect instruments and equipment to ensure they are clean and ready for further processing or storage.

DISINFECTION

Disinfection is not a sterilising process. It is a process intended to destroy pathogenic microorganisms (with the exception of spores) or render them inert. Much of the equipment used in health care is disposable, which helps to reduce cross-infection. However, non-disposable equipment must be disinfected or sterilised after each use and after it has been cleaned manually. Examples of disinfectants are alcohols, chlorines, household bleach, glutaraldehydes and phenols. Different grades of disinfectants are used for different purposes. For example, only instrument grade disinfectant should be used with medical instruments. Disinfectants can be caustic and toxic to tissues. Each health care institution has its own policy in relation to disinfection techniques.

Terminal disinfection refers to the cleaning procedures performed after the transfer, discharge or death of an individual who has been in isolation. Most Australian states and territories require that the body of a person who had a contagious illness be placed in a special impervious plastic wrap or bag before being transferred from an isolation room. The contents of the client's room and all items of equipment used in the care of the individual are cleaned and disinfected. The method used should be sufficiently thorough to destroy all pathogenic microorganisms. Most health care facilities have personnel who are experienced in, and responsible for, terminal disinfection procedures.

Sterilisation is a process that is intended to destroy all types of microorganisms, including highly resistant bacterial spores. A sterile article is one that is totally free from all microorganisms. Sterility is an all-or-none state, because a single living cell renders an article unsterile. Any item that penetrates into body tissues or the bloodstream, such as needles, invasive diagnostic instruments or fluids for parenteral administration, must be sterile. Dressing materials that come into direct contact with the body surface, such as gauze placed over a wound, must also be sterile.

METHODS OF STERILISATION AND DISINFECTION

Sterilisation by steam under pressure (moist heat) at 121–134°C (autoclaving)

Steam is the most dependable sterilising agent because it releases a large amount of heat when it condenses on the articles being sterilised. Steam also provides moisture for destroying microorganisms through coagulation of cellular protein. An autoclave is an appliance used to sterilise instruments or other objects with steam under pressure. Autoclaving is suitable for metal, glass and some specific rubber items, cotton fabric, nylon, polycarbonate and polypropylene. It is unsuitable for substances that are impermeable to moisture, such as oils and waxes. Materials used to wrap items for autoclaving must be permeable to steam and provide an effective barrier against external contamination.

Sterilisation by dry heat at 160°C

Although the need to use dry heat as a method of sterilisation has declined because of the availability of many commercially sterilised items, a dry heat oven may still be used to sterilise non-stainless instruments, glass reusable syringes and some sharp instruments. To be effective the temperature in the hot air oven must be maintained consistently at 160°C for a minimum period of 120 minutes plus penetration time or according to manufacturer instructions.

Sterilisation by chemical vapours

Sterilisation by ethylene oxide or formaldehyde is generally restricted to articles that cannot withstand autoclaving or dry heat, such as instruments with plastic components, electrical leads and electronic devices.

Radiation sterilisation

The industrial sterilisation of pre-packaged medical devices commonly uses either gamma radiation emitted by cobalt-60 isotope, or a beam of electrons produced in a machine. As efficiency of this process depends only on absorption of the dose required to destroy the microbial contaminants, irradiation is extremely reliable.

Thermal disinfection

Thermal disinfection is a process using heat and water at temperatures and times that destroy pathogenic, vegetative agents, but not bacterial spores. It is therefore a satisfactory way of disinfecting items that can withstand heat and moisture but do not require sterilisation. Pasteurisation is a thermal disinfection process using hot water at a temperature of 75°C for an instrument/water contact time of at least 30 minutes or a comparative heat/time ratio such as 70°C for a contact time of 100 minutes (Australian Government Department of Health and Ageing 2004). Thermal disinfection is a convenient and cost-effective way to disinfect articles in the home. The quality of the water can be an issue in some areas and use of distilled, pre-boiled or deionised water might be necessary. Specially designed thermal disinfecting machines are commonly used in health care facilities to disinfect articles such as toilet utensils, bed clothing, mops and brushes.

Chemical disinfection

Chemicals are effective disinfectants, as they attack all types of microorganisms, act rapidly, are stable in light and heat, are inexpensive, are not harmful to body tissues and do not destroy the article being disinfected. The effectiveness of chemicals may be reduced by:

- An excessive number of microorganisms
- Inaccessible microorganisms (e.g. in crevices or in deposits of organic material on the article)
- Concentration too low or contact time too short
- Inappropriate pH
- Inactivation by organic matter, detergent, cotton or synthetic materials.

If an inappropriate chemical is used, or if it is used incorrectly, the article will not be disinfected. Gram-negative bacteria such as *Pseudomonas* may multiply in the chemical solution. These organisms have frequently been associated with HAIs. Disinfectants containing phenols, quaternary ammonium compounds or chlorhexidine have a narrow spectrum and their effectiveness is limited to non-sporing bacteria and some viruses. Chlorine and iodine compounds, glutaraldehyde and formaldehyde are broad-spectrum disinfectants, which means they are effective against a broad range of pathogens, including tubercle bacilli and hepatitis viruses.

In most health care institutions there is a central sterile supply department responsible for cleaning, packing and sterilising reusable equipment. Nurses required to operate a steriliser, such as an autoclave, should be provided with adequate information on how to use the equipment safely and efficiently.

Many articles are packaged before being sterilised, which helps to ensure that sterility is maintained until they are used. Maintenance of sterility is assisted by double wrapping individual items or by enclosing single-wrapped items in a plastic bag after they have been sterilised. Industrially sterilised items should be stored in the container (e.g. carton) provided by the manufacturer. It is important to note that the porous wrappings used during steam or gas sterilisation are only effective as barriers to contamination if they remain dry and intact. Before any packaged sterile item is used, the expiry date on the package must be checked. Heat-sensitive tape that changes colour or displays a pattern when exposed to high temperatures is used on sterilised packages as a visual indicator that the item is sterile.

Environmental controls

Environmental controls include those relating to the preparation of food, and general cleaning procedures. Floors are generally cleaned with a vacuum cleaner designed to prevent dust being released into the air. Spillages of blood or any other body fluid in general areas are cleaned with hospital grade chemical disinfectant in accordance with the routine infection containment policies and practices of the health care facility. A spills kit should be available for cleaning in areas which have a higher infectivity risk, for example operating rooms, mortuaries and laboratories (Australian Government Department of Health and Ageing 2004). All surfaces, such as bedside lockers and over-bed tables, should be cleaned daily to eliminate dust and food debris. A chemical disinfectant may be used to clean these and other items of furniture. Ward areas and utility rooms such as pantries, bathrooms, toilets and pan rooms should be cleaned daily. Floors and all bench surfaces are cleaned and a non-abrasive substance used to wipe the bath after each use. Rubbish containers should be equipped with close-fitting lids and must be emptied frequently and never left with material overflowing from them. Cleaning is generally a non-nursing duty, but nurses have a responsibility to ensure that cleaning is carried out effectively and in line with infection control policies. Nurses also have a responsibility to ensure that linen is handled carefully; for example, bedclothes should not be flicked or shaken, as these actions liberate dust and microorganisms into the environment. Soiled linen should be rolled up or folded and placed immediately into the appropriate receptacle. All health care workers should wear clean washable clothing that is changed daily.

Actions should be taken to keep all areas free from the possibility of vector transmission (flies, other insects and animals) by placing rubbish and soiled linen immediately into the appropriate containers, by disposing of food scraps correctly, by keeping any food or fluid covered, and by emptying toilet utensils (bedpans and urinals) immediately.

SAFE HANDLING OF BLOOD AND BODY SECRETIONS

There is potential for contamination from blood or body secretions when handling soiled linen, pathology specimens, equipment or rubbish. Infective or potentially infective articles include wound dressings, suction or drainage tubing and containers, intravenous therapy apparatus, needles and syringes, bedpans, urinals and other toilet utensils. Rubbish includes sharps, infectious waste, human tissues, general waste and radioactive waste. Rubbish should be segregated and disposed of according to type, such as general, infectious, cytotoxic and radioactive. Standard precautions should be followed in relation to avoiding exposure to blood and body secretions or excretions. Gowns and gloves, for example, should be worn by anyone handling contaminated articles, and linen soiled with blood or body substances should be placed and transported in an impermeable (leak-proof) bag. The infection control guidelines recommend the use of a single bag, provided that it is sturdy and impervious and that the items to be discarded can be placed in the bag without contaminating the outside of the bag. Double-bagging is not performed routinely but this is necessary when the outside of a bag is visibly contaminated. Linen bags and rubbish bags should never be overfilled and should be tied securely before being transported.

Spills management

There should be systems in place for dealing with blood and body substance spills. The management of spills depends on a range of factors and the following should be considered:

- The likely pathogen involved in the spill
- The size of the spill
- The type of spill
- The type of surface
- The area involved
- Whether or not bare skin is likely to come into contact with the spill
- Correct dilution of the disinfection agent designated to be used to clean the spill.

HANDLING AND DISPOSAL OF SHARPS

Sharp instruments represent the major cause of accidents involving potential exposure to blood-borne disease. Sharps must not be passed by hand between workers. Needles or any other sharp implement should not be recapped, bent or disconnected from syringes but disposed of intact. All sharp instruments and needles are disposed of immediately after use by placing them into a special sharps puncture-proof container. There should be a sharps container available at the place the sharp is used. The person using the sharp should be the person to dispose of it into the container. If a sharp is dropped onto the floor or bed it should be picked up and placed into the container using forceps (see Chapter 26 for further discussion about safe disposal of sharps).

SPECIMEN COLLECTION AND TRANSPORT

Standard precautions should be followed when handling laboratory specimens. If additional precautions are needed, for example, if the specimen is from a client diagnosed with a particularly virulent, unusual or epidemiologically important pathogen, such as CJD, advice should be sought from an expert in the pathology laboratory. The nurse should wear gloves when collecting specimens. Enrolled Nurses (ENs) may be required to obtain specimens such as a midstream specimen of urine (MSU) or a stool (faecal) specimen. Other specimens that may be requested include blood samples and swabs from wounds or body orifices such as the nose, throat or vagina. Personnel from a pathology department often obtain these specimens from clients. ENs are advised to check their code of practice and the policies of the employing agency in regard to collecting pathology specimens from clients. All specimen containers should be sealed tightly to prevent spillage and contamination of the outside of the container. Details should be written on the container label. The container should be placed in a sealed plastic bag, also clearly labelled, and taken as soon as possible to the pathology department.

TRANSPORTING CLIENTS

It may be necessary to transport clients with infections to surgery or centres for diagnostic tests. Clients infected with microorganisms transmitted by the airborne route should only leave their rooms if it is essential to do so. Respiratory secretions should be contained by asking the client to wear a mask. The client should also be provided with tissues and a bag in which to seal them if necessary. The person transporting any client who is infectious should wear appropriate barrier protection. The nurse needs to take precautions to prevent, contain or be ready to clean or cover any leakage of body excreta (e.g. faeces, vomitus, sputum, urine), blood and other body fluids, and exudates from infected wounds or skin lesions.

The nurse provides the client with a gown to wear as a robe en route and explains as sensitively as possible how the client can assist with preventing transmission of infection during the transfer and throughout any procedure. The client may be transported in a wheelchair or on a stretcher or hospital trolley. These may be protected with extra layers of linen or disposable protectors. Any person in another area who is to be in contact with the infectious client, such as ambulance officers and surgical staff, should be informed of the precautions necessary before the transfer. Information concerning the isolation precautions should also be clearly documented on the client's chart. Equipment should be cleaned according to infection control guidelines.

BARRIER AND ISOLATION PRECAUTIONS

A client with a highly transmissible infection is nursed using isolation precautions. The client is nursed in a single room and those involved in providing care use special barrier precautions, which include the appropriate use of gowns, gloves, masks, eyewear and other protective devices or clothing. Clients who are infected with the same pathogen may sometimes be nursed together; isolation precautions are used with the clients sharing a room (cohort nursing). Although health care facilities develop and implement their own isolation policies, isolation precautions are based on the following general principles:

- Each step in the care plan is carefully devised to minimise the risk of cross-infection, as one act of carelessness can result in a spread of infection. Before any nursing activity is performed, the technique to be used should be planned carefully so that the risk of cross-infection is minimised. Once the nurse's hands have become contaminated, possessions such as watches, pens, scissors or any part of the uniform must not be handled. To reduce the risk of acts of carelessness, items such as pens and scissors should be kept in the client's room. To avoid the need to use personal watches for measuring the client's vital signs, the room should be equipped with a wall clock that has a second hand
- People should avoid touching their hair, nose, mouth or eyes while caring for a client in isolation
- Protective clothing such as gowns, masks and gloves are put on before entering or immediately on entering the room. Disposable gowns are preferable; non-disposable gowns may be used once then placed in the appropriate container for decontamination and reprocessing
- Hands should be washed on entering the room, after contact with the client or contaminated articles, and before leaving the room. Correct hand-washing technique is the most effective way of preventing cross-infection
- Items used during care of the client should be disposable when possible. Reusable items should be kept in the room and, when they are removed for decontamination and reprocessing, bagged and labelled as 'infective'. In some circumstances it is necessary to use a double-bagging technique to ensure transmission of infective microorganisms is controlled.

When articles need to be removed from the room two people are required. The nurse inside the client's room places the contaminated articles into a bag and seals the bag securely. Another person outside the door holds open a clean bag to receive the contaminated bag. Once this has been done, the person outside the room seals the clean bag securely. If the bag is not coloured distinctively, a label is placed on the outside of the bag to signify that the contents are contaminated. Both persons wash and dry their hands after handling the bag(s).

PROTECTIVE ISOLATION

Some immunocompromised clients need to be protected from contracting infections and must be protected from microorganisms carried into the room by those who enter. No one with an active infection such as a common cold is allowed in the room. Anyone who does enter is required to wear gown, mask, gloves and disposable coverings on the head and feet. When possible the client is nursed in a room with its own ventilation system.

The infection control officer, team or committee within a health care facility plays a major role in developing specific isolation precautions. Nurses must know when and how those precautions should be implemented. A card is generally fixed to the door of the client's room, stating that additional precautions are required and requesting that any visitor speaks with the nurse before entering. This then provides the nurse with the opportunity to explain the precautions that need to be implemented.

PREPARATION FOR ISOLATION

Before isolation precautions are implemented, the client and significant others require thorough explanations about the precautions and the reasons for them. The information provided must be clear and comprehensive to prevent spread of infection through ignorance or carelessness. The information should be provided sensitively to reduce any feelings of embarrassment, resentment or apprehension that the client may experience. Clients nursed in isolation may feel that they are a nuisance, are unclean or are afflicted with some disease that makes them unacceptable to others. Such clients may also be anxious that no one will come into their room to care for or visit them.

Because isolation may lead to withdrawal or sensory deprivation, the individual is reassured that measures will be implemented to provide adequate stimulation. The client should be provided with any means of diversion or intellectual stimulation that they need, such as a television set, telephone, books and magazines, craft projects or other forms of activity that may be of interest. Ideally the room should have an outside view as a means of reducing the client's feeling of being isolated.

The client's room should be set up with equipment that

will remain in that room; for example, there should be a thermometer, stethoscope and sphygmomanometer that will be used only for that client. These items must remain in the room, and used only with the client being nursed in that room. Lined rubbish containers with lids, a soiled linen receiver and liquid soap dispensers are also placed in the room.

PREPARATION FOR DISCHARGE TO THE HOME ENVIRONMENT

When clients are discharged from a health care setting the nurse has a responsibility to ensure that the client and family members have the knowledge and ability to control and prevent the onset or the spread of infection at home. Several social, demographic and cultural factors influence this knowledge and ability.

FACTORS AFFECTING KNOWLEDGE AND ABILITY TO PREVENT AND CONTROL INFECTION

Factors that influence the ability of clients to absorb and retain information imparted to them include their age, educational level, language and cognitive abilities. Factors that influence a client's ability to perform the infection prevention and control measures include their physical abilities, financial status and living conditions. Additionally a client's cultural beliefs may impact on perceptions concerning the cause of infection and the need to comply with the recommended control measures. Assessing all these factors is essential when the nurse prepares a client for discharge home.

Living conditions and financial situation

Clients live in a range of different environments — some are homeless, others will live in extremely poor conditions and in poverty. Some of the most disadvantaged clients the nurse will encounter are Indigenous people, many of whom, among others, live in rural and remote areas where housing is inadequate and there is a lack of clean water because there is no mains water supply. Some live in overcrowded and unsanitary conditions where leakages of sewage are common (Human Rights and Equal Opportunities Commission Report 2006).

The lack of water and the lack of money impact on the ability of these people to:

- Maintain bodily hygiene
- Keep the home clean, or wash clothes and bed linen
- Purchase medications, equipment, linen or other essential items
- Purchase and safely prepare nutritious food.

See Chapters 9 and 10 for further information concerning issues that impact on health risks for Indigenous people.

Cultural beliefs

One of the most significant issues in infection control is an understanding of bacteria and viruses, how they spread and how they cause illness. Generally this understanding of the cause of illness is accepted and understood in Western cultures, but some other cultures may have quite different perceptions. According to a person's cultural beliefs, illness may be perceived as being a natural punishment for wrongdoing, caused by God's will or by magical, mystical or spiritual intervention (Queensland Government Multicultural Health Resources 2003). Without the belief and understanding that illness is the result of bacterial or viral invasion there is little incentive for compliance with infection control measures dictated by Western understandings. The nurse who tries to explain Western perceptions to clients from other cultures may find language and cultural barriers difficult to overcome, and the help of an interpreter familiar with the culture and language of the client is strongly recommended.

GOING HOME WITH AN INFECTION

Generally the advantage of the home environment is that there is less exposure to the organisms that cause nosocomial infections and therefore, when poverty and clean water are not primary issues, the home usually presents less risk of infection than a hospital. Before being discharged home, the client should be provided with the necessary education verbally and in written form. Some general points for client education in relation to preventing infection are identified in Clinical Interest Box 25.3.

If a client goes home with an infection, education appropriate to the specific type of microorganism and mode of transmission of the infection is essential. Education might need to include advising the client to:

- Launder the clothes, towels and bed linen of the person with the infection separately to those of the rest of the household
- Use a solution of chlorine bleach and hot water for laundering, as this will destroy most organisms. If possible, hang laundered items in the fresh air and sunshine to dry, or dry in a dryer at the highest possible temperature, as most organisms do not survive in hot dry conditions
- Use a 1:10 solution of chlorine bleach and water for cleaning the bathroom and toilet facilities, kitchen surfaces or equipment used by the person with the infection (e.g. wheelchair, commode, bedpan, urinal)
- Wash dishes on the strongest cleaning cycle of the dishwasher. If there is no dishwasher, soak dishes in scalding water after washing them with gloves on, then allow them to air dry. If the infective organism is transmitted via the respiratory or gastrointestinal tract, treat dishes with a 1:10 solution of chlorine bleach and water
- Tie up soiled dressings or other contaminated materials in plastic bags and mark with a biohazard sign. Contact the local hospital, council or community health nurse for advice on safe disposal
- Use a heavy plastic container with a secure lid for the

CLINICAL INTEREST BOX 25.3
Preventing infections in the home: general discharge education

Nursing diagnosis
- Knowledge deficit relating to transmission of microorganisms and causes of infection

Objectives
- Client will be aware of and implement ways to prevent occurrence or transmission of infection at home
- Client will demonstrate correct hand-washing technique

Nursing interventions: teaching
- Reinforce need for daily personal hygiene, including mouth care
- Advise the client to keep the home environment as clean and uncluttered as possible, using household bleach (1:10 solution) as a disinfectant
- Advise that fresh air should be allowed to circulate in the home regularly
- Advise that frequent damp dusting and vacuuming reduces the number of microorganisms in the environment
- Advise client to perform frequent hand washing, especially before preparing food, eating and after visits to the toilet or contact with body fluids
- Advise client to avoid sharing personal care items such as razors, cups and toothbrushes
- Ensure that client understands the need to keep food refrigerated until use, to discard food that is beyond the use-by date, and to cook food thoroughly
- Educate client on preventive health care (e.g. immunisations, nutrition, exercise, relaxation and stress-management techniques)

Evaluation
- Client will be asked to describe techniques that will reduce risk of infection
- Client's hand-washing technique will be observed

disposal of needles, syringes or other sharp objects used in caring for the person with the infection
- Use clean disposable gloves for wound care (the nurse educates about correct hand washing, use of gloves and aseptic technique needed before discharge. The discharge plan may need to include arranging for the Hospital-in-the-Home nurse or the district or community health nurse to conduct a follow-up visit)
- Dedicate a separate area in the home for all 'clean' items. Ensure no contaminated item enters this 'clean zone'.

Nurses frequently visit clients in their own home and often need to perform aseptic procedures such as wound dressings. They sometimes need to perform sterile procedures such as catheterisations. Nurses may find it challenging in some homes to conduct such procedures without the advantages that the hospital provides, but the principles of asepsis must always be followed.

SURGICAL ASEPSIS

Surgical aseptic techniques are aimed at totally eradicating microorganisms from an area. They are most often practised in the operating room, obstetric areas and major diagnostic or special treatment areas such as a burns unit or an intensive care unit. In the operating room, nurses follow a process to ensure that asepsis is maintained. The sequential steps of the process are to:
- Put on shoe coverings
- Put on a mask
- Put on a cap to cover the hair
- Put on protective eyewear
- Carry out a surgical hand wash
- Put on (with assistance) a sterile gown
- Put on sterile gloves.

A surgical aseptic technique may also be used by the nurse in a general medical or surgical unit or in a client's home, for example, when performing a urinary catheterisation or redressing wounds. On these occasions it is not always necessary for the nurse to follow the above process in full; for example, often only sterile gloves, a mask and a sterile field are needed, provided that the principles of surgical asepsis are maintained. To reduce the risk of microorganisms being transmitted via the respiratory route, talking by the nurse conducting any sterile procedure is kept to the absolute minimum.

PRINCIPLES OF SURGICAL ASEPSIS

Principles of surgical asepsis are applied when nurses create a sterile field, add supplies or liquids to a sterile field or don sterile gloves. The principles of surgical asepsis are that:
- Sterility is preserved by touching a sterile item only with another one that is sterile (e.g. picking up a sterile dressing with sterile forceps)
- Only sterile objects may be placed on a sterile field
- Once a sterile item touches something that is not sterile it is contaminated (e.g. if the nurse touches a sterile dressing with an ungloved hand)
- A sterile object held out of the range of vision or below a person's waist is considered contaminated
- Prolonged exposure to air leads to contamination of a sterile field or object
- The edges of a sterile field are considered to be contaminated
- If a sterile field becomes wet it is considered contaminated
- Whenever there is the slightest doubt about an article being sterile it is considered unsterile and discarded.

CREATING A STERILE FIELD

The nurse creates a sterile field by using the inner surface of the cloth or wrapper that contains the sterile items as a work surface. This area is where the nurse places sterile equipment. The nurse must not contaminate the inner area. Before undertaking a procedure that needs a sterile field the nurse should:
- Remove objects from the area to be used
- Assemble all equipment needed
- Wash hands

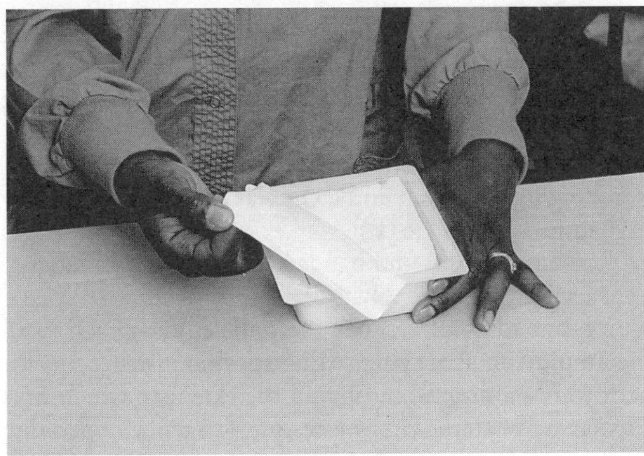

Figure 25.8 | Opening a commercially prepared sterile package *(Potter & Perry 2008)*

- Check the date or sterilisation indicator tape on all sterile packages to be used.

Sterile items that have been packaged commercially are generally designed so that the outer paper or plastic wrapper can be torn away simply without contaminating the inner contents. The outer wrapper should be removed by tearing away from the body (Figure 25.8).

Items sterilised within the facility may have an outer wrapper of thick strong paper or cloth. To open these items the nurse follows this procedure:

- Place the package in the centre of a flat surface at or above waist level (Figure 25.9A)
- Remove tape that seals the item
- Position the package so that the outermost (distal) triangular flap can be moved away from the front of the body (Figure 25.9B)
- Touch no more than 2.5 cm of the edge of the wrapper
- Smoothly open the first triangular side flap, keeping the arms flat and away from the inner sterile area. Ensure the opened flap lays flat on the working surface (Figure 25.9C)
- Standing away from the package, take hold of the outside surface of the last flap, pull the flap back towards the body, allowing it to fall flat on the working surface (Figure 25.9D).

Adding sterile items to a sterile field

Sterile items can be added directly from their packaging onto the sterile field or by transferring them with sterile forceps. A packet containing a sterile item must be opened in such a way that the sterilised item does not come in contact with the non-sterile outer wrapper (Figure 25.10). The item may be gently allowed to fall onto a sterile field, with care taken not to contaminate the sterile field with the wrapper, or it may be retrieved directly from its packaging by a person holding sterile forceps or wearing sterile gloves.

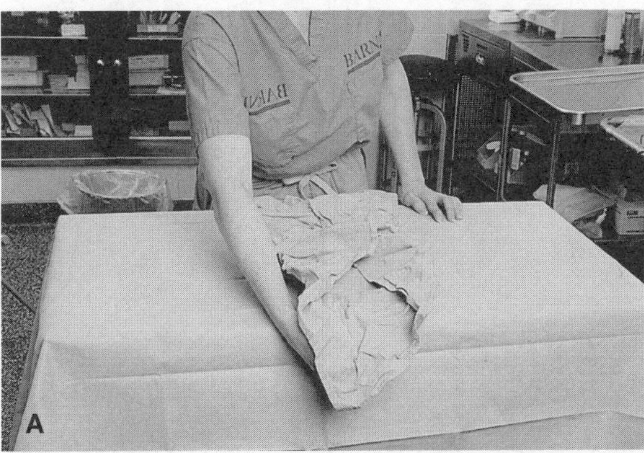

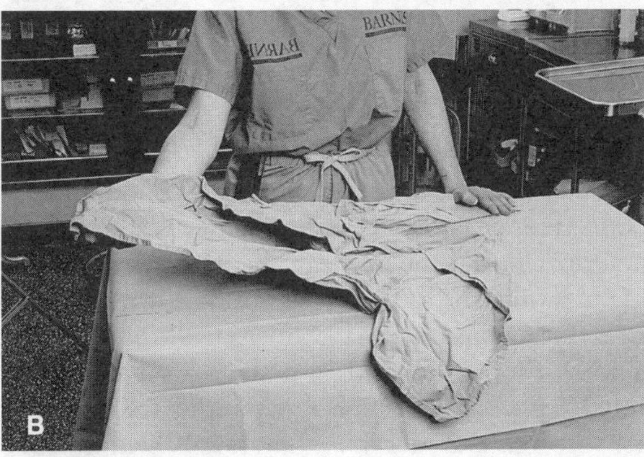

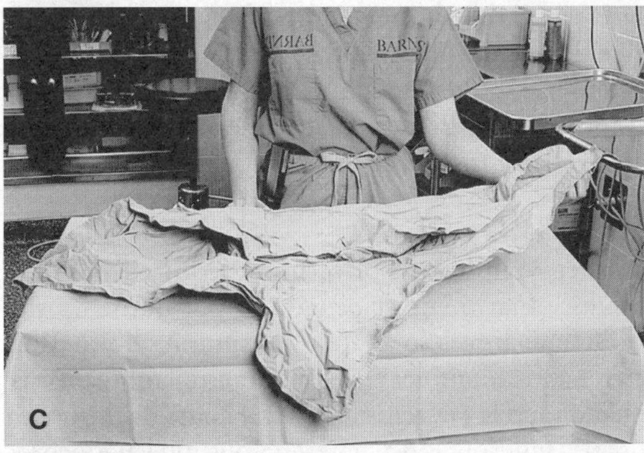

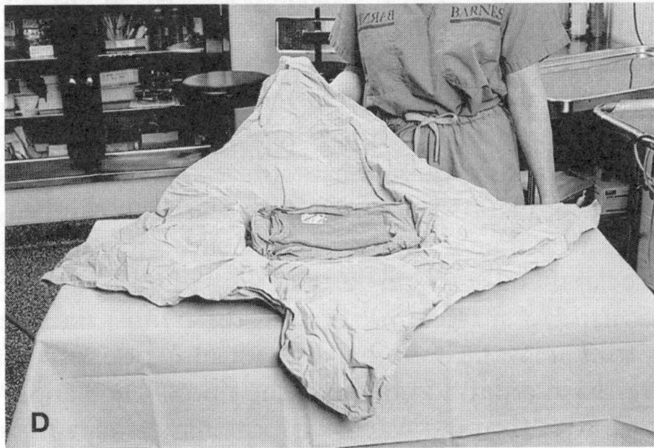

Figure 25.9 | Opening a hospital sterilised package
A: Opening the outer top flap of the sterile package. **B**: Opening the first side flap. **C**: Opening the second side flap. **D**: Opening the back and final flap *(Potter & Perry 2008)*

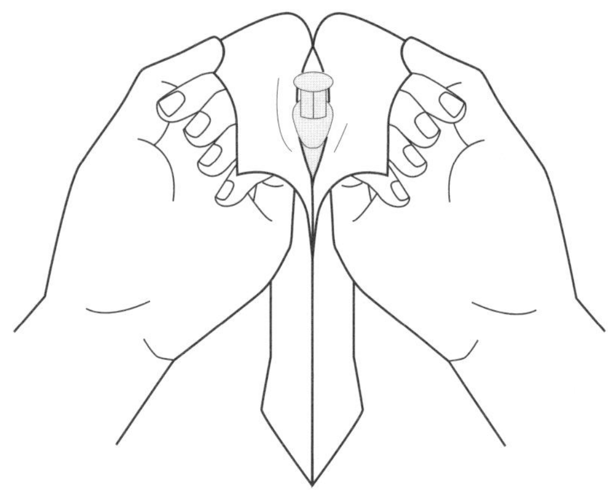

Figure 25.10 | Opening a single sterile item (deWit 2005)

Adding sterile solutions

A bottle containing a sterile solution is contaminated on the outside and sterile on the inside; the neck is considered contaminated, but the inside of the lid is sterile. To avoid contamination, the cap is placed upside down on a surface or held during pouring. Before opening the bottle the label should be checked to verify it is the correct solution and within the expiration date. Before pouring the solution the nurse discards 1–2 mL. The container is held in front of the nurse and the nurse avoids touching any sterile areas in the field. To pour the solution into a sterile container on the sterile field, the bottle of solution is held at a height to prevent splashing and to prevent the outside of the bottle from touching the sterile field.

SURGICAL SCRUB

A surgical hand wash or scrub is required before any procedure that involves penetration of normally sterile tissues. The aim is to achieve maximum elimination of bacteria and to prevent the growth of microorganisms on the hands and lower arms for several hours by the use of an antiseptic solution. It is a more vigorous and lengthy process than the normal routine or aseptic non-surgical hand wash. Before a surgical hand wash in areas such as the operating room, the nurse puts on shoe covers, a surgical cap to cover the hair, and a mask; all jewellery is removed from the arms and hands because it harbours microorganisms; and all traces of nail polish are removed because if chipped or worn longer than 4 days, it too harbours microorganisms (Association of Operating Room Nurses 2006).

During a surgical hand wash the hands, nails and forearms are washed thoroughly with antiseptic soap from fingertip to at least 5 cm above the elbow. The hands are kept under running water with the hands kept higher than the elbows at all times. The Australian Government Department of Health and Ageing (2004) infection control guidelines recommend a 5-minute scrub for the first surgical procedure of the day and a 3-minute scrub for those that follow. The recommended time relates to the time actually spent scrubbing the skin. It does not include rinsing or drying time. Procedures and policies may vary concerning which antimicrobial agent is to be used. Guidelines for the standard steps involved in a surgical hand wash are provided in Table 25.7. The procedure involves:

- Cleaning the nails (Figure 25.11A)
- Using light friction and a circular motion to wash the hands (Figure 25.11B)
- Rinsing the arms and hands keeping the hands above the elbows (Figure 25.11C).

Nurses are advised to check the policies and practices of the employing agency regarding specific instructions for performing a surgical scrub and the extent to which ENs participate in sterile procedures in the agency's operating suite or other specialised units.

STERILE GOWNS

Nurses must wear a sterile gown when assisting at a sterile field in an operating theatre or areas such as the delivery room of an obstetric unit. Assisting in sterile procedures is dependent on the nurse first having received specialised education and being evaluated as competent in all relevant areas of practice and being delegated by a senior Registered Nurse (RN) to do so. The EN should also remain mindful of the scope of practice designated by the professional bodies that govern EN practice in the geographical location where the nursing work is to be performed.

The sterile gown acts as a barrier to the transfer of microorganisms from skin surfaces into the air, and this reduces the risk of wound contamination. The sterile gown is put on after a mask and surgical cap and after performing a surgical hand wash. The nurse needing to don a sterile gown should follow this sequence:

1. Apply a mask and surgical cap (plus protective eyewear if needed)
2. Perform surgical hand wash
3. Pick up sterile gown at the inner neckline
4. Hold the gown away from the body
5. Allow the gown to unfold while holding it high enough to prevent contact with the floor
6. Insert an arm into each sleeve without touching the outer surface of the gown and without allowing the outside of the gown to contact any surface
7. Have another person pull at the inside of the gown to adjust the fit and tie the gown closed at the back.

After the gown has been put on, only the front of the gown and only the area from the waist to neck and the front of the sleeves are considered sterile. The back and sides of the gown and below the waist are considered contaminated, as are the collar, the undersides of the sleeves and underarm area, because these areas cannot be kept in constant view to ensure they remain sterile (Crisp & Taylor 2005). ENs who are interested in perioperative nursing are recommended to undertake courses dedicated to this specialised area. Chapter 44 provides information specific to perioperative nursing.

TABLE 25.7 | GUIDELINES FOR A SURGICAL HAND WASH (SURGICAL SCRUB)	
Review and carry out the standard steps in Appendix 4	
Action	**Rationale**
Prepare articles needed (e.g. cleansing agent, sponge pad or brush, sterile paper towel)	Once the hand wash begins, the hands cannot touch any non-sterile item without negating the time already spent on washing the hands
Check hands: • All rings, watch, bangles etc removed • No cuts, sores, lesions or skin infections present	 Unsterile items harbour microorganisms Nurses who have damage/wounds/infection on the hands cannot perform surgical scrub adequately because friction is necessary when scrubbing for surgical procedures
Using foot pedal controls, adjust the water flow and temperature to comfortably warm	Water flow/temperature can be controlled without contaminating hands on the taps
Wet arms and hands from at least 5 cm above the elbow to the fingertips. Keep hands higher than elbows. Rinse thoroughly under the water	When hands are higher than elbows, microorganisms cannot drain downwards over the clean hands
Apply antimicrobial cleansing agent to palm and work up a lather. Clean under nails with a nail stick under running water (Figure 25.11A). Discard nail stick	Running water and lather aid thorough cleansing of nails
When using a pre-packaged scrub kit (brush or sponge pad and nail cleaner) do not put the brush or pad down until hand wash is completed. Hold nail cleaner until all nails have been cleaned and then discard. If the pad or brush is not already infused with cleansing agent, wet it and apply antimicrobial detergent	Once scrub has begun, the pad or brush would become contaminated if it was placed on an unsterile surface
Starting at tips of fingers use light friction and a circular motion to wash thoroughly around the fingers and nails (Figure 25.11B), then the back of the hands, the palm and wrists of each hand. The brush or pad should be held perpendicular to the fingers and nails	Use of friction and antimicrobial detergent over this time period is effective in reducing microorganism count to minimal levels
Continue use of friction and circular motion to clean all surfaces of both arms. The brush or pad should be kept parallel to the arm	Washing a wide area lowers risk of nurse contaminating sterile gown that is put on after surgical scrub
Scrubbing should continue for a minimum of 5 minutes for the first surgical scrub of the day and 3 minutes for those that follow	These times are recommended by Australian Government Infection Control Guidelines (Department of Health and Ageing 2004) but time of scrub may be determined by the type of antimicrobial agent being used
Rinse each arm and hand under running water, allowing gravity to let water flow from fingertips down the hand to the wrist, forearm and elbows and away into the sink from the elbow area (Figure 25.11C)	Rinsing in this manner maintains the hands as the cleanest area after the procedure. Rinsing rids area of resident microorganisms
Discard brush or pad. Stop water flow using foot pedal control	Foot controls prevent the need to touch contaminated taps that would contaminate the hands
Keeping hands above elbows, dry hands with a sterile towel. Standing slightly away from the sterile field and bending slightly at the waist, pick up the towel by one corner and allow it to drop open	Leaning forward prevents accidental contact of body with sterile towel or scrub attire
Blot dry one hand from fingers towards elbow using a rotary movement	Starting with the fingers maintains the hands as the cleanest area
Do not go back over an area once it is dried	Moving back over a previously dried area contaminates it
Carefully reverse the towel or use a second towel to repeat drying process for the other hand and arm. The arms and hands should be kept above waist level	Touching the damp part of the towel with the dried hand will contaminate the hand Keeping the hands above the elbow protects the scrubbed area Careful and thorough drying prevents hands from becoming chapped and assists the process of putting on sterile gloves
Discard towel carefully and proceed to putting on a sterile gown, then sterile gloves	Towel must be discarded appropriately to reduce risk of accidental contamination
(adapted from deWit 2005)	

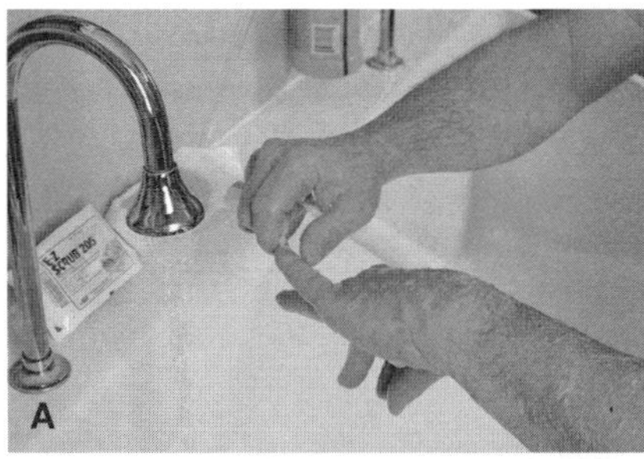

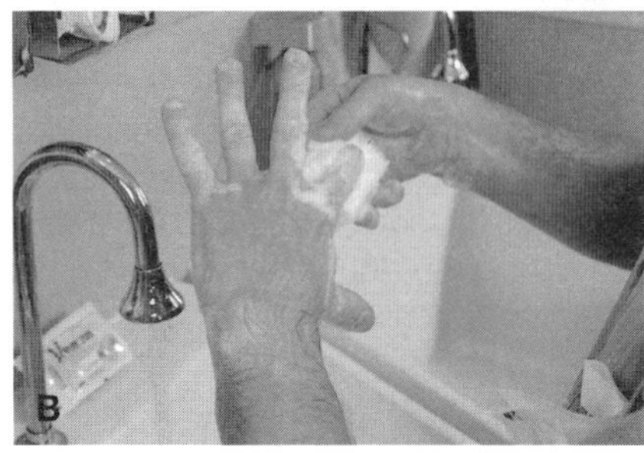

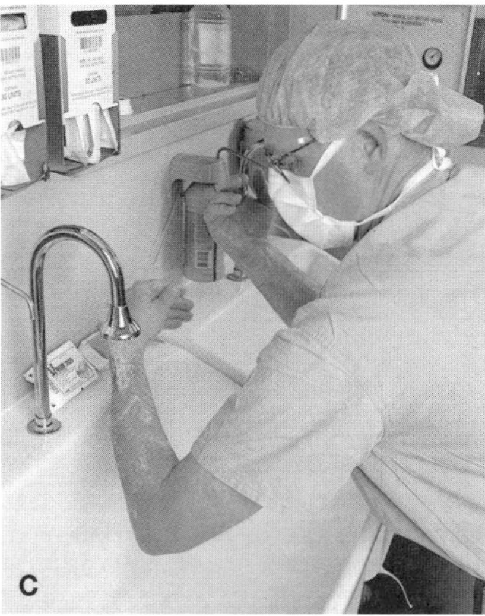

Figure 25.11 | Performing a surgical scrub
A: Surgical hand wash procedure: cleaning the nails. **B**: Using light friction and a circular motion to wash the hands. **C**: Rinsing the arms and hands, keeping the hands above the elbows *(deWit 2005)*

APPLYING AND REMOVING STERILE GLOVES

Sterile gloves are available in different sizes and it is important that gloves fit firmly but not too tightly. There are two sterile gloving techniques — open and closed. Open gloving is used for procedures carried out by nurses at the bedside, such as inserting urinary catheters. Figure 25.12 illustrates the procedure for open gloving. Closed gloving is the method used when sterile gloves are worn in conjunction with sterile gowns. Guidelines for the open-gloving technique are provided in Table 25.8.

Sterile gloves are removed and disposed of in the same way as non-sterile gloves (Figure 25.7). After removing the gloves, hands should be washed to remove all traces of glove powder and reduce the risk of latex allergies developing. Washing the hands after removing gloves is necessary to adhere to standard precautions.

INFECTION PREVENTION AND CONTROL FOR HEALTH CARE WORKERS

New Zealand and each state and territory in Australia has legislation relating to the transmission of infection. All the legislation relates to common goals and principles and contains the following elements in some form:

- **Exposure-control plan**. These are designed to minimise or eliminate employee exposure. The plan describes how to avoid exposure to infectious agents, such as when to use protective equipment, and what should be done in the event of an exposure occurring; for example, exposure to hepatitis or HIV via a needle-stick injury. In Australia, influenza vaccination should be offered to health care workers in accordance with National Health and Medical Research Council recommendations (NHMRC 2007)
- **Compliance with standard precautions**. Personal protective clothing and equipment must be provided at no cost to employees and should be readily available
- **High-risk exposure**. Needle-stick or mucous membrane exposure to blood or infectious body fluids must be reported immediately. Appropriate preventive treatment for HIV and hepatitis viruses must be put in place as soon as practicable after the exposure or suspected exposure
- **Housekeeping**. Routine cleaning and decontamination procedures must be established
- **Education**. Education programs, written policies and guidelines must be provided for all personnel in relation to infection prevention and control activities for their own and client safety (Australian Government Department of Health and Ageing 2004).

ROLE OF THE INFECTION-PREVENTION AND CONTROL NURSE

Responsibilities

Many health care facilities employ one or more members of staff to be responsible for the area of infection prevention and control. In a hospital often a committee is responsible. Individual nurses may be members of the committee. The role of the infection prevention and control committee is to maintain surveillance of nosocomial infections throughout the hospital. The infection prevention and control nurse's role is to facilitate the implementation of policies established by the committee. The combined roles of the nurse and the committee include:

- Monitoring for outbreaks of infection within the facility
- Monitoring antibiotic-resistant organisms
- Ensuring that staff are advised on all aspects of safe aseptic practice
- Educating staff and clients on infection prevention and control policies and procedures
- Reviewing infection control policies and procedures
- Recommending appropriate isolation procedures
- Researching laboratory reports and records for incidence of infections and establishing a close working relationship with the hospital microbiologist and all departments to investigate unusual events
- Identifying and rectifying infection control problems (equipment and procedures)
- Reviewing client records for community-acquired infections that may be reportable to the health department
- Gathering statistics regarding the epidemiology of iatrogenic infections
- Coordinating immunisation programs for staff and maintaining health-screening records
- Conferring with support services such as the 'housekeeping' department within the facility.

The infection prevention and control nurse is responsible for reviewing laboratory and radiology reports, case notes, autopsy reports and documentation of staff infections, and for reporting all relevant information to the infection prevention and control committee. The committee authorises the distribution of data to relevant people within the establishment.

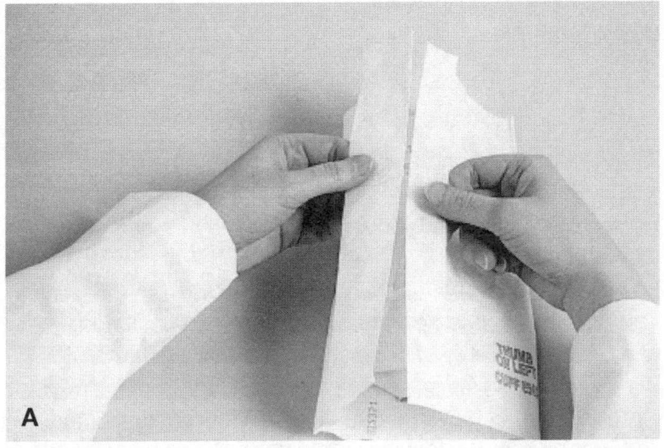

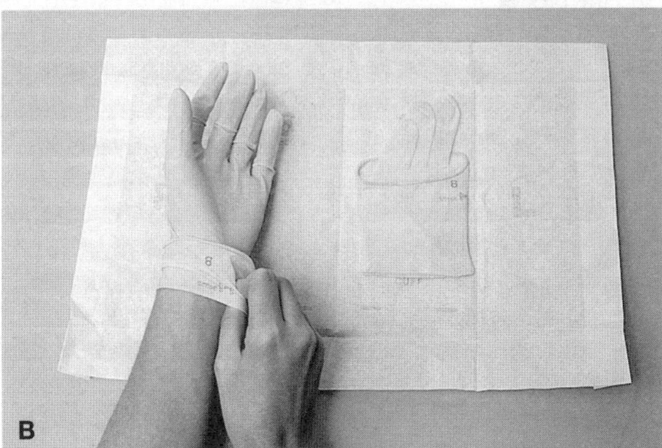

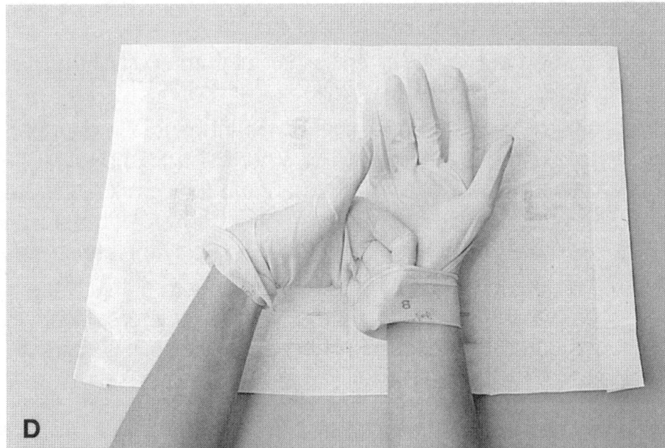

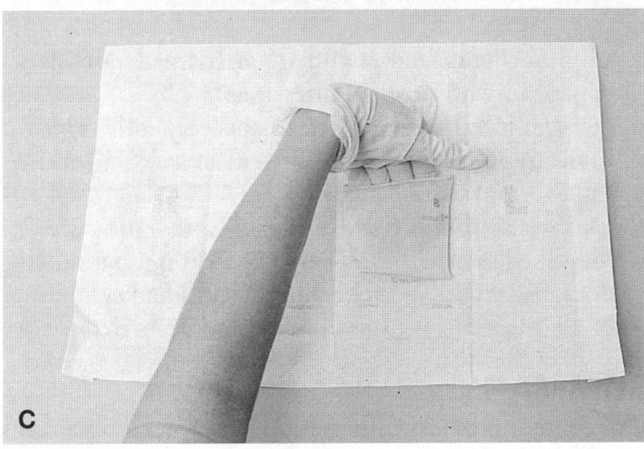

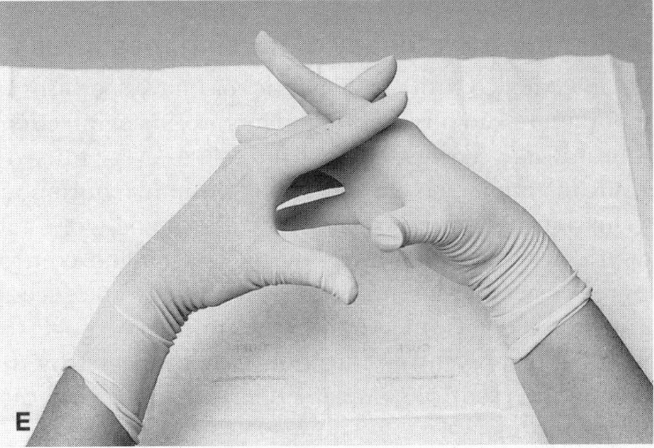

Figure 25.12 | Open gloving

A: Opening the inner wrapper. **B**: Finger position for pulling on the first glove. **C**: Sliding the gloved hand under the cuff of the second glove. **D**: Pulling on the second glove with the thumb of the dominant hand in the abducted position. **E**: Easing the gloves into the correct position *(Potter & Perry 2008)*

TABLE 25.8 | GUIDELINES FOR OPEN-GLOVING TECHNIQUE

Review and carry out the standard steps in Appendix 4

Steps	Rationale
Wash and dry hands	Reduces risk of transmitting microorganisms
Remove outer glove bag by peeling sides away. Slide correct-size gloves, covered by inner paper wrapper, onto a clean dry flat surface above waist level	Maintains asepsis
Wash and dry hands again	Hands are contaminated after touching outer wrapper of gloves. Removes bacteria from skin surfaces, minimising risk of transmitting infection
Carefully move inner wrapper away to expose sterile gloves (Figure 25.12 A). Keep gloves on inside surface of the inner wrapper. Position gloves with wrist opening nearest to the body	Maintains sterility of gloves
Identify the right and left gloves. Prepare to glove dominant hand first	Gloving dominant hand first makes managing the process easier and reduces risk of contamination by fumbling
Use thumb and first two fingers of non-dominant hand to pick up first glove. Lift at least 12 cm off wrapper	Keeping glove held well above work surface reduces risk of contamination
Grasp the folded over part of the cuff (each glove has a cuff about 5 cm wide that is folded back to reveal inside of glove). Take care to touch only the inside surface of the glove	Inner part of cuff that has been handled lies next to the skin; thus, sterile exposed part of glove is not contaminated
Insert fingers of other hand into the held glove and pull the glove up over the dominant hand without touching the outer surface of the glove (Figure 25.12 B)	If outer surface of glove touches the skin it is contaminated and the procedure will need to be repeated with fresh sterile gloves
With gloved hand slide fingers underneath the cuff of the second glove (Figure 25.12 C)	Inner side of cuff of second glove protects the sterile fingers of the first glove, maintaining sterility
Ease second glove up over non-dominant hand. Be careful not to touch outside of glove or other gloved hand with bare skin. Keep thumb of dominant hand abducted back (Figure 25.12 D). Once hand is settled in glove, slide cuff carefully up over the wrist, being careful to touch only the sterile sides	Prevents contamination
Adjust fingers in gloves by pulling glove fingers out with the opposite hand to straighten and adjust until fitted neatly. Hands can be interlocked to help ease gloves into correct position (Figure 25.12 E)	Gloves must fit correctly and comfortably to ensure hand dexterity during procedures

(adapted from Potter & Perry 2008)

Evaluating the efficacy of nursing measures

The infection control nurse and the committee perform an important role in surveillance and monitoring of infections in health care settings but it is the role of every nurse to ensure infection rates are kept to a minimum. Continuous evaluation determines the efficacy of nursing work and identifies if and when infection prevention and control strategies need to be increased or modified. The success of nurses is determined by whether or not the goals for reducing or preventing infection have been met by the nursing interventions implemented. Signs that indicate success include:

- No local signs of infection around portals of entry (e.g. wounds, IV or wound-drain insertion sites, gastrostomy or jejunostomy feeding tubes)
- Susceptible clients do not develop signs or symptoms of respiratory, urinary tract or other infections (e.g. surgical clients recover and are discharged without contracting nosocomial infections)
- Signs of infection are detected at a very early stage, indicating that nurses are efficient in assessing and monitoring their clients
- Outbreaks of infection in a health care setting are identified at a very early stage, indicating that nursing documentation and reporting of signs and symptoms of all infections is prompt, clear and accurate.

SUMMARY

This chapter provides information about microorganisms, the way infections develop and are transmitted, the ways the body defends against them, and why some clients are more susceptible to infection than others. It provides the EN with information about how to practise nursing in a way that incorporates standard and additional precautions, the prevention and control strategies recommended by the Department of Health and Ageing in Australia. Infection prevention and control principles are applicable to every area of nursing practice. The principles and practices covered in this chapter provide nurses with the essential information to ensure that they protect themselves, their clients and other health care workers from pathogenic microorganisms.

REVIEW EXERCISES

1. What is meant by 'normal flora'?
2. What are the conditions under which most pathogens thrive?
3. Provide three examples of how pathogens are transmitted.
4. Describe the body's natural defences against infection.
5. Explain the difference between actively and passively acquired immunity.
6. What is meant by the term iatrogenic infection?
7. List five factors that influence susceptibility to infection in an older client.
8. Provide six examples of occasions when nurses must wash their hands.
9. Explain the difference between disinfection and sterilisation.
10. Explain what you understand by the terms standard precautions and additional precautions.

CRITICAL THINKING EXERCISES

1. Mrs Smith is 30 years old and has been admitted to hospital with viral pneumonia. What are the nursing interventions necessary to control transmission of the infection?
2. Mr Andrews is in hospital following a motorbike accident. He has a fractured pelvis and grazes to his right arm and leg. He is confined to bed and has a urinary catheter. He tells you he is HIV positive. What infection control measures are appropriate when caring for Mr Andrews?
3. What are the organisms that a nurse may be frequently exposed to? How can nurses protect themselves against pathogenic organisms?

REFERENCES AND FURTHER READING

Association of Operating Room Nurses (ACORN) (2006) *Standards for Perioperative Nurses*. ACORN, Sydney

Australian Government Department of Health and Ageing (2004) *Infection control guidelines for the prevention of transmission of infectious diseases in the health care setting*. Commonwealth of Australia Publication, Canberra ACT. Available: www.health.gov.au/internet/wcms/publishing.nsf/Content//icg-guidelines-index.htm/$FILE/part1.pdf [accessed 20 March 2008]

Australian Government Department of Health and Ageing (2008) *Immunise Australia Program*. Available: www.immunise.health.gov.au [accessed 21 March 2008]

Boyce J, Pittett D (2002) Guidelines for Hand Hygiene in Health Care Settings: Recommendations of the Healthcare Infection Control Practices Advisory Committee and the HICPAC/SHEA/APIC/IDSA Hand Hygiene Task Force. In: *Morbidity and Mortality Weekly Report*, 51 (RR16:1): 1–44. 25 October 2002. Centers for Disease Control and Prevention. Available: www.cdc.gov/handhygiene [accessed 21 March 2008]

Brown TL, Burrell LJ, Edmonds D, Martin R, O'Keeffe J, Johnson P, Grayson ML (2005) Hand hygiene: A standardised tool for assessing compliance. Australian Infection Control. Available: http://www.debug.net.au/HandHygiene%20compliance%20tool.pdf [accessed 21 March 2008]

Bryant B, Knights K, Salerno E (2006) *Pharmacology for Health Professionals*. Harcourt Australia, Sydney

Crisp J, Taylor C (eds) (2005) *Potter & Perry's Fundamentals of Nursing*, 2nd edn. Elsevier Australia, Sydney

deWit S (2005) *Fundamental Concepts and Skills for Nursing*, 2nd edn. Elsevier Saunders, Philadelphia

Ebersole P, Hess P (2001) *Geriatric Nursing and Healthy Ageing*. Mosby, St Louis

Herlihy B (2007) *The Human Body in Health and Illness*, 3rd edn. Saunders, Philadelphia

Herlihy B, Maebius NK (2000) *The Human Body in Health and Illness*. WB Saunders, Philadelphia

Higgins C (2007). *Understanding Laboratory Investigations for Nurses and Health Professionals*. Blackwell Publishing, Hoboken, NJ

Human Rights and Equal Opportunities Commission (2006) *Statistical Overview of Aboriginal and Torres Strait Islander Peoples in Australia*. Online. Available: www.hreoc.gov.au/social_justice/statistics/index.html [accessed 17 March 2008]

Jarvis WR (2007) *Bennett and Brachman's Hospital Infections*. Lippincott, Williams and Wilkins, Hagerstown, MD

King LR, Belman B, Kramer SA (2001) *Clinical Pediatric Urology*. Informa Healthcare, London

Lashley FR, Durham JD (2007) *Emerging Infectious Diseases: Trends and Issues*. Springer Publishing, New York

Lucet J, Rigaud M, Mentre F (2002) Hand contamination before and after different hand hygiene techniques: a randomized clinical trial. *Journal of Hospital Infection* 50: 276–80

National Health and Medical Research Council (2007) *The Australian Immunisation Handbook*, 9th edn. Commonwealth Government of Australia, National Capital Printers, Canberra. Online. Available: http://www.health.gov.au/internet/immunise/publishing.nsf/content/handbook-9-c3.9 [accessed 20 March 2008]

National Occupational Health and Safety Commission (2003) *National Code of Practice for the Control of Work-related Exposure to Hepatitis and HIV (Blood-borne) Viruses*, 2nd edn. Commonwealth of Australia, Canberra. Online. Available: http://www.ascc.gov.au/NR/rdonlyres/14850412-BF2D-4E22-B4F7-076CBD4383F6/0/HIV_2Ed_2003.pdf [accessed 20 March 2008]

Potter PA, Perry AG (2008) *Fundamentals of Nursing*, 7th edn. Mosby, St Louis

Queensland Government Multicultural Health Resources (1998) Multicultural health: resources and support tools. *Cultural Diversity. A guide for health professionals*. Online. Available: www.health.qld.gov.au/multicultural/health_workers/cultdiver [accessed 10 May 2008]

Ritter H (2005) Clinical microbiology. In: Carrico R (ed.) *APIC text of infection control and epidemiology*. Association for Professionals in Infection Control and Epidemiology, Washington DC

Schneeberger P, Smits M, Zick R, Wille J (2002) Surveillance as a starting point to reduce surgical-site infection rates in elective orthopaedic surgery. *Journal of Hospital Infection* 51: 179–84

Springhouse Publishing Company Staff (2007) *Nursing: Perfecting Clinical Procedures*. Lippincott, Williams and Wilkins, Hagerstown, MD

Wilson J (2000) *Clinical Microbiology: an Introduction for Healthcare Professionals*. Baillière Tindall, Edinburgh

Wilson M (2005) *Microbial Inhabitants of Humans: Their ecology and role in health and disease*. Cambridge University Press, Cambridge UK

World Health Organisation (2007) Health Topics — Infectious Disease, World Health Organisation, Geneva. Online. Available: http://www.who.int/en [accessed 15 October 2007]

ONLINE RESOURCES

Immunise Australia: www.immunise.health.gov.au

Queensland Government Multicultural Health Resources: www.health.qld.gov.au/multicultural/health_workers/support_tools.asp

Chapter 26
SAFETY AND PROTECTION

OBJECTIVES

- Define the key terms/concepts
- Identify common safety hazards in health care facilities and in the home environment
- Identify the factors that may affect the ability of individuals to protect themselves against environmental hazards
- Apply relevant principles in planning and implementing safety precautions within a health care facility
- State the safety measures that must be implemented to prevent thermal injuries, harm from sharp objects, poisons and falls
- Understand the implications of environmental pollution on world health
- Outline the guidelines that need to be adhered to when considering physical restraint as part of a client's care management
- Understand the implications of physical restraint on the wellbeing of clients and their families
- Gain awareness of the occupational health and safety (OHS) strategies that protect the nurse in the workplace
- Understand the importance of health promotion in reducing the risk of injury and harm in the environment

KEY TERMS/CONCEPTS

aggression in the workplace
biohazard
body mechanics
falls
fire prevention
hazard
immunisation
no-lift policy
occupational health and safety (OHS)
poisons
pollution
restraint
restraint minimisation
safety
sharps
thermal injury

CHAPTER FOCUS

Safety is a basic need of every individual throughout their lifespan. People are constantly exposed to environmental hazards that endanger safety and, while many individuals are able to maintain a safe environment independently, factors such as age or illness may reduce the ability to protect against them without assistance. Most incidents that cause harm are preventable, and nurses require the knowledge and skill to identify the potential hazards in any situation within any environment where client care takes place. Maintaining a safe environment includes preventing accidents such as falls, scalds, burns, cuts and ingesting poisons and preventing fires, injury from chemical hazards and harm from cross-infection. It is an integral part of nursing care to carefully assess clients to determine their ability to protect themselves against accidents and hazards and to become aware of clients who are particularly at risk of being harmed by them. The planning, implementation and evaluation of safety measures to prevent harm to clients is an integral part of all aspects of nursing care. Identifying and minimising threats to safety in the workplace is an essential component of a process directed towards providing and maintaining a safe environment and protecting all of those within it.

LIVED EXPERIENCE

I have worked in aged care for over 5 years now and I love it. Before the no-lift policy came in I thought I was going to have to give it up because I was getting backache and by the end of the day it was quite bad. The no-lift policy has made such a difference — I'm still busy but the work seems so much lighter now that we don't manually lift the residents. At the end of the day, yes, I'm tired, but I feel really good about the work I do and I rarely get any problem with my back now.

Maureen, 27, Enrolled Nurse, residential aged care

Safety may be defined as freedom from danger and the risk of psychological or physical injury. For clients to be safe and feel safe the nurse needs to ensure that there is a safe environment in which to work and provide client care. Nurses work with clients in a range of environments that include hospitals, clinics, schools, long-term care facilities and clients' homes. A safe environment maintains protection of clients, staff and all other people who may be within it. A safe environment is one in which:

- The risks of injury or accident are minimised; for example, risk of falls is reduced by signs indicating when a floor is wet, smoke alarms, water temperature regulators, non-slip floors and support rails
- Health hazards such as excessive noise, air pollution or the transmission of infection are reduced or eliminated; for example, by the use of protective earmuffs, effective ventilation methods and infection prevention and control strategies
- Physical hazards are reduced; for example, lifting equipment is provided, corridors are kept clear of rubbish, equipment such as wheelchairs and electric hoists are maintained in optimal, safe condition.

FACTORS AFFECTING THE SAFETY OF CLIENTS

Nurses must assess the environment for threats to their clients and their own or other people's safety, then plan and implement the measures necessary to reduce, or when possible totally eliminate, actual or potential hazards and the risk of harm.

Part of assessment means identifying individuals who are most at risk from hazards in the environment. All clients should be assessed for factors that may affect their ability to recognise hazards and to protect themselves from harm. Clients who are receiving medical or nursing care may be either temporarily or permanently affected by a physical, psychological or emotional impairment that interferes with the ability to recognise, avoid or protect themselves against environmental dangers.

The ability to avoid danger depends on being aware of it, and to be aware people must be able to perceive, interpret and react appropriately to sensory stimuli. People are provided with information about their surroundings through the senses. For example, the sense of smell warns of the presence of smoke or noxious fumes. Any alteration to the efficiency of any one of the five senses (taste, smell, hearing, vision or touch) may significantly reduce the ability of clients to detect and protect themselves from danger. This then may significantly increase the potential for a mishap or accident. In addition to impaired sensory organs, other factors affect the ability of clients to perceive and protect themselves from harm, including age, reduced mobility or cognitive awareness, reduced capacity for communication and intellectual, mental or psychological impairment.

AGE

The very young and very old are at particular risk of accidental injury, but each stage of human development poses its own risks to safety. Very young infants are totally dependent on others for their safety. They must be protected against infection, accidents and exposure to extremes of temperature. Toddlers and young children have not learned to distinguish between safety and danger and are therefore constantly exposed to hazards as they explore and learn about the environment. They are vulnerable to accidents because many hazards are not obvious to them; for example, they may ingest poisonous substances such as cleaning fluids if the substances are not stored out of reach in childproof containers; they may wander into a swimming pool that is not safely behind a childproof fence; they may place plastic bags on their heads if bags are left within reach.

School-age children are exposed to a wide range of new experiences. They begin to participate in more activities away from home, such as playing a sport, visiting at a friend's house or riding a bike around the local park. Nurses can play an active role, alongside parents and teachers, in teaching and reinforcing safety measures such as what to do if approached by a stranger, observing road safety rules and wearing protective sports clothing, such as a safety helmet when riding a bicycle, skateboard or scooter.

Adolescents are at the challenging developmental stage of moving from dependence to independence and allowing their own adult personality to emerge. This is a stressful process for many adolescents and, in an attempt to cope with the tension and emotional discomfort that sometimes occur, they may participate in risk-taking behaviour. This may be the time when they start smoking, drinking alcohol and/or consuming other types of drugs. The risks to safety often result from these behaviours because they damage the body and impair the ability to make rational decisions. Smoking and consuming alcohol and other drugs are known risks to health, but they also increase the potential for incidents such as drug overdose, falling, drowning or vehicle accidents. Adolescence is also the time when physical changes promote the desire for sexual activity. If appropriate precautions are not planned and taken, sexual activity presents the possibility of sexually transmitted infections, unplanned pregnancy and emotional distress.

Not all adolescents take part in these behaviours. Many have a strong grasp on, and accept and practise, the rules and laws that are designed to protect everyone in the community; for example, don't drink and drive, don't drink alcohol and swim, wear a seatbelt in the car. Young people in the years leading up to and during adolescence can be kept safe from these specific dangers if they receive appropriate information and guidance about how to say no to drugs, choices about abstinence from sexual activity or how to practise safe and effective birth control. They need to be able to discuss and ask questions about these issues in an environment where they feel comfortable to do so. Nurses are frequently in the position to practise health promotion by teaching safety measures, answering questions and facilitating discussion with adolescents in the health care setting.

Young and middle-aged adults tend to be at a level of risk according to their lifestyle practices. For example, a high-fat diet, smoking and lack of exercise increase the risk of respiratory and cardiovascular disorders and cancer. The types of leisure activities indulged in, particularly sports, are often linked to injury in this age group. Workplace injuries are also common, particularly in males and particularly among tradesmen. The risk of being involved in a motor vehicle accident also remains significant (Australian Bureau of Statistics 2005).

As a normal part of ageing, older adults may experience physiological changes, including decreased muscle strength, diminished sensory acuity and slowed reflexes. Many older people adapt successfully and modify lifestyle practices to accommodate the physical changes of ageing, but statistics indicate that getting older does increase the risk of accident and injury. For example, injury from falls becomes much more common in adults over age 65. The rate of individuals needing medical attention as a result of falls is higher in residential care and hospital settings than in the community generally (National Ageing Research Institute 2004).

ELDER ABUSE

Abuse of older people is a safety issue that nurses need to be aware of when assessing clients. Elder abuse, particularly of those who have dementia, is sometimes related to the actions of family carers who are so tired and stressed by the hard and constant work of caring that their tolerance level reaches zero. Carers are often ashamed or too embarrassed to ask for help, and clients often do not have the courage or privacy needed to speak out about what is happening to them (Faye & Sellick 2003). Nurses must be alert for signs and symptoms of abuse when assessing clients (see Chapter 23) and recognise when family carers might need interventions such as regular periods of respite.

REDUCED MOBILITY

Mobility enables people to protect themselves against many environmental hazards and maintain their own safety. The inability to initiate, coordinate or perform motor activities reduces the capability to physically move away from dangerous situations and potential injury. Individuals who are unsteady on their feet, for example, as a result of a neurological disorder, a debilitating illness or from the effects of medication, are more vulnerable to injury from loss of balance and falling.

IMPAIRED COGNITION OR MENTAL AWARENESS

Impaired awareness or consciousness can reduce the ability to perceive, interpret and react to people, objects or situations in ways that maintain safety. For example, a person with Alzheimer's dementia may walk across a busy road or touch a hot oven because they fail to perceive these things as potentially harmful. The risk of injury to self or to others is significantly increased if a person is confused, disoriented or suffers from memory lapses; for example, clients with head injuries, those under the influence of chemical substances and those with dementia or serious psychiatric illnesses. They need the nurse and all members of the health care team to work together to ensure that they are protected from harm or from harming others.

IMPAIRED CAPACITY FOR COMMUNICATION

Clients who are unable to perceive danger because they misinterpret environmental cues or do not understand, see or hear verbal or written warnings or instructions are at greater risk of injury. Clients who have a language barrier or experience any communication impairment, such as aphasia for example, may not have the ability to report dangers they observe or to ask for help.

INTELLECTUAL, MENTAL OR PSYCHOLOGICAL IMPAIRMENT

Any alteration in the brain's ability to interpret what is happening in the environment places a client at greater risk of harm. Interference with developmental processes or changes in brain function can also cause behaviour that is not based on clear and logical decision making. This may result in clients being a threat to their own safety.

Sometimes clients may have a condition that leads them to harm themselves. Examples of self-harming behaviour include self-inflicted wounds such as cuts or burns, ingesting or injecting poisonous substances, or inserting objects into body orifices. Close monitoring is required in such cases to protect the client from self-harm (see Chapter 45). Behaviours such as these have been associated with what mental health nurses might call 'disabling distress' — behaviour that results from serious unresolved anxiety (Watkins 2001). Any circumstance or condition that increases anxiety may interfere with a person's normal pattern of behaviour. It does not, in most situations, lead to self-harm, but it is not uncommon for anxiety to lead to feelings of utter panic. People who are anxious or experiencing feelings of panic can sometimes react to situations with such intensity that clear thinking and logical responses to what is happening are impossible. These individuals may experience levels of anxiety so severe that it affects their perception of, and ability to react appropriately to, the threat of harm. (Chapter 13 discusses nursing responses to anxiety and panic.)

RISK ASSESSMENT AND MANAGEMENT

The goal of nursing practice in relation to the need for safety is to prevent injury or harm. Nurses need to assess potential risks then plan interventions that can prevent accidents that are often the cause of injury or harm to clients. The nurse assessing potential risks to safety in relation to young children or at-risk clients living at home needs to check the entire house and garden area. Organisations responsible for community health frequently have assessment tools designed to aid the assessment of home safety. Clinical Interest Box 26.1 provides an example of one part of an assessment tool used to assess home safety. The example provided relates to checking for safety risks in a home kitchen.

Nursing interventions need to be considered in relation to the level of risk that a client faces and the impact of the intervention on social benefits and enjoyment of life. People balance risk against the pleasure or sense of achievement they will gain when they make choices about what activities they will pursue throughout life: there is a level of risk in many leisure and work activities. Whenever possible, clients should continue to be given the opportunity to consider the risks they face and make informed choices about which interventions are in their best interests. For example, a nurse visiting a client at home may be very concerned about the number of times the client has tripped over a lively pet dog. The nurse may consider the potential for serious injury is high but, even when the risks and possible outcomes are explained, the client may choose to live with the risk of tripping over the dog again and suffering an injury rather

CLINICAL INTEREST BOX 26.1
Example of a home safety assessment tool

Gainford Park Community Health Centre
Home safety assessment
Client:
Primary (family) carer:
Client's address:
Date:
Community nurse/health worker conducting assessment:

Area 1: Kitchen	Yes/No		Action/Details
All household, cleaning products, medications, alcohol and other dangerous substances are stored in original containers and out of reach in child-resistant cupboard			
All sharp and other potentially dangerous objects are stored out of reach (e.g. knives, glassware, plastic bags)			
All electrical appliances and their cords are out of reach and maintained in safe condition (e.g. cords not frayed)			
All family members are aware of safety measures (e.g. saucepan handles facing rear of stove, using back burners for cooking, not leaving tea-towels hanging on oven door, not leaving tablecloths hanging down, or leaving matches, oven gas lighter or gas guns in reach)			
Small food items (e.g. nuts, dried beans) are stored in sealed containers out of reach			
Floor mats are removed or rendered non-slip			
Fire extinguisher/blanket correctly located; family aware of correct method of use			
Power points are fitted with safety caps			
Stove, microwave oven, refrigerator and dishwasher in securely fixed position			
Hot water temperature set at reduced level			
Family aware of need to monitor potential hazards: • Chairs, stepping stools that could be used for climbing • Microwave oven • Hot water taps, basin, sinks that can be reached/operated by at risk person			

than losing the pleasure and sense of security provided by the pet.

Often risk assessment presents difficult decisions; for example, the person who has swallowing difficulties and is at risk of choking may prefer to take the risk of eating and drinking substances they enjoy, even when they increase the risk of choking. Decisions are especially difficult when the person who is at risk is deemed not competent to make an informed decision, as may be the case with people who have intellectual or cognitive impairment (Clinical Interest Box 26.2). The nurse should discuss risk assessment issues with other members of the health care team and clearly document all related discussions with the client in situations such as these.

It is the nurse's role to assess the client and the client's environment for hazards that are a potential cause of injury, whether the environment is in the home or in a health care facility. Infective microorganisms present a significant threat in health care settings (the safety and protection measures needed to deal with this risk are addressed in Chapter 25). Some of the other most common causes of injury or harm result from thermal injuries, contact with sharp objects, poisons and pollutants, and falls.

CLINICAL INTEREST BOX 26.2
FRANK AND MARY'S STORY

Frank cared for his wife, Mary, coping very successfully for more than 10 years as her Alzheimer's dementia gradually worsened. For the whole of the 42 years they had been married, Mary had gone for a walk almost every day. She walked for an hour or more each morning. She continued to do this as her memory became less reliable and she occasionally got lost. Frank and other neighbours sometimes had to drive around the district until they found her.

Frank became increasingly worried about Mary's safety as she became more confused, particularly after she was knocked down on a pedestrian crossing by a car and suffered some nasty bruising. She spent a couple of days in hospital after this incident and when she came home Frank tried to keep her happy in the house or garden, or by walking with her.

Frank found walking with Mary difficult, as she liked to walk a long way and she wanted to walk alone; she shouted at him, yelled out and repeatedly tried to push him away. She even gesticulated angrily at him when he walked behind her at a distance, which he continued to do for over 6 months. Frank worried constantly that Mary would walk in front of a car again before he could reach her and stop her.

The problem was that if Mary did not go for her walk she was very agitated and cried a lot during the day and did not sleep very much during the night. She would spend the rest of the day after a walk happily pottering about in the house and garden, and she hardly stirred at all during the night.

Frank and Mary had two daughters and one son. Together with the health care team they all discussed the risks for Mary and the impact of forcibly stopping her from walking. It was discussed how, if Mary were able to decide for herself, she would choose to take the risk of another injury in order to enjoy the lifetime habit of regular long walks. Although some of the health care team were unsure, there was no conflict within the family about the decision.

Mary continued her daily walks for another 18 months until she could no longer physically manage to do so. During this time she sustained a range of minor injuries, once when she walked into the path of a cyclist, and falling twice, on the second occasion fracturing an arm. After Mary died, Frank reflected on the choice that was made. He was quite certain that, if faced with the same difficult decision, he and his family would make the same choice again.

(story told by Frank, 77, carer of Mary, who had Alzheimer's dementia and died aged 76)

COMMON CAUSES OF INJURY

THERMAL INJURIES

Protection from burns and scalds includes protecting clients from the threat of fire and also from everyday risks of thermal injury. Burns or scalds can result from exposure to flame, hot liquids or objects, electrical or gas appliances, or from overexposure of the skin to the direct hot rays of the sun. Serious damage may also occur when the body tissues are exposed to extreme cold. (See Chapter 48 for information about the first aid management of burns, scalds and heat and cold trauma after exposure to the natural environment.)

Any client with impaired circulation or loss of physical sensation or who is confused or taking medications that alter mental awareness is at increased risk of a thermal injury, of which injuries by heat are the more common. The tissues of the very young and the elderly are less robust than those of other age groups and this places them at particular risk of damage by thermal injury. Measures to reduce the risk of thermal injuries include:

- Checking the temperature of any object applied to the client's body for therapeutic purposes; for example, hot packs or wheat or ice packs
- Placing a barrier between the client's skin and the therapeutic item and monitoring the client closely throughout the treatment
- Educating the client on the safe use of heat and cold treatments if they are to be continued after discharge; for example, advising to avoid lying on or going to sleep with a hot or cold pack in place
- Ensuring that heaters and other gas or electrical appliances are equipped with appropriate safety guards and are positioned away from flammable substances
- Ensuring that appliances are checked regularly and maintained adequately and that any faulty equipment or frayed cords are reported immediately
- Ensuring that any electric device a client brings to the hospital from home is checked by the hospital engineering staff for safe functioning before it is used on the premises
- Supervising potentially at-risk clients to prevent

CLINICAL INTEREST BOX 26.3
Safety measures recommended for senior citizens to prevent fire inside the home

- Smoke alarms situated correctly throughout the house
- Smoke alarms being checked every month to ensure they are in working condition
- Changing the batteries in smoke alarms routinely on the day that daylight saving ends
- Keeping keys in the main doors in preparation for a quick exit in an emergency
- Checking electric blankets for safety, storing them flat when not in use, and switching them off before going to bed
- Installing fire screens in front of open fires
- Extinguishing all candles and cigarettes before going to bed or leaving the house
- Avoiding drying clothes in front of a heater
- Cleaning the lint filter in the clothes dryer every time before it is used
- Establishing and practising an emergency fire evacuation procedure; for example, know two ways to get out of every room, decide on a meeting place outside the house, and practise the plan regularly
- Basic rules include: keep low, crawl if possible, when there is smoke
  - Never go back into a burning house
  - Wait at the designated meeting place until the fire brigade arrives

(Country Fire Authority, Community Safety Department 2003)

accidental contact with hot appliances that could cause a thermal injury
- Checking and, if necessary, reducing the temperature of hot food or beverages before giving them to vulnerable clients. Supervising or assisting with food and drinks whenever there is a risk of an accidental scald or burn
- Warning clients when food or drinks are hot
- Checking the bath and shower water temperature is regulated at a safe level.

Many fires and thermal injuries occur in the home. Clinical Interest Box 26.3 identifies safety measures recommended for senior citizens to prevent fire in the home.

Children are at particular risk of thermal injury. Not all people recognise areas of risk and the nurse can play an important role in health promotion by educating clients and families about safe practices; for example, the nurse may need to educate parents about ways to prevent thermal injuries to children (Box 26.1).

Box 26.1 | Protecting children and other vulnerable individuals from thermal injury in the home environment

- Turn off and place all electrical or other appliances out of reach after use; for example, hot iron, curling tongs. Never allow cords to dangle within a child's reach
- Install a hot water temperature regulator, set at a level that will not inflict a scald or burn
- Install protective devices such as stove, open fire, heater and radiator guards
- Place electrical wires so they are hidden and out of reach
- Position protective covers over electric power outlets and strategically place furniture to prevent child access to the outlets. Teach children as early as possible that it is dangerous to touch the outlets or insert things into them
- Install a circuit breaker to protect against overloading the home's electrical system
- Reduce the risk of hot fluid spills by keeping containers out of reach; for example, by turning the handles of saucepans away from the edge of the stove and by not using a tablecloth that hangs down over the table, as this allows children to pull hot drinks or objects over the edge
- Ensure that young children are not left unattended when there is a risk of injury from heat; for example, in the bathroom or kitchen or in rooms in which there are open fires or heaters
- Place electrical appliances such as frypans, toasters and sandwich makers towards the back of kitchen benches. Teach children as early as possible what 'hot' means and which items are hot and dangerous in the home
- Provide children with safe non-flammable clothing
- Keep matches out of reach and teach children about the dangers of playing with matches
- Install and maintain smoke alarms in working condition
- Plan and practise safe action in the event of a fire; for example, contacting the fire service, evacuating the home
- Avoid heat exhaustion and sunburn; for example, never leave children in a locked car or out in the sun without skin protection or adequate fluids

Reducing the risk of fire in health care facilities

Fire is a constant risk in a health care institution because of the presence of many highly combustible materials such as oxygen and cleaning solvents. Employers at health care institutions have a responsibility to conduct programs in fire prevention and safety for all staff members. Fire drills and in-service updates are held periodically in health care institutions so that all personnel can practise the emergency procedures. This usually includes an annual practice of the evacuation procedure for the facility. Nurses have a responsibility to be aware of fire prevention precautions and to practise fire safety and evacuation measures when the opportunity is offered. Nurses should refer to the facility's fire safety policies and protocols regarding their specific responsibilities in the event of a fire. The knowledge needed to promote fire safety includes knowing the:

- Location and type of fire extinguishers in the unit and how to use them
- Location of fire exits
- Method used to sound the alarm

- Actions to reduce the spread of fire
- Designated safe assembly areas
- Evacuation procedure to remove clients from a fire area.

Three elements are necessary to start and maintain a fire — combustible material, heat and oxygen. A combustible material is anything that will burn, such as paper, textiles, flammable liquids or furniture. Heat sufficient to ignite the combustible material may originate from a lighted match, a live cigarette, a spark or from friction. If the other two elements are present, there is sufficient oxygen in the atmosphere to support combustion. Fire extinguishers contain water or a chemical, and act by either cooling the burning substance or by cutting off the supply of fuel or oxygen. There are various types of fires (such as flammable liquid fires or electrical fires), with different types of fire extinguishers used for each. Every nurse should be familiar with the use of each type of fire extinguisher.

While methods of extinguishing fires are commonly aimed at reducing heat and excluding oxygen, methods of preventing fires are directed towards controlling combustible materials and heat. Measures to prevent fire include:

- Permitting smoking only in designated areas. This requires a client, if permitted to smoke, being directed to the designated area and provided with an ashtray
- Supervising any client who is smoking while disoriented or unsteady
- Informing and encouraging staff and visitors not to smoke, in accordance with regulations
- Displaying clear warning signs indicating that smoking is forbidden and dangerous where oxygen is stored or in use
- Keeping all areas free from an accumulation of combustible materials; for example, stacks of cardboard containers
- Keeping all fire exits clear and clearly labelled. Doors leading to and from emergency exits must never be locked or propped open
- Storing all chemicals and flammable gases or liquids; for example, anaesthetic agents, alcohol-based substances or grease, according to strict safety guidelines
- Ensuring that electrical appliances are checked and maintained by an electrician at regular intervals
- Having a detailed fire and evacuation plan specifically designed for each facility, with which all staff are familiar.

SHARP OBJECTS

The sharp objects most likely to cause cuts or puncture wounds in a health care setting are needles used for testing a client's blood glucose level or for administering an injection, and glass ampoules that contain medication. Measures to prevent injury from needles include:

- Placing a used needle directly into a receptacle without replacing the needle cap
- Placing the used needle carefully into a rigid puncture-proof container specifically designed for the disposal of needles and other sharps such as glass ampoules and scalpel blades. The container should be appropriately labelled with an international biohazard sign. If available, needles can be disposed of using a needle-destruction kit, designed to reduce the handling of used needles
- Using forceps to retrieve a needle that is accidentally dropped
- Securing the safety seal on the full sharps container before it is removed from the work area for safe destruction.

In the event of an injury from a sharp object, such as a needle-stick injury, the incident is reported immediately and documented on an incident report form (see Chapter 20). The level of risk of an infection being transmitted via the needle-stick injury is assessed and the individual treated in accordance with the policies of the health care facility. (See Chapter 25 for information concerning protective measures after possible exposure to blood-borne microorganisms.)

Measures to prevent injury from glass ampoules include:

- Placing a small gauze pad around the neck of the glass ampoule to protect the fingers as it is opened
- Snapping the neck of the ampoule firmly and quickly away from the body to protect the nurse's hands and face in the event of the neck of the ampoule shattering
- Disposing of the used glass ampoule into the designated sharps container.

Sharp items or instruments such as scissors should never be left unattended in the vicinity of a client or carried in the nurse's pocket. Every care must be taken to avoid discarding sharps into the soiled linen container or any place other than the designated sharps container. Injuries from sharp objects range from minor cuts to serious wounds causing life-threatening blood loss. Most accidents involving sharp objects can be avoided by using basic safety measures. Box 26.2 lists some general preventive measures to reduce the risk of injury by sharp objects.

POISONS AND POLLUTANTS

A poison is any substance that is detrimental to the functioning of the body. This includes a huge range of substances such as drugs, household cleaning and gardening materials, and biological hazards such as chemicals, radioactive materials and any material contaminated with infective organisms. The functioning and structure of the body may be harmed when only very small amounts of some particularly potent poisonous substances are ingested, inhaled, injected or absorbed into the body through the skin or mucous membranes. There are antidotes to some but not all poisons. In addition to preventing the transmission of pathogenic organisms that are toxic when they enter the body (see Chapter 25), prevention of poisoning includes safe storage, use and disposal of materials that are a biohazard; safe storage, administration and disposal of medications;

Box 26.2 | General preventive measures to reduce the risk of injury by sharp objects

- Safe storage of all sharp objects, eg, knives, scissors, garden tools, out of the reach of children and at-risk adults
- Careful selection of toys, tools and other items to ensure that there are no sharp edges that can cause damage to a vulnerable person. Avoid long, pointed toys
- Fitting safety glass with clear eye-level markings in all full-length glass panel doors and windows
- Clearing up broken glass immediately and disposing of it safely. In the home this may be best achieved using a dustpan and brush to sweep it up. If the garbage is collected and crushed mechanically it can be tipped directly into the household garbage bin. Alternatively, it can be wrapped carefully in a thick layer of newspaper and sealed securely before it is placed in the bin

and keeping the local environment, and the world, free from toxic pollutants.

Safe storage, use and disposal of materials that are biohazards

Accidents involving chemical and hazardous substances usually result from incorrect use of the substance. For example, a substance intended for cleaning may cause serious harm if it is ingested or spilled on the skin. In the home all potentially harmful substances such as medications, detergents, bleaches, pesticides, petrol or kerosene must be kept in their original containers, clearly labelled and stored in a safe, preferably locked, place that is well out of the reach of at-risk individuals. Measures to prevent injury from hazardous substances in the workplace include:

- Monitoring and maintenance of a register of hazardous substances on the premises
- All chemical containers being clearly labelled
- Strict observance of the policies and regulations regarding the use of hazardous substances
- Ensuring a material safety data sheet (MSDS) is stored with each hazardous substance on the premises: an MSDS is the primary source of safety information for users of hazardous chemicals in the workplace, and manufacturers are obliged to provide them when hazardous substances are supplied (National Occupational Health & Safety Commission [NOHSC] 2003)
- Storing volatile substances separately from each other and away from populated areas
- Observing the Commonwealth *Poisons and Therapeutic Goods Act 1966*. Under this Act, any container that holds a poisonous substance must carry a prominent label with a clearly printed warning. The wording that must be used depends on the 'schedule' to which the substance belongs (see Chapter 28 for information regarding poison schedules)
- Observing strict policy guidelines for dealing with radioactive materials in the health care facility. When caring for clients receiving radiation therapy, especially if they have radioactive implants, nurses must wear a tracking device to record the length of time they are exposed to the radiation. The time determined to be within safe limits should never be exceeded. Protective devices such as lead aprons should be worn and the distance between the source of radiation and the nurse should be maintained at the maximum possible. International warning signs should be displayed at the entry point of any place where radiation is a hazard
- Strictly adhering to all policy precautions regarding the safe disposal of infectious material (see Chapter 25)
- Strictly adhering to all policy precautions regarding the safe disposal of radioactive material. The Australian Radiation Protection and Nuclear Safety Agency (ARPNSA) was founded in 1997 to coordinate the work of individual agencies in protecting the community from the risks of radiation during the disposal of radioactive wastes. Hospital policy is usually in line with the recommendations of the ARPNSA. In the event of any leak or risk of leak the ARPNSA will institute measures to protect those at risk, to treat those affected and to clean up areas of contamination (Crisp & Taylor 2005).

Safe storage, administration and disposal of medications

Safety precautions with medications in the health care facility include:

- Locking the area in which medications are stored, to make it inaccessible to unauthorised persons
- Recognising that the pharmacist is responsible for the contents of most medical substances supplied
- Recognising that only the pharmacist may attach or alter a label, fill a container or transfer medication from one container to another. If a label on a container is illegible, the container must be returned to the pharmacist for clarification
- Observing the safety precautions for the administration of all medications (see Chapter 28).

Accidental poisoning with prescription or other drugs is not uncommon in the home. Children and older adults are particularly at risk. General safety advice includes:

- Storing all drugs and dangerous substances in original, clearly labelled containers and *never* transferring noxious substances to other containers, such as soft drink bottles
- Limiting the use of medications when possible
- Using all medication under the supervision of a medical officer
- Returning unwanted or discontinued medications to a pharmacist as soon as they are finished with

- Having the contact numbers for emergency services — for example, ambulance service and Poisons Information Centre — readily at hand (e.g. kept close to the telephone)
- Not inducing vomiting as a first aid measure unless advised to do so by a poisons expert.

Additional safety precautions to protect children from poisoning by drugs include:

- Referring to medications as drugs, never lollies
- Replacing childproof lids on medicines after use and storing all medications safely out of reach, preferably in a locked cupboard
- Providing information about the hazards of prescription and non-prescription drugs, including the overuse of paracetamol, aspirin and alcohol as soon as children are old enough to understand
- Discussing strategies to help school-age and older children to say 'no' when subjected to pressure to participate in using illegal drugs or alcohol.

Older adults are at particular risk of poisoning by prescribed medications, evidenced by them being admitted to hospital with adverse drug reactions more often than younger adults. They are at higher risk of poisoning by medications because age alters the rate at which medications are absorbed, metabolised and excreted from the body. If the process is significantly slow, drug toxicity can occur. This problem can be exacerbated because body weight is often lost as people age, resulting in altered distribution of drugs around the body and the need for a lower dose than has been prescribed (Bryant, Knights & Salerno 2006).

Older adults generally consume more prescription and over-the-counter drugs than other people and they frequently take a combination of many different drugs on a daily basis. Sometimes older people are referred to specialist medical officers and are prescribed medications by more than one of them. This results in what is known as *poly-pharmacy*, a potentially dangerous indiscriminate use of multiple medications at the same time (Bryant et al 2006). Nurses can help prevent poisoning by prescribed medication in older adults by keeping these factors in mind, and actively:

- Observing for and promptly reporting any signs of toxicity; for example, tinnitus, gastric disturbance, mental status changes, visual disorders
- Advocating for frequent reviews of client medication regimens
- Encouraging older clients to ask questions of the medical officer, Registered Nurse (RN) or pharmacist about prescribed and non-prescribed herbal or other drugs
- Encouraging older people to discuss with the medical officer the possibility of withdrawing medications that may no longer be essential
- Ensuring that non-pharmacological approaches are considered whenever appropriate
- Checking that the client has understood instructions about taking medications and, if necessary, seeking the help of an RN to clarify instructions.

Enrolled Nurses (ENs) can participate in medication-related interventions only in accordance with the code of practice in their geographical area and only in accordance with their level of knowledge and expertise.

Measures to assist older clients taking medications safely at home include the use of a controlled dispenser that contains the medications for each day and time in a separate section (Figure 26.1).

When an older client has visual impairment it will help if instructions for taking the medications are clearly printed in large bold letters. If clients are confused it may be necessary for the medications to be taken under the supervision of a family member and kept out of reach at other times.

Environmental pollution

To be healthy the world and local environments need to be free of pollutants. Pollutants are poisonous. Pollution occurs as a result of harmful chemicals or waste materials being allowed to contaminate the air, the soil or the water. Noise is also considered a pollutant when, as a result of the noise levels being so high or so constant, it causes distress, or even physical damage, to the body's hearing mechanisms.

Air pollution

Globally the air is polluted primarily by the accumulation of toxic fumes from homes, commercial and industrial activities and motorised vehicles. Air pollutants disperse throughout the world's atmosphere. In areas where the concentration of pollutants is high, many people living in that particular area may become sick. A range of respiratory disorders, including lung cancer, is associated with air pollutants (Socha 2003). If the air continues to be polluted at the current rate there are warnings that the Earth will heat up (global warming) because of a serious depletion of the ozone layer that protects it from the sun's burning rays (Traudt 2003). If nurses want to take part in the fight to protect the world and its people from the effects of air pollution, ozone depletion and slow global warming they must, alongside other members of the community, lobby governments to enforce strict clean air laws locally and internationally.

At a local level nurses can practise health promotion measures to improve air pollution. Health promotion includes educating clients about the importance of:

- Using low-fuel-consumption cars and using them less often by walking, cycling, car pooling or using public transport
- Recycling waste materials; for example, newspapers, metal, plastic and glass containers
- Making homes energy efficient; for example, by buying only energy-efficient appliances
- Planting trees (they reduce carbon dioxide levels and produce oxygen)

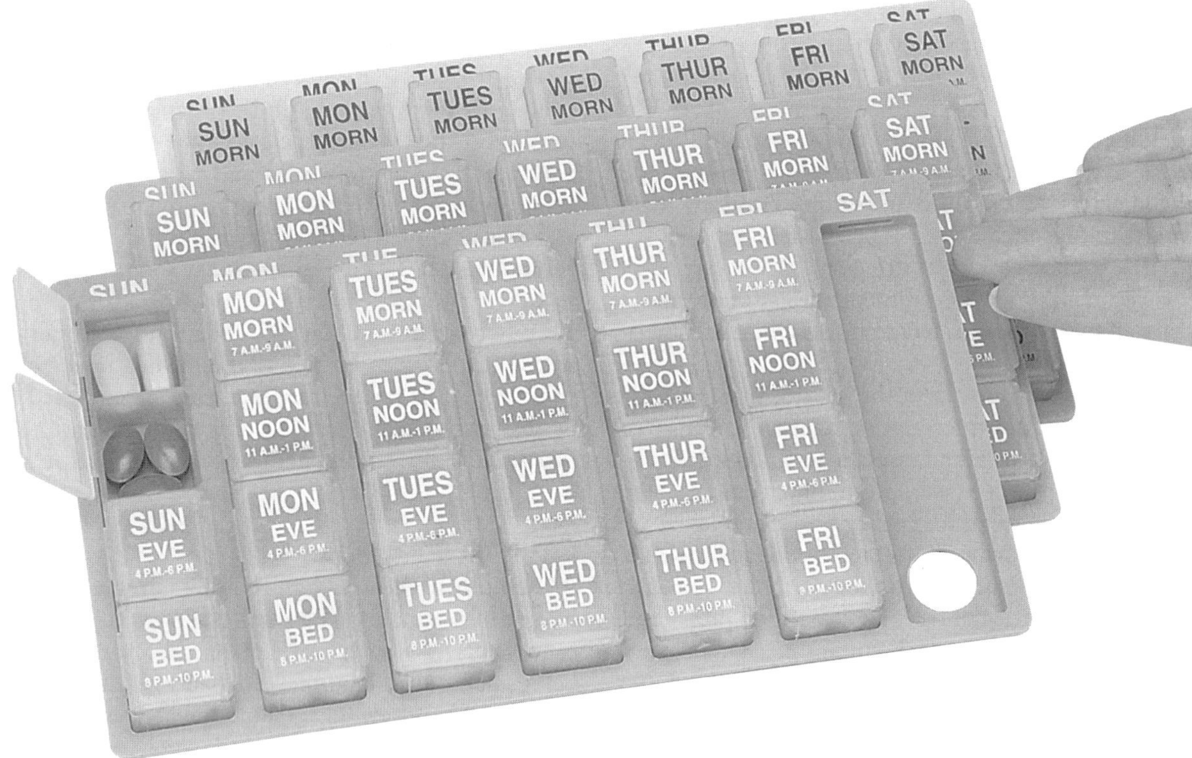

Figure 26.1 | A controlled medication dispenser *(Potter & Perry 2008)*

- Not purchasing Styrofoam, aerosol sprays and other products that contain chlorofluorocarbons (CFCs)
- Avoiding cigarette smoking.

Soil and water pollution

Water and soil can be polluted by the incorrect and unsafe disposal of toxic wastes, such as radioactive materials, or by the misuse of toxic chemicals, such as weed- or insect-controlling chemicals used for crop spraying. Water filtration units help to protect the community by filtering out harmful pollutants from water supplies. In most areas the responsibility for the health of the community in relation to the quality of the air, soil and water is that of an environmental protection agency (EPA). It is commonly the EPA that checks the quality of local water and issues warnings when contamination problems arise, for example, when it is necessary to boil all drinking or cooking water and when the level of pathogens such as *Escherichia coli* in sea water make swimming unsafe.

FALLS

Individuals are susceptible to falling if they have impaired mobility, motor or cognitive function or sensory disabilities, or if they are experiencing alteration to mental status from any cause, including the effects of head injury, drugs or alcohol. Falls are the most frequent cause of injury for older clients in an acute-care facility (deWit 2005) but every client in every care setting should be assessed for the risk of having a fall. Table 26.1 provides an example of a falls risk assessment tool.

General safety measures to prevent falls include:

- Ensuring that floors are free of clutter, slippery substances and loose rugs. Spills should be wiped up immediately, floor coverings should be maintained in good repair and rugs should have a non-slip backing or be removed from the area. Large, clearly worded warning signs should be displayed when floors are wet or slippery
- Installing handrails in corridors, stairways, bathrooms and toilets. These provide support for individuals who are weak or unsteady when walking and also provide support when a client is sitting down or getting up; for example, sitting on the toilet or getting out of the bath
- Placing a non-slip mat on the floor at the base of the bath or just outside the shower cubicle. A chair should be available in the bathroom for clients to sit on; for example, during a shower or while dressing or undressing. Floor tiles in any area should be of the non-slip variety
- The nurse remaining with and supporting at-risk clients during hygiene and toileting procedures and whenever there is a risk of the client falling
- The nurse frequently checking more independent clients during hygiene and toileting procedures and ensuring that every client is aware of the position of the call button in the shower or toilet area

TABLE 26.1 | FALLS RISK-ASSESSMENT TOOL

Place a tick in front of the items that apply to the patient.

General information
- ❑ Age over 70
- ❑ History of falls*
- ❑ Confusion at times
- ❑ Confused most of the time*
- ❑ Impaired memory or judgment
- ❑ Unable to follow directions*
- ❑ Needs assistance with elimination
- ❑ Visual impairment
- ❑ Feels physically weak*

Medications
- ❑ Receiving central nervous system suppressants (narcotic, sedative, tranquilliser, hypnotic, antidepressant, psychotropic, anticonvulsant)
- ❑ Receiving medication that causes orthostatic hypotension (antihypertensive, diuretic)*
- ❑ Medication that may cause diarrhoea (cathartic)
- ❑ Medication that may alter blood glucose levels (insulin, hypoglycaemics)

Gait and balance
- ❑ Poor balance when standing*
- ❑ Balance problems when walking*
- ❑ Swaying, lurching, or slapping gait*
- ❑ Unstable when making turns*
- ❑ Needs assistive device (walker, cane, holds onto furniture)*

* Note: A tick on any starred item indicates a risk for falls. A combination of four or more of the un-starred items indicates a risk for falls.
(deWit 2005)

- Adjusting the height of the bed to meet the needs of individual clients, enabling them to get into and out of the bed safely and independently whenever possible
- Placing any items that the client might need within easy reach; for example, when the client is in bed or sitting on a chair. Items required should be on the locker or over-bed table that is positioned close to the client. This avoids the risk of a fall from the bed caused by the client stretching while attempting to reach for a needed item
- Ensuring that all walking aids, for example, crutches and frames, are fitted with non-slip tips to prevent them skidding on the floor. Clients who are using walking aids should be supported adequately and supervised until they are able to use the aids safely. All walking aids should be positioned at the correct height for the individual client
- Ensuring that clear lighting is available in all areas and that a nightlight is provided in the client's room
- Placing the signal device within the client's easy reach so that assistance can be summoned if necessary; for example, to get out of bed
- Keeping all areas free of items that could cause a person to fall; for example, electrical cords, cleaning equipment, linen, dressing or medication trolleys
- Ensuring that ambulant clients wear shoes or slippers that are well fitting and have non-slip soles. The cord from a dressing gown should not be allowed to trail, as it could cause the person to trip
- Doors should remain fully open or closed, as people are more likely to bump into a door that is ajar
- Side rails on cots should remain elevated whenever an infant or very small child is left unattended.

Careful consideration is needed to determine the most appropriate preventative measures to use when clients are at risk of falling out of the bed. Traditionally, bed rails have been used for at-risk clients, such as those with dementia or other forms of cognitive impairment. Currently, alternative safety devices such as 'low-low' beds, concave or water mattresses, and the positioning of pillows or mattress bumpers to reduce movement to the edge of the bed are usually considered better options, as the use of bed rails and other forms of restraint have their own inherent safety risk; for example, a client climbing over the top of a bed rail risks a more severe injury because of falling from a greater height. Each client needs to be assessed individually for risks to their safety and the care plan should reflect this individual assessment, but there are some general precautions that protect clients from falls in a health care facility (Clinical Interest Box 26.4).

In some circumstances even the most careful nursing interventions are unable to prevent the risk of injury or harm to clients. In such cases, as a last resort, it becomes necessary to consider the use of restraining devices to protect clients.

PROTECTIVE DEVICES AND OTHER FORMS OF RESTRAINT

Physical restraints, sometimes called protective devices, are used to limit the freedom of movement of a client to varying degrees. Protective or restraining devices are only appropriate if they are used to protect the client from harm or from harming others; for example, a confused postoperative client who is continually trying to remove his urinary catheter may, for his own safety, need to be prevented from doing so. When absolutely essential, soft material wrist restraints have been used to maintain client safety in such situations but whenever possible a less restrictive measure should be implemented. The problem may be solved by the use of hand mittens, for example, or by giving the client a soft football-shaped piece of foam covered with stockingette, which may keep the hands occupied and focus concentration away from the catheter.

It is never appropriate to use a protective device to restrain a client for the convenience of nursing staff, for example, so that the nurse can continue with other work free from

CLINICAL INTEREST BOX 26.4
General precautions to protect clients from falls in a health care facility

- Orientate the client and family to the area: the client's room, the bathroom and toilet
- Assess the client's risk of falling (see Table 26.1)
- Ensure that the client can reach and understands how to operate the signal device (call bell) and reassure that, if necessary, it is alright to call out for help
- Answer call bells promptly so that clients do not feel the need to get out of bed and go to the toilet unaided
- Maintain the bed in the low position except when providing direct client care
- Ensure the brakes on beds and wheelchairs are in the on position so they do not move when clients get into or out of them
- Explain and encourage the use of support rails along corridors, in the bathroom and toilet
- Ensure that the client has snug-fitting non-slip footwear
- Take extra care with cognitively impaired or confused clients
- Have the client in a room close to the nurses' station to enable frequent observation, or sit the client close to the nurses' station, where the constant company and activity provide a focus of interest and stimulation that may prevent unsafe wandering
- Frequently check the client, stay if the client is restless or agitated and up and about
- Provide diversion activities that the confused client will enjoy and that will deter from unsafe wandering; for example, a box of photographs to look through
- Use extra safety measures, such as a mattress placed on the floor by the bed if the client tends not to call for help and is at high risk of falling out
- Regularly walk with the restless client: exercise promotes sound sleep, reducing the risk of nocturnal wandering and falls during the night
- Toilet the client on a regular basis (according to an individually assessed normal toileting pattern) to reduce the risk of the client trying to get out of bed without help

(adapted from deWit 2005)

interruption by a confused or agitated client. Physical restraints have been used in the past in the management of clients who were confused, combative or at high risk of falling when unattended, but the use of restraints is stressful for clients and their families and may cause more harm than it prevents. Contemporary nursing practice recognises that physical restraint is an invasion of basic human rights. In addition, evidence indicates that negative effects from the use of physical restraints include damage to nerve and muscle function, risk of asphyxiation, increased agitation, confusion and distress and an increase rather than a decrease in the incidence of falls (Joanna Briggs Institute 2002a). The use of any restraint requires that the client's rights and choices be of paramount consideration in the decision-making process. Whenever possible the nurse should gain the client's permission before placing in position protective restrictive items such as side rails on a bed or a safety strap on a wheelchair.

Protective devices include the use of:

- Side rails on a client's bed
- Security or safety belt on trolleys or wheelchairs
- Soft material ties (extremity immobilisers) that prevent movement of the hands and feet
- Padded coverings for the hands; for example, hand mitts
- Vest or jacket chest restraint that secures a client in an upright position in a wheelchair

Nurses have a responsibility to:

- Check that there is a written medical officer's order to use the protective device
- Apply the device so that it is secure and effective but comfortable
- Check that the device is not impeding circulation of the client's blood to the restricted limb
- Remove the device at least every 2 hours, change the client's position and ensure comfort
- Ensure that active or passive exercises are performed at least every 2 hours on all joints and muscles affected by the device
- Ensure all hydration, nutrition, toileting and other comfort and care needs are met while the device is in place
- Remove the protective device immediately it is no longer necessary, after gaining permission from the medical officer concerned to do so.

An extensive review of the use of restraint in Australia indicates that, despite the growing concern regarding its use, a significant proportion of clients and residents continue to be subjected to physical restraint. The study identified that the use of restraint is considerably greater in residential care than in acute care and that the three most common devices used to restrain clients are wrist, waist and chest restraints (Joanna Briggs Institute 2002a). The main reasons for continuing to use physical restraints were identified as maintaining the client's safety; managing agitation and aggression; behaviour control, such as preventing wandering; and providing physical support. It was also identified that they were at times used to help achieve work organisation goals; maintain a comfortable social environment, for example, to stop residents from bothering others; and to facilitate treatment, for example, to prevent clients tampering with medical devices or removing dressings or catheters (Joanna Briggs Institute 2002a).

The study identified that some residential aged-care agencies now operate successfully within a restraint-free environment, but *restraint minimisation* strategies still need to be developed and evaluated in many residential and acute care settings. Some of the suggestions for restraint alternatives identified in the research undertaken by the Joanna Briggs Institute (2002b) are provided in Clinical Interest Box 26.5. Nurses are recommended to read more extensively on matters concerning appropriate nursing actions to promote restraint-free care. The Joanna Briggs Institute research articles are available via the internet.

CLINICAL INTEREST BOX 26.5
Suggestions to promote restraint minimisation

Reducing risk of wandering
- Bed, chair or wrist alarms
- Exit door alarm
- Electronic movement sensors
- Planned night-time activities for those who wander at night
- Daytime recreational and social activities
- Activity areas at the end of each corridor

Reduce incidence of agitation and aggression
- Easy access to safe outdoor areas
- Structural design of units modified to enhance visibility of residents
- Rocker and recliner chairs
- Outlets for industrious or anxious behaviour; for example, physical, occupational and recreational therapies
- Soothing music
- Diversions such as television or radio

(adapted from Joanna Briggs Institute 2002b)

Not all forms of restraint are physical. It is also restrictive to control a person's access to their own resources — for example, their own money or personal belongings — or to control a client's personal choices. This includes the selection of what may be watched on television or with whom they can socialise. In addition, medication that interferes with a person's behaviour or functioning, such as those that reduce agitation, delusional thoughts, manic behaviour or sexual desire, can be viewed as a chemical form of restraint (Clinical Interest Box 26.6 outlines forms of restraint in order of degree of restrictiveness).

It is an important area of research for nurses to identify and then advocate for alternatives to restraint. Restraint practices must be implemented only as a last resort and with extreme caution. The intervention should always be the least possible restraining measure necessary to prevent harm to the client. The use of restraint is governed by legal requirements, and nurses need to be familiar with, and follow, the laws relevant to their geographical location. The nurse must also be familiar with, and follow, the policies and procedures for the appropriate use and monitoring of restraints that have been documented by the employing facility. General guidelines for the use of restraint or restrictive measures include the following:
- The least restrictive measure possible should be implemented
- The client should be cared for in the least restrictive environment possible
- Restraint should be used constructively; for example, to continue the safe administration of medical treatment (not to discipline or punish)
- The aim of the restraint must be to benefit the client
- A medical officer must provide a written order indicating the type of restraint to be implemented and the specific behaviour for which it is to be used. It cannot be used as a response to any other behaviour
- A medical officer must regularly review the need for the restraint to continue and the review should be timely; for example, the *Victorian Mental Health Act 1986* states that a client who is physically restrained or in a seclusion room must be reviewed as clinically appropriate, but at least every 15 minutes by an RN, and reviewed by the medical officer at least every 4 hours
- Family members must be consulted and consent obtained
- Reasons to restrain or continue restraint are clearly documented
- Restraints used may only be of an approved type
- Supporting medical and nursing documentation must be provided.

Young and old clients living in residential care settings can suffer serious social restrictions and a loss of quality of life if nurses do not advocate on their behalf for their rights to enjoy social interaction. Residents or clients requiring long-term support from the health care system, for example people with learning or other intellectual disabilities, need and should have, as far as is possible, the same things in life that are important to other people (Marsland 2003).

CLINICAL INTEREST BOX 26.6
Forms of restraint, in order of restrictiveness

1. Restricting body extremities; for example, securing hands, wrists or ankles to the arms or legs of a chair or to bed rails, using body restraining vests
2. Restricting body movements by other means; for example, safety belts or vests
3. Restricting movement in the environment by secluding a client in a dedicated seclusion room. The *Western Australian Mental Health Act 1996* (p. 64) describes this as a room that is not within the control of the person to leave
4. Restricting movement in the environment by restriction within a ward or unit
5. Restricting activities of daily living; for example, selection of preferred foods, television programs, social activities or choice of visitors or people to meet or socialise with
6. Denial of purposeful or meaningful activities, such as access to preferred leisure or work pursuits
7. Restricting choice of treatment; for example, in some cases people with mental health, intellectual or cognitive impairment are given treatment not of their choosing that is mandated by the legal system (courts)
8. Restricting access to personal belongings; for example, use of own money
9. Restricting the expression of personal feelings or views; for example, censoring expressions of emotion (expressions of anger or frustration may be controlled and vocabulary normally used may be censored, e.g. swearing). This form of restriction and control is more common in mental health nursing than in other areas

(adapted from Olsen 1998)

Nurses have a responsibility to develop care plans for these clients or residents that include opportunities to make friends, meet and socialise with a range of different people and to be stimulated by a range of experiences. Although some residents and clients may be seriously confused or intellectually impaired, they usually retain the capacity to enjoy social interaction and activities that stimulate the senses. Nurses can protect the rights of clients to enjoy the least possible restrictive environment by promoting, planning and participating in visits to places that provide such stimulation, such as a park, the ocean, the zoo or places to enjoy music or other performances. Social interaction for older residents can also be enhanced by promoting visits by local school children and other local groups to residential aged-care facilities.

OCCUPATIONAL HEALTH AND SAFETY

In Australia and New Zealand, as in other countries, organisations are encouraged by law to maintain safety in the workplace. In each jurisdiction of Australia (Commonwealth, state or territory) there is a principal Occupational Health and Safety (OHS) Act that aims to ensure that every employee is at the lowest possible risk of disease or injury from any factor within workplaces or from the activities conducted within them. In New Zealand the *Health and Safety in Employment Act 1992* serves the same purpose. These Acts impose obligations on all people who may influence the health and safety of others in the workplace by their actions or lack of actions. The key principle in these Acts is the 'duty of care' responsibility of employers to provide a safe place of work for employees. Employers are required to:

- Promote the health and safety of all employees in the workplace
- Provide methods of doing the required work that are safe and without risk to health
- Prevent industrial accidents, injuries and diseases
- Protect the health and safety of employees in relation to any work activity undertaken
- Promote successful recovery or maximum rehabilitation for any injured employee.

Specific additional regulations are developed to give more detailed guidance concerning the prevention or management of specific hazards in the workplace; for example, there are more detailed regulations concerning smoking, the use and management of asbestos, noise levels, and the handling of anything that is heavy or dangerous, such as poisons.

To support the Acts and Regulations there are codes of practice that give employers practical guidelines about how to implement and therefore comply with them. The Australian Safety and Compensation Council (ASCC) has recently released a set of standards and guidelines designed to improve existing health and safety practices in Australian workplaces and to make them consistent throughout the whole of the country (ASCC 2005).

Employers have an obligation to implement safety programs and policies in accordance with legal Acts, codes of practice and national guidelines to ensure that working conditions are as safe as possible. They normally achieve this by adopting a systematic approach to safety that involves allocating specific people to be responsible for each particular area of risk. Often there is a multidisciplinary OHS committee, whose aim is to create and maintain a safe environment. The committee and associated subcommittees collectively work towards setting and maintaining high standards of safety for staff and clients (see Chapter 25 on the precise role of the infection prevention and control committee, for example). Personnel who are accountable for safety programs have an obligation to:

- Identify existing and potential hazards
- Assess the level of risk constituted by every identified hazard
- Determine measures to eliminate or minimise and control the level of risk
- Implement prevention and control measures
- Ensure that all staff are aware of the measures and carry out their personal responsibilities
- Monitor the effectiveness of prevention and control measures implemented.

Nurses can expect that safety awareness educational programs will be provided by the employing agency so that they have all the information necessary to practise nursing in a way that is in accordance with safety regulations and the agency's own policies. For example, education for nurses and other hospital personnel would normally include that instigated by the infection prevention and control committee and the fire safety and prevention committee. Nurses can also expect that they will receive information during their nurse education and at their place of employment concerning how to lift and move clients without risking their own health or safety.

THE NO-LIFT POLICY

Injury caused by the manual lifting of clients was identified as a workplace hazard for nurses several years ago. In 1994 the Australian Nursing Federation (ANF) started work on identifying how to reduce this health hazard. The result was the introduction of a no-lift, no-injury program — a set of principles and practices to guide the safe handling of clients. The aim of the program was to eliminate the manual lifting of clients in all but exceptional or life-threatening circumstances. A no-lift policy has been systematically introduced throughout health care facilities in Australia and New Zealand, with significant success in reducing both the incidence and the severity of injuries to nurses caused by lifting clients in the workplace. It has additional benefits in that it has reduced the potential for client injuries related to falls and reduced the incidence of skin tears and bruising among residents in aged-care facilities. It has also promoted independence and mobility in clients generally (Harulow 2002). Safety principles for

CLINICAL INTEREST BOX 26.7
Safety principles for lifting and moving clients

Assessment

- Assess the level of risk involved in lifting or moving the client
- Determine the safest and most effective method to employ
- Re-assess what is needed before each lift, as a client's condition can change rapidly
- Ensure the lift or move is within your skill level and physical capability

Preparation and planning

- Use a lifting machine or other handling equipment, such as slide sheets or lifting belts, every time they can lower the risk of injury, unless there are reasons why to do so would be detrimental to the client's condition
- Check that the equipment is in good working order and gather additional people to help as needed
- Ensure that there is enough space, free of obstacles, in which the client and any machine necessary can be safely manoeuvred

Nursing interventions

- As appropriate, use mechanical lifting devices and hoists or rigid or sliding fabric devices to assist with lifting, moving or transferring clients. This includes when moving clients from bed to chair, bed to trolley, bed to bathroom, on and off the toilet or moving them up, down, side to side or around the bed or on any other occasion when they need to be re-positioned and the risk of injury can be reduced by using a safety device
- Ensure that the wheels of beds, wheelchairs, commodes or trolleys are locked before transferring clients to or from them

lifting and moving clients are outlined in Clinical Interest Box 26.7.

While the principles are set out here, the skills of safely moving and lifting clients cannot effectively be gained from a textbook — they must be taught by practical demonstration and practised. Many health care agencies reinforce the skills nurses learned as nursing students by conducting their own educational programs; some require that nurses and others involved in client care attend these programs on a regular annual basis. Given that the primary objective of the no-lift policy is to protect residents, clients and staff from injury and to assist in providing quality care, all nurses have a responsibility to comply with the policy and to maintain associated competencies by attending the educational programs offered. Health care workers who deliberately fail to comply with a workplace no-lift policy unnecessarily risk their health and employment future and may also expose themselves to legal action (Clinical Interest Box 26.8)

While the no-lift policy is designed to protect nurses from injury, it is also imperative to their safety that nurses follow the principles of correct body posture and mechanics.

CLINICAL INTEREST BOX 26.8
A case of non-compliance with the no-lift policy

In relation to the no-lift policy the Australian Nursing Federation cited the example of two nurses who made the decision to ignore the policy at their place of employment and together attempted to reposition a resident using an unauthorised 'top and tail' type of lift. During the lift all three fell on the floor. As a result one of the nurses sustained a back injury and the resident suffered a skin tear.

The resident's family lodged a formal complaint against the nurses. The WorkCover Authority in the state of Australia where the nurses were employed rejected one nurse's claim for medical expenses and lost wages, on the basis that the nurse had attended the training in no-lift techniques provided by the employer and that the nurse understood the procedures and was aware that appropriate equipment was available. The nurse eventually resigned.

(Marshall 2001)

BODY POSTURE AND MECHANICS

Fatigue, muscle strain and injury can result from improper use or positioning of the body during activity or rest. Correct posture is achieved when all parts of the body are in alignment, and is important whether an individual is sitting, lying, standing or moving. The normal spinal curves should be maintained and the joints should be supported in their normal positions. Correct posture and alignment reduces strain on all muscles and joints, and enables internal organs to function without interference, for example, by facilitating full lung expansion.

Body mechanics is the term used to describe the physical coordination of all parts of the body to promote correct posture and balanced movement. The practice of correct body mechanics promotes economical expenditure of energy, resulting in less fatigue, and reduces the risk of muscle and joint injury. The general principles of body mechanics are based on the laws of physics as they are applied to the human body, and include:

- Keeping the base of support wide. A wide base of support (Figure 26.2) provides greater stability and is achieved by placing the feet apart with the toes pointed in the direction of movement. The body weight should be distributed evenly between both feet and the knees should be flexed slightly to provide added stability
- Keeping the centre of gravity low. The centre of gravity (Figure 26.2) is located in the pelvic area
- Keeping the line of gravity vertical. The line of gravity, or gravital plane (Figure 26.2), is an imaginary line running from the top of the head down through the centre of gravity and further down to the base of support. For maximum efficiency and stability, the line of gravity should remain perpendicular to the ground

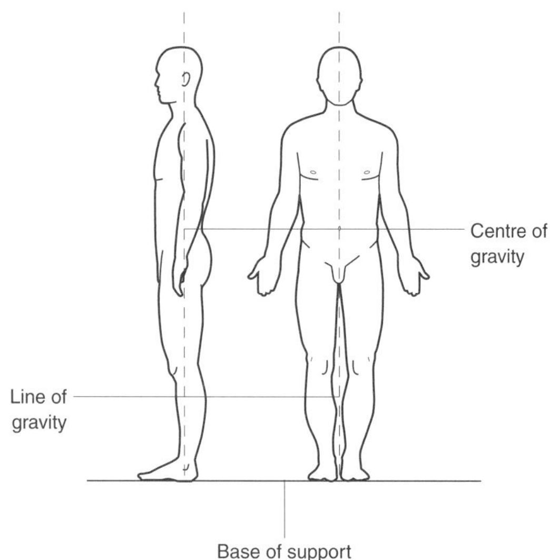

Figure 26.2 | Body mechanics — correct standing posture

- Using the large and strong muscles of the body. Large muscles do not become fatigued as quickly as small muscles. The body's large muscles are located in the shoulders, upper arms, hips and thighs. To avoid using the small muscles of the back, the knees should be flexed; for example, when picking something up from the floor, as this action involves the use of buttock and thigh muscles
- Holding heavy objects close to the body. Less effort is expended when a heavy object is held close to the body than when it is held with the arms extended
- Using body movement to manage heavy weight. When an object is being lifted, less energy is used if the lifter's weight is transferred during the movement and used to counteract the weight being lifted (mechanical or other lifting aids should be used whenever possible)
- Pushing or sliding objects. It is easier to push or slide an object than it is to lift it, because lifting necessitates moving against the force of gravity. Friction between an object and the surface on which the object is moved affects the amount of energy required to push or slide the object. This is the rationale for using smooth silky slide-sheets to move clients in and around the bed.

Knowledge of the principles of body mechanics and skill in applying them are important in ensuring that energy is used efficiently and muscle strain prevented. To promote safety and comfort during all work and leisure activities it is important that nurses apply all the principles of body mechanics:

- Avoid unnecessary bending, stretching and twisting
- Face the direction in which movement is to occur
- Use both arms and hands
- Turn the whole body when the direction of movement is changed
- Move with smooth even actions and avoid sudden jerking movements
- Obtain adequate assistance to move a heavy person or object, and use a lifting device
- Stand directly in front of the person or object to be moved, with the knees flexed to minimise back flexion.

In addition to using correct body mechanics themselves, nurses can promote the comfort and safety of clients by providing education about how to apply them when sitting, standing or walking and when pushing or pulling objects.

To sit correctly the buttocks should be positioned well back in the chair to promote spinal alignment. The feet should be flat on the floor, and the hips flexed slightly to reduce strain on the lower back. If the chair has arms, the elbows should be flexed and the forearms placed on the armrests to avoid shoulder strain. A variety of ergonomically designed chairs are available that promote correct body alignment and reduce muscle and joint strain.

To stand correctly the feet should be 15–20 cm apart with equal weight on both legs to minimise strain on the weight-bearing joints. The knees should be flexed slightly, the buttocks and abdomen retracted, the shoulders back and the neck straight.

To walk correctly, the correct standing position is assumed and then one leg is advanced a comfortable distance. The heel should touch the floor first, followed by the ball of the foot and then the toes. During this sequence the other arm and leg should be advanced to promote balance and stability.

To push or pull correctly it is necessary to stand close to the object and place one foot slightly ahead of the other. The elbows are flexed and the hands placed on the object. To push, smooth continuous pressure is applied by leaning into the object and transferring the weight from the back leg to the front leg. To pull, smooth continuous movement is used and the object is moved by leaning away from it. The weight is transferred from the front leg to the back leg and once the object is moving it should be kept in motion, as stopping and starting uses more energy.

Nurses are advised to wear suitable shoes for all workplace activities. Shoes that have low heels, flexible non-slip soles and closed backs promote body alignment and help to prevent accidents.

Health care facilities are obligated to provide educational programs for nurses in a range of health and safety areas, including programs concerned with fire safety, back safety and the no-lift policy. Many of them make such training programs compulsory for staff on an annual basis. Every individual employee has a responsibility to ensure that they are aware of the safety precautions and policies of the employing agency and to observe the standards set by the committees or others that are accountable for safety programs. Such programs are designed to create and maintain a safe environment, and prevent accidents or injury from any source.

IMMUNISATION FOR NURSES

Nurses are advised to take advantage of every opportunity provided to enhance their safety in the workplace. Many health care agencies and educational institutions offer immunisation programs to protect student nurses and nursing staff from the threat of infectious diseases. This is in accordance with the infection control guidelines provided by the Australian Government Department of Health and Ageing (2004) and the immunisation programs outlined by the Australian National Health and Medical Research Council (NHMRC 2007). It is recommended that nurses accept these offers or contact their own general practitioner to protect themselves from risk against any disease that poses a potential threat, such as hepatitis or tuberculosis. It is also recommended that any possibility of contamination by infectious body fluids or material of any sort be reported promptly and the suggested post-incident precautions be implemented as soon as possible (see Chapter 25).

AGGRESSION IN THE WORKPLACE

Some health care agencies have implemented educational programs to provide staff with skills to prevent and manage outbursts of aggression directed towards them by clients. While not a lot is known about how often this occurs in Australian and New Zealand health care settings, the risk to nurses' safety is a concern (Lam 2002). It is recommended that nurses undertake these specialised programs because the risk created by aggression in the workplace is reduced when staff have specific training in preventing aggression and developing conflict resolution skills (Essex 2001; Grenade & Macdonald 1995).

Nurses are sometimes faced with aggression in the form of workplace bullying and harassment. This may stem from managers, supervisors, co-workers or others in the workplace. This is behaviour that (usually intentionally) intimidates, offends, degrades or humiliates one or more workers, and may or may not be conducted in front of others (ANF 2007). Every workplace should have policies and processes in place to deal with reports of bullying or harassment but, unfortunately, this destructive workplace behaviour often goes unreported because those affected are too intimidated to come forward for assistance. Protective measures for nurses include:

- The ability to seek legal protection:
  - — the Commonwealth *Occupational Health and Safety Act 1986* offers some legal protection against acts of bullying and harassment. It stipulates that employers are legally bound to ensure the health and safety of employees and that workplace bullying and harassment are acts that can negatively affect the health and safety of employees
  - — the Commonwealth *Equal Opportunity Act 1984* offers some legal protection from acts of workplace discrimination. This covers bullying or harassment in relation to acts of racism or sexism and situations in which there is excessive scrutiny of a person's work, denial of access to training, being set up to fail or unfairly being denied opportunities for promotion.
- The ability to lodge an unfair dismissal claim if the nurse is dismissed for making a complaint or 'whistle blowing', meaning raising publicly an issue of bullying or harassment
- The ability to make a WorkCover claim if able to prove that personal stress has resulted from verbal abuse, intimidation or humiliation, all of which are deemed occupational violence
- The ability to access assistance from professional organisations that defend the rights of nurses. For example, the ANF has a policy relating to harassment, bullying and discrimination in the workplace, and has established methods of supporting nurses who experience unresolved acts of workplace harassment, bullying and discrimination (ANF 2007).

SUMMARY

Nurses have a professional responsibility to ensure that they are aware of policies and practices relating to safety and the prevention of harm in the workplace. In particular, nurses should be informed about infection prevention and control measures, fire risk prevention and management precautions and evacuation procedures, safe administration and storage of medications (see Chapter 28) and safe practice in all client care activities, including no-lift techniques.

Safety is a basic need of every individual throughout each stage of life. The very young and very old are at higher risk of harm than others but there are risks to safety associated with every age group. It is the role of the nurse to assess each client for factors that may increase their risk of harm and to assess any environment in which client care occurs for potential hazards. Some of the more common hazards include the risk of infection, thermal injury, harm by sharp items, poisons and falls. The nurse plans, implements and evaluates all necessary safety precautions and follows policy guidelines to ensure their own safety and that of every person in the workplace environment. As a last resort nurses may need to use restraints to protect clients from harm. Restraint is an invasion of human rights and is only appropriate when it is for the client's benefit and no other alternative is effective. Restraint should only be used according to strict legal and policy guidelines and nurses have a responsibility to involve themselves in identifying and advocating for the use of restraint minimisation measures in all areas of nursing practice.

Employers have a responsibility to ensure that nurses and all staff are informed about every area of safety concern, including infection prevention and control, fire prevention and management, the use of correct body mechanics and no-lift techniques. Nurses have a responsibility to promote safety in all health care settings, which include the clients' homes, schools, clinics, residential care settings and hospitals. Nurses also have a role in health promotion and can achieve this by educating clients about actions for personal protection, minimising hazards in the home and keeping the environment free from pollution. Quality nursing care incorporates consideration of safety and protection from harm in all environments and in all interactions with clients or residents.

REVIEW EXERCISES

1. What are five factors that may compromise the abilities of clients to protect themselves from health hazards in the home or in the health care environment?
2. State six nursing interventions that will reduce the risk of a client with impaired mobility from falling in the acute care hospital environment.
3. What actions could you recommend to a mother of a toddler that will reduce the child's risk of suffering a burn or scald in the home environment?
4. What actions could you recommend to a daughter caring for a mother who has dementia, which will reduce the risks to her mother from medications and other hazardous substances that are in the home environment?
5. What activities could you suggest to a client who wants to contribute to reducing the global problem of air pollution?
6. What are the nursing responsibilities in the event of a fire in the work environment?
7. What are the main principles guiding the safe moving and lifting of clients in the health care setting?

CRITICAL THINKING EXERCISES

1. Mr Cladell, 83, lives in an aged-care facility. He has Alzheimer's dementia but ambulates freely within the unit despite considerable physical frailty. Over the past 2 weeks he has fallen three times, but, fortunately, suffered relatively minor injuries (bruising). He had never fallen previously.
   a) What physical reasons might there be for Mr Cladell falling?
   b) What aspects of the environment might be related to his falls?
   c) Outline specific interventions that may be needed to reduce Mr Cladell's risk of injury from falls.
2. Mrs Kingsley, 72, is in an acute-care hospital after a collapse at home. She is receiving intravenous fluids to improve her hydration status. She has pulled her IV line out on one occasion and, although it has since been securely bound to her arm, she continues to pull at the IV line and is quite agitated. It has been suggested that an extremity restraint be used.
   a) Consider the merits of this action and consider what better alternatives there might be.
   b) Outline the measures needed before this restraint should be applied.
   c) What are the nursing responsibilities in relation to caring for Mrs Kingsley if the restraint is applied?

REFERENCES AND FURTHER READING

Australian Bureau of Statistics (2005) Ausstats 4364.0. *National Health Survey*. ABS, Canberra

Australian Government Department of Health and Ageing (2004) *Infection Control Guidelines for the prevention of transmission of infectious diseases in the health care setting*. Commonwealth of Australia Publication, Canberra ACT. Online. Available: www.health.gov.au/internet/wcms/publishing.nsf/Content//icg-guidelines-index.htm/$FILE/part1.pdf [accessed 20 March 2008]

Australian Nursing Federation (ANF) (2007) *Harassment, bullying and discrimination in the workplace policy.* Online. Available: www.anf.org.au/anf_pdf/P_Harassment.pdf [accessed 20 March 2008]

Australian Safety and Compensation Council (ASCC) 2005 *National OHS Strategy 2002–2012.* Australian Government, Canberra

Barraclough S, Gardner H (2007) *Analysing Health Policy: a problem-oriented approach*. Elsevier Australia, Sydney

Bryant B, Knights K, Salerno E (2006) *Pharmacology for Health Professionals*. Elsevier Australia, Sydney

Country Fire Authority, Community Safety Department (2003) *Secure Seniors Home Safety Checklist*. City of Greater Dandenong, Vic

Crisp J, Taylor C (eds) (2005) *Potter & Perry's Fundamentals of Nursing*, 2nd edn. Elsevier Australia, Sydney

Daly C (2007) *Transitions in Nursing: Preparing For Professional Practice*, 2nd edn. Elsevier Australia, Sydney

deWit S (2005) *Fundamental Concepts and Skills for Nursing, 2nd edn*. WB Saunders, Philadelphia

Ebersol P, Hess P, Luggen A (2007) *Toward Healthy Ageing.* Mosby, St Louis

Essex C (2001) NHS staff must be trained in how to prevent aggression. *British Medical Journal*, 323: 168

Faye B, Sellick M (2003) *Advocare's Speak Out Survey 'SOS' on Elder Abuse*. Advocare Inc. Perth, WA. Online. Available: www.advocare.org.au [accessed 10 May 2008]

Grenade D, Macdonald E (1995) Risk of physical assault among student nurses. *Occupational Medicine* 45: 236–58

Harulow S (2002) No lift, no injury goes from strength to strength. *Australian Nursing Federation Professional News* (April) Online. Available: www.anf.org.au/02_anf_news_professional/news_professional_0204.html [accessed 10 May 2008]

Joanna Briggs Institute (2002a) Physical Restraint Part 1: Use in acute and residential care facilities. In: Evidence based practice information sheets for health professionals. *Best Practice* 6(3): 1–5

—— (2002b) Physical Restraint Part 2: Minimisation in Acute and Residential Care Facilities. In: Evidence based practice information sheets for health professionals. *Best Practice* 6(4): 1–6

Kongstvedt PR (2007) *Essentials of Managed Health Care*. Jones and Bartlett, Boston

Lam L (2002) *Aggression Exposure and Mental Health Among Nurses. Australian e-journal for the advancement of mental health* 1(2) Online. Available: www.auseinet.com/journal/col1iss2/lam.pdf [accessed 10 May 2008]

Marshall K (2001) On the Record. *Australian Nurses Federation, Victorian Branch. Newsletter* (March): 9

Marsland D (2003) Evaluating the quality of support services for people with learning disabilities. In: Gates B (ed) (2003):

Learning Disabilities: Towards Inclusion, 4th edn. Harcourt, Edinburgh

National Ageing Research Institute (2004) *An analysis of Research on Preventing Falls and Falls Injury in Older People: Community, Residential Aged Care and Acute Care Settings*. Report to the Australian Government Department of Health and Ageing, Canberra

National Health and Medical Research Council (NHMRC) (2007) *The Australian Immunisation Handbook*, 9th edn. Commonwealth Government of Australia National Capital Printers, Canberra. Online. Available: http://www.health.gov.au/internet/immunise/publishing.nsf/content/handbook-9-c3.9 [accessed 20 March 2008]

National Occupational Health & Safety Commission (NOHSC) 2011 (2003) *National Code of Practice for the Preparation of Material Safety Data Sheets*, 2nd edn. Commonwealth of Australia, Canberra., MSDS Code 2022(2003)

Olsen D (1998) Toward an ethical standard for coerced mental health treatment: least restrictive or most therapeutic? *Journal of Clinical Ethics* 9 (3): 235

Perry AG, Potter PA (2002) *Clinical Nursing Skills & Techniques*, 5th edn. Mosby, St Louis

Runciman B, Merry A, Walton M (2007) *Safety and Ethics in Healthcare: A Guide to Getting It Right*. Ashgate Publishing, London

Socha T (2003) *Air Pollution and Effects*. http://healthandenergy.com/air_pollution_causes.htm [accessed 10 May 2008]

Springhouse Publishing Company Staff (2007) *Nursing: Perfecting Clinical Procedures*. Lippincott, Williams and Wilkins, Hagerstown, MD

Traudt J (2007) *Indoor Safety and Comfort*. Online. Available: http://healthandenergy.com/indoor_safety_and_comfort.htm [accessed 10 May 2008]

Watkins P (2001) *Mental Health Nursing: the Art of Compassionate Care*. Butterworth–Heinemann, Oxford.

Chapter 27

HYGIENE AND COMFORT

OBJECTIVES

- Define the key terms/concepts
- State the significance of personal hygiene to the maintenance of health
- Identify factors that influence hygiene practices
- Identify complications that may result if personal hygiene is neglected
- Perform nursing procedures for client hygiene accurately and safely
- Identify the factors that may interfere with client comfort
- Identify the importance of a well-made bed and comfortable positioning of clients to the promotion of health and wellbeing
- Apply appropriate principles to select supplementary equipment used in conjunction with bed making
- Apply appropriate principles when planning and implementing measures to promote comfort
- Describe the positions that clients may be required to assume in bed

KEY TERMS/CONCEPTS

divided bed
occupied bed
operation bed
personal hygiene
positioning of client for comfort
positioning of client for examinations and treatment
principles in promoting comfort
principles of bed making
supplementary equipment
unoccupied bed

CHAPTER FOCUS

Hygiene is the science of health and its preservation and can also be described as cleanliness that is conducive to the preservation of health. Personal cleanliness helps the individual to maintain a positive body image and helps protect the body against disease such as infection. Comfort may be described as ease or wellbeing; for people to feel comfortable their physiological, psychological and spiritual needs must be met. This chapter introduces nurses to knowledge and skills required to assist clients with their hygiene and physical comfort needs.

LIVED EXPERIENCE

The thing that I value most is the nurse who is calm and organised, gets all of my things ready before helping me get undressed for my shower. There is nothing worse than being left cold and shivering while the nurse runs to get something that was forgotten. It makes a difference, too, having my mouth cleaned thoroughly, especially after I've eaten, and having my hair brushed properly. It's so frustrating not being able to do everything for myself anymore. I wonder if the nurses really know what a huge difference it makes to my life to feel clean and fresh and tidy and to get that way with a minimum of fuss.

Glenda, age 50, with multiple sclerosis

Many factors influence whether or not a client is comfortable; they relate to physical, emotional and spiritual needs being met. To most people, physical comfort means being clean, dry, warm and free of hunger and pain. Emotional comfort relates more to being relatively free from stress and feeling satisfied with interpersonal relationships; in particular, people are more likely to be emotionally content when they feel loved and are able to love others. Spiritual comfort is connected to a sense of purpose and satisfaction in life that may or may not be entwined with religious meaning. The nurse considers all these interrelated elements when caring for clients' comfort. This chapter deals with the physical elements of comfort, specifically in relation to hygiene care and moving and positioning clients. Management of pain is dealt with in depth in Chapter 35. Information about assisting clients with stress and spiritual comfort is provided in Chapters 11 and 13.

FACTORS AFFECTING PERSONAL HYGIENE

Personal hygiene refers to the measures people take to keep their bodies clean. Neglect of personal hygiene can have a detrimental effect on physical and psychological health and the comfort of an individual. Many factors influence people with regard to personal hygiene practices. It is important for nurses to appreciate that emphasis on cleanliness varies according to an individual's personal preference, cultural or religious values, and lifestyle. Other factors that may affect an individual's hygiene practices include:

- Stage of development
- Level of independence
- Physical and intellectual capabilities
- Emotional state
- Economic status
- Knowledge of the significance of hygiene
- Availability of facilities (e.g. water)
- Environment or climate.

Nurses should respect individual preferences and cultural norms and whenever possible enable clients to follow their usual routine of personal cleansing. For example, if a client prefers to bath rather than shower or to shower in the evening rather than the morning, or to shower every second day, these practices are best continued. Maintaining routine and normality can help limit the stress of illness.

Many clients will be able to attend to their own hygiene, while others will require partial or total assistance from the nurse. Some clients — those who are unconscious, for example — will be unable to participate in planning their own hygiene care. In these instances it is the responsibility of the nurse to ensure that suitable nursing care plans are devised to meet hygiene needs. Assessing clients' abilities to care for their own hygiene needs safely and effectively includes identifying factors such as loss of balance, poor vision, decreased sense of touch or limitations in mobility. In the case of some older people with dementia, the ability to remember, plan and carry out self-care activities will need to be assessed. It is important for the nurse to recognise that an inability to care for personal hygiene needs without assistance, and the lack of privacy that accompanies intervention by another person, can be very embarrassing for the client. The associated loss of independence can be demoralising and depressing. A calm, sensitive, caring and professional approach can help reduce these effects. The nurse who is providing care in the client's home needs to be mindful that, for some, even necessary visits by helpful professionals may feel like an invasion of the sanctity that home normally provides.

Wherever care is provided, the nurse's role is to ensure that the client maintains high standards of personal hygiene for efficient body function and sense of wellbeing. It is important for the nurse to be aware of the function and care requirements of areas such as the skin, hair, mouth, eyes, nose, ears and nails to help clients maintain high standards of personal hygiene in each of these areas. Assisting with hygiene provides an ideal opportunity for the nurse to observe and assess the client for any abnormalities or changes in health status. It also provides a time to talk informally together, which can provide the nurse with insights about the client's psychological and spiritual wellbeing. The nurse must, on every occasion, seek the consent of the client before starting to provide any personal care and assistance.

SKIN AND SKIN CARE

The skin is a semipermeable layer that protects underlying tissues and organs from injury or invasion by microorganisms. It is waterproof, controls the rate at which water is lost from the body by evaporation, helps regulate body temperature, and produces keratin, melanin, sweat and sebum. The skin also plays an important role in perception of sensation through the sensory nerve endings it contains, which are sensitive to touch, pressure, pain and temperature. (See Chapters 37 and 42 for more information about the skin and sensory abilities.)

If the skin is not washed regularly dirt, sebum, dried sweat and dead skin cells collect, providing an ideal medium for the growth of bacteria and fungi. Bacteria decompose the dirt and dried sweat producing an unpleasant body odour, and infections such as boils are more likely if the skin is not cleansed adequately.

Skin undergoes many changes during a person's life span and, as a result, care needs may vary according to the client's age or stage of development. In addition, characteristics of normal skin may vary according to ethnic or racial background.

INFANTS

In infancy the skin is soft and smooth and less resistant to injury or infection. It is very sensitive to heat or cold, so it is vital that the temperature of bath water is tested before bathing. Mild non-irritating soaps and lotions should be used on the skin and, as the infant has no bladder or bowel control, thorough cleansing of the genital and anal areas is necessary to prevent excoriation. After washing, the infant's skin should be patted dry with a soft towel paying particular attention to skin creases and folds. Cradle cap, a crusting on the scalp, which may occur as a result of an accumulation of sebum, can usually be prevented by regular gentle washing and drying of the scalp and hair (Barker 2007; Pantley 2003).

ADOLESCENTS

Adolescence is accompanied by many changes that are due to hormonal activity. Sweating from the axilla usually occurs at this stage and the adolescent may need education concerning the importance of having a regular shower or bath. Education can also include information about the function of deodorant and antiperspirant. Acne is a common problem, and skin hygiene, together with a balanced diet, is important in preventing secondary skin infections.

THE MIDDLE YEARS

Middle age is often associated with further skin changes, particularly during the female climacteric or menopause. Because of a decrease in circulating ovarian hormone levels, the skin may become drier and the pubic and axillary hair may become sparse. Some women experience thinning and dryness of the external genitalia, which may be accompanied by pruritus. Lubricants are available to reduce the discomfort this can produce.

OLDER ADULTS

Older age is associated with increasing changes in the dermis, with the result that skin is thinner, less elastic and dry. The decreased production of sebum and associated dryness mean that the skin of older people is less able to tolerate soap. To help counteract the dryness, a mild soap or soap-free washing lotion can be used. Oil may be added to the bath water, or a moisturising lotion applied after a bath or shower. To prevent skin irritation caused by dry skin some older people choose to change from a daily shower or bath to every second day or less frequently (Clinical Interest Box 27.1).

CLINICAL INTEREST BOX 27.1
Hygiene and the elderly

My skin just won't tolerate being washed every day now, even when I use plenty of cream, my legs are still flaky and itchy, so now I only have a shower every other day. You know, I just stand at the sink and wash the essential bits, under my arms and the private bits down below. A 'top and tail' I call it. Even when I do shower I can't use soap on my legs.

(Mrs Bolton, age 72)

NURSING OBSERVATIONS OF THE SKIN

The skin should be observed for:

- Colour. Particular note should be taken of any abnormalities such as pallor, jaundice, cyanosis or altered pigmentation. Areas of red, deep pink or mottled skin that does not become paler with fingertip pressure may be a sign that a pressure ulcer is developing. (See Chapter 37 for information on the development and prevention of pressure ulcers.)
- Hydration. Deviations from normal include excessive dryness or oiliness, increased sweating and fluid retention (oedema)
- Texture. The skin may be smooth and supple or contain rough scaly patches. It is also important to observe if the skin appears thin and fragile
- Turgor. Picking up and then releasing a small fold of skin is the simplest way to assess skin turgor. Adequately hydrated skin returns rapidly to its previous state, whereas the skin of a client who is dehydrated is slow to respond. The skin of an older client may also resume its shape more slowly because of reduced elasticity
- Lesions. The skin should be observed for the presence of bruises, blisters, inflammation, rashes, localised swellings such as cysts, petechiae, bites, scratch marks or puncture marks.

Abnormalities and changes are reported and documented and appropriate nursing care implemented in response to nursing observations.

Care of the skin includes maintenance of cleanliness and protection from injury. The skin must be protected against injury by gentle handling and the use of appropriate bed linen and equipment. Cleansing involves the use of soaps and lotions that do not cause irritation or dryness, and careful drying of the skin, particularly in folds or creases. If the client wishes, and it is not contraindicated, deodorants, powders and perfumes may be used to enhance the feeling of freshness and to improve morale. Cleansing of the skin may be achieved by several means and the method selected depends on the client's level of mobility and independence. Some clients will be able to have a bath or shower, while more dependent clients may require a bed or trolley bath. Whichever method of cleansing is used the nurse must ensure the client's privacy, comfort and safety. It is now sometimes a reality that male and female clients are accommodated in the same ward or unit area and some even share bathroom and toilet facilities. This can increase the client's discomfort and concerns about privacy, especially during hygiene and toileting procedures. The nurse will need to be sensitive to the concerns of clients faced with this situation and make every possible effort to reassure them that every effort will be made to maintain their personal privacy (Crisp & Taylor 2005; deWit 2005; Springhouse Staff 2007).

BATHING AND SHOWERING

A client may have either a bath or a shower, depending on individual preference and general condition. Both methods of cleansing refresh the client, stimulate circulation and promote relaxation. They also provide an opportunity for the nurse to observe the condition of the client's body, including assessment of mobility and strength.

NURSING OBSERVATIONS AND ASSESSMENT

If clients are able to attend to personal hygiene needs safely and independently, they may be left to bath or shower in private. It is the responsibility of the nurse to ensure that the bathroom has been prepared for use, and that the client has all the necessary items. The nurse should ensure that the client knows where the signal bell is and how to use it to call for a nurse.

It is the nurse's responsibility to assess how much assistance a more dependent client requires. Some clients may need help to get in or out of the bath or shower, while others will require the nurse to remain with them throughout the entire procedure. The nurse should remain with, and provide assistance for, any client who is weak, frail, unsteady or confused. Some clients may require a waterproof chair to sit on during the shower. For example, a chair would be helpful for a postoperative client who can walk to the shower but is at risk of becoming easily fatigued.

DEVICES TO ASSIST WITH BATHING OR SHOWERING

There are several other devices designed to assist the nurse with bathing or showering clients. These include handrails, bath seats, mechanical hoists, mobile baths and shower trolleys.

Handrails fixed to the wall at the side of the bath or shower can be used for support by clients who are able to stand. Bath benches or seats fit across the top of a bath, allowing clients who find it difficult to get in and out of the bath to sit with their feet in the water and be sponged down or, if there is a shower nozzle fitted over the bath, to be showered. Bath seats are commonly used in the home. Grab rails are often fitted on the wall adjacent to the bath to assist clients who are frail or weak.

A mobile hydraulic or electronic lifting device consists of a sturdy metal frame with a wide base of support from which a seat or sling is suspended. The lifting device is on wheels, which makes it relatively easily moved by one person when it is empty. A rechargeable battery is used to power an electronic device that enables even heavy clients to be moved with ease. A hydraulic pump is used to lift the client. A mobile lifting device can be wheeled to the bed and the seat or sling lowered to bed level so that the client can be transferred safely. The design and use of lifting devices varies according to the manufacturer, but safety and the client's sense of security are best maintained by having two nurses present when a client is being lifted with any mechanical device. One nurse can then operate the device while the other supports and guides the client during the lift and transfer to the bathroom.

It is generally easier to remove the client's clothing before the lift and transfer to the bathroom, but being moved around in a lifting device can feel extremely undignified and distressing. The utmost care must be taken to ensure that the client's privacy and dignity are maintained, in particular the client's private body areas must be securely covered from view during transfer to the bathroom. The prospect of being lifted in a machine can be very frightening and may increase existing feelings of vulnerability. It may help reduce anxiety if clients are given an opportunity to see how the hoist works before the first occasion on which it is used to lift and assist them.

When the client is correctly and safely positioned in the seat or sling, two nurses wheel the machine to the bathroom. The client can be lowered effortlessly into the bath by mechanically adjusting the height of the seat or sling. The client remains on the seat or sling throughout the procedure. Mechanical hoists facilitate safe client transfer in and out of the bath and they eliminate strain on the nurse's back. Mechanical hoists with fabric slings can also be used to transfer clients between bed and chair or bed and trolley. Any client that requires the use of a mechanical lifting machine must never be left unattended in the device or in the bath. Clients who may require the use of a mechanical lifter include those who are heavy or extremely weak, frail or helpless. As hoists are made in a variety of styles, the nurse must check the manufacturer's instructions concerning the use of each machine, in particular the safe application of the fabric slings.

Hoists are large pieces of equipment. When clients require them in the home, structural alterations to the house may be necessary to facilitate their use. Government-funded care packages sometimes provide for this need. In some situations nurses teach family members who are providing home-based care for dependent relatives how to use the hoist safely.

Fixed bath chairs are fixed to the floor at the side of the bath. They are equipped with a hydraulic mechanism for lowering and raising the seat. The client sits on the seat, which is manoeuvred over the edge of the bath and then lowered into the water. The client remains on the seat while being bathed and during transfer out of the bath.

Mobile baths are available in some health care facilities. A mobile bath can be moved to the client's bedside. The client is transferred from the bed into the bath and transported to the bathroom. The bath is filled and the client bathed in the usual manner.

Shower trolleys are designed for use in the normal shower area. Using a hoist, the client is positioned onto the trolley and wheeled to the bathroom. A foot pump is then used to blow up an inflatable edge that surrounds all sides of the trolley. This converts the trolley into a shallow bath. A drainage hose underneath the trolley is directed to the drainage hole of the shower recess and the client is washed by the nurse using the shower nozzle.

Whenever and wherever mechanical aids are used,

nurses must be familiar with the operational safety aspects of each one. A full explanation about the aid being used, reassurance about its safety, and maintaining the client's personal privacy and dignity during use are important components of reducing stress and embarrassment for the client. Examples of some aids that are available are illustrated in Figure 27.1.

CLIENTS REQUIRING SPECIAL CONSIDERATION

Clients who are weak, frail, unsteady or confused will require the nurse's assistance to bath or shower. Key aspects of assisting a client are outlined in Table 27.1. A client may feel faint and collapse in the bath or shower. If this occurs the nurse should immediately drain the bath or turn off the shower. Towels should be used to cover the client for warmth and dignity and extra towels should be placed under the client's legs and feet to increase venous return. The nurse should summon immediate assistance and remain with the client, ensuring that the airway is clear. (See Chapter 48 for full emergency care actions in situations in which a person has fainted.)

Some clients will require special consideration when bathing or showering; for example, special attention is needed for clients who have drainage or intravenous (IV) tubing, wound dressings, plaster casts or specific skin disorders. There may also be special needs associated with surgical or other interventions.

A client with IV tubing

Careful handling is necessary to avoid kinking or dislodging any tubing, and precautions must be taken to prevent the IV insertion site becoming wet. Mechanical IV pumps may be switched to battery mode during the time a client is showering. The pump can be switched off for a short period of time while the client's clothing, such as night attire or hospital gown, is removed and replaced with a clean one.

Intravenous tubing and the flask or bag containing the IV fluid should be positioned above the level of the client's heart to maintain flow of the fluid into the vein. Lowering the container causes a reversal of pressures that may result in the infusion stopping and blood from the client's vein flowing into the IV tube.

A 1

2

3

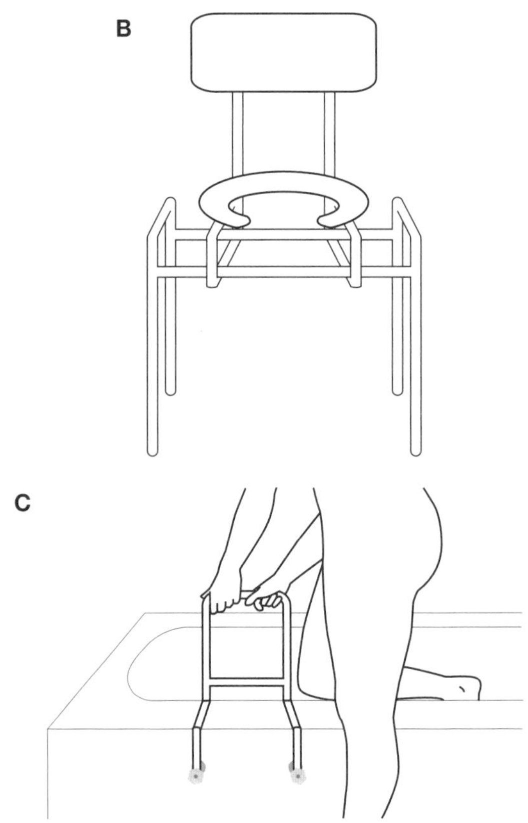

Figure 27.1 | Devices to assist bathing and showering. **A**: Mechanical lifting device. 1) Lower client, transport to bathroom in this position and raise clear of bath. 2) Position over bath. 3) Lower client and perform bathing **B**: Shower chair. **C**: Handrail attached to the side of the bath

TABLE 27.1 | GUIDELINES FOR ASSISTING A CLIENT TO BATH OR SHOWER

Review and carry out the standard steps in Appendix 1

Action	Rationale
Prepare the bathroom:	
• Adjust temperature and exclude draughts	Avoids chilling
• Ensure bath or shower is clean	Prevents cross-infection
• Ensure there is a non-slip mat or strips in the bottom of the bath or shower recess and a bathmat on the floor	Provides non-slippery areas, thus preventing falls
• Place a chair beside the bath or shower, or in the shower if needed (unless a mechanical hoist is used)	Provides a seat for the client while undressing and dressing or showering
• Ensure that all the required items are assembled in the bathroom and within easy reach	Avoids the nurse needing to leave the area at any stage
Assess the client's mobility and strength, and gain assistance if necessary to assist client to the bathroom	Adequate assistance is necessary to promote safety and comfort
Offer the client use of toilet facilities before procedure	Helps to promote comfort
Adjust the water flow and temperature (if not automatically regulated) before client begins cleansing. Water temperature of 38–41°C is comfortable and safe for most clients. Turn on cold water first, then hot water when filling bath. Turn hot water off first	Prevents scalding. Water that is too hot may cause peripheral vasodilation and faintness
Help the client sit down and undress	Reduces the risk of falls
Observe the condition of the client's skin	Detects any abnormalities
Using mechanical devices if appropriate, assist the client into the bath or shower. Offer a chair to sit on in the shower	Promotes safety, prevents falls
Ensure that the client is positioned away from the taps	Reduces risk of scalds
Encourage the client to participate as much as able, ensuring that all body areas are washed and that the skin is rinsed free of all soap	Promotes independence and adequate cleansing
When the client has completed washing, drain the bath or turn off the shower	Facilitates easier and safer exit from the bath or shower
Assist the client from the bath or shower and ensure that drying is thorough	Prevents excoriation, promotes comfort
While being dried the client should be seated or standing, holding supporting rails if able	Reduces fatigue, promotes safety
Enquire if the client wishes to use powder or deodorant. Avoid excessive amounts of powder	Powder can accumulate and 'cake' on the skin
Ensure that the client is dressed without delay	Helps to minimise fatigue and prevent chilling
Ensure that the client's oral hygiene and hair-care needs are attended to. Assist a male patient with a facial shave as required	Promotes comfort and self-esteem
Escort the client back to their room and allow a rest period if required	Restores energy after the exertion of the bath
Ensure that the client is comfortably positioned with all requirements within reach	Helps to promote comfort, sense of security and safety
Attend to the bathroom: • Air room if possible • Ensure that bath or shower is clean • Remove any soiled linen • Return personal articles to the client's unit	Ventilates the room and removes steam, prepares area for further use and minimises risk of cross-infection
Report and document	Client's condition is evaluated so that appropriate care can be planned and implemented

A client with a urinary catheter or wound-drainage tubing

Drainage tubing and the container receiving the drainage fluid must be positioned below the area where the tubing is inserted to promote drainage and to prevent backflow.

A client with a wound dressing or bandage

The Enrolled Nurse (EN) should check the nursing care plan, providing it is current, or ask the nurse in charge if the dressing or bandage is to be removed before the bath or shower. If wound coverings or bandages are to remain in position they must be protected from moisture.

A client with a plaster cast on a limb

A waterproof cover must be applied securely over the limb to protect the plaster from moisture.

A client with a skin disorder, or who has had perineal or rectal surgery

A substance to be added to the bath water may be prescribed, such as salt or pinetar preparation. The nurse should also ascertain whether a lotion or cream has been prescribed for application following the bath. The nurse must be aware of the policies, guidelines and scope of practice for ENs in the geographical area of employment in relation to the application of any cream or lotion that contains medication. Where the application of medicated creams or lotions is within the nurse's scope of practice, gloves should be applied before they are administered because they are absorbed through the skin.

BATHING THE CLIENT IN BED

Clients who are confined to bed or whose condition does not enable them to have a bath or shower may be provided with equipment for washing in bed, or may be given a bed bath by the nurse. If clients are able to wash unaided they are provided with all necessary items, the upper bedclothes turned down, and a towel placed over them for warmth and privacy. The nurse will need to help with washing and drying the back and any other parts of the body the client is unable to attend to independently. When each bath is completed and each client's hair and teeth have been attended to, the nurse remakes the bed.

A complete bed bath involves washing the entire body of a client in bed. It is performed by the nurse when a client is unable to wash unaided. Clients who may require a bed bath include those who have a debilitating illness or are paralysed or unconscious. A bed bath is also frequently needed after surgery. Depending on the client's level of mobility, either one or two nurses perform the procedure. Health care facilities commonly adopt their own specific guidelines concerning how to perform a bed bath. An alternative to the traditional sponge bowl method is the bag bath method (Clinical Interest Box 27.2).

The following description of conducting a bed bath explains a more common approach. The basic equipment required for a bed bath is:

> **CLINICAL INTEREST BOX 27.2**
> **Bag bath method of washing a client in bed**
>
> This method involves the use of a bag containing 10 pre-moistened disposable cloths, each one used for a different area of the client's body. A bag bath is convenient because it is made ready quickly by warming in the microwave oven and it avoids the use of a bowl filled with water. Bowls, if not cleaned satisfactorily, are a source of microorganisms. Therefore bag baths can reduce the risk of infection. However, they are an expensive option and are not used as commonly as other methods.

- Wash bowl with warm water
- Soap (on a soap dish)
- Two bath towels
- Two face washers
- Items for oral hygiene (e.g. toothbrush, toothpaste, denture cup, water)
- Hair brush and/or comb
- Powder, deodorant, body lotion (optional)
- As indicated:
  — clean bed linen
  — clean night clothes
  — nail brush
  — shaving equipment, make-up
  — container for soiled linen.

Key aspects related to performing a bed bath or sponge are:

- Throughout the bed bath the nurse should promote the privacy, safety and comfort of the client, while ensuring that all hygiene needs are met
- During the bed bath the nurse assesses the status of the client's skin, hair, nails and level of mobility. The bed bath also provides time to talk with the client without interruption and it is often during this time that issues of concern are raised
- Clients should be encouraged to help themselves as much as they are able, to promote independence
- Clients who have not been bathed in bed before may be embarrassed about the exposure of their bodies and their loss of independence. It is the responsibility of the nurse to demonstrate sensitivity and to ensure adequate privacy throughout the procedure. The client's privacy and warmth is maintained by exposing only the area that is being washed: this is achieved by using a dry towel to cover other areas of the client's body
- The nurse who is to perform the bed bath must be aware if there are any limitations of movement or positioning for the client. For example, a client who has had a total hip replacement must not lie on the affected side and a client who is experiencing difficulty in breathing may need to remain sitting up throughout the bed bath to prevent further respiratory distress
- When dressing a client who has some impairment of an arm or leg (e.g. paralysis), the affected limb should be placed into the garment first so that maximum use may be made of the flexibility of the unaffected limb
- If a client is experiencing pain (e.g. after surgery) ensure that prescribed analgesia is given before the bed bath is performed
- Ensure that the water is the correct temperature and changed throughout the procedure when it becomes cool, too soapy, dirty or after washing the genital area
- If clients have a range of movement that permits it, when cleaning nails it may be helpful to place their hands and/or feet in the bowl of water. This is more

refreshing for clients and enables the nails to be cleansed more effectively

- Ensure that all soap is rinsed off the skin, as residual soap may cause dryness
- Special care should be taken to ensure that all skin folds and creases are washed and thoroughly dried; for example, under breasts, in the groin area, between the buttocks, fingers and toes. If these areas are not dried properly the skin may become excoriated and painful
- If the client's skin is very dry, bath oil may be used instead of soap, or a moisturising lotion applied after the bed bath
- Throughout the bed bath the client's skin should be observed for areas of redness, breaks, bruises and other deviations from normal. (See Chapter 37 for information concerning skin changes and identifying signs of developing pressure ulcers [decubitus ulcers].) Deviations should be reported and documented. Nursing measures should be implemented as appropriate
- If the client has an indwelling urinary catheter or has had certain types of perineal or vaginal surgery, special care should be taken with perineal hygiene
- During the bed bath the client's joints should be put through the full range of motion, unless this is contraindicated. Movement improves circulation, maintains joint mobility, and preserves muscle tone.

Table 27.2 provides the complete guidelines for performing a bed bath.

Perineal care

Many clients prefer to wash their own perineal area, and privacy should be provided for them if they are able to do so. The nurse may provide a degree of privacy by holding the covering towel or sheet up and away from the client's body, forming a tent while the client washes their genital area beneath it. If the client is unable to wash the perineum unaided the nurse is advised to put on gloves and to place an underpad beneath the client to protect the mattress. Only the area to be washed should be exposed. If faecal material is present it should be enclosed in a fold of underpad or tissue or removed with disposable wipes or tissues. The anus and buttocks are then cleansed and dried and the soiled underpad removed and replaced with a clean one. The perineum should be washed and rinsed thoroughly and patted dry. Care should be taken to wash a female client's perineum from front to back to minimise the risk of contamination from the anal area. Frequent perineal care may be needed for menstruating women. If needed, a fresh perineal pad should be put in place at the completion of the perineal wash.

Care should be taken to retract the foreskin of uncircumcised adult male clients so that the head of the penis can be cleaned effectively. Once the area is cleaned the foreskin should be returned to its natural position. The scrotum should be lifted and the area below washed, rinsed and dried thoroughly. Retraction of an infant's or child's foreskin is not recommended. The foreskin is resistive to retraction until separation of the foreskin and glans penis occurs naturally at about age 3–5 years. After this it is recommended that the child's foreskin be checked only very occasionally for retraction. It is recommended that the child's mother undertake this during the routine bath at home (Leifer 2007; Pantley 2003). Therefore, under normal circumstances the nurse will not need to retract the foreskin of children during their hygiene care. However, if the tip of a child's penis shows signs of irritation this should be reported and documented. Normally this will clear up within a few days if a protective ointment, such as oil of vitamin E or an antibiotic ointment is applied after gentle cleansing (Peron 1991).

If there is a urinary catheter in situ, the area around it should be carefully washed with soap and water. When the perineal wash is completed the underpad is removed and the client made comfortable.

Providing intimate care can cause embarrassment to the nurse and to the client, but this should never result in personal hygiene being neglected. A professional, dignified and sensitive manner can help with uncomfortable feelings. Chapter 12 addresses issues of embarrassment during intimate care (Crisp & Taylor 2005; deWit 2005).

BATHING AN INFANT

Bath time should be an enjoyable occasion for the infant, and the bath should be completed as quickly and safely as possible. Preparation for a bath includes:

- Ensuring that the room is warm and draught-free
- Warming the towels and clothing
- Assembling all the items required: baby bath half-filled with water at 38°C; bath thermometer; two towels; a face washer; cotton wool swabs and cotton tipped applicators; mild soap or cleansing lotion; a clean set of clothing and napkins; baby oil, cream or powder; clean linen for the cot; a receptacle for soiled linen; hair brush; nail scissors; and gown or apron
- Preparing an area (e.g. on the bench or table beside the bath) on which the infant can be placed while being undressed, dried and dressed. A towel should be placed on the bench to provide a soft and warm area on which to place the infant.

The procedure for bathing the infant is as follows:

- Wash hands and put on gown or apron
- Lift the infant from the cot and place on the prepared area beside the bath
- Undress the infant, except for the nappy, which is left on
- Wrap the infant in a towel, and wash the face with cotton wool swabs moistened with warm water. Items such as cotton swabs should not be inserted into the nose or ears (Leifer 2007). The inside of the ears should be left alone, but the outer ear should

TABLE 27.2 | GUIDELINES FOR PERFORMING A BED BATH

Review and carry out the standard steps in Appendix 1

Action	Rationale
Offer the client use of toilet facilities before starting the procedure	Helps promote comfort during the procedure
Clear the top of the locker or over-bed table	Provides space for bath equipment
Shut windows and doors and/or draw the screens around the bed and close blinds	Promotes privacy and warmth
Adjust the bed to a suitable height	Facilitates the procedure and prevents strain on the nurse's back
Assemble all the items necessary at the bedside	Nurse must remain with the client throughout the procedure
Ascertain whether the assistance of a second or more nurses or a mechanical lifting device is necessary	Promotes comfort and safety
Wash and dry hands	Prevents cross-infection
Remove the upper bed covers and place them on a chair. Place a towel over the client	Facilitates the procedure and promotes warmth and privacy
Remove the client's upper nightclothes	Exposes the body for adequate cleansing
Position the client lying back on one or two pillows, unless contraindicated	Allows a relaxing position, facilitates the procedure and prevents it from causing discomfort or distress
Begin to wash and dry the client (using one towel to protect the bedclothes) in the following suggested order: • Face and neck • Arms and hands • Axillae, chest and breasts • Abdomen • Legs and feet • Genitals and groin (change water now) • Back and buttocks	Logical progression that ensures that all areas of the body are washed
Roll the client onto one side of the bed to wash the back. Straighten or replace the bottom bed sheets	Avoids moving the client again unnecessarily
Roll the client onto the other side and fit the bottom sheet into position over the mattress	To complete making the bottom part of the bed
Dress the client in clean nightclothes	Promotes warmth and comfort
Replace pillows and assist the client into position	Promotes comfort
Attend to the client's hair and oral hygiene and a facial shave if necessary	All hygiene needs must be attended to
Replace the upper bedclothes and remove the towel	Promotes comfort and warmth
Replace equipment (e.g. the client's personal items in the locker, and the signal device in easy reach)	Ensures that the surroundings are tidy and that client has easy access to their belongings
Disinfect wash bowl and tooth mug after use, in accordance with agency protocol	Infection control
Remove soiled linen container	
Wash and dry hands	
Note client's response, document the procedure and report observations	Appropriate care can be planned and implemented

be cleansed with moistened cottonwool. Pat the face gently to dry

- With the infant on the bench, unwrap the towel and remove the nappy. The infant should be washed in a top-to-toe direction, turning the surface of the washcloth as the bath progresses. The genitalia should be washed from front to back to prevent faecal matter from coming into contact with the urethra, as this would risk the onset of a urinary tract infection. A mild soap may be needed for heavily soiled areas. The type of soap used varies with each health care agency. Alkaline soaps should be avoided because they alter the pH of skin (Leifer 2007). Particular attention should be paid to the skin folds, axillae, groin and between the fingers and toes
- The nurse lifts the infant by sliding the left arm under the infant's neck and shoulders to hold the infant's left upper arm. The nurse's right arm is placed under the infant's buttocks to hold the left leg. The infant is gently lowered into the water, and the nurse's left arm

and hand remain in position to support and control the infant's movements. (A left-handed nurse would probably be more comfortable reversing these arm positions.)
- Using the right hand the nurse rinses off the infant's body. The infant should be allowed some time to splash and kick in the water
- The nurse then lifts the infant from the bath and returns the infant to the prepared bench. The infant is dried quickly but thoroughly. Where skin areas come in contact with each other there is a possibility of chafing, and particular care is needed when drying these areas, which include the folds of the neck, behind the ears, the axillae and the groin. Oil or cream may be applied sparingly (e.g. to the buttocks). The type of oils and creams used varies with different health care facilities. The use of baby powder is not recommended because it may irritate the respiratory tract (Leifer 2007)
- The infant is then dressed before becoming cold. The nappy is placed on first, then the singlet, then the gown, and then the hair is gently brushed.

The infant is then returned to the cot, which is made up with clean linen. A second nurse may be available to make the cot while the infant is being bathed, or the infant may be placed in an infant chair while the cot is made up. The infant should be placed in the cot lying on the back — the position recommended to reduce the incidence of sudden infant death syndrome (SIDS) (Barker 2007; Leifer 2007; Pantley 2003). Very young infants feel more secure if they are wrapped in a light blanket before the upper bedclothes are placed over them. The nurse should ensure that the sides of the cot are pulled up and fastened securely.

The used items are then attended to and the bath cleaned before it is used again. After washing the hands the nurse reports and documents anything of concern relating to the infant. (Areas that should be observed and assessed and abnormalities that may occur in infants are outlined in Chapter 23). As the infant grows rapidly in the first 12 months, the procedure is adapted to suit the child's developmental level and, as the child grows, most of the actual washing is done in the bath, with the nurse supporting the infant as needed. Infants and young children must never be left unsupervised in a bath. Nurses have an important role in providing support and reassurance for new mothers, particularly when instructing them how to bath their babies.

HAIR CARE

Hair is modified epithelium and provides protection for underlying structures; for example, the hair on the head protects the scalp, and the eyelashes protect the eyes. Hair that is not washed and brushed tends to become tangled, greasy and malodorous. The scalp can become encrusted with sebum and dried sweat, which causes a feeling of discomfort. In an attempt to relieve the discomfort the individual may scratch the scalp and cause breaks in the skin that provide a portal of entry for microorganisms.

Hair care includes beard and moustache care as well as shaving, brushing, combing and shampooing head hair. Brushing and combing the hair stimulates scalp circulation, removes shed skin cells and distributes the natural oils that give the hair a healthy sheen. Shampooing removes grease, dirt, blood or other substances and prevents an offensive odour. Appearance is important to most people, so hair that is well groomed generally promotes morale and a positive body image. The frequency of hair care depends on the length and texture of the hair, the client's usual practice and general condition. Hair should be brushed or combed at least twice daily and shampooed according to personal preference or as necessary. During long periods of hospitalisation, clients may desire the services of a hairdresser to cut or style their hair, but hair should not be cut or restyled unless the client gives permission. Brushes and combs should be washed regularly and never shared between clients.

NURSING OBSERVATIONS AND ASSESSMENT OF THE HAIR AND SCALP

As part of client assessment the nurse should observe for and report any abnormalities such as excessive dryness, hair fragility or dandruff, alopecia (hair loss) or pediculosis capitis (head lice). The scalp should be observed for redness, heavy scaling, flaking or lesions. Some clients will be able to care for their hair independently, while others will require the nurse's assistance. Clients may have their hair shampooed during a bath or a shower, or it may be done with the client sitting in front of a sink. If the client is confined to bed the hair may be washed with the client in bed or lying on a trolley.

WASHING THE CLIENT'S HAIR IN BED

Certain devices are available to facilitate hair washing in bed, such as a shampoo tray (Figure 27.2A). If specially designed equipment is not available, a waterproof sheet can be placed under the client's head and arranged so that the water can drain into a bucket at the side of the bed (Figure 27.2B). Clients who can be moved from the bed onto a trolley may be wheeled to a sink and positioned so that the neck is supported on a pillow and the head extended over the sink (Figure 27.2C).

The method of giving the client a shampoo is usually determined by the facilities available and the client's condition. A suggested procedure for shampooing the hair of a client confined to bed is outlined in Table 27.3. The basic equipment for shampooing the hair consists of:
- Shampoo of the client's choice
- Conditioner if desired
- Two bath towels
- One face washer
- Protection for the bed (e.g. a waterproof sheet)

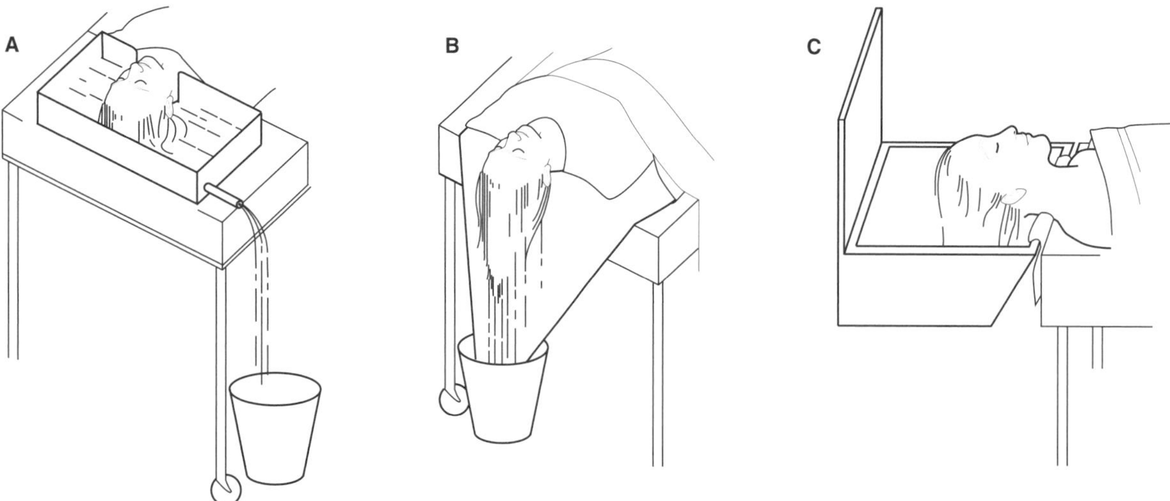

Figure 27.2 | Hair washing in bed. **A**: Using a shampoo tray. **B**: Making a trough from a waterproof sheet. **C**: Client on a trolley with the head over a sink

- Warm water (directed with handheld nozzle or jug)
- Brush and comb
- Hair dryer if available
- Shampoo tray or equipment for fashioning a trough
- A receptacle for soiled water.

If a client is too ill or cannot tolerate a shampoo with water, a dry shampoo may be used. Several commercially prepared substances are available that are applied to the hair then brushed out.

MANAGEMENT OF PEDICULOSIS

Pediculosis is a condition in which hair is infested with lice. Lice (or pediculi) are minute parasites that suck blood from the skin and inject a toxin that causes itching, which may result in excoriation from scratching. The lice lay eggs (or nits) which attach themselves along the shaft of the hair with a cement-like substance that makes removal difficult. Pediculosis can occur wherever there is hair, and the three varieties of lice infestation are pediculi corporis,

TABLE 27.3 | GUIDELINES FOR WASHING A CLIENT'S HAIR IN BED

Review and carry out the standard steps in Appendix 1

Action	Rationale
Arrange the equipment in a convenient location	Facilitates the procedure
Position the client lying flat, if not contraindicated	Facilitates the procedure
Protect the client and bed linen with waterproof sheet and/or towels	Prevents client and bed from becoming wet
Place shampoo tray under the client's head, or fashion a trough (Figure 27.2B)	Facilitates drainage of water
Place a dry face washer across the client's eyes	Protects eyes from water and shampoo
Wet the hair thoroughly, apply shampoo and lather gently	The hair needs to be adequately cleansed and the scalp stimulated
Rinse the hair thoroughly	Shampoo must be rinsed off the hair and scalp to prevent dryness
Repeat the shampoo and rinsing if necessary	Hair must be adequately cleansed
Apply conditioner if the client wishes, comb through and then rinse off	Conditioner helps to keep the hair soft and glossy
Remove the tray or trough and wrap a towel around the client's head. Rub the hair dry or use a hair dryer	It is important to dry the hair quickly to avoid chilling the client
Comb or brush the hair	Removes any tangles and helps promote comfort
Change any wet bed linen or nightclothes, and assist the client into position	Helps promote warmth and comfort
Disinfect used equipment, wash and dry hands	Prevents cross-infection
Note the client's response, document the procedure and report observations	Appropriate care may be planned and implemented

infesting body hair; pediculi pubis, infesting pubic hair; and pediculi capitus, infesting head hair. Signs and symptoms that pediculi have infested the hair include pruritus, excoriation of the skin from scratching, and visible lice or nits. Untreated pediculosis can result in secondary skin infection such as dermatitis. The lice also spread from person to person on clothing, bedding, combs and brushes. It is important to note that pediculosis is not necessarily a sign of poor personal hygiene, as the parasites survive equally well on clean hair. The nits and lice can be destroyed by the use of a prescribed lotion or shampoo. With the available preparations, one single application is often effective. Sometimes a second treatment is recommended about 1 week later, in case any remaining nits have hatched into lice. The bed linen, personal clothing, hair brush and comb belonging to the person infested with lice must also be treated to prevent reinfestation. To avoid transmitting the parasites to others, the nurse should wear gloves and perform thorough hand washing after the treatment.

SHAVING

Many men shave every day; if so, this should be continued during illness. Shaving promotes client comfort by removing whiskers that may itch and irritate the skin. A facial shave can be performed using an electric or blade razor. Because the skin can be cut or nicked with a blade razor, an electric one is preferable. If a client is unable to shave independently the nurse will need to assist or perform the procedure for the client. Electric razors should be checked for function and cleanliness before use, and brushed free of whiskers after use. If the razor head is adjustable the appropriate setting will need to be selected. The nurse proceeds as follows:

- The electric razor is moved in a circular motion, pressed firmly against the skin, and each area of the client's face shaved until it is smooth
- If a blade razor is used the blade should be checked to see that it is clean, sharp and rust free. Many blade razors are disposable and used once only
- When using a blade razor it is best to use hot water and soap or shaving cream to lather the skin. Shaving is easier if the skin is held taut and the razor drawn over the skin in firm strokes
- When using a blade razor it is best to shave in the direction the hair is growing and to rinse the razor frequently to remove soap and whiskers
- Short gentle strokes are best around the nose and mouth to avoid irritation of these sensitive areas
- If the client wishes, aftershave lotion may be applied.

Some females develop a growth of facial hair, and this is usually removed by depilatory creams, tweezers or wax. Shaving should be avoided, as it encourages the growth of hair.

EYE, EAR AND NASAL CARE

ASSESSMENT AND CARE OF THE EYES

The eyes are the organs of sight through which visual information about the environment is transmitted to the brain for interpretation. If the eyes are not cleansed adequately, secretions may accumulate. The conjunctiva of the eyes should be observed for inflammation or pallor, and the sclera observed for signs of jaundice. Any discharge, discomfort or pain, and the presence of contact lenses, prostheses or spectacles should be noted. Under normal circumstances the eyes are kept clean by face washing and showering. If the eyes become irritated or infected, some clients may require extra care, which consists of cleansing, usually with sterile, soft gauze swabs, to remove secretions from the eyelids and to reduce discomfort. As eye bathing is sometimes required as part of the client's hygiene needs, guidelines for the procedure are outlined in Table 27.4.

When bathing the eyes the nurse uses an aseptic technique to reduce the risk of introducing microorganisms. (See Chapter 25 for information concerning aseptic technique and the prevention and control of infection.) The eyes are always cleansed from the inner to the outer canthus (Figure 27.3) and according to the guidelines in Table 27.4. The procedure must be carefully performed to prevent any injury to the eyes.

Clients who may require special eye care include those whose corneal reflex is impaired, due to unconsciousness or facial paralysis, for example, and those whose eyes are irritated or infected. Clients with conjunctivitis, a common condition caused by infection, allergies or irritating substances such as dust or smoke, may also require special eye care. Swabbing or bathing the eyes is sometimes referred to as an 'eye toilet' and the basic equipment consists of:

- Sterile dressing pack
- Extra sterile gauze swabs
- Sterile normal saline solution
- A receptacle for soiled swabs
- Disposable gloves
- A towel.

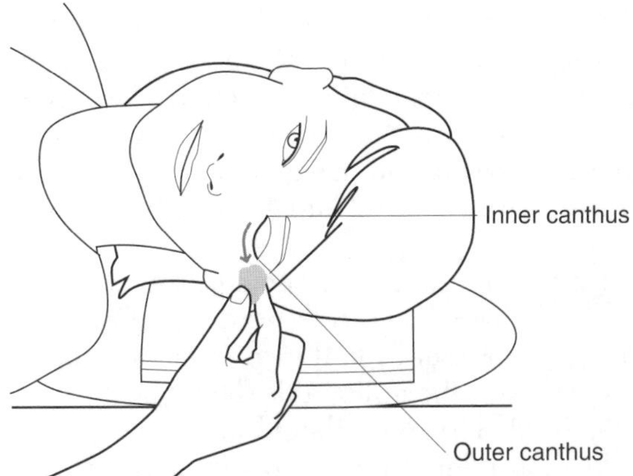

Figure 27.3 | Swabbing the eyes

TABLE 27.4 | GUIDELINES FOR PERFORMING AN EYE TOILET

Review and carry out the standard steps in Appendix 1

Action	Rationale
Assemble the equipment and place in a convenient location	Items should be readily accessible during the procedure
Ensure adequate lighting	Facilitates observation of the client's eyes
Ensure adequate privacy	Reduces embarrassment
Position the client with the head slightly to one side	Facilitates the procedure and prevents fluid running down the face
Wash and dry hands	Prevents cross-infection
Place a towel under, and kidney dish beside, the client's cheek. Observe for abnormalities	Protects the client and bedding. Additional treatment may be indicated
Using sterile technique, open sterile pack and add sterile solution and extra gauze swabs if required	Reduces the risk of cross-contamination
Perform hand wash procedure and don gloves	Gloves are applied to prevent cross-infection
Beginning with the least affected eye, ask the client to close the eye	Prevents contamination from infected eye being transferred to unaffected eye
Moisten gauze swabs and cleanse eyelids, from inner canthus to outer canthus (see Figure 27.3)	Prevents injury to the eyeball and prevents fluid and debris from entering the nasolacrimal duct. For safety reasons, forceps are not used
Use a clean gauze swab for each wipe and continue until the eye is clean	Prevents cross-contamination
Repeat the procedure for the other eye	
After cleansing, instil any prescribed drops or ointment	Drops or ointment may be prescribed to treat irritation or infection
Wipe any moisture from the client's face, remove the towel and reposition the client if necessary	Helps promote comfort
Remove equipment, dispose of soiled swabs, wash and dry hands	Prevents cross-infection
Report and record the procedure	Appropriate care may be planned and implemented

Table 27.4 provides the guidelines for performing an eye toilet but it should be noted that, provided that the principles of asepsis are maintained, it may not always be necessary, or agency policy, to use a sterile dressing pack each time an eye toilet is performed.

ASSESSMENT AND CARE OF THE EARS

Lack of aural hygiene can lead to an accumulation of dirt and wax, which may result in discomfort and temporary hearing loss. The ears are cleaned as part of normal hygiene practices, for example during a shower. They should be assessed for any discharge or complaints of tinnitus, discomfort or pain, and the use of a hearing aid should be noted. (See Chapter 42 for relevant information about hearing aids.)

Clients who are dependent on others for their hygiene needs should have their ears cleansed with the face washer during the shower or bath. If there is an accumulation of debris or wax in the orifice, this should be documented and reported. The nurse should not insert any object, including cotton-tipped applicators, into a client's ear canal as part of routine hygiene. Applicators may compact the cerumen, making the ear more difficult to clean (deWit 2005). Excessive cerumen or dry wax necessitates ear irrigation. This is undertaken only after examination and authorisation by a medical officer.

ASSESSMENT AND CARE OF THE NOSE

Secretions from the mucous membrane that lines the nose may accumulate, causing discomfort and providing a medium for the growth of microorganisms. The nose should be assessed for the presence of any discharge other than the normal mucus secretion, for bleeding, swelling of the mucosa, or any obstruction.

Blowing the nose is the most effective way of removing secretions from the nostrils. If clients are unable to perform this function, as a result of being unconscious or due to presence of an intranasal tube, for example, the nurse may be required to clean the nostrils. This is commonly achieved using small cotton-wool-tipped applicators moistened with a solution such as water and sodium bicarbonate. An applicator is inserted gently into the nostril, rotated and withdrawn, and the technique is repeated until the nostrils are clean. Sometimes a water soluble cream is applied around the nostrils to prevent soreness.

MOUTH CARE

Poor oral hygiene leads to dental decay and unhealthy mucous membranes, providing a potential source of infection as well as being a source of discomfort for the individual. If food particles are not removed from the mouth and teeth an unpleasant taste and halitosis (bad breath) can result. The mouth should be inspected for obvious dental decay, pallor, inflammation, or the presence of ulcers on the mucosa. The lips should be observed for hydration, pallor or cyanosis, and the presence of cracks or vesicles. Dentures, partial plates, bridges and crowns should be noted.

ORAL HYGIENE

Oral hygiene involves measures to keep the mouth and teeth clean and in healthy condition. Care of the mouth includes brushing the teeth, mouth rinses and regular visits to the dentist. The measures necessary to maintain the mouth and teeth in a healthy condition include:

- An adequate fluid intake to stimulate the flow of saliva. Saliva helps maintain a healthy mouth by washing away shed epithelial cells, food debris and microorganisms. Saliva also keeps the mouth lining moist and acts as a mild antiseptic that inhibits the growth of microorganisms, and maintains the pH balance inhibiting caries formation.
- A well-balanced diet that provides the tissues with the nutrients necessary for growth and repair. Foods that require chewing stimulate saliva flow as well as blood circulation to the gums and should be included when possible
- Brushing and flossing the teeth to remove plaque and food debris massages the gums, while tongue brushing and cleansing prevent mouth odour and infection
- Rinsing the mouth with non-alcoholic based mouthwashes to remove unpleasant tastes or odours
- Regular visits to the dentist to allow inspection of the teeth for decay, cleaning, and treatment of any cavities and other abnormalities.

If oral hygiene is neglected, complications may occur, including:

- Dental decay and halitosis
- Reduced nutrition due to inability to chew and diet restrictions
- Coated tongue and subsequent dulling of taste, which may lead to loss of appetite
- Inflammation of the oral mucosa (stomatitis), inflammation of the tongue (glossitis), inflammation of the gums (gingivitis), and periodontitis (inflammation of ligaments, gums and bones supporting the teeth)
- An accumulation of food particles, dead epithelial cells and microorganisms on the teeth, tongue and lips (sordes) and materia alba (white deposits on the neck of the teeth and adjacent gums)
- The spread of oral infections to other parts of the body such as the parotid glands, eustachian (auditory) tubes and respiratory tract
- Dryness of the mucosa, resulting in cracking or ulcers
- Social isolation.

AT-RISK CLIENTS

Clients with reduced flow of saliva or those whose normal chewing or swallowing actions are impaired are particularly prone to developing an unhealthy condition of the mouth. Examples include clients who:

- Experience dyspnoea, which results in mouth-breathing and consequently a dry mouth
- Are febrile or dehydrated
- Are not taking food or fluids orally or whose fluid intake is restricted
- Are receiving certain medications that cause dryness of the mouth
- Have impaired movement of the mouth, such as facial paralysis or surgical immobilisation of the jaw
- Have a nasogastric tube or airway in position, which may irritate or damage the mucosa or lead to an accumulation of debris in the mouth
- Wear partial or full dentures, which allow food particles to accumulate in the mouth
- Are unable to care for their oral hygiene adequately because of their physical or emotional state
- Are ventilator dependent.

ASSISTING THE CLIENT WITH ORAL HYGIENE

Many clients are able to attend to their oral hygiene but others may require encouragement and some assistance. The nurse should offer clients the opportunity to brush their teeth before breakfast, after meals and in the evening. The nurse should ensure that each client has a toothbrush and toothpaste and should assist them to the bathroom if necessary.

Some clients with cognitive or memory impairment may need repeated prompting to enable them to complete the task of cleaning their teeth. Clients may not clean effectively or may refuse to clean their teeth at all; for example, clients with Alzheimer's dementia may not understand what it is they are being asked to do. They may get frustrated, irritated, agitated and even aggressive as a result. Sometimes the problem may be resolved by temporarily distracting the client with another activity and returning later to cleaning the teeth. It may be helpful to follow the routine for cleaning the teeth conducted previously, for example the same time of the day, after breakfast or after getting dressed. It may even help to have a familiar mirror, towel or other object from home. It should be remembered that the client has a damaged brain, the challenging response is due to this damage and the person is not being deliberately difficult. A calm, quiet consistent approach and gentle encouragement is often the key to managing challenging responses, but different techniques work with different clients. Nurses need to find the key to gaining cooperation with each individual person. This may not be easy and a team approach is usually more effective in problem solving.

For clients confined to bed, the nurse should provide teeth-cleaning equipment consisting of a toothbrush, toothpaste, a mug of cold water, a container for used water and a towel. Clients who are accustomed to using dental floss as part of their normal hygiene should be encouraged to continue the practice.

Clients who are unable to brush their teeth will require the nurse's assistance with this procedure. Clients are taken to the bathroom, or teeth-cleaning equipment is brought to the bedside. The client should be assisted into a comfortable sitting position and the clothing protected by a towel. The nurse should apply toothpaste to a dampened toothbrush and gently but thoroughly brush the client's teeth using an up-and-down movement. Water is provided for the client to rinse the mouth, and a container is positioned to receive the used rinsing water. The mouth is then rinsed, but leaving some paste helps protect the teeth. Finally the lips are wiped dry, the toothbrush and toothpaste put away, and the mug and container removed for cleaning.

Some clients wear partial or full dentures, which, like natural teeth, require effective care to remove deposits and to prevent mouth odour. Care of dentures involves removing, brushing and rinsing them after meals. If it is the client's usual practice, dentures may be soaked in a commercial denture cleaner before brushing. All dentures should be removed at night, so the nurse should ensure that they are put in a container and placed in a safe position. Many clients are very reluctant to be seen without their dentures, so it is important to pull curtains and close doors to provide privacy when necessary. If clients are not able to care for their dentures independently it is the nurse's responsibility to attend to this.

To remove a partial denture the nurse, wearing disposable gloves, exerts equal pressure on the clips each side of the plate ensuring that pressure is not placed on the borders, because they may easily bend or break. A full upper denture may be removed by breaking the seal of the denture from the palate. This can be achieved by taking hold of the denture at the front or side with the thumb and index finger. A lower denture is removed by holding it in the centre, and turning it slightly before lifting it out of the mouth. A gauze square may be used to provide a firm grip on the dentures. Dentures should be gently placed in a denture container and taken to the bathroom for cleaning and rinsing. When handling dentures care must be taken to avoid damage.

It is a safety measure to place a washcloth in the basin before cleaning the dentures in case they are dropped. Before they are replaced the client's mouth is rinsed, and preferably the gums brushed to remove any debris. When clients are unable to insert their own dentures the nurse should assist. Moistening the dentures facilitates easier insertion and aids correct positioning into the mouth to keep them firmly in place. Clients should be encouraged to wear their dentures to facilitate eating and speaking and to prevent changes in the gum line that may affect denture fit.

If normal oral hygiene practices are not possible, the mouth and teeth must be cleaned by other means. Special mouth care is often required if the client:

- Is unconscious
- Is not taking oral food or fluids
- Experiences any impairment to mouth movement (e.g. facial paralysis)
- Has developed sordes
- Has a mouth infection
- Has a very dry mouth (e.g. as a result of mouth breathing, dehydration, or the effect of certain medications).

In these instances the client's mouth is cleansed either by the use of mouth rinses or by carefully swabbing all areas. The latter procedure is often referred to as a 'mouth toilet'. A variety of substances may be used to clean and refresh the mouth. The nurse should refer to the health care facility's policy manual for information on the equipment, substances and method to be used. Special care by swabbing the mouth is performed according to the client's needs and carried out at intervals ranging from every 2 hours to three or four times a day.

A suggested procedure for performing special mouth care (swabbing) is outlined in Table 27.5. The basic equipment consists of:

- Cotton-wool-tipped applicators
- A receptacle for soiled items
- Cleaning solution (e.g. sodium bicarbonate and water, or diluted hydrogen peroxide)
- A tongue depressor
- A container for dentures
- A towel
- Lip cream.

(Crisp & Taylor 2005; Darby 2006)

NAIL CARE

Care of the nails involves keeping them clean, shaped and trimmed. Regular care of the nails is important because dirty fingernails can carry microorganisms, which may be transferred to food or passed to other people. People who have dirty nails can also infect themselves by scratching. Many clients will be able to care for their nails independently, while others will require assistance. For example, clients who have limbs encased in plaster, are unconscious, confused or vision impaired may need the nurse to assist with nail care.

ROUTINE NAIL CARE

Nails should be kept clean and trimmed according to the policy of the health care agency and the client's personal

TABLE 27.5 | GUIDELINES FOR PERFORMING SPECIAL MOUTH CARE (SWABBING)

Review and carry out the standard steps in Appendix 1

Action	Rationale
Assemble the equipment and place it in a convenient location	Nurse must remain with the client throughout the procedure
Ensure adequate lighting	Visualisation of the mouth is essential
Ensure adequate privacy	Reduces embarrassment
Position the client so the head is turned to one side	Reduces the risk of aspiration of fluid
If the client is unconscious, suction equipment should be available	To remove excess fluid from the mouth, and prevent aspiration
Place a towel under the client's cheek	Protects client and bedding
Wash and dry hands, don gloves	Prevents cross-infection
Remove any partial or total dentures	Allows access to all areas of the mouth
Use the tongue depressor to help keep the client's mouth open, and inspect the mouth	The nurse must be able to see inside the mouth to detect any abnormalities
Gently and thoroughly swab all surfaces of the teeth, tongue and mouth	All debris and secretions must be removed
Ensure any prescribed substances are applied to ulcers or infected areas	Assists healing
Clean dentures thoroughly before replacing them in the mouth	All aspects of oral hygiene must be attended to
Apply a lubricant to the lips	Prevents soreness and cracking
Wipe any excess solution from the client's face, remove the towel and reposition the client if necessary	Promotes comfort
Remove equipment, dispose of soiled items, wash and dry hands	Prevents cross-infection
Report and document the procedure	Appropriate care may be planned and implemented

preference. Personal preference dictates whether fingernails are long and pointed, rounded or cut square. Preference may be influenced by the person's occupation. Nurses, for example, generally keep their fingernails short and smoothly rounded to avoid the risk of scratching their clients.

Nails can be kept clean by removing any visible dirt with a blunt instrument such as an orangewood stick. A metal nail file is not used because it can make the nails rough and trap dirt (deWit 2005). After washing, the cuticles should be gently pushed back and cuticle cream applied to keep them soft. Cuticle cream is not commonly provided by health care agencies but all-purpose hand cream may be available. Some clients will have their own hand-care products. Nail care is generally carried out after a shower or bath, but nails that are particularly dirty or thickened are easier to attend to if the client's hands or feet are soaked in warm soapy water for 5–10 minutes beforehand. Whenever nails are being trimmed, extreme care must be taken to prevent any damage to the nail beds and surrounding tissue.

AT-RISK CLIENTS

Clients who have diabetes or any circulatory disorder that affects the lower limbs are at high risk of infection, which can start easily in a damaged nail bed. It is therefore often the policy of the institution that such clients have foot and nail care undertaken only by a podiatrist. The podiatrist is also often required to care for the feet of older people whose nails have become thickened and distorted with age or for those with conditions such as corns, calluses or ingrowing toenails. Nail clippers are used in preference to scissors for trimming nails. Toenails should be cut straight across. Nails not trimmed in this way tend to grow inwards, creating a risk for pain and infection in the surrounding soft tissue.

NURSING OBSERVATIONS AND ASSESSMENT

While undertaking nail care the nurse observes for:

- Discolouration, such as pallor or cyanosis
- The presence of inflammation around the nail edges
- Signs of brittleness or cracks
- Deviations from normal shape, such as a spoon-shaped or concave appearance.

Pallor or cyanosis of the nails may indicate heart disease, while brittleness and/or a spoon-like shape may indicate the presence of an iron-deficiency anaemia. Any change or abnormality should be reported and documented. During nail care the nurse can take the opportunity to educate clients, or those that care for them at home, on how best to provide nail care. Education can also include how to inspect the hands and feet for lesions, dryness, or signs of inflammation or infection, and the importance of reporting any change or abnormality promptly to the community nurse or medical officer.

HYGIENE SUMMARY

Personal hygiene needs must be met to keep the body clean, to maintain healthy functioning and to promote a positive body image. Neglect of personal hygiene needs causes discomfort and may lead to infection and other serious complications. Continuous assessment of the client's total body is important for planning and implementing appropriate, high-quality nursing care. It is the nurse's responsibility to ensure that all clients have access to the facilities necessary for meeting their hygiene needs. Dependent clients require assistance from the nurse in meeting these needs and the nurse should ensure that the client's dignity, comfort and safety are promoted throughout all hygiene care procedures. The nurse also has an important role to play in educating clients and those that care for them at home about all aspects of hygiene that promote optimal health.

PROMOTING COMFORT

Human comfort depends on meeting a wide range and complex interaction of needs. Nutritional, fluid, elimination, oxygen and temperature regulation needs must be met for the human body to function efficiently and comfortably. The nurse's role incorporates monitoring and meeting these needs. In addition, the nurse promotes the comfort of clients by promoting ease of movement, rest and sleep and freedom from pain. (See the relevant chapters in Unit 9 for specific information relating to these areas.)

Physical and emotional comfort are interdependent, and if either aspect is disrupted the other is commonly affected. For example, if clients are experiencing some form of physical discomfort such as pain, they may develop emotional tension and become withdrawn, anxious or depressed. Conversely, an anxious person may develop physical symptoms such as headaches, loss of appetite or gastrointestinal disturbances. Therefore, for clients to be comfortable, they must be free from physical discomfort and emotional tension. An important nursing responsibility is assessing factors that are interfering with clients' comfort, then planning and implementing measures that promote their physical and emotional ease. Discomfort can result from stimuli of physical or psychosocial origin. Freedom from anxiety is important in helping the client to develop a sense of wellbeing and emotional security. (See Chapter 13 for information concerning how to help a client manage anxiety.) To promote the physical comfort of clients the nurse should assist in meeting all care needs. This includes ensuring that clients are wearing comfortable clothing, that the surrounding environment is conducive to comfort, and that clients are nursed in the most comfortable position possible.

CLOTHING AND COMFORT

A person's comfort is enhanced if they are able to wear clothes of their own choice. Many people feel uncomfortable and undignified if they are required to wear clothing such as a hospital gown provided by the health care facility. For this reason, clients returning from surgery or other procedures are changed into their personal attire as soon as their condition allows. Some residents living in aged-care facilities or special accommodation do not have adequate clothing of their own. In this case the nurse should ensure that the clothes supplied by the agency are appropriately selected to meet the residents' individual needs. For example, for an older person living in an aged-care facility the choice of clothes should be appropriate in terms of age, gender, temperature and other environmental conditions. They should be clean, fit well and, in the case of clients who are very frail or confused, be easy for them to manage, for example, velcro fastenings for ease of dressing and toileting.

COMFORT AND THE ENVIRONMENT

A suitable physical environment is one in which there is adequate lighting, fresh air, ventilation, warmth and cleanliness. Ideally it is free from excessive noise and unpleasant sights and smells. In addition, there should be sufficient space for the client's personal belongings, and facilities available for visitors. In the case of residents in long-term accommodation the environment should be as home-like as possible, have attractive window views to the outside world and an outdoor area that is safe and accessible. Ideally, residents will have a single room. If not the facility should provide a room where residents can spend private time with visitors if they wish. The environment should also provide a relaxed happy atmosphere and opportunities to enjoy activities that enhance quality of life, such as outings, concerts and games. For those who are able, the environment should provide the chance for residents to participate in simple everyday activities such as watching television, gardening, crafts or cooking. Comfort can be enhanced by promoting a psychological climate in which the client is encouraged to communicate any fears or anxieties. A physical environment that reduces the client's privacy and independence is unsuitable and can be a source of stress and discomfort.

EQUIPMENT TO PROMOTE COMFORT

Provision of a comfortable bed

A comfortable position is, to a significant extent, dependent on the client's bed. The prime objective of bed making is the promotion of comfort, as a bed that is made incorrectly may disrupt rest and sleep and may be a contributing factor to the development of complications such as decubitus ulcers. Beds may be made up in a variety of ways to meet the client's needs, and each health care facility commonly adopts its own method of bed making. Although the techniques may vary slightly, the principles of bed making remain the same.

Various types of bed are available, most of which can be adjusted manually, mechanically or electronically. Most beds may be raised or lowered horizontally, and some can also be adjusted to alter the position of the head, foot or centre. Some beds have a movable section that can be adjusted to form a backrest, against which pillows may be placed to provide support for the client. Beds are fitted with wheels, which enables them to be moved easily when necessary, and a brake device that prevents inadvertent movement. There are several special types of beds, frames and mattresses that are used for particular circumstances.

Frames (Figure 27.4) are available that may be either fitted to the bed or used in place of a more conventional bed. The Balkan frame, for example, is made from wood or metal, extends lengthwise above the bed, and may be used in conjunction with traction apparatus. The Bradford frame consists of a metal frame across which canvas slings are stretched, and may be used to nurse a person who has a fracture or disease of the hip or spine. The Stryker frame consists of two canvas-covered frames attached to a metal frame and may be used to facilitate changing the position of a person with a spinal cord injury or paralysis. Figure 27.4 illustrates the Balkan, Bradford and Stryker bed frames. The circolectric bed consists of one circular and two flat frames that are operated mechanically, and may be used to move a dependent person into various positions.

Mattresses are commonly made of rubber and covered with a waterproof material, which facilitates cleaning and therefore helps to prevent cross-infection. Other styles of mattress are available, including those made from foam rubber. Clients with specific needs, such as those who are more vulnerable to the development of decubitus ulcers, may be nursed on special mattresses. These include the water mattress, the egg-crate style (Figure 27.5A), the alternating pressure or ripple mattress (Figure 27.5B), and a mattress that is divided horizontally into three sections. The type of mattress selected must meet the client's needs, provide comfort and support, and should help prevent development of complications such as decubitus ulcers.

Pillows are available in a variety of materials, most of which are enclosed in a protective waterproof covering over which a pillow slip is placed. The number of pillows used depends on the needs of the client, and should be sufficient to provide maximum comfort and support.

Sheets are commonly available in two styles: the long sheet is similar to a conventional single-bed sheet; the draw sheet is a narrow sheet that may be placed across the bottom sheet. Because of their design, draw sheets are easy to replace under a client without disturbing the other bedclothes. A waterproof sheet may be placed under the draw sheet to protect the bottom sheet against moisture, for example, if a client is incontinent or is required to use toilet utensils in bed. In some care settings, special reusable incontinence bed protectors with tuck-in flaps are available and may be used instead of a draw sheet. These maintain a client's comfort because they are double or multi-layered and very absorbent. They have an integral waterproof barrier, which means that the side on which the client lies remains dry. They are commonly referred to as 'Kylie sheets'.

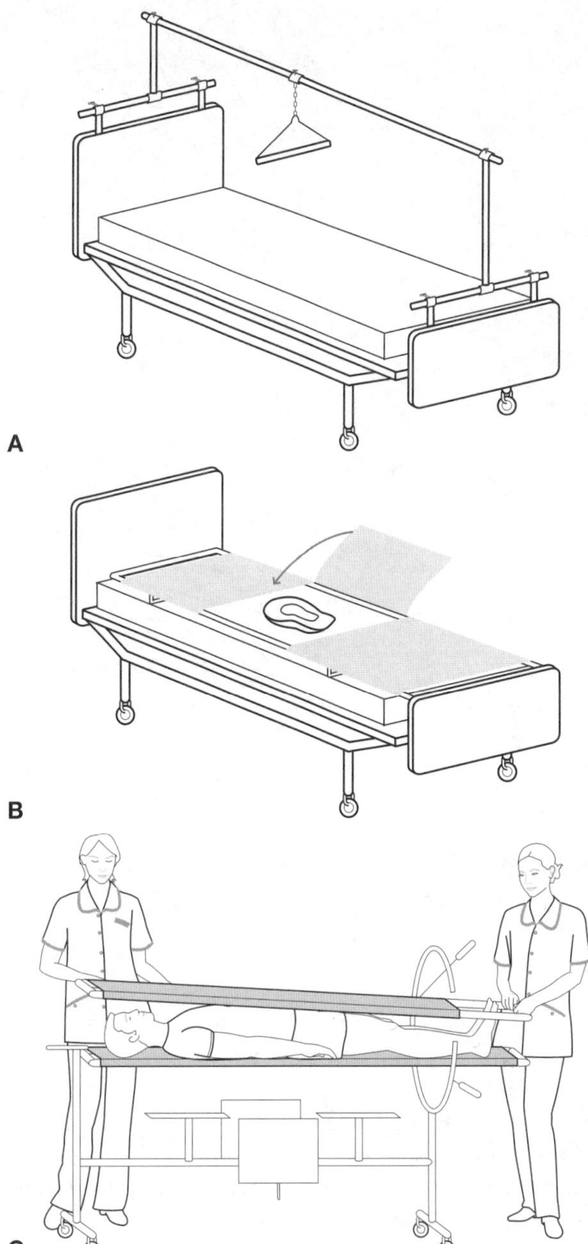

Figure 27.4 | Bed frames and special beds. **A**: Balkan frame. **B**: Bradford frame (note the removable strip in the centre to allow insertion of a bedpan). **C**: Stryker frame. The client is turned to the prone or supine position. Body alignment is not changed during repositioning

The frequency with which bed linen is changed depends on the health care facility's policy, but any bedclothing that becomes wet, soiled or excessively wrinkled should be replaced promptly if the client's comfort is to be maintained.

Blankets are available in wool or loosely woven cotton and should be light, warm and able to withstand frequent laundering. Quilts or bedspreads are commonly made from a cotton fabric that is easily laundered. Some health

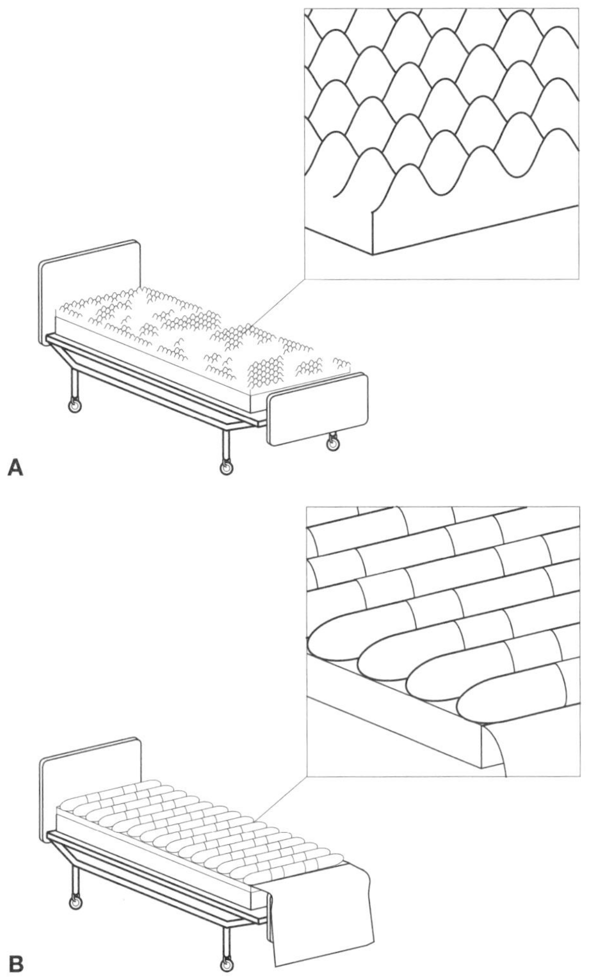

Figure 27.5 | Special mattresses. **A**: An egg-crate mattress. **B**: A ripple mattress

care facilities may use Continental-style quilts in place of blankets and a bedspread.

The use of supplementary items is also an important aspect of nursing care in maintaining comfort.

Supplementary equipment

A variety of supplementary equipment is available that may be used to enhance comfort, provide added support or promote safety.

Bed cradle. A bed cradle is a frame designed to keep the upper bedclothes off all or part of a client. The cradle may be large enough to extend from one side of the bed to the other, or small enough to place over one leg. The cradle is positioned directly above the area of the client's body which is to be free of the upper bedclothes, and the top sheet and blankets are brought up over the cradle. A bed cradle may be used for a client with a burn, an uncovered or painful wound or a plaster cast. The cradle protects the area by elevating the bedclothes, and facilitates observation of the area by the nurse or medical officer (Figure 27.6A).

Fracture board. A fracture board, or bed board, can be placed under the mattress to provide a firm surface and greater support for the back and legs. Fracture boards may be used for clients who have an injury or disease affecting the spine or lower limbs (Figure 27.6B), but with the introduction of solid-based rather than spring-based beds, the need for fracture boards has decreased.

Foot board. Various styles of foot board are available. These are placed towards the end of the bed to support the client's feet in a neutral position. A foot board may also be used to keep the weight of the upper bedclothes off the client's feet (Figure 27.6C). For comfort, a pillow may be placed between the feet and the foot board.

Sheepskin. A sheepskin may be placed over the bottom sheet to provide a soft surface for the client (Figure 27.6D). Friction between the skin and bottom sheet is reduced, and air circulates between the wool fibres to help keep the skin dry. A sheepskin may be used to promote client comfort, particularly for those with reduced mobility or who are emaciated. The use of a sheepskin helps prevent the development of decubitus ulcers. For maximum effectiveness, the client's skin should be in direct contact with the wool surface. A surgical gown that opens at the back may be used for modesty by covering the front of the body.

Heel or elbow protectors. Made from sheepskin, foam rubber or inflatable plastic material, these protectors are designed to fit the shape of the heel or elbow (Figure 27.6D). They are commonly used to prevent the development of decubitus ulcers on these areas, as they reduce friction between the skin and the bed linen.

Bed rails. Many beds are fitted with built-in side rails that can be raised (Figure 27.6E). Historically, side rails have been used to prevent clients, such as those at risk of seizures or who are restless or confused, from falling from the bed. However, bed rails are a form of restraint and currently their use is being evaluated carefully. Whenever possible, the use of bed rails is replaced by less restrictive, safe alternatives, such as the use of very low beds and bed bolsters (Ebersole, Hess & Luggen 2007). This change is in line with a policy of careful risk assessment and the use of the minimal restraint possible for any client in any situation. (See Chapter 26 for issues concerning restraint and safety.) At times when bed rails are required they may be covered with padded slips to prevent restless clients from damaging themselves, for example, by sustaining bruises, skin tears or other damage as a result of limbs hitting the rails.

Trapeze. An overhead trapeze bar or hand grip is a swinging bar suspended from an overhead pole, which may be used by a client to facilitate movement in bed (Figure 27.6F).

Rope. A length of rope or similar material may be attached to the foot of the bed and positioned on top of the quilt. By holding on to the end of the rope, the client is able to pull themself up into a sitting position.

Sandbag. A sandbag is commonly a waterproof bag filled with sand, used to maintain part of the body in alignment; for example, sandbags may be used to immobilise a fractured leg before splinting or surgery.

Wedge-shaped pillow. A wedge-shaped pillow is placed between the legs to maintain abduction, for example, after total hip replacement.

The nurse must ensure that any supplementary equipment is positioned and used correctly to promote the client's comfort and safety.

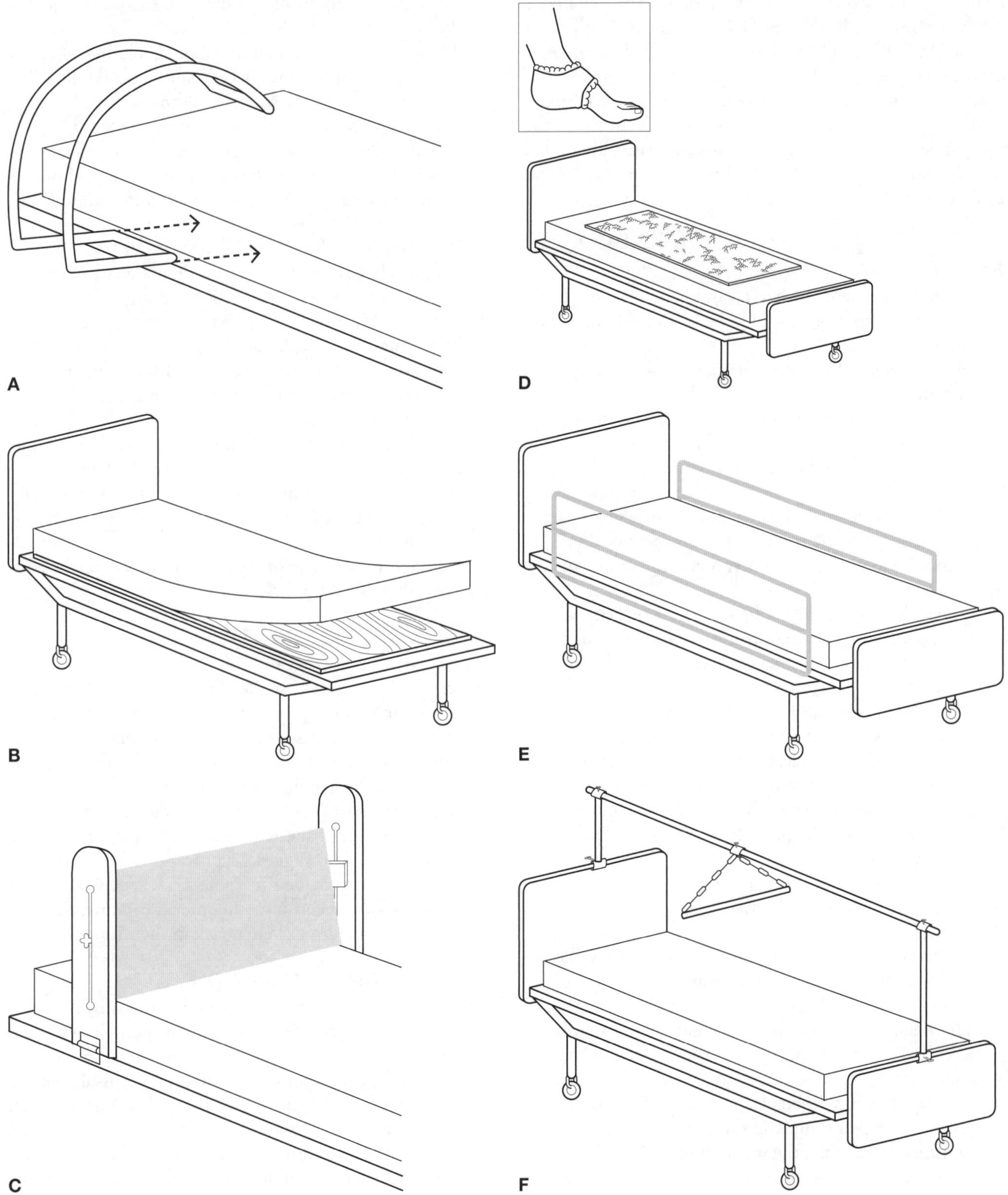

Figure 27.6 | Supplementary equipment used in bed making. **A**: Bed cradle. **B**: Fracture board **C**: Foot board. **D**: Sheepskins. **E**: Bed rails. **F**: Overhead trapeze

BED MAKING

MAKING AN UNOCCUPIED BED

An unoccupied bed is the term used to describe a bed that is either temporarily vacated by the client, for example, during a shower, or a bed that is being made up after a client's discharge from the health care facility. The unoccupied bed can be made up as a 'closed' or an 'open' bed. To make a closed bed, the upper bedding is tucked in at the bottom and sides. To make an open bed, the upper bedding is folded up at the bottom and sides. The advantage of the open style is that the upper bedding can be quickly folded lengthwise, or into a pack to facilitate ease of transferring a client from a trolley into the bed.

KEY PRINCIPLES RELATED TO BED MAKING

- All the equipment, such as clean linen and the soiled-linen container, should be collected before the procedure is started.
- Measures should be implemented to prevent cross-infection:
  - — the nurse's hands should be washed and dried before and after making the bed
  - — all linen should be held away from the body. This limits the risk of contaminating clean linen with any microorganisms on the nurse's clothing. It also limits the risk of contamination of the nurse's clothing with microorganisms from soiled linen
  - — bedclothes should not be shaken or flicked, as this permits easy transmission of microorganisms to other people or other surfaces via the airborne route
  - — soiled linen should immediately be placed into a soiled-linen container. It should never be placed on top of clean linen (it may contaminate the clean linen), on the floor (it may collect microorganisms from the floor surface) or anywhere other than in the appropriate designated container
  - — beds should not be made while procedures involving the use of sterile equipment are being performed nearby, as disturbed dust particles can travel and contaminate a sterile field. (See Chapter 25 for further information concerning infection prevention and control.)
- The nurse should don gloves to remove any solid faecal matter before placing the soiled linen in the container. Using toilet paper to envelop the faeces, the faecal matter should be placed in a bedpan, covered, taken to the pan room and flushed as normal.
- During bed making, the nurse should observe the principles of body mechanics to prevent back strain.
- When positioning the bottom sheet, the nurse should ensure that it is put on with the hem facing down. Sheets must be free from rough areas, wrinkles or creases, to promote comfort and to avoid damage to the client's skin.
- To maintain bedclothes in position, the corners are mitred (Figure 27.7). Mitred corners help to prevent the bedclothes becoming loose and uncomfortable for the client.
- To facilitate efficient bed making, bedclothes to be replaced are folded and placed on a chair. Folding the bedclothes avoids excessive wrinkling and facilitates ease of replacement. Alternatively, the bedclothes may be placed over a 'bed-stripper', which is a frame attached to the foot of the bed. Bedding that is not being replaced is rolled up and placed into the soiled-linen container.
- If a waterproof draw sheet is used, it must be completely covered by a cotton draw sheet to prevent it making contact with the client's skin.
- A vertical pleat or fold should be made in the upper bedclothes, to provide room for the client's feet. This technique prevents the bedclothes from pressing down on the feet, which can result in a condition known as foot drop.
- When a bed is to be made up after a client's discharge from the health care facility, the entire bed and fittings are cleaned beforehand. The bed should then be allowed to air before being made up with clean bedding.

A suggested procedure for making an unoccupied bed is outlined in Table 27.6.

MAKING AN OPERATION BED

An operation bed (Figure 27.8) is a version of an open unoccupied bed and is made up to receive a client after surgery or anaesthesia. An operation or surgical bed is also sometimes referred to as a surgical or post-anaesthetic bed. The upper bedding is arranged into a pack, which can be easily removed to facilitate efficient transfer of the client from a trolley into the bed. Once the client is in the bed, the upper bedding pack is unfolded and carefully placed over the client. The suggested procedure for making an operation bed is provided in Table 27.7. (See Chapter 44 for information concerning other preparation required for receiving postoperative clients back in their room.)

MAKING AN OCCUPIED BED

The term 'occupied' is used to describe a bed that is being made while the client is sitting or lying in it. When making an occupied bed the nurse must be aware of any restrictions in the client's movement or position, such as a painful wound or a urinary catheter. The nurse should ensure that the client's safety and comfort are maintained throughout the procedure. In addition to following the key principles relating to making a bed, before starting to make an occupied bed the nurse should:

- Assess the need for assistance. Two or more nurses may be necessary to move the client safely and

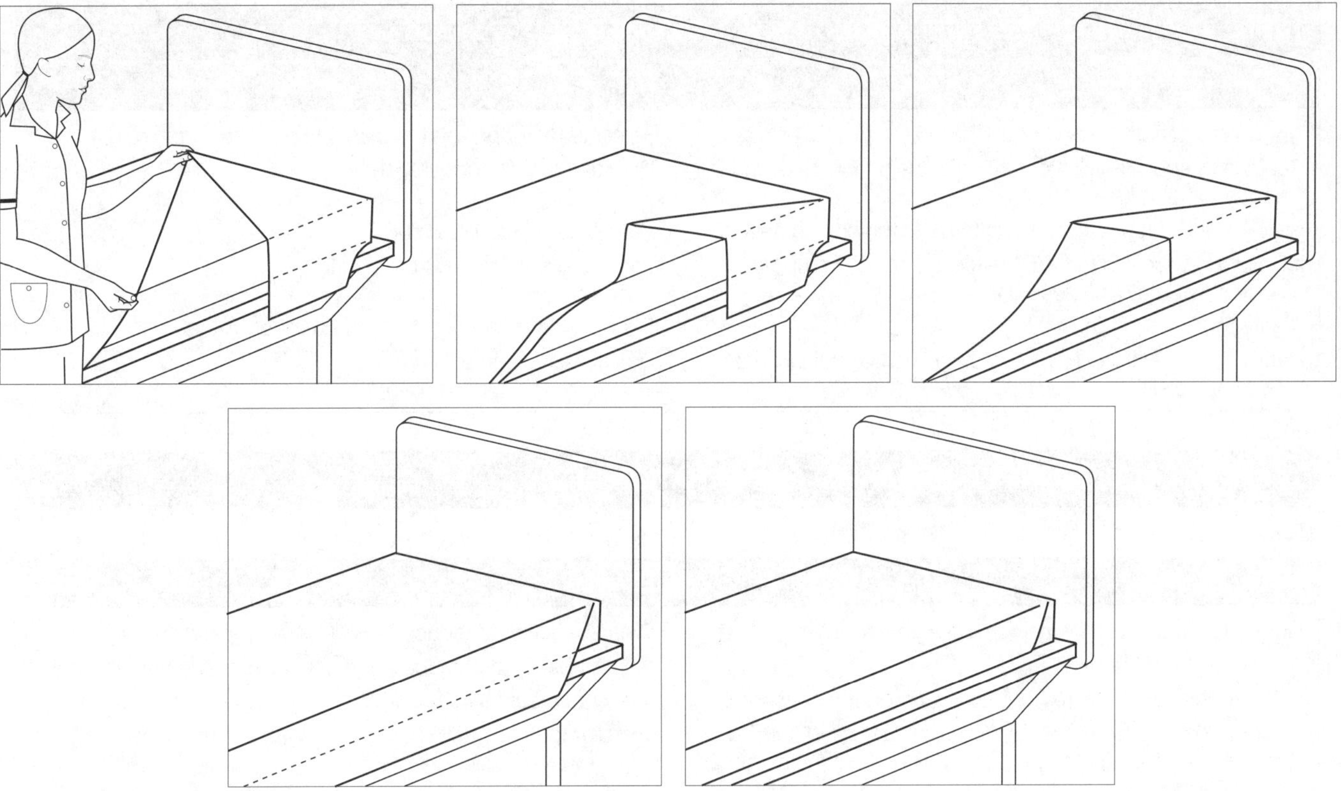

Figure 27.7 | Mitred corners

TABLE 27.6 | GUIDELINES FOR MAKING AN UNOCCUPIED BED

Review and carry out the standard steps in Appendix 1

Action	Rationale
Wash and dry hands	Prevents cross-infection
Place clean linen and soiled-linen container near the bed	Facilitates access during the procedure
Ensure that there is a chair on which to place the bedclothes, or use the bed-stripper attached to the foot of the bed	Bedclothes must be kept free of the floor to prevent contamination
Move the bedside locker and over-bed table if necessary	Provides more space in which to work
Adjust the height of the bed	Appropriate height of the bed prevents strain on the nurse's back
Place pillows on the chair. Place any soiled pillow slips in the container	Prevents cross-infection
Loosen the upper bedclothes	Facilitates ease of removal
Remove each item of upper bedclothes separately, fold and place on the chair or bed-stripper	Folding reduces wrinkling and facilitates replacement
Loosen the bottom bedclothes, fold and place on the chair. Any soiled items are placed in the soiled-linen container	Prevents cross-infection
Roll, rather than fold, the waterproof sheet	Folding may damage waterproof material
Pull the mattress well up to the head of the bed	Prevents gap between the head of the bed and the mattress
Starting with the bottom sheet, replace each item separately	Bedclothes are easier to adjust or remove if they are replaced and tucked in separately
If a draw sheet is used, position it about 25 cm from the head of the bed	The draw sheet needs to go under the client's buttocks
The bedclothes should be centred and, unless being made up as an open bed, tucked in around the mattress	Facilitates correct placement of the bedclothes

(Continued)

TABLE 27.6 | GUIDELINES FOR MAKING AN UNOCCUPIED BED — cont'd

Action	Rationale
Turn the top sheet back over the blankets	Protects the upper part of blankets (e.g. from spilt fluids)
Replace the quilt, mitre the bottom corners, and allow the edges to hang freely	Provides a neat appearance
Replace and arrange the pillows to meet the client's needs	Promotes comfort and support
If a client is to return to bed, the top corner of the upper bedclothes may be folded back	Facilitates easy access for the client
Adjust the height of the bed	Enables the client to get in and out of bed safely
Replace any furniture. Remove soiled-linen container, wash and dry hands	Prevents cross-infection

TABLE 27.7 | GUIDELINES FOR MAKING AN OPERATION BED

Review and carry out the standard steps in Appendix 1

Action	Rationale
Collect clean bedclothes and soiled-linen container	Clean bedclothes reduce the risk of postoperative infection
Adjust height of the bed	Correct height of the bed prevents strain on the nurse's back
Loosen all bedclothes, remove, and place in the container	Prevents cross-infection
Place a clean bottom sheet, waterproof sheet and draw sheet on the mattress. Tuck ends and sides of the sheets under the mattress	Waterproof and draw sheet protect the bottom sheet (e.g. from wound drainage)
Lie the top sheet and blankets on the bed, fold the top and bottom back. Fold each side to the centre, then fold in half. Fold the top and bottom to the centre, then fold in half	Creates a pack which can be removed quickly before the client re-enters the bed, and then unfolded over them
Place the pillows on a chair in the room	Pillows are placed on the bed when the client's needs are determined
A heating pad may be placed in the bed under the pack	Warms the bed before the client's return
Adjust the height of the bed	Prepares the bed to receive the client from the trolley
Place all the required equipment (e.g. emesis bowl) within easy reach	Prepares the room for the client's return
Wash and dry hands	Prevents cross-infection

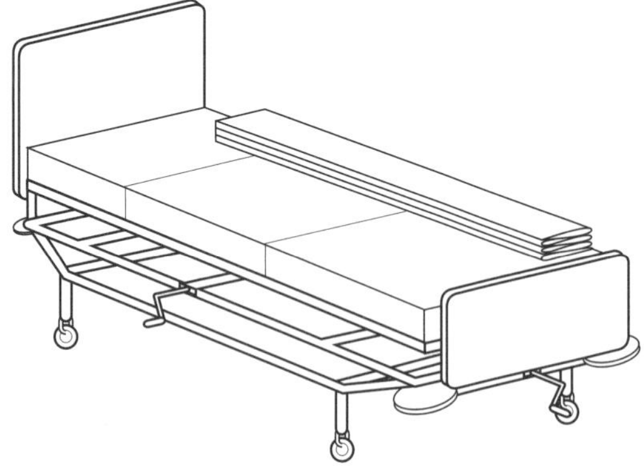

Figure 27.8 | Operation bed

painlessly and to complete the procedure quickly to avoid the client becoming fatigued. The client must be adequately supported and kept warm during the procedure. Some clients must be moved keeping the body in total alignment; e.g., some clients with spinal injuries or who have had spinal surgery must avoid twisting. In these circumstances clients must be log-rolled so that the body is moved as one unit. At least three people are required to log-roll the person and keep their body in alignment. Standing on the side of the bed to which the client is to be turned, one nurse supports the client's head, another supports the trunk, while the third nurse supports the legs. Before starting movement, a pillow is placed between the client's legs. At a given signal, the individual is rolled in one coordinated, smooth movement towards the nurses (Figure 27.9)

- Consider if it is preferable to make the occupied bed from top to bottom, rather than from side to side. It is often easier and less disruptive for a client (e.g. one who has distressed breathing or a leg in traction) if the nurses adjust the bottom sheet in this manner. The suggested procedure for making an occupied bed is provided in Table 27.8.

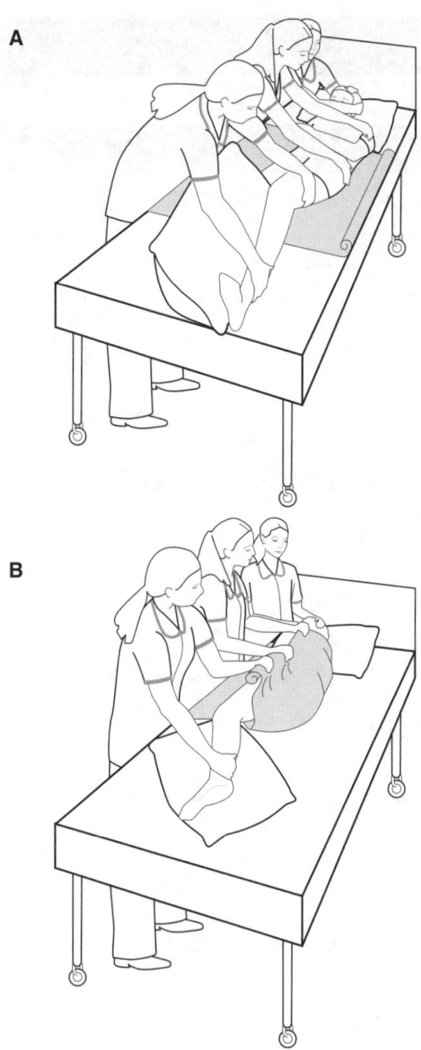

Figure 27.9 | The log-roll method of moving a client

The technique used to make an occupied bed should be one that causes minimal disturbance to the client. Commonly, the bed is remade after attention to the client's daily hygiene needs. It may be necessary to make an occupied bed more frequently, for example, if the bedclothes become wet, soiled or disarranged. When possible, two nurses should work together to make the bed, for the promotion of client comfort and safety. At times it may be necessary for more than two nurses to make an occupied bed, for example, to help when a client has multiple injuries. The use of a slide sheet is helpful when moving clients in and around the bed. It reduces the risk of injury to nurses and to clients. (Chapter 26 provides information relating to the use of slide sheets and safety when moving clients.)

Making an occupied bed provides the nurse with an ideal opportunity for communicating with and observing the client. During the procedure the nurse is able to assess certain aspects of the client's condition, such as emotional state, skin colour, the presence of pain, the ability to move, or distress associated with exertion. Observations made should be documented and any deviations from normal should be reported immediately to the nurse in charge. When the condition of clients permits, they may be able to move themselves during bed making, by using an overhead hand grip.

MAKING A DIVIDED BED

A divided bed is sometimes referred to as a split, or traction, bed. Making a divided bed involves arranging the upper bedding into two sections. This style of bed is commonly used for a client who has traction equipment applied to a lower limb. A divided bed allows the leg in traction to be free from the weight of the upper bedding, while the rest of the client's body is covered. Because the upper bedding is arranged in two sections, the client's torso and unaffected leg may be kept covered without interference to the traction apparatus. A lightweight cover may be placed over the leg in traction to ensure adequate warmth.

The foot of the bed is elevated to counterbalance the traction, and a fracture board is commonly placed under the mattress to provide a firm and supportive surface. A trapeze or overhead bar should be provided to facilitate the client's movement. When changing or straightening the bottom sheet it is sometimes easier and less disruptive for the client in traction if nurses work from the top to the bottom of the bed, rather than from side to side.

Certain adverse effects may be associated with prolonged bed rest and immobility; it is therefore important that the nurse implements preventive measures to reduce such effects.

COMFORTABLE POSITIONING

Clients assume, or are assisted into, the position they find the most comfortable, unless a specific posture is indicated for therapeutic reasons. If a client is able to move without assistance, the nurse should ensure that the bed pillows are positioned for support and comfort and that there are adequate bedclothes. A signal device and the client's personal requirements should always be within easy reach. A specific position may be necessary to prevent deformities, relieve pressure and strain, to assist circulation or breathing, or to enable various examinations or treatments to be performed. Some clients will be able to assume a position independently, while others will require the nurse's assistance. The nurse should be aware of measures to promote the client's safety and comfort and should be able to assist a client into specific positions. Correct positioning can promote comfort, maintain and help restore body functioning and help to prevent the complications associated with bed rest and immobility.

KEY ASPECTS RELATED TO POSITIONING

- To minimise the risk of back strain nurses are advised to observe the principles of body mechanics and the no-lift policy when assisting clients to move (see Chapter 26).

TABLE 27.8 | GUIDELINES FOR MAKING AN OCCUPIED BED	
Review and carry out the standard steps in Appendix 1	
Action	**Rationale**
Collect clean linen and soiled-linen container before starting to make the bed	Nurse must remain with the client during the procedure
Move the bedside locker and over-bed table if necessary	Provides more space in which to work
Ensure there is a nearby chair on which to place the bedclothes, or use the bed-stripper	Bedclothes should be kept free of contamination from the floor
Adjust the height of the bed	Appropriate height of the bed prevents strain on the nurse's back
Leaving sufficient pillows to support the client, place the remainder on the chair	The client's comfort and safety must be promoted
Remove each item of upper bedclothes separately. Bedclothes to be replaced are folded and put on the chair or bed-stripper	Reduces wrinkling and facilitates replacement
Cover the client with a procedure blanket before removing the top sheet	Promotes comfort
Place soiled items into the soiled-linen container	Prevents cross-infection
Remove accessories such as a bed cradle or foot board	Facilitates bed making
Support the client and gently turn them onto one side of the bed	Provides sufficient room to adjust or change the bottom sheet(s)
If only one nurse is making the bed, the side rail away from the nurse should be elevated	Promotes safety
Loosen the bottom sheets on the unoccupied side and roll each one towards the centre of the bed	Provides access to one side of the mattress
Brush out any debris (e.g. crumbs or pieces of plaster) from the exposed mattress. Eliminate any creases from the mattress cover	Foreign objects, or creases in the cover, cause discomfort
Working at the unoccupied side of the bed, either unroll, pull the bottom sheets taut, and tuck in around the mattress OR If using a fresh sheet, place on the bed and unfold it so that the centre laundry crease lies at the centre of the mattress. Tuck in at the top, bottom and side. Roll the excess to the centre of the bed	Provides a smooth surface under the client
Carefully turn the client to the other side of the bed, providing adequate support as they are moved. If appropriate, elevate side rail	Comfort and safety must be promoted
From the opposite side of the bed, either remove any soiled sheets and place in the soiled-linen container OR Untuck and roll sheet(s) to the centre of the bed	Prevents cross-infection
Ensure that side of the mattress is free from debris and creases, unroll and tuck the sheet(s) in around the mattress	Completes the making of the base of the bed
Assist the client back into the centre of the bed, arrange the pillows to meet comfort needs and assist the client into position	Promotes comfort
Replace any accessories, put on the top sheet and remove the procedure blanket	Promotes comfort and privacy
Replace the blankets and quilt, ensuring that they are positioned to cover the client's chest and shoulders	Promotes warmth and comfort
Make foot pleats in the upper bedclothes and avoid tucking them in too tightly	Provides room for foot movement
Place the signal device and the client's requirements within easy reach. Adjust the height of the bed	Facilitates access
Replace any furniture. Remove the soiled-linen container, wash and dry hands	Prevents cross-infection

- The client should be provided with information about the importance of correct positioning and the reasons why a specific position may be indicated. To provide some exercise and to promote independence the client should be encouraged to participate in regular changes of position unless active movement is contraindicated.
- All parts of the client's body should be maintained in proper alignment, with equal weight distribution, and the joints in a functional or neutral position. Muscle tension and strain are prevented when the joints are maintained in a slightly flexed position.
- Adequate support should be provided to maintain the natural curves of the client's vertebral column.
- To promote safety and comfort, adequate assistance should be obtained to move a heavy, very frail or dependent client. The client's body should be handled gently to prevent pain or injury. Appropriate lifting devices are used when necessary to assist clients into position.
- Supplementary equipment should be used when needed (e.g. a sheepskin may be used to relieve pressure).
- To prevent prolonged pressure on any area of the body, the client's position should be changed at least every 4 hours. Each time a client's position is changed, the nurse should observe the status of the client's skin to detect any signs of the consequences of prolonged pressure.
- The client should be encouraged to participate in some form of exercise unless this is contraindicated. Exercise helps to promote circulation and muscle tone; if the client is unable to move independently, all joints should be put through the full range of motion.

There are various positions that an individual may assume, or be required to assume.

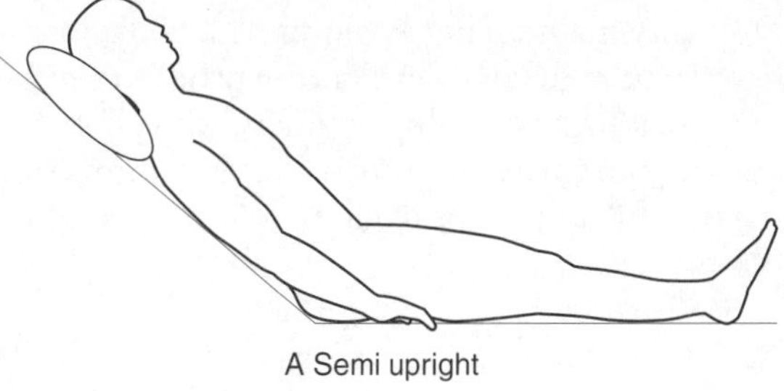

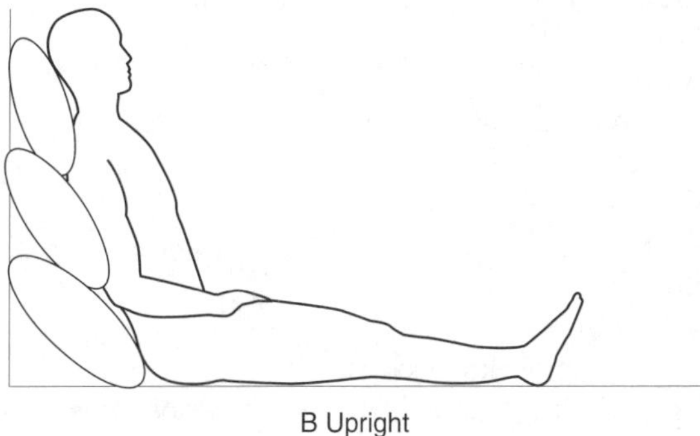

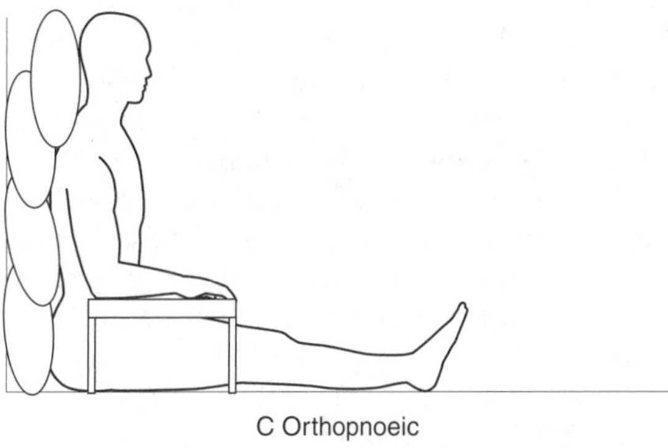

Figure 27.10 | Sitting positions. **A**: Semi-upright, or semi-Fowler's, position. **B**: Upright, or Fowler's, position. **C**: Orthopnoeic position

SITTING POSITIONS

There are three variations of a sitting position:

1. The semi-upright, or semi-Fowler's, position, in which the client sits at an angle of about 30 degrees, supported by pillows, which are placed against the backrest of the bed (Figure 27.10A)
2. The upright, or Fowler's, position, in which the client is in a full sitting position, with pillows placed to support the upper body (Figure 27.10B)
3. The orthopnoeic position, in which, from an upright position, the individual leans onto an over-bed table (Figure 27.10C).

A particular one of these sitting positions may be indicated:

- After abdominal or thoracic surgery. Less tension is exerted on an abdominal wound, therefore comfort is promoted. Drainage by gravity from body cavities is facilitated (e.g. when there has been a drainage tube inserted after surgery)
- To facilitate breathing and reduce dyspnoea. Because the diaphragm is able to flatten, maximal chest expansion is promoted and the risk of lung congestion is decreased. Leaning forward, as in the orthopnoeic position, helps to increase lung capacity and therefore alleviate distressed breathing
- To facilitate independence, as a sitting position enables the client to see and participate in ward activities. The activities of daily living (e.g. eating and drinking or using toilet utensils) are also facilitated in this position.

The disadvantages of a sitting position include:

- Difficulty maintaining the position, which may become tiring or uncomfortable
- Difficulty in sleeping
- Prolonged pressure on the buttocks and sacral area, which increases the risk of decubitus ulcers

- Difficulty maintaining a comfortable body temperature: in cold weather it may be hard to bring the bedclothes up to the shoulders, while in hot weather the client may experience discomfort from the number of pillows required to maintain a sitting position.

POSITIONS FOR SPECIFIC SITUATIONS

There are a variety of other positions suitable for a range of different circumstances. These include:

- Supine
- Prone
- Semi-recumbent
- Lateral
- Sim's
- Coma
- Dorsal
- Lithotomy
- Genupectoral (knee–chest).

Figure 27.11 illustrates this range of positions.

Supine (dorsal recumbent) position

In a supine position, the client lies flat on their back with a pillow under their head. Limbs should be positioned in normal alignment. A foot board, firm pillow or other aid may be necessary to maintain the correct position of the feet. A supine position may be indicated:

- To facilitate relaxation of the abdominal muscles (e.g. during medical examination of the abdomen). After abdominal surgery, clients may be placed in the supine position to relieve tension on the abdominal area
- For several hours after a lumbar puncture. Re-establishment of normal circulation of the cerebrospinal fluid is facilitated, and lying flat helps to prevent a severe headache, which may occur from a change of pressure in cerebrospinal fluid.

The disadvantages of a supine position include:

- Restriction of chest expansion. The lungs are unable to inflate fully, secretions accumulate and congestion of the lungs may occur
- Difficulty may be experienced when toilet utensils are being used. This may lead to incomplete emptying of the bowel or bladder, which may result in constipation or urinary tract infection
- Depression may result from loss of independence and the difficulties associated with activities of living (e.g. eating and drinking). A client in a supine position may also experience difficulty in seeing, or participating in, ward activities
- Increasing the work of the heart, as lying flat increases venous return (preload).

Prone (anterior recumbent) position

In a prone position, the client lies on the abdomen with the head supported on a small pillow and turned to one side. A small pillow may be placed under the abdomen to maintain the natural curve of the spine, or to relieve pressure on the breasts. A pillow may be placed under the ankles to maintain the feet in the correct position and to facilitate slight flexion of the knees. (Alternatively, the client may be positioned so that the toes are extended over the end of the mattress.) The client's arms should be positioned comfortably, for example flexed beside the head or extended alongside the torso. A prone position may be indicated:

- To relieve pressure on the posterior surface of the body. If a client has, for example, a burn or decubitus ulcer on the back, a prone position will alleviate pressure on the damaged area and therefore permit healing and relieve pain
- To provide access to the posterior surface of the body for medical examination
- To promote drainage from the respiratory tract. Drainage by gravity is further facilitated when the foot of the bed is elevated.

The disadvantages of a prone position include:

- Restriction of chest expansion. Lung congestion is more probable, as the lungs are unable to inflate fully and secretions accumulate
- Difficulty may be experienced in performing the activities of living; for example, eating, drinking or emptying the bladder or bowel
- Depression, from loss of independence and an inability to participate in ward activities.

Semi-recumbent position

In a semi-recumbent position, the client lies on the back, with three or four pillows supporting the head, neck, and shoulders. There are no specific indications for this position, but the client may find it the most comfortable one to assume. To reduce shearing forces, which are a predisposing factor in the formation of decubitus ulcers, the nurse must ensure that the client is correctly positioned.

Lateral position

In a lateral, or side-lying, position, the client lies on the side, with the head supported on a pillow. The arms are placed comfortably in front of the body and, depending on the purpose of the position, the legs may be flexed or extended. If the client is required to assume a lateral position for a prolonged period, a pillow may be placed along the back to facilitate maintenance of the position. The limbs should not assume a dependent position and may be supported; for example, the upper arm and leg may be flexed and supported on pillows. A lateral position may be adapted for specific purposes; for example, the left lateral position, in which both legs are flexed, is commonly used for examination or treatment involving the rectum. During a lumbar puncture, the client is positioned laterally with both knees flexed and drawn towards the abdomen, and the head flexed towards the chest. A lateral position may be indicated:

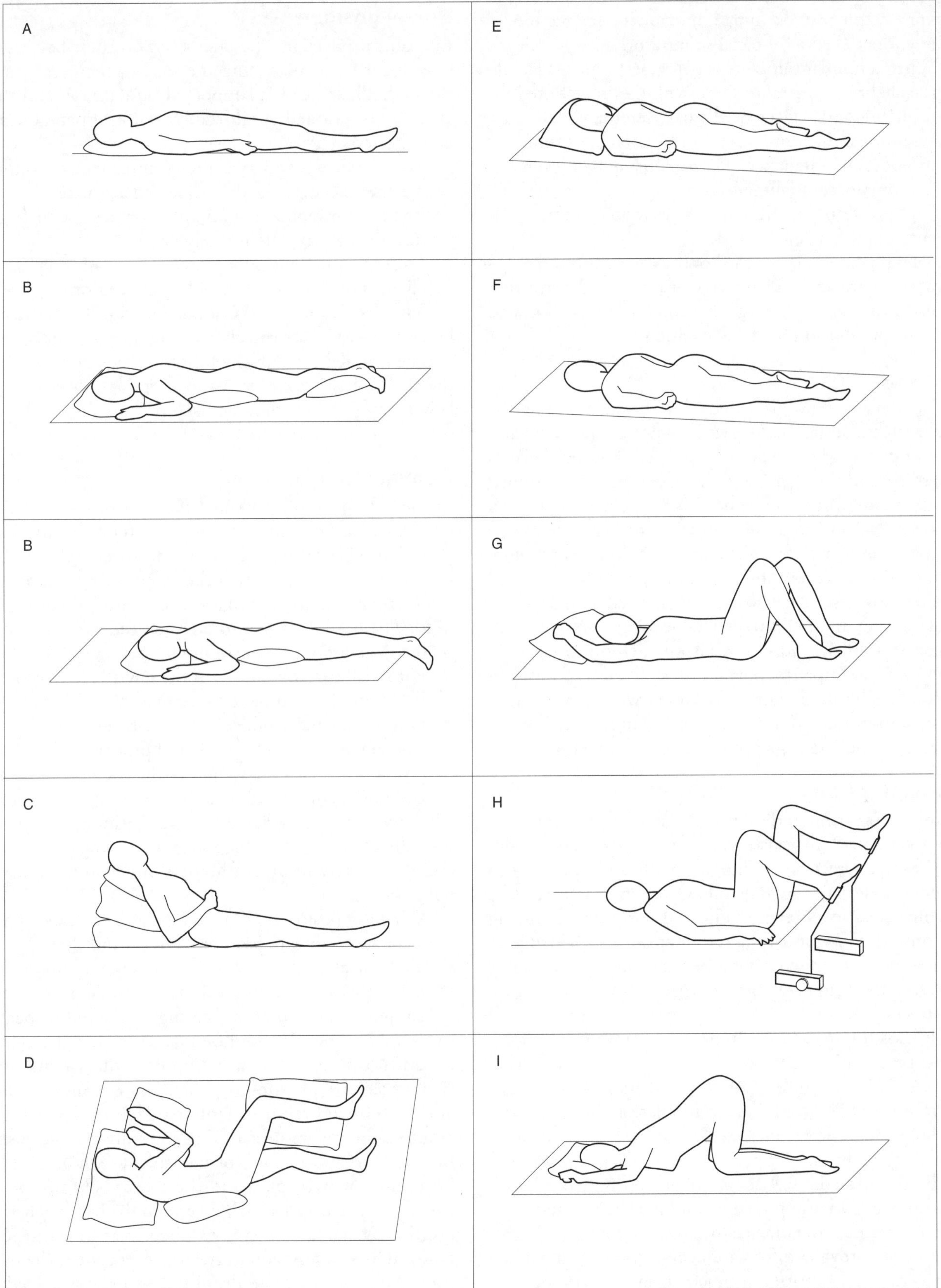

Figure 27.11 | Various positions. **A**: Supine. **B**: Prone. **C**: Semi recumbent. **D**: Lateral. **E**: Sim's. **F**: Coma. **G**: Dorsal. **H**: Lithotomy. **I**: Genupectoral (knee–chest)

- For treatment or examination involving the rectum (e.g. the insertion of rectal suppositories)
- When a lumbar puncture is being performed. Placing the client in a lateral position with the spine flexed facilitates entry of the needle between the vertebrae
- To nurse an unconscious client. A lateral position promotes maintenance of a clear airway by preventing the tongue from falling back and causing obstruction. This position also prevents oral secretions from entering the trachea.

If a lateral position is assumed over a long period, the disadvantages are an increased risk of postural deformities, decubitus ulcers and various other complications associated with the prolonged use of any position.

Sim's position

In the Sim's, or semi-prone, position the client lies on the side with the upper leg drawn up towards the chest and the buttocks towards the edge of the bed. The lower arm is placed behind the client, and the upper arm is positioned comfortably in front. The head is supported on a small pillow. Women can adopt this position when having a vaginal examination but the dorsal position is used more commonly for this purpose. The Sim's position is not used frequently but women who have experienced frontal vaginal sexual assault may find this preferable to the dorsal position (Matteson 2001) and it may also be helpful for women with physical impairments that make the dorsal position uncomfortable or unmanageable. Some women might find the Sim's position less embarrassing than the dorsal position when a vaginal examination is being performed.

Coma position

In the coma position, the client is placed in a position that is basically the Sim's position but without a pillow under the head. Correct positioning of the head is essential to promote a clear airway, and a pillow may impede breathing. A coma position may be indicated temporarily during unconsciousness, such as after an episode of fainting. A clear airway is facilitated with the head on one side, as this prevents the tongue or oral secretions from obstructing the trachea.

If used for an extended time, the disadvantages of the coma position include:

- Restriction of chest expansion. The lungs are unable to inflate fully, secretions accumulate and the risk of lung congestion is increased
- Likely occurrence of postural deformities such as limb contractures. Also, prolonged pressure on the shoulder and arm placed behind the client may result in damage to the brachial plexus.

Chapter 48 provides information concerning the use of the coma (recovery) position in an emergency situation.

Dorsal position

In a dorsal position, the client lies on their back, with knees flexed and apart, and the soles of their feet flat on the bed. Their head is supported on a pillow and their arms are positioned comfortably. A dorsal position may be indicated:

- To introduce a urinary catheter into a female, as the urethral meatus is made visible and accessible
- To perform vaginal examinations or treatments (e.g. insertion of vaginal ointment)
- To administer an enema or rectal suppositories, if the client is unable to assume a lateral position.

The disadvantage of a dorsal position is that it may be embarrassing for the client. The dorsal position may also be adapted to form the lithotomy position, in which the client's legs are elevated and supported by stirrups. A lithotomy position may be used during gynaecological surgery or during the birth of a baby.

Genupectoral position

In the genupectoral, or knee–chest, position, the client kneels so that body weight is supported on the knees and chest. The client is positioned on the knees with the chest resting on the bed, and with the elbows either supporting some of the weight, or with the arms extended beyond the head. The head is turned to one side and supported on a pillow. A genupectoral position may be indicated:

- For specific examinations of the lower colon, as the insertion of instruments is facilitated
- During the management of a specific obstetric emergency: if the umbilical cord prolapses, this position prevents the weight of the baby pressing on and obstructing the flow of blood through the cord.

The disadvantages of a genupectoral position include that it is difficult, uncomfortable and embarrassing to maintain; and that it may result in the person becoming dizzy or faint, and falling.

Whatever position the client assumes, the nurse should implement measures to promote comfort and safety. Pillows should be arranged for maximum comfort and support and placed so that the client's head, neck, shoulders and spine are supported at a comfortable angle. The pillow behind the head and neck should be placed so that the client's head is not pushed forward. Supplementary equipment such as sheepskins should be used to enhance comfort and to relieve pressure. Upper bedclothes should be arranged for maximum covering and warmth, and tucked in loosely to allow room for movement. A foot board or firm pillow may be placed in the bed to help sustain the client's position, and to help maintain the feet in a neutral position. When a person is required to assume a specific position for examination or treatment purposes, the nurse should ensure adequate draping and privacy to reduce embarrassment and promote comfort.

It is also important to ensure that the client is correctly positioned when sitting in a chair. A variety of chairs is available and a style should be chosen to meet the client's needs. A chair should be comfortable and support the client adequately. Specially designed chairs may be indicated for some clients; for example, a chair with an elevated seat is used after hip surgery, to prevent strain on the joint. When sitting in a chair, the client's spine and buttocks should be well aligned to the contours of the chair. Both feet should be flat on the floor, or (at times) it may be necessary to support one or both feet on a footstool or chair. Limbs should be supported in a position of comfort, and pillows used when necessary; for example, to support an arm when an intravenous infusion is in progress or a plaster cast has been applied. The client should be adequately dressed and light coverings should be provided to promote warmth and privacy.

SUMMARY

It is the role of the nurse to ensure that clients are physically clean, well groomed and, as far as is possible, free of physical discomfort and psychological stress. Nurses must be competent in their responsibilities and practices in assisting clients with all areas of hygiene, in bed-making procedures and the use of supplementary equipment, and in the correct positioning of clients to ensure the best possible level of comfort. Ensuring that clients are clean, fresh and comfortable promotes relaxation, rest and sleep, which are essential for healing and wellness. The nurse who successfully assists clients to meet all hygiene and comfort needs plays an essential role in promoting their physical and psychological wellbeing.

REVIEW EXERCISES

1. Which factors may influence an individual's hygiene practices?
2. When assessing a client, what should be observed by the nurse in regard to the client's skin, hair, nails, mouth, eyes, ears and nose?
3. List the factors that influence whether a client may be sponged, bathed or showered.
4. What must a nurse take into consideration when showering a client with a urinary catheter, intravenous drip or a plaster cast on a limb?
5. What items would a nurse need to gather when preparing to sponge a client in bed?
6. What would determine the nurse's choice to give a client special mouth care or mouth toilet?
7. What differences occur when making a bed that is either unoccupied or occupied?
8. How is the client positioned when lying supine, prone, semi-recumbent or lateral?
9. How is the client positioned when sitting semi-upright, upright or in the orthopnoeic position?

CRITICAL THINKING EXERCISES

1. Mr Stewart, 27, sustained a fractured tibia and fibula of his right leg as a result of a motorcycle accident. He was taken straight from the accident to the emergency department and then surgery, and has not washed since before the accident. He has arrived on the ward direct from the operating suite, with a plaster cast on the injured leg, and in a considerable amount of pain. What needs to be done to meet his comfort and hygiene needs?
2. Mr Gauchi, 75, has advanced-stage lung cancer, is extremely lethargic and has a very dry mouth as a result of constant mouth breathing. How would you perform his bed bath and remake his bed without causing him any further distress? What would be the best position for him in bed and what other matters need attention for his comfort?

REFERENCES AND FURTHER READING

Barker R (2007) *Baby love*, 3rd edn. New Holland Publishers, Chatswood Australia

Crisp J & Taylor C (eds) (2005) *Potter & Perry's Fundamentals of Nursing*, 2nd edn. Elsevier Australia, Sydney

Darby M L (2006) *Mosby's Comprehensive Review of Dental Hygiene.* Mosby Elsevier Philadelphia

deWit S (2004) *Fundamental Concepts and Skills for Nursing*. Elsevier Saunders, Philadelphia

Ebersole P, Hess P & Luggen A (2007) *Toward Healthy* Ageing. Mosby, St Louis

Leifer G (2007) *Introduction to Maternity and Pediatric Nursing*. Elsevier Health Science Division, Philadelphia

Lowdermilk D L (2007) *Maternity and Women's Health Care*, 9th edn. Evolve Elsevier, Philadelphia

Matteson P (2001) *Women's health during the childbearing years: a community-based approach*. Mosby, St Louis

Pantley E (2003) *Gentle Baby Care*. McGraw-Hill Professional, Columbus OH

Peron J (1991) Care of the intact penis. *Midwifery Today*, 24, 17 November

Springhouse Publishing Company Staff (2007) *Medical-Surgical Nursing Made Incredibly Easy*, 2nd edn. Wolters Kluwer Health Lippincott Williams & Wilkins, Philadelphia

Chapter 28
MEDICATIONS

OBJECTIVES

- Define the key terms/concepts
- Identify the different formulations of medications
- Identify a drug by its three names (generic, trade and chemical names)
- List the drug administration routes
- Discuss factors affecting drug absorption
- Define 'first-pass metabolism' and discuss its impact on drug dosage
- Discuss the role of plasma proteins in drug distribution
- Compare enzyme induction and enzyme inhibition
- List the organs involved in drug excretion
- Discuss the reasons for therapeutic drug monitoring
- Define drug action, desired outcome, side effects, toxic effects, allergic reaction and drug interactions
- Discuss the legal and other responsibilities of the Enrolled Nurse (EN) regarding drug administration
- Demonstrate an ability to correctly calculate drug dosages
- Demonstrate knowledge of the correct administration of drugs via:
  - the enteral route (oral and nasogastric)
  - the parenteral route (subcutaneous and intramuscular)
  - the intravenous route
  - the ear and eye
  - rectal and vaginal routes
  - inhalation
  - transdermal and topical application
- Demonstrate an understanding of the actions of the different drug groups in order to monitor drug effectiveness
- Show an understanding of safe handling of hazardous substances
- Discuss the importance of discharge planning and education in client compliance with drug therapy

KEY TERMS/CONCEPTS

absorption
administration routes
allergic reaction
compliance
distribution
drug action
enzyme induction
enzyme inhibition
excretion
first-pass metabolism
generic name
metabolism
pharmacodynamics
pharmacokinetics
pharmacology
poisons Acts
poisons Regulations
poisons schedules
protein bound
side effects
therapeutic drug monitoring
trade, or proprietary, name

CHAPTER FOCUS

The use of medication is an important part of many clients' treatment regimens. It is therefore vital for the nurse to have both the knowledge and the skills to administer medications safely and correctly.

LIVED EXPERIENCE

I couldn't believe it — when I went to pack Mum's drugs up to take them into the hospital with her, I filled a shopping bag with them. So many pills and bottles. Some from her doctor, some from the health shop, Gaviscon and Mylanta from the supermarket . . . such a mixture and she really didn't know what she was supposed to be taking half of them for. Now she's been assessed properly and she's down to only three lots of tablets. The nurse spent some time with her and me explaining what they were for and gave us both written information as well. Mum now says that she thinks feeling dizzy and being so confused all the time was due to taking so many different drugs, and she's so much better now that I think she was right about that.

Angela, daughter of Mavis, age 74

Administering medication is one of the nurse's most important responsibilities and should be treated with the importance it deserves. It is not merely another task to be completed quickly before another is undertaken. Medication administration offers nurses the opportunity to increase their knowledge and skills, to observe the client for expected and unexpected actions, and to ensure that clients have been adequately educated about medications. The topics included in this chapter provide the nurse with a basis for being equipped to safely and competently administer medications to clients.

PHARMACOLOGY

'Pharmakon' is the Greek word for drug, and pharmacology is the study of the actions, uses and adverse effects of drugs. The term drug has several definitions, which include it being any substance that may be used medicinally in a range of forms and administered to the body by different methods to prevent, diagnose or treat a disease or condition, or 'any natural or synthetic substance that alters the physiological state of a living organism' (Taylor & Reide 1998). Furthermore, drugs can be divided into medicinal drugs (or medications), which are substances used in the treatment, prevention and diagnosis of a disease; and non-medicinal drugs (or social drugs), which are substances used for recreational use and include caffeine, alcohol, nicotine, cannabis, heroin and cocaine. The distinction between the two is not always clear-cut, as some non-medicinal substances can be used in a medicinal way (e.g. caffeine is included in some preparations to treat migraine) and some medicinal substances can be used in non-medicinal ways (e.g. opioid analgesics such as pethidine and morphine can be used recreationally for their mind-altering properties).

Pharmacology can further be subdivided into pharmacokinetics, which is the way the body affects the drug with time (e.g. absorption, distribution, metabolism and excretion), and pharmacodynamics, which are the effects of the drug on the body (e.g. actions and side effects). Before considering these two areas of pharmacology, it is important to consider drug nomenclature, as well as drug formulations and administration routes.

DRUG NOMENCLATURE

The nurse should be aware that each drug has various names — its chemical, generic and trade names. The chemical name provides an exact description of the drug's chemical composition. This is usually only used by chemists and pharmacologists. Occasionally a drug's generic name may describe its chemical compositions, as with lithium carbonate or potassium chloride.

The generic name is given by the manufacturer who first develops the drug. Even generic names are not standardised and nurses should be careful when using textbooks published in countries other than the one where they are practising nursing. Examples of different names used in different countries include adrenaline (Australia) and epinephrine (US); pethidine (Australia) and meperidine (US). Generic names are written with a lower-case first letter.

The trade (or proprietary) name is the name under which a manufacturer markets a drug. An example is the diuretic, frusemide, marketed as Urex, Lasix, Frusid and Uremide. Trade names are written with an initial capital letter.

DRUG FORMULATIONS AND ADMINISTRATION ROUTES

A drug may be presented in a variety of forms (Table 28.1) and administered via several different routes.

Routes of administration of drugs include:

- Enteral — this involves both the oral route, and nasogastric and percutaneous endoscopic gastrostomy (PEG) tube routes. (See Chapter 31 for information about nasogastric and PEG tubes.) The advantage of the enteral route is that it is simple, cheap and convenient. Disadvantages include that drugs may be affected by food or gastric pH, and that it is not useful in critically ill clients as the gut may not be functioning
- Intravenous (IV) — drug delivery IV is rapid, as the absorption phase is bypassed. It is the route of choice in an emergency situation. However, one disadvantage is that because the drug delivery is fast, it is very difficult to retrieve if a mistake is made; for example, if the wrong drug is administered
- Intramuscular (IM) — drug absorption IM is generally fast because of the vascular nature of muscle. However, this can be slowed by the addition of oily substances (termed a depot preparation). A disadvantage of this route is that administration can be painful, especially if treatment is prolonged over a period of time and muscles are used a number of times

TABLE 28.1 | DRUG FORMULATIONS

Capsule	Gelatine container enclosing a drug in liquid, powder or granule form
Tablet	A drug mixed with a base compound and compressed into a variety of shapes. Tablets are sometimes coated, which delays release of the drug until the tablet reaches the intestine. Tablets are coated if the drug could cause gastric irritation or if it would be destroyed by gastric juice. Another form of tablet is 'slow release' (or sustained release), which contains a drug that is released over a prolonged period
Granules	Small rounded pellets that are usually coated
Lozenge	Small tablet containing a medicinal agent in a flavoured fruit or mucilage base, which dissolves in the mouth to release the drug
Mixture	Aqueous vehicle in which drugs are dissolved or suspended
Suspension	Liquid in which insoluble particles of a drug are dispersed
Elixir	Sweetened, flavoured alcoholic solution containing a drug
Linctus	Sweetened syrup containing a drug
Tincture	Alcoholic solution containing a drug
Emulsion	Mixture of oil and water containing a drug
Syrup	Concentrated sugar solution containing a drug
Cachet	Envelope of rice paper that encloses a drug
Injection	Sterile aqueous or oily solutions and suspensions containing a drug, which are administered parenterally
Suppository	Solid preparation containing a drug, which melts when inserted into the rectum
Pessary	Solid preparation containing a drug, which is administered vaginally
Drops	Aqueous or oily solution containing a drug. Drops may be instilled into the eye, ear or nose
Cream	Aqueous or oily emulsion for topical application
Ointment	Semi-solid greasy preparation for topical application
Paste	Similar to ointment but contains a high proportion of powders. Pastes have a very stiff consistency and will adhere to lesions at body temperature
Liniment	Oily or alcoholic preparation for topical application
Paint	Liquid preparation for application to the skin or mucous membranes
Lotion	Aqueous, alcoholic or emulsified vehicle for topical application
Powder (dusting)	Medicated substance for topical application

- Subcutaneous (SC) — drug absorption SC is relatively slow because of the poor blood supply in subcutaneous tissue. Adrenaline added to a subcutaneous preparation will make the absorption even slower because adrenaline causes constriction of blood vessels
- Intradermal (ID) — except for local anaesthetics, drugs are not commonly given via this route. Substances such as serums or vaccines are sometimes administered intradermally and this route is used for allergy testing; for example, Mantoux tests are performed intradermally
- Intrathecal (IT) injections are given directly into the central nervous system (CNS) via the cerebrospinal fluid, bypassing the blood–brain barrier. (See Chapter 41 for an explanation of the blood–brain barrier.) Epidural injections are given into the space between the arachnoid mater and the dura mater and are often used as local anaesthetics during surgical procedures involving the pelvic region
- Intra-articular injections are given directly into articular joints, usually involving corticosteroids to reduce joint inflammation. Disadvantages to this route is that it can be painful and often is required to be done under radiological imaging to ensure that it is administered into the joint cavity
- Transdermal — drugs given via this route require low doses over long periods of time. Transdermal preparations include hormones, antiemetics, anti-anginal agents and nicotine patches
- Topical — preparations include antiseptics, creams and lotions. Some preparations have systemic as well as local effects, as a small amount is absorbed systemically
- Inhalation — the large surface area of the lungs facilitates rapid absorption. Agents given via this route include oxygen, anaesthetic agents, mucolytic agents and bronchodilators
- Mucous membranes — some drugs administered via this route have both local and systemic effects. Drugs designed to be absorbed through the mucous membranes can be administered sublingually (e.g. sprays, lozenges), intra-nasally (e.g. sprays, drops, metered sprays), rectally (e.g. suppositories), vaginally (e.g. pessaries and creams) or via the conjunctiva of the eyes (e.g. drops and inserts):
  - advantages of the rectal route include its suitability in clients who are nauseous or vomiting, have

swallowing problems or are unconscious; and the slow absorption of anti-inflammatory preparations, which makes this route ideal for overnight administration, unlike oral preparations, the affects of which have often worn off by the following morning

— disadvantages of the rectal route include suppositories causing anal or rectal irritation, especially with prolonged use; self-administration may be difficult for some clients, and the presence of faecal matter in the rectum interferes with drug absorption

— vaginal preparations, if required to be left in situ, are best inserted at night when the client is in bed and ready to sleep. This limits leakage of the medication and provides the best opportunity for absorption. One advantage of this route is that the client is often able to self administer.

PHARMACOKINETICS

Pharmacokinetics describes the way the body affects the drug over time and relates to the processes of absorption, distribution, metabolism and excretion (Figure 28.1).

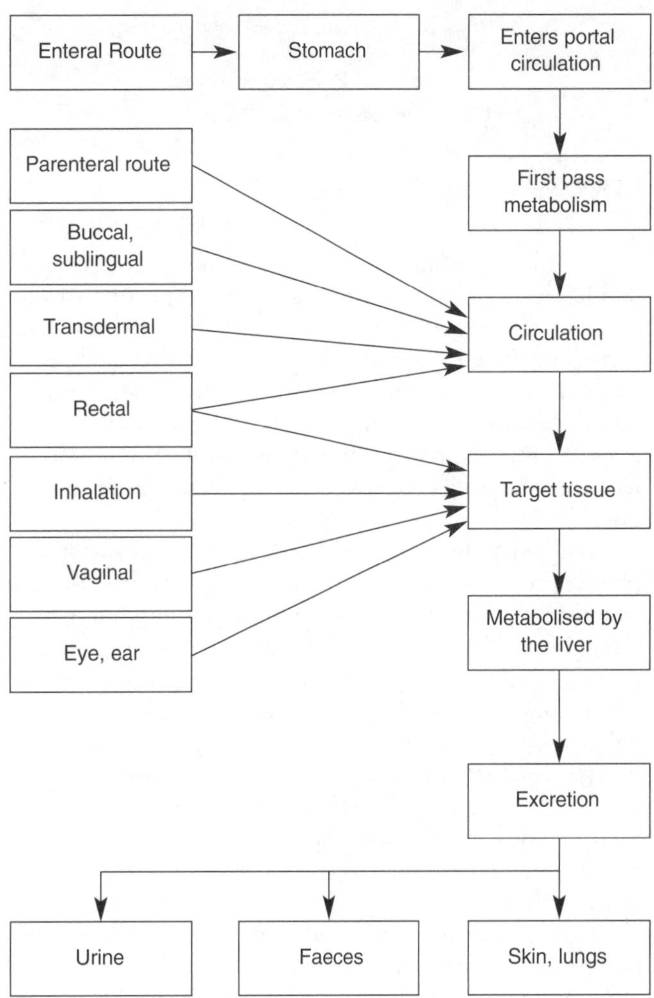

Figure 28.1 | Pharmacokinetics simplified

ABSORPTION

Absorption is the movement of a drug from the site of administration into the bloodstream. The rate and amount of drug absorbed depends on three factors:

1. Degree of blood flow to the area: a drug will be absorbed rapidly from a highly vascular area
2. Solubility of the drug: to be effectively absorbed across the cell membrane, a drug should be lipophilic (fat-loving). Acidic drugs are readily absorbed in the stomach, while alkaline drugs are better absorbed in the intestine. However, because most drugs pass rapidly through the stomach, most absorption takes place in the intestine
3. Route of administration: the route of administration affects the speed with which a drug takes effect. An oral medication has to undergo absorption in the gastrointestinal tract before it reaches the bloodstream and can take effect. It is therefore slower acting than if the same drug was given by injection. A drug given by injection avoids the need for absorption because it bypasses the gastrointestinal tract. The fastest effect from a drug occurs via the IV route because the drug is injected directly into circulating blood.

FIRST-PASS METABOLISM

Medication is absorbed from the gastrointestinal tract and enters the hepatic portal system, where it reaches the liver and is metabolised. Some drugs are almost entirely metabolised during this hepatic first pass, resulting in only very small amounts being available for therapeutic use. These drugs are better given via another route. An example of this is glyceryl trinitrate (Anginine), which is used to treat angina pectoris. If given orally, almost 96% is destroyed in this hepatic first-pass metabolism. Given sublingually, the drug bypasses the liver and is able to reach the target organs to have therapeutic effect. First-pass metabolism is also the reason why oral doses and parenteral doses are not equal — giving drugs via the parenteral route bypasses the first-pass metabolism and means that smaller doses can be given to achieve the same therapeutic effect.

DISTRIBUTION

After the drug has been absorbed into the general circulation it will then be distributed to different tissues for drug action to occur. To be transported in the blood, the drug molecules become protein bound (i.e. bind loosely to blood proteins); however, there is always some unbound (or free) drug. Equilibrium exists between the bound and unbound drug but only the unbound drug molecules are able to bind with the tissue (Figure 28.2).

The blood plasma contains a variety of plasma proteins (e.g. albumin, corticosteroid-binding globulin (CBG) and glycoproteins), which are able to bind to drugs to produce a drug–protein complex. If plasma proteins are deficient,

D_u + Pr D_bPr (where D_u = unbound drug,
↓ Pr = protein,
D_bPr = protein-bound drug)

D_u binds to tissue receptors → Action

Figure 28.2 | Drug–plasma protein binding

for example, if a client has a condition such as liver disease, malnutrition or extensive burns, a greater portion of the drug remains unbound and is available to bind to the tissue, increasing the effects of the drug and requiring a decrease in the dose. Conversely, if there is an increased level of plasma proteins, in a client who has multiple myeloma, for example, there is an increase in the amount of bound drug, reducing the drug's effectiveness, requiring an increase in dose.

Drugs may also compete for the same binding site on the plasma protein when more than one drug is administered concurrently. The drug with the higher affinity (or greater attraction) will be bound and displace the other(s) from the protein-binding site, resulting in the plasma concentration of the now unbound drug increasing. For example, aspirin will displace phenytoin from the plasma protein, resulting in an increased level of unbound phenytoin and, potentially, phenytoin toxicity. The effect is the same as giving an increased dose of the drug (Figure 28.3).

The blood–brain barrier of the central nervous system is generally very selective and allows very few drugs to pass through it. However, some conditions alter the permeability of the blood–brain barrier. For example, meningitis renders it permeable to penicillin, which is otherwise unable to pass through. The placental barrier is not as effective, and many drugs are able to cross the placenta to the fetus. Drugs that can reach the fetus in this way have the potential to cause significant damage, including congenital malformations. Unless absolutely necessary, drugs should not be taken during pregnancy and especially not during the first trimester, when organ development in the fetus occurs.

METABOLISM

Metabolism is the process whereby a substance is chemically altered, making it hydrophilic (water-loving) so that it can be readily excreted. The metabolism of drugs into inactive forms for excretion involves enzymes that are mainly found in the smooth endoplasmic reticulum in the liver. However, some enzymes are also found in the plasma, intestine and other organs. The main enzymes involved are those of the cytochrome P-450 family (several different types numbered from a to d). There are two types of enzymes involved in metabolism. During Phase I metabolism, enzymes modify the drugs by a series of chemical processes such as oxidation, reduction, hydrolysis and addition or removal of an active group from the drug molecule. During Phase II metabolism, the metabolite from Phase I, or a drug, may be directly conjugated (joined to another substance) by the enzymes, making the end product soluble for excretion.

Normally, these enzymes are present in small amounts. However, in some circumstances the amount of enzymes can alter, thereby also altering the rate of metabolism. For example, alcohol stimulates production of hepatic enzymes in habitual drinkers, resulting in the alcohol being more rapidly metabolised than in a non-drinker. This process of causing the amount of enzymes to be increased is called enzyme induction. Alcohol can also cause the levels of other enzymes involved in drug metabolism to increase, leading to the drug being more rapidly metabolised and therefore having a reduced therapeutic effect. Enzyme induction can be due to environmental pollutants, including benzopyretics in cigarette smoke, pesticides and some drugs, such as warfarin and phenytoin. Enzyme inhibition is the opposite effect and is the decreased synthesis of enzymes, resulting in the slowing down of the metabolic steps and an increased therapeutic effect. Some drugs are known enzyme inhibitors and include cimetidine, erythromycin, diltiazem, verapamil and ketaconazole. Figure 28.4 illustrates the process of drug metabolism simplified.

DRUG EXCRETION

After metabolism, drug excretion may be through the kidneys, lungs, exocrine glands, liver and/or intestine. The chemical composition of the drug determines the organ(s) of excretion, for example, 100% of frusemide, 80% of digoxin and 50% of salbutamol are excreted in the urine. The kidneys are the main organs for drug excretion and, if a client's renal function is impaired, the client is at risk of drug toxicity. Drugs that depend on renal function for excretion are eliminated more slowly in the very young and in older people. Gaseous compounds such as general anaesthetic agents are eliminated via the lungs. Alcohol is also partially excreted via the lungs and this is the basis of the police random breath testing to detect drink-drivers.

Some drugs, penicillin for example, exit unchanged in the urine, while others must undergo transformation in

P_u + Pr ↔ P_bPr (where P_u = unbound phenytoin, Pr = protein, P_bPr = bound phenytoin–protein complex)

Add aspirin, which has a greater affinity for the protein (where A_u = unbound aspirin)

(P_u + Pr ↔ P_bPr) + A_u → P_u + P_u' (previously bound phenytoin) + Pr ↔ A_bPr (bound aspirin–protein complex)

↓

P_u + P_u' = more phenytoin available to bind to tissue receptor site, resulting in more potent drug effect and possibly adverse effects.

Figure 28.3 | Displacement of phenytoin from its protein-binding site by aspirin

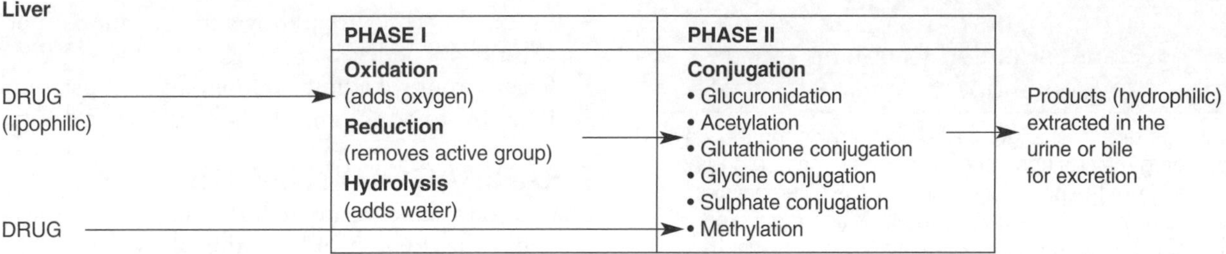

Figure 28.4 | Drug metabolism simplified

the liver before being excreted by the kidneys. Many drugs enter the hepatic circulation to be broken down by the liver and excreted into the bile and then into the bowel. The liver has a large metabolic capacity so, in people with liver disease, drug elimination is generally not affected until a large portion of the liver's functional capacity is lost.

IMPORTANCE OF THERAPEUTIC DRUG MONITORING

For drugs to be therapeutic, a certain blood level needs to be reached and maintained. It is therefore a priority that medications are administered on time. If they are administered late, the level of the medication in the blood may drop below a therapeutic level; for example, if the level of an antibiotic is too low it provides an opportunity for microorganisms to multiply. If the blood levels are too high, toxicity and serious consequences might occur. The main aim of therapeutic drug monitoring is to optimise drug therapy by achieving adequate drug levels, while minimising toxicity. This is especially important in clients at the extremes of age. Clinical Interest Box 28.1 outlines some signs and symptoms of toxicity commonly seen in older clients. Clinical Interest Box 28.2 identifies changes related to ageing that influence pharmacokinetics.

Drug levels are measured to:

- Individualise the dose to the client; for example, lithium (a mood-stabilising drug commonly used to modify or prevent recurrent episodes of mania or depression [Healy 2005]), phenytoin (a drug used to control convulsive seizures and sometimes cardiac arrhythmias) and warfarin (an anticoagulant used to manage or prevent the formation of a thrombus [blood clot] [Tiziani 2006]). With each of these drugs the optimal dose is highly individual, the effects need careful monitoring, and the dose may need to be adjusted periodically
- Avoid toxicity; for example, digoxin, vancomycin. Digoxin is a drug that slows and strengthens the heartbeat. Therapeutic levels of digoxin are very close to toxic levels, leaving only a narrow margin of safety. Before each dose of digoxin the client's heart rate and rhythm should be checked and the drug withheld and the senior nurse and/or medical officer notified if the client's heart rate is less than 60 beats/min (adult client) or there is any arrhythmia or other concern.

Concerns that may indicate toxicity include slow or irregular heartbeat, anorexia, nausea, vomiting, diarrhoea, drowsiness and extreme tiredness,

CLINICAL INTEREST BOX 28.1
Indicators of drug toxicity in older adults

Skin
- Rashes
- Pruritus
- Urticaria
- Photosensitivity (e.g. abnormal responses to sunlight)

Gastrointestinal tract (GIT)
- Discomfort and pain; for example, pancreatitis
- Nausea and vomiting
- Blood in stools or vomitus
- Diarrhoea

Cardiovascular system
- Abnormalities in cardiac rhythm; for example, palpitations, tachycardia
- Hypotension or hypertension
- Congestive cardiac failure
- Depression of bone marrow activity (causing anaemia, leukopenia or other abnormalities of the blood)

Central nervous system
- Increasing confusion and irritability
- Alterations in gait; for example, stumbling
- Tremors
- Unusual drowsiness or insomnia
- Blurred vision or other vision abnormalities
- Slurred speech
- Ototoxicity (changes in hearing and balance)
- Intolerance to heat or cold (changes in temperature regulation)
- Anticholinergic effects (ranging from dry mouth and hot dry skin to serious mental impairment and seizures)

Renal system
- Electrolyte imbalance
- Urine retention
- Polyuria
- Fluid retention

Respiratory system
- Dyspnoea
- Asthmatic responses

Biliary system
- Jaundice
- Impaired liver function
- Clotting changes

(Ebersole & Hess 2005: 295)

CLINICAL INTEREST BOX 28.2
Changes related to ageing that influence pharmacokinetics

Many age-related changes to the body impact on the way that a drug may be absorbed, distributed, metabolised and excreted from the body. Because of these differences, all drug therapy should be given cautiously and monitored carefully in the older client. Age-related changes that may affect the pharmacokinetics of a drug include:

- Altered nutritional habits and ingestion of non-prescription drugs that may alter drug absorption; for example, ingestion of antacids and laxatives
- Changes in the quantity and quality of digestive enzymes
- Increase in gastric pH
- Decrease in gastric motility
- Decrease in intestinal blood flow
- Delayed gastric emptying
- Decreases in total body water and lean body mass and increase in body fat, which may all lead to an altered distribution of the drug
- Decreased levels of plasma proteins and therefore decreased protein binding of drugs
- Changes in the Phase I metabolism in the liver, involving the microsomal enzymes
- The liver's ability to recover from injury such as hepatitis is reduced with age
- Hepatic function may also be affected by severe nutritional deficiencies
- Decreased cardiac output and reserve
- Decreased blood flow to liver and kidneys
- Congestive cardiac failure reduces both the capacity of the liver to metabolise drugs as well as reducing the hepatic flow
- Creatinine clearance decreases with age, resulting in a longer half life of many drugs and the subsequent risk of accumulation
- Decreased renal excretion

weakness, confusion, abdominal pain, blurred vision or visual disturbances (Tiziani 2006). Vancomycin is a powerful antibiotic reserved for the treatment of severe infections that are not responding to other antibiotics. This drug can produce severe adverse effects that include rash, itching, fever, tachycardia, nausea, vomiting, diarrhoea and, sometimes, hearing loss or kidney damage (Tiziani 2006) The effects of toxicity are often extremely unpleasant, may cause permanent damage or, if undetected and/or untreated, may prove fatal

- Ensure effective blood levels; for example, prophylactic anticonvulsants to avoid convulsive seizures, gentamicin to ensure adequate antimicrobial cover
- Check client compliance
- Check that comorbidities that may alter drug metabolism and elimination are not having an effect on blood levels; for example, renal impairment, hepatic failure, shock, sepsis
- Ensure that concurrent drug administration is not affecting blood levels
- Change route of administration; for example, from IV or IM to oral administration, or change dosage.

PHARMACODYNAMICS

Pharmacodynamics relates to how a drug acts on the body, including the strength and duration of its effects.

DRUG ACTION

The extent of the response to a drug depends on its concentration at the site of action, which in turn depends on dosage, absorption, metabolism and elimination. More than any other factor, the route of administration determines the onset of drug effect. Drugs that are administered directly into the bloodstream provoke a rapid response, whereas drugs administered orally or topically must be absorbed into the bloodstream before they can take effect. Drugs act by affecting or controlling changes in biochemical or physiological processes in the body. Drugs produce their actions in one of three ways: altering body fluids, altering cell membranes, or interacting with receptor sites.

Most drugs act at specific cell receptor sites. A specific drug forms a complex with only one type of receptor but may produce multiple effects because of the location of those receptors in cells of different tissues or organs. For example, the anticholinergic drug atropine sulphate not only reduces the production of saliva, bronchial, nasal and gastric secretions, but it also increases heart rate, stimulates ventilation, and raises intraocular pressure. A 'selective' drug acts at a receptor in a particular type of body tissue and produces little effect on similar receptors in other organs. For example, the bronchodilator salbutamol has specific selectivity for receptors in bronchial smooth muscle but produces little or no stimulation of similar receptors in cardiac muscle.

A drug may produce more than one effect:

- The desired action is the physiological response the drug is expected to cause
- Side effects (also called adverse effects or adverse reactions) are secondary effects caused by most drugs. For example, a side effect of acetylsalicylic acid (aspirin) is increased bleeding time; and a common side effect of morphine is nausea
- Toxic effects develop after prolonged administration of high doses of medication, or when a drug accumulates in the blood because of impaired metabolism or excretion
- Allergic reactions are unpredictable responses to a drug that acts as an antigen, triggering the release of antibodies (see Chapter 25). Allergic reactions may be mild, such as urticaria and pruritus, or they may be severe; for example, severe wheezing and respiratory distress, or life-threatening anaphylactic reaction
- Idiosyncratic reactions are those where the client's

body either overreacts or underreacts to a drug, or when the reaction is unusual and there is no known cause
- Drug interactions occur when one drug modifies the action of another drug; for example, a drug may either increase or decrease the action of other drugs. A drug may be synergistic (enhances the effects of another drug) or it may be antagonistic (opposes the effects of another drug).

NURSING CARE AND ADMINISTRATION OF MEDICATIONS

The nurse's role in drug administration is a complex one, requiring both knowledge and skill. To promote safe and correct drug administration, the nurse requires knowledge about the drugs being administered, including:
- Indications for use
- Routes of administration
- Range of dosages
- Desired effects and possible adverse effects
- Safe handling of hazardous substances
- Storage
- Legislation, and health care facility policies.

The nurse also requires certain skills to:
- Administer drugs by various routes
- Calculate the correct amount of drug to administer
- Evaluate the effects of drugs
- Educate clients about drug therapy
- Teach self-administration
- Record the drugs administered and the client's response to them.

LEGAL ASPECTS OF DRUG ADMINISTRATION

Before a drug can be administered safely, the nurse needs to be aware of the legal aspects of drug administrations. This includes knowledge of the laws governing the possession, use and dispensation of drugs and of the directives of the nurse's registering body on the administration of medications to clients. It also means observing the employing health care facility's occupational health and safety (OHS) regulations that are designed to promote safe storage, handling and use of drugs (see Chapter 26). Currently, the states and territories of Australia differ on the regulations governing administration of medication by an Enrolled Nurse (EN). In Tasmania an EN whose qualifications have been determined as appropriate for the purpose of administration of medications and whose practising certificate has been endorsed may administer medications listed in schedule 2, 3 and/or 4 of the Poisons List Order 2001 (Nurses Board of Tasmania 2007). In Queensland, the Health (Drug & Poisons) Regulation 1996 (section 58A) was amended in 2006 to enable the EN with medication endorsement to administer controlled Schedule 8 drugs (Controlled Drugs) under the supervision of a Registered Nurse (RN) or doctor (Queensland Nursing Council 2006). Other states and territories are currently moving towards, or have established, specific guidelines regarding limited medication administration by the EN. Each EN will need to ascertain the regulations specific to the state or territory of Australia in which nursing is practised.

Legal Acts concerning poisons and the poisons regulatory bodies in New Zealand and each state and territory in Australia (Table 28.2) deal with the control of all drugs, from prescription medication through to agricultural poisons and research drugs. The laws and regulations apply to sale, supply, storage, dispensing and labelling. The drugs and poisons schedules divide drugs into groups according to their mode of action, therapeutic use, potency, potential for abuse and addiction, and safety. While there is currently no national drugs and poisons schedule in Australia, and each state and territory has its own version, the recommendations of the National Drugs and Poisons Schedule Committee in the form of the Standard for the Uniform Scheduling of Drugs and Poisons (SUSDP, Table 28.3) are usually incorporated into the legislation and regulations of each state and territory. An agreement between Australia and New Zealand has led to harmonisation of trans-Tasman scheduling, and the two countries now have compatible schedules, labelling and packaging requirements (Bryant & Knights 2006).

ADMINISTRATION OF DRUGS

Before administering medications in any form or by any route the nurse must check that the client does not have any drug allergies. The nurse also observes the client who is starting a new medication for any signs of allergy or adverse reaction, and reports and records such responses promptly to the medical officer and the nurse in charge. If the situation arises that a client chooses not to take a prescribed medication, this must be recorded on the client's medication chart and also reported to the client's medical officer and the nurse in charge. The principles of asepsis (see Chapter 25) are employed during the preparation and administration of all medications.

To ensure that medications are administered correctly and safely, the nurse must observe the seven rights of drug administration (Reiss, Evans & Broyles 2002):
1. The right client
2. The right medication
3. The right dose
4. The right route
5. The right time
6. The right documentation
7. The client right to refuse medication.

Before any medication is administered the client medication chart (Figure 28.5) must be checked thoroughly and systematically to determine the name of the drug, the route, the dosage, and the date and time for administration of the medication prescribed.

The nurse compares the label of the drug container with the client medication chart three times:

TABLE 28.2 | AUSTRALIAN LEGISLATION INVOLVED IN THE REGULATION OF DRUGS

Jurisdiction	Drug regulation legislation	Additional drug offences Acts
Commonwealth (Cth)	*Therapeutic Goods Act 1989* (Cth) *Therapeutic Goods Regulations 1990* (Cth) *National Health Act 1953* (Cth)	*Customs Act 1901* (Cth) *Crimes (Traffic in Narcotic Drugs and Psychotropic Substances) Act 1990* (Cth) *Narcotic Drugs Act 1967* (Cth) *Criminal Code Act 1995* (Cth) *Criminal Code (Serious Drug Offences) Amendment Act 2004* (Cth)
Australian Capital Territory (ACT)	*Poisons and Drugs Act 1978* (ACT) *Poisons Act 1933* (ACT) *Poisons Regulations* (ACT) *Drugs of Dependence Act 1989* (ACT) *Drugs in Sport Act 1989* (ACT) *Drugs of Dependence Regulations 2005* (ACT)	
New South Wales (NSW)	*Poisons and Therapeutic Goods Act 1966* (NSW) *Poisons and Therapeutic Goods Regulation 1994* (NSW)	*Drug Misuse and Trafficking Act 1985* (NSW)
Northern Territory (NT)	*Poisons and Dangerous Drugs Act 1983* (NT) *Therapeutics Goods and Cosmetics Act 1986* (NT) *Poisons and Dangerous Drugs Regulations 1996* (NT)	*Misuse of Drugs Act 1990* (NT)
Queensland (Qld)	*Health Act 1937* (Qld) *Health (Drugs and Poisons) Regulation 1966* (Qld)	*Drugs Misuse Act 1986* (Qld)
South Australia (SA)	*Controlled Substances Act 1984* (SA) *Controlled Substances (Poisons) Regulations 1996* (SA) *Drugs of Dependence (General) Regulations 1985* (SA)	*Drugs Act 1908 (SA)*
Tasmania (Tas)	*Poisons Act 1971* (Tas) *Poisons Regulations 1975* (Tas) *Alcohol and Drug Dependency Act 1968* (Tas) *Therapeutics Goods Act 2001* (Tas) *Therapeutics Goods Regulations 2002* (Tas)	*Misuse of Drugs Act 2001* (Tas)
Victoria (Vic)	*Therapeutic Goods (Victoria) Act 1994* (Vic) *Drugs, Poisons and Controlled Substances Act 1981* (Vic) *Drugs, Poisons and Controlled Substances Regulations 1995* (Vic)	
Western Australia (WA)	*Poisons Act 1964* (WA) *Poisons Regulations 1965* (WA)	*Misuse of Drugs Act 1981* (WA)

TABLE 28.3 | STANDARD FOR THE UNIFORM SCHEDULING OF DRUGS AND POISONS (SUSDP)

Schedule	Label	Description	Examples
Unscheduled substances			
	—	Unscheduled substances are those not requiring control by scheduling. They are not considered to be poisons. It is important to note that many therapeutic preparations are unscheduled substances and may be purchased in supermarkets and health food stores	Most antacids, some analgesics, laxatives, contact lens products, infant formulas, vitamins, sunscreens, topical antiseptics and many herbal remedies
Schedule 1 Poisons	—	This schedule is not currently used. It was formerly used for substances requiring proof of age, identity and the signature of the purchaser. It has been suggested that some complementary and alternative medicines be moved into this Schedule so that they can be subject to control	

TABLE 28.3 | STANDARD FOR THE UNIFORM SCHEDULING OF DRUGS AND POISONS (SUSDP) — cont'd

Schedule	Label	Description	Examples
Pharmaceutical substances			
Schedule 2 Poisons	Pharmacy medicine	Available to the public only from pharmacies, or where a pharmacy service is unavailable, from persons licensed to sell Schedule 2 poisons. A pharmacist's advice is available if required	Most cough and cold preparations, some antihistamines, mild analgesics, worm tablets, anti-angina sprays, anti-inflammatory agents, topical antifungals, histamine H_2-receptor antagonists for gastro-oesophageal reflux and decongestant eye drops
Schedule 3 Poisons	Pharmacist only medicine	Only available to the public from a pharmacist or from medical, dental or veterinary practitioners, but without need for a prescription. The safe use of these substances requires professional advice. The storage must not be accessible to the public	Metered-dose asthma aerosols, topical corticosteroids, adrenaline, histamine H_2-receptor antagonists for gastro-oesophageal reflux, and topical antifungals for vaginal use
Schedule 4 Poisons	Prescription only medicine Prescription animal ready	May be used or supplied only under prescription from a medical, dental or veterinary practitioner. Must be stored in a dispensary. In some Australian states and territories, specially qualified nurses (Nurse Practitioners), optometrists and podiatrists may prescribe a limited range of Schedule 4 drugs	Many drugs: all new drugs, antibiotics, insulins, antidepressants, hormones (including contraceptives), most cardiovascular and central nervous system drugs, vaccines, anti-glaucoma eyedrops and most injections
Agricultural, domestic and industrial substances			
Schedule 5 Poisons	Caution	Substances with a low potential for causing harm, which can be minimised by the use of appropriate packaging with simple warnings and safety directions on the label. For sale by a pharmacist, Poisons Licence holder or general dealer. Must not be stored or supplied in a drink or food container	Household poisons, ether, naphthalene, petrol, some head lice preparations and borax
Schedule 6 Poisons	Caution or poison (depending whether for internal or external use)	More dangerous chemicals than Schedule 5, with a moderate potential for causing harm. Extra storage and packaging controls and warning labels are required	Household and garden pesticides and solvents, some iodine preparations
Schedule 7 Poisons	Dangerous poison	Substances with a high potential for causing harm at low exposure and which require special precautions during manufacturing, handling, storage or use. A permit is required to buy these chemicals and the purchaser must be over 18 years of age. These poisons should be available only to specialised or authorised users who have the skills necessary to handle them safely. Special regulations restricting their availability, possession, storage or use may apply	Arsenic, strychnine, cyanide and commercial pesticides

(Continued)

TABLE 28.3 | STANDARD FOR THE UNIFORM SCHEDULING OF DRUGS AND POISONS (SUSDP) — cont'd

Schedule	Label	Description	Examples
Controlled drugs and prohibited substances			
Schedule 8 Poisons	Controlled drug	Substances that may produce addiction or dependence. Possession without authority is illegal. The tightest controls are used to reduce abuse, misuse and dependence. Prescriptions are only valid for 3 months. Drugs must be stored in a locked cabinet and records kept for 3 years	Opioids (e.g. morphine, methadone, high-dose codeine) and CNS stimulants (e.g. dexamphetamine)
Schedule 9 Poisons	Prohibited substances	Substances for which the manufacture, possession, sale or use is prohibited except in special circumstances. Drugs that may be abused or misused and drugs possibly required for teaching, research or analytical purposes, but which are too toxic for therapeutic use	Heroin and most recreational drugs (except alcohol and tobacco)

(adapted from Australian Health Ministers Advisory Council 2001)

1. Before removing the container from the trolley or cupboard
2. Before removing the drug from the container
3. Before returning the container to the trolley or cupboard.

To identify a client correctly, before a drug is administered, the nurse:

- Checks the drug order form against the client's identity bracelet
- Asks the client to state his or her name
- Addresses the client by name.

Special care should be taken when identity bracelets are not worn (e.g. in residential care settings) or where the client is unable to state his or her own name, because of dementia or mental disturbance for example. One safety measure that has been implemented in some aged-care residential settings is to have a current photograph of each resident that can help with identification.

Most medication errors occur when a nurse fails to follow the recommended safety guidelines, or when the nurse is distracted while preparing or administering medications. To prevent drug administration errors the nurse should:

- Check the date and time to be given
- Read drug labels carefully
- Be aware that many drugs have similar names
- Check the expiry date on the drug label
- Check the decimal point on prescriptions and drug container labels
- Not administer a drug if the prescription or drug label is illegible (or if the nurse has any doubt at all about the order)
- Be proficient in calculating dosages
- Use administration equipment (e.g. a medicine glass or syringe) with distinct markings
- Not administer any drug prepared by another person (unless the nurse was present throughout the whole time it was being prepared)
- Not prepare medications in advance of the prescribed time for administration
- Not leave prepared medications (e.g. a loaded syringe or oral medication in a medicine cup) unattended
- Have the drug checked by an RN (nurses need to check the laws and regulations governing the geographical area of their work, concerning who may administer which drugs and what rules need to be observed in the process)
- Give full attention to the task.

ERRORS IN ADMINISTRATION

Errors can arise for many reasons. Information on ways to avoid errors in administration is provided throughout this chapter, and also in Clinical Interest Box 28.3. Each health care facility has its own protocol for dealing with medication errors, and the nurse must understand and adhere to that protocol.

If the nurse does make a medication error (e.g. administering the wrong drug, wrong dose or via the wrong route) or if a nurse identifies an error made by another nurse, the incident must be reported immediately to the nurse in charge. The nurse has a professional and ethical responsibility for reporting any error, no matter how minor or trivial it may seem at the time. Measures to counteract the effects of the error may be necessary, such as administering an antidote (with a medical officer's order) or monitoring the drug's effects over time. The nurse is also responsible for completing an incident report form describing the nature of the incident. The incident report provides an objective analysis of why the incident occurred and is a means for

Medication chart

Use gummed label when available

Surname	Medical record no.	Sex
Fore names	Birth date	
Patient's address		

Ward/clinic
Dr in charge
Dr requesting

Print all drug names, doses and directions.

Regular and PRN drugs

Drug (approved name)		Dose	Date / Time										
Special directions (eg diluent, volume, etc.)		Route											
		Start date											
Doctor	Pharmacist	Cease date											
Drug (approved name)		Dose											
Special directions (eg diluent, volume, etc.)		Route											
		Start date											
Doctor	Pharmacist	Cease date											
Drug (approved name)		Dose											
Special directions (eg diluent, volume, etc.)		Route											
		Start date											
Doctor	Pharmacist	Cease date											
Drug (approved name)		Dose											
Special directions (eg diluent, volume, etc.)		Route											
		Start date											
Doctor	Pharmacist	Cease date											

Figure 28.5 | Example of a client medication chart (Paterson 1996)

CLINICAL INTEREST BOX 28.3
Safe medication management guidelines

- All medications must be kept in a locked cupboard or medication trolley, the key of which is kept by an RN at all times. Some preparations (e.g. suppositories, vaccines and insulin) require refrigeration and are stored in a lockable refrigerator. Nothing else should be stored in this refrigerator. Drugs or preparations for external use are stored apart from those intended for internal use.
- Drugs of addiction (e.g. Schedule 8 [Victoria]) are kept in a separate locked cupboard that is firmly fixed to a wall. It is customary for this cupboard to be within another locked cupboard. The key is kept in the possession of an RN at all times.
- A register must be maintained of all drugs of addiction, and the records must contain full details of all receipt of drugs and all disposal of drugs, whether by administration to a client, return to the pharmacy department, or by any other means. The nurse who administers the drug and the nurse who checks the drug both sign their names in the register.
- Health care facilities implement a protocol that conforms to the relevant state or territory regulations whereby certain drugs (usually drugs of addiction such as morphine) are checked at regular intervals (e.g. every 8 hours). Two nurses, one of whom should be an RN, count the drugs together and document their findings in a register. The number of drugs in the containers is compared with the number of drugs already recorded in the register. Both nurses sign the register to indicate that the count is correct. If the count is not correct, the health care facility protocol should be followed.
- Drugs of addiction and restricted substances can be supplied only with a written order by a medical officer or dentist.
- A qualified pharmacist has complete responsibility for all containers issued from the pharmacy department. No one else is permitted to label a container, alter the wording on a label or transfer the contents of one container to another.
- There should be a written medical officer's order for all drugs administered to clients. Verbal orders, including telephone orders, are open to misinterpretation. A written prescription must contain the date of prescribing, the client's full name, the name and dosage of the drug, the route of administration, the frequency of administration, and the signature of the medical officer who is writing the prescription. If the nurse has any doubt about the meaning of an order, the medical officer must be contacted immediately for clarification (before the drug is administered).
- An RN must check every dose of medication to be administered by an undergraduate student nurse. Nursing regulations dictate that an RN must accompany student nurses during administration of a drug.
- A nurse should administer only a medication that has been prepared personally; for example, the nurse should not administer any medication that has been prepared by someone else and not witnessed personally.
- The nurse who administers a drug to be taken orally must remain with the client until the drug has been swallowed.
- If the nurse is checking a drug that is to be administered by another nurse (e.g. a drug of addiction or intravenous antibiotic), in addition to the safety measures already stated, the checker must observe the dose being measured, reconstituted and drawn up, and then witness the drug being administered.
- After administering any drug the nurse records it immediately on the appropriate medication record form. Prompt recording prevents errors. Details recorded on the client's medication chart include the name of the drug, dosage, route and exact time of administration. The nurse who administers the drug must sign the record sheet.

the facility's safety personnel to monitor such events and to implement measures to prevent recurrence. The incident, measures taken and outcomes should also be recorded in the client's medical notes (see Chapter 20 for information on nursing documentation).

DRUG CALCULATIONS

Competence in calculating the required dose of prescribed drugs is one of the important factors in preventing errors in their administration. To promote accurate and safe administration of drugs, the nurse must understand the system of weights and measures used in prescriptions and be able to correctly calculate dosages.

SI UNITS

The International System of Units (SI units) for mass and volume are kilograms (kg) and litres (L). Smaller measures of mass commonly used are:

- grams (g): 1000 g = 1 kg
- milligrams (mg): 1000 mg = 1 g
- micrograms (mcg, μg): 1000 mcg = 1 mg.

Smaller units of volume commonly used are millilitres (mL: 1000 mL = 1 L) and microlitres (μL). See Appendix 2 for information concerning other units of measurement.

The strength of a pharmaceutical preparation used in electrolyte replacement therapy is normally expressed in millimoles (mmol) per tablet or millimoles per given volume of solution (e.g. mmol/L). A millimole is one thousandth of a mole, which is the molecular weight of a substance expressed in grams. For example, sodium has a molecular weight of 23, so a mole of sodium weighs 23 g, a millimole of sodium weighs 23 mg, and a 1 mM aqueous solution of sodium chloride, for example, contains 1 mmol of sodium chloride (containing 23 mg of sodium) in 1 L of water. Millimoles are also used to express the concentration of substances other than electrolytes and are used widely in laboratories, for example, in haematology reports.

PERCENTAGES

The strength of a pharmaceutical substance may be expressed as a percentage (parts per 100 parts) using one of the following combinations of weight and volume:

- Percentage weight in volume (% w/v). For example, 10% w/v indicates that 10 g of the active ingredient is present in 100 mL of product
- Percentage weight in weight (% w/w). For example, 10% w/w indicates that 10 g of the active ingredient is present in 100 g of product
- Percentage volume in volume (v/v). For example, 10% v/v indicates that 10 mL of the active ingredient is present in 100 mL of product
- Percentage volume in weight (% v/w). For example, 10% v/w indicates that 10 mL of the active ingredient is contained in 100 g of product.

EXPRESSING THE STRENGTH OF ACTIVE INGREDIENTS IN PHARMACEUTICAL PRODUCTS

Solid dose forms

In most instances, the strength of the active ingredient present in each solid form, such as a tablet, is expressed in grams, milligrams or micrograms. Strengths of some solid dosage forms are expressed in units of activity. For example, a vitamin capsule may contain 100 IU (international units). Products used for electrolyte replacement are expressed in grams or milligrams, and also in millimoles. For example, the strength of a potassium chloride tablet might be expressed as containing 600 mg of potassium chloride, or as containing 8 mmol of K^+ (potassium) and Cl^- (chloride).

Liquid dose forms

Liquid oral dose forms

The amount of an active ingredient in liquid oral preparations is expressed as w/v. For example, a liquid preparation may contain 250 mg (of the active ingredient) in 5 mL.

Liquid parenteral dose forms

Small-volume injections generally bear a label expressing the strength of the product as w/v. Care must be taken to note the total volume contained in the ampoule. For example, the label may indicate 25 mg/1 mL but the ampoule may contain 2 mL, therefore the total amount of active ingredient in the ampoule is 50 mg. The strength of some small-volume injections may also be expressed as percentage weight per volume (% w/v).

The strength of some other injections, such as adrenaline, is frequently expressed as 1 in 1000. This indicates that 1 g of active ingredient is contained in 1000 mL of product, thus 1 mL of the solution contains 1 mg of adrenaline.

The strength of certain substances, such as insulin, is expressed in units of activity per given volume, for example, 100 units per 1 mL, and is prescribed in units, for example, 10 units of Actrapid insulin.

Large-volume parenteral products

Large-volume parenteral products contain labels indicating the strength of the product in percentage terms. For example, a solution of sodium chloride for intravenous infusion may contain 0.9% w/v, which means 0.9 g sodium chloride in 100 mL solution.

CALCULATING DOSAGES

Although the introduction of unit doses and prepared solutions has meant that the need for nurses to undertake calculations has decreased, there are certain situations in which the nurse does need to perform basic calculations in connection with administration of drugs and other pharmaceutical products. The calculation of dosages must be performed with total accuracy, therefore the nurse must be competent in dealing with decimals, fractions, percentages, ratios, and proportions.

Formulae for calculating drug doses include:

Liquid drugs

$$\text{Volume of stock to be administered} = \frac{\text{Dose required} \times \text{Volume in stock strength}}{\text{Amount in stock strength}}$$

Example. A medical officer prescribes fentanyl 100 micrograms intramuscularly (IM). The medication in stock is available in ampoules containing 50 micrograms per mL.

Dose required = 100 micrograms
Stock strength = 50 micrograms/mL
Volume in stock strength = 1 mL
Amount in stock strength = 50 micrograms

$$\text{Volume of stock to be administered} = \frac{100 \text{ micrograms} \times 1 \text{ mL}}{50 \text{ micrograms}}$$

= 2 mL to be administered

Solid drugs

$$\text{Amount of stock to be administered} = \frac{\text{dose required}}{\text{stock strength}}$$

Example. A medical officer prescribes oral morphine 15 mg. The medication in stock is available as tablets containing 28 mg.

Dose required = 15 mg
Stock strength = 28 mg

$$\text{Amount of stock to be administered} = \frac{15 \text{ mg}}{28 \text{ mg}}$$

= ½ tablet to be administered

Drugs measured in units

$$\text{Amount of stock to be administered} = \frac{\text{Number of units required} \times \text{Volume in stock strength}}{\text{Number of units in stock solution}}$$

Example. A medical officer prescribes subcutaneous insulin 10 units. The insulin is available in 100 units per mL.

Number of units required = 10
Number of units in stock solution = 100
Volume in stock strength = 1 mL

$$\text{Amount of stock to be administered} = \frac{10 \times 1 \text{ mL}}{100}$$

= 0.1 mL to be administered

Calculation of paediatric dosages (Tiziani 2006)

Clarke's body weight rule

$$\text{Child's dose} = \frac{\text{Adult dose} \times \text{Weight of child (kg)}}{\text{Average adult weight (70 kg)}}$$

Clarke's body surface area rule

$$\text{Child's dose} = \frac{\text{Adult dose} \times \text{Surface area of child}}{\text{Surface area of adult (1.7 m}^2\text{)}}$$

It should be noted that preparing medications for infants and children requires additional skills. Nurses caring for children are recommended to consult paediatric textbooks for further information. Table 28.4 provides general guidelines concerning administering medications to infants and children.

MEDICAL ABBREVIATIONS

When writing prescriptions, the medical officer frequently uses abbreviations that are derived from Latin. Many medical officers have given up using these abbreviations because they can be easily misinterpreted, and it is safer to use the English terms. Abbreviations are also used when referring to strength of medications such as grams (g) and milligrams (mg). The abbreviation for micrograms using the Greek letter μ (mu), that is, μg, is not recommended, as it may lead to errors; mcg is the preferred abbreviation. Table 28.5 illustrates some of the common abbreviations that may still be written on prescriptions or drug forms.

ADMINISTERING MEDICATIONS

ADMINISTERING ORAL MEDICATIONS

Oral medications may be presented in solid or liquid form. The nurse must know whether solid medications must be swallowed whole, chewed, sucked, or whether the medication may be crushed for administration. Powdered medications, and some drugs in granule form, are mixed with a liquid before administration. Enteric-coated or sustained-release preparations must never be crushed,

TABLE 28.4 | GENERAL GUIDELINES FOR ADMINISTERING MEDICATIONS TO CHILDREN

Action	Rationale
Wash and dry hands	Prevents cross infection
Oral medications	
When possible use liquid rather than tablet form	Children find it difficult to swallow tablets
Offer a pleasant tasting drink or treat after medication is swallowed	Removes unpleasant after-taste, makes compliance more likely with next dose
Mix medication with tiny amount of pleasant tasting substance, such as honey (unless contraindicated by pharmacist) to help persuade a reluctant child to take medication	Makes the experience less negative, improves compliance
Avoid mixing the medication in food	The food may not all be consumed and the full dose of medication will not be ingested
Measure liquid doses using a small measuring cup: hold the measuring cup at eye level	Ensures correct amount is poured
Discard any excess amount poured from the bottle	Prevents contamination of unused medication in the bottle
Use a small plastic syringe (1 or 2 mL) to measure very small amounts	It is difficult to accurately measure tiny amounts of liquid any other way
Administer liquids to young infants via a syringe without a needle	Liquid can be administered into side of mouth between cheek and gums to reduce possibility of it being spat out
Injections	
Select site for intramuscular injection where muscle is developed	Careful site selection is imperative to avoid pain and bruising because infants and children do not have well-developed muscles
Have at least two people present during administration, at least one familiar person if possible	One person needs to hold the child securely. Children may be frightened and move suddenly and with vigour, making administration difficult or causing the needle to dislodge. A familiar face is reassuring
Use distraction techniques such as a toy that makes a noise, or a conversation	Distraction can help focus away from a frightening event and may reduce the perception of pain
Administer the injection firmly and quickly	Reduces pain and length of time child is fearful
Ensure that child is awake and held closely	Administering pain to a sleeping child causes awakening to trauma. The distress may instil fear of going to sleep

(Crisp & Taylor 2005)

TABLE 28.5 | COMMON ABBREVIATIONS USED IN PRESCRIPTIONS

Abbreviation	Latin term	English meaning
ac	ante cibum	Before meals
bd or bid	bis die or bis in die	Twice a day
mane	mane	In the morning
nocte	nocte	At night
pc	post cibum	After meals
po	per ora	By mouth, orally
pr	per rectum	Rectally
prn	pro re nata	As required
pv	per vaginam	Vaginally
qqh	quaque quarta hora	Every four hours
qid	quattuor in die	Four times a day
stat	statim	Immediately
tds	ter die sumendum	Three times a day
tid	ter in die	Three times a day

chewed or opened. They must be swallowed whole. Enteric coatings are used to:

- Prevent chemically sensitive drugs such as penicillin G and erythromycin from being decomposed by gastric secretions
- Prevent the side effects of nausea and vomiting caused if the drug is broken down in the stomach
- Prevent the drug from being diluted before it reaches the bowel
- Allow a delayed effect on the release of the drug (Bryant & Knights 2006).

Effervescent powders and tablets should be taken immediately after dissolving. All liquid preparations should be shaken before they are poured. Any mixture that stains the teeth should be taken through a straw, and the client should rinse out the mouth after each dose.

In certain circumstances oral drugs may be administered through a nasogastric or PEG tube. Clinical Interest Box 28.4 provides tips to ensure safe administration of medications via a nasogastric or PEG tube. Further information about nasogastric and PEG tubes can be found in Chapter 31. The pharmacist should be consulted before crushing any tablets and administering them orally or via a nasogastric or PEG tube. It is often the case that the medication is manufactured and available in a preferable formulation, for example liquid instead of solid.

Some medications are administered by buccal or sublingual application. These routes are indicated for drugs that tend to be destroyed by gastric juice, or those that are rapidly detoxified by the liver. Buccal tablets are placed in the space between the upper molar teeth and gums. Clients should be advised to alternate cheeks with each administration to prevent mucosal irritation occurring. Sublingual tablets are placed under the tongue. Both forms remain in place while they dissolve. The client should be advised not to chew or swallow such tablets. Before administering any oral medication the nurse must ascertain if any clients have a nil by mouth status, such as may apply to clients who are to have certain tests or surgery.

CLINICAL INTEREST BOX 28.4
Tips for administering medications via a nasogastric or PEG tube

- Do not crush or open any medications without first checking with the pharmacist
- Crush the medication using a mortar and pestle
- Mix with a small amount of water
- Stop and restart feeding, as required by specific medication, to allow for the most effective absorption. Again, check with the pharmacist if you are unsure
- Check the fluid status of the client; that is, check to see if there is a fluid restriction that may determine the amount of fluid used to flush the line before and after drug administration
- Check the position of the nasogastric or PEG tube
- Flush the tube with water (20–30 mL)
- Administer the medication either by gentle syringing or by allowing to flow by gravity. Each medication should be administered separately
- Flush the tube with water between each medication and after the last medication
- Restart the tube feeding when appropriate
- Document the medication on the medication chart. Document the fluid administered on the client's fluid balance chart
- Administering medication via a nasogastric or PEG tube is the main reason that tubes become blocked, so nurses must ensure that flushing is thorough and that they never mix medications together to instil via a feeding tube because this causes the clumping responsible for blocking the tube

(deWit 2005)

Suggested guidelines for safely administering oral medications are provided in Table 28.6. The equipment required comprises a drug order sheet and medication record, a medicine glass, the prescribed medication, and a glass of water, with a drinking straw or spoon if necessary.

ADMINISTERING DRUGS BY INJECTION

Drugs are given by injection for a variety of reasons, including:

- The drug may be one that is not absorbed when given orally
- The drug may be one that is destroyed by digestive juices
- A rapid onset of action may be required
- Very precise control over dosage may be needed
- The client may be unable to take drugs orally.

Drugs may be administered by injection subcutaneously (SC), intramuscularly (IM), or intravenously (IV). The administration of an injection is an invasive procedure

TABLE 28.6 | GUIDELINES FOR ADMINISTERING ORAL MEDICATIONS*

Action	Rationale
Check the drug order sheet for the client's name, name of medication, dose, route, time of last administration and frequency of administration	Promotes correct and safe administration of the drug
Wash and dry hands	Prevents cross-infection
Prepare the client's medication by first reading the label on the container, including the expiry date, and checking it with the written drug order	Prevents preparation errors
Solid dose forms	
Calculate the correct dose (if necessary)	Ensures correct dose is given
Tip the required number of tablets or capsules into the lid of the container and transfer into the medicine glass. Do not touch the drug	Maintains cleanliness of drugs
Liquid dose form	
Calculate the correct dose (if necessary)	Ensures correct dose is given
Shake bottle thoroughly	Promotes mixing of the contents
Hold the bottle with the label against the palm of the hand	Mixture will be poured away from the label, to avoid smearing
Remove bottle cap and place it upside down	Prevents contamination of the inside of the cap
Hold the medicine glass at eye level and pour the prescribed dose (marking on the glass should be even with the fluid level at the base of the meniscus). Discard any excess	Ensures accuracy of measurement
Wipe lip of bottle with tissue or paper towel. Replace cap	Prevents contamination of contents and prevents bottle cap from sticking
Add water to the medication if necessary (only if prescribed)	Water should not be added unless prescribed, as dilution of the medication may reduce effectiveness
Check the label of the container again	Reading the label again reduces risk of errors
Check the client's identity band and ask them to state their name	Confirms the client's identity
Explain the purpose of the medication and its action	Understanding improves compliance with drug therapy
Assist the client into a sitting or side-lying position when possible	Prevents aspiration during swallowing
Administer the medication. Offer the client a glass of water, unless this is contraindicated	Most solid drugs are swallowed more easily with liquids
Remain with the client until the medication is swallowed	The nurse assumes responsibility for ensuring that the client receives the prescribed medication
Wash and dry hands	Prevents cross-infection
Record each drug administered on the medication record	Prompt documentation prevents errors
Report immediately if the client refuses medication, or if unable to swallow a whole tablet or capsule	Appropriate care can be planned and implemented

* Safe medication management guidelines, outlined in Clinical Interest Box 28.3, should be incorporated into relevant aspects of this procedure and the nurse must act only within the laws and policies governing nursing practice in the geographical area of employment

that must be performed using aseptic technique. When a needle pierces the skin there is a risk of infection. Infection is avoided by hand washing, preventing contamination of the solution, preventing needle and syringe contamination, and by preparing the skin before injection.

A variety of syringes and needles is available, most of which are single use and disposable. Syringes (Figure 28.6) are available in a range of sizes, varying in capacity from 1 to 50 mL. A syringe consists of a cylindrical barrel with a tip designed to fit the hub of a needle, and a close-fitting plunger. The barrel of the syringe is calibrated into millilitres and tenths of a millilitre or, in the case of an insulin syringe, into units. Needles (Figure 28.6) are available in various lengths and gauges, with different sizes of bevels. A needle has three parts: The hub, which fits onto the tip of a syringe, the shaft, and the bevel or slanted tip. Needle gauge is determined by the lumen of the needle: as the diameter of the lumen increases, the gauge decreases. For example, a 16-gauge needle is substantially larger in diameter than a 22-gauge needle.

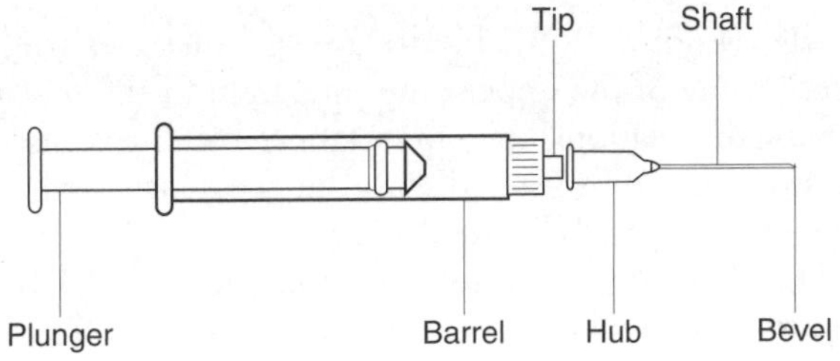

Figure 28.6 | Component parts of a syringe and needle

Selecting an appropriate syringe and needle depends mainly on the prescribed route, viscosity of the medication, amount of medication to be administered, and the client's body size and amount of fat. Generally a 2–3 mL syringe is adequate for SC, IM and most IV injections. Subcutaneous injections are generally given through a small-diameter needle (e.g. 25-gauge) while IM injections usually require a 21–23-gauge needle. Intravenous injections are generally administered through a 20-gauge needle.

Medications for injection are presented as liquids in glass ampoules or rubber-capped vials, or in powder form requiring reconstitution before administration. An ampoule is made of clear glass, with a constricted neck that must be snapped off to allow access to the medication. Ampoules contain volumes from 1 mL to 10 mL or more. A vial is a single- or multiple-dose glass container with a rubber seal at the top, which is protected by a metal cap until it is ready for use. Multiple-dose vials are not recommended because of the risk of cross-infection between clients. Vials contain medications in either liquid or powder form. Sterile water (often labelled 'water for injection') and sodium chloride 0.9% (normal saline) are commonly used as diluents to dissolve drugs in powder form. The vial label or the manufacturer's information specifies which diluent to use, as well as any other recommendations for administration (e.g. compatibilities, how fast to administer). These instructions should be consulted before the preparation and administration of the medication. Table 28.7 illustrates the procedure for the preparation of medications from ampoules and vials.

TABLE 28.7 | PREPARATION OF MEDICATIONS FROM AMPOULES AND VIALS

Ampoules	Vials
Tap the top of the ampoule lightly with a finger to dislodge any fluid above the neck of the ampoule	Remove the metal cap to expose the rubber seal
Place a gauze square around the neck of the ampoule to protect the fingers as the glass is broken	Wipe the surface of the seal with an alcohol swab, to remove any dust or grease
File the neck of the ampoule if necessary. Snap the neck in a direction away from the hands, to prevent shattering the glass towards the fingers or face	To prepare a powdered drug, assemble needle and syringe and draw up the amount of diluent recommended on the label of the vial or in the manufacturer's information, and gently inject into the vial. Gently shake or roll the vial between the hands to dissolve the powder
Assemble needle and syringe. Remove needle cover	Before drawing up the solution, assemble the needle and syringe and remove the needle cover. Draw back on the plunger to draw air into the syringe, equivalent to the volume of medication to be aspirated
Insert the needle (attached to the syringe) into the centre of the ampoule opening, being careful not to touch the needle on the rim of the ampoule, to prevent needle contamination	With bevel pointing up, insert the tip of the needle through the centre of the rubber seal
Aspirate the medication by pulling back on the syringe. Keep the needle lip below the surface of the medication to prevent aspiration of air bubbles	Inject the air from the syringe into the vial. Hold the plunger, as it may be forced backwards by air pressure within the vial
To expel air bubbles from the syringe, remove the needle from the ampoule and hold syringe with the needle pointing up. Draw back slightly on the plunger and then push the plunger up to eject the air (but avoid dispersing medication into the environment). Holding the syringe and needle upright, tap the syringe barrel to dislodge remaining air bubbles. It is important to expel air bubbles because if air is injected it may gain entry to the bloodstream and block a blood vessel	Holding the syringe and plunger, invert the vial. Hold the vial in the non-dominant hand
Place a new needle on the syringe for administration of the next medication	Allow air pressure to gradually fill the syringe with medication. Keep the tip of the needle below fluid level. Pull back slightly on the plunger if necessary
	Remove the needle from the vial by pulling back on the barrel of the syringe
	Tap the syringe barrel to remove any air bubbles
	Place a new needle on the syringe to administer the medication

Some medications are available in disposable, single-dose pre-filled syringes that relieve the nurse of the need to calculate and prepare doses of the medication. It may be necessary to advance the plunger a small way to expel some medication if the dose ordered is less than that in the syringe. The nurse still needs to check the name, strength and amount of the medication. Particular care is needed because many pre-filled syringes look the same but contain very different drugs. Some medications are available in an injection system that requires a device similar to the plunger in a standard syringe to be screwed into the end of a pre-filled vial with an inbuilt needle. After use the whole injection unit is discarded into the appropriate sharps safe container. This device is designed to minimise the risk of needle-stick injury (Crisp & Taylor 2005).

Injection sites

Subcutaneous injection (SC) involves injecting medication into the loose connective tissue under the dermis. Only small volumes of medication (up to 2 mL) and only medications that will not damage subcutaneous tissue are administered by this route. Subcutaneous sites that are commonly used are the upper outer aspect (middle third) of the upper arm, the upper anterior thighs, and the abdomen below the costal margins to the iliac crests (Figure 28.7). Subcutaneous injections are administered with the needle inserted at an angle of 45 degrees (Figure 28.8) or 90 degrees, depending on the size of the needle used.

Intramuscular injections (IM) involve injecting medication into deep muscle tissue. Muscle is less sensitive to irritating or viscous drugs, and up to 3 mL can be injected into muscle without causing severe discomfort (2 mL for elderly or frail clients or children). The sites chosen are areas where there is minimal risk of the needle penetrating a large blood vessel or nerve. Intramuscular sites that are commonly used are the middle third of the anterior lateral aspect of the thigh (vastus lateralis muscle), the upper outer quadrant of the buttock (gluteal muscle), and the upper outer aspect (middle third) of the upper arm (deltoid muscle) (Figure 28.9). Figure 28.10 illustrates the IM injection site of the upper outer quadrant of the buttock, showing the relationship to the sciatic nerve. Intramuscular injections are administered with the needle inserted at an angle of 90 degrees (Figure 28.11).

The Z-track method of injection (Figure 28.12) is a technique used when irritating preparations such as iron are given IM. A new needle is attached to the syringe after preparing the drug so that no solution remains on the outside of the needle. The subcutaneous tissue is drawn to one side before inserting the needle, to promote absorption and prevent skin staining and pain. The Z-track method of injection deposits medication into the muscle without tracking residual medication through sensitive tissues.

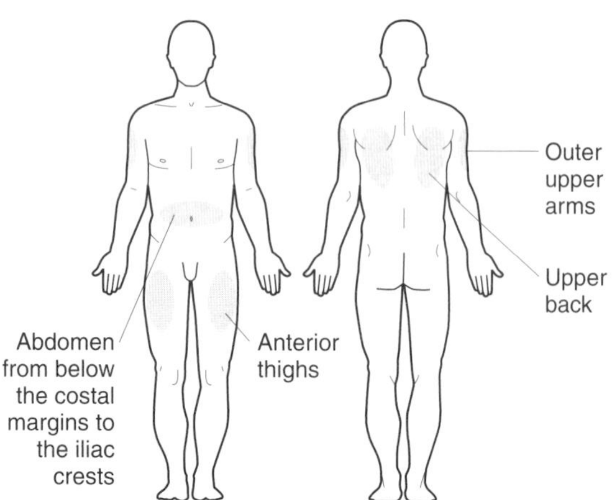

Figure 28.7 | Common sites for subcutaneous injections

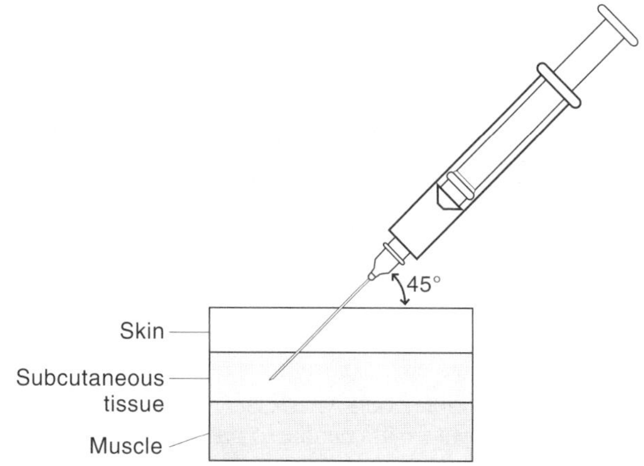

Figure 28.8 | Insertion of needles: subcutaneous injections

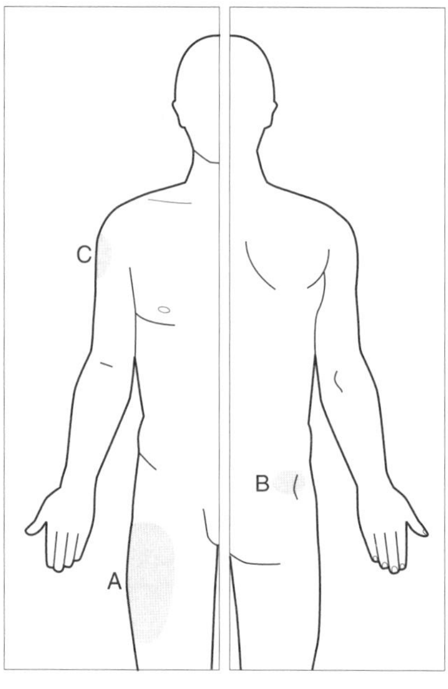

Figure 28.9 | Sites for intramuscular injections. **A**: Vastus lateralis muscle. **B**: Gluteal muscle. **C**: Deltoid muscle

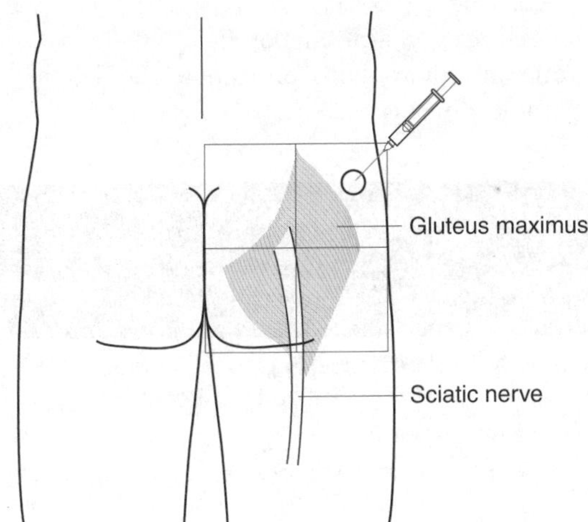

Figure 28.10 | Intramuscular injection site of the upper outer quadrant of the buttock, showing the relationship to the sciatic nerve

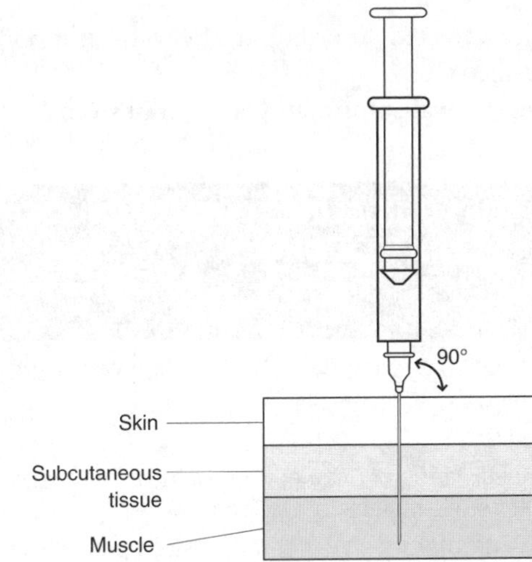

Figure 28.11 | Insertion of needles for intramuscular injections

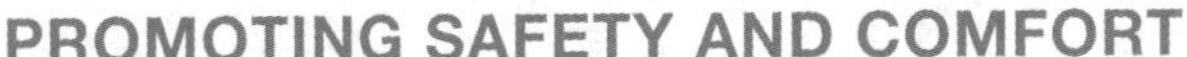

PROMOTING SAFETY AND COMFORT

To ensure correct SC or IM administration of an injectable medication and to minimise the client's discomfort, the nurse should:

- Position the client comfortably to reduce muscular tension
- Use a sharp needle in the smallest suitable length and gauge
- Select the correct injection site, using anatomical landmarks
- Ensure the rotation of injection sites to prevent all injections being given in the same area. This may be achieved by asking the client the site of the last injection and/or documenting the site in the client's clinical notes or care plan or on the medication chart
- Insert the needle smoothly and quickly
- Hold the syringe steady while the needle remains in the tissues
- Aspirate the syringe before injecting a medication, to check that the needle has not entered an artery or vein
- Press on, or gently massage, the area for several seconds after administration, unless contraindicated.

Injection sites should be assessed as free of any bruising, hardness, signs of inflammation or other abnormality.

Suggested guidelines for administering subcutaneous and intramuscular injections are outlined in Table 28.8. The equipment required comprises:

- Drug order sheet and medication record
- Kidney dish and cover
- Syringe, selected according to the volume of medication to be administered

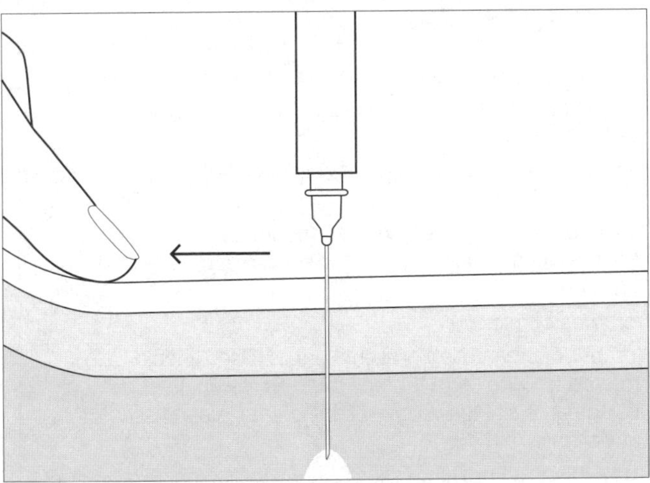

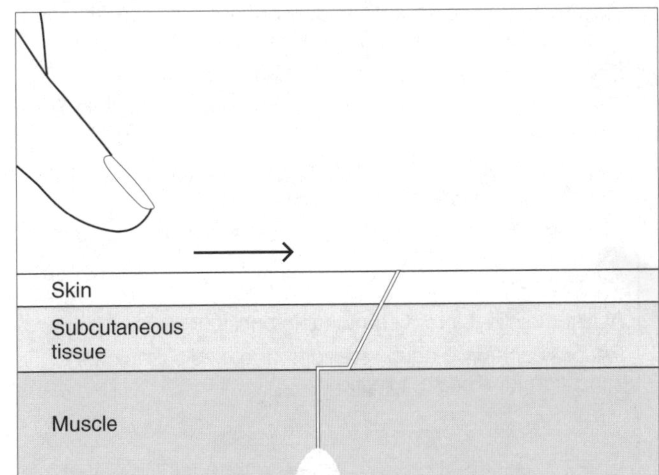

Figure 28.12 | Injection by the Z-track method. The tissue is tensed laterally at the injection site before the needle is inserted, which pulls the skin, subcutaneous tissue and fat into a Z formation. After this tissue has been displaced the needle is inserted straight into the muscular tissue. After injection the tissues are released while the needle is withdrawn and, as each tissue layer slides by the other, the track is sealed

- Needles, selected according to the route and body size of the client
- Antiseptic swabs; for example, alcohol swabs
- Prescribed drug in ampoule or vial
- Cotton swab for applying pressure to the site
- Disposable gloves.

TABLE 28.8 | GUIDELINES FOR ADMINISTERING SUBCUTANEOUS AND INTRAMUSCULAR INJECTIONS*

Action	Rationale
Explain procedure to the client, and the purpose of the medication	Reduces anxiety. Understanding improves compliance with drug therapy
Ensure privacy	Prevents embarrassment
Gain the assistance of another nurse if the client is a child, or an adult who is restless or irrational	Promotes safety during administration
Check the drug order sheet for the client's name, name of medication, dose, route, time of last administration and frequency of administration	Promotes correct and safe administration of the drug
Wash and dry hands	Prevents cross-infection
Calculate the dose and prepare the medication from the ampoule or vial, having checked the label and expiry date. Have two nurses check according to safe administration guidelines	Promotes safety during administration
Check the client's identity band and ask them to state their name and, if possible, the site of the last injection	Confirms the client's identity and prevents all injections being given into the same site
Select an appropriate injection site and assist the client into a comfortable position	Comfort promotes relaxation and therefore helps to reduce anxiety
Relocate the site using anatomical landmarks. Check site for any masses, lumps, signs of infection, scars or skin lesions	Insertion of medication into the correct site avoids injury to underlying structures. Masses, scars, etc will interfere with drug absorption
Cleanse the site with an antiseptic swab and allow to dry	Removes microorganisms from the skin
Remove the needle cap and hold the syringe in the dominant hand. Hold the client's skin between the thumb and forefinger and either pull it taut or pinch it up	A needle penetrates tight skin more easily than it does loose skin. Pinching the skin up may be necessary when an SC injection is given to an obese client, or when an IM injection is given to an client with small muscle mass
Insert the needle quickly and firmly, at a 45° or 90° angle for SC injection, and at a 90° angle for IM injection	Quick firm insertion minimises anxiety and discomfort
Slowly pull back on the plunger. If blood appears in the syringe, the needle is withdrawn and the injection repeated at another site, using a fresh dose, syringe and needle	Checks whether needle has penetrated a blood vessel
If no blood appears inject the medication slowly	Slow injection reduces tissue trauma and pain
Place an antiseptic swab over the injection site and withdraw the needle	Support of tissues minimises discomfort as the needle is withdrawn
Dispose of syringe into kidney dish without recapping or place directly into a sharps safe disposal container	Recapping used needles may result in a needle-stick injury
Massage the area gently. Do not massage an SC heparin injection site	Massage improves dispersal and absorption of the drug. Massaging a heparin injection site may result in severe bruising
Assist the client into a comfortable position	Promotes comfort
Record each drug administered on the medication chart, including the site of injection	Prompt documentation prevents errors. Sites should be rotated for long-term therapy such as insulin, as repeatedly using same site leads to thickening of skin and tissue atrophy
Discard syringe and needle into an appropriately labelled rigid-walled sharps container without recapping the needle	Proper disposal prevents sharps injury to personnel or visitors
Wash and dry hands	Prevents cross-infection

* Safe medication management guidelines, outlined in Clinical Interest Box 28.3, should be incorporated into this procedure and the nurse must act only within the laws and policies governing nursing practice in the geographical area of employment

ADMINISTERING DRUGS VIA THE INTRAVENOUS ROUTE

Intravenous (IV) medications may be administered in a number of different ways, including:

- As a mixture in a large volume (e.g. 500 or 1000 mL) of compatible IV fluid. Potassium chloride and some vitamins are administered in this manner
- As an IV bolus (also called an IV push). A bolus is a small volume introduced either into an already existing IV infusion or into an IV access port (this may also be referred to as a medication or heparin port). This method is convenient if the client has a fluid restriction. However, because the small volume is introduced directly into the circulatory system, there is little margin for error if a mistake is made. It is difficult, if not impossible, to 'retrieve' the medication once it has been administered
- As a mixture in a small volume (e.g. 50–100 mL) of compatible fluid in a secondary fluid container separate from the primary infusion. This may be administered as either a piggyback infusion or tandem infusion or into a burette (volume-control administration set).

The client will already have an existing infusion line or an intermittent venous access port. The advantages of the intermittent venous access port include increased client mobility, comfort and safety, cost benefit in not having continuous IV therapy, and nurse convenience in not having to monitor flow rates.

Nurses must be aware of their responsibilities and limitations to their scope of practice in relation to the law (e.g. the relevant Nurses or Health Professions Regulation Act) and the rules stipulated by the nursing regulatory bodies in the geographical area of employment. They must also practise according to the policy of the employing hospital or other agency regarding the administration of IV medications. Table 28.9 provides guidelines for the administration of IV medications.

TABLE 28.9 | GUIDELINES FOR THE ADMINISTRATION OF INTRAVENOUS MEDICATIONS*

Action	Rationale
General procedures for administration of all IV medications	
Calculate the correct dose and prepare the medication according to Table 28.7: Preparation of medications from ampoules and vials	Promotes correct and safe administration of the medication
Collect all necessary information about the medication, including action, purpose, normal dose, side effects, any special administration information and compatibility of fluids and medication	Promotes correct and safe administration of the drug and enables the nurse to monitor the therapeutic effects of the medication
Ensure the correct medication is given by checking the 'five rights'. Two nurses must complete the checking procedures for IV drugs — nurses must adhere to regulations regarding the qualifications of nurses eligible to prepare and check	Promotes correct and safe administration of the medication
Explain the procedure to the client, and the purpose of the medication	Reduces client anxiety. Understanding improves compliance with drug therapy and keeps the client informed of planned therapy
Check cannula insertion site for any signs of redness, warmth, swelling or pain/tenderness on palpation	Ensures safe administration of medication into venous system rather than into surrounding tissues
Assess the patency of the IV infusion line or intermittent access port	Ensures safe administration of medication
If necessary, check vital signs before, during and after infusion of medication	Allows nurse to monitor client's response to medication
Wash and dry hands, put on disposable gloves	Prevents cross-infection
Safely dispose of uncapped needle and syringe after use	Prevents accidental needle-stick injuries
Record medication administration promptly on medication administration sheet	Prevents medication errors from occurring; for example, dose being duplicated
Report any adverse reactions to medical officer and nurse in charge; document in client's medical notes	Allows medical officer to stop or change medication promptly if an adverse reaction occurs and to treat symptoms of adverse reaction
Record volume of fluid in medication bag (used for piggyback/tandem administration) or burette on client's intake/output form	Prevents circulatory overload

(Continued)

TABLE 28.9 | GUIDELINES FOR THE ADMINISTRATION OF INTRAVENOUS MEDICATIONS* — cont'd	
Action	**Rationale**
Large-volume infusions (e.g. potassium chloride)	
Before adding medication, ensure that it is compatible with the IV fluid	Prevents chemical reaction occurring, which may result in clouding or crystallisation of the IV fluid
Clean injection port with alcohol swab and allow alcohol to dry	Prevents introduction of microorganisms
Insert syringe and add required medication to the IV infusion bag via the medication injection port	Correct addition prevents infection, as medication port is self-sealing to prevent the introduction of microorganisms
After withdrawing syringe, gently mix contents of infusion	Ensures even distribution of medication throughout the infusion fluid
Complete a medication additives label, with details of medication added to fluid, date, time, and nurses' signatures	Informs all staff of the contents of the infusion
Ensure infusion rate is correct. A volumetric pump or burette may be added (according to hospital policy)	Prevents circulatory overload
As well as preparing medication, prepare two syringes with 1 mL normal saline each, for flushing line before and after medication	Prevents blockage of line
Clean injection port with alcohol swab and allow alcohol to dry	Prevents introduction of microorganisms
Insert needle with normal saline into rubber diaphragm of injection port. Pull syringe plunger back gently, looking for blood return	Determines position of cannula
Slowly inject 1 mL normal saline into port	Clears needle and port of blood and checks patency of the access line
Remove needle and clean injection port with alcohol swab and allow alcohol to dry	Prevents introduction of microorganisms
Inject medication slowly over several minutes (or as directed by manufacturer's information)	Ensures that medication is given at the correct rate. Rapid administration may cause pain or phlebitis or be fatal
Withdraw syringe, clean injection port with alcohol swab and allow alcohol to dry	Prevents introduction of microorganisms
Slowly inject 1 mL normal saline into port	Flushes medication into venous system
Remove cap from needleless port and flush with 1 mL normal saline by inserting syringe into valve	Clears reservoir of blood and checks patency of access port
Remove syringe and insert medication syringe into valve. Inject medication slowly over several minutes (or as directed by manufacturer's information)	Ensures that medication is given at the correct rate. Rapid administration may cause pain or phlebitis or be fatal
Withdraw syringe and flush with 1 mL of normal saline. (Some agencies have a policy to follow this with a heparin solution — check policy)	Flushes medication into venous system. Heparin is an anticoagulant that prevents the formation of a blood clot that could block the cannula
Replace sterile cap over valve	Prevents access of microorganisms
Intravenous bolus into existing infusion line	
Select injection port closest to client	Allows for easier aspiration for blood return to check placement
Clean injection port with alcohol swab and allow alcohol to dry	Prevents introduction of microorganisms
Connect syringe to IV line by either inserting needle into injection port (needle system) or removing cap of needleless injection port and connecting syringe tip directly	
Occlude infusion line above port by pinching tubing. Gently pull back on syringe plunger to aspirate blood	Checks position of cannula and ensures medication to be administered is into venous system
Inject medication slowly over several minutes (or as directed by manufacturer's information), continuing to occlude tubing above port	Ensures medication is given at the correct rate. Rapid administration may cause pain or phlebitis or be fatal
Release tubing and regulate infusion rate if necessary	Occluding tubing may affect the infusion rate
If using a needleless system, replace injection port cap with a new sterile cap	Prevents introduction of microorganisms

TABLE 28.9 | GUIDELINES FOR THE ADMINISTRATION OF INTRAVENOUS MEDICATIONS* — cont'd

Action	Rationale
Piggyback/tandem infusion	
Connect infusion tubing to medication bag and allow solution to fill tubing	Tubing should be filled with solution and free of air to prevent air embolus
Hang medication bag and connect tubing to infusion port (e.g. stopcock, needleless system, tubing port) on the primary infusion line after having wiped port with alcohol swab	Prevents introduction of microorganisms
Regulate flow rate using regulator clamp	Ensures medication is introduced at the correct rate to maintain therapeutic levels
When completed, remove and discard secondary infusion bag in a safe and appropriate manner	
Ensure primary infusion is running at the correct rate	Secondary infusion may have interfered with the flow of the primary infusion
Burette	
Fill burette with desired amount of fluid from infusion bag	
Clean injection port on top of burette with alcohol swab	Prevents introduction of microorganisms
Inject medication into port and gently mix with fluid in burette	Ensures even distribution of medication throughout fluid
Regulate infusion rate to allow medication to infuse at the required rate	Ensures medication is introduced at the correct rate to maintain therapeutic levels
Label burette with medication administration label containing name of medication, total volume, time of starting administration and patient details	Ensures all staff are aware of medication infusion occurring; prevents other medication being added to burette at same time
When infusion is complete, remove label from burette and return infusion to previous rate	Alerts staff that medication infusion is complete
If more than one medication is to be administered, ensure that burette and line are 'flushed' in between the medications	Prevents incompatible medications coming into contact with each other

* Safe medication management guidelines, outlined in Clinical Interest Box 28.3, should be incorporated into this procedure and the nurse must act only within the laws and policies governing nursing practice in the geographical area of employment

ADMINISTERING EYE AND EAR MEDICATIONS

Instilling eye drops and ointments

Eye drops or ointment prescribed may include those that combat infection, dilate or constrict the pupil, act as a local anaesthetic, stain the cornea, reduce inflammation or reduce intraocular pressure. Key aspects regarding the use of ophthalmic medications include checking the:

- Name, strength and amount of drops or ointment to be instilled
- Frequency, and time of last administration
- Eye into which the eye medication is to be instilled (e.g. left, right or both eyes)
- Expiry date on the container, and discarding the medication if the expiry date has passed.

Eye drops are supplied in a squeeze bottle with a nozzle top through which the drops are delivered. To prevent cross-infection a separate container of drops or ointment is supplied for each client. Single-dose packaging is preferred, as contamination of the medication is likely to occur if a container such as dropper bottle is used repeatedly. Guidelines for instilling eye drops and ointment are presented in Table 28.10. The equipment required comprises:

- Drug order sheet and medication record
- Disposable gloves
- Prescribed drops or ointment
- Normal saline (if required)
- Two or three gauze swabs
- Paper bag for used swabs
- Sterile eye pad and tape if required.

The use of gauze swabs rather than cotton wool balls is recommended when cleansing the eyes before administering eye drops. Cotton wool is not recommended because it contains particles that may irritate and damage they eye (Elliott, Aitken & Chaboyer 2007).

Instilling ear drops

Ear drops prescribed may include those that combat infection or soften wax. Guidelines for instilling ear drops are presented in Table 28.11. The equipment required comprises:

- Drug order sheet and medication record
- Disposable gloves
- Prescribed drops, warmed to body temperature
- Two or three cotton wool swabs
- Cotton-tipped buds (if required)
- Paper bag for used swabs.

TABLE 28.10 | GUIDELINES FOR INSTILLING EYE DROPS OR OINTMENT*

Action	Rationale
Explain the procedure and ensure privacy	Reduces anxiety
Check the drug order sheet for the client's name, name of medication, dose, route, time of last administration and frequency of administration. Check the expiry date of the medication	Promotes correct and safe administration of the drug
Assist the client to a position with the head tilted well back (if possible)	Facilitates correct instillation of medication
Wash and dry hands thoroughly	Prevents cross-infection
If eye contains any discharge or crusting, it should be cleaned with normal saline and gauze swabs before instilling drops or ointment	Discharge or crusting prevents good absorption of medication
Gently pull down the lower lid to form a pouch	Facilitates correct instillation of medication
Remove the cap of the container and hold the dropper or tube slightly away from the eye	Avoids contacting any part of the eye and contaminating the nozzle
If drops are being instilled, the prescribed number is dropped into the pouch of the lower lid	Medications should be instilled correctly; for example, into the pouch of the lower lid and not directly onto the eyeball
If ointment is being instilled, the first 1.25 cm is discarded onto a swab. Directing the nozzle of the tube near the lid, a ribbon of ointment is squeezed into the pouch of the lower lid	Reduces the risk of instilling contaminated ointment
Request the client to close the eyelid gently. Wipe away any excess with a gauze swab. Request that the client blink gently several times	Facilitates even distribution of the medication over the eye's surface
Apply an eye pad if required	A pad may be prescribed for comfort or protection
Assist the client into a comfortable position	Promotes comfort
Remove and attend to the equipment appropriately. Wash and dry hands	Prevents cross-infection
Record each drug administered on the medication record	Prompt documentation prevents errors
Report and document the procedure	Care can be evaluated

* Safe medication management guidelines, outlined in Clinical Interest Box 28.3, should be incorporated into relevant aspects of this procedure and the nurse must act only within the laws and policies governing nursing practice in the geographical area of employment

ADMINISTERING DRUGS VIA THE RECTAL ROUTE

Medication may be given rectally in the form of suppositories or retention enemas. The rectal route may be used when drugs cannot be taken orally, for example, when clients are vomiting or unconscious, or when a local action is required. Some clients will be able to insert suppositories themselves without the assistance of a nurse, which may prevent embarrassment. Other clients will need the nurse to administer the suppository. The nurse should be aware of the different types of suppositories and enemas available. Types of medications that may be administered rectally by suppository include analgesics and antiemetics. Suppositories prescribed to promote a bowel action are composed of various substances, such as glycerine. Evacuant suppositories act by softening and lubricating the faeces to facilitate easier passage and excretion, or by increasing peristalsis through the irritation of intestinal sensory nerve endings. Suggested guidelines for administering rectal suppositories are presented in Table 28.12. The equipment required comprises:

- Drug order sheet and medication record
- Prescribed suppository/suppositories
- Disposable gloves
- A small disposable sheet to protect bed linen
- Water-soluble lubricant
- Receiver (e.g. paper bag) for used articles
- Appropriate toilet facilities; for example, bedpan, toilet paper
- Soap, face washer and towel for client use after bowel motion or insertion of suppository.

INSTILLING VAGINAL MEDICATIONS

Vaginal medications are available as creams or pessaries. Both forms are generally administered with an inserter or applicator, allowing the medication to be placed high in the vaginal vault for maximum effect. Vaginal pessaries are presented in conical, oval or cylindrical shapes and are supplied in individual foil or plastic wrappers. Vaginal anti-infective medications are prescribed to treat vaginal infections, and vaginal hormone preparations are prescribed to treat conditions such as senile vaginitis.

TABLE 28.11 | GUIDELINES FOR INSTILLING EAR DROPS*

Action	Rationale
Explain the procedure and ensure privacy	Reduces anxiety
Check the drug order sheet for the client's name, name of medication, dose, route, time of last administration and frequency of administration. Check the expiry date of the medication	Promotes correct and safe administration of the drug
Assist the client to lie on the side opposite to the affected ear side	Facilitates instillation of the drops into the ear
Wash and dry hands thoroughly	Prevents cross-infection
Inspect the ear for any wax or drainage. Wipe out gently using a cotton bud, ensuring that wax is not forced inward	Any occlusion will prevent drops from being evenly distributed
Gently pull the auricle up and back. For a child under 3 years, the earlobe is pulled down and back	Straightens the ear canal
Ensure that the drops are at room temperature. Instil the prescribed number of drops so that they fall against the sides of the canal and not on the tympanic membrane	Cold drops may cause vertigo and nausea. Avoids discomfort
Gently massage or apply pressure to the projection in front of the meatus (the tragus)	Ensures that the drops flow into the canal
Wipe the outer ear free of excess drops	Promotes comfort
If prescribed, place a cotton wool swab loosely into the meatus, or instruct the client to lie with affected ear upward for 10 minutes	Prevents the medication from leaking out
Dispose of equipment appropriately. Wash and dry hands	Prevents cross-infection
Record each drug administered on the medication record	Prompt documentation prevents errors
Report and document the procedure	Care can be evaluated

* Safe medication management guidelines, outlined in Clinical Interest Box 28.3, should be incorporated into relevant aspects of this procedure and the nurse must act only within the laws and policies governing nursing practice in the geographical area of employment

TABLE 28.12 | GUIDELINES FOR INSERTING A RECTAL SUPPOSITORY

Action	Rationale
Explain the procedure	Reduces anxiety
Assemble the equipment and follow the nursing policies related to checking medications	The correct type, size and quantity must be administered
Ensure adequate privacy	Reduces embarrassment
Place the client in a left lateral position with the right leg flexed	Anatomical site of the lower colon means that this position is the most effective for the introduction and retention of suppositories
Ensure that the person is adequately covered, with only the buttocks exposed	Promotes warmth and comfort
Wash and dry hands and put on disposable gloves	Prevents cross-infection
Lubricate finger of glove and suppository	Facilitates insertion of suppository
Gently insert the suppository by directing it with the finger, through the anus about 3.5 cm into the rectum	Suppository must pass the internal anal sphincter and come in contact with rectal mucosa
During insertion, encourage the client to take deep breaths through the mouth	Helps to relax the anal sphincters
Encourage the client to retain the suppository for the correct length of time. A suppository administered to cause a bowel action should be retained for at least 20 minutes	Client must be aware whether the suppository is to be retained to allow any medication to be dissipated, or whether to expect a bowel action. Suppositories to promote a bowel action must be retained long enough to be effective
Ensure the client has easy access to toilet facilities and the signal device; for example, nurse call bell	Reduces anxiety related to accidental expulsion of the suppository or faeces

(Continued)

TABLE 28.12 | GUIDELINES FOR INSERTING A RECTAL SUPPOSITORY — cont'd

Action	Rationale
Dispose of used equipment appropriately, wash and dry hands	Prevents cross-infection
If a bowel action results, the faeces are observed and the observations reported and documented	Helps to assess the effectiveness of the treatment and detects any abnormalities
Attend to the client's hygiene and position	Helps promote comfort
If a prescribed medication was used, ensure that each drug administered is recorded on the medication record	Prompt documentation prevents errors
Report and document the procedure	Appropriate care may be planned and implemented

Unlike the rectum, the vagina does not have a sphincter and therefore creams may run out. To help avoid this, vaginal preparations should be instilled at night whenever possible, when the client is in bed ready for sleep. Sanitary pads are recommended to prevent staining or soiling of underwear. The use of tampons is not recommended.

Clients who require vaginal medication may prefer to self-administer to avoid embarrassment. The nurse may be required to perform the technique or to instruct the client in how to instil vaginal medications. A suggested procedure is outlined in Table 28.13. The equipment required comprises:

- Drug order sheet and medication record
- Prescribed pessaries or cream
- Inserter or applicator
- A small disposable sheet to protect bed linen
- Disposable gloves
- Receiver (e.g. paper bag) for used articles
- Perineal pad.

ADMINISTERING DRUGS BY INHALATION

Drugs can be inhaled to produce a local or systemic effect via the respiratory tract by steam inhalation, nebuliser, atomiser or aerosol spray. Most commonly, drugs are delivered to the lungs as sprays from pressurised aerosol dispensers, or as dry powder from an inhaler.

Aerosol inhalers are widely used to administer bronchodilators. The drug and its inert propellant are maintained under pressure in a small canister. When the valve is

TABLE 28.13 | GUIDELINES FOR INSTILLING VAGINAL MEDICATIONS*

Action	Rationale
Check the drug order sheet for the client's name, the name and dose of medication, frequency and time of last administration. Check the client's identity. Check the label and expiry date of the medication	Promotes correct and safe administration of the medication
Explain the procedure and the purpose of the medication	Reduces anxiety. Understanding improves compliance with drug therapy
Ensure privacy and assist the client into the dorsal recumbent position, with legs flexed and extended apart	Position provides easy access to and adequate exposure of the vaginal canal
Wash and dry hands and don disposable gloves	Prevents cross-infection
Attach the applicator to the tube of cream or place the pessary in the applicator	Promotes correct and safe administration of the medication
Gently retract the labial folds	Exposes the vaginal orifice
Insert the applicator into the vagina in an upward and backward direction, about 7.5 cm. Push the plunger to deposit the medication	Proper placement ensures equal distribution of medication along the walls of the vaginal cavity
Withdraw the applicator, wipe any residual cream from the labia, and apply a perineal pad	Promotes comfort; perineal pad prevents staining of clothing
Encourage the client to remain in the recumbent position for 20–28 minutes after administration	Allows medication to melt and be absorbed into the vaginal mucosa
Wash applicator in warm soapy water, rinse and dry. The applicator is stored for future use by that client only. Remove gloves. Wash and dry hands	Prevents cross-infection
Record administration on the medication record	Prompt documentation prevents errors

* Safe medication management guidelines, outlined in Clinical Interest Box 28.3, should be incorporated into relevant aspects of this procedure and the nurse must act only within the laws and policies governing nursing practice in the geographical area of employment

activated, a measured quantity of propellant carrying the drug is released through the mouthpiece. A spacer may be used to ensure maximal benefit from inhalation and can be particularly beneficial for young children or clients who find it difficult to manage aerosol inhalation without one. The bronchodilator is released into the plastic spacing device and then inhaled. A dry powder inhaler (e.g. Rotahaler Inhalational Device, Diskhaler Inhalational Device) may be used if a client is unable to coordinate aerosol inhalation. When the mouth is placed on the mouthpiece, the client inhales through the device causing drug particles to be drawn into the respiratory tract.

A nebuliser adds moisture and/or medications to inspired air, using the aerosol principle. Nebulisation is often used for administering bronchodilators or mucolytic agents. A high-pressure gas source (air or oxygen) is used to draw up the medication from a chamber. Small-volume nebulisers are generally used for administering medications. Before administering the medication, sufficient sterile 0.9% w/v sodium chloride solution must be added to the medication. To prevent cross-infection, each client should be provided with their own nebuliser and mask for use on repeated occasions. The mask and nebuliser should be cleaned at regular intervals and disposed of when treatment is discontinued or the client is discharged.

A suggested procedure for using a hand-held inhaler is outlined in Table 28.14. The equipment required comprises the drug order sheet and medication record, and the prescribed drug and inhaler.

APPLYING TRANSDERMAL MEDICATIONS

Certain medications can be applied to the skin to supply drugs directly into the bloodstream for prolonged systemic

TABLE 28.14 | GUIDELINES FOR USING HAND-HELD INHALERS*

Action	Rationale
Check the drug order sheet for the client's name, the name and dose of medication, frequency, and time of last administration. Check the label on the inhaler, including the expiry date and the client's identity	Promotes correct and safe administration of the drug
Wash and dry hands	Prevents cross-infection
Explain the procedure and the purpose of the medication	Understanding improves compliance with drug therapy
Assist the client to assume an upright position	Position facilitates entry of the medication into the respiratory tract
Load the inhaler with the canister of medication. Twist to break the capsule	Prepares the inhaler for administration of the medication
Remove the mouthpiece cap	
Shake the inhaler	
Instruct the client to hold the inhaler with the mouthpiece at the bottom	Ensures correct administration of drug
Instruct the client to breathe out slowly and fully	Enables subsequent deep inhalation to be performed
Instruct the client to place the mouthpiece well into the mouth, close the lips firmly around it and tilt the head back slightly	Tight seal is necessary to prevent the escape of medication into the air
The client inhales quickly and deeply through the mouthpiece while administering a metered dose by pressing the canister downwards	Draws the medication into the lungs
The client removes the inhaler, holds the breath for as long as possible, then breathes out slowly through the mouth	Allows medication to reach the alveoli. Allows increased absorption and diffusion of the drug, and better gas exchange
The technique is repeated if necessary until the prescribed dose has been inhaled or a different inhaler is also required. Time between inhalations depends on which medications are being inhaled	Time between inhalations allows deeper penetration of the second inhalation
Replace the cap on the mouthpiece	Prevents contamination of mouthpiece
Wash and dry hands	Prevents cross-infection
Encourage the client to drink, eat or brush teeth immediately after use	Prevents hoarseness, irritated sore throat or oropharyngeal candidiasis
Record administration on the medication chart	Prompt documentation prevents errors

* Safe medication management guidelines, outlined in Clinical Interest Box 28.3, should be incorporated into relevant aspects of this procedure and the nurse must act only within the laws and policies governing nursing practice in the geographical area of employment

effect. The medications are applied via an adhesive disc which releases a known amount of drug per time (e.g. 5 mg over 24 hours). Transdermal medications include glyceryl trinitrate (known as nitroglycerin in the US) (to relieve angina pectoris), nicotine (for nicotine withdrawal) and oestrogen (for hormone replacement therapy). Drugs administered transdermally avoid being broken down by the liver before they have had a chance to take effect.

Adhesive discs, which are applied to the skin, are composed of an adhesive layer, a rate-limiting membrane, a drug reservoir and a waterproof external layer. The discs are applied to a dry, hairless area of the body. The waterproof external layer enables the client to shower or bathe without adversely affecting the drug's action. Drugs applied in this manner can exert their effects for as long as 24–72 hours. Client education should include the correct application of the transdermal disc, the frequency of application, the need to rotate application sites to prevent skin irritation occurring, correct storage of the discs, the need to wash the hands after application and correct disposal of the discs after use. Education should particularly stress the importance of keeping the discs out of reach of children. Hands should be washed immediately after applying the discs to avoid the nurse absorbing any of the drug transdermally through the hands.

TOPICAL APPLICATIONS

Topical preparations such as those used in the treatment of dermatological conditions may be formulated as an ointment, lotion, cream, jelly, powder, paint, paste or spray. Drugs may be applied to the skin by painting, spreading or spraying medication over an area, applying moist dressings, or by soaking body parts in a solution. Drugs applied to the skin have local effects, with the exception of transdermal preparations that are designed to produce systemic effects. To avoid medication being absorbed through the skin of the hands, the nurse should wear disposable gloves for protection or use an applicator during administration of topical medications. To prevent accumulation, any residual medication on the skin should be removed before reapplication. When applying a prescribed topical preparation, the manufacturer's directions must be followed.

MONITORING THE EFFECTS OF MEDICATIONS

The nurse plays a vital role in monitoring the effects of prescribed medications. Evaluating the client's response is essential and the nurse is required to assess, report and record all responses to medication. This includes the desired effects and any adverse reactions. To monitor the effects of any medication the nurse must first have a clear understanding of the purpose of the drug and its desired effects. Table 28.15 lists the major actions of common drug classes and provides the nurse with a guide to the expected effects of various groups of drugs. For example, the nurse needs to be aware that an analgesic drug is administered for the purpose of alleviating pain, an anti-inflammatory drug to relieve inflammation and an antipyretic to lower body temperature. Documentation should therefore include whether or not the drug has successfully achieved the desired effects, for example if the pain has been successfully relieved by the analgesic.

Whenever medication of any sort is administered there is always a possibility that side effects or adverse reactions may occur. Adverse reactions to a drug may be due to overdose, idiosyncrasy, toxic effects, allergy or drug interactions. Early detection of the manifestations of an adverse reaction and immediate, factual and concise reporting of these manifestations allows prompt action to be taken. Manifestations of an adverse reaction will depend on the type of medication administered and on each individual. It is important for the nurse to refer to either the manufacturer's information or a reliable textbook to have all of the information concerning possible adverse reactions. The nurse should be informed and knowledgeable about every medication before it is administered and document and report any adverse or side effect immediately to the nurse in charge and medical officer.

SAFE HANDLING OF HAZARDOUS SUBSTANCES

Cytotoxic drugs (used in chemotherapy) may be prescribed in the treatment of malignant disease. Cytotoxic drugs, which are toxic agents used to inhibit the growth of malignant cells, may be administered orally, IV or by regional perfusion. As cytotoxic agents are harmful to normal as well as malignant cells, extreme care is required during their preparation and administration.

Although the EN is not required to prepare or administer cytotoxic drugs, they may nonetheless assist in the care of a client receiving chemotherapy. It is essential therefore that the nurse is aware of, and understands, the related safety guidelines. Clear guidelines, which are developed by health authorities and are available in health care facilities, set down procedures to be followed in the preparation and administration of cytotoxic agents. In addition, the guidelines specify how to deal with spillages, extravasation (leakage of antineoplastic agents into the client's subcutaneous tissues), and the safe disposal of used equipment and the client's body wastes. Nurses who are pregnant should avoid contact with any cytotoxic agent, especially during the first trimester, when fetal organs are developing.

A material safety data sheet (MSDS) should be available with every hazardous substance used in a health care facility. The MSDS is the primary source of safety information provided for people using hazardous substances in the workplace. It provides essential information, direct from the manufacturer, about what to do in the event of leakage, spillage or any type of accident or incident involving the chemical (Arnold 2003). (See Chapter 26 for further information about safety and hazardous substances.)

TABLE 28.15 | MAJOR ACTIONS OF COMMON DRUG CLASSES

Drug class	Action
Drugs acting on the cardiovascular system	
Antianginal agents	Relax smooth muscle and reduce myocardial oxygen demand, thereby reducing angina
Antihypertensive agents	Reduce high blood pressure
Antiarrhythmic agents	Prevent, alleviate or correct cardiac arrhythmias
Antiplatelet agents	Decrease platelet aggregation to prevent thrombus formation
Cardiac glycosides	Increase force of myocardial contraction
Diuretics	Promote the formation and secretion of urine
Fibrinolytic agents	Activate the endogenous fibrinolytic system to dissolve intravascular blood clots
Lipid-regulating agents	Reduce blood cholesterol level
Vasodilators	Dilate blood vessels, improving circulation
Drugs acting on the respiratory system	
Antiasthma agents	Prevent asthma symptoms
Bronchodilators	Relax bronchiole smooth muscle to relieve bronchospasm and improve ventilation
Cough suppressants; expectorants and mucolytics	Depress the cough centre in the medulla oblongata; break up mucus, enabling expectoration
Drugs acting on the nervous system	
Analgesics	Alter the perception of pain
Antianxiety agents	Prevent or relieve anxiety
Antidepressants	Prevent or relieve depression
Antiepileptics	Also called anticonvulsants. Prevent or reduce the severity of epileptic seizures
Antimigraine agents	Prevent or relieve migraine headaches
Antimuscarinic agents	Also known as anticholinergics. Inhibit the transmission of parasympathetic nerve impulses, resulting in reduced muscle spasm, decreased secretion of sweat, saliva and nasal, bronchial and gastrointestinal secretions
Antipsychotic agents	Counteract or reduce symptoms of psychosis
Dopaminergic agents	Either stimulate dopamine receptors or replenish supply of dopamine. Commonly used in the treatment of Parkinson's disease
General anaesthetics	Used to induce and maintain anaesthesia during surgery
Local anaesthetics	Block nerve conduction
Muscle relaxants	Reduce contractility of muscle fibres, thereby reducing muscle spasm
Neuromuscular-blocking agents	Have an action at the muscle receptor end-plate and are used as an adjunct to general anaesthetics to relax muscle
Opioid analgesics	Alter perception of pain, induce euphoria, depress respiratory and cough reflexes
Parasympathomimetic agents	Central nervous system stimulants. Either mimic action of acetylcholine or block acetylcholine breakdown at receptor sites, thereby increasing total amount of acetylcholine
Sedatives and hypnotics	Depress the central nervous system
Stimulants	Excite the central nervous system
Sympathomimetic agents	Mimic noradrenaline and have effects including cardiac stimulation and relaxation of bronchial smooth muscle
Drugs acting on the endocrine system	
Androgens	Control development of and maintenance of male sex organs and male secondary sex characteristics

(Continued)

TABLE 28.15 | MAJOR ACTIONS OF COMMON DRUG CLASSES — cont'd	
Drug class	**Action**
Drugs acting on the endocrine system — cont'd	
Antidiabetic agents	Regulate the metabolism of glucose
Antithyroid agents	Inhibit synthesis of thyroid hormone (thyroxine)
Calcium-regulating agents	Lower blood calcium levels
Corticosteroids	Hormones that influence or control key processes in the body, including carbohydrate and protein metabolism, electrolyte and water balance
Hypothalamic and pituitary hormones	Used as replacement therapy
Oestrogens	Control development and maintenance of female sex organs, secondary sexual characteristics and mammary glands
Progestogens	Convert the endometrial proliferative phase to the secretory phase in preparation for a fertilised ovum
Thyroid agents	Replace thyroid hormones
Drugs acting on the gastrointestinal tract	
Anorectic and weight loss agents	Suppress hunger sensation
Antacids	Neutralise gastric acidity and reduce pepsin activity
Antidiarrhoeal agents	Relieve diarrhoea
Antiemetics	Prevent and relieve nausea and vomiting
Antiulcer agents	Assist in the healing of gastric and duodenal ulcers
Laxatives	Promote peristalsis and evacuation of the bowel by increasing the bulk of faeces by softening the stool or by lubricating the intestinal wall
Prostaglandins	Inhibit gastric secretion
Topical rectal agents	Reduce pain associated with haemorrhoids
Drugs acting on the genitourinary system	
Diuretics	Promote the formation and secretion of urine
Prostaglandins	May cause contraction or relaxation of smooth muscle in blood vessels, bronchi, uterus or gastrointestinal tract
Sex hormones	Sex hormones are prescribed for a variety of reasons, including the development or control of male or female sex organs and secondary sex characteristics. Common uses include oral contraceptives, hormone replacement drugs to treat primary amenorrhoea, delayed onset of puberty or to relieve the symptoms of menopause. Sex hormones may also be used therapeutically to treat osteoporosis, to promote sex drive and fertility, and in treatment related to breast or prostatic cancer. The sex hormones include anabolic steroids, androgens, antiandrogens, oestrogens and progesterones
Drugs acting on the musculoskeletal system	
Analgesics	Prevent and reduce pain
Non-steroidal anti-inflammatory drugs (NSAIDs)	Reduce inflammation
Disease-modifying anti-rheumatic drugs (DMARDs)	Treat rheumatoid arthritis
Antigout agents	Reduce pain and inflammation associated with gout or alter production or distribution of uric acid
Muscle relaxants	Reduce contractility of muscle fibres, reducing muscle spasm
Drugs acting on the immune system	
Antihistamines	Reduce the effects of histamine released from cells
Corticosteroids	Hormones that influence or control key processes in the body, including carbohydrate and protein metabolism, electrolyte and water balance
Immunomodifiers	Modify the immune system
Vaccines, immunoglobulins and antisera	Vaccines induce a specific active artificial immunity. Antisera contain antibodies (immunoglobulins) against a specific disease to confer passive immunity

TABLE 28.15 | MAJOR ACTIONS OF COMMON DRUG CLASSES — cont'd

Drug class	Action
Drugs acting on the blood	
Anticoagulants	Prevent or delay the coagulation of blood
Antiplatelet agents	Decrease platelet aggregation to prevent thrombus formation
Fibrinolytic agents	Activate the endogenous fibrinolytic system to dissolve intravascular blood clots
Haemostatics	Treat or prevent haemorrhage by inhibiting fibrin clot breakdown
Lipid-regulating agents	Reduce blood cholesterol level
Vasodilators	Dilate blood vessels, improving circulation
Drugs acting on the skin	
Dermatological agents	Prevent or treat skin infections; cleansers; moisturising agents; sunscreen agents; topical anaesthetics; topical analgesics
Anti-infective agents	
Antihelmintics	Treat worm infestations
Antibacterial agents	Inhibit the growth of or destroy bacteria
Antifungal agents	Inhibit the growth of or destroy fungal infections
Antimalarial agents	Prevent or treat malaria
Antimycobacterial agents	Treat tuberculosis and Hansen's disease (leprosy)
Antiprotozoal agents	Treat protozoal infections
Antiviral agents	Prevent or treat viral infections
Drugs used in neoplastic disorders	
Antineoplastic agents	Also called cytotoxics. Prevent the proliferation of malignant cells by attacking them at various stages of the cell cycle
Corticosteroids	Hormones that influence or control key processes in the body, including carbohydrate and protein metabolism, electrolyte and water balance
Immunomodifiers	Modify the immune system

CONTINUATION OF MEDICATION AFTER DISCHARGE

Before discharge from a health care facility with medications, the nurse must ensure that the client:

- Has been instructed adequately and is able to demonstrate safe self-medication techniques
- Understands the medication regimen, including the purpose of the prescribed medications, the frequency of administration and any contraindications
- Understands the importance of any related blood tests
- Understands the importance of not stopping medications abruptly without first discussing the matter with the general practitioner or other medical officer
- Is advised to consult the medical officer about any untoward effects from the medication
- Understands the importance of notifying other health professionals about the medication regimen; for example, the visiting community health nurse
- Understands the reasons for not sharing medications with others
- Knows how to store the medications correctly and safely
- Knows how to discard out-of-date or unwanted medications safely
- Knows how to dispose of used syringes and needles safely if used.

Alternatively, if the client is unable to complete the above, then a family member or friend should be instructed in the safe administration of the medication, covering all the points listed above. Another alternative is a visiting nurse, who may be required to call on the client at home and assist in the administration of, or monitoring of, the drug therapy. The nurse may also be able to gain an understanding of any difficulties the client is experiencing, offer information that may help the client deal with them, and monitor the client's compliance with the medical officer's directions. Sometimes clients do not comply with the prescribed medication regimen after they return home. There are a variety of reasons why this may occur (Clinical Interest Box 28.5). Clinical Interest Box 28.6 provides suggestions to help the nurse enhance client compliance with medication regimens after discharge.

CLINICAL INTEREST BOX 28.5
Non-compliance with medication — issues for the nurse to consider

How many of us have been guilty of not completing a course of antibiotics because we 'feel better' or forget to take them and decide we are better anyway, or keep a few of those antibiotics for the next time it happens, to save going to the medical officer again? Non-compliance with drug therapy can be due to both deliberate and unintentional reasons. Some reasons for non-compliance with drug therapy are that clients:

- Do not understand the information given to them
- Disregard the information given to them, perhaps because they do not believe in, or have a fear of, using drugs or believe another sort of remedy is more likely to be effective. Attitudes and beliefs about drugs can be influenced by cultural background and past experiences with drugs
- Alter the drug regimen to fit with lifestyle; for example, only eating meals twice a day so only taking a drug twice a day instead of as ordered, that is, three times a day with meals
- Decrease dose or stop medication because of adverse effects
- Take double doses to make up for missed doses
- Stop medication because there is no change in condition ('It isn't doing me any good')
- Find them too expensive
- Perceive that they do not need them anymore
- Receive unclear directions (given in a rush, too much jargon, given rapidly in English when English is not the first language of the client)
- Have problems with changing routine; for example, their medication routine differs from their previous regimen
- Have difficulty implementing the regimen; for example, multiple medications to be taken at several different times of the day
- Simply forget to take them.

Several nursing interventions may enhance the ability and willingness of clients to comply with the prescribed medication regimen (Clinical Interest Box 28.6).

CLINICAL INTEREST BOX 28.6
Nursing actions to enhance client compliance with medication regimens after discharge

Giving information

- Ensure the client understands English clearly; if they do not, arrange for an interpreter
- Assess the client's memory and cognitive function for understanding and retention of information
- Ensure the client can hear you; for example, hearing aid in place and switched on
- Ensure the client will be able to concentrate; for example, is not uncomfortable, needing the toilet, in pain, thirsty, hungry or anxious
- Ensure a quiet, calm private area is available so that client is not distracted while you are providing information and so that the client's medical condition remains confidential
- Provide verbal and written instructions to the client and family member when appropriate. Other visual material may be available (video instructions are available for education about certain medications, such as insulin)
- Ask the client to repeat instructions back to you to check the accuracy of their understanding, and encourage them to ask any questions they have about the purpose of the medication and when and how to take it. If necessary, arrange for a visiting nurse to check on the client's ability to cope with more complex medications, such as insulin injections and disposal of sharps. In the home sharps can be safely disposed of in an empty plastic milk container that has a screw top cap and a 1:10 bleach:water solution in the bottom of it. The environmental biohazard waste-management strategies in the local area should be followed when disposing of the full container
- Ensure adequate time is given to educating the client about medication. Avoid giving instructions just as the client is ready to leave the hospital. Provide time for client to practise and demonstrate their ability with devices such as needles and syringes or nebulisers and inhalers

Willingness to follow the medication regimen

- Discuss the client's feelings, attitudes and beliefs about the medication prescribed. If the client indicates an unwillingness to carry out the medication after being provided with reasons to comply, refer this information to the medical officer and nurse in charge. Alternative therapies may be possible
- Discuss how the regimen fits in with the client's lifestyle and how any adverse effects might cause a problem to planned activities

Ability to follow the medication regimen

- Ensure that the client will be able to read labels on medication pots and bottles. If vision is a problem, contact the pharmacy about printing bigger labels or providing additional large print information
- Check that motor skills will allow the client to successfully use the medication; for example, that they can open the childproof lid on the container, or are able to pour out liquid medication or instil their own eye or ear drops
- Evaluate the client's social situation; for example, is the cost of the medication a problem, or can the client get the prescriptions filled without trouble?

This is certainly not an exhaustive list. Make a list of your own and see how many more you can add to it.

SUMMARY

As part of the holistic care of the client, the nurse may be required to administer and monitor the effects of medications; it is therefore essential to have the necessary knowledge to ensure the safety of all clients who are receiving medications. Of particular importance is an understanding of the legal responsibilities involved in administering medication. Nurses must be willing to accept that responsibility and work within the boundaries dictated by the nursing registering bodies governing the geographical area of their work. To promote accurate and safe drug administration the nurse must understand the system of weights and measures used in prescriptions, know the meanings of abbreviations and be competent in performing the correct calculation of dosages.

The nurse must have a basic understanding of how drugs are transported in the body, how they act, how they are metabolised and how they are excreted. Furthermore, it is important to have an understanding of the actions of the various drug groups so that the nurse will know what the desired effects of the drug are and will therefore be able to monitor the client's reaction more adequately.

Drugs are presented in a variety of forms, for example, tablets, capsules, mixtures and injectable solutions, which are administered via a variety of different routes. The nurse should not only be competent in administering medication via these routes, but also in monitoring both the desired effects and any side effects that may occur.

The nurse must observe the seven rights of drug administration (right client, right medication, right dose, right route, right time, right documentation, client right to refuse) at all times and understand the procedure if a medication error does occur. To maintain a safe working environment it is important that the nurse understands the guidelines regarding safe handling of hazardous substances. The nurse has an important role in ensuring that the client understands all aspects of any prescribed drug regimen before being discharged from a health care facility. Nurses must follow the principles of asepsis during the preparation and administration of medications via any route and must constantly assess and promote the client's safety and comfort throughout the administration of any drug therapy.

REVIEW EXERCISES

1. What are the three different names a drug may have?
2. Name the six major routes of drug administration.
3. Drug absorption depends on three factors. Name them.
4. What is first-pass metabolism?
5. What is the role of the plasma proteins in drug distribution?
6. What is the difference between a 'bound' drug and an 'unbound' drug?
7. Define the terms 'enzyme induction' and 'enzyme inhibition'.
8. How would decreased renal function affect drug excretion?
9. Why is therapeutic drug monitoring important?
10. Explain the differences between side effects, toxic effects and allergic reactions.
11. What do the Poisons Act and Poisons Regulations of each state and territory deal with?
12. What are the 'seven rights' the nurse must observe when administering a drug?
13. How does the nurse identify the correct client?
14. What does the nurse do if there is any doubt about a drug order?
15. What is the procedure to follow if a drug error occurs?
16. What are the three most common ways of administering a parenteral drug?
17. Name the common sites for subcutaneous injections.
18. Name the common sites for intramuscular injections.
19. Why is it important to discard used injection needles without recapping them?

CALCULATION EXERCISES

1. Convert the following to milligrams (mg):
   a) 0.96 g
   b) 42.8 g
   c) 0.005 g
2. Convert the following to grams (g)
   a) 568 mg
   b) 59 mg
   c) 9 mg
3. Convert the following to micrograms (mcg)
   a) 0.591 mg
   b) 0.47 mg
   c) 0.08 mg
4. Convert the following to milligrams (mg)
   a) 67 mcg
   b) 3 mcg
   c) 258 mcg
5. Your client is prescribed 450 mg soluble aspirin orally. Stock on hand are 280 mg strength tablets. How many tablets would you administer?
6. Warfarin tablets are available in strengths of 1 mg, 2 mg, 5 mg and 10 mg. Choose the best combination of tablets for each of the following warfarin dosages:
   a) 4 mg
   b) 8 mg
   c) 12 mg
7. Mr Smith is ordered 0.125 mg digoxin orally daily. Digoxin tablets are available in 62.5 mcg strength. How many tablets should you administer to Mr Smith?
8. Mr Jones has epilepsy and has been ordered phenobarbitone 140 mg IM stat for seizures. Stock ampoules contain 200 mg/mL. What volume should be administered?
9. Kylie is a 10-month-old infant weighing about 10 kg. She is ordered atropine 10 mcg/kg as a premedication. What volume is required if the atropine ampoule contains 0.1 mg/mL?
10. Your client is prescribed penicillin syrup 250 mg orally 6-hourly. Penicillin syrup is available as 250 mg/5 mL. Calculate the total amount (in mL) that your client will receive in a 24-hour period.

ANSWERS

1. a) 960 mg b) 42,800 mg c) 5 mg
2. a) 0.568 g b) 0.059 g c) 0.009 g
3. a) 591 mcg b) 470 mcg c) 80 mcg
4. a) 0.067 mg b) 0.003 mg c) 0.258 mcg
5. 1.5 tablets

6. a) 2 × 2 mg b) 1 × 5 mg, 1 × 2 mg, 1 × 1 mg
   c) 1 × 10 mg, 1 × 2 mg
7. 2 tablets
8. 0.7 mL
9. 1 mL
10. 20 mL

CRITICAL THINKING EXCERCISES

1. Mrs Brown has been started on warfarin 2 mg orally nocte and will be discharged from hospital in the next few days. What information would you include in your client education for Mrs Brown?
2. There are many factors that can result in a client not being compliant with drug therapy. What are some of the reasons for non-compliance? Outline some nursing actions that you could apply before a client is discharged to reduce the risk of non-compliance with drug therapy.

REFERENCES AND FURTHER READING

Arnold N (2003) *New NOHSC National Code of Practice for the Preparation of Material Safety Data Sheets. Risk Review*. Online. Available: www.noel-arnold.com.au/content/risk-reviews/riskreviews_article.php?relevant_id=187 [accessed 30 October 2007]

Australian Health Ministers Advisory Council (2001) Standard for the Uniform Scheduling of Drugs and Poisons No 16. AGPS, Canberra

Bryant B, Knights K (2006) *Pharmacology for Health Professionals*, 2nd edn. Mosby, Sydney

Crisp J, Taylor C (eds) (2005) *Potter & Perry's Fundamentals of Nursing*, 2nd edn. Elsevier Australia, Sydney

deWit S (2005) *Fundamental Concepts and Skills for Nursing*, 2nd edn. WB Saunders, Philadelphia

Ebersole P, Hess P (2001) *Geriatric Nursing & Healthy Ageing*. Mosby, Missouri

—— (2005) *Gerontological Nursing & Healthy Ageing*. Mosby, Missouri

Ebersole P, Hess P, Touhy TA, Jett K, Luggen A (2008) *Toward Healthy Ageing: Human Needs & Nursing Response*, 7th edn. Mosby Elsevier, St Louis

Elliot D, Aitken L, Chaboyer W (2007) *Critical Care Nursing*. Mosby Elsevier, Sydney

Galbraith A, Bullock S, Manias E (2006) *Fundamentals of Pharmacology*, 5th edn. Addison Wesley, Melbourne

Gatford J, Phillips N (2006) *Nursing Calculations*, 7th edn. Churchill Livingstone, Melbourne

Healy D (2005) *Psychiatric Drugs Explained*, 4th edn. Elsevier, Edinburgh

Katzung BG (2007) *Basic and Clinical Pharmacology*, 10th edn. McGraw Hill Medical, New York

Neal M (2002) *Medical Pharmacology at a Glance*, 4th edn. Blackwell Science, Oxford

Nurses Board of Tasmania (2007) *Standards of Medication Management for Nurses and Midwives (May 2007)*. Online. Available: www.nursingboardtas.org.au/ [accessed 29 October 2007]

Paterson R (1996) *Pharmacological Aspects of Nursing Care in Australia*, 2nd edn. Nelson, Melbourne

Queensland Nursing Council (2006) *Enrolled nurse medication policy amendment (2006): Controlled S8 drugs*. Online. Available: www.qnc.qld.gov.au [accessed 29 October 2007]

Reiss BS, Evans ME, Broyles BE (2002) *Pharmacological Aspects of Nursing Care*, 6th edn. Thomson Delmar Publishing, New York

Royal College of Nursing Position Statement — Enrolled Nurse [under review]. Online. Available: www.rcna.org.au/UserFiles/en-div2_nurse_feb_2003-_under_review_25nov04.pdf [accessed 29 October 2007]

Taylor M, Reide P (1998) *Mosby's Crash Course — Pharmacology*. Mosby, London

Tiziani A (2006) *Havard's Nursing Guide to Drugs*, 7th edn. Mosby, Melbourne

Chapter 29

COMMUNICATION

OBJECTIVES

- Define the key terms/concepts
- Identify the components of the communication process
- State the factors that influence effective communication
- Identify the factors that act as barriers to effective communication
- Identify and implement the skills that facilitate therapeutic communication
- Identify ways to minimise communication difficulties for clients who have visual, hearing, speech or cognitive impairments

KEY TERMS/CONCEPTS

barriers to communication
channels of communication
decoding
empathy
encoding
levels of communication
reminiscence therapy
therapeutic communication skills
validation therapy
verbal/non-verbal communication

CHAPTER FOCUS

Communication is an interactive process involving the verbal or non-verbal transference of information between people. Effective and empathic communication is basic and essential to the provision of quality care in nursing and vital to the development of a therapeutic relationship between a nurse and client. This chapter has a particular emphasis on the crucial communication issues affecting the development of the therapeutic relationship.

LIVED EXPERIENCE

When I had viral meningitis I was put in a room by the nurses' station, I was all by myself and I was so scared. My head hurt so much I thought I was going to die. I remember one nurse — Sue — she came in often and kept reassuring me that the pain would pass and that I would be all right. She was always calm, always explained everything she was doing. She's the nurse I remember because she understood how I was feeling, probably because she was really the only one that ever seemed to have time to listen.

John, 34, reflecting on his experience of a serious illness
3 months after his recovery

Communication involves the ability to interact with people at a variety of levels and in a range of situations. Effective communication is important in all areas of everyday life; the quality of relationships between people depends on it. Nurses need to communicate effectively with everyone in the health care environment, and therapeutically with clients. The ability of nurses to communicate therapeutically is a critical factor in how clients experience illness. Nurses need to be skilful in what they do for clients but at the same time they need to be communicating with them in ways that are supportive and helpful and promote feelings of trust. While the focus of this chapter is on therapeutic nurse–client interactions, the skills involved will enhance communication in all relationships between people.

The nurse who has effective communication skills:

- Listens attentively to others
- Assists clients to communicate their needs
- Clearly communicates information to clients, their relatives and other members of the health care team
- Accurately relays information to personnel in other health care agencies
- Responds empathically to feelings experienced by clients and their relatives.

All communication is a two-way process in which messages are conveyed by verbal and/or non-verbal means by one person, and received by another. All behaviour conveys some message and is therefore a form of communication. For example, even a client refusing to speak or acknowledge the presence of a nurse conveys a message that the nurse will attempt to interpret (decode). Non-verbal communication includes the messages sent by facial expression, gestures, body posture and appearance, and those that are written (see Chapter 20 for information concerning written communication in nursing).

Communication is an ongoing dynamic series of events in which meaning is generated and transmitted. Communication occurs when a person responds to a message and assigns meaning to it. Meanings are mental images that are created to develop a sense of understanding. During interactions people respond to messages they receive and create meanings for those messages. If the intended meaning of a message is misunderstood by the recipient, communication has not occurred effectively.

Communication takes place at many different levels and, depending on their area of practice, nurses may need competence in all of them. While the various levels are outlined briefly, the focus of this chapter is primarily on communication at the interpersonal level, between nurse and client in the therapeutic relationship.

LEVELS OF COMMUNICATION

The most basic level at which communication occurs is the intrapersonal level. Others include the interpersonal, small-group, organisational, public and mass communication levels.

Intrapersonal communication is a process that occurs within individuals. For example, if a person looks outside and sees that it is raining and thinks 'I had better bring the washing in', the person is communicating intrapersonally. Thus, intrapersonal communication involves an ongoing dialogue of thoughts. A dialogue of thoughts is a process that can help in deciding about future plans, resolving internal conflict and evaluating personal behaviour and relationships with others.

Interpersonal communication usually refers to communication that occurs between two people (a dyad). It can occur face to face, or via means such as a telephone. Interpersonal communication is at the heart of nursing practice.

Small-group communication occurs between three or more people interacting with one another. Small-group communication usually occurs face to face, but it may also develop through the use of a communication medium, for example when several people hold a conference via a telephone or video link-up. There is generally a common purpose for a group of people interacting.

Organisational communication refers to a system of disseminating and transferring information within an organisation, for example when hospital management personnel are communicating with medical officers and staff at ward level to determine bed availability for clients waiting for admission. This level of communication often encompasses the other three levels of intrapersonal, interpersonal and small-group communication.

Public communication involves interaction with large groups of people, for example when a speaker addresses an audience.

Mass communication occurs when a small number of people send messages to a large, anonymous audience through the use of some specialised media, such as film, television, radio, newspapers, magazines or books.

Communication with clients in health care settings is often at the interpersonal level, between two people only, commonly the nurse and the client. It has a different purpose from communication in social situations. Social communication is initiated for the purpose of friendship and enjoying the company of others. Mutual needs are met through social interaction. The aim of the communication between a nurse and client is to establish a therapeutic relationship to benefit the client, even when the contact is brief. In any therapeutic relationship the needs of the other person are always placed ahead of personal needs.

Therapeutic communication is client focused, purposeful and time limited. It involves the nurse coming to know and respond to the client as a unique person, and the client coming to trust the nurse. Within a therapeutic relationship the nurse and client communicate comfortably during times of the most intimate nursing care or emotional significance. Throughout the relationship the nurse remains continually sensitive to the client's feelings and needs. A therapeutic relationship is purposeful in that it involves the nurse assisting clients identify, adapt to or resolve health problems.

ELEMENTS OF THE COMMUNICATION PROCESS

Communication is a multidimensional and complex process in which ideas, thoughts, values, knowledge or feelings are shared and interpreted. During the process people simultaneously send and receive numerous messages at many different levels. To simplify understanding of this complex process, models of communication have been developed. Figure 29.1 is an example of one such model. It depicts the basic elements of communication and shows that communication is an active process between sender and receiver. The process of communication involves:

- A sender
- A receiver
- A message
- A channel
- Feedback
- Variables (influences).

The sender is the individual who initiates the communication. The receiver is the person to whom the message is transmitted. The role of sender and receiver may alternate between participants at any time during the period messages are being transmitted.

The message is the information that is transmitted by the sender, and may be comprised of both verbal and non-verbal information.

The channel is the means by which the message is conveyed, for example, through the visual, auditory, olfactory or tactile routes. The sender's facial expressions and body gestures visually convey a message to the receiver; for example, a facial grimace or tense body posture sends a visual message to the nurse that the client may be in pain. The spoken word is conveyed via the auditory channel and touching a person while communicating uses the tactile channel. A nurse can convey a message of caring and compassion to a distressed client by a simple touch of the hand. The olfactory route is particularly important in nursing. Unpleasant odours can indicate a variety of conditions, including incontinence of urine or faeces or the onset of a urinary tract or other infection; a smell of acetone on a client's breath can indicate a serious lack of insulin in the body (diabetic ketoacidosis).

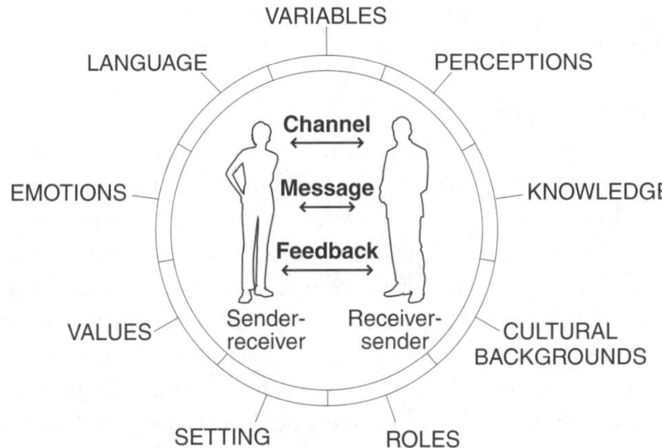

Figure 29.1 | The communication process

Feedback helps the sender recognise whether the meaning of the message conveyed has been perceived as intended. The receiver's verbal and non-verbal responses convey feedback to the sender to reveal the receiver's understanding of the message. Feedback helps to clarify communication as it guides people in adjusting the messages they send to one another. Effective communicators continuously seek feedback from the people with whom they are communicating, to determine whether the information they are transmitting is being received and understood as intended — that there are no misinterpretations of the meaning of the messages.

Variables are the factors that influence the quality and effectiveness of the communication. They include factors such as the setting in which communication takes place, the presence of distractions such as background noise, and the language, perceptions, values, knowledge, cultural background, role and emotions of each person taking part in the communication. Variables can enhance the effectiveness of communication between people but they are often barriers. A setting that does not provide adequate privacy may be a significant barrier when a nurse and client are attempting to communicate about the client's personal concerns.

When communication is occurring and information is being transmitted from one person to another, two processes must take place: encoding and decoding. Encoding refers to the cognitive processes that occur in the mind of the person who is to send the message. These thoughts must be translated into a code, such as verbal language, to be transmitted to the person who is to receive the message. Decoding refers to the cognitive processes used by the receiver of the message to make sense of what is seen or heard. Generally the sender and the receiver encode and decode messages in a cyclic pattern while communication is taking place. Clinical Interest Box 29.1 illustrates the communication process in action.

FACTORS THAT INFLUENCE THE COMMUNICATION PROCESS

Even during a simple act of interpersonal communication between two people, many factors can influence how effectively messages are conveyed and understood. These factors are frequently referred to as the variables (Figure 29.1); they relate to anything that influences or interferes with how the sender transmits a message, how the recipient perceives (interprets) the meaning of the message and the route or channel of communication.

PERCEPTION

Perception is a process by which the meanings of messages are interpreted. The way messages are perceived is related to a combination of a person's social and cultural influences, gender, educational background and knowledge, and past

CLINICAL INTEREST BOX 29.1
The communication process in action

Mr Smith, who has been in hospital for several days, is about to be discharged home. Before he is discharged, the nurse in charge must make certain that Mr Smith understands he has to attend an appointment with the medical officer in 2 weeks time. The nurse in charge (the sender) thinks about the best way to pass on the information (the message), and decides (encodes) to write the time and date of the appointment on a card in addition to telling Mr Smith. Thus, both spoken and written words (auditory and visual channels) are used to transmit the message. Mr Smith (receiver) listens to the nurse in charge and looks at the appointment card. Because the words used are familiar to him, he is able to understand (decode) the information. He confirms he has understood the message by asking, 'You mean I need to come back here and see the medical officer again at 11 o'clock on Tuesday 2nd October?' (feedback to the nurse).

experiences. This complex mix of influences means that no two people are likely to perceive the same message in exactly the same way. Some of the strongest influences on the way messages are sent and their meanings perceived are the attitudes, values and beliefs that individuals hold (Stein-Parbury 2005; Williams 2007).

ATTITUDES, VALUES AND BELIEFS

Attitude is the way one person behaves towards another. A person's attitude can be positive, or negative and unpleasant. An unpleasant attitude in the workplace makes other people feel uncomfortable and it is detrimental to the wellbeing of clients. Attitude can be influenced by what is happening in a person's life. For example, a fight with a friend may create feelings of anger or distress. Such feelings can be reflected in a negative, even hostile, attitude towards others, which can change the way messages are transmitted and received. Nurses have a professional responsibility to maintain a positive attitude towards clients at all times, so every effort must be made to put personal concerns and feelings aside when communicating with clients, relatives and other health professionals in the workplace.

Attitude towards others is also related to the values and beliefs that a person holds about the ideas or practices of other people in society, and they are not always consciously recognised. For example, cultural values commonly lie outside conscious awareness and are often simply taken for granted as being the right values (Stein-Parbury 2005). It is natural for people's values and beliefs to differ within and across social and cultural groups. Nurses will encounter many situations in which their own cultural values and beliefs differ from those of clients (see Chapter 9). Tolerance and understanding of differences in views and cultural practices helps to facilitate therapeutic relationships between nurses and their clients. For example, a nurse who holds strong values and beliefs about no sex without marriage will need to demonstrate acceptance that personal views are not shared when caring for a pregnant, single, female client. If the nurse is unable to accept this and put personal views to one side, it will be difficult to communicate with the client in a therapeutic manner.

While a nurse's personal values can create interference in therapeutic relationships if they are imposed on clients or used in judgment, they can also serve to enhance therapeutic effects. For example, a nurse who holds beliefs that all people have positive qualities and that every individual is a worthwhile person will find that such beliefs enhance the establishment of effective therapeutic relationships (Antai-Otong 2007; Stein-Parbury 2005).

DIFFERENCES IN KNOWLEDGE

When the level of knowledge between two people is different, communication can be difficult. For example, an individual's level of knowledge may be so far above that of the person being spoken to that the meaning of the message may be lost entirely. The nurse must take care to express messages in words and phrases that will be understood. For example, a nurse who is familiar with nursing or medical language, especially jargon, may forget that a client may not be, and if words or phrases are used that are not part of the client's vocabulary the message may be misinterpreted. The use of specific language that is familiar to members of a subculture or profession may confuse, frighten or alienate people who are not part of that subculture or profession. For example, not every male client will know what the nurse means when asked, 'Do you need a bottle?' The word bottle is nursing jargon used to describe a portable male urinal but it could easily be perceived as meaning something entirely different.

PAST EXPERIENCES

Past experiences can have a powerful effect on a person's perceptions of the meaning of messages. For example, a client who has had a previous traumatic and painful experience in hospital may discount, distrust or disbelieve messages from the nurse that pain after surgery will be controlled. The nurse can help by talking with the client about the past experience and explaining fully every measure that will be implemented to ensure adequate pain relief.

EMOTIONS

Emotions strongly influence how a person relates to other people, and the power of emotion in communication should not be underestimated. Nurses must also be aware that if they become too emotionally involved with the suffering experienced by a client, they may be unable to effectively meet that client's needs. This aspect is one of the most difficult situations faced by nurses, as on the one hand nurses must become emotionally involved to assist clients, while on the other hand personal emotions cannot be allowed to adversely affect client care. All nurses need to be aware of their emotions, and many find it helpful to talk with other experienced nurses about what they are feeling and experiencing.

It is also important to realise that, if people cultivate 'emotional distance' in an interpersonal interaction, they prevent any deep sharing of meaning and may even arouse animosity. For example, if a client feels that a nurse is treating them as an 'interesting case' or a 'problem' rather than as a person, they are likely to feel resentful, and therapeutic communication is not likely to occur.

Another way by which emotions influence communication is when the receiver of a message becomes irritated or annoyed by any distracting mannerisms of the sender, such as irritating gestures, persistent coughing or throat clearing. Being distracted by annoying mannerisms can cause the listener to lose concentration on the message being conveyed.

It is not unusual for clients to be anxious or upset, and strong emotions interfere with the ability to absorb the information in messages such as those given by medical officers or nurses. There would be little point, for example, in a medical officer informing a client about treatment plans immediately after telling her that her breast biopsy revealed a malignant breast tumour. It would not be surprising if the client's anxiety level increased to such an extent on hearing the diagnosis that it prevented her from absorbing any of the following information about the proposed treatment. The nurse can help in this situation by ensuring the information is repeated when the client is less anxious or distressed and by providing the information in written form for the client to absorb more effectively at a later time.

RELATIONSHIPS AND ROLES

The style and type of communication that occurs between people depends on the quality and type of relationship that exists between them. Individuals communicate in ways that they perceive are appropriate to particular relationships and the roles they have within them. For example, a woman might communicate passively and non-assertively with the medical officer and the nurse but may be assertive with her husband, dominating with her children and bossy towards her colleagues at work.

There are numerous different types of interpersonal relationships, including those between friends, acquaintances, work colleagues, family members and partners. It is usually only when there is enough trust in a relationship that totally honest communication occurs, when ideas, judgments and emotions can be revealed without fear of reprisal, humiliation or rejection.

The nurse–client relationship is unique: trust in the nurse needs to develop quickly and trust is essential if the relationship is to be therapeutic. Clients in hospital may not say what they are thinking or feeling if there is a lack of trust in the nurse; often this means that the client has a fear of being judged. A therapeutic relationship means demonstrating unconditional acceptance of all clients, without judging (Stein-Parbury 2005; Williams 2007). The nurse accepts the client as a worthwhile person even if the client's behaviour is challenging. As a nurse's communication skills develop they become increasingly effective and therapeutic, but even when they have been learned and practised they may still be difficult to apply in some particularly challenging situations. Clinical Interest Box 29.2 provides examples of situations where communicating effectively with clients can be challenging.

ENVIRONMENTAL SETTING

Effective communication is more likely to occur if it takes place within a setting that is conducive to listening and concentrating. An area that is at a comfortable temperature, private and free from noise and other distractions is suitable, whereas an area where there is noise or a lack of comfort or privacy may create tension and confusion, making effective

CLINICAL INTEREST BOX 29.2
Communication challenges in nursing

- Chatty, lonely clients who want someone to talk to all the time
- Clients or others who are too angry and hostile to listen to explanations
- Clients who are excessively demanding, constantly wanting someone to wait on them or meet their requests
- Silent, withdrawn clients who do not express any feelings or needs
- Sad, depressed, despondent clients who have slow mental and motor responses
- Irritable, annoyed clients or relatives who blame nursing staff unfairly
- Sensory impaired clients who cannot hear or see well
- Clients who have cerebral impairments and cannot articulate or understand words well
- Gossiping, catty or manipulative people who violate confidentiality and cause friction
- Bitter, complaining people who are negative about everything
- Mentally impaired clients who are frightened or distrustful
- Confused, disoriented clients who are bewildered and uncooperative
- People who speak very little English
- Anxious, nervous people who cannot cope with what is happening
- Grieving, crying, distressed people who are suffering a major loss
- Screaming, kicking toddlers, who fight against treatment
- Unresponsive or comatose clients who do not communicate at all
- Flirtatious, sexually inappropriate advances
- Loud, obscene or poorly behaved individuals causing a disturbance
- People violating a rule (e.g. smoking or using mobile phones in a restricted area)
- Clients who are dying and want to talk about it

(adapted from Potter & Perry 2008: 342)

communication difficult. For example, background noise and the movements of other people in the environment may distract the listener, and even missing one or two vital words in a sentence can result in the meaning of a whole sentence being lost.

Ideally clients should be able to communicate with health professionals and other people in a private room, but this is sometimes difficult to achieve in busy health care facilities. Nurses should, whenever possible, talk with clients about personal issues in a private area. Clients can be accompanied to an interview room or even a quiet garden area to gain privacy. The very least that nurses can do if the client does not have a single room is to close the curtains surrounding the bed, speak quietly and avoid discussing personal details while visitors are in the area.

Two other factors, physical discomfort and pressure of time, are particularly important in nurse–client interactions because they can seriously interfere with the quality of therapeutic communication.

PHYSICAL DISCOMFORT

Communication is likely to be less effective if one or both participants are experiencing fatigue, pain or other physical discomfort. Like its emotional counterpart, physical discomfort can distract a person so that it is not possible to concentrate on what is being said. The nurse who is about to engage in a therapeutic dialogue with a client is advised to ensure that the client is free of pain, lying or sitting in a comfortable position and not needing to go to the toilet. It is also important to consider that some medications, including those administered for pain relief, can affect a client's memory and the ability to concentrate or to think clearly.

PRESSURE OF TIME

Because most people have many pressures on their time, the urge to speed up communication is increasing. Nurses need to overcome feelings of urgency to complete other tasks while communicating with clients. This is not always easy, but even a few minutes of attentive listening can be very therapeutic for a client. Not all interactions with clients need to be lengthy but it does take time to explain, to listen, to reduce fears or anxieties and to assimilate facts. A client who is sensitive to the nurse's need to get on with other things is unlikely to raise any issues of concern that need to be talked about. It is one of the major challenges in contemporary nursing practice to prioritise tasks and manage time so that the psychological as well as the physical needs of clients are met.

THE ROUTE OR CHANNEL OF COMMUNICATION

The meaning in a message is at greater risk of being misconstrued if the channel of communication is not the most appropriate. For example, the oral route may not effectively communicate a long and involved message — it may be better transmitted in written form. It is sometimes difficult to relay messages of caring and concern with words; a gentle touch can be more eloquent than the spoken or written word in many situations.

FORMS OF COMMUNICATION

Communication is the process of sharing information and understanding, using verbal and non-verbal methods. Verbal communication involves the use of words and how they are delivered. Words can be written or spoken (vocal). Non-verbal communication involves facial expressions, body posture and gestures, touch and the use of space.

VOCAL COMMUNICATION

In addition to the words used, vocal communication involves the tone and pitch of the voice, the rate and volume of speech and the use of pauses, all of which provide information about the speaker's message.

The words

Messages are only understood if the words used are familiar to the sender and the receiver. Nurses in Australia and New Zealand often care for clients for whom English is not a first language, and it may be necessary to get help from an interpreter. Even within a cultural or subcultural group the meaning of many words can be ambiguous and one word can have two meanings in the same culture, so that remarks can easily be misunderstood. For example, if a 5-year-old client was being prepared for a surgical operation and the nurse told him he would be going to the theatre in 2 hours' time, imagine his distress when he arrived in the operating room to have his tonsils removed, when he thought that he was being taken to see a film!

Sounds

In addition to words, sounds made by the voice can deliver very strong messages about a person. Sounds can convey pain (groans, moans), distress and sadness (crying, sobs), boredom or despair (sighs), excitement or fear (screeches and screams) or a range of other emotions. The meaning of a sound can easily be misinterpreted, as most sounds can express more than one emotion. A moan might not always express pain — it may be a moan of pleasure or disappointment. The nurse must always validate the meaning of a sound with the client; for example, the nurse might ask, 'That sounds like you have pain, Mrs Jacobs. Do you have pain?'

Tone and pitch

The tone and pitch of the voice can have a powerful effect, sometimes more so than words. No matter what words are being said, a loud aggressive voice will send a strong message. A nurse's tone and pitch of voice and the inflections used add meaning to words. Tone and pitch of voice can display anger, apathy, disgust, enthusiasm, excitement and other emotions. An individual can often determine more about another person from the way in which the words are spoken than from the actual words used. Loud, rapid, forcefully spoken words can intimidate and communicate aggression, a patronising tone can communicate condescension or contempt, and expressionless speech can communicate lack of interest. A client and nurse can discern much about each other from their respective voices. Of particular importance, the tone and pitch of clients' voices can convey messages about their emotional feelings and energy levels.

Rate and volume

Rate and volume of speech are best kept at a moderate level. Speaking too fast, too slowly or too loudly is not conducive to comfortable conversation, and messages may be lost or misinterpreted. Nurses frequently care for clients with hearing and cognitive impairments; such clients need to be consulted and assessed to determine the most successful rate and volume of speech to facilitate therapeutic communication.

The use of pauses

Pauses can provide time for clients to think about what they want to say, but pauses that are too long may seem awkward or uncomfortable. In normal conversation the style of communication that individuals use is generally not thought about consciously. When engaged in therapeutic relationships, nurses need to consciously evaluate the way they communicate and develop a conscious awareness of the tone, pitch, rate and volume at which they speak. Other basic aspects of vocal communication that are helpful to be aware of are the need to:

- Be brief: short pieces of information make understanding easier — the fewer words the less the risk of misinterpretation
- Keep the messages clear, simple and direct: complicated information leads to confusion and unnecessary words detract from clarity; for example, additions such as, 'you know', 'OK', 'and that' or 'um' are best avoided
- Enunciate words clearly: make messages clearly heard; mumbling makes them incoherent
- Use examples to clarify meaning: an example often makes it easier for the message to be understood. For example, the nurse might clarify, 'By aids to help you at home I mean things like a seat that fits across the bath, grip rails in the bathroom for you to hold onto and perhaps a ramp instead of steps at your back door.'
- Time the delivery of the message appropriately: timing is important when giving information of any sort. Trying to tell a client about what will happen in surgery just as the pathology nurse is taking a blood sample would demonstrate poor timing, as the client's concentration would not be totally focused on the message.

NON-VERBAL COMMUNICATION

In nearly every interaction, words are accompanied by simultaneous non-verbal messages that the sender may not be consciously aware of. Non-verbal communication refers to messages transmitted without using words. They include those transmitted via:

- Facial expressions
- Body movements and gestures
- Eye behaviour
- Touch
- Use of space
- Personal appearance.

It is generally accepted that non-verbal messages form the most significant component of communication. Research conducted by Professor Albert Mehrabian (1972) first identified that in conversations messages transmitted and received are about 7% words, 38% tone and pitch of voice and 55% non-verbal clues. These percentages have not been contradicted by any other research, neither has the proposition, identified by Mehrabian (1972), that most non-verbal messages are about emotions and that they are mostly automatic, and so more reliable than words because they are not as easy to fake (Mehrabian 1972). Perhaps that is why there is a saying that 'actions speak louder than words'.

During interpersonal communication with clients it is essential for the nurse to look as well as listen. Concentrating only on words means that much of what could be discerned is being missed. Non-verbal communication comes from many sources and it is easy to miss something significant. For example, while watching a person's foot tapping, a significant hand gesture or eye movement may not be noticed. Generally, non-verbal messages are not received in isolation and they are interpreted subconsciously but nurses need to develop the skills of consciously considering verbal and non-verbal messages, together and in context, and validating the meanings perceived in the messages.

Facial expressions

Facial expressions convey emotional states, and so a great deal of information can be obtained about clients' feelings by observing their facial expressions. For example, a frown or an eyebrow raised in disbelief reveals something of how a client is reacting to what is being said. Some specific facial expressions of emotion seem to be universal across cultures. They are those that convey surprise, fear, disgust, anger, happiness and sadness (Ekman 1997). Facial expressions provide the nurse with continual non-verbal feedback from most clients, but some people have expressionless mask-like faces that reveal little or nothing of what they are thinking or feeling. This may be a client's usual demeanour but sometimes it is due to the effects of an illness such as Parkinson's disease, Alzheimer's dementia or severe depression. In such cases the nurse must detect the client's mood from other clues such as body posture, activity level, appetite or simply by asking how the client is feeling.

Facial expressions can attempt to mask true emotions, for example, a client may smile to hide feelings of sadness, anxiety or boredom. This may be so as to not worry loved ones, not to concern the nurse, or to keep feelings private. Facial expression may be incongruent with what a person is saying; for example, a client may be smiling while talking about a very sad event, such as the death of their child. In such cases the client would be described as having 'an inappropriate affect' (Varcarolis 2006).

Clients are often very sensitive to the facial expressions of the nurse and it is imperative that, even though it is sometimes difficult to control, nurses make every effort not to facially express feelings of shock, alarm, repulsion or any other negative emotion in front of the client. Imagine the effect on a client with a stoma, an amputation or serious burns who detects repulsion on the face of a nurse. Additionally, nurses need to develop awareness of the effect their facial expressions may have on clients during procedures and interactions of any sort. For example, frowning in concentration while dressing a wound may be interpreted by the client as the nurse being worried and concerned about the look of the wound.

Body movements and gestures (body language)

The way individuals move, walk, sit or stand communicates information about their mood, attitude, state of mental and physical health, and self-esteem. An upright posture together with decisive, quick and purposeful movements communicates a sense of wellbeing and self-confidence. A slumped posture, hesitant movements and a slow shuffling or stumbling gait may indicate depression, physical illness or impairment or that a person is drug affected or fatigued.

Gestures are motions of the limbs or body made to express thoughts or feelings, to emphasise or clarify what is being said or to replace the spoken word. For example, a shrug of the shoulders can replace the words, 'I don't know' and pointing to an object is easier than explaining where or what it is. Some basic communication gestures convey the same message in almost every culture. For example, nodding the head is almost universally used to indicate 'yes', or affirmation.

Conversely, a specific gesture may be meaningless or assume a different meaning in another culture. For example, the 'V' sign made with two fingers may mean victory, the number two, or something rather rude. Even within one culture the meaning may be different according to whether the gesture is made with the palm facing out or facing in. In most European countries the V sign means victory when gestured with the palm facing away from the body and a rude 'shove it' when the palm is facing towards the body of the person gesticulating (Haynes 2002). It is not uncommon for an acceptable gesture in one culture to be considered rude in another. For example, pointing at an object with the index finger is considered impolite in the Middle and Far East. In Indonesia it is common and more acceptable to use an open hand or thumb (Haynes 2002). (See Chapter 9 for more information on cultural difference.)

Although body language can communicate much about how a client is feeling, it is a mistake to interpret a single movement, gesture or facial expression in isolation. For example, a person with arms folded across the chest and stomping about might simply be protecting himself from the cold, but if this was accompanied by sobbing, shouting or facial grimacing it may indicate severe pain, distress or anger. All non-verbal clues need to be observed together when considering what is really happening.

When a person's actions or gestures do not match spoken words, the messages are said to be incongruent. This means that the body movements or gestures are conveying one message, while the verbal words are conveying a different message. When a client conveys incongruent messages it is important that the nurse tries to clarify what is happening even though it may at first feel awkward doing so. Clinical Interest Box 29.3 provides an example of how a nurse can explore incongruence between verbal and non-verbal messages.

Eye behaviour

Eye contact is one of the most crucial aspects of communication. How often people make eye contact or how long they hold a gaze can make a vital difference to the quality of an interaction. Eye contact and behaviour can convey openness and sincerity, and an individual's emotional state and level of interest in a person or what is being said, and a failure to make eye contact can reduce the effectiveness of communication. Causes for failing to make eye contact include shyness, nervousness, low self-esteem, embarrassment or defensiveness.

CLINICAL INTEREST BOX 29.3
Exploring incongruence between verbal and non-verbal communications

Andrew, 40, was admitted to hospital for overnight observations after being concussed in a motor vehicle accident the day before. The nurse was concerned because, although there seemed to be no problems from his concussion, she had observed Andrew limping and grimacing when he was walking around. When she asked if he had any pain he said no. The nurse began exploring the incongruent messages being received by saying, 'I am concerned about you because even though you say you have no pain you seem to have trouble walking'. After talking with Andrew for only a short while he admitted he had considerable pain in his foot, but did not want to tell anyone because he could not afford any more time in hospital and thought it was probably only bruising that would get better without treatment. X-rays revealed that Andrew had broken two bones in his foot, which, without correct treatment, could have resulted in permanent disability.

In some cultures the norms about what eye contact means, how often it should occur and with whom, are quite different to those of the white Anglo Saxon population. According to their cultural norms, people try to balance their eye contact somewhere between staring and avoiding all contact. Some of the differences in eye behaviour include that Japanese people tend to gaze at the neck rather than at the face when conversing; Southern Europeans tend to have a high frequency of gaze that may be offensive to others; people from Arab countries tend to use prolonged eye contact to gauge trustworthiness; in Asia, Africa and Latin America people avoid eye contact as a sign of respect (Stern 2004), and eye contact can make Aboriginal people feel awkward, so they may look the other way during conversations (Kimberley Interpreting Service 2003). Nurses therefore need to consider cultural differences when using eye contact with clients.

Looking down on a client from a higher position can be intimidating. When clients are in bed it is preferable for the nurse, or any other health professional, to sit down and make eye contact at eye level because communicating at eye level indicates equality in a relationship. Conversely, rising to the same eye level as a person who is angry, bossy or intimidating in any way may reduce feelings of vulnerability because it helps to establish a more equal sense of power (Crisp & Taylor 2005).

Touch

Touch (tactile communication) is one of the most powerful and personal forms of expression. A person's first comfort in life comes from touch, and so, frequently, does their last, as touch may communicate with a dying person when words cannot. There is no way to practise nursing without touching and, in nursing, touch may be the most important of all non-verbal communications. Touch occurs in everyday procedures such as taking vital signs and assisting clients with showers or baths. It also occurs at times of joy, fear, stress and loss (see Chapter 14 concerning loss and grief). How nurses use touch in client care conveys a great deal about the way they feel towards their clients and their illnesses.

Some people, including nurses, appreciate the significance of touch as a therapeutic act so much that they perform the techniques of relaxation massage or the 'laying on of hands'. Massage, performed skilfully and sensitively, can produce relaxation and can communicate caring. Laying on of hands involves placing the hands on or near the body of an ill person in an attempt to heal (Rankin-Box 2001). In nursing, touch can be used therapeutically to transmit positive feelings of understanding, compassion or reassurance. To be effective, tactile communication must be used at the appropriate time and place. Not all people like to be touched and all individuals consider a certain amount of space around them as private. Touch can be seen as an invasion of that privacy unless it is desired. Touch must be used at the right time and in the right way, otherwise the message may be misinterpreted. Nurses always need to assess and be sensitive to how comfortable the client is with being touched.

Space

The concept of 'space' is important in communication, as it determines the distance a person usually keeps between themself and other people. The individuals involved and the context or situation dictate acceptable distance zones. People surround themselves with their own 'informal' personal space, which is invisible and mobile. There are four categories of space or zone (Figure 29.2).

The intimate zone (between 15 cm and 45 cm from the body surface) is the most important to a person, who guards it as if it were personal property. Usually only those who are emotionally close to the person are permitted to enter this zone, such as spouses, partners or lovers, parents, children, close friends and relatives. The personal zone (between 46 cm and 1.2 m) is about the distance individuals keep between them at friendly gatherings and social functions. The social zone (between 1.2 m and 3.6 m) is the distance individuals keep between themselves and strangers or people who are not well known to them. The public zone (over 3.6 m) is a comfortable distance at which an individual generally chooses to stand when addressing a large group of people.

Individuals have their own personal tolerance for touch, closeness and distance, which is often also influenced by cultural conditioning. For example, some Asian people may feel very uncomfortable if they are touched on the head because the head is the repository of the soul in the Buddhist religion (Haynes 2002). When two people are communicating, each person makes personal

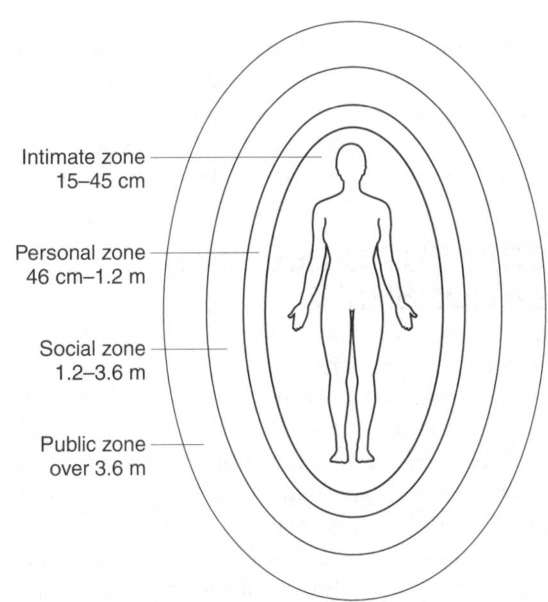

Figure 29.2 | Zone differences

space decisions and attempts to maintain an 'acceptable' boundary of personal space. Sometimes the personal space expectations of each person conflict and the result is spatial invasion. Spatial invasion makes people very uncomfortable and precipitates a communication reaction of either fight or flight, neither of which is helpful in promoting communication. Most people have experienced a situation when, during a conversation with another person, that person moves in uncomfortably close to make a point. The first person often feels this as an invasion of personal space and responds first by pulling the head away. If this first non-verbal cue is not received, the person may even step back and move away.

The nature of nursing practice means that nurses frequently invade a client's intimate or personal space. Many clients will be uncomfortable with this closeness, and nurses should be sensitive to how each client is responding. Conversely, such necessary closeness when handled sensitively may promote rapport between a nurse and a client.

Personal appearance

Personal appearance has a strong influence on the initial perceptions and first impressions people form about others. Physical characteristics, degree of cleanliness, manner of dress, style of hair and make-up are some of the things that provide the information from which impressions are formed. The adornments that a person wears or carries, such as jewellery, handbag or briefcase, provide additional information, as do the objects with which they decorate their environment. People tend to judge others by their appearance, a habit that can be detrimental, as it can lead to incorrect assumptions. For example, the social or financial status of a person may be incorrectly inferred from the clothing worn.

The appearance of clients provides nurses with general impressions of their state of physical and emotional health that are useful, but these impressions need to be validated by verbal information and objective measurements. Clients also form a general impression from the initial appearance of a nurse, and well-groomed nurses are likely to create a favourable impression of professionalism.

THERAPEUTIC HELPING RELATIONSHIPS

Communication is neither innately nor intuitively derived, but is an activity that must be learned. Therapeutic communication requires knowledge of the concepts and theories of the communication process, as well as skill in applying them. Therapeutic communication requires practice, time and effort, and a desire to improve. Communication can generally be improved if people increase their understanding of the process of communication; develop heightened self-awareness, particularly in relation to personal attitudes, values and beliefs; and develop increased sensitivity to others.

The following guidelines can facilitate effective communication:

- Be clear about the message to be conveyed, and how and why it will be conveyed
- Use the most appropriate medium (channel) for conveying a message
- Use language that is appropriate for the recipient's level of intellectual understanding, emotional status and culture
- Choose the right timing and length of message for each occasion
- Use specific skills to gain and interpret feedback from the other person
- Use active listening skills to listen for what is said
- Use keen observation skills to determine what is not being said; for example, be aware of non-verbal communication
- Observe for clues and contradictions in the verbal and non-verbal messages from the other person
- Encourage and wait for questions, and answer them clearly and honestly
- Ask appropriate questions and actively listen to the response
- Be sensitive to individual differences in communication behaviour and, as far as possible, adjust the style of communicating to accommodate these differences
- Identify and minimise the barriers to effective communication.

SKILLS TO FACILITATE THERAPEUTIC COMMUNICATION

Therapeutic communication techniques in nursing are those that:

- Convey respect and acceptance of clients, no matter what situation they are in or illness they have
- Encourage the expression of the views, feelings and ideas of others
- Demonstrate a non-judgmental attitude towards the situations, views, feelings and ideas of others.

They include the skills of active listening, asking questions, providing feedback, paraphrasing, clarifying, reflecting, using silence and summarising.

ACTIVE LISTENING

Active listening is not an automatic ability. It is a skill that develops with practice and perseverance. Active attentive listening is as important to the process of therapeutic communication as speaking and it could be said that the art of therapeutic conversation lies in the ability to listen with perception.

Active listening requires attention and concentration, to hear not only the words but the feelings or meanings that are often hidden behind the words. Active listening involves being tuned in and ready to receive messages. Nurses can demonstrate readiness to listen by minimising environmental distractions and adopting a posture of involvement that includes:

- Sitting at a comfortable distance away from the client
- Facing the client
- An open relaxed posture (arms not folded and legs not crossed)
- Leaning slightly forward
- Making eye contact.

Active listening incorporates simultaneously listening for the content, or facts, of the message, and the feelings in or behind the message. Sometimes feelings are expressed openly, for example, 'I'm really fed up and I am scared that this ulcer on my leg will never heal', but often feelings are only hinted at, implied or talked around. Sometimes it is the way something is said that reveals how a client is feeling; for example, 'My doctor was here just now; he said everything is going fine, according to plan', might be said in a way that reveals the client is happy about the news, or in a way that indicates the client doubts the truth of the news. Sometimes feelings are deliberately concealed or expressed only non-verbally.

Active listening requires the nurse to:

- Stay mentally alert
- Focus on the speaker's ideas
- Pay close attention to what is said
- Avoid interrupting the other person's speech or being anxious to butt in
- Avoid thinking about what to say next while listening
- Remain alert for an unexpected remark
- Keep an open mind.

Communication strategies that indicate active listening include eye contact, nodding or smiling to encourage the speaker to continue, prompting the speaker by using expressions such as 'go on' or 'then what?', and asking questions to clarify what has been said.

ASKING QUESTIONS

Nurses ask questions to gain information from clients. The responses provide the data from which care is planned and implemented. The type of questions asked depends on the situation and the type of response required. Some questions call for simple and direct responses, while others are more probing in nature. Types of questions used during nurse–client interactions include those that are closed, open-ended, primary, secondary, summary and reflective.

Closed questions

Closed questions are those designed to elicit a simple 'yes' or 'no' or a very short and factual answer. Closed questions often start with 'who', 'where' or 'when'. For example, 'When did you last see your medical practitioner?' is a closed question, and the expected response to this question would be merely a date. Closed questions limit options. They are not designed to elicit extensive detail or to discover or explore feelings or attitudes.

Open-ended questions

Open-ended questions are designed to evoke a long answer. They enable a person to choose how much or how little information to reveal. Open-ended questions often start with 'why', 'what' or 'how'. Open-ended questions are more effective in encouraging a person to elaborate on a topic, as such questions cannot be answered with a simple 'yes' or 'no'. This style of questioning invites the person to reveal personal perceptions, views, thoughts and feelings. For example, 'What were your reasons for choosing to move from Alice Springs to Melbourne?' is an open-ended question. The nurse should always allow the client to fully answer each question before moving on to a follow-up question or changing the topic.

Primary questions

Primary questions are those that introduce new topics or areas, while secondary questions are used to probe for more information. Secondary questions are sometimes referred to as follow-up or focused questions. They aim to get more complete or accurate data. Both primary and secondary questions may be closed or open-ended.

Summary questions

Summary questions summarise a series of questions and answers to make sure that an accurate understanding has taken place, for example, 'Let me see if I have understood what you have told me. You had a heart attack when you were aged 47, the following year you were diagnosed with diabetes, and now you are having problems keeping your blood sugar levels within the recommended range?'

Reflective questions

Reflective questions are sometimes used to help correct real or suspected inaccuracies, for example, 'Didn't you say that you had your heart attack before you were diagnosed as having diabetes?'

'Why' questions and leading questions

It may hinder the development of a therapeutic relationship to use questions beginning with 'Why?' because they may seem judgmental. For example, 'Why don't you want a shower?' can sound accusatory to a client. It is better to ask, 'I'm concerned that you don't feel up to a shower; how are you feeling?'

It is also recommended that the use of leading questions be avoided. Leading questions are rhetorical because they have an implied answer and are often used to confirm what nurses think they know. For example, clients might find it easier to answer 'Yes' to a leading question such as 'You're all right, aren't you?'; while they might feel obliged to answer 'No' to the question 'You don't need any more pain relief, do you?' Clients might interpret such leading questions as the nurse not caring or not being interested in how they are really feeling, or not having the time to be concerned.

When clients are admitted it is usual for the nurse to ask a range of questions. Most interviews comprise a mixture of closed and open-ended questions, but nurses need to be sensitive to the fact that overuse of closed questions can seem like an interrogation. Being bombarded with multiple closed questions as a nurse completes an admission form can feel dehumanising because it does not provide an opportunity for clients to talk about issues that might be important and of concern to them. It is often a more relaxed and friendly approach to ask questions less directly. A gentle command could be used instead; for example, 'Tell me about your health over the last few years' may elicit most or even all the information needed but gives some control to the client. Skilful questioning, using mostly open techniques, can be a way of beginning a meaningful relationship with a client.

FEEDBACK — PARAPHRASING, CLARIFYING AND REFLECTING

Other techniques that help the communication process are clarifying, paraphrasing and reflecting. All these are methods of providing feedback. Feedback is a very important component of the communication process. If a listener is not providing any feedback, the sender has no way of knowing whether a message has been received or how well it has been understood.

Facial expression and body language can provide some feedback from the listener to the sender, or the person who is sending the message can obtain feedback by asking the listener to verbally express their understanding of what was said, or to demonstrate understanding. For example, after a nurse has taught a client how to use an aerosol inhaler, the client can be asked to demonstrate understanding by showing the nurse that they can use it effectively. Alternatively, the listener can describe their perceptions of a sent message by using the skills of clarifying, paraphrasing and reflecting, all of which give the sender the opportunity to correct any misperceptions.

Paraphrasing

Paraphrasing is a technique whereby the listener reiterates what the sender has said in their own words, more briefly whenever possible. Paraphrasing is a means of sending feedback to the sender of the message that lets the person know whether or not the meaning of the message was received as intended. Paraphrasing can be very effective for checking understanding of the content of a message, whereas reflecting works particularly well to reiterate the client's feelings. It takes practice to paraphrase accurately. Clinical Interest Box 29.4 provides an example of an incorrect and a more accurate paraphrasing of a client statement.

CLINICAL INTEREST BOX 29.4
Paraphrasing

Client statement
'I've smoked 20 cigarettes a day all my life and it's never been an issue before. I don't even have much of a cough, so I don't understand why that anaesthetist has told me to stop.'

Example of incorrect paraphrasing
'You think smoking doesn't harm you and you don't want to stop?'

Example of more accurate paraphrasing
'You're not convinced of the need to stop smoking?'

Clarification

Clarification is used in situations in which there is a lack of sense about what a client means, to the degree that it makes the use of paraphrasing impossible. Clarifying reinforces that the nurse is trying to gain an understanding, and the nurse should not continue until clarification has been managed. The nurse must be careful not to put blame for lack of clarification onto the client; for example, saying, 'You're not being very clear about how this happened' would be unhelpful, might alienate the client and would not facilitate a therapeutic relationship. It would be better for the nurse to take responsibility and say, 'I'm having some trouble following what you mean'. Clinical Interest Box 29.5 provides other statements the nurse can use to aid clarification without blaming the client.

When needing to clarify it is possible to ask a direct question such as 'What do you mean?', but this is best avoided because it may sound critical and accusatory to clients. Whatever way clarification is sought the tone and pitch of voice, facial expression and body language used can make a difference to how the client feels about not being understood (Stein-Parbury 2005).

Reflecting

Reflecting is another skill that can be used to check that a message received has been correctly interpreted. Reflection is the mirroring of feelings the nurse believes have been expressed by clients. The feelings are reflected by the nurse's words as a way to check that perception of a client's feelings is correct. For example, a client may say 'Just look at me, I've lost so much weight since I've been in hospital'. The nurse might reflect back the feelings perceived by using a reflective question, 'You're anxious about how much weight you

CLINICAL INTEREST BOX 29.5
Statements to aid clarification without blaming the client

- I'm having a bit of trouble grasping what you mean
- I'm having a bit of trouble understanding
- I'm a little confused about . . .
- I feel a bit unsure of what you meant
- I'm a bit at sea trying to follow what happened
- Could you run that by me again — I lost the flow a bit

have lost?'. The client may confirm with a 'yes' or correct a misperception by saying, 'Oh no, I feel good — I've been trying to get to this weight for years.'

Reflecting feelings is especially important in nursing because it conveys that the nurse recognises and accepts a client's emotions as a valid part of the illness experience. For example, a client may say, 'This hip of mine doesn't seem any better now than before the operation'. The nurse may reflect, 'You seem pretty frustrated (anxious/worried) about your lack of progress'. This validates the client's feelings and at the same time provides permission for the client to talk more about what is being experienced. Reflected feelings should be stated tentatively, no assumptions should be made about what a client is feeling unless stated directly, and often they are only implied or hinted at. It is quite difficult to select the right words to describe a feeling and the intensity of it. The nurse should not proceed with dialogue about a client's feelings until the client has verified that the nurse's perception of what the client is feeling is correct. Care is also needed not to underestimate or overestimate the intensity of the feelings that a client is experiencing (Stein-Parbury 2005).

It is often helpful and therapeutic for a client to be able to share what they are feeling with the nurse. But not all clients want to talk about what they are feeling. They may prefer to keep those feelings under control or share them with someone else — a partner, close family member, friend or priest, for example. The nurse must respond sensitively to the messages given out by clients when they initiate discussion of feelings, and clients should never feel coerced into talking about feelings they prefer to keep contained.

THE USE OF SILENCE

Silence, used correctly as a communication tool, can be as effective and as supportive as words. There are instances where words seem inadequate when a person wishes to convey thoughts and feelings to another person. In such instances, it may be most helpful simply to sit quietly with the person and share the silence. Just to be with another person at moments of grief, sorrow, conflict or joy may be more helpful than trying to fill the silence with useless words or clichés (Clinical Interest Box 29.6).

In some situations silence is not productive and can cause discomfort. Silence can be used to indicate approval or disapproval of a situation, or it may be used to punish or hurt another person. In such instances silence causes barriers to communication and may cause a person to feel inferior or rejected. There are times in nursing when silence is not therapeutic. During interviews with clients there may be times when the nurse cannot think how to respond to what a client has said. It is understandably difficult to know how to respond when a client says something such as 'I don't want this baby' or 'I know I'm going to die' or 'my life will never be the same now'. If what is called 'a stumped silence' ensues after personal information or strong views or feelings have been revealed, the client may feel awkward and perceive that the nurse is expressing negative judgment or disapproval. Rather than have an uncomfortable stumped silence it is better to use the skill of paraphrasing or reflecting feelings, touching gently or saying something such as 'I wish I knew what to say to help'. Nurses need to develop awareness of stumped silences and practise communication strategies that help avoid them, and ways to use silence therapeutically.

CLINICAL INTEREST BOX 29.6
Case study example of the therapeutic use of silence with a withdrawn client

Mary, a 19-year-old nursing student, was assigned to care for Sue, a 48-year-old woman with a history of recent myocardial infarction and associated stress. Sue refused to have visitors and refused to speak with any of the staff. After discussion with the care team, Mary included in her plan of care that she would 'spend 10 minutes, every shift, simply being with Sue'. The objectives were to develop trust and to promote communication, particularly in relation to Sue's feelings about her condition.

Each day Mary announced to Sue that she was concerned about her and would stay for 10 minutes if that was OK. Sue would shrug, then turn on the radio and turn to face out the window. Mary would say that she would return again the next day for 10 minutes. By the Friday of the first week of placement, Sue smiled when Mary entered the room, Mary commented on the radio program, but Sue failed to respond.

On the Monday of the second week of placement, Mary entered and made her usual announcement of purpose and duration and Sue started to cry. When she offered to go and get her a tissue, Sue said, 'Please don't go'. For the rest of the time Mary sat and held Sue's hand in silence. By the Wednesday, when Mary entered the room Sue greeted her with a slight smile and said, 'Hello'. Communication began and Sue started to talk, just briefly, about some of her fears.

SUMMARISING

Summarising is a way of briefly highlighting the key aspects of a conversation. It is a skill most often used before terminating an interaction or nurse–client interview. In addition to clarifying, paraphrasing and reflecting feelings, it is another method of allowing the nurse to check understanding of what has been shared and discussed, and to have that understanding confirmed or corrected by the client. Summarising is a helpful strategy in that it also informs the client that the interaction is coming to a close and provides the opportunity for the client to raise any issues of concern not yet discussed. For example, the community health nurse might summarise an interaction in a client's home:

> So, to sum up, your mum has now been diagnosed with Alzheimer's dementia. As well as looking after your own home and your two children you are currently doing all the shopping, cooking and cleaning for your mum, and this is without help from anyone. We have agreed that I will

arrange a visit from the Aged Care Assessment Services to see what help is available.

After waiting for points to be clarified and the summary to be confirmed or corrected, the nurse might then ask, 'Is there anything else you would like to ask or tell me before I go?' This is important because it is not uncommon for clients or relatives to present the most significant aspect of what has been happening to them just as the interview is about to end. This is probably because the significant aspects are often those that are embarrassing or that elicit the most intense emotions. These things are not easy to share and, as the nurse summarises, clients realise that the opportunity to do so will soon be gone. The nurse should factor this possibility into the time allocated for interactions. Summarising and permitting the client to raise issues not previously mentioned enables the client and the nurse to feel a sense of satisfactory completion at the end of the interaction.

Summarising can also be useful at the beginning or midway through an interaction. Sometimes it is helpful for the nurse to summarise the content of a previous interaction, for example, 'When we last spoke you told me you were anxious about who was looking after your home and your dog while you were in hospital and that you were going to contact your neighbour about keeping an eye on things. How have things worked out?' This serves to focus the interaction into the area needing further exploration.

Midway through an interaction it may be helpful to summarise before moving on to a new topic; for example:

> Before we talk about what will happen after your surgery, just let me see if I have things clear. You haven't had anything to eat or drink since 6 o'clock this morning. You haven't taken your medication that was due at lunchtime, and you are worried because you were so unwell after your last anaesthetic. The only other thing is that you want me to make sure the anaesthetist is coming so that you can talk to him about that.

In addition to confirming or correcting the content of the interaction as perceived by the nurse, this can help clients recall what has been said so far and prompt questions they might wish to ask while the issues are fresh in their mind. Whether the summary is at the beginning, midway or at the termination of an interaction, sufficient time should be allowed for the client to expand on a point, clarify misperceptions or add something new.

The skills of listening, understanding, exploring, intervening and summarising and the effective use of verbal and non-verbal techniques combined are the basic building blocks on which all successful relationships are based. Nurses adapt these basic skills according to the context in which interactions take place and according to the individual needs of each client. As the ability to adapt communication skills grows with increasing experience, nurses tend to function more strongly from a position of 'being with' rather than 'doing to' the client.

CONVEYING EMPATHY

Empathy refers to the ability to recognise and understand the essence or reality of a client's experience and to relay that understanding to the client. Empathy is considered to be different from sympathy. Sympathy is seen by some as subjectively sharing the feelings of the other person whereas empathy is seen as 'feeling with' and knowing the other person's experience without equating the intense feelings with past personal experience. In nursing, empathy is often viewed as a more desirable response than sympathy, but more research is needed to determine what type of responses are of most comfort to clients (Stein-Parbury 2005).

Empathy can be communicated by touch, by direct, clear and accurate statements that reflect understanding of the core of a client's experience, and by skills such as reflecting feelings. These are the communication aspects of empathy, but how to feel it cannot be learned from textbooks, as it is an intrinsic characteristic. Nurses need self-awareness of their inherent capacity for empathy so that they can strengthen it through practice and learn how to communicate it using a unique personal style rather than a textbook formula (Stein-Parbury 2005).

Expressions of empathy foster feelings of trust. If a person is able to demonstrate an understanding of how another person is feeling, rapport is established between them, and this promotes mutual trust. Trust is a belief that a person will respect another's needs and will behave towards them in a responsible and predictable manner. When people trust each other they feel more comfortable in their relationship, and communication is more effective.

FOSTERING HOPE

Fostering hope is an essential component of a therapeutic relationship. Hope is vital to a client's sense of psychological wellbeing. It creates positive feelings that can strengthen the endeavour to get well and provide a sense of purpose in even the most difficult circumstances, including sudden or chronic illness, serious impairment or even impending death (McIntyre & Chaplin 2002). The nurse can nurture hope by commenting on the positive aspects of what a client has achieved or by helping the client to focus on remaining abilities rather than on those that are lost. (See Chapter 43 for further information about nurturing hope.)

SELF-DISCLOSURE

Self-disclosure refers to the skill of sharing personal experiences, feelings, thoughts, ideas and views with clients in a way that is comforting. It can be comforting because it communicates understanding of the client's situation and feelings and reinforces that the experience is not unique (Crisp & Taylor 2005). Self-disclosure should only be used when it is helpful to the client, the purpose is to benefit the client, and the focus will not remain on the nurse after self-disclosure has occurred. For example, the nurse might say, 'I had a premature baby 2 years ago and was overwhelmed with the constant demands. I was lucky I had a lot of support. What sort of support will you have with your baby?' Self-disclosure can be used as a means of prompting and encouraging clients to express their own fears, feelings and experiences. It also sends a message that the nurse trusts the client with personal information, which may help the client to feel comfortable enough to reciprocate that trust (Stein-Parbury 2005).

THE USE OF HUMOUR

Fun and laughter can be very therapeutic, but humour needs to be used with caution and, initially, tentatively when people are ill or upset and vulnerable, because not all people share or appreciate the same sort of humour. Humour has the potential to:

- Release tension and reduce anxiety
- Reduce embarrassment
- Reduce depression by stimulating the release of endorphins from the hypothalamus
- Stimulate immune system functioning
- Reduce pain by decreasing serum cortisol levels (Crisp & Taylor 2005).

The use of humour can promote rapport between nurse and client and facilitate communication that is relaxed and comfortable. However, it should be used to benefit the client and never as a mechanism to hide behind when nurses are ill at ease in particular situations. (See Chapter 13 for further information concerning the therapeutic use of humour.)

COMMUNICATING WITH CHILDREN, ADOLESCENTS AND OLDER ADULTS

In addition to the skills previously explained, there are some additional aspects to consider when communicating with children, older adults and clients' relatives and friends.

OLDER ADULTS

Older adults may need more time to respond during conversation or to answer questions because they have a large repertoire of experiences to draw on and sorting through them requires time. The process of retrieving a memory of an event and the words needed to express themselves may be slower than in previous years. This may be due to memory impairment associated with normal ageing. It may be mild, and many older people adapt to this change, but at times of stress, tiredness or when situations are demanding, the slowed ability to recall events and words may be much more noticeable. The nurse needs to be patient and allow older clients adequate time to respond. If sure of a word the client is searching to remember, it may help, after waiting a few moments, to provide it.

Older adults sometimes find it takes longer to absorb new knowledge, especially if the information does not connect to familiar concepts. Older and younger clients alike find it more difficult to absorb information while anxiety levels are high. Giving new information to older clients while they are ill, upset or anxious is likely to mean that they will be unable to recall it (Ebersole et al 2008). Nurses also need to consider that many older clients will have age-related changes to hearing and vision that also impact on communication.

CHILDREN

Ability with language and the processing of concepts and thoughts differs according to a child's age and developmental level. The nurse needs to adapt the style of communication according to these differences. Table 29.1 presents some basic guidelines for communicating effectively with children.

ADOLESCENTS

As when communicating with anyone, all the skills that enhance effective communication are employed when talking with adolescents. Adolescents may be very sensitive to feelings of being judged or criticised, so it is important to be open minded when listening attentively to their feelings, ideas and opinions. It is helpful for adolescents to have expectations clearly explained and it enhances self-esteem when praise is given appropriately. (Chapter 12 provides further information to assist the nurse when interacting with adolescents.)

COMMUNICATING WITH CLIENTS' RELATIVES, FRIENDS AND SIGNIFICANT OTHERS

The loved ones and friends of a sick person will often need support to help them cope with that person's illness. A person's illness can be a very disruptive episode in the lives of their significant others. They may need to discuss their concerns and share the frustrations of the illness. Table 29.2 provides some general guidelines for communicating effectively with relatives, friends or others who are emotionally close to a sick client.

BARRIERS THAT INTERFERE WITH THERAPEUTIC COMMUNICATION

Several aspects of communication can impair effective communication, hinder the development of trust in a therapeutic relationship and damage an existing one. In addition to the inappropriate use of humour mentioned earlier, some other communication pitfalls act as barriers to therapeutic relationships that nurses need to be aware of and avoid. They are not hard to fall into inadvertently, but also they are not hard to avoid once aware of them. Using the basic communication skills previously outlined, together with avoiding the pitfalls, will enhance every relationship and facilitate therapeutic relationships between nurses and clients. Because of the emotional content of many nurse–client interactions, the potential for nurses to inadvertently put up barriers if they are not aware

TABLE 29.1 | GUIDELINES FOR COMMUNICATING EFFECTIVELY WITH CHILDREN

Action	Rationale
Address parents first at the initial meeting, then the child	It is courteous to address the parents and the child at the start of the interview, but the focus should then move to communicating directly with the child
Put children at ease; for example, by asking their name, stating yours and talking about their friends/toys/pets/school	A child who is relaxed generally communicates quite freely
Talk directly to children (do not continually direct remarks or questions to the parents)	Demonstrates respect for the child. Sometimes in their anxiety parents tend to answer for their child; talking directly to the child helps to avoid this and demonstrates respect for the child and the child's feelings and opinions
Talk at eye level	Standing above a child is intimidating
Ask children questions that they can answer on their own. If parents are present, the nurse should look to them for confirmation or reply only when necessary	Establishes a relationship with the child and begins to develop trust
Explain any procedures or activity to be performed in terms the child can understand. Include the child in the discussion when a plan of care is being explained to the parents	Children are more likely to accept interventions if they know what to expect
Talk with a child as you would an adult; for example, be honest, do not disregard any information the child offers. Provide older children with the chance to speak without the parents present	Demonstrates respect for the child
Answer a child's questions honestly whenever possible. For example, if a child asks if a procedure is going to hurt, it is much better to be honest	If a child has been told that a procedure will not hurt, and it does, trust in the nurse will be reduced
Respect a child's confidences. If a child reveals information necessary for a parent to know, explain why this is so and suggest the child tells the parent. Otherwise seek the child's permission to talk to the parent about the matter	Failing to respect a confidence destroys trust

TABLE 29.2 | GENERAL GUIDELINES FOR COMMUNICATING EFFECTIVELY WITH RELATIVES AND FRIENDS

Action	Rationale
Introduce yourself to the relatives and inform them that you are helping to look after their loved one	It is a common courtesy to greet all visitors regardless of whether or not they need support or information
Provide them with opportunities to express any concerns and anxieties	Simply having concerns heard can reduce stress
Include them in discussions about the individual's care when appropriate; for example, only when certain that the client approves	Relatives have often been providing care at home for clients before their admission to hospital and will often continue care after the client is discharged from hospital. It is rude and dismissive of their care work to exclude them from care planning decisions
Offer opportunities to assist with care activities as appropriate	Often relatives like to feel useful, needed and involved
Answer their questions as appropriate (be aware of confidentiality issues) or refer questions to the nurse in charge	The unknown is often very stressful. Information is important in planning for what is still to come
Demonstrate warmth; for example, by touch, close proximity, body posture and facial expressions. This is of particular relevance when relatives are confronted with a loved one who is seriously ill or dying	When a loved one is sick or dying it helps to know others empathise

CLINICAL INTEREST BOX 29.7
Barriers to effective communication

- Stereotyping, labelling or pre-judging the speaker
- Talking, not listening
- Becoming distracted or daydreaming
- Asking leading questions
- Asking 'Why?' questions
- Asking too many probing (perceived as prying) questions
- Listening only to content; not hearing feelings
- Not attending to non-verbal cues
- Overuse of closed questions
- Finishing the other person's sentences
- Offering false reassurance or using clichés
- Criticising and judging
- Preaching or moralising
- Interrupting
- Advice giving
- Jumping to conclusions
- Incongruent body language
- Being defensive
- Changing the subject inappropriately

of them is high. Sometimes nurses unknowingly use communication barriers as a way of protecting themselves from uncomfortable feelings. Examples of these include changing the subject inappropriately and offering false reassurances and using clichés. A list of barriers that block effective communication is provided in Clinical Interest Box 29.7.

CHANGING THE SUBJECT INAPPROPRIATELY

People sometimes change the subject when they are uncomfortable with, or unwilling to discuss, a specific topic. For example, a client may say to a nurse, 'I feel so weak, I don't think I am going to be around for much longer'. If the nurse feels unable to deal with the feelings the client has raised, they may abruptly switch the conversation to a more comfortable area by saying, 'You shouldn't dwell on that. Let's get you washed — where are your things for the shower?' The client gets the message, accurate or not, that the nurse is not sensitive to their concerns. The nurse misses the opportunity to be helpful because the client is denied the opportunity to discuss their feelings, and therapeutic communication between the two is blocked.

FALSE REASSURANCE

A nurse may try to alleviate emotional discomfort with a client's concerns, or an inability to cope with what a client is expressing, by giving false reassurance. Such responses are often automatic, trite, and in the form of clichés or platitudes, such as, 'You'll be right' or 'Don't worry, it'll work out'. These do nothing to allay anxiety. In fact, the client may become more anxious, wondering if the nurse is trying to hide something about their condition. As with inappropriate changes of topic, responses that offer false reassurance can make clients feel that their anxieties are being dismissed and do not matter, and that as a person they are of no importance to the nurse. Because platitudes and clichés are often automatic, the nurse may need to rescue the situation if one has been uttered without thinking. For example after saying, 'Don't worry, you'll be right' the nurse might rescue the situation by saying, 'Still that's easy for me to say, isn't it? You sound as though you are really worried that things are not going well.'

It is, of course, appropriate to provide comforting reassurance when it is needed, but reassurance should always be based on honesty, and the client's feelings should be explored and clarified. It would, for example, be appropriately reassuring to say, 'Don't worry, it is usual to be weak after the operation you have had, and it is usual to get stronger within a few days'. Nurses need to listen for the feelings being expressed by clients, and respond appropriately to those feelings and anxieties, no matter how disturbing they may be. It is only by doing so that nurses can communicate caring and offer the comfort that clients need. It is one of the challenges of nursing to develop a range of skills to respond therapeutically to the many intimate and intense emotions expressed by clients. Many nurses choose to undertake courses specifically designed to develop self-awareness and extend basic counselling skills.

Examples of other pitfalls that are communication blockers and not uncommon in nurse–client interactions are being defensive and offering advice or a personal opinion.

BEING DEFENSIVE

A defensive response is most often the result of a nurse feeling judged negatively or unfairly when a client complains, or feeling the need to defend other members of the health care team who are being criticised. For example, when a client says something of this nature: 'I've been waiting ages for someone to redress this leg ulcer, this is the third time I've asked for it to be done.' It might be tempting to retaliate and say, 'Well, it's not my fault, we're short-staffed and we've been run off our feet today'. Retaliation such as this is a defensive and antagonistic response and likely to annoy the client further. It brings the focus on to the feelings of the nurse rather than those of the client. By being defensive rather than demonstrating an understanding of the client's point of view, the nurse becomes an adversary rather than a therapeutic helper. It is more helpful to reflect the client's feelings with a reply such as, 'Yes, I'm sorry, it's upsetting to have been waiting so long'.

Being defensive when criticised implies that the client does not have the right to show feelings or state an opinion. When clients complain, the nurse can defuse negativity and anger by listening uncritically to what the client has to say. It is often appropriate for the nurse to explore whether or not there are deeper concerns underlying the cause of a client's complaint. In a therapeutic relationship the nurse might choose to facilitate the client expressing deeper feelings or concerns by tentatively saying something such as, 'You sound as if you feel you are not getting the care you need'.

In certain situations clients may not be in control of their angry feelings. (Chapter 45 focuses on mental health and incorporates strategies that can help the nurse to cope with and help clients who are aggressive or demonstrate other unacceptable ways of communicating.)

OFFERING ADVICE OR GIVING AN OPINION

When a client asks a nurse for advice such as, 'What would you do?' it is appropriate and therapeutic to share information about available options and provide an opportunity to discuss them. When advice or a personal opinion is offered, the focus moves onto the nurse. This may mean that the client is swayed to do what the nurse considers best and may not consider all the options effectively in relation to themselves and their own life situation. What may be the right decision for one person may not be the right or best decision for another. It is empowering and therefore therapeutic for clients to have control of decisions and make their own informed choices. Providing information about alternatives and educating clients are important components of a nurse's role, but providing advice is different and can cause problems. For example, giving advice or a personal view about treatment options may lead to a client accepting that advice as expert advice and later blaming the nurse for a real or perceived negative outcome.

Using the communication skills of active listening, asking questions, clarifying, paraphrasing and reflecting, and avoiding the communication pitfalls are important in all interactions with clients and others. Clinical Interest Box 29.8 provides analysis of a transcribed nurse–client interaction that identifies the use of some therapeutic communication skills and some non-therapeutic communication blockers.

STRATEGIES THAT ENHANCE INTERACTIONS WHEN CLIENTS HAVE SPECIAL REQUIREMENTS

A variety of conditions can impede the ability to communicate effectively. Clients with these conditions have special requirements. Some of the more common of these conditions include alterations in vision, hearing and speech ability, cognitive impairment or a total inability to communicate, generally associated with unconscious or dying clients. Clients who do not speak the same language as the nurse also have special requirements, and it may be necessary to communicate through an interpreter. Working with an interpreter and other cross-cultural communication issues are discussed in Chapter 9. A useful resource for nurses in relation to a range of cross-cultural issues is D'Avanzo's (2008) text on cultural health assessment.

ALTERATIONS TO VISION

Some clients will have partial or total inability to see what is in the environment. When clients have reduced vision it can interfere with the ability to see another person's body language, so verbal communication must be particularly clear, and touch used as effectively as possible. Each visually-impaired person experiences vision loss differently, so careful individual assessment is necessary to determine needs. The aims of care for every client with reduced vision includes promoting a sense of security, ensuring safety and comfort and facilitating effective therapeutic communication. Table 29.3 provides some general guidelines for facilitating effective communication with clients who have reduced vision. Entering a new environment for the first time can be a frightening experience, and even more so when vision is reduced, so effective and clear communication explaining who and what is in the environment, especially potential dangers, is vital.

ALTERATIONS TO HEARING

The client who is experiencing hearing loss, either temporary or permanent, needs assistance to adjust to the physical and psychosocial implications. The main way to assist the client with impaired hearing is to maintain and improve the ability to communicate. General guidelines to facilitate effective communication with hearing-impaired clients are outlined in Table 29.4. If a client has a hearing aid it must be maintained in good working condition and used correctly (see Chapter 42).

ALTERATIONS TO SPEECH

Imperfect articulation of speech (dysarthria) is related to neurological damage that causes alterations to the muscles (primarily of the mouth and tongue) involved in the act of forming words. People with a condition called receptive aphasia (often resulting from damage to the temporal lobe of the brain or a central lesion) are unable to understand what someone else is saying. For example, the person may hear the word fork and recognise it as a familiar word but be unable to attach the word to the object it represents. If clients have expressive aphasia (often caused by damage to the frontal lobe of the brain) it means they are unable to clearly express what they want to say or what they are feeling. For example the client may say the word 'yes' when meaning 'no' or may cry instead of laugh. Often clients have receptive and expressive aphasia together. This is very frustrating for them and the nurse has an important role in communicating in a way that promotes rehabilitation. When caring for clients experiencing speech difficulties, the nurse usually collaborates closely with a speech therapist. Table 29.5 provides guidelines for communicating therapeutically with clients experiencing speech difficulties.

A range of practical communication aids can help clients with speech, hearing or visual impairments. Some examples are provided in Clinical Interest Box 29.9.

CLINICAL INTEREST BOX 29.8
Interview transcript analysis of a nurse–client interaction

Mrs Lee is a widow who lives at home alone. She has arthritis and is recovering from a fractured neck of femur (hip), which was the result of a fall. She uses a walking frame to get around indoors. The community health nurse is with Mrs Lee, visiting on a regular weekly check-up call. She has greeted Mrs Lee with a smile and has chatted briefly about the weather while checking her blood pressure. Now she is sitting near and facing her client so that they can communicate at eye level.

Speaker	Communication	Response type
Nurse	Mrs Lee, how have you been since I was here last?	Open question
Mrs Lee	Fine [big sigh, head lowered, no eye contact]	
Nurse	You say you have been fine, but that was a very big sigh. How are you feeling?	Testing incongruence between body language and verbal communication
Mrs Lee	Oh, OK, I suppose, but I'm just tired	
Nurse	You don't have much energy?	Paraphrasing
Mrs Lee	No	
Nurse	Well, don't worry, it's probably just a reaction to this awful wet weather. Tell me what you have been doing this week	False reassurance and inappropriate change of topic
Mrs Lee	Not much, just watching TV mostly	
Nurse	Um-hmmm [nodding head]	Prompt to continue
Mrs Lee	Oh yes, my daughter came to visit on Thursday. She kept talking about me selling the house and going to live with her and her husband. She's got three children	
Nurse	You sound as though you are not happy about doing that	Reflecting feelings
Mrs Lee	I don't know really. I just hadn't even thought about it	
Nurse	[Nurse waits silently]	Effective use of silence
Mrs Lee	I don't think I could cope with the kids	
Nurse	Why not?	'Why?' question could be interpreted as judgmental. Use of an open question; for example, 'What makes it difficult?' would be a better response
Mrs Lee	It's just that, well, I do love them but they get on my nerves sometimes — too noisy for me	
	[Nurse does not respond, neither of them speak or make eye contact]	Stumped silence Open question
Nurse	Do you think you will stay here then, or go to your other daughter, or have you considered a hostel, a nursing home, a retirement village, or what?	Multiple questions that could confuse. Use of an open question; for example, 'What are you thinking you would like to do?' might be a better response
Mrs Lee	What would you do if you were me?	
Nurse	Well, if it was me I would look closely at all the options before making a decision. What are you thinking you might do?	Sensibly avoided giving advice
Mrs Lee	Well, I'd rather stay here but I'm fed up because I'm struggling to keep the place clean and I get bored by myself all the time	
Nurse	Let me get this right: you've thought about going to live somewhere else but you would rather stay here. You get a bit miserable by yourself and you're worried about not being able to look after the house like you used to	Seeking clarification and confirmation by summarising
Mrs Lee	Yes, that about sums things up	
Nurse	How would you feel about having someone come and help with the cleaning?	Open question
Mrs Lee	That would be good, yes, but I can't have someone come too early in the day. It takes me a long time to get dressed and ready in the mornings	
Nurse	After what time would it be OK?	Closed question
Mrs Lee	After 10 o'clock	

(Continued)

CLINICAL INTEREST BOX 29.8 — cont'd
Interview transcript analysis of a nurse–client interaction

Speaker	Communication	Response type
Nurse	All right, how about I organise someone from the Home and Community Care Service to come and talk to you about it?	Open question
Mrs Lee	Yes, please do	
Nurse	I wonder too, how you would feel about starting going to the Day Centre again, perhaps once or twice a week?	Probing question
Mrs Lee	No thanks, why would I want to go back there? No one cares about you there	
Nurse	Well, I only asked	Defensive — provoking increased annoyance: a non-therapeutic response
Mrs Lee	Then don't!	
Nurse	I'm sorry. I am concerned that you said you were fed up and bored. I thought it might help.	Defusing angry feelings
	Did something happen there that you didn't like?	Promoting exploration
Mrs Lee	I had a good friend there, we played cards together. Then one time she didn't come and it wasn't until I asked about her that anyone bothered to tell me she had been taken into hospital. When she didn't come back after a few weeks, I stopped going and I've never been back	
Nurse	You were really upset that no one told you what had happened to her?	Reflecting feelings and acknowledging client's right to feel disgruntled and upset
Mrs Lee	Yes [with tears in her eyes]	
Nurse	You really miss your friend	Reflecting feelings
Mrs Lee	Yes	
Nurse	Is there anything I can do to help?	Focused question
Mrs Lee	Well, I would like to know what happened to her and if she is all right. Could you call the Day Centre and see if by any chance she ever returned there?	
Nurse	Yes, in fact I am due to visit a client there later today. I will see what I can find out. I will let you know when I visit next week.	Clearly stating information
Mrs Lee	I'd appreciate that	
Nurse	You know, that was pretty stupid not continuing to go to the Day Centre — your friend might have got better and gone back there	Judging and moralising: non-therapeutic communication
Mrs Lee	I doubt it, but that would make me feel very silly. Don't you want to ask me something else?	
Nurse	No, I don't think so	
Mrs Lee	Well, you can't find out much without knowing her name, can you?	
Nurse	[Laughing] Now that makes me feel pretty silly	Therapeutic use of humour
Mrs Lee	Her name is Julie Wilcox	
Nurse	Mrs Lee, I've checked your blood pressure and that was fine. We've talked about getting you some help with the housework and I will get someone from Home and Community Care Service to ring and make an appointment to come and talk to you about that. I am also going to see if I can find out what happened to your friend Julie Wilcox. I will try and have some news for you when I come again next week, but I can't promise anything. Is there anything else you want to talk about today?	Summarising Appropriately not making promises she cannot be certain of keeping Providing Mrs Lee with opportunity to raise other issues
Mrs Lee	Well, I do get lonely and I think I do need to do something about going back to the Day Centre even if Julie isn't there. If I don't start getting out soon I will end up a really miserable cranky old crone. Will you ask if there is a place for me there?	
Nurse	Yes, of course I will, happily, because I really couldn't cope with a cranky old crone! Would you like me to get you some information about other clubs and activities in this area too? You might have some choices about what you would like to do	Therapeutic use of humour, positive reinforcement for client's decision to begin socialising again
Mrs Lee	Thank you, yes, I really think I would like that	

TABLE 29.3 | GUIDELINES FOR FACILITATING EFFECTIVE COMMUNICATION WITH VISUALLY-IMPAIRED CLIENTS

Action	Rationale
Address the client by name as you approach	Alerts the client to your presence
Introduce yourself each time you enter the client's room or area	Reduces stress when client knows who is there
Tell the client when you are leaving the room or area. If the client enters an area where you are, alert them to your presence	Courteous to let the client know when you are leaving the room or when they have entered the presence of someone unseen
Orientate the client to others who are in the area	Facilitates communication with others, reduces sense of isolation
Orientate client to what items and sounds are in the area	Reduces stress from the unknown
Leave things where they are	Reduces risk of injury from trips or spills, increases client's sense of security
Use a normal tone of voice	There is sometimes a tendency to speak loudly to visually-impaired people, but it is of no help and can be irritating
Address the client by name when addressing questions or remarks towards them. In a group situation, each person should address each other by name as they speak to one another	Alerts the client to who is being spoken to
Give step-by-step explanations of procedures as they are performed	Reduces fear of what is happening and prepares client for the physical feelings associated with the procedure
Ensure the call bell is always within reach	Increases safety and sense of security
Do not assume a visually-impaired person needs assistance — ask before initiating help	Many visually-impaired people have adapted to their condition and function independently. They may resent an assumption that help is needed when it is not
If the client needs assistance moving around an area: • Stand just in front of the client with your elbow bent at a 90° angle • Have the client grasp your elbow and follow	This method of assisting visually-impaired clients is safe because the nurse is looking towards the front. It is respectful because the client actively follows rather than being pulled by the arm or hand, which might feel degrading
• Alert client to potential dangers such as stairs, changes in levels, and other barriers	Maintains safety; for example, prevents accidental falls
• Guide the client's hand to handrails or other useful aids that might facilitate them moving around more independently	Independence promotes a sense of wellbeing
To assist the client to sit in a chair, place one of their hands on the back or arm of the chair and give them time to locate the seat area	Assists the client to sit down with minimal assistance. Demonstrating understanding of how to communicate information enhances therapeutic relationship
Explain the location of food and beverages on the table. The clock face technique can help describe food on the plate; for example, the potato is at nine o'clock	Communicating this information clearly aids independence and enhances mealtime pleasure. Communicating the practical information establishes a trusting relationship that prepares the way for communication of other deeper and more personal issues

ALTERATIONS TO COGNITIVE ABILITIES

The first step in communicating with a cognitively impaired client is to assess the level of impairment. This may range from a minor difficulty in remembering the meaning of words or simple phrases to a total inability to comprehend what is being said, or to express thoughts and ideas. The nurse adjusts communication techniques according to the needs of individual clients. Depending on the level of impairment it may or may not be necessary to:

- Speak more slowly
- Make gestures more pronounced
- Remind clients who you are each time you address them
- Use very simple one-step-at-a-time instructions; for example, when assisting clients to get dressed or clean their teeth
- Ask only very simple closed questions
- Give very clear and basic explanations.

When people cannot comprehend what is being said or cannot find the words to express their own thoughts, it can be very frustrating and embarrassing for them and also challenging for the nurse. It can sometimes take patience and effort to include cognitively impaired clients

TABLE 29.4 | GENERAL GUIDELINES TO FACILITATE EFFECTIVE COMMUNICATION WITH HEARING-IMPAIRED CLIENTS

Action	Rationale
Reduce or eliminate background noises	Minimises competing sounds
Ensure adequate lighting	The client can see facial expressions and body language clearly to receive non-verbal messages
Approach from the front or the side, not from behind	Approaching from behind can startle the client
If necessary gain the client's attention by gently waving your hand in their line of vision or lightly tapping their shoulder	Communication is not possible until the client is actively concentrating on the communicator
Face and look directly at the client when speaking. Allow a clear view of your face by placing yourself near a light source	Clear vision is essential to read facial expressions and body language. Shadows and glares affect the client's ability to see your face clearly
Ensure spectacles, if they are worn, are clean	Clients who can lip-read need a clear view of the communicator's lips
Check hearing aids are in place and working effectively	Clients do not always wear hearing aids all the time
Speak towards the client's ear that has the most hearing capacity	This uses remaining hearing ability to advantage
Speak clearly and at normal or only slightly higher volume than normal. Speak at normal rate unless the client indicates that speaking slowly is a help: do not shout or overexaggerate speech	Louder sounds mean a higher pitch of voice is used. A higher pitch means that vowels are accentuated and consonants become concealed. Therefore a loud voice or shouting does not help. If a louder voice is used, a lower tone and pitch must be used
Rephrase if words are not understood	Rephrasing the statement with different words may make lip-reading easier
Keep your hands away from your mouth and avoid chewing or smoking while speaking	Covering the mouth reduces the ability to lip-read
Clearly state the topic of conversation	Client can focus on the topic — knowing words likely to be included in the conversation may facilitate easier recognition of words associated with the topic
Do not turn or walk away from the client while still talking	Reduces client's ability to decipher messages from facial expressions or to lip-read
Consciously use gestures and body movements to help clarify meanings	A large proportion of communication occurs via facial expressions and body language
If there continues to be difficulty, use written communication or other communication aids	Resorting to other methods of communication is less frustrating for the client than not receiving messages at all or receiving them inaccurately

in conversations, and nurses should be wary of excluding them, for example, by speaking to each other over or across the client. Excluding cognitively impaired clients from conversations reinforces feelings of low self-worth; conversely, including them promotes feelings that they are valued and worthwhile. Disorders that cause dementia, such as Alzheimer's disease, are among the most common causes of cognitive impairment.

Table 29.6 provides general guidelines to facilitate communication with clients who are experiencing some of the more severe symptoms of a dementing illness. These include significant memory loss, decreased sense of personal identity, loss of language and communication skills, disorientation and difficulty with visual perception. Clients with a dementing illness are most commonly in the older age group and so frequently experience the additional difficulties of reduced hearing and vision associated with the normal ageing process. This means that, in addition to using dementia-specific communication skills, the nurse must use the communication skills specifically relevant to vision and hearing impairment. In particular this means that the nurse must be aware of which clients need to wear hearing aids or glasses, as the clients themselves may no longer remember that they need them or how to put them on.

Validation therapy and reminiscence therapy

Validation therapy and reminiscence therapy are two communication tools that are particularly helpful when working with people who have progressive dementia (as opposed to those experiencing symptoms of dementia that can be treated and cured, such as those caused by vitamin deficiency or drug toxicity).

Validation therapy is a process of communicating with seriously disoriented people that supports their feelings in whatever time or location they believe themselves to

TABLE 29.5 | GUIDELINES FOR COMMUNICATING THERAPEUTICALLY WITH CLIENTS EXPERIENCING SPEECH DIFFICULTIES

Action	Rationale
Face directly and make eye contact. Listen attentively, allow time for responses. Do not take over and complete sentences for the client	The aim is to help clients relearn how to speak — they need to work hard at this and they need the practice. They may give up if nurses deter efforts by pre-empting what they are about to say
Use short phrases and simple, closed questions	This encourages progress
Let the client know that you do not understand: never pretend that you do	Honesty demonstrates respect for the client. The client can sense when not understood and feels patronised and upset if the nurse is not honest about it
Be consistent, use the same words and gestures each time you give an instruction or ask a question	Consistency promotes success in communicating effectively and this encourages further practice
Clearly match up items with words	Aids rehabilitation
Use a communication picture board only as a back-up resource	The aim is to encourage the client to practise verbal expression
Take care not to exclude clients from conversations	It takes patience to communicate with and encourage speech-impaired clients, it may be easier to exclude them but it is not therapeutic and it does not promote rehabilitation
Ensure only one person is speaking at a time	The client will have difficulty focusing on more than one speaker and may become dejected when unable to follow and join in conversation
Do not shout or speak loudly	A raised voice does not help and can cause distress

CLINICAL INTEREST BOX 29.9

Communication aids for clients with speech, hearing or visual impairments

Communication aids to help visually-impaired people

- Magnifiers
- Talking books (audio-taped novels, etc)
- Braille books and documents
- Guide dogs
- Enlarged-print books
- Modified telephones
- Canes

Communication aids to help hearing-impaired people

- Hearing aids
- Telephone, radio and television amplifying devices
- Telephone typewriter devices
- Picture boards
- Television caption devices
- Shake awake clocks

Communication aids to help people with impaired speech

- Call bells and alarms
- Sign language
- Pen and paper or magic slate
- Electronic voice devices
- Communication board with commonly used words, letters or pictures that indicate needs (e.g. a drink, toilet)
- Use of eye blinks for simple responses (e.g. one blink indicating yes, two blinks indicating no)
- Artificial voice box (vibrating device helpful for clients who have had a laryngectomy)

be in. It is a therapy founded by Naomi Feil in 1963 and currently used extensively in dementia care. Used to full effect, it helps people with progressive dementia, such as the Alzheimer's type, to retain their dignity, self-worth and sense of identity, justify their life and resolve life's unfinished business, thus reducing their stress (Feil 2002).

As dementia worsens, the person's grasp on the real world slips further and further away. The person lives in a world that exists only in their own mind, a mind stripped of recent memories. The world that is the person's reality may be one much further back in their life, where they are much younger and loved ones that have died still live. Or it may be a very strange, confusing and distorted world of some other description. Attempting to orient the person to the reality of the real world generally increases confusion and frequently causes distress. Instead nurses need to develop the skill of being able to step into the personal world of the client with dementia and validate the reality

TABLE 29.6 | GENERAL GUIDELINES TO FACILITATE COMMUNICATION WITH CLIENTS WITH DEMENTIA

Action	Rationale
Ensure that you can be seen and heard before addressing the client by name. Sit, stand or kneel so you gain eye contact. Touch the client gently to attract attention if necessary	Client may not respond if simply called by name without the other cues
Minimise distractions	Damage to the brain leaves little ability to screen out extraneous noise
Introduce yourself each time you communicate with the client, if necessary	The client may not remember who you are from one encounter to the next
Be aware of how you present yourself	When words are not understood, facial expression, body language and appearance are what the client responds to most. A smile rather than a frown is appealing
Be aware of the feelings you transmit and the atmosphere you create; for example, keep tone of voice warm and low, move about calmly	Feelings of tension, irritability or a sense of being rushed will upset and may frighten a disoriented and confused client. A calm relaxed approach helps the client remain relaxed. Relaxed clients are more likely to agree to what the nurse is asking of them. A nurse who is rushed or agitated will create the opposite effect
Begin your conversation socially; for example, talk about a reassuring topic such as the weather — don't rush into asking the client to do things, and always ask, do not order	Helps to gain the client's trust. Gaining trust before asking the client to agree to tasks, such as having a shower, facilitates co-operation. The client is more likely to agree when asked rather than directed to do something
Keep messages short, simple and specific. Give one message at a time	The client may have only minimal understanding of words
Use questions that require a yes/no answer, rather than open-ended questions	A question such as, 'Is this the dress you would like to wear today?', is less complicated to understand and answer than, 'What would you like to wear today?'
Use statements more than questions	Asking questions that a client cannot remember how to answer may trigger a negative response, and the client might interpret questions as 'prying' and feel resentful. Statements may be more acceptable and they tend to elicit interest; for example, 'That cat looks hungry.'
Back up words with gestures. Show as well as tell; for example, point to clothes that are placed ready to put on	Aids understanding
Pause between sentences and allow plenty of time for the information to be understood. Wait for a response	Allows time for a damaged brain to process messages
Repeat or rephrase the message if there is no response — several times if necessary	Some words may be recognised when others are not
Look and listen for other cues when speech doesn't make sense; for example, facial expressions and gestures can reveal emotions	Detecting the client's underlying feelings provides clues as to an appropriate response
Respond by reflecting feelings	Reflecting feelings; for example, 'That makes you feel angry, doesn't it?' shows understanding even if you are not sure of what caused the emotion. Being understood has a positive effect on self-esteem
Break tasks down into small steps	Everyday tasks are made up of a series of complicated actions stored in the memory. The client may feel overwhelmed at not being able to remember how to manage a complete task; for example, to get undressed. But may manage independently if prompted what to do at every step; for example, undo buttons, take this arm out of the sleeve, etc. This approach enables tasks to be completed successfully and can be satisfying and pleasurable for nurse and client
Use touch therapeutically, provided that the client does not indicate a dislike of being touched	Touch is a powerful medium to impart caring and can be reassuring when words are not understood. An arm around the shoulder or a squeeze of the hand can convey more than words. A hand or foot massage can have a calming effect

of that world (Sherman 1999). Stepping into the client's personal world is one aspect of validation therapy that can easily be implemented with only a little practice. Clinical Interest Box 29.10 provides an example of validation as therapy.

Reality orientation is a form of rehabilitation, used to orientate a confused person. It has limited use in dementia care and is most effective when used to repeatedly name people, objects and places. Reality orientation may be helpful when clients who have early-stage Alzheimer's dementia are struggling to remain oriented to time, person and place. However, to try to use reality orientation when clients are far removed from real time and place can cause serious distress. It means arguing with the client's reality, which can lead to agitation, aggressive outbursts and distress (Sherman 1999).

Reminiscence therapy is a way of stimulating memories of pleasurable events that may be recent or from long ago. When stimulated, such memories can help reinforce a person's sense of self. Some people with dementia will be able to recollect an outing from the day before; others may not, but many will be able to remember events or people from much earlier times. Photographs of holidays, family members or pets, music, objects associated with past hobbies or jobs, or particular smells, are some of the things that can be used to stimulate memories that can then become a focus for conversation. The smell of eucalyptus, lavender or mint, for example, can stimulate memories of the bush, a garden or cooking. The look, smell and feel of a horse's saddle can kindle memories for someone who was once a jockey. Sometimes reminiscing can cause feelings of loss and sadness, and the nurse needs to be sensitive to this. Reflecting the client's feelings, and comforting, are appropriate, for example, 'You miss your garden', said with a gentle touch or a hug if accepted. After doing this it may be best to distract the client away from what triggered the sadness.

Working with people who have dementia or other types of cognitive impairment requires special knowledge and skill. While there are courses for nurses that focus on these specialty areas, some simple strategies are easily implemented and can be therapeutic and soothing for people with cognitive impairment. These include listening to familiar songs or music, enjoying favourite foods or an aromatherapy bath. Even simply walking with a client with dementia can be very beneficial because it can distract a client who is anxious and can often demonstrate concern and affection more effectively than words.

CLINICAL INTEREST BOX 29.10
Validation as therapy

Anne's husband, Bob, has Alzheimer's-type dementia. The community nurse was visiting their home when Anne told her how Bob had been up all night three nights in a row, how he had just kept on and on saying that the army was coming. He kept getting out of bed, going to the window and shouting out for the army to turn back. Anne explained how she repeatedly tried to calm him, telling him the war had ended long ago, that the army had disbanded and there were no soldiers coming. But no sooner had she got him back to bed he was up again, even more agitated than before.

On the third night, feeling exhausted, Anne told how she tried something different. She explained how she had picked up the phone and asked to speak to the General. She and 'the General' had a conversation about his new orders to turn the troops back and to hide up in the hills until notified it was safe to return. With the news that the General and the army had turned back and were retreating to the hills, Bob enjoyed a glass of milk, closed the curtains got into bed and slept peacefully for the rest of the night.

Anne had worked out for herself that, while reality orientation did not help Bob, stepping into his world and validating what was happening there eased his mind and solved a problem.

CLIENTS WHO ARE UNABLE TO RESPOND

Some clients are unable to communicate at all, for example, those who are not conscious. It may be difficult at first to speak to a person who does not respond and with whom you have no eye contact and from whom you receive no feedback of any sort; however, it becomes easier with only a little practice. Even when clients are unable to respond it should be assumed that they can hear when spoken to and feel when touched. Table 29.7 provides guidelines for communicating with unresponsive clients.

Effective communication with clients who have special needs involves assessing and responding to the individual needs of each client. Planning effective measures includes adapting basic therapeutic communication techniques and adding extra communication strategies relevant to the client's particular impairment. These strategies need to be implemented and other appropriate communication aids accessed, including other health professionals, such as speech therapists. The success of care is evaluated by how well the client feels able to communicate needs, feelings and thoughts. Signs that the client is withdrawn, anxious, aggressive or frustrated indicate that therapeutic communication may not be at a high level. When a nurse feels frustrated or irritable with a client it may indicate the same thing, and that means communication techniques need to be reviewed and improved.

Communication is an important issue for all clients with sensory, speech or cognitive impairments because of the effect it can have on socialisation and psychological wellbeing. Being inhibited in the ability to communicate can have a negative impact on a person's sense of identity and self-image. Nurses play a vital role in ensuring that clients with such impairments are rehabilitated to the maximum possible level of functioning, educated about the communication aids available, and cared for in a way that reinforces their value and worth as individuals.

TABLE 29.7 | GUIDELINES FOR COMMUNICATING WITH UNRESPONSIVE CLIENTS

Action	Rationale
Say who you are and why you are in the room and call the client by name during all procedures and care activities	The client may have awareness of a presence in the room. It is a way of demonstrating respect for the client
Orientate the client to date, time and place	It may be that the message is received even though the client does not respond
Explain what you are going to do and why	It may be that the client is aware of things happening but is not able to work out what they are
Explain the cause of sensations; for example, 'There is a fan blowing cool air towards your body' or 'I'm putting your foot into a bowl of warm water'	Not understanding the cause of bodily sensations and being unable to ask could provoke the client's anxiety
Avoid talking about the client to others while in the client's room, especially if saying something that the client would not want to hear	Unresponsive clients may be able to hear and if they recover they may remember what was said
Consider the use of other channels of communication; for example, aromatherapy uses the olfactory channel	Stimulating the senses of an unresponsive client may promote recovery and might be a means of providing pleasurable feelings

COMPLICATIONS IN NURSE–CLIENT RELATIONSHIPS

Complications can occur in any relationship, and decisions have to be made about how to respond to them. Complications in nurse–client relationships that require a professional response include physical attraction, offers of gifts, and transference and counter-transference.

PHYSICAL ATTRACTION

Physical attraction can occur between a nurse and a client but nurse–client relationships must be established and maintained as therapeutic only. Entering into social or personal relationships with clients may be seen as an abuse of power and constituting professional misconduct. When the nurse goes beyond the established therapeutic relationship and enters into a social or personal relationship with a client, a professional boundary is violated. Boundary violations occur if the nurse accepts gifts or if self-disclosure or physical contact lacks therapeutic value. Sexual contact of any kind is never therapeutic and never acceptable within the nurse–client relationship (Stuart & Laraia 2001).

OFFERS OF GIFTS

Personal gifts can be a means of showing appreciation or a way to bribe or manipulate the nurse. There are ethical and moral concerns in accepting money or personal gifts from clients or their relatives and it is generally best to diplomatically refuse if they are offered. If a client or relative is persistent it is advisable for the Enrolled Nurse (EN) to refer to the Nurses Board guidelines for the state or territory they practise in and inform, and seek advice from, the nurse in charge. The situation may be resolved by a request for appreciation to be shown by donating money to a related charity of which there are a great many. They include the Alzheimer's Association, Multiple Sclerosis Association, Arthritis and Epilepsy Foundations and the Schizophrenia Fellowship. Alternatively, money may be donated to a hospital via its fundraising committee. It is not unusual for gifts, such as a box of chocolates or flowers, to be accepted when offered as a thank you to the entire care team.

TRANSFERENCE AND COUNTER-TRANSFERENCE

Transference is a subconscious response in which clients associate the nurse with someone significant in their lives. Feelings and attitudes about that person are transferred to the nurse. For example, a male client may relate to a female nurse as if she were his mother, because she has one or more mannerisms the same as the mother. The client may have negative feelings about his mother and become aggressive towards the nurse without provocation. The significant trait that defines transference is the inappropriate intensity of the client's response. The responses and reactions of the client are an attempt to reduce anxiety (Stuart & Laraia 2001).

The nurse deals with transference by being prepared to listen to the client and deal with what may be irrational and highly charged feelings. The nurse uses the therapeutic techniques of exploration, clarifying and reflecting to help the client gain self-awareness and begin problem solving.

Counter-transference is initiated by the nurse's subconscious emotional response to a specific client. The response is irrational, inappropriate, highly charged and is generated by certain qualities of the client. It is simply the nurse's own transference. For example, it may occur when a nurse's feelings of rejection are triggered by a particular client's appearance and/or mannerisms that resemble those of an unfaithful ex-boyfriend. Transference and counter-transference involve intense feelings that may be positive or negative and that are not justified by the real situation. Nurses need to be alert to when powerful feelings towards clients (or received from clients) are unjustified. Failure to recognise that this is happening interferes with the ability to be therapeutic. While the occurrence of transference and counter-transference tend to be identified more frequently and discussed more openly in the area of mental health nursing than in general areas, wherever the nurse is working it is advisable to share what is happening with other health professionals. A team approach to managing the issues promotes protection for the nurse and client.

SUMMARY

Communication is a process of sharing experiences, ideas, attitudes, values and feelings. It occurs at different levels, and communication at the interpersonal level is at the heart of nursing care. Messages between people are communicated via visual, auditory, tactile and olfactory channels. The individual attitudes, values and beliefs, levels of knowledge, past experiences and current physical and emotional status are some of the many variables that influence the effectiveness of communication between people. Interpreting verbal and non-verbal messages, the use of open and closed questions, clarifying, paraphrasing and reflecting feelings are some of the skills nurses need when communicating with clients and others in the workplace. Additional skills are needed to communicate effectively with clients who have special needs, such as those who are experiencing sensory and cognitive impairments. The ability to use the skills of validation therapy and reminiscence therapy are tools that help nurses communicate therapeutically with clients who are seriously disoriented as a result of progressive dementia. The nurse needs to be aware of and respond professionally when complications such as the offer of a personal gift, physical attraction or transference and counter-transference occur within nurse–client interactions. The most important skills of actively listening to clients and exploring what the illness experience really means to each individual facilitate understanding and so foster the development of a helpful and therapeutic relationship.

REVIEW EXERCISES

1. State six ways that you can convey to a client that you are listening attentively to what they are saying.
2. Identify the variables that influence effective communication.
3. State six barriers to effective therapeutic communication between client and nurse.
4. Explain what is meant by a defensive response.
5. Outline four specific measures that can enhance communication with a client who is:
   a) visually impaired
   b) hearing impaired
   c) speech impaired.

CRITICAL THINKING EXERCISES

1. Why is communication an essential determinant in the success or failure of a nurse–client relationship?
2. Describe the differences between verbal and non-verbal communication. Which has the most influence on the quality and effectiveness of communication between a nurse and client, and why?
3. Mrs Jackson, 89, has dementia of the Alzheimer's type. She is a resident in the aged-care facility where you work. How would you, the EN, respond to Mrs Jackson when she starts to cry and pace anxiously about, saying that she has been waiting for the bus to take her to work, it hasn't come and she's going to be late?

REFERENCES AND FURTHER READING

Antai-Otong D (2007) *Nurse-Client Communication: A Life Span Approach*. Jones and Bartlett, Boston

Boyd MA (2007) *Psychiatric Nursing: Contemporary Practice*, 4th edn. Lippincott, Williams and Wilkins, Hagerstown, MD

Crisp J, Taylor C (eds) (2005) *Potter & Perry's Fundamentals of Nursing*, 2nd edn. Elsevier Australia, Sydney

D'Avanzo C (2008) *Mosby's Pocket Guide to Cultural Health Assessment*, 4th edn. Mosby Elsevier, St Louis

Daly C (2007) *Transitions in Nursing: Preparing For Professional Practice*, 2nd edn. Elsevier, Sydney

Ebersole P, Hess P, Touhy TS, Jett K, Luggen A (2008) *Toward Healthy Ageing*, 7th edn. Mosby Elsevier, St Louis

Ekman P (1997) *The Expression of Emotions in Man and Animals*, 3rd edn. Oxford University Press, Oxford

Feil N (2002) *The Validation Breakthrough: Simple Techniques for Communicating with People with Alzheimer's type Dementia*, 2nd edn. MacLennan & Petty, Sydney

Haynes J (2002) *Communicating with Gestures*. Online. Available: www.everythingsl.net/inservices/body_language.php [accessed 10 May 2008]

Kimberley Interpreting Service (2008) How to work with Aboriginal interpreters. Online. Available: www.kimberleyinterpreting.org.au/l_workwith.html [accessed 10 May 2008]

Lewenson SB, Truglio-Londrigan M (2007) *Decision-Making in Nursing: Thoughtful Approaches for Practice*. Jones & Bartlett, Boston

McIntyre R, Chaplin J (2002) Hope: the heart of palliative care. In: Kinghorn S, Gamlin R (eds), *Palliative Nursing: Bringing Comfort and Hope*. Baillière Tindall, Edinburgh

Mehrabian A (1972) *Non-Verbal Communication*. Aldine-Atherton, Chicago

Potter PA, Perry AG (2008) *Fundamentals of Nursing*, 7th edn. Elsevier Mosby, St. Louis

Rankin-Box D (2001) Healing. In: Rankin-Box D (ed.), *The Nurse's Handbook of Complementary Therapies*, 2nd edn. Baillière Tindall, Edinburgh

Rosdahl CB, Kowalski MT (2002) *Textbook of Basic Nursing*, 8th edn. Lippincott, Philadelphia

Sheldon LK (2005) *Communication for Nurses*. Jones & Bartlett, Boston

Sherman B (1999) *Dementia with Dignity: a Handbook for Carers*, 2nd edn. McGraw-Hill, Sydney

Shmerling L (1996) *Communication in the Workplace*. Macmillan, Melbourne

Stein-Parbury J (2005) *Patient and Person: Interpersonal Skills in Nursing*. Elsevier/Churchill Livingstone, Sydney

Stern MA (2004) *Communication Tip: Maintaining Eye Contact*. Online. Available: www.matthewarnoldstern.com/tips/tipps16.html [accessed 10 May 2008]

Stuart G, Laraia M (2001) *Principles and Practices of Psychiatric Nursing*, 7th edn. Mosby, St Louis

Varcarolis E (2006) *Foundations of Psychiatric Mental Health Nursing: A Clinical Approach*. WB Saunders, Philadelphia

Williams C (2007) *Therapeutic Interaction in Nursing*. Jones and Bartlett, Boston

ONLINE RESOURCES

Communicating with gestures: www.everythingsl.net/inservices/body_language.php (can also access via www.everythingESL.net and then searching for Communicating with gestures)

Unit 9

Health promotion and nursing care of the individual

Chapter 30

MEETING FLUID AND ELECTROLYTE NEEDS

OBJECTIVES

- Define the key terms/concepts
- Describe the differences between units of matter, including atoms, molecules and isotopes
- List five common elements or electrolytes in the body
- Explain diffusion, osmosis and active transport mechanisms in the body
- Explain radioactivity in terms of effect and half-life
- Explain the concept of homeostasis
- State the factors affecting fluid and electrolyte balance
- Describe the methods used to assess fluid and electrolyte status
- Describe how the kidneys help to maintain fluid and electrolyte balance
- State the factors affecting acid–base balance
- Describe how the lungs help to maintain the acid–base balance
- Apply appropriate principles in planning and implementing nursing actions to:
  - — maintain fluid and electrolyte balance
  - — monitor fluid input and output
- State the clinical features of over-hydration and under-hydration
- Plan and implement nursing care for a client who is:
  - — experiencing fluid loss (dehydration)
  - — experiencing fluid retention (oedema)
  - — receiving intravenous therapy

KEY TERMS/CONCEPTS

acid
acidosis
aldosterone
alkaline
alkalosis
antidiuretic hormone
base
buffer
dehydration
diffusion
electrolyte
element
extracellular
fluid balance
fluid retention
fluid volume deficit
fluid volume excess
homeostasis
insensible loss
interstitial
intracellular
intravascular
ion
isotonic
isotope
matter
molecule
oedema
osmosis
over-hydration
pH
radiation
sensible loss
under-hydration

CHAPTER FOCUS

This chapter gives a brief overview of the physics and chemistry involved in homeostasis of the body. It also focuses on the fluid and electrolyte needs of clients over the lifespan and how a client's wellbeing can be affected by alteration in fluid input or output. Nurses are required to assess, maintain and educate clients to maintain their fluid and electrolyte balance according to their specific needs. Fluid requirements vary according to age, height, sex, metabolism and the presence of any underlying conditions. Nurses must be able to accommodate for all these different factors when they plan, care and educate clients.

A basic knowledge of two sciences, physics and chemistry, is helpful in many aspects of nursing. This chapter therefore addresses some aspects of physics and chemistry that help to provide a valuable framework in the study of physiology and understanding of the rationale behind many nursing and medical practices. Although the boundary between the two sciences is often indistinct, physics may be defined as the study of the laws and properties of matter relating particularly to motion and force, while chemistry may be defined as the science dealing with the elements, their compounds, and the chemical structure and interactions of matter.

The concepts of atoms, atomic structure and bonding

provide the link between physics and chemistry. Both physics and chemistry are interrelated and interdependent, and one action rarely happens in isolation. Therefore, this chapter outlines some of the physical and chemical principles that are commonly applied in nursing practice. This chapter also discusses the acid–base and the fluid and electrolyte balances that are essential components of the body's homeostatic processes.

LIVED EXPERIENCE

My whole family was so worried when my grandfather was admitted to hospital for a bad case of gastroenteritis. Grandad was only 70 years old and the day that he was admitted to hospital, he became very confused. He didn't know who Grandma was, and she began to cry. He was wandering around, not really recognising anyone. We thought that maybe he had dementia, but we knew it didn't come on that quickly. When we told the nurses that Grandad was not normally confused, they allayed our fears by telling us that because he had lost so much fluid through diarrhoea and vomiting that this had led to an imbalance with all his body fluids, and would soon be corrected after they had put an IV drip in and replaced all his fluids. They were right! Within a couple of days, Grandad was back to his normal self!

D'Arcy, 18-year-old grandson

SCIENCE IN NURSING

In health the body maintains a precise osmolarity and fluid balance within body compartments; the volume and constituents of body fluids varying only slightly in order to maintain a stable internal physical and chemical environment. When there is a disturbance in fluid and electrolyte balance, the body attempts to compensate by various adaptive mechanisms. If the imbalance is too great or prolonged, the body's compensatory mechanisms may deplete the ability to maintain homeostasis and health.

The physiological processes involved in the maintenance of fluid, electrolyte and acid–base balance are:

- Distribution of fluid and electrolytes within the body
- Movement of fluid and electrolytes
- Balancing of fluid input and output
- Mechanisms that regulate fluid and electrolyte balance
- Maintenance of the body's acid–base balance.

WATER

The two largest constituents of the body fluids are water and electrolytes. The four main functions of water in the body are:

1. A vehicle for the transportation of substances to and from the cells
2. To aid heat regulation by providing perspiration for cooling by evaporation
3. To assist maintenance of hydrogen ion (H^+) balance in the body
4. To serve as a medium for the enzymatic action of digestion.

Water is critical to maintaining a state of homeostasis because water is the medium in which most metabolic and chemical reactions in the body take place. Without sufficient water, cells cannot function and death results (deWit 2001).

MATTER

To assist in understanding normal body function and dysfunction, knowledge of certain chemical principles is important. An understanding of chemistry is the basis for the study of homeostasis, which is described later in the chapter.

All living and non-living materials are generally classified as matter. Matter can be defined as a substance that occupies space and has mass, or weight. All matter is composed of either the same or different kinds of atoms. A collection of atoms with the same atomic number represent a pure substance termed an element. Atoms, in turn, are composed of particles termed electrons, protons and neutrons. Protons and neutrons consist of smaller units such as the quark and are held together by electromagnetic forces. The human body, like all other matter, is composed of different elements and atoms. Some atoms form electrolytes or ions, while others combine to form molecules that form structures of the body's cells and tissues.

ATOMS

An atom is composed of a central dense core of positively charged heavy particles termed protons and an equal number of lighter neutrons that bear little charge and are considered neutral. The nucleus is surrounded by a cloud of negatively charged electrons that are held in place by the positive electromagnetic force of the nucleus. The number of positively charged protons in each neutral atom normally equals the number of negatively charged electrons and therefore an atom is neither positive nor negative in its overall electrical charge under normal conditions. The number of neutrons may vary, but they do not affect the charge of the atom.

Atoms differ from each other in the number of particles they contain and, to aid in the identification of atoms, each one is assigned an atomic number. The atomic number of an atom is equal to the number of protons in its nucleus. For example, the hydrogen atom has one proton, so its

TABLE 30.1 | SOME NATURALLY OCCURRING ELEMENTS

Name	Symbol	Atomic number
The first 20 elements, by increasing atomic weight		
Hydrogen	H	1
Helium	He	2
Lithium	Li	3
Beryllium	Be	4
Boron	B	5
Carbon	C	6
Nitrogen	N	7
Oxygen	O	8
Fluorine	F	9
Neon	Ne	10
Sodium	Na (Latin: *natrium*)	11
Magnesium	Mg	12
Aluminium	Al	13
Silicon	Si	14
Phosphorus	P	15
Sulphur	S	16
Chlorine	Cl	17
Argon	Ar	18
Potassium	K (Latin: *kalium*)	19
Calcium	Ca	20
Some other well-known elements		
Iron	Fe (Latin: *ferrum*)	26
Copper	Cu (Latin: *cuprum*)	29
Zinc	Zn	30
Selenium	Se	34
Silver	Ag (Latin: *argentum*)	47
Tin	Sn (Latin: *stannum*)	50
Iodine	I	53
Barium	Ba	56
Gold	Au (Latin: *aureum*)	79
Mercury	Hg (Latin: *hydragyrum*)	80
Lead	Pb (Latin: *plumbum*)	82
Some heavier naturally radioactive elements		
Radium	Ra	88
Uranium	U	92
Plutonium	Pu	94

atomic number is 1, the helium atom has two protons, so its atomic number is 2; thus, the larger the atomic number the larger and the heavier the atom is. Table 30.1 lists some common elements and their atomic numbers.

ISOTOPES

An isotope is an atom that has gained one or more extra neutrons in its nucleus. The atomic weight remains unchanged, as it is the sum of only the protons, but the mass of the atom increases by the mass of the neutron(s) added to the atom. For example, one isotope of carbon has six neutrons in the nucleus, another has seven, and another has eight. All have six protons, so all are carbon atoms. Isotopes are named according to the number of protons and neutrons in the nucleus: thus, the isotopes above are named carbon-12 (^{12}C), carbon-13 (^{13}C) and carbon-14 (^{14}C). Many isotopes are radioactive and are used in medicine for diagnostic and therapeutic procedures, for example iodine-131 (^{131}I).

ELEMENTS

Matter that is composed entirely of the same kind of atoms — that is, each with the same number of protons — is known as an element. There are 112 different elements that are known to exist, some of which do not exist in nature but have only been observed in physics laboratories. Each is classified by its own individual atomic number and particular chemical properties. Every element (and thus each kind of atom) is named and has been given a unique symbol that is used as a 'shorthand' for that element (see Table 30.1). When arranged into a table with a series of rows (or 'periods') based on increasing atomic weights, from lightest to heaviest, elements with similar properties, such as being a metal or an inert gas, become grouped in vertical columns (see the periodic table of the elements in any chemistry textbook). Elements can combine naturally with each other to form new substances; for example, one atom of sodium (Na) combines with one atom of chlorine (Cl) to form a salt, sodium chloride (NaCl); similarly one atom of Carbon (C) combines with two atoms of oxygen (O_2) to form carbon dioxide (CO_2).

Table 30.2 lists the common elements that make up the human body and their relative concentration within it. More than 95% of the body is made up of the elements oxygen, carbon, hydrogen and nitrogen, while the remaining 5% is comprised mainly of calcium and phosphorus with other elements in very small quantities.

MOLECULES

A molecule is the smallest unit of matter that can exist alone and exhibit the characteristic chemical properties of an element or a combination of elements. A molecule is composed of two or more atoms held together by electromagnetic forces (chemical bonds). A molecule can consist of atoms of the same kind (e.g. an oxygen molecule [O_2]) or of different kinds (e.g. water [H_2O]). A molecule can consist of as few as two atoms (e.g. carbon monoxide (CO) or many atoms (e.g. the 63,000,000,000-odd atoms in the molecules that contain our genetic material, deoxyribonucleic acid [DNA]). Adding or removing an atom or changing its location in a molecule alters the molecule and subsequently its chemical and physiological characteristics.

Molecules may be classified into two basic types: organic and inorganic. Organic molecules contain the element

TABLE 30.2 | ELEMENTS IN THE BODY

Element	Atomic symbol	Percentage of body mass (approximate)
Oxygen	O	65
Carbon	C	18
Hydrogen	H	10
Nitrogen	N	3
Calcium	Ca	1.5
Phosphorus	P	1
Potassium	K	0.4
Sulphur	S	0.3
Sodium	Na	0.2
Magnesium	Mg	0.1
Chlorine	Cl	0.2
Iron	Fe	0.1
Iodine	I	0.1
Copper	Cu	Trace
Zinc	Zn	Trace
Cobalt	Co	Trace
Fluorine	F	Trace

Trace = less than 0.01%

carbon. All known living things are carbon-based life forms. Inorganic molecules may or may not contain carbon and are smaller and simpler than organic molecules.

COMPOUNDS

A compound is a substance composed of two or more molecules of the same type, which cannot be separated by physical means. A compound has different properties from those of its individual elements.

MIXTURES

A mixture is made up of two or more different types of elements or compounds that have been mixed without forming a new compound. Therefore, the elements present in the mixture retain their individual properties, and the components of a mixture can be separated by physical means such as settling or filtering.

IONS AND ELECTROLYTES

An ion is an atom or molecule that has lost or gained one or more electrons. Elements or compounds that dissolve in a solvent, such as water, to form separate ions are known as electrolytes. By dissociating, an ion loses or gains an electron or electrons from the electron cloud and becomes electrically charged. If an electron is lost, the previously neutral atom becomes more positive, as the positively charged protons are no longer balanced by the same number of negatively charged electrons. Conversely, if an atom gains an electron, a previously neutral atom becomes more negatively charged. The number of electrons gained or lost is denoted by a number after the chemical symbol of the element or compound; for example, Ca^{++} is a calcium ion that has lost two electrons, while OH^- is a hydroxide ion that has gained one electron. Movement of positively and negatively charged ions across a membrane produces an electric current or potential, for example, the electrical nerve signals in the brain. Positively charged ions are called cations, and negatively charged ions are called anions.

Electrolytes are chemical substances that, when dissolved or melted, dissociate into ions and can conduct an electric current. Electrolytes are a major constituent of all body fluids and affect the functioning of many physiological processes. Electrolytes are essential to the normal function of all cells and are involved in metabolic activities, fluid homeostasis and in creating charge differences on which the functioning of nerves and muscles depend.

The maintenance of electrolyte balance in the body depends on homeostatic mechanisms that regulate the absorption, distribution and excretion of water and the solutes dissolved in it. Many conditions can cause an electrolyte imbalance; for example, prolonged diarrhoea may cause a loss of many electrolytes.

ACIDS AND BASES

An acid is any substance that releases hydrogen ions (H^+) when dissolved in water. Acids have chemical properties essentially opposite to those of bases. Examples of acids found in the body include hydrochloric, lactic, pyruvic, carbonic, citric, folic and fatty acids. A base is any substance that accepts hydrogen ions in chemical reactions. Alkalis are bases that are soluble in water. Examples of bases found in the body include hydrogen bicarbonate and sodium hydroxide.

THE MEANING OF pH

The pH scale is used to express the concentration of hydrogen ions (H^+) in acids or bases. The 'p' stands for potential or power, and the 'H' stands for hydrogen. Therefore, pH represents the potential, or power, of hydrogen ions present. The pH of a solution is determined by measuring the amount of H^+ present. The scale is numbered from 0–14; the lower the number on the scale, the more H^+ is present, therefore the more acidic the solution is. A pH of 7 indicates a neutral solution, while a pH above 7 is termed basic, or alkaline, and a solution below 7 is acidic. Each integral step in the pH scale (i.e. 14, 13, 12 … to zero pH) represents a tenfold increase in H^+ ion concentration; thus, the pH scale is an inverse logarithmic scale of the amount of hydrogen ions present.

ACID–BASE BALANCE

The pH of arterial blood is maintained between 7.35 and 7.45; however, the normal cellular metabolism of nutrients in the human body continuously produces acids, which are released into the capillaries. As acid enters the capillaries the blood becomes more acidic. The blood in venules is approximately 7.36, making venous blood more acidic than arterial blood.

The body's capacity to form, excrete and 'buffer' acids and bases is known as the acid–base balance. The acid–base balance is critical to the survival of the human body. Variations outside the normal arterial range of a pH of 7.35–7.45 indicate serious dysfunction in the body. The normal metabolism of nutrients by cells produces large amounts of hydrogen ions (H^+) that form acids. The concentration of hydrogen ions in the cells and tissues must, however, be kept low to prevent cellular damage. To maintain pH within normal limits, the body excretes acids at the same rate that they are produced and buffers any excess hydrogen ions.

BUFFER SYSTEMS

A buffer is a chemical substance that resists changes in the pH of solutions. Buffers react with a relatively strong acid or base and decrease the acidic or basic strength of the solution. Buffer systems provide the body fluids, especially the blood, with protection against changes in acidity or alkalinity.

For example, CO_2 is an end product of cellular metabolism and when combined with water, forms carbonic acid ($CO_2 + H_2O \rightarrow H_2CO_3$), which drains back into the circulation. Excess carbonic acid in the blood is rapidly decomposed into carbon dioxide and water ($H_2CO_3 \leftrightarrow CO_2 + H_2O$) and the CO_2 is excreted by the lungs to maintain the pH at normal physiological levels. Conversely, if water is being lost from the blood, it is replaced by the ionisation of carbonic acid, and a rise in pH is prevented. Thus, carbonic acid acts as a buffer in the blood. An example of the buffering action of bicarbonate ion is its reaction with lactic acid. Lactic acid is produced from glucose during muscle contraction, and the dissociation of lactic acid tends to lower the pH. As lactic acid is a stronger acid than carbonic acid, its conjugate base (lactic ion) is weaker. The stronger base (bicarbonate ion) combines with the hydrogen from lactic acid forming dissociated carbonic acid.

ACIDOSIS AND ALKALOSIS

Acidosis is a condition in which the blood becomes acidic ($pH < 7.35$) due to an increase in hydrogen ion concentration as a result of an accumulation of an acid, or the loss of a base. Alkalosis is a condition characterised by an increased pH, above 7.45, due to a decrease in hydrogen ion concentration as a result of a loss of acids or the accumulation of a base.

An acid–base imbalance occurs when there is a deficit or excess of carbonic acid or base bicarbonate. In some situations in which a client cannot efficiently excrete enough CO_2, for example, in a client with pneumonia, the buffer system may be unable to keep the pH within the normal range. In this situation the excess CO_2 will make the blood more acidic, reducing the pH. If the pH falls below 7.35 the condition is termed acidosis; if the pH rises above 7.45 the condition is termed alkalosis.

Normally the body can soak up or neutralise acids as they are formed (buffering). This is done by:

- Blood: initial buffering of acids occurs in tissue, blood cells and the plasma
- Lungs: rapidly alter blood pH by increasing or decreasing the respiratory rate, increasing the removal of carbon dioxide
- Kidneys: excrete additional acids that cannot be excreted by any other method; they also reabsorb bicarbonate back into the bloodstream after acids have been excreted.
- A pH above or below the normal pH of arterial blood (7.35–7.45) may result in severe dysfunction and potential death.

CAUSES OF pH DISTURBANCES

Respiratory causes

Respiratory acidosis occurs with hypoventilation, when the body is unable to ventilate enough CO_2 out of the lungs, as may occur in airway obstruction, emphysema, asthma or opiate overdose. (The kidneys compensate, e.g. by retaining bicarbonate.) Respiratory alkalosis occurs with hyperventilation, when rapid respirations blow off too much carbon dioxide, resulting in alkalosis of a respiratory nature, as may occur in panic attacks. (The kidneys compensate, e.g. by excreting more bicarbonate.)

Metabolic causes

Metabolic acidosis occurs when the body is unable to excrete enough acids because of a problem with malabsorption, such as diarrhoea; metabolism, for example, diabetes (ketone acids [see Clinical Interest Box 30.1]); or organ failure, such as kidney failure. (The lungs compensate, e.g. by increasing ventilation and increasing excretion of acidifying CO_2.)

Metabolic alkalosis occurs when too much acid is lost,

> **CLINICAL INTEREST BOX 30.1**
> **Diabetic ketoacidosis**
>
> Clients with diabetes who have not been administered enough insulin or are unwell, or those with undiagnosed diabetes, are at risk of developing diabetic ketoacidosis. Without adequate insulin the body uses its muscle and fat for metabolism, producing ketone acids. To rid the body of acids, emesis and later hyperemesis occurs, resulting in a loss of not only acid but fluid and other electrolytes as well. The ketone acids can severely affect the pH of the blood, causing a metabolic acidosis. The body tries to compensate by excreting acid by the lungs (compensatory respiratory alkalosis), kidneys and skin.
>
> Hyperglycaemia causes an osmotic-induced polyuria and a subsequent fluid and electrolyte imbalance and may result in severe dehydration. If insulin is not administered and the correct rehydration therapy instigated, in severe cases the condition can result in cerebral oedema, coma and death.

for example by vomiting, nasogastric drainage, or use of some diuretics. (The lungs compensate, e.g. by decreasing ventilation and decreasing excretion of acidifying CO_2.)

COMPENSATION

A change in pH by one system of the body will tend to cause an opposite compensatory change in pH, known as respiratory or metabolic compensation. If respiratory acidosis exists, the body will compensate by producing a metabolic alkalosis. If metabolic alkalosis exists, the body will compensate by producing a respiratory acidosis.

CHEMICAL ENERGY

Chemical reactions, whereby one substance is changed into another substance or substances, are accomplished by a transfer of energy. Chemical reactions that take place in the body cells result in the release of energy. The major source of energy for the body is the food that is consumed. The energy that the cell extracts from the metabolic breakdown of food is stored in adenosine triphosphate (ATP) molecules until needed. ATP is an organic compound produced in all cells and which can readily liberate its energy. When energy is required for cellular activity, one of the phosphate bonds of the ATP molecule is broken, releasing energy, and forming adenosine diphosphate, which is then recycled to form ATP for further energy storage. ATP provides the energy necessary for most physiological processes to take place efficiently. Energy is required by all cells to:

- Synthesise large molecules from smaller ones (anabolism)
- Act together to cause muscles to contract
- Support the electrical energy of nerves
- Effect active transport
- Supply heat.

Most of the chemical reactions in the body require the assistance of catalysts to influence the rates at which chemical reactions proceed. The body's catalysts are a group of proteins known as enzymes.

HOMEOSTASIS

Homeostasis is the term that refers to the processes by which the internal environment of the body is maintained within narrow physiological parameters. Homeostasis can also be defined as the tendency of the body to maintain the stability of the internal environment. Homeostasis is dynamic and active, as the body constantly and actively pursues the maintenance of a stable internal environment.

Homeostatic mechanisms are the mechanisms by which the body is able to control the state of the internal environment. They are the processes and means by which the body is able to adapt to stresses (anything that threatens or upsets homeostasis) and yet maintain its inner balance. Any stress situation that arises activates protective homeostatic mechanisms that endeavour to compensate for that stress. Without homeostatic mechanisms to maintain the internal environment, the body cannot survive. When the ability of the body to maintain homeostasis is overwhelmed, illness, and sometimes death, occurs.

Much of nursing practice is aimed at maintaining or restoring the client's homeostasis. Many of the topics discussed in this and other chapters relate to the state of homeostasis; for example, acid–base balance in body fluids, energy production, fluid and electrolyte balance, and body temperature regulation. Homeostatic regulation of the body is achieved by the cooperative action of most organs and tissues, including the lungs, kidneys and cardiovascular system, and the pituitary, suprarenal and parathyroid glands.

For these mechanisms to maintain homeostasis, the body must be able to detect changes and to react appropriately to those changes. The ability of the body to detect changes is through the process of feedback. Two types of feedback exist. Negative feedback brings the body's internal environment back to its optimal state. Negative feedback is a decrease in function in response to a stimulus; for example, if the blood glucose level rises above normal, action is instituted by several control systems (such as the islets of Langerhans in the pancreas) to restore the blood glucose level to normal.

Positive feedback directs the body's internal environment away from its optimal state. Positive feedback is an increase in function in response to a stimulus; for example, during childbirth one uterine contraction induces further contractions, which continue to increase in intensity and frequency until the baby is born. Many positive feedback situations are undesirable and can, for example, result in the over-production of a normal body chemical, thus compounding the problem.

FLUID AND ELECTROLYTES

DISTRIBUTION OF FLUID AND ELECTROLYTES

An average healthy adult body of 70 kg consists of about 40 L of water. Fluid contained in the body is divided into two compartments: the intracellular fluid compartment (ICF) comprises the fluid located inside cells (about 25 L) and makes up about 60% of total body fluid. The extracellular fluid compartment (ECF) comprises the fluid located outside the cells (about 15 L). The ECF is divided up further into sub-compartments:

- The intravascular fluid part of blood (plasma) — about 3 L
- The interstitial fluid — fluid that surrounds the cells — about 12 L
- Transcellular fluid — fluid contained elsewhere in the body, such as in lymphatic vessels and ducts, cerebrospinal fluid in the brain and spinal cord, serous fluid secreted into potential spaces such as the abdominal and pleural cavities, synovial fluid contained in joint cavities, and gastrointestinal secretions such as mucus.

The fluid contained in each of these different compartments varies in composition, but each contains various salt and mineral electrolytes, whose molecules dissociate in water into electrically charged ions capable of conducting a weak electrical charge, and non-electrolyte substances such as glucose and urea, which do not dissociate in water or develop electrical charges. The predominant electrolytes in extracellular fluid are sodium and chloride, while the predominant electrolytes found in intracellular fluid are potassium and phosphate.

MOVEMENT OF BODY FLUIDS AND ELECTROLYTES

Fluid and electrolytes are constantly moving between the cells and the extracellular compartments through the processes of diffusion, osmosis and active transport.

Diffusion

Diffusion (Figure 30.1) is the movement of a substance, or solute, such as sodium (an electrolyte) or oxygen (a molecule) from an area of greater concentration to an area of lower concentration, resulting in an even distribution of the substance in a gas or a fluid, or through a semipermeable membrane such as the cell wall. Many substances in the body move by diffusion, such as electrolytes, amino acids and glucose. Sometimes diffusion of fluids occurs through a membrane, such as the movement of oxygen from alveoli in the lungs through the capillary membrane into the bloodstream. The rate at which diffusion occurs depends on several factors, including:

- Size of the molecules — larger molecules move less rapidly because of impacts from other substances
- Viscosity of the solution — the more viscous a solution is the slower the rate of diffusion
- Concentration — the greater the difference in concentration between the two regions the faster the rate of diffusion
- Temperature — the higher the temperature the more rapid is the rate of diffusion.

Osmosis

Osmosis (Figure 30.2) is the net movement of water through a semipermeable membrane, such as the cell wall, from an area of high water concentration to an area of low water concentration (i.e. from an area of lower solute concentration to an area of higher solute concentration), the movement continuing until the concentrations of both solutions equalise. The rate at which osmosis occurs depends upon several factors, including:

- The concentration of solute
- The temperature of the solution
- The electrical charge of the solute
- The difference between the osmotic pressures exerted by the solutions.

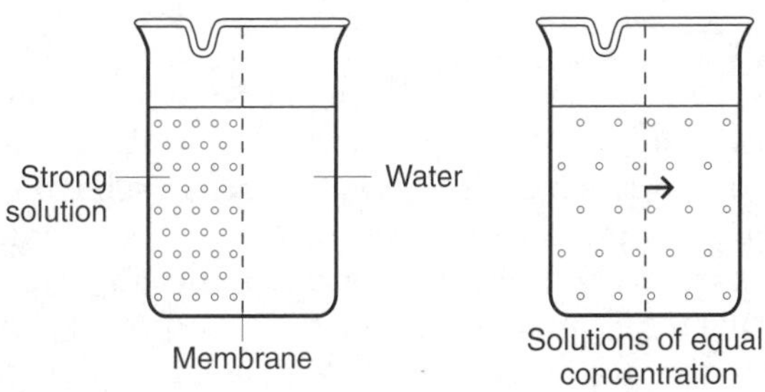

Figure 30.1 | Diffusion

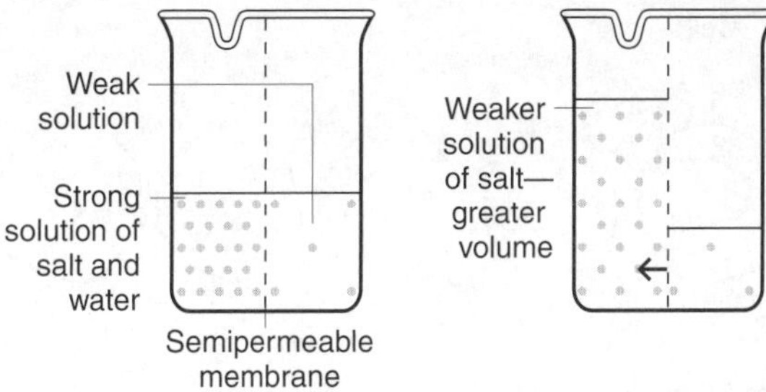

Figure 30.2 | Osmosis

Active transport

Active transport is the movement of substances from an area of lower concentration to an area of higher concentration. An example is the sodium–potassium pump in cell membranes. To maintain normal cell function, the cell has to maintain a highly concentrated intracellular amount of potassium (160 mEq/L) in comparison to the extracellular potassium concentration of 5 mEq/L. Sodium, on the other hand, is maintained at a relatively low intracellular concentration of 15 mEq/L and relatively high extracellular concentration of 143 mEq/L. Energy stored by the cell in the form of ATP is required to power the pump to maintain this difference, or cell death will ensue.

Cellular transport mechanisms

It is important to understand the mechanisms by which substances are actively moved in and out of the body cells. The transport mechanisms that move substances in and out of cells are diffusion, osmosis, active transport, phagocytosis, pinocytosis and filtration.

Phagocytosis

Phagocytosis ('cell eating' [Figure 30.3]) is the process by which certain cells engulf and dispose of microorganisms and cell debris. One example of this is the ingestion of

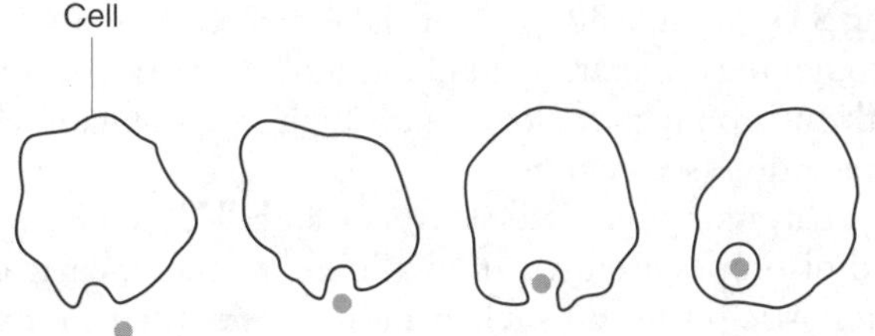

Figure 30.3 | Phagocytosis

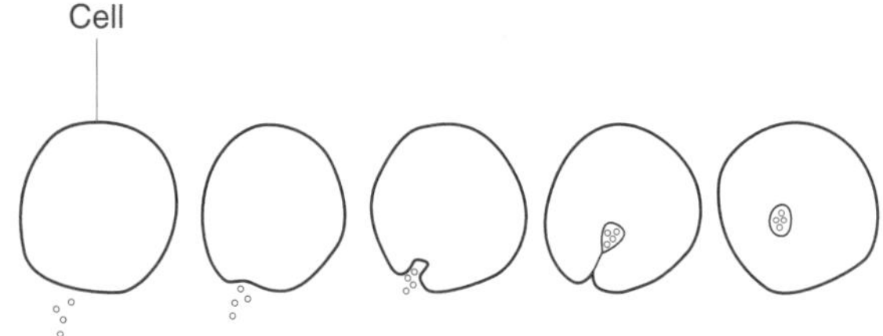

Figure 30.4 | Pinocytosis

bacteria by leukocytes (white blood cells). The leukocytes ingest foreign substances by flowing around them in amoeboid fashion and engulfing them. That part of the cell membrane around the foreign matter is pinched off, forming a vesicle (small sac).

Pinocytosis

Pinocytosis ('cell drinking' [Figure 30.4]) is a similar process to phagocytosis, and is the process by which extracellular fluid is taken into a cell. The cell membrane develops an indentation filled with extracellular fluid, then closes around it, forming a vesicle or vacuole of fluid within the cell. Pinocytosis is the only mechanism by which large molecules such as proteins can be transported into a cell.

Filtration

Filtration involves the removal of particles from a solution by allowing fluid and some substances to pass through a membrane. In the body, filtration involves hydrostatic pressure, which forces liquid with ions and small molecules dissolved in it through a membrane, leaving behind larger molecules. Filtration, like diffusion, is a passive process, with substances moving from a higher-pressure area to a lower-pressure area. Filtration, which occurs in the capillaries and in the glomerulus of the kidneys, is a one-way process, as distinct from diffusion, which occurs in both directions.

RADIATION

Radiation is the emission of energy in the form of rays or waves. Nuclear radiation refers to particles or waves that emanate from the nucleus of an atom. Radioactivity is the result of nuclear instability; if there are too many or too few neutrons in a nucleus, it is unstable (radioactive) and breaks up. Radioactivity therefore refers to giving off radiation as the result of the disintegration of the nucleus of an atom. Natural radioactivity is a property exhibited by all chemical elements with an atomic number greater than 83 (see Table 30.1). Artificial radioactivity is achieved through the bombardment of naturally occurring isotopes with subatomic particles or with high levels of gamma or X-radiation (see below).

Many isotopes are radioactive and are called radioisotopes. Radioisotopes are used in medicine for therapeutic and diagnostic purposes, such as radiotracers, used to locate abnormalities such as tumours within the lungs, brain or bones; therapeutic measures used to destroy tumours; and palliative measures to relieve pain in advanced cancer. Radiation therapy can be administered externally through the use of X-ray machines or radioisotopic sources, or internally through the implantation of radioisotopes into the body. Internal radioisotope therapy can be:

- Intracavity — radioactive isotopes are placed in a body cavity or body organ
- Interstitial — radioactive isotopes are implanted directly into the malignant tumour tissue
- Systemic — radioisotopes are injected intravenously.

HALF-LIFE

All radioactive material decays. The half-life of any radioactive material is the time required for half of the mass of material to decay. Not all the nuclei of a radioactive element break up or decay simultaneously — individual nuclei decay at different times. Half-lives of radioisotopes range from seconds to many years; for example, the half-life of fluorine (^{18}F) is 110 minutes, whereas the half-life of carbon-14 ($^{14}_{6}C$) is 5570 years. In the case of medical radioisotopes, the half-life must be known for accurate dose calculations.

TYPES OF RADIOACTIVITY

Three basic types of radiation are alpha particles, beta particles and gamma rays. Alpha radiation has poor penetration ability and is rarely used in therapeutic radiation therapy. Alpha particles are identical to helium nuclei (two protons and two neutrons held together). Beta radiation is generally emitted from radioactive isotopes and is used for internal source radiation. Beta particles are electrons emitted after the break up of particles in the nucleus of atoms. Gamma radiation consists of waves rather than particles, of very short wavelength and therefore high frequency and high energy, which penetrate deep areas of the body. Therapeutically, gamma sources are used more than any other form of radioactive emission.

X-rays (or Roentgen rays) are produced, for medical applications, by machines. X-rays are produced when electrons travelling at high speed strike certain materials — particularly heavy metals. They can penetrate most substances and are used to investigate the integrity of body structures, to therapeutically destroy diseased tissues and to make photographic images for diagnostic purposes, for example, in fluoroscopy.

LASER

Laser is an acronym for light amplification by stimulated emission of radiation. By exciting a large number of electrons to a high energy level in a gaseous, solid or liquid medium, the electrons emit very narrow beams of light. The beams are all of one wavelength and parallel to each other, allowing the beam to be focused to a microscopic point. It is therefore used for many medical and surgical procedures, such as for skin cancers and eye and brain surgery.

FLUID BALANCE

FLUID INTAKE

Daily recommended intake is considered to be a minimum of 2500 mL of water daily, which is obtained from fluid ingestion (about 1500 mL), food ingestion (about 750 mL is obtained from the fluid content of meat, fruit and vegetables) and from metabolism (about 250 mL is formed by the cellular metabolism of nutrients).

FLUID OUTPUT

Water is continually lost from the body, with the average loss per day being via:

- Sensible loss (loss that can be easily measured) such as:
  - — urine (about 1500 mL/day)
  - — faeces (about 100 mL/day)
- Insensible loss (loss that cannot be easily measured) such as:
  - — skin (in perspiration) (about 400 mL/day)
  - — lungs (in expired air) (about 300 mL/day).

Fluid continuously shifts between the different compartments and sub-compartments of the body to ensure that each compartment is maintained with the exact amount of fluid and electrolytes required. The body regulates its fluid balance and volume by altering input and output to maintain adequate hydration to supply the fluid requirements of the blood, tissues and cells. To accomplish this, the body's numerous homeostatic mechanisms ensure that the fluid input is equal to or greater than output. The balance between fluid input and fluid output is maintained within a narrow range, unless body dysfunction causes an imbalance.

REGULATION OF FLUID INPUT AND OUTPUT

Thirst

The primary regulator of fluid intake is the body thirst mechanism. Thirst results from a decrease in fluid input, excessive fluid loss or excessive sodium intake. The thirst centre, located in the hypothalamus, is highly sensitive to changes in the concentration or osmolarity of the blood. (A fluid that is more concentrated is said to have a higher osmolarity.) A change in the blood osmolarity of 1–2% or a 10% decrease in blood volume stimulates osmoreceptors in the hypothalamus to trigger the sensation of thirst. Actions such as mouth breathing or eating dry or salty foods can be misinterpreted by the body as thirst. Situations such as these can cause additional fluid intake even though the osmolarity of the blood or the blood volume is normal.

Antidiuretic hormone

As the name suggests, antidiuretic hormone (ADH) is a hormone that reduces the production of urine, or diuresis. If blood osmolarity increases or blood volume decreases, osmoreceptors in the hypothalamus relay messages to the neurohypophysis (posterior pituitary gland) causing secretion of ADH. ADH causes sodium and therefore water to be reabsorbed from urine filtrate, and urine output falls. Thus, while the thirst mechanism controls fluid input, ADH controls fluid output.

Aldosterone

If osmolarity or blood volume continue to decrease, specific cells located in the afferent arteriole of the glomerulus in the kidney, known as the juxtaglomerular apparatus, start secreting renin. Renin converts angi-tensinogen (a plasma protein) to angiotensin I, which is in turn converted in the lung to angiotensin II. Angiotensin II stimulates glomerulosa cells in the adrenal cortex to secrete aldosterone. Aldosterone and oestrogen enhance NaCl reabsorption in the renal tubules and increase water reabsorption, thus increasing fluid retention and blood volume.

Progesterone

Progesterone decreases NaCl reabsorption and subsequently reduces water reabsorption by directly inhibiting aldosterone's effect on the renal tubules.

Atrial natriuretic peptide (ANP)

An elevation in blood volume or blood pressure causes atrial natriuretic peptide hormone (ANP) to be released from cells located in the atria of the heart. ANP directly causes excretion of NaCl and consequential diuresis.

Glucocorticoids and mineralocorticoids

Steroid-based hormones secreted from the adrenal cortex in disease or stress increase renal tubular reabsorption of NaCl and cause fluid retention.

SYSTEMS REGULATING FLUID AND ELECTROLYTE BALANCE

At the systemic level the body's fluid volume, electrolyte concentration and composition are regulated by:

- The cardiovascular system, comprised of the heart, blood and blood vessels, which regulate the volume and pressure of blood that the kidneys receive by changing cardiac output. Cardiac output is altered by vasoconstriction, vasodilation, and increasing blood volume or heart rate. Alterations in the blood volume or pressure are monitored by the baroreceptors and chemoreceptors in arteries and arterioles to ensure that sufficient blood reaches the vital organs
- The gastrointestinal tract, which assists in fluid balance by absorbing fluid, electrolytes and nutrients, which assist other systems in regulating electrolytes
- The kidneys, which regulate blood volume and composition by the selective reabsorption of water and electrolytes, and through the removal of waste
- The lungs, which maintain the composition of the blood's oxygen and carbon dioxide levels, therefore playing an important role in regulating the acid–base

balance in extracellular fluid. The lungs are also responsible for a percentage of insensible fluid loss through ventilation
- The endocrine system:
  - — the hypothalamus influences the production of pituitary hormones, and therefore indirectly plays an important role in the fluid balance and electrolyte content of the body
  - — the pituitary gland secretes ADH to increase the active transport of sodium out of the urine filtrate. Water passively diffuses out of the tubules to follow the sodium back into the bloodstream, directly reducing urine output
  - — the parathyroid and thyroid glands, which secrete hormones that maintain the level of calcium in the blood by regulating calcium and phosphorus absorption and storage in bone
  - — the adrenal glands, which secrete hormones (e.g. aldosterone, progesterone and oestrogen) and steroids that alter the reabsorption or excretion of sodium, water and potassium.

FACTORS AFFECTING FLUID AND ELECTROLYTE BALANCE

Several factors may disturb the body's fluid and electrolyte balance, resulting in over-hydration (water excess) or under-hydration (water deficit). Imbalances can be categorised into two types of conditions, according to the cause: a deficit or excess of essential body substances such as water, sodium, potassium or calcium; or an abnormal shift of fluid from one fluid compartment to another.

Water deficit syndromes

Water deficit syndromes result from depletion of water or an excess of solutes outside the cell. Both may result in loss of fluid from the cells themselves, causing cell shrinkage and dehydration. Causes include:
- Decreased fluid intake as a result of unavailability of fluids, or secondary to other conditions; for example, unconsciousness
- Increased fluid output secondary to other conditions; for example, diarrhoea, vomiting, excessive urine output, hyperventilation, excessive perspiration, diabetes insipidus, prolonged fever, burns, haemorrhage or inadequate replacement of aspirated or drained fluids
- Increased solute load secondary to other conditions; for example, hyperglycaemia associated with uncontrolled diabetes mellitus; excessive intravenous infusion of highly osmotic or concentrated solutions of glucose or sodium bicarbonate; or excessive oral intake of solutions with a high osmolarity, causing fluid shifts into the intestine.

Water excess syndromes

Water excess syndromes result from either fluid overload or solute deficit, and both result in cellular oedema. Oedema is the movement of excess amounts of fluid from the vascular compartment into interstitial tissues, as in peripheral oedema, resulting in swelling of the affected tissue and, in severe cases, weeping of water from the skin; into cavities, as in ascites, or into the airways, as in the affected alveoli of pulmonary oedema. Causes include:
- Excessive ingestion of water in a short time
- Excessive administration of intravenous fluids or hypotonic solutions
- Disturbance of homeostatic mechanisms; for example, water retention resulting from kidney, cardiac or liver failure
- Insufficient sodium; for example, from use of diuretic medications
- Inappropriate ADH secretion due to cerebral infections, head injury or increased intracranial pressure.

Clinical Interest Box 30.2 outlines further risk factors that can lead to fluid, electrolyte and acid–base imbalances.

Fluid volume imbalances

Water moves freely between compartments and sub-compartments of the body, depending on the osmolarity of each compartment. A change in osmolarity in one compartment will be compensated for by a change in osmolarity in another compartment. For example, if a client loses fluid through excessive vomiting, fluid is drawn into the cells of the gastric mucosa from the interstitial spaces, and this interstitial fluid is replenished from the bloodstream to maintain homeostasis. If the interstitial tissue becomes more concentrated with solutes, fluid from cavities and cells is drawn into the interstitial space to maintain the blood's osmolarity. An imbalance can occur when fluid is not replaced fast enough to prevent cells being damaged by dehydration. Other such situations include depletion of

CLINICAL INTEREST BOX 30.2
Risk factors for fluid, electrolyte and acid–base imbalances

Age Very young; very old
Gender Women
Environment Diet; exercise; hot weather and sweating
Chronic diseases Cancer; cardiovascular disease, such as congestive heart failure; endocrine disease such as Cushing's disease and diabetes mellitus; malnutrition; chronic obstructive pulmonary disease; renal disease
Trauma Crush injuries; head injuries; burns
Therapies Diuretics; steroids; intravenous (IV) therapy; total parenteral nutrition (TPN)
Gastrointestinal losses Gastroenteritis; nasogastric suctioning; fistulas

(Potter & Perry 2008)

extracellular volume from the plasma to interstitial fluid (this condition can result from severe burns, fever, haemorrhage, diarrhoea or vomiting), and excess extracellular volume caused by conditions such as cardiac, renal or hepatic failure, or excessive intravenous administration of normal saline.

When fluids are either lost or retained in excessive amounts there is an accompanying loss or retention of electrolytes, so that both fluid and electrolyte balances are disturbed. When there is a fluid and electrolyte imbalance, cells may not receive adequate nourishment, waste products may accumulate because of inefficient removal and there may be disturbances to physiology that depend on the transmission of electrical energy, with potential impairment to normal physiology such as skeletal and cardiac muscle contraction, consciousness, reflexes or temperature regulation.

NURSING PRACTICE AND MEETING FLUID AND ELECTROLYTE NEEDS

Assessing a client's fluid and electrolyte status is essential to enable appropriate care to be planned and prevent or correct any imbalances. Assessment is made by obtaining information from the client about their usual pattern of fluid input and output. The nurse should ascertain the types of fluid the client prefers and the amount they usually consume. The nurse should also note any recent alterations in the client's intake, or loss of fluids, through vomiting or diarrhoea, for example. The nurse should observe for early signs of fluid retention or dehydration so that appropriate therapy can be implemented. Information on the signs and symptoms of fluid retention and dehydration is provided later in this chapter.

Key aspects related to helping a client meet their fluid and electrolyte needs, and therefore maintain fluid balance, are ensuring adequate intake of fluid and food, measuring and recording fluid input and output and observing for the signs and symptoms of imbalance.

ENSURING AN ADEQUATE INTAKE OF FLUID AND FOOD

To maintain normal fluid and electrolyte balance, adequate nutrition is essential. Information on helping clients meet their nutritional needs is provided in Chapter 31.

Sufficient fluid intake must be maintained throughout all stages of development in the life cycle. Infants and young children have a higher percentage of total body water and a higher metabolic rate than do adults, therefore they require a larger fluid intake than is proportional to their body weight (see Clinical Interest Box 30.3). With increasing age there is a gradual decrease in efficiency of the fluid and electrolyte regulating mechanisms because of conditions such as arteriosclerosis and reduced hormone production. As a result, the older person may become more prone to electrolyte disturbances than a younger adult.

If a client's fluid output exceeds their fluid input, this is termed a negative fluid balance; conversely, if a client's input exceeds their output, this is termed a positive fluid balance. Fluids may need to be increased or decreased in accordance with medical advice.

CLINICAL INTEREST BOX 30.3
Paediatric gastroenteritis

Treatment of gastroenteritis in the young requires special attention to fluid and electrolyte balance. Fluids such as flat lemonade and mineral water are often used by clients' significant others for rehydration. This treatment has potential life-threatening consequences. Lemonade has a high sugar content, and sugar acts as an osmotic agent, drawing water into the gastrointestinal tract from the body's fluid compartments. This fluid loss results in increased diarrhoea and dehydration. Sugar is also utilised by bacteria in the gastrointestinal tract as a form of nutrition, resulting in increased gas production by the bacteria, causing gaseous distension and abdominal pain.

Hydration in the young needs to be assessed by a medical officer. Clients often require rehydration with products such as Gastrolyte, by oral or nasogastric administration, and in more severe cases intravenous therapy may be required.

Fluid requirements increase in response to various factors including a high environmental temperature, strenuous physical activity, fever, and clinical conditions such as hyperthyroidism, diabetes insipidus, hyperglycaemia, burns or gastroenteritis. Fluid input may need to be restricted to below the normal daily requirements as part of the management of specific renal, liver or cardiac diseases. If fluid intake is unrestricted, the nurse should ensure that the client is provided with appropriate amounts according to their age and metabolic needs.

Some clients may need encouragement to consume their normal volume of fluid or an increased volume requirement of fluid above their normal daily fluid requirements. This may be accomplished by:

- Constructing a plan that distributes the fluid throughout a 24-hour period
- Providing assistance to clients who experience difficulty in pouring fluid or holding a cup or glass
- Explaining the importance of consuming the normal or increased fluid volume
- Providing the client's preferred types of fluid if not contraindicated
- Ensuring that all fluids are presented attractively and at the correct temperature
- Encouraging smaller amounts of fluid at more frequent intervals
- Ensuring that about 75% of the total volume of fluid is taken by early evening so that sleep is undisturbed
- Ensuring that toilet facilities are easily accessible
- Documenting input and output to assess and maintain the client's fluid and electrolyte balance.

Clients may need to have their fluid input severely limited to minimise the potential for fluid retention and pulmonary or systemic oedema. Clients with severe liver, renal or cardiac failure may have their daily input restricted to

500–750 mL/day plus their sensible loss from the previous 24 hours. Clients with less severe symptoms may need to restrict their daily intake to 1500 mL. It is essential that clients and all those involved in their care are aware of any specified amount. Clients may be assisted to restrict fluid intake by:

- Explaining to the client and significant others the importance of consuming only the volume ordered
- Planning to distribute fluid evenly throughout the day, including fluid to swallow medications
- Encouraging small amounts at regular intervals to avoid thirst
- Providing thirst-quenching fluids; for example, water, and avoiding sweetened drinks that increase thirst
- Notifying ancillary staff; for example, dieticians and kitchen staff, of changes
- Ensuring that the client's mouth does not become dry, by regular attention to oral hygiene.

If not contraindicated, the client may be permitted sweets or sugar-free gum to stimulate production of saliva to keep the mouth moist.

MONITORING FLUID INPUT AND OUTPUT

It may be necessary to monitor fluid input and output if a client has an existing or potential problem related to fluid or electrolyte balance. Fluid status may be monitored by a variety of methods and investigations.

Weighing

Weighing, together with maintaining a record of fluid input and output, is a commonly used method of assessing fluid status. Weight gain may result from a positive fluid balance, while weight loss may occur with negative fluid balance. One millilitre of water weighs 1 g, therefore if a client's fluid intake exceeds their fluid output by 1000 mL in 24 hours, their body weight will increase by about 1000 g (1 kg).

The client should be weighed daily at the same time, wearing the same type of clothing and using the same set of scales. Weight can be measured with a standing scale or chair or bed scale and the measurement should be recorded on the appropriate form. The measurement can be affected by bowel and urine elimination pattern and this should be taken into account.

Fluid balance charts

The function of a fluid balance chart (Table 30.3) is to show an accurate record of all fluid input and output over a 12- or 24-hour period. The frequency of measuring and documenting fluid input and output depends on the client's condition and the institution's policies. For example, clients with an intravenous line may need fluid documented ½-hourly to 24-hourly. Terms such as strict fluid-balance charting indicate that the nurse is required to maintain extreme diligence in ensuring that all fluid, diet, urine and faeces are measured and recorded. Clients with less acute conditions may only be required to have their urine, faeces and fluid intake recorded. An accurate recording of input and output is essential, as the results are used by medical officers to assess the client's condition and progress and as a guide for prescribing fluid and drug treatment.

Key aspects related to maintaining an accurate record of fluid balance

- Measure and record all intake immediately to avoid omission or errors. Include all fluids taken orally and those administered by an alternative route (intravenously, nasogastric, gastrostomy, etc) in millilitres (mL).
- Measure and record all fluid output immediately in millilitres. It is possible to measure accurately urine, vomitus, gastric aspirate, and wound drainage if the client has a drain tube connected to a bag or bottle. Although significant amounts of fluid may be lost in perspiration, lymph exudation and soiled garments and bed linen during vomiting, sweating and incontinent episodes, it is not possible to measure these losses accurately. Instead, an explanatory note is entered on the chart, or comparative weights of dry and wet or soiled bed linen can be helpful.
- Request an ambulant person to use a bedpan or urinal so that urine output can be measured and tested if required. When a client wishes to pass a bowel action as well as urine, they can be provided with a bedpan for each or a bedpan and a bottle, so that an accurate measurement of their urine may be more easily obtained. An alternative method of measuring faeces is to place a previously weighed washbowl under the toilet seat and compare the weights before and after.
- Empty and measure urine from urinary drainage bags at regular intervals; for example, 1–4 hourly.
- Record each entry in black ballpoint into the appropriate column on the chart.
- Determine the total input and output in a given period by adding up the columns at the end of the specified period; for example, every 1–24 hours, depending on the complexity of the client's condition.
- Document on the chart a continuing negative or positive fluid balance. If the total output exceeds the input there is a negative balance, while a positive fluid balance occurs when the total input exceeds the output.

OBSERVING FOR SIGNS AND SYMPTOMS OF IMBALANCE

The client is observed for signs or symptoms that indicate a fluid and electrolyte imbalance, which can result in either over-hydration or dehydration. Over-hydration is an excess

TABLE 30.3 | SAMPLE FLUID BALANCE CHART

Fluid balance chart										**Client identification label**			
Date	**Input**						**Output**						
										Other			
Time	Oral	Enteral	IV	IV	IV	Total	**Time**	Urine	Faeces	Gas asp	Wound		

of water in the body and may result from increased fluid input or decreased fluid output, due to a specific cardiac, liver or renal condition, for example. Excess fluid in the body may accumulate in certain parts of the body and can be related to the client's body position. For example, in a recumbent position fluid tends to accumulate in the sacral area, which is the lowest point. If the person is ambulant or sitting for prolonged periods, the lower legs and feet may become oedematous. Oedema may occur as a result of an increase in blood hydrostatic pressure, increased blood volume or reduced plasma oncotic pressure.

Typical signs may include the clinical features of peripheral oedema and or pulmonary oedema:

- Rapid weight gain
- Dilute urine with a low specific gravity
- Swollen peripheries, possibly including feet, ankles and legs as well as fingers and hands
- Periorbital and facial swelling
- 'Pitting' oedema (tissue that remains indented when digital pressure is applied and then removed)
- Bounding pulse and distended neck veins
- Reduced gastric motility, constipation and swollen abdominal organs
- Ascites (excess fluid in the peritoneal cavity)
- Headaches, irritability, lethargy and mood changes, due to cerebral oedema
- Irritating cough that is more frequent when supine or at night, dyspnoea, rales, hypoxaemia, orthopnoea or clear frothy or blood-tinged sputum.

Under-hydration (or dehydration) is a deficit of water in the body and may result from a decreased fluid input, an increased fluid output or an inability of the kidneys to adequately concentrate urine. Cellular dehydration results in:

- Thirst
- Weight loss
- Dry skin and mucous membranes
- Increased pulse rate and reduced pulse pressure
- Decreased blood pressure
- Poor tissue turgor; for example, sunken eyes and abdomen
- Oliguria, with concentrated urine of increased specific gravity, or anuria
- Irritability and confusion and increasing lethargy.

NURSING MANAGEMENT OF A CLIENT WITH FLUID AND ELECTROLYTE IMBALANCE

As previously described, the major manifestations of fluid and electrolyte imbalance are over-hydration or under-hydration. When either of these conditions occur, nursing care must be planned and implemented to help restore homeostasis and to promote comfort. Clinical Interest Box 30.4 discusses the consequences of dehydration in the elderly.

CLINICAL INTEREST BOX 30.4
Dehydration and the elderly

The older adult who suffers from nausea, vomiting or diarrhoea is especially prone to dehydration. If the person has a fever, this adds to the fluid loss. The person may also become confused. Offering the client small amounts of liquid or an electrolyte solution frequently, if it can be tolerated, helps prevent additional problems.

(deWit 2005: 424)

CARE OF A CLIENT WITH FLUID RETENTION

Oedema impairs the function of cells and vital organs and increases the possibility of cell death. The accumulation of excess fluid makes oedematous tissue vulnerable to pressure and damage from external sources, and susceptible to infections through the oedematous skin, such as cellulitis and septicaemia from oedematous gastrointestinal-tract mucosa, for example.

Key aspects related to the care of a client with oedema

- Medical treatment is implemented to treat the underlying conditions causing the fluid retention. Medications such as diuretics, which promote the formation and excretion of urine, may be prescribed.
- Restricting fluid input until homeostasis has been achieved.
- Measuring and recording all fluid input and output.
- Daily or twice-daily weighing.
- Assessing for hydrational status by observing for pitting oedema, oliguria, dry mouth, etc.
- Elevating the oedematous area to facilitate lymph drainage.
- Placing the client in a position of comfort when possible.
- Maintaining skin integrity. As oedema can restrict blood circulation and lead to the formation of decubitus ulcers and thrombi, positions should be changed every 2 hours. Pressure-relieving devices, for example, sheepskins or ripple mattresses, may be used to reduce pressure on oedematous areas. Oedematous parts of the body should be handled and moved carefully to avoid skin damage.
- Ensuring that any dietary restrictions prescribed, such as low sodium diets, are adhered to. If sodium intake is reduced, the sodium and water already in the tissues tend to re-enter the blood to be excreted in the urine, thus reducing oedema.
- The nurse should continue to assess the client's fluid status to evaluate the effectiveness of the actions that have been implemented.

CARE OF A CLIENT WITH A FLUID DEFICIT

Excessive loss of any fluid from the body may cause dehydration. It results from a variety of disorders, may be mild and readily corrected by oral fluid replacement, or may be severe, leading to shock, acidosis and death. To prevent serious complications, medical treatment is implemented to treat the underlying conditions causing the fluid loss and dehydration.

Key nursing actions for a client with dehydration

- Administering prescribed medications; for example, antiemetics, to prevent vomiting.
- Initiating oral rehydration as prescribed, or via a nasogastric tube or gastrostomy tube (if this is the client's normal method of fluid intake), to replace lost fluids. If unable to tolerate the fluid via the oral route it may be necessary to administer fluid via nasogastric or intravenous routes. Information on intravenous therapy is provided later in this chapter.
- Monitoring the client's fluid status by measuring, testing and recording all fluid input and output and reporting declining output.
- Maintaining the integrity of skin and mucous membranes, which may become dry and more susceptible to breakdown; thus, careful attention to skin and oral hygiene is essential.

Two of the common causes of dehydration are vomiting and diarrhoea resulting in excess loss of fluid. (Chapter 33 discusses care of the client who is vomiting, while care of the client with diarrhoea is covered in Chapter 33.)

Maintenance of fluid and electrolyte balance is essential for homeostasis, and when an imbalance occurs actions must be taken to restore homeostasis. The major sources of fluid and electrolytes are the foods and fluids a person consumes. If a mild imbalance occurs, adjustment to the diet or fluid intake may be sufficient to rectify the imbalance. If the loss of fluid and electrolytes is too great to be corrected by oral intake or if the ingestion of substances orally is contraindicated, administration by an alternative route is necessary. Intravenous infusion can provide the client with the fluids and electrolytes necessary to maintain normal body function. Intravascular therapy may also be used to administer total parenteral nutrition (TPN), blood or blood products, and drugs. (Information on TPN is provided in Chapter 31, and Chapter 28 discusses drug administration.) This chapter addresses the techniques involved in the intravenous administration of fluids and electrolytes.

INTRAVENOUS THERAPY

Management of a client who is receiving intravenous therapy is to maintain the intravenous equipment and to prevent complications occurring during and after completion of the intravenous (IV) infusion. Insertion of an intravenous infusion is performed by a registered medical officer, or a Registered Nurse (RN) qualified in IV cannulation. It is the nurses' responsibility to be fully aware of the nursing regulations and policies regarding all aspects of IV therapy.

Before insertion of a cannula, the most appropriate site is selected, which depends on several factors, including the condition of the client's veins, avoiding areas that may be oedematous, infected or otherwise impaired; and general comfort considerations (Figure 30.5). Other site determinants include:

- A vein in the non-dominant arm is preferably used
- The initial site should be in the most distal part of the vein, to allow more proximal replacement in the same vein in the event of cannula blockage, infiltration or phlebitis. A commonly selected site is one of the superficial veins on the dorsum of the hand

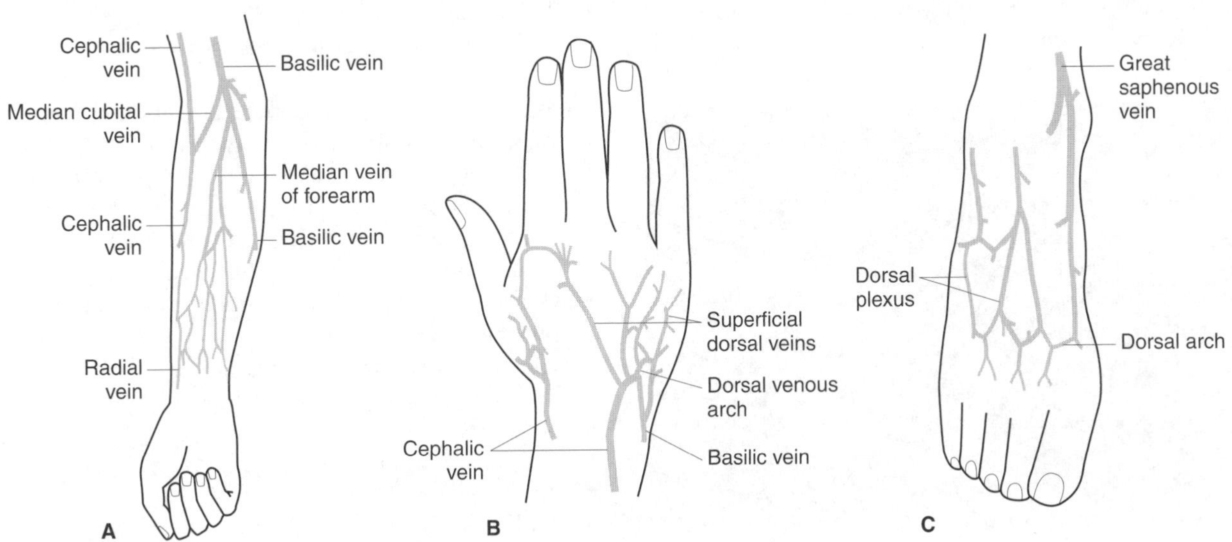

Figure 30.5 | Common IV sites *(redrawn from Potter & Perry 2008)*

- If the site chosen is near a joint, extension and splinting of the limb may be necessary; for example, by back slab (Figure 30.6)
- In some cases local anaesthetic cream may be applied topically or local anaesthetic solution may be administered by a local injection before cannulation.

The medical officer determines the type and amount of fluid to be administered, according to the needs of the client. Intravenous solutions are packaged in plastic containers, which collapse as they empty, or in glass bottles that require an airway to vent the bottle as the fluid runs through the tubing to the client (Figure 30.7). There are numerous types of fluids that can be administered intravenously; most consist of water with added glucose and electrolytes such as sodium chloride, potassium and calcium.

TYPES OF INTRAVENOUS SOLUTIONS

- **Hypotonic** — these solutions promote osmosis of some water from the extracellular fluid into cells. An example of a hypotonic solution is sodium chloride solution of less than 0.9% w/v concentration.
- **Hypertonic** — these solutions promote osmosis of water out of cells into the extracellular fluid. An example of a hypertonic solution is sodium chloride solution of greater than 0.9% w/v concentration.
- **Isotonic** — these solutions do not promote osmosis but increase the extracellular fluid volume. Two examples of isotonic solutions are 0.9% w/v sodium chloride solution, and 5% w/v glucose (dextrose) solution.

INSERTION OF A PERIPHERAL INTRAVENOUS INFUSION

Equipment

As there is a variety of equipment available for the IV administration of fluids and electrolytes, the nurse should refer to the institution's policy manual for information about the type of equipment currently in use. The basic

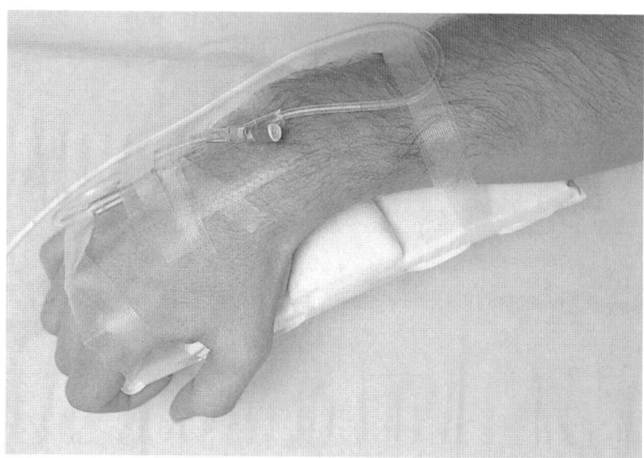

Figure 30.6 | Back slab, or IV arm board *(Potter & Perry 2008)*

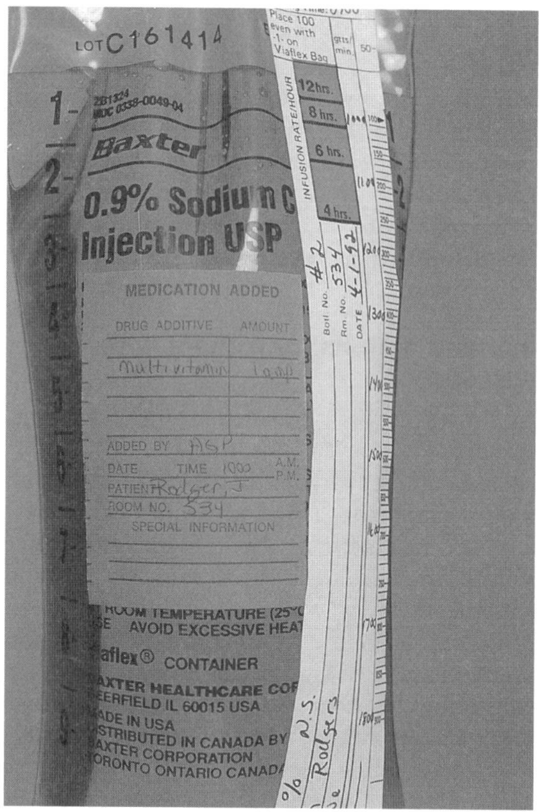

Figure 30.7 | IV infusion bag *(Potter & Perry 2008)*

equipment necessary for the insertion of a peripheral IV infusion may include:

- Sterile dressing pack
- Gloves
- Goggles
- Flask or bottle of IV solution
- Pole or stand to hang the flask
- Intravenous pump
- Intravenous giving set
- Three-way extension set
- Selection of IV cannulas, syringes and saline ampoules
- Skin preparation (antiseptic, e.g. chlorhexidine solutions or swabs, depending on institution's policy)
- Local subcutaneous anaesthetic agents or topical local anaesthetic, 2.5 mL syringe and 25-gauge needle or insulin hypodermic syringe with needle attached, and clear self-occlusive dressing (e.g. Opsite)
- Gauze swabs for placement under cannula hub to prevent ulceration
- Clear occlusive dressing (e.g. Opsite IV 3000 and or hypoallergenic tape [Figure 30.8])
- Scissors
- Arm board and or bandage
- Tourniquet
- Additional lighting.

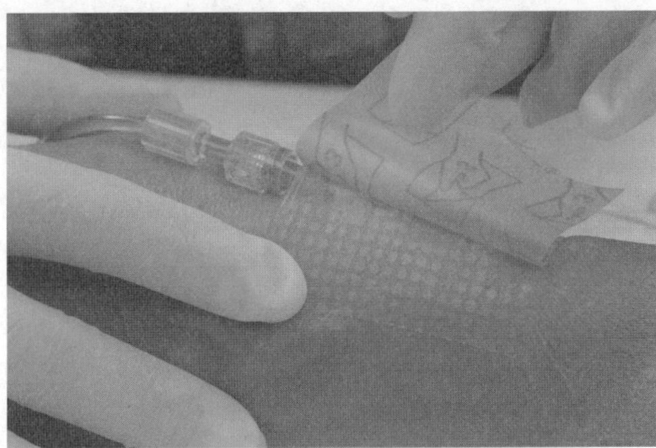
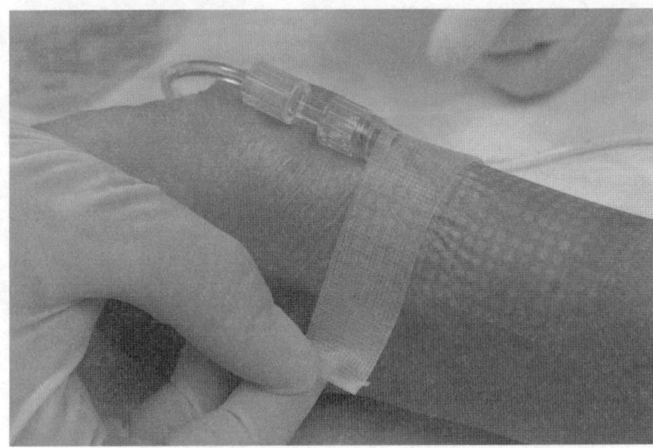

Figure 30.8 | IV cannula held in place with clear adherent dressing *(Potter & Perry 2008)*

Procedure

Before insertion of an IV cannula and the start of the infusion, the nurse should ensure that the client is positioned comfortably with the insertion site exposed. The nurse should ensure that adequate lighting is available and that all the equipment has been assembled in a convenient location. The nurse's hands should be thoroughly washed and dried in preparation for assisting the medical officer with the equipment. (Standard precautions are required if there is potential contact with contaminated body fluids.) The IV solution must be checked against the medical order and signed by two RNs, or a medical officer and a RN, to confirm the correct fluid infusion. Any additives or other information is written onto a self-adhesive label and attached to the IV bag. The nurse must adhere to the nursing regulations and policies relating to the checking and administration of IV solutions. The procedure is performed using aseptic technique and sterile equipment. The IV administration set must initially have the flow regulator turned off before it is attached to the flask and then hung on the pole or stand (Figure 30.9 and 30.10).

The drip chamber is squeezed to allow a small quantity of fluid to partially fill the chamber, after which the fluid is run through the tubing, ensuring that all air bubbles are removed; the tubing is then clamped. The tourniquet is applied 10–20 cm above the intended puncture site to dilate the vein. The site is prepared by cleansing the skin with an antiseptic solution. The IV cannula is inserted into the vein and, after its position has been verified, the tourniquet is released and the cannula is attached to the skin with a clear occlusive dressing or a hypoallergenic tape. The giving set may be attached to an infusion pump connecting the tubing to the client (Figure 30.11); if no pump is used the tubing is connected to the cannula or a three-way tap. The clamp is regulated to administer the fluid at the required infusion rate. If necessary the limb may be supported on a board, which is secured in position with tape and/or a bandage. A board or back slab is commonly used when the puncture site is close to a movable joint, to provide stability and to reduce the risk of phlebitis or dislodgement.

After the infusion has been established the nurse

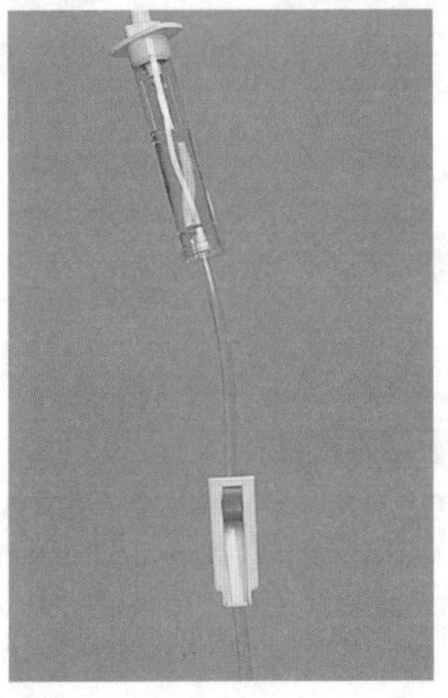
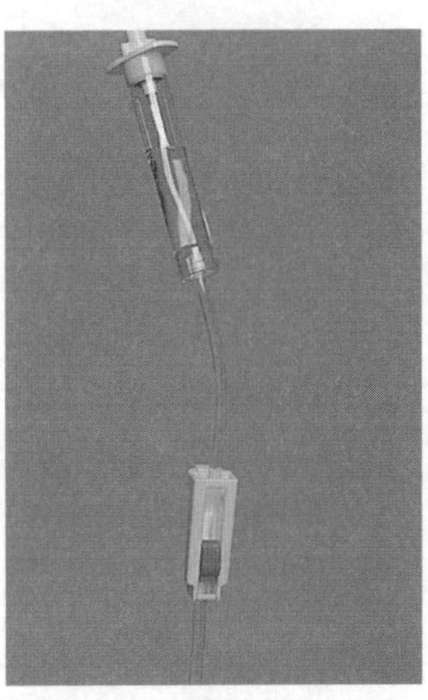
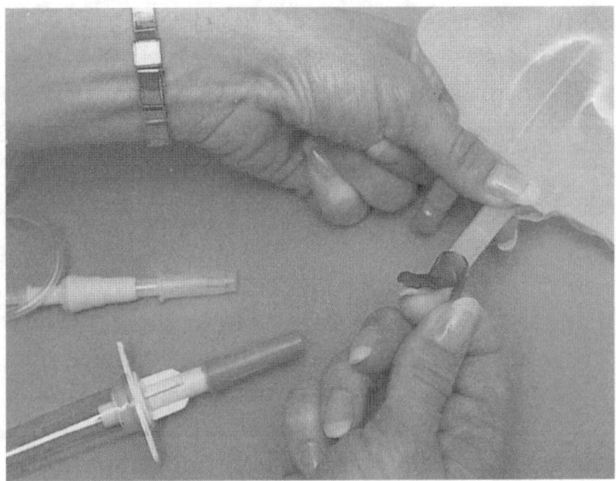

Figure 30.9 | IV administration set with flow regulator turned off (*left*), and on (*centre*) *Right*: removing the protective plastic sheath covering the IV solution bag before attaching the administration set *(Potter & Perry 2001, 2008)*

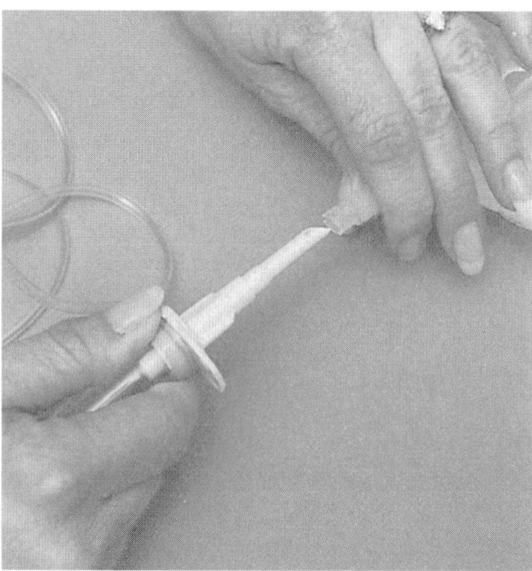

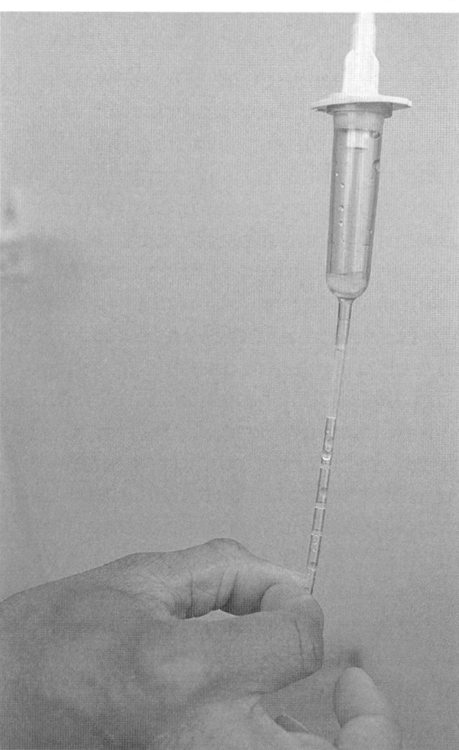

Figure 30.10 | IV administration set. Top: inserting the administration set into the tubing port of the IV bag. Below: removing air bubbles by firmly tapping the IV tubing where the air bubbles are located *(Potter & Perry 2001, 2008)*

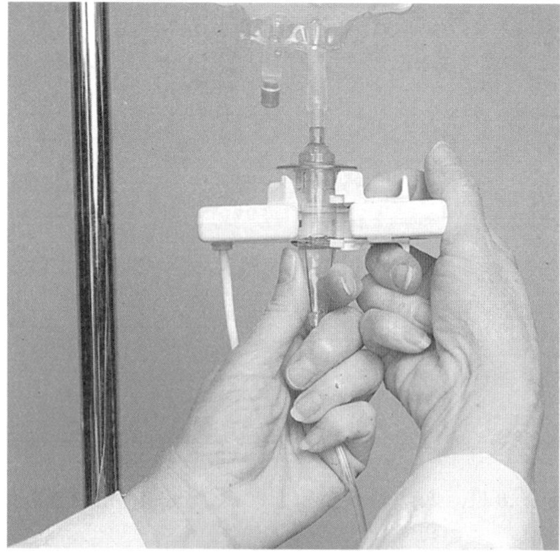

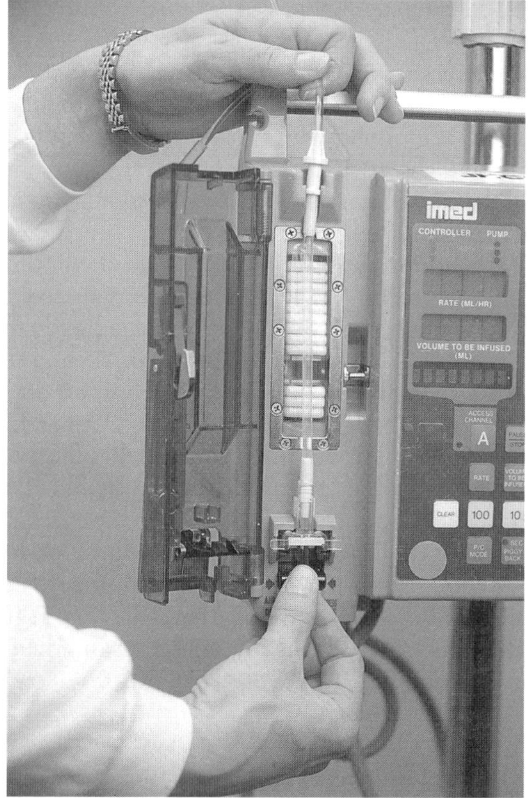

Figure 30.11 | IV infusion pump. Top: fitting the electronic eye to the administration set. Below: placing the IV tubing in the control box *(Potter & Perry 2001, 2008)*

should promote the client's comfort by positioning them comfortably and, if necessary, supporting the limb in which the infusion is inserted on a pillow. A signal device such as a bell or buzzer and any other items required should be easily accessible. All non-essential equipment, sharps and waste are removed or disposed of in the appropriate manner. The procedure is documented, recording details that include the fluid type, flow rate, time initiated and location of the IV cannula.

CARE OF AN INDIVIDUAL WITH AN INTRAVENOUS INFUSION

The nurse has a responsibility to promote the general comfort of the client, to ensure that the infusion is administered as prescribed and to observe for and prevent complications. Key aspects related to the care of a client with an IV infusion are described as follows:

- Ensure that the flow rate is set as prescribed and adjusted when necessary to deliver the correct amount of fluid within the prescribed time. Various methods of determining the number of millilitres per minute are used to distribute the total amount of solution equally over the time period prescribed for the infusion.

- A calibrated burette (e.g. macrodrip or microdrip volume control set) may be incorporated into the infusion system. Such devices enable very small or precise amounts of fluid to be administered and may also be used when medications are to be given IV. A formula is used to determine the number of drops per minute at which the solution should flow. To calculate the flow rate, the following formula is used:

$$\frac{\text{Volume (mL)}}{\text{Time (hours)}} \times \frac{\text{Drop factor (drops/mL)}}{\text{60 min}} = \text{Drops per minute (dpm)}$$

- When calculating the rate it is essential to know the calibration of the drip rate for each manufacturer's product, as these vary from 10 drops/mL to 60 drops/mL
- The flow rate should be checked every 15 minutes to ensure that the drip rate is stable, then every hour or at the time intervals specified in the institution's policy on IV infusions
- Check the level of solution to determine the volume of fluid remaining in the flask. It is important to ensure that a flask does not empty completely, as this can interfere with the flow rate and permit air to enter the tubing, which could lead to an air embolism. Air emboli may result in sudden decrease in blood pressure, rapid weak pulse, cyanosis and loss of consciousness
- Check the insertion site every 24 hours for signs of infection, inflammation or infiltration (see Clinical Interest Box 30.5). Infection at the insertion site is indicated by redness, warmth, swelling and tenderness. The vein may become injured or irritated and phlebitis may occur. Signs and symptoms that indicate phlebitis are pain, swelling and inflammation along the course of the vein; the vein may also feel hard and warm to touch. Infiltration occurs if the needle becomes displaced, causing IV solution to flow into the surrounding tissues. Signs and symptoms of infiltration are cool skin in the site area, swelling and discomfort at the site, oedema of the limb, sluggish flow rate, and absence of blood in the tubing when it is lowered
- Observe the client for signs of over-hydration or circulatory overload, caused by excessive or too rapid fluid administration. Signs and symptoms of circulatory overload are elevated blood pressure, venous dilation, especially of the neck veins, coughing, tachypnoea and shortness of breath
- Check the information on the label of the flask when each new flask is started and at the start of each shift. It is essential that the client receives the prescribed solution; the nurse should therefore follow the nursing protocol regarding checking of IV solutions
- The type, volume and expiry date of the solution is checked. Glass containers are inspected for chips and cracks and the seal over the opening is observed to ascertain if it is intact. Plastic containers should be squeezed gently to detect leaks. The solution is examined for particles, abnormal discolouration, and cloudiness. The container is not to be used if any doubt exists, and the intact container is retained for further investigation
- Throughout the course of the infusion, document details of the flow rate, the type and amount of fluid and additives being administered, and the client's fluid input from other sources and fluid output. The vital signs (temperature, pulse, ventilations and blood pressure) are also measured regularly and documented.

CLINICAL INTEREST BOX 30.5
Complications of intravenous therapy

Administration of intravenous fluids can commonly result in phlebitis and/or infiltration (caused by the cannula moving against the vein wall), as can administration of hypertonic fluids or fluids with a high or low pH. Infection-control guidelines recommend removal or replacement of the IV cannula after 72 hours to prevent phlebitis, bacterial invasion or infiltration and to prevent scarring to the vein.

Nurses must be aware of the scope of their role in relation to the management of IV infusions. Of prime importance is careful observation of the client and the IV equipment used during the infusion, and accurate reporting of the observations to a medical officer or nurse in charge. Complications that may occur when a client has an IV infusion, and which must be recognised and reported immediately, are:

- A flow rate that is too slow or too fast, or cessation of flow
- Infection, pain or infiltration at the insertion site
- Phlebitis of the vein being used for the infusion
- Circulatory overload
- Air embolism.

Other complications include air emboli, cannula breakage, vegetative growths in the cannula lumen, circulatory overload and electrolyte imbalances.

DISCONTINUATION OF AN INTRAVENOUS INFUSION

An IV infusion is discontinued when ordered by the medical officer on completion of therapy, if infection or infiltration occurs, or if it is necessary to restart the infusion in another site. The flow of solution is stopped and all tape removed from the client's skin. The cannula is gently and smoothly withdrawn from the vein, and a gauze swab placed over the insertion site and digital pressure is

CLINICAL INTEREST BOX 30.6
Nursing diagnoses for clients with fluid, electrolyte and acid–base alterations

- Body temperature, altered, risk for
- Cardiac output, decreased
- Fluid volume deficit, at risk for
- Gas exchange, impaired
- Oral mucous membrane, altered
- Tissue integrity, impaired
- Breathing pattern, ineffective
- Fluid volume deficit
- Fluid volume excess
- Mobility, impaired
- Skin integrity, impaired
- Tissue perfusion, altered, peripheral

applied until the bleeding stops. The site is cleansed with antiseptic, and an adhesive bandage applied. The tip of the cannula is inspected and may be sent to the laboratory in a sterile container for culture and microscopy if septicaemia is suspected or if it forms part of the institution's policy. The appearance of the insertion site, the time the infusion was discontinued and the reasons why it was stopped are documented. Clinical Interest Box 30.6 lists some possible nursing diagnoses for clients with fluid, electrolyte and acid–base imbalances.

SUMMARY

Nursing practice encompasses the use of physical and chemical principles and concepts. This chapter has outlined some of these principles and concepts to provide the nurse with information that will help in the study of physiology and assist in understanding the rationale behind many nursing actions.

Water is distributed throughout the body as either intracellular fluid or extracellular fluid. An essential part of the body's homeostatic processes is the maintenance of both acid–base and fluid and electrolyte balance. Fluids and electrolytes, including acids and bases that are ingested or produced by metabolic activities of cells, are constantly moving between the fluid compartments to maintain a pH and an osmotic equilibrium through the processes of diffusion, osmosis, pinocytosis, phagocytosis and active transport.

Fluid is normally lost from the body, as urine and faeces, termed sensible loss, and perspiration and expired humidity, termed insensible loss. The body's many regulating mechanisms assist it to maintain pH and fluid and electrolyte balance under normal and stressful conditions, and can result in an imbalance if variations are not adequately corrected.

Assessing clients in regard to their acid–base and fluid and electrolyte status is necessary for planning and implementing appropriate corrected nursing care. The nurse assists clients to meet their fluid and electrolyte needs by ensuring an adequate intake of food and fluid and by monitoring their fluid input and output. The nurse should recognise the signs and symptoms of fluid and electrolyte imbalance and of clinical conditions that may predispose a client to a change in acid–base balance, and understand the key aspects of caring for a client with an imbalance.

Certain clients may need either more or less than the normal amounts of fluid, and clients who are unable to have fluids orally may require an IV infusion, nasogastric or gastrostomy tube. The nurse caring for a client with an infusion must be aware of the extent of their role and function, to promote safety and comfort during insertion and while the infusion is in progress. The client's need for fluids and electrolytes is continually assessed so that appropriate nursing actions may be planned, implemented and evaluated.

REVIEW EXERCISES

1. Explain the difference between acidosis and alkalosis.
2. Give one cause of each of the following acid–base disturbances: respiratory acidosis; metabolic acidosis; respiratory alkalosis; and metabolic alkalosis.
3. List three transport mechanisms the cell uses to obtain substances.
4. Describe the two fluid compartments and what each represents.
5. Differentiate between the terms intracellular, interstitial and intravascular.
6. List two hormones and the effects that they have on fluid and electrolytes.
7. Discuss why it is essential to know what type of pH disturbance exists before treatment.
8. A client who is dependent on insulin but fails to take enough insulin will develop what form of pH disturbance?
9. Explain in terms of hydrostatic pressure and oncotic pressure why a client with congestive cardiac failure will develop oedema when administered fluid in excess of their daily requirements.
10. Describe the immediate nursing care of a client with a fluid volume deficit.
11. Explain the potential complications that a client with a fluid volume excess may experience.
12. Describe the appearance of phlebitis due to the presence of an IV cannula.
13. Describe what nursing measures would be taken to minimise harm to a client undergoing IV therapy.
14. An old practice, which is today considered dangerous and therefore not used, was the administration of flat lemonade to infants, children and adults for the treatment of gastroenteritis. Explain the effect, in terms of osmosis, this would have in the digestive tract on the movement of water and electrolytes and the potential effect on a client.

CRITICAL THINKING EXERCISES

1. An 18-month-old infant is admitted for gastroenteritis and is 5% dehydrated. The infant has been refusing all oral rehydration fluids. What could you do to ensure that the infant is rehydrated with the correct fluids? If the infant is not rehydrated adequately, what are they at risk of?
2. Mrs Jones, 74, has severe congestive cardiac failure and the clinical features of peripheral and pulmonary oedema. She claims to have taken her diuretics regularly but she continues to drink 2 L or more of fluid a day. How do you plan, educate and provide care for her to ensure that, when she is discharged home, she will only consume the ordered daily volume?
3. Mr Parkes is admitted in accident and emergency at 2200 hours, for right upper-lobe pneumonia. On reaching the ward at 2300 he is febrile, tachycardic, tachypnoeic and has a hacking cough. He has an IV line in situ with a 1 L bag that appears almost empty. What nursing diagnosis would be appropriate?

REFERENCES AND FURTHER READING

Baumberger-Henry M (2008) *Fluids & Electrolytes Made Incredibly Easy*, 2nd edn. Lippincott Williams & Wilkins, Ambler

Coulston AM & Boushey CJ (2008) *Nutrition in the Prevention and Treatment of Disease*. Academic Press, Amsterdam, Boston

Crisp J, Taylor C (eds) (2005) *Potter & Perry's Fundamentals of Nursing*, 2nd edn. Elsevier Australia, Sydney

deWit SC (2001) *Fundamental Concepts and Skills for Nursing*. WB Saunders, Philadelphia

—— (2005) *Fundamental Concepts and Skills for Nursing*, 2nd edn. WB Saunders, Philadelphia

Hargrave-Huttel RA (2001) *Medical Surgical Nursing*, 4th edn. Lippincott, Philadelphia

Kapit W, Meisami ME (2000) *The Physiology Coloring Book*, 2nd edn. Benjamin Cummings, California

Kok F, Bouwman L & Des F (2008) *Personalized Nutrition: Principles and Applications*. Taylor & Francis, London

Marieb EN (2006) *Human Anatomy and Physiology*, 6th edn. Benjamin Cummings Longman Inc, San Francisco

Potter PA, Perry AG (2001) *Fundamentals of Nursing*, 5th edn. Mosby, St Louis

—— (2008) *Fundamentals of Nursing*, 7th edn. Mosby, St Louis

Tortora GJ, Grabowski SR (2000) *Principles of Anatomy and Physiology*, 9th edn. Wiley & Sons, New York

ONLINE RESOURCES

pH of the Blood: Acid–Base Balance: www.usyd.edu.au/su/anaes/lectures/acidbase_mjb/acidbase.html

Acid–base balance: www.mtsinai.org/pulmonary/books/physiology/chap7_1.htm

www.dbhs.wvusd.K12ca.us/webdocs

Acid–base terminology: www.acid-base.com/terminology.ssi#Term

Chapter 31
NUTRITION

OBJECTIVES

- Define the key terms/concepts
- Identify the three major groups of nutrients
- List the six groups of vitamins required for health
- List the eight major elements or electrolytes required for health
- Identify the functions and common food sources of the essential nutrients
- Describe the physical characteristics associated with a usual nutritional status
- Identify factors and disorders that may affect a client's nutritional status
- Identify commonly used assessment techniques to measure a client's nutritional status
- State the components of a healthy balanced diet
- Describe the components of the food guide pyramid
- State the principles of good nutrition
- Describe how the healthy balanced diet can be adapted to meet specific dietary beliefs and or requirements
- Apply appropriate principles to meet nutritional needs throughout the lifespan, during episodes of illness or alterations in physiological or psychological status
- Assist in meeting a client's nutritional needs accurately and safely in relation to assisting at mealtimes and caring for a client requiring enteral and parenteral feeds

KEY TERMS/CONCEPTS

anorexia nervosa
basal metabolic rate (BMR)
body mass index (BMI)
bulimia nervosa
carbohydrates
catabolism
disaccharides
dysphagia
enteral
enzymes
essential amino acids
fat-soluble vitamins
monosaccharides
non-essential amino acids
polysaccharides
recommended daily allowances (RDAs)
total parenteral nutrition (TPN)

CHAPTER FOCUS

This chapter focuses on the nutritional needs of clients over the lifespan and how a client's wellbeing can be affected by an alteration in the quantity and quality of absorbed nutrients. Nurses are required to assess and educate clients to maintain nutritional health status and provide information on how to undertake care for clients related to nutrition. Nutritional requirements vary according to age, height, sex, religion, culture, socioeconomic factors, and physical and psychological status. Nurses must be able to accommodate for all these different factors when they plan, care and educate clients.

LIVED EXPERIENCE

When I was admitted to a hospital with diverticulitis recently, I was unable to eat or drink anything orally for 5 days. By the sixth day, when I was able to start on clear fluids, I found I had lost my appetite! One of the student nurses who was looking after me suggested I clean my teeth and use a mouth wash to freshen my mouth, as she said this would help to stimulate my appetite. Guess what? This worked! Even though I wasn't thrilled with the broth and jelly, I found I could taste it and by the time I was able to resume my usual diet, my appetite was fully back!

Chrissie, 56 years

NUTRITION

While eating has psychosocial and cultural significance in life, the major roles of food intake are to provide nutrients necessary for the development and growth of cells and the replacement of substances required by cells to maintain efficient body function. Information about the ingestion and digestion of food and the absorption of nutrients, is provided in Chapter 33. After the digested nutrients have been absorbed into the blood and lymph, they are distributed to the cells for further chemical processing, which releases the energy necessary for body function. The process of metabolism converts the nutrients into chemical forms that produce energy and rebuild body tissue. The two phases of metabolism are anabolism (or constructive phase), when simple substances derived from the nutrients are converted into complex substances that can be used by the cells; and catabolism (or destructive phase), when these complex substances are reconverted into simpler forms to release the energy necessary for cell function.

The term nutrition is used to describe all the processes by which the body uses food for energy, maintenance and growth. Nutritional requirements vary in response to changes throughout the lifespan. Factors that increase the body's metabolic demand include the periods of rapid growth during infancy and adolescence, pregnancy and lactation, increased physical activity, and periods of stress, disease or trauma. Metabolic requirements diminish with reduced energy demands, decreased physical activity and age.

Adequate nutrition is partially dependent on the ability of the body to ingest and digest food, to absorb nutrients from the intestine and to excrete waste products. In addition, the quality and quantity of food consumed has an important influence on a client's current and future health status. A diet containing the essential nutrients for each stage of the lifespan is vital to maintain wellbeing.

Many factors influence a client's pattern of eating, and include:

- Availability of food
- Economic status
- Influences such as family, or advertising
- Food fads and fallacies
- Cultural and ethnic beliefs and values
- Social and emotional aspects of food
- Physical or psychological status of the client, such as an allergy or intolerance to specific foods or nutrients, difficulty in chewing or swallowing, level of independence, disorders that interfere with nutrition and result in maldigestion, malabsorption, or loss of nutrients, leading to emotional states such as depression or anxiety.

NUTRITION ASSESSMENT

A client's nutritional status is assessed by obtaining information about their appetite, food preferences, height and weight and level of activity, and from observing their general appearance. Observation of a client's general appearance provides information about their general state of health and their nutritional status. Some characteristics of altered nutritional status are presented in Table 31.1. Assessing the client's eating pattern and their nutritional status may identify problems or risk factors.

In addition to the physical characteristics associated with poor nutritional status, psychological symptoms may be evident. A client with a poor nutritional status may experience irritability, lethargy, apathy or inability to concentrate. It is possible, however, that these symptoms and the physical signs presented in Table 31.1 may be

TABLE 31.1 | CHARACTERISTICS OF ALTERED NUTRITIONAL STATUS

General	Cachexia, hepatomegaly, splenomegaly, cardiomegaly, weight loss or gain
Hair	Dull, dry or brittle hair; hair thinning or loss
Nails	Brittle, broken, ridged or spoon shaped. Pale nail bed
Skin	Dry or scaly, bruising or petechiae unrelated to trauma, ulceration, abnormal colour changes, dermatitis
Oral mucosa	Pale mucous membrane, ulceration and cracking, ketone-smelling breath
Lips	Angular stomatitis, cheilosis
Tongue	Swollen or smooth tongue, atrophic papilla, cracking or fissuring
Gums	Spongy and/or bleeding gums, gum recession
Teeth	Mottled, dental caries, absent teeth
Conjunctiva	Pale to reddish-pink
Vision	Diminished visual acuity or loss
Cardiac	Tachycardia, cardiomegaly, palpitations, angina
Muscles	Muscle wasting, atrophy, diminished strength or tone, constipation
Skeleton	Curvature of arms or legs, altered gait, shortened stature, fractures
Neurological	Altered mood or affect, reduced concentration span, coordination, sensory or motor activity and reflexes, vision loss
Urine	Ketonuria, urobilinogen, haemoglobinuria, haematuria

related to an underlying condition and/or the client's nutritional status.

Certain groups of clients may be more at risk of a poor nutritional status, including those who are:

- Suffering emotional or physical stress
- Alcohol, drug or nicotine dependent
- Pregnant or lactating
- Older or the young
- Unaware of nutritional values
- Strict vegetarians
- Following 'fad' diets.

To maintain or promote an appropriate intake of food and therefore a good nutritional status, clients should be encouraged to follow the principles of a balanced healthy diet that provides the body with essential nutrients.

HEALTHY BALANCED DIET

A healthy balanced diet is one that consists of foods taken regularly, in sufficient quantities, from each of the basic food groups. A healthy balanced diet is a diet that is composed of 60% carbohydrate, 20% protein and 20% fat. The recommended number of daily servings from each of the five food groups varies slightly according to the client's stage of development. The five food groups and the recommended daily allowances (RDAs) are:

1. **Milk and dairy products**. The major nutrients provided by foods from this group are protein, fat and calcium; 300–600 mL of milk, or equivalent substitutes such as cheese and yoghurt, should be consumed daily. During pregnancy or lactation the amount should be increased to 900 mL of milk or equivalent substitutes daily
2. **Meat, fish and eggs**. The major nutrients provided by foods from this group are protein, fat and iron. One to two servings from this group is the RDA
3. **Fruits and vegetables**. The major nutrients provided by foods from this group are carbohydrate, fibre, water-soluble vitamins and water. The RDA is at least four servings of either fruits or vegetables, or a combination of both
4. **Breads and cereals**. The major nutrients provided by foods from this group are carbohydrates, protein, vitamins, iron and fibre. Depending on energy requirements, at least four servings daily are recommended
5. **Fats (butter, margarine, oils)**. The major function of foods in this group is to provide a vehicle for the fat-soluble vitamins: A, D, E and K. The RDA of fats is 15–30 g.

Nutritional needs of infants and children

Throughout all stages of development, a healthy balanced diet is necessary to provide the nutrients required for the body's needs. For information on maternal and newborn nutrition, see Chapter 49.

Solids are generally introduced when an infant is about 6 months old, but this varies according to the infant's needs and development. The term educational diet is sometimes used to describe the gradual introduction of solids. The aim of introducing solids is to wean the infant off milk to prevent such problems as failure to thrive, malnutrition and anaemia, and also to educate the palate to different tastes and textures; eating therefore becomes largely a learning process. Rice cereal, pureed stewed fruit and vegetables are suitable first foods. Because food allergies can be a problem during infancy, it is important that single-ingredient foods are introduced one at a time. If an infant has an adverse reaction to a food, it can then be readily identified and eliminated from the diet. By 6–8 months of age, chewing movements begin and the infant can be introduced to coarser-textured foods.

When the infant begins to grasp objects and put them in their mouth, they may be ready to be introduced to finger foods. When an infant can take fluids from a cup, at about 7–8 months of age, fruit juice may be introduced. Giving fruit juice from a bottle should be discouraged, as this may contribute to the development of jaw and tooth deformity and dental caries, and excessive volumes of fruit juice may result in diarrhoea.

At about 12 months of age the infant should be eating a range of basic foods. The diet should consist of bread and cereals, fruit and vegetables, meat and/or other protein foods, milk and/or milk products and small amounts of butter or margarine. Salt, sugar and fatty foods should be avoided.

The toddler and pre-school child

During this stage of development a child's rate of growth is slower than in infancy and this is normally reflected by a decrease in appetite, although appetite is generally unpredictable during these years. Children should be encouraged to eat a variety of nutritious foods, which should be served at regular times in a calm and relaxed atmosphere. Because young children are active, snacks between meals are important. The foods offered for snacks should contribute to the nutritional needs of the child, while foods with poor nutritional value should be avoided. Small hard foods, such as nuts, raw carrots, etc, are potentially dangerous for the young child, as they may be inhaled and obstruct airways. The toddler and preschool child should be having, each day:

- 4–5 servings from the bread and cereal group
- 3–4 servings from the fruit and vegetable group
- 1–2 servings from the meat and protein group
- 600 mL of milk, or equivalent in dairy cheese or yoghurt
- 5–10 g of butter or margarine.

The school-age child

During the first 12 months of life a foundation is laid down for good dietary practices. By the time the child is of school age, eating patterns are usually firmly established. As the child grows and develops, their tastes can change — foods that were previously enjoyed may be refused, while the child may acquire a taste for other foods, due in part to social interaction and their changing physiological needs and subsequent sensory changes.

Nutritional requirements are similar to those for children of preschool age, although kilojoule needs are diminished in relation to body size. However, fat and protein reserves are being laid down for the increased growth needs of the adolescent period, and the school-age child should be encouraged to consume a healthy balanced diet consisting of foods from each of the five food groups and should be discouraged from consuming foods that have poor nutritional value. If the child consumes an excessive quantity of food and/or food that is high in kilojoules, and does not exercise, they may be at risk of childhood obesity and subsequent development of conditions such as adult-onset diabetes and cardiovascular disease. Iron-deficiency anaemia is another nutritional problem associated with school-age children due to inadequate amounts of iron in the diet.

Adolescence

From 10 years of age, children's bodies are developing rapidly to prime the body for reproduction. A pre-puberty growth spurt occurs earlier in girls than in boys, as they store more fat, which initiates adolescence faster (see Chapter 16 for further information). During this time there can be major changes in their selection and volume of food; hormones alter senses such as taste to enable the adolescent to adapt to obtain changing nutrient requirements. Some clients at this age may be vulnerable to self, peer and social influences that may alter their perception of appearance and self-worth and drastically modify their eating habits (see 'Eating disorders', later in this chapter).

ENERGY REQUIREMENTS

In addition to the consumption of foods from the five food groups that provide the essential nutrients, dietary requirements need to be considered in terms of energy requirements. Energy is needed for all the chemical and physical activities of the body, such as muscular activity, production of glandular secretions and the synthesis of substances in cells. The amount of energy required by a client is the amount necessary to maintain physiological processes and depends on factors such as age, sex, climate, body build, height and weight, level of physical activity, and usual function or dysfunction.

Energy requirements are increased during periods of rapid growth, for example, during pregnancy, infancy and adolescence and when a person engages in a high level of physical activity. Certain types of body dysfunction, such as hyperthyroidism — a disorder of the thyroid gland — can also increase the amount of energy required. Energy requirements are decreased when a client's level of physical activity is low, with certain metabolic conditions, such as hypothyroidism, and during stages of development when there is little growth, such as old age.

The two units of measurement that specify the energy value of food are calories and joules. A calorie is defined as the amount of heat required to raise 1 gram of water by 1°C. A joule, which is the standard international (SI) unit of energy and heat, is equivalent to the amount of work performed when a 1 kg mass is moved 1 m by the force of 1 newton. One calorie is equal to 4.184 joules. As joules are very small units, it is more convenient to measure food energy in terms of kilojoules. One kilojoule (kJ) is 1000 joules. (For further units of measurement, see Appendix 2.)

The energy value of the three major types of nutrients are:

1. 1 g protein produces about 17 kJ
2. 1 g carbohydrate produces about 17 kJ
3. 1 g fat produces about 38 kJ.

Energy expenditure varies with the level of physical activity a client engages in and ranges from about 5 kJ/min during sleep to about 120 kJ/min during heavy physical activity. When the intake of kilojoules is increased or energy expenditure is decreased, weight gain occurs. Conversely, loss of weight occurs when the intake of kilojoules is decreased or energy expenditure is increased.

Basal metabolism is the term used to describe the minimal maintenance of all normal body functions at rest and in the absence of disease. The amount of energy required to support basal metabolism is measured when a client is awake but at complete rest and has not eaten for at least 12 hours. The measurement is expressed as basal metabolic rate (BMR), according to the number of kilojoules consumed per hour per square metre of body surface area (or per kilogram of body weight). The BMR is one diagnostic test commonly used to estimate nutritional needs. Variations in the BMR between clients of the same weight and height may be due to alteration in body composition, such as muscle mass as opposed to fatty tissue, and the presence of certain disease states.

Appendix 7 gives reference ranges for acceptable weight for height for Australians. This table is based on body mass index (BMI) which is calculated using the following formula:

BMI = Weight in kilograms divided by height in metres^2

For example, the BMI of a male who is 6 feet (1.83 metres) tall and weighs 115kg is:

$$\frac{115}{1.83^2} = \text{BMI of 34}$$

The value obtained when this formula is used should be rounded to the nearest whole number. A BMI value below 20 is common in certain ethnic groups, such as people of Asian descent, and in athletes, but otherwise indicates that a person is underweight. A BMI of 20–25 is within the healthy weight range. A BMI of 25–30 may indicate more muscular build or overweight, while a value of 31–40 is defined as moderate to severe obesity and a value above 40 signifies morbid obesity.

GLYCAEMIC INDEX

Glycaemic index (GI) classifies carbohydrate foods according to how rapidly glucose is released from them and absorbed into the blood. It has traditionally been used to treat clients with diabetes mellitus but is now being used for establishing optimal diets for the general populace. The lower the GI the slower the rate of absorption and the slower the rate of insulin release. Complex carbohydrates such as starch provide lower GI nutrients and result in a more stable blood glucose level.

Some simple carbohydrates, such as those found in fruits, have a lower GI value than some complex carbohydrates, such as those found in rice and potatoes. Foods with low-GI values have been used to treat hypercholesterolaemia and obesity. Low-GI foods include multigrain breads, bran, legumes, milk, yoghurt and fruits. High-GI foods, of which there are more than 70, include rice, potatoes, wholemeal and white bread, and some cereals. Further health benefits may be gained by including foods that are high in fibre.

NUTRIENTS

Nutrients are chemical substances in food that provide energy, build and maintain cells or regulate body processes. The essential nutrients are:

- Carbohydrates
- Proteins
- Lipids (fats)
- Water
- Fibre
- Vitamins
- Mineral salts.

CARBOHYDRATES

Carbohydrates are a group of organic compounds that includes sugar, starch and cellulose. They are composed of one or more monosaccharide (single-sugar) units. Sugars can be classified as either simple or complex and are divided into groups according to the complexity of their molecular structure. Simple sugars, or monosaccharides, include glucose, fructose and galactose. Disaccharides, which are a combination of two sugars, include sucrose, lactose and maltose. For example, glucose and fructose combine to form sucrose. Complex sugars or polysaccharides are a combination of many sugars and include starch, glycogen and cellulose. Before carbohydrates can be utilised by the body cells, disaccharides and polysaccharides must be converted by chemical digestion into glucose.

Carbohydrates provide energy, assist in the metabolism of fat and act as a protein sparer (if there is insufficient carbohydrate in the diet, protein is converted to glucose and used for energy). Carbohydrate foods also supply indigestible cellulose, which adds bulk to the intestinal contents, resulting in stimulation of peristalsis. The major food sources of carbohydrates are:

- Sugars, present in fruits, honey, cane sugar, milk and cereals
- Starch, present in vegetables, cereals and foods made from cereals (e.g. bread and pasta)
- Cellulose, present in vegetables, fruits and cereals (complex carbohydrates).

PROTEINS

Proteins are a group of nitrogenous compounds composed of chains of amino acid subunits. Twenty-two amino acids have been identified in humans. Eight of these — the essential amino acids — the body is unable to make, and they must be obtained from dietary sources. The remaining 14 non-essential amino acids can be synthesised by the body. Before proteins can be utilised by the cells, they must be broken down by physical and chemical digestion into their constituent amino acids. According to the number and type of amino acids present, proteins are classed either as complete (containing all essential amino acids) or incomplete (lacking one or more essential amino acids).

Proteins build and repair tissue and supply energy (protein that is not needed for growth and repair of tissues is converted into glucose and stored in the liver and muscles as a reserve store of energy). The major food sources of protein are meat, fish, eggs, cheese, milk, poultry and soya beans (complete [or first-class] protein); and cereals, lentils, legumes and nuts (incomplete [or second-class] protein).

LIPIDS (FATS)

Lipids are a group of substances that are insoluble in water and are composed of fatty acids and glycerol. Fatty acids are classed as saturated or unsaturated. Saturated, or solid, fats are chiefly of animal origin, such as butter, and contain a full complement of hydrogen. Unsaturated, or soft or liquid, fats are chiefly of vegetable origin, such as margarine, and are capable of adding more hydrogen to their molecular structure.

Before fats can be utilised by the body cells they must be broken down by chemical digestion into their constituent fatty acids and glycerol. Fat supplies energy and may be used in the tissues or stored in adipose tissue, which functions to support and protect nerves and organs from trauma, insulate the body to prevent excessive heat loss or gain, and as a reserve store of fuel. Fats also supply the fat-soluble vitamins A, D, E and K as well as stimulating adolescence, fertility and mood, and suppressing appetite through the action of hormones such as leptin, secreted by adipocytes.

The major food sources of fat are animal fats, present in meat, butter, cream, egg yolk, cheese and fish oils; and vegetable fats, present in margarine, cocoa and oils such as olive, safflower, corn and peanut.

WATER

Water is a chemical compound obtained by the body from food and fluid and as a result of the metabolism of protein, fat and carbohydrate in the tissues. Water constitutes about 60% of the total body weight and is present as intracellular fluid and extracellular fluid. Water is also the basis of all body secretions and excretions.

Water is necessary for the digestion, absorption and metabolism of food, for the production of secretions and for the maintenance of body fluids. Water is also necessary for the regulation of body temperature by evaporation of sweat, and for the elimination of waste products through the kidneys, bowel, skin and lungs.

Water is present in all body fluids and as part of the cellular structure of solid foods. Foods vary in water content; fruit and vegetables contain about 80–90% water, meat contains about 70%, and bread contains about 35%.

FIBRE

Dietary fibre, often referred to as cellulose, is the fibrous parts of food that the digestive system has difficulty in digesting. Fibre creates bulk in the stools, which enhances defecation and is used to prevent or minimise symptoms of certain disorders, such as haemorrhoids, diverticular disease, formation of gallstones, simple constipation and intestinal cancer. Foods with a high fibre content are fruits, vegetables and wholegrain products. Clinical Interest Box 31.1 provides discussion on the effects of constipation on the older client.

VITAMINS

Vitamins are a group of organic compounds that, with few exceptions, must be obtained from dietary sources. Although they have no energy value, they are essential for normal metabolic and physiological bodily function. The term vitamin was first used in 1912, and letters of the alphabet were assigned to them as they were discovered. Now that more is known about their composition, the chemical name for a vitamin is frequently used.

Vitamins are classed as being either water or fat soluble. The water-soluble vitamins are easily destroyed during the preparation and prolonged cooking of food. If they are consumed in excess of the body's need, they are excreted in the urine. Fat-soluble vitamins are oxidised by exposure to air, light and high temperatures. As fat-soluble vitamins are not soluble in water, any excess is stored in the body, and a condition known as hypervitaminosis may occur, which may result in organ failure.

Excessive intake of vitamin A over long periods can result in hypervitaminosis A, a condition characterised by yellow discolouration of the skin (often mistaken as jaundice), loss of appetite and dry itchy skin. Excessive intake of vitamin B may result in allergic-type reactions. Hypervitaminosis D may occur if excessive amounts of vitamin D are taken and is characterised by nausea, vomiting, diarrhoea, general irritability and severe impairment of kidney function. In normal circumstances a healthy balanced diet will provide the body with sufficient quantities of all vitamins without the need for supplemental vitamin ingestion. Table 31.2 describes the functions and effects of vitamin deficiencies.

CLINICAL INTEREST BOX 31.1
Constipation and the older client

Constipation can occur at any age but is common in the elderly, associated with diminished exercise, fibre and fluid intake, as well as diminished neurogenic gastrointestinal regulation. Measures to avoid constipation are required to reduce the incidence of conditions such as diverticulosis, megacolon, carcinoma, strokes and heart attacks. A nutritional assessment of dietary intake is required, as is examination for any underlying pathologies, such as those causing disorders such as iron-deficiency anaemia from per-rectal bleeding, for example. The clinical features of this anaemia include constipation, lethargy, easy exhaustion, pale conjunctivae and pagophagia (craving for ice). Iron is obtained in large quantities from meat, and many older clients may be unable to obtain and consume or absorb the required amounts. Iron-replacement therapy may be required; however, supplemental iron can result in constipation, false-positive occult blood test and gastrointestinal upset.

MINERAL SALTS

Mineral salts are a group of compounds that play an important role in metabolism, maintenance of blood pressure, cardiac function, fluid and electrolyte balance, acid–base balance and the regulation of other body processes. Storage and processing of food does not alter its mineral content, although mineral salts may be lost when food is soaked or cooked in water. The elements that mineral salts contain are classed as either major or trace elements; trace elements are present in only minute quantities in the body. A mineral salt that has the property of being a conductor of electrical current is referred to as an electrolyte. The functions and effects of mineral salt deficiencies are listed in Table 31.3.

DIETS TO MEET CLIENT NEEDS

A person's normal diet depends on their age, pattern of eating and the food they choose. Dietary requirements may change during illness; for example, a client may avoid eating foods that cause adverse reactions such as indigestion, nausea or diarrhoea. The client's diet may also need to be adapted as part of their treatment during certain conditions and disease states.

While acknowledging the factors that influence a client's choice of foods and observing any restrictions to their diet in the management of disease processes, nurses should encourage the consumption of healthy balanced meals, following the principles of good nutrition. The principles of good nutrition are that:

- A variety of foods from each of the basic food groups should be eaten each day
- The intake of fat, sodium, sugar and alcohol should be limited
- The intake of complex carbohydrate and dietary fibre should be high
- Adequate amounts of water should be consumed

TABLE 31.2 | VITAMINS AND HEALTH

Vitamin	Functions	Sources	Effects of deficiency
Vitamin A (retinol or carotenes)	Sustains normal vision in dim light, promotes healthy growth of epithelial tissue and bone and therefore raises resistance to infection	Cod liver oil, liver, kidney, egg yolk, milk and dairy products, yellow fruits and yellow and green vegetables	Night blindness, keritonisation of epithelial tissue (and therefore less resistance to infection), stunted growth, zinc deficiency
Thiamine (B1)	Nerve function Energy and carbohydrate metabolism	Yeast extract, wholegrain cereals, meats, leafy green vegetables	Polyneuritis, beriberi, Wernicke–Korsakoff syndrome, muscular and mental development
Riboflavin (B2)	Energy and protein metabolism, cellular respiration, healthy skin and mucous membranes	Liver, yeast extract, milk and dairy products, eggs, green leafy vegetables	Fissures at the corner of mouth (cheilosis), angular stomatitis, glossitis, dermatitis, failure to thrive
Niacin (B3)	Energy utilisation; metabolism of fat, carbohydrate and protein; nervous system function	Liver, bran, meat, fish, yeast extract, legumes	Pellagra (diarrhoea, dermatitis, dementia); glossitis, anaemia
Pantothenic acid (B5)	Metabolism of carbohydrates, protein and fat; formation of haemoglobin and acetylcholine	Offal, yeast, fish, meat, egg yolk, apricots	Fatigue, sleep disturbances, headaches, personality changes, irritability
Pyridoxine (B6)	Protein metabolism, nervous system function, formation of red blood cells	Liver, fish, meat, wholegrain cereals, bananas, avocado, egg yolk, peanuts	Neuritis, depression, anaemia, EEG and ECG changes, cheilosis, renal stone formation
Cyanocobalamin (B12)	Formation of red cells and nucleic acids	All foods of animal origin	Pernicious anaemia, CNS atrophy, vision loss
Biotin	Synthesis of fatty acids, metabolism of carbohydrates and fat, gluconeogenesis	Liver, brewer's yeast, fish, offal, soya beans	Lethargy, dermatitis, EEG and ECG changes, hypercholesterolaemia
Folic acid (folacin, folate)	Metabolism, DNA and RNA synthesis, formation of haemoglobin	Liver, citrus fruit, offal, nuts, leafy green vegetables	Macrocytic anaemia, malabsorption
Vitamin C (ascorbic acid)	Formation of collagen, assists in wound healing, maintenance of capillaries, production of neuro-transmitters, aids absorption of iron	Citrus fruits, tropical fruits, berry fruits, tomatoes, potatoes, green vegetables	Delayed healing, bleeding tendencies, scurvy, reduced nervous and muscle function
Vitamin D (calciferol)	Calcium and phosphorus metabolism, immune function	Cod liver oil, fish, butter, margarine, egg yolk, sunlight on the skin	Rickets, osteomalacia
Vitamin E (alpha-tocopherol)	Antioxidant action protects the cell membrane, prevents heart disease and delays the ageing process (not yet confirmed)	Wheatgerm, vegetable oil, wholegrain cereals, nuts, legumes	Muscle degeneration, haemolytic anaemia in the newborn, infertility, malabsorption
Vitamin K (menadione)	Formation of clotting factors II, VII, IX and X; assists in regulating calcium metabolism	Liver, leafy green vegetables, egg yolk, synthesised by bacterial flora in the gastrointestinal tract	Bleeding tendencies

- Food should be prepared and cooked in such a way that the nutrient value is not lost
- Dietary intake and energy expenditure should be adjusted to achieve and maintain the appropriate weight for age and height
- Breastfeeding for babies is recommended
- People should become aware of the information contained on the labels of prepared and packaged foods. Notice should be taken of the expiry date, the presence of preservatives and other additives. The listing of ingredients on the container denotes the relative quantities of each, with the major ingredient listed first. The remainder are listed in order of decreasing quantities.

TABLE 31.3 | MINERAL SALTS AND HEALTH

Mineral	Functions	Sources	Effects of deficiency
Major elements found in mineral salts			
Calcium (Ca)	Formation of bones and teeth, muscle contraction, normal blood clotting, activator for enzymes and neurotransmitters	Milk, yoghurt, cheese, sardines, salmon, sesame seed paste	Osteoporosis, tetany and severe muscle spasms, osteomalacia
Phosphorus (P)	Formation of DNA, bones and teeth; nerve and muscle function	Milk, cheese, meat, fish, eggs	Anaemia, weight loss, abnormal growth
Sodium (Na) Potassium (K) Chloride (Cl)	Act closely together in the maintenance of osmotic pressure balance between intra- and extracellular fluid; nerve and muscle function, maintenance of acid–base balance	Salt, fruits, vegetables, monosodium glutamate	Cell and tissue fluid abnormality, arrhythmias, muscular weakness
Magnesium (Mg)	Activator of enzymes; nerve and muscle function	Cereals, nuts, leafy green vegetables, dried beans	Anorexia, nausea
Iodine (I)	Formation of thyroxine	Seafoods, vegetables, iodised salt	Goitre, myxoedema and hypothyroidism, still births and spontaneous abortions, mental and growth retardation, cretinism
Iron (Fe)	Formation of haemoglobin, necessary for the transport of oxygen	Liver, red meats, eggs, leafy green vegetables	Iron-deficiency anaemia, pagophagia, lethargy and exhaustion, poor tissue regeneration
Minor (trace) elements found in mineral salts			
Zinc (Zn)	Metabolism, collagen formation, component of certain enzymes, healthy skin and hair	Wheatgerm, oysters, meat, cheese, wholegrain cereals	Impaired healing, poor condition of the skin, growth retardation, fatigue, hair loss, behavioural changes
Copper (Cu)	Aids iron absorption; nerve function	Shellfish, nuts, wholegrain cereals	Neutropenia, hypochromic anaemia, vascular disorders
Cobalt (Co)	Synthesis of vitamin B12	Leafy green vegetables	Pernicious anaemia due to vitamin B12 deficiency
Sulphur (S)	Constituent of amino acids	Protein foods	Deficiency is rare
Selenium (Se)	Antioxidant	Fish, liver, cereals	Muscular dystrophy, delayed growth, renal and cardiac degeneration

CLINICAL INTEREST BOX 31.2
High rates of malnutrition in elderly

A ground-breaking Australian study involving UNSW has revealed alarming levels of malnutrition in the elderly, with close to 80% malnourished or at risk when first admitted to hospital.

However, early intervention with a dietitian proved doctors could dramatically reduce length of hospital stay and health costs.

The findings follow a one-year study by a team of gastroenterologists, geriatricians and dietitians at Sydney's Prince of Wales Hospital. The results will be presented at Digestive Diseases Week in Washington on May 19.

The study, led by President of the Gut Foundation, Professor Terry Bolin together with the Prince of Wales Department of Geriatric Medicine and Department of Nutrition and Dietetics, showed that when arriving for admission to hospital 80% of elderly patients were malnourished or 'at risk' but their hospital stay could be halved by implementing a nutritional care program. Professor Terry Bolin said:

> What this study has shown is that the prevalence of malnutrition among the elderly in the community is high but we have simple and effective remedies. Malnutrition has significant impact on mortality, morbidity, length of hospital stay and readmission. The benefit of early action could potentially save our health system hundreds of millions of dollars.

The study is believed to be the first randomised study of its kind examining malnutrition in a clinical setting with control and intervention groups.

(University of New South Wales 2007)

Clients may choose, or may be prescribed, certain specific diets, as follows.

HEALTHY BALANCED DIET

A healthy balanced diet is one without dietary restrictions or modifications. A client may select the foods they prefer within the principles of good nutrition and diets based on age, health and cultural or religious beliefs. Some clients choose to follow a diet in which specific foods or nutrients are restricted or increased, as part of a commitment to a healthy lifestyle. Other people will follow a diet based on cultural or religious commitment.

Nutrition Australia uses different food 'models' to depict a healthy approach to eating based on the Australian Dietary Guidelines. An example is the 'Healthy Eating Pyramid' (Figure 31.1) and includes:

- Foods to be eaten in small amounts such as sugar, butter, margarine and oil
- Foods to be eaten in moderate amounts, such as milk, cheese, yoghurt, lean meat, poultry, fish, nuts and eggs
- Foods to eat most such as cereals, bread, vegetables, legumes and fruit.

Another example is the 'Healthy Eating Pyramid for Lacto-ovo Vegetarians' (Figure 31.2).

VEGETARIAN DIETS

Clients may choose to follow a vegetarian diet for health, ecological or religious reasons. Vegetarian diets exclude all flesh foods, such as meat, fish and poultry, and have an intake high in plant foods. The lacto (milk)–ovo (egg) vegetarian diet includes milk, other dairy products and eggs, while a lacto vegetarian diet includes milk and other dairy products but excludes eggs. The vegan diet (strict vegetarian) excludes all animal-derived products and consists of plant foods only.

RELIGIOUS AND CULTURAL DIETS

Certain religious or cultural groups have particular rules concerning the choice, preparation and storage of specific items in the diet; however, clients may vary in their adherence to religious dietary doctrines. Some examples of the religious dietary restrictions are:

- Seventh-Day Adventist: a lacto-vegetarian diet is commonly followed and stimulants such as coffee, tea and alcohol are not permitted

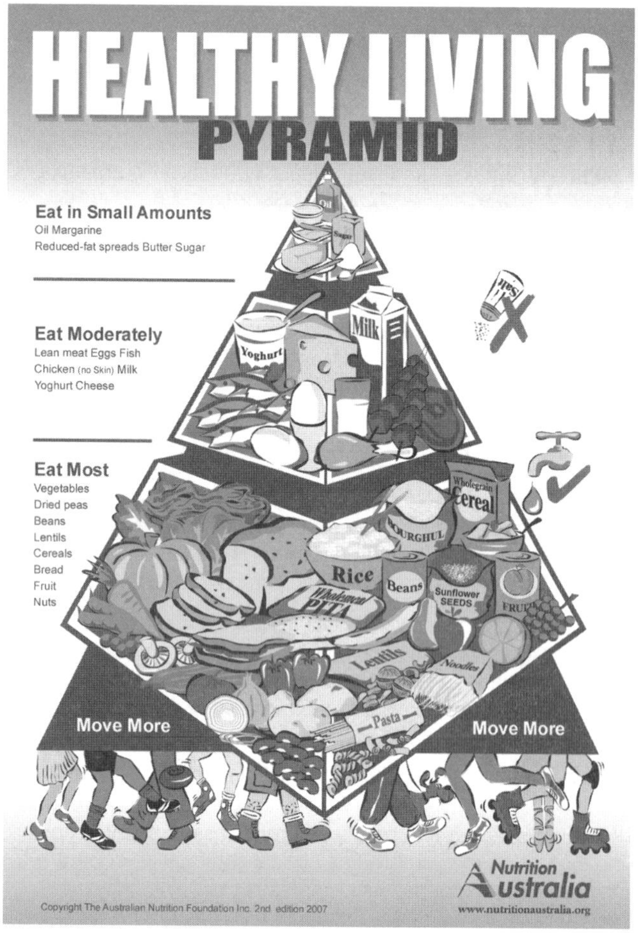

Figure 31.1 | Healthy Eating Pyramid *(Nutrition Australia)*

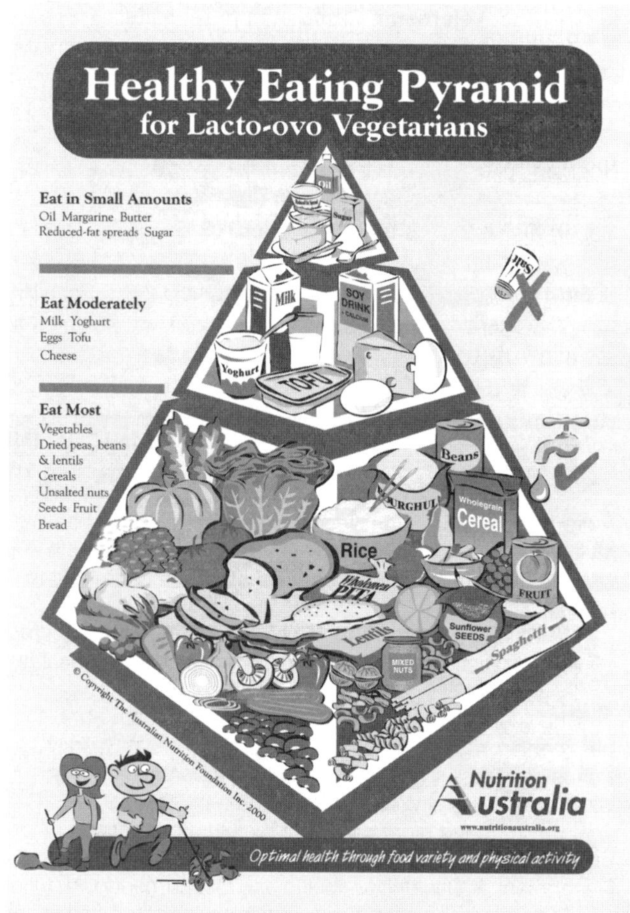

Figure 31.2 | Healthy Eating Pyramid for Lacto-ovo Vegetarians *(Nutrition Australia)*

- Roman Catholic: Ash Wednesday and Good Friday are specified days on which abstinence from meat is obligatory. In addition, Roman Catholics are required to fast for 1 hour before taking Holy Communion
- Mormon (Church of Jesus Christ of Latter Day Saints): meat, although not forbidden, is eaten infrequently. Drinks containing caffeine (e.g. tea, coffee and cola) are not permitted. Tobacco is also forbidden.
- Judaism (Jewish faith): foods must be 'kosher' (prepared according to Jewish law) and only certain parts of an animal may be eaten. All pork, shellfish and predatory birds are prohibited. Meat and dairy products are never eaten at the same time and are required to be stored and prepared separately. Certain periods of fasting are observed such as Yom Kippur, a 24-hour fast. Passover, lasting 8 days, prohibits the consumption of leavened (yeast containing) bread. Cooking is not permitted on Saturdays (the Sabbath)
- Islam (Moslem, Muslim): all pork and pork products, alcohol and caffeine are forbidden. Any meat consumed must be from animals slaughtered according to strict rules (Halal). Ramadan, a period of fasting, forbids eating or drinking of any substance from sunrise to sunset for one lunar month
- Hinduism (Hindu): people of the Hindu faith abstain from eating beef products and follow a vegetarian diet. Stimulants are forbidden.

THERAPEUTIC DIETS

A specific diet may be prescribed to rectify a nutritional deficiency, to decrease specific nutrients, or to provide modifications in the texture or consistency of food. If a therapeutic diet is prescribed, it is important that the client understands the reasons for any restrictions or modifications. Information about various therapeutic diets is provided in Table 31.4. Figure 31.3 shows part of a sample nursing care plan for a client on a restricted diet.

NURSING PRACTICE AND NUTRITIONAL NEEDS

Each institution has its own system for delivering meals, and the nurse should ensure that both the client and their immediate environment are prepared in readiness for meal times.

ASSISTING CLIENTS AT MEALTIMES

Key aspects related to providing clients with meals

- Nursing care should be planned to ensure that there are no unpleasant sights, sounds, smells or treatments being performed during mealtimes, as these could interfere with appetite.
- Clients should be offered the use of toilet facilities, and their hygiene needs should be attended to before meals arrive in the ward.
- Ambulant clients may need assistance to a table; non-ambulant clients should be assisted into a comfortable position. Eating areas should be cleared of unnecessary items to provide space for the meal tray.
- When the meals arrive the nurse should ensure that each client receives the correct meal, prepared in the correct manner according to their dietary, ethnic, cultural or religious requirements and that all the necessary items (e.g. correct eating utensils), are provided.
- Medications that are required before, during or after the meal are administered (e.g. insulin).
- During mealtimes the nurse should assist as necessary (e.g. by cutting food, opening packets, or pouring fluids).
- If a client is not able to eat what has been provided, measures should be taken to obtain an alternative meal type or other form of nourishment.
- The nurse should observe and chart the client's intake of food and inform nursing, medical or dietitian staff if the client's intake declines.
- Following the meal, the nurse should ensure that the client has the opportunity and equipment to perform normal hygiene (e.g. cleaning of hands, face and teeth or dentures).

Certain clients may experience difficulty or be unable to feed themselves for a variety of reasons, including age, general weakness, paralysis, or limitation of movement due, for example, to the presence of arm splints, intravenous lines or casts. A client who is dependent may experience embarrassment if they require assistance at mealtimes; the nurse should therefore endeavour to make mealtimes as normal and enjoyable as possible.

Key aspects related to assisting an adult client at mealtimes

- Ensure that the client is comfortable before starting a meal.
- Elimination and hygiene needs should be attended to before a meal is started.
- The client may require to be assisted into a comfortable position and the table adjusted to the appropriate height.
- The meal should be placed where it can be seen and smelt, to stimulate the appetite.
- Condiments (e.g. salt and pepper) should be provided and may be added to the food, provided the client is not on a salt-restricted diet.
- The nurse should ascertain whether the client prefers one food at a time or a combination (e.g. meat alone, or combined with a vegetable). It is also important to ensure that food or fluids are not too hot or cold.
- Suitable utensils should be selected (e.g. a client may prefer to eat using a spoon rather than a fork). The amount of food placed on the utensil should be easily managed by the client. The utensil should be placed

TABLE 31.4 | THERAPEUTIC DIETS

Diet	Description	Indications
Clear liquid	No solids permitted and only fluids that leave no residue, are non-irritating and non-gas forming are allowed, e.g. water, black tea or coffee, clear soups and fruit drinks	Obstruction or irritation of the gastrointestinal tract Preparation for colonoscopy Postoperatively before starting on solids
Full liquid	All fluids, plus foods that become liquid at room temperature, e.g. jelly and ice-cream, are permitted	Progression from clear liquids Before starting on solids Inability to chew or swallow solids
Soft	Semi-solid easily digested foods are permitted, e.g. soup, cooked cereal, milk pudding, mashed or pureed vegetables and fruit, eggs, soft meats and fish	Advancing from a liquid diet Clients with chewing or swallowing difficulties Certain gastrointestinal disorders
Low fibre	Foods that can be absorbed easily and leave no colour or residue are permitted, e.g. clear soup, tender meat, fish or chicken, eggs, refined cereal products, jelly, ice-cream	As part of preparation for colonoscopy Colitis Before and after surgery on the lower colon
High fibre	Foods that contain residue that adds bulk to the faeces and stimulates peristalsis, e.g. fruit, vegetables, nuts, wholegrain products	Prevention of cancer Prevention and treatment of constipation Hypercholesterolaemia
Low kilojoule	The number of kilojoules is reduced below the usual daily requirement. Foods that are low in fat or refined carbohydrate are permitted	Weight reduction
High kilojoule	The number of kilojoules is increased above the usual daily requirements. Foods that are high in carbohydrate, protein and fat are included	Weight gain. To replace and repair damaged tissue, e.g. after severe burns
Low cholesterol	Foods that are high in fat and cholesterol are restricted, e.g. butter, cream, whole milk, cheese, egg yolk, meat	Prevention or treatment of heart disease, atherosclerosis, high serum cholesterol levels
Low fat	Foods that are high in fat are restricted, e.g. butter, cream, whole milk, cheese, fatty meat	Liver or gallbladder disorders Irritable bowel syndrome Weight reduction
Low protein	The amount of protein is restricted and fat and carbohydrate is increased	Kidney or liver failure
High protein	The amount of protein is increased and foods high in complete protein are included, e.g. meat, fish, eggs, cheese, milk	To replace and repair damaged tissue
High iron	Foods that are rich in iron are included, e.g. liver, red meat, green leafy vegetables	Prevention and treatment of iron-deficiency anaemia
Controlled carbohydrate (diabetic)	The amounts of carbohydrate, kilojoules and protein are controlled to meet nutritional needs, to control blood sugar levels and to maintain an appropriate body weight	Diabetes mellitus
Controlled sodium	Foods that are high in sodium are omitted and no salt is added to food	Cardiovascular disease. Certain kidney diseases, liver failure, fluid retention (oedema)
Gluten restricted	Foods that contain gluten are eliminated, e.g. wheat, rye, oats, malt, barley. Rice and corn are permitted	Coeliac disease
High vitamin	A balanced healthy diet that includes foods that are high in one or more deficient vitamins	Vitamin deficiency diseases, e.g. night blindness Anaemia, e.g. vitamin B12, folate Beriberi Scurvy Rickets

gently into the front of the mouth, to avoid injury or stimulation of the gag reflex.

- The food should be presented at a rate that meets the client's needs, giving them sufficient time to chew and swallow each mouthful and to maintain dignity.
- Sips of fluid should be offered during the meal. A flexible straw, rather than a cup or glass, may be easier for some clients to manage.
- To maintain dignity and to promote independence, the client should be encouraged to be as independent

Date initiated	Plan	Nursing interventions	Insert title name signature & date	Revision date	Comments
Day 1	Decrease total calories ingested	Medical officer contacted____________ Dietitian contacted ____________ Dietary history obtained ____________ Total daily calories ordered____________ Diet type ordered Diet kitchen contacted Occupational therapist required Yes No Physiotherapist required Yes No Psychologist required Yes No Fluid balance chart required Yes No Circle requirements Diet Fluids PU PR other, e.g., strict____________			
	Lose weight as evidenced on weight chart	Recordings of weight Frequency of weighing required ________ Weight ________ at ________ am/pm Other requirements, e.g., weigh in light clothing ____________			
	Increase activity level	Enter daily routine and activities ____________			

Figure 31.3 | Part of a sample nursing care plan for a client on a restricted diet

as possible and may be encouraged, but never forced, to eat a meal.

- Allow the client to wipe their mouth with a serviette during the meal, or assist if necessary.
- On completion of the meal, the client's hygiene and comfort needs should be met. The nurse should report and document the intake of food and fluid.

Key aspects related to assisting a child at mealtimes

Mealtimes in a hospital should be pleasant unhurried occasions and the environment should be one that enables the child to enjoy mealtimes. Some guidelines are:

- Mealtimes should be free from distractions
- Servings need to be small to minimise the psychological reaction to a large-sized serving
- Adequate time should be allowed for the meal to be eaten without hurrying
- The child should be prepared for the meal. Toilet needs should be attended to, hands and face washed, serviette or bib provided, distractions such as toys put away, and the child made comfortable in bed or seated on a chair at a table
- Painful or emotionally distressing procedures should not be performed immediately before or after a meal, and activities should be timed so that a child does not become too tired to eat a meal
- Meals should be served attractively, in amounts appropriate to the age and the condition of each child
- Children should be encouraged to feed themselves, even though they may do it in a 'messy' fashion
- Assistance should be given if the child is unable to manage or to use distractive therapy to maintain input
- Some children may need coaxing, but a child must never be forced to eat.

Uneaten food should be removed without comment and the nurse in charge informed. If the child's illness is causing anorexia, other forms of nutrition may be offered. Refusal to eat may be an attempt by the child to gain more attention, or it may be that the foods are different in appearance, presentation, availability of condiments, or timing, to the meals they are used to eating. Every attempt should be made to provide nutritious foods that the child enjoys. In a clinical setting, a lot of patience may be required to assist a child to eat a healthy balanced diet, particularly if their carers are not present, they are apprehensive of their setting, are in pain, used to different foods, or if their diet is of poor standard at home.

Children should be observed for any adverse reaction to food and the nurse in charge and or medical officer informed if a child vomits before, during or after a meal; develops diarrhoea; or develops what may be an allergic reaction to a food, such as a rash, pruritus, or breathing difficulties.

CLINICAL INTEREST BOX 31.3
Gastro-oesophageal reflux and failure to thrive

Failure to thrive is a term used in paediatrics to describe a newborn, infant, toddler or child who fails to gain weight when measured against percentile charts for age, head circumference and height. In infancy failure to thrive can be associated with mild to severe alterations in nutritional state as a consequence of numerous clinical disorders.

A common condition is gastro-oesophageal reflux (GOR), which can be due to lax cardiac sphincter muscle or changes in coordination of oesophageal peristalsis. GOR can cause oesophagitis from intermittent bathing of oesophageal tissue in stomach acid. Common symptoms may also include food refusal, diminished intake, prolonged feeding times, distractibility, sleep disorders and continued crying, which may lead some to diagnose an infant as a 'colicky baby'. Diagnosis is made by history and monitoring oesophageal pH over a 24-hour period. Treatments may include thickening agents, positioning up to 30 degrees from the horizontal, peristaltic medications and gastric acid inhibitors.

Key aspects related to assisting a client with chewing or swallowing difficulties

Some clients who experience difficulty in chewing or have dysphagia due, for example, to glossitis, stomatitis, cerebral vascular accidents or dental conditions, are at risk of malnutrition because of limitations to the types of foods they can chew and swallow safely. Clinical Interest Box 31.3 provides an example of how gastro-oesophageal reflux can affect the nutritional status in children. Clients may require modifications to the consistency of food. Depending on the cause and degree of difficulty, the client's needs may be met by:

- Referral to a speech pathologist to ascertain the cause of the problem by observing the client's swallowing reflex and by investigations such as salivagrams, fluoroscopy or barium swallows
- Providing meals comprised of soft foods or thickened fluids
- Initiating the swallowing reflex by gentle pressure on the tongue with the feeding utensil
- Offering all food and fluid carefully and monitoring to avoid or detect aspiration
- Placing the food into the unaffected side of the mouth in clients with a facial paralysis (e.g. Bell's palsy) or after a cerebrovascular accident. The nurse should ensure that food does not accumulate in the cheek of the affected side.

Key aspects related to assisting a client with visual impairment at mealtimes

- It is important to encourage independence; the nurse should therefore consult the client about the type of assistance that would be most beneficial. For example, clients may find it helpful if the nurse describes the meal by referring to the plate as a clock face. The nurse should state where each food on the plate may be located (e.g. the meat at 2 o'clock, the potatoes at 4 o'clock and the beans at 6 o'clock).
- To avoid injury the client should be made aware of the proximity and location of hot articles (e.g. cups of tea or coffee) and the nurse should ask if assistance to pour the fluids is required.
- If the client is unable to feed themself, they should be asked to indicate when they are ready for the next mouthful.
- Self-feeding should be encouraged at all ages to promote independence and dignity. When a client is being fed, the nurse should perform the procedure in a relaxed and confident manner, with due regard for maintaining their dignity. A variety of self-help devices are available to assist clients in feeding themselves (Figure 31.4). Such devices may be helpful for a client who has limited arm mobility, limited grasp or reduced coordination, and include:
  - — Plate guards, which attach to one side of the plate and are used to assist a client to place food on the eating utensils
  - — Angled or swivelling utensils (e.g. forks and spoons that are angled to assist clients with a limited range of arm or hand movement)
  - — Utensils with built-up handles. The thicker handles are beneficial for clients with diminished grasp or who experience joint pain or discomfort (e.g. arthritis)
  - — Cuffs, which are placed over a client's hand, with a spoon or fork inserted into the slot in the cuff. A cuff may be beneficial for a client with diminished grasp or movement.

COMMON DISORDERS ASSOCIATED WITH NUTRITION

Although many disorders are related to a specific nutrient deficiency, the common disorders of nutrition may be classified as malnutrition, obesity, eating disorders and nutrient loss as a result of vomiting or diarrhoea.

MALNUTRITION

Malnutrition occurs as a consequence of continued poor nutrition status and may be described as the condition in which nutrients are being used or lost by the body in excess of the intake and absorption or utilisation of nutrients. Identifying factors that put a client at risk is an important factor in ensuring that all clients have their individual nutritional needs met. People who are at risk of malnutrition include those who:

- Are experiencing increased metabolic demands or protracted loss of nutrients; for example, due to burns, surgery, inflammatory conditions or infections, vomiting, diarrhoea, physical or psychological trauma, hormonal imbalance or prolonged pyrexia

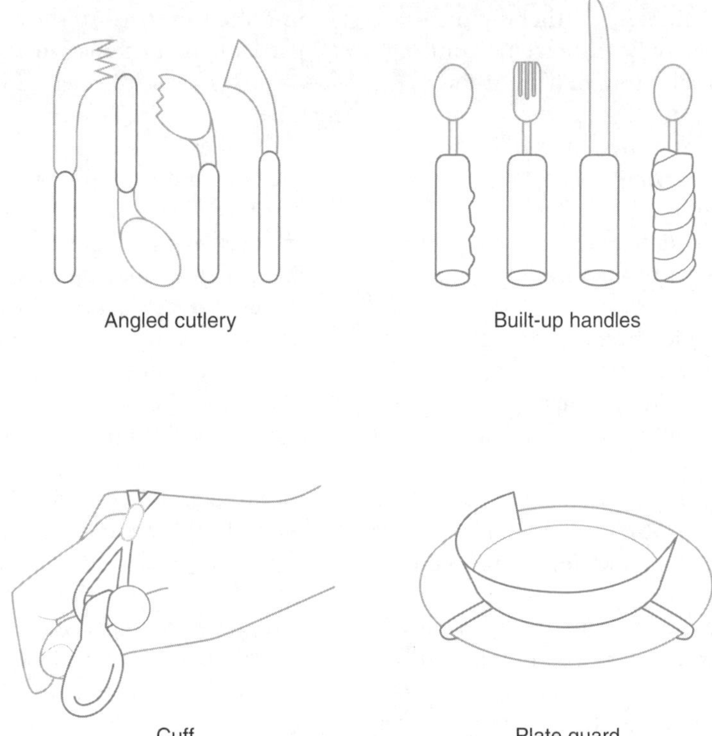

Figure 31.4 | Feeding aids

- Are not consuming oral food or fluid for more than a few days
- Have a BMI value below 20 or who have recently experienced a loss of more than 10% of their normal body weight
- Are alcohol or drug dependent
- Are receiving medications or treatments that have an anti-nutrient or have catabolic properties (e.g. immunosuppressants or antitumour agents)
- Have a disorder that results in defective digestion, utilisation or absorption of nutrients (e.g. gastrectomy, diabetes mellitus, Crohn's disease).

Malnutrition results in impaired growth and development, lowered resistance to infection, damage to tissues and delayed healing and anaemia. Treatment includes identifying the cause and providing adequate nutrients.

OBESITY

Obesity is the condition in which there is an excess of body fat, and is determined by calculating the client's BMI. Obesity results from excessive kilojoule intake, metabolic disturbances, side effects of drugs such as steroids, an inadequate expenditure of energy, or from a combination of factors. Obesity may have serious consequences, including cancer, premature cardiovascular disease, breathing difficulties, hypertension, diabetes mellitus, gall bladder disease or psychosocial problems.

Principles of treatment include reducing dietary intake and any causative drugs or hormones, while planning exercise, dietary and behaviour modification and the administration of medications such as appetite suppressants, hormonal therapy or oral substances containing, for example, cellulose. Surgical intervention is sometimes indicated in instances of morbid obesity. A variety of surgical procedures is available and most are aimed at reducing the capacity of the stomach.

EATING DISORDERS

The two most recognised disorders of eating are anorexia nervosa and bulimia nervosa. Anorexia nervosa is characterised by self-imposed starvation and consequent emaciation. Body image, with a consequential loss of weight, becomes the client's prime focus and is the result of a belief that their body is too fat, even when extreme emaciation is evident. Bulimia nervosa is characterised by episodes of 'bingeing' on large quantities of food, followed by purging with laxatives or self-induced vomiting.

The causes of both disorders are difficult to determine, but most experts agree that they result from an interaction of biological, psychological and sociocultural factors. Treatment, which is difficult and varied, includes behaviour modification, psychotherapy and, in some cases, hospitalisation until the desired weight is achieved.

NUTRIENT LOSS AS A RESULT OF VOMITING

Vomiting, if prolonged, may result in significant nutrient deficiency, dehydration and electrolyte disturbance. To correct the imbalance, oral, enteral, IV therapy or total parenteral nutrition (TPN) may be indicated. Vomiting is not a disease itself but is a symptom of disease and may occur as a result of:

- Diseases of the stomach, intestines, liver, biliary system, pancreas or peritoneum
- Hypersensitivity to certain foods
- Ingestion or presence of irritants
- Acidosis, either metabolic or respiratory
- Pain
- Adverse reaction to, or a side effect of, certain medications
- Hormonal changes during early pregnancy
- Disturbances of equilibrium (e.g. travel sickness, vestibulitis)
- Disorders of the central nervous system (e.g. concussion, cerebral oedema, brain tumours)
- Psychological factors (e.g. apprehension, unpleasant sights or smells).

Vomiting (emesis) is the expulsion of the stomach or small intestinal contents and is a reflex action caused by stimulation of the emesis centre in the medulla oblongata. When this centre is stimulated the glottis and nasopharynx close, the cardiac sphincter of the stomach relaxes and contractions of the diaphragm and abdominal muscles occur. As a result of the increased intra-abdominal pressure, the stomach or intestinal contents are forced upwards and are expelled through the mouth. Vomiting may be preceded by a feeling of sickness (nausea) and accompanied by salivation, sweating and pallor. In conditions such as intestinal or sphincter obstruction, 'projectile' vomiting may occur, in which the vomited material is ejected with great force.

Vomiting should be assessed in terms of the nature of vomiting (effortless or projectile) and the characteristics of the material vomited (vomitus). Observations made of the vomitus may assist in determining the cause of vomiting and include observations of the:

- Consistency: the vomitus may consist of fluid, partially digested or undigested food
- Colour: vomitus may vary in colour from clear to yellow, to brown or green. The presence of bile tends to colour vomitus yellow or green and may indicate propulsion of the contents of the small intestine into the stomach
- Presence of blood: blood may be present as bright red streaks or clots, or may have a 'coffee grounds' appearance. The latter occurs when blood has been partially digested by gastric acid secretions. Vomiting of blood is called haematemesis. Forceful vomiting may induce blood-stained vomit (e.g. Weismann's tear)
- Odour: vomitus is usually sour smelling, but a 'faecal' odour indicates reflux of bowel contents due to an intestinal obstruction (e.g. paralytic ileus)
- Quantity: if possible, vomitus should be measured in millilitres to assess the amount of fluid being lost, particularly if haematemesis is present.

Key aspects related to care of a client who is vomiting include:

- If the client is sitting, place an emesis bowl under the chin and position a towel to protect clothes and bedding
- If the client is lying down, lift and turn the head to one side to reduce the risk of aspiration
- Ensure privacy, as clients will feel distressed and embarrassed by the incident
- Ensure dentures do not become dislodged
- The nurse should stay with the client to provide comfort and support, to ensure aspiration is recognised or prevented, and to splint a wound or area of pain to reduce further pain or dehiscence of wounds, if present
- The vomitus should be removed as soon as the episode is over to reduce the risk of a recurrence caused by the sight, smell or thought of the vomitus
- Soiled linen or clothing should be changed and removed immediately from the room
- Hands and face should be washed to refresh the client and to remove any vomitus
- Oral hygiene should be attended to by cleaning teeth, plates or dentures and providing a suitable mouth rinse to eliminate any unpleasant aftertaste
- The client should be assisted into a position of comfort and permitted to rest quietly
- The nurse should report and document the incident so that appropriate nursing or medical actions may be implemented. An antiemetic medication may be prescribed by a medical officer and administered to reduce nausea and to prevent further vomiting.

ALTERNATIVE METHODS TO MEET NUTRITIONAL NEEDS

An alternative method of meeting nutritional needs may be indicated when a client is unable to consume food or fluid orally. Alternative methods include total parenteral nutrition (TPN), intravenous therapy, and tube feeding via orogastric, nasogastric, nasoduodenal, nasojejunal, gastrostomy, gastroduodenal or gastrojejunal tubes.

TOTAL PARENTERAL NUTRITION (TPN)

Sometimes referred to as hyperalimentation, TPN involves the parenteral administration of a complete nutritional preparation that contains high concentrations of essential nutrients and may include intralipid solutions, containing fats. This method of feeding may be indicated when it is not possible for the client's nutritional needs to be met via the digestive tract.

Hypertonic solutions are administered through a catheter that has been inserted into a large vein, such as the subclavian vein. The solution containing nutrients enters directly into the bloodstream. TPN solutions administered by this route provide a medium for rapid bacterial growth and, because the tubing provides access for the entry of microorganisms, contamination and septicaemia must be prevented. The catheter is inserted by a medical officer using sterile equipment and technique. Care of the equipment throughout the course of treatment requires strict asepsis.

Management of a client who is receiving TPN is the responsibility of the Registered Nurse (RN), and the client must be monitored continually to prevent or detect possible complications. Complications that may result from TPN include:

- Hyperglycaemia or hypoglycaemia
- Fluid and electrolyte imbalance
- Catheter-related septicaemia
- Infection of the catheter site
- Extravasation of blood from the vein as a result of catheter trauma
- Air emboli
- Liver failure
- Diarrhoea or constipation.

The nurse may be required to assist with the care of a client receiving TPN and must be aware of the scope of their role in promoting safety and comfort.

INTRAVENOUS THERAPY

Intravenous therapy involves the introduction of a solution or solutions into a peripheral or central vein. Information about intravenous therapy is provided in Chapter 30.

ENTERAL TUBE FEEDING

Naso-enteric tubes are orogastric, nasogastric, naso-duodenal or nasojejunal tubes used to administer a range of nutritional feeds to a client for a variety of reasons, including:

- Malabsorption (e.g. inflammatory bowel disorders)
- Surgery (e.g. oral or throat surgery)
- Central nervous system disorders (e.g. paraplegia, unconsciousness, pharyngeal paralysis)
- Metabolic disorders (e.g. hyperinsulinaemia, hypoglycaemia)
- Food refusal or dysphagia, when the client is too ill or weak to eat normally.

The nurse should be aware of the policies and regulations regarding their role and responsibilities in checking the location of the tip of the enteral tube, and infection-control policies, in their health care setting. For information on insertion of a nasogastric tube refer to Table 31.5.

TABLE 31.5 | PROCEDURE FOR INSERTING A NASOGASTRIC TUBE

Review and carry out standard steps in Appendix 1

Action	Rationale
Validate the medical orders in the patient record	Ensures correct procedure is about to take place
Explain the procedure to the clients	Reduces anxiety and gains client's consent and cooperation
Critically think through your assessment data and problem solving, e.g. provide privacy, comfort measures, pain relief	Evaluating each aspect and its relationship to other data will help identify specific problems and modifications of the procedure that may be needed for the individual
Prepare equipment	
Locate and gather the equipment including suction equipment or equipment related to providing nutrition as indicated prior to beginning the procedure. In addition to the tube, you will need the following: • Clean gloves • Water-soluble lubricant • Emesis basin • Tape or adhesive bandage (such as a Coverlet) • Tissues • Bath towel • A glass of water and straw • Large syringe with an adapter or a bulb syringe • Stethoscope • Rubber band and safety pin	Ensures all equipment is at client's bedside to maximise efficiency, reduce apprehension on the client's part and increases the confidence in the nurse
Assist the client into the high Fowler's position unless contraindicated	Facilitates tube insertion and reduces risk of gastro-oesophageal reflux and aspiration
Wash and dry hands	Prevents cross infection and contamination of tubing
Don appropriate equipment and clothing as per infection control protocols	Minimises risk of cross infection

(Continued)

TABLE 31.5 | PROCEDURE FOR INSERTING A NASOGASTRIC TUBE—cont'd

Action	Rationale
Implementation	
Explain the procedure and why it is needed	Ask the patient if either nostril is obstructed (history of broken nose, deviated septum, or nasal surgery)
Raise the bed to the appropriate working position based on your height and assess the patient's nostrils	Ask the patient to breathe through one nostril while occluding the other will help ascertain if one nostril has an occlusion
Measure the portion of tube to be inserted by extending it from the tip of the patient's nose to the earlobe and from the earlobe to the xyphoid process	Determines the insertion length of the tube to ensure the tube is inserted an adequate distance so that the distal tip rests in the stomach
Mark the tube with tape at this point	The use of lubricant will ease insertion by decreasing friction
Lubricate the first 6–10 cm of the tube with water-soluble lubricant. *Note*: Some small-bore tubes self-lubricate when dipped in water	Insertion of the NGT can stimulate the Gag reflex
Grasp the tube with your right hand and gently insert it into the nostril, guiding it straight back along the floor of the nose. Have an emesis basin and tissues in the patient's lap	Flexing the head forward allows the NGT to follow the posterior wall of the nasopharynx and enter the oesophagus rather than the trachea
Next, ask the patient to tilt the head slightly forward	The muscular movement of swallowing helps advance the NGT
Have the patient sip water (if not contraindicated) and swallow while you gently but steadily advance the tube	
When the tube has been advanced as far as the tape marker, secure the tube to the patient's nose using tape or the adhesive bandage	Ensures the tube does not move out of the stomach
Place a vertical strip down the bridge of the nose Cut the lower end of the tape into two 'tails' and wrap them around the tube	
Check for proper placement of the NGT. Follow the protocol for the techniques required at your facility (auscultation, aspiration, X-ray)	Ensures the NGT is in the correct location and not in the trachea
Lower the bed, make the client comfortable and dispose of used equipment Wash or disinfect your hands To provide enteral nutrition, see Table 31.6 Care required before starting a feed	Increases the client's psychological comfort and reduces the material that can be media for growing bacteria
Report and document the procedure and any complications	Documentation increases the communication between health care professionals and complies with legal requirements for reporting change

Nasogastric tubes

Feeds given by a nasogastric tube inserted via the nares into the stomach (Figure 31.5) are normally administered to clients who experience short-term difficulties in nutrition, or when surgically placed tubes such as gastrostomy tubes (see below) may be contraindicated by the client's physical condition.

Nasoduodenal and nasojejunal tubes

Tubes placed into the duodenum or jejunum are used for clients with gastric disorders that contraindicate gastric placement, such as severe reflux, partial or total gastrectomy, and malabsorption.

Gastrostomy tubes

Feeding via a gastrostomy tube may be indicated if there has been recent surgery or an obstruction in the upper part of the digestive tract, or as a long-term treatment for feeding difficulties. A gastrostomy tube is a hollow tube, often composed of silicone, inserted through the abdomen into the stomach by a surgeon either through an external approach, via an incision through the abdominal wall, or endoscopically via the mouth through the stomach and through the abdominal wall. The opening around the tube may be sutured to prevent leakage or accidental removal (Figure 31.6), or held in place by the use of an inflatable balloon and a flange or similar device that applies pressure to hold the tube against the inside wall of the stomach.

Gastrostomy (percutaneous endoscopic gastrostomy [PEG]) and jejunostomy (percutaneous endoscopic jejunostomy [PEJ]) devices are used for long-term nutritional support, generally more than 6–8 weeks (Kozier et al 2000). Fluid enteral feeds are normally introduced 24 hours later through the tube, into the lumen of the

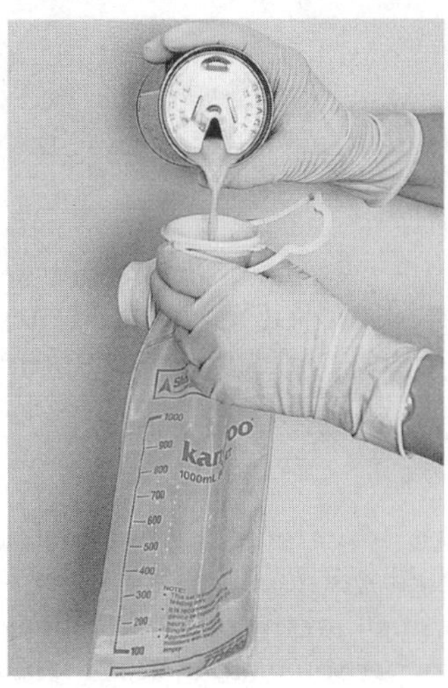

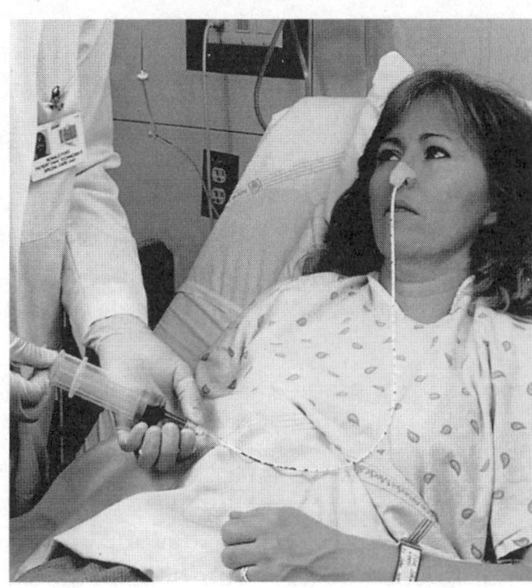

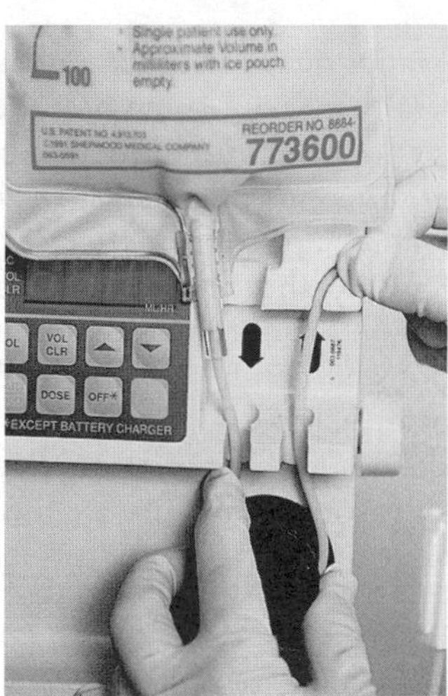

Figure 31.5 | Administering enteral feeds via nasogastric tubes *(Potter & Perry 2001, 2008)*

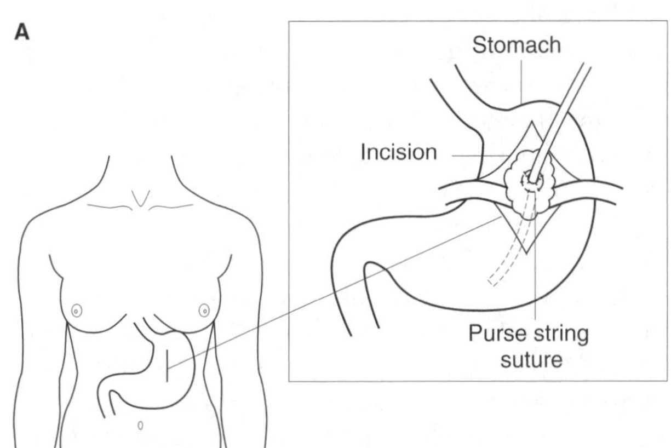

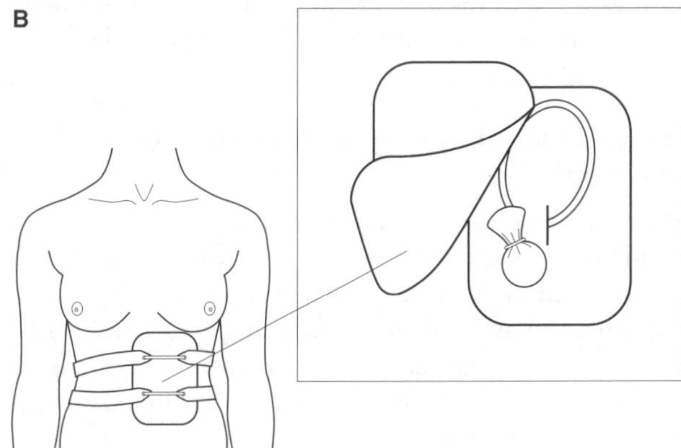

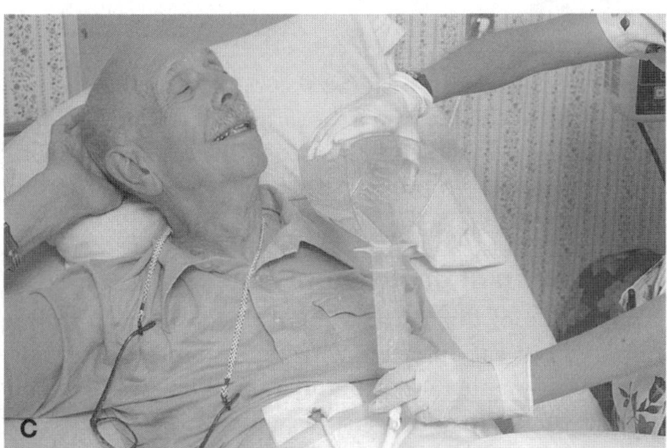

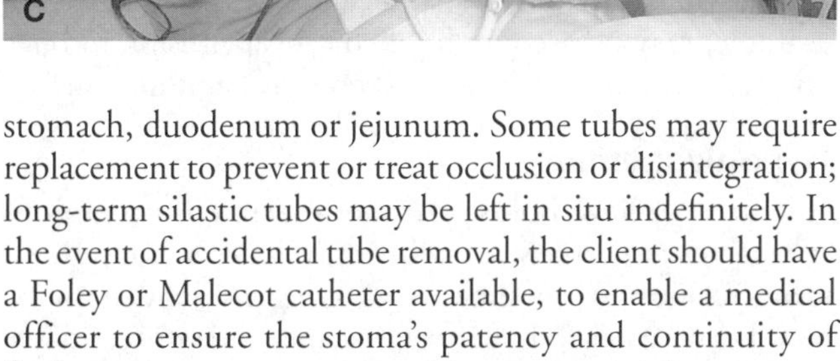

Figure 31.6 | Gastrostomy feeding. **A**: Gastrostomy incision and procedure. **B**: When not in use the end of the tube is covered by sterile gauze then covered by a pad held in place with straps. **C**: Pouring the feeding formula into a syringe connected to the gastrostomy tube *(deWit 2001, 2005)*

stomach, duodenum or jejunum. Some tubes may require replacement to prevent or treat occlusion or disintegration; long-term silastic tubes may be left in situ indefinitely. In the event of accidental tube removal, the client should have a Foley or Malecot catheter available, to enable a medical officer to ensure the stoma's patency and continuity of feed.

Prepared enteral feeds are administered either by:

- Intermittent or bolus feeds, in which a solution is administered at regular intervals (e.g. every 4 hours). Administered to clients who are able to tolerate volumes at a rate they could normally drink orally. A syringe or giving set is attached to the end of the nasogastric tube and filled with the feed or fluid, which is allowed to flow in slowly by gravity or by the use of an enteral feeding pump. The rate of administration can be adjusted; for example, by the height at which the syringe or set is held at, or by adjusting the enteral pumping rate
- Continuous feeds, in which a gravity infusion set or a controlled enteral feeding pump is used that can deliver the fluid at a regulated rate over a predetermined time. Continuous feeds are administered to clients who have experienced difficulty in tolerating bolus doses, or for clients with malabsorption, reactive hyperinsulinaemia, diarrhoea or other metabolic problems.

Depending on the institution and the nutrition required, the enteral feed may come pre-packaged, for example in cans, and will not require refrigeration, while other solutions stored in containers such as waxed cardboard or made in-house do require refrigeration.

The nurse should be aware of the policies and regulations in their health care setting regarding their role and responsibilities in checking the location of the tip of the nasogastric tube.

Guidelines for administering enteral feeds via a naso-enteric or gastro-enteric tube are listed in Table 31.6.

CARE SPECIFIC TO GASTROSTOMY TYPE TUBES

For clients who may be discharged home or to encourage independence with enteral tubes in situ, the client may be taught how to test, administer and perform the care required independently. Part of the education involves discussing some of the complications and how to deal with them, as described below.

Care and cleaning of gastrostomy tube and equipment

Abdominal distension. Determine tube position by testing the aspirate with pH-sensitive paper. Before administering an enteral feed or fluid, gas may be vented (released) from the stomach to avoid distension. Venting is achieved by removing a spigot, unscrewing a cap and/or releasing an obstructive clamp, or by inserting a catheter and raising the tube to a vertical position.

Hanging times. In a warm environment, feeds can be contaminated by pathogens. The maximum hanging times are 2–4 hours for immunocomprimised clients, and 4 hours in a clinical setting. For clients at home the time can be extended to about 6–8 hours, depending on the type of feed and the client's condition.

Cleaning. Feeding equipment, syringes, etc, can be washed with warm soapy water and left to air dry and can be used for 3 days. The equipment should be washed again in warm soapy water immediately before each use.

Skin care

The area around the gastrostomy site requires daily cleaning with warm soapy water to remove build-up of secretions from the stoma site and to prevent infection. The tube and the surrounding pressure device should be rotated in the stoma daily to prevent adhesion or ulceration of the surrounding skin. The skin around the site should be inspected for redness, oozing, swelling or bleeding.

COMMON PROBLEMS ASSOCIATED WITH GASTROSTOMY TUBES

Tube blockage

Occasionally tubes can become blocked because of inadequate flushing, feeds being too thick or the administration of certain crushed medications. To unblock the tube, a volume of 10–20 mL of sterile water can be administered into the tube or by 'milking' (squeezing and stretching the tube).

Bleeding

Bleeding may indicate the presence of an infection or trauma to the tube. Bleeding is stopped by localised pressure or 'stomahesive' dressing, and the incident documented and reported.

Redness

Localised redness with or without swelling may indicate inflammation from acidic gastric contents due, for example, to the tube being too small for the stoma, the flange being too loose on the skin, or perishing or bursting of the balloon in the stomach. Any ooze can be checked for acidity using pH-sensitive paper. If acid is detected, a waterproof cream can be applied to prevent further irritation of the skin by acid. The use of dressings to soak up the fluid or topical antacids may cause further skin breakdown. The size of the tube and the flange's location needs to be checked daily to prevent migration. An indelible pen can be used to mark the lower limit of the tube, and the measurement is recorded on the care plan. In some cases a client may require a tube to be replaced with a larger-diameter one.

Complications with tubes or flanges are reported to a medical officer or a stomal therapist. In some situations, particularly after surgery, primary and or secondary peritonitis may be caused by inadequate pressure from the flange and balloon and subsequent poor sealing of underlying tissues.

Diarrhoea

If the feeds are administered too rapidly or the client is intolerant to the feed, diarrhoea may develop. This may be minimised by slowing the rate of the feed or changing the feed type. If symptoms persist a medical officer should be contacted.

Granulation of gastrostomy site

Granulation of the surrounding tissue occurs as a healing response but can interfere with the comfort of the tube. To prevent granulation the stoma should be washed daily and the tube turned daily. Application of silver nitrate, for example, may be used under medical supervision to burn off the 'proud flesh' (tissue with excessive granulation).

Hypoglycaemia

Clients who have bolus feeds administered too rapidly, excessive quantities, or who may have a lax pyloric sphincter are at risk of the feeds entering the duodenum too rapidly and causing hyperinsulinaemia and consequential hypoglycaemia.

Clinical Interest Box 31.4 lists some possible nursing diagnoses relating to clients with altered nutrition.

TABLE 31.6 | CARE REQUIRED BEFORE STARTING AN ENTERAL FEED

Review and carry our the standard steps in Appendix 1

Action	Rationale
Check medical/dietitian orders to ascertain type, frequency and amount of fluid to be administered, and time period	Ensures correct quantities are given to meet the client's nutritional needs
Explain the procedure to the client	Reduces anxiety/apprehension and gains client's consent and co-operation
Assist the client, if required, into a high Fowler's position unless contraindicated	Facilitates digestion and reduces the risk of gastro-oesophageal reflux and aspiration
Prepare equipment	
Wash and dry hands	Prevents cross-infection and contamination of enteral feed or tubing
Don appropriate equipment or clothing as per infection-control guidelines	Minimises risk of cross-infection
Feed is warmed to room temperature	Administration of cold fluids may cause abdominal discomfort
Feeds shaken	Eliminates any separation of the constituents
Assemble and place equipment in a convenient location	Facilitates access during the procedure and minimises contamination of enteral feed or tubing
Feeding using a syringe	
Remove the spigot or cap from the end of the enteral tube and attach the syringe and gently aspirate. With some gastrostomy devices a special connector may be required to connect to a syringe or giving set	Prevents the tube collapsing or trauma to the mucosa
Measure aspirate of stomach contents	Establishes whether the previous feed has been absorbed
Determine tube position by testing aspirate with pH-sensitive paper, abdominal X-ray or use of a portable global-type positioning system radiological device such as the Cathlocater, which provides a rapid bedside method of accurately proving the tip position	The position of the tube must be verified by a Registered Nurse (RN) or medical officer before starting the feed Administration of the solution through a malpositioned tube through the nasal route can cause feed to enter the lungs, pleura, brain, oesophageal wall or duodenum pH is measured by pH-sensitive paper and should be between 0 and 4 to better ensure correct placement in the stomach. (The pH may rise if the client is treated with antacid or gastric acid inhibitors.) Aspirates of naso-duodenal or jejunal tubes would normally have a higher pH, e.g. > 7.0 False pH readings may affect accurate determination of enteral tube tip placement
Return volumes less than 150 mL (adult). Notify medical officer if volumes greater than 150 mL (adult)	Aspirate is usually replaced in the stomach, as it contains important digestive substances and proteins that aid in, e.g. vitamin B12 transport. Residual volumes > 150 mL may indicate malabsorption or partial or total bowel obstruction
Connect the syringe to the enteral tube before filling, and refill to ensure that the syringe does not completely empty of feed	Prevents entry of air into the gastrointestinal tract and subsequent abdominal distension and discomfort
Regulate the rate by changing the height of the syringe to allow the feed to flow slowly by gravity	A feed administered too rapidly may cause nausea and discomfort or dumping syndrome (hyperinsulinaemia). Correct height of the syringe ensures that the feed will flow without slowing or stopping
Administer the total volume ordered unless the client is unable to tolerate the volume	Ensures that only the prescribed volume is administered, to prevent discomfort, reflux, vomiting or aspiration and to maintain client's nutritional status

(Continued)

TABLE 31.6 | CARE REQUIRED BEFORE STARTING AN ENTERAL FEED—cont'd

Action	Rationale
Feeding using an intermittent or continuous enteral giving set	
Follow steps on previous page up to end of 'Prepare equipment' section	
For intermittent or continuous enteral feeds, pre-fill the giving set to remove air from the tubing and hang the bag at the desired height	Prevents entry of air into the gastrointestinal tract and subsequent abdominal distension and discomfort. Correct height of bag or giving set ensures that the feed will flow without slowing or stopping
If using a pump, thread tubing through the pump guides and set rate, limits and alarms	Pre-setting alarms will allow the nurse to refill the giving set to ensure nutritional goals are reached
When using a giving set or pump, ensure that there is sufficient feed in the giving set for the prescribed time or volume	Preventing the bag or giving set from emptying will prevent air from entering the stomach or the intestine causing gastric distension and discomfort
Securely connect the giving set to the tube. Note: a special connector tube may be required for some gastrostomy tubes. Tape or a pin may be required to connect the tubing together or to the client's clothes	Prevents accidental disconnection of the giving set and subsequent loss of nutrients and gastric contents
Administer the total volume ordered, unless contraindicated. If using a pump, set the required volume alarm to register completion at the prescribed time or volume	Ensures that only the prescribed volume is administered to prevent discomfort, reflux, vomiting or aspiration and to maintain client's nutritional status
Disconnecting the feed	
On completion of the feed (both naso- or gastro-enteral tubes) clamp the tube and remove the syringe or giving set.	Maintains the patency and reduces bacterial colonisation of the tube Volumes of water are, e.g. 5–10 mL for infants and children, 10–50 mL for adults, depending on fluid restrictions. Refer to institution's protocols. Prevents leakage of solution or stomach secretions Note: the immunocomprimised or infants may require sterile water for flushing
Introduce a small amount of water after administration of the feed	Ensure that gastric contents do not leak from inadequately sealed tubes
Disconnect the syringe and securely reinsert the spigot or cap	Assists in digestion and reduces the risk of reflux and regurgitation
Encourage the client to remain sitting up for about 30 minutes after completion of a bolus feed	Prevents blockage of tube or pathogen invasion
Remove and attend to the equipment, rinsing giving sets and syringes	Giving sets may be used for periods of up to 3 days, depending on the clinical institution's policies and the client's condition
Report and document the procedure and any complications	Enable appropriate care to be planned

CLINICAL INTEREST BOX 31.4
Nursing diagnoses relating to clients with nutrition alterations

- Aspiration, risk for in enteral nutrition
- Constipation
- Diarrhoea
- Fluid volume deficit
- Fluid volume excess
- Impaired skin integrity
- Infant feeding pattern, ineffective
- Infection
- Knowledge deficit
- Nutrition, altered: less than body requirements
- Nutrition, altered: more than body requirements
- Self-care deficit feeding

SUMMARY

Nutrition is necessary for the development and growth of cells and for the replacement of substances required by the cells to maintain efficient body function. A diet that contains the essential nutrients is essential throughout each stage of the lifespan, and people should be encouraged to follow the principles of good nutrition and to eat a balanced healthy diet. Food provides energy that is necessary for all the chemical and physical activities of the body. Energy requirements vary according to age, sex, body composition and presence of ailments or conditions. Each nutrient performs a specific function, and a nutrient deficiency may result in body dysfunction.

Many factors influence a client's eating pattern, and choice of foods and illness may necessitate certain changes in dietary intake. Modification to the consistency of food may be indicated, or a specific diet may be prescribed for therapeutic purposes. The nurse should assist clients to meet their nutritional needs and the nurse may need to assist or feed a client who is unable to feed themselves. If a client is unable to consume food or fluid orally, an alternative method of meeting their nutritional needs may be necessary.

Problems associated with nutrition should be identified so that appropriate medical, nursing and dietitian care can be planned and implemented to meet the client's nutritional needs.

REVIEW EXERCISES

1. What is the usual preferred diet for an adult client?
2. How many kilojoules are required per day for adequate nutrition?
3. Describe what essential amino acids are.
4. List the fat-soluble vitamins.
5. Differentiate between lacto-vegetarian and vegan dietary requirements.
6. Describe what the glycaemic index diet refers to.
7. What condition does faecal halitosis indicate?
8. What complications can a client with a gastrostomy tube be afflicted by?
9. Discuss the care of a client with a gastrostomy tube that is leaking acid onto the skin.
10. What volume of fluids would an infant normally ingest to maintain normal growth and development?
11. What is the correct method for differentiating whether a nasogastric tube is located in the stomach or duodenum?

CRITICAL THINKING EXERCISES

1. An 8-week-old infant is admitted for failure to thrive, food refusal and poor oral intake, and irritability. On numerous occasions the baby had posseted (vomited a small amount) both during and after feeds. The mother has had two previous births, and both babies were successfully breastfed and had no feeding, sleep or growth problems. The mother appears tired and states that she is apprehensive that the infant is not taking enough fluid orally and that the infant's and her sleep is now increasingly being disrupted. What would you discuss with her and her medical officer?
2. Mrs Jones is admitted by her medical practitioner for continued weight loss, which she has noticed over a period of 2 months. Her original weight was 70 kg but has now dropped to 52 kg, although she reports that she is eating the same amount, if not more food than before. Recently she has noticed some problems with swallowing and excessive loss of hair. Her pulse is elevated and she appears anxious and is warm to touch. The provisional diagnosis is hyperthyroidism. What care would you arrange to assist in planning, regaining and then maintaining her weight?
3. Mr Rogers, 72, has had frequent bouts of constipation and is being treated with iron-replacement therapy for blood loss from diverticulitis. What diet and care would you recommend to reduce the constipation but maintain iron stores, without affecting the severity of the diverticulitis?
4. Miss Peters, 24, who is also a strict vegan, is hospitalised for severe abdominal pain and dysmenorrhoea. She asks you for jugs of ice to chew on, although she is allowed clear fluids. You suspect pagophagia as a result of blood loss. What other signs or symptoms may reinforce your diagnosis of anaemia and what plan would you devise to prove the anaemia and improve her blood count?

REFERENCES AND FURTHER READING

Baumberger-Henry M (2008) *Fluids & Electrolytes Made Incredibly Easy*, 2nd edn. Lippincott Williams & Wilkins, Ambler

Bender DA (2008) *Introduction to Nutrition and Metabolism*, 3rd edn. Taylor and Francis, New York

Coulston AM & Boushey CJ (2008) *Nutrition in the Prevention and Treatment of Disease*. Academic Press, Amsterdam; Boston

deWit SC (2001) *Fundamental Concepts and Skills for Nursing*. WB Saunders, Philadelphia

—— (2005) *Fundamental Concepts and Skills for Nursing*, 2nd edn. WB Saunders, Philadelphia

Edmunds M (2002) *Introduction to Clinical Pharmacology*, 3rd edn. Mosby, New York

Gibney MJ, Voster H, Kok FJ (2002) *Introduction to Human Nutrition*. Blackwell Publishing, Melbourne

Grosvenor MB, Smolin LA (2002) *Nutrition from Science to Life*. Harcourt Inc, Orlando

Kok F, Bouwman L & Des F (2008) *Personalized Nutrition: Principles and Applications*. Taylor & Francis, London

Kozier B, Erb G, Berman AJ, Burke K (2000) *Fundamentals of Nursing: Concepts, Process and Practice*, 6th edn. Prentice-Hall Inc, Upper Saddle River, New Jersey

Mann J, Truswell AS (2007) *Essentials of Human Nutrition*, 3rd edn. Oxford University Press, New York

Mitchell MK (2003) *Nutrition Across the Life Span*, 2nd edn, WB Saunders Co, Philadelphia

Potter PA, Perry AG (2001) *Fundamentals of Nursing*, 5th edn. Mosby, St Louis

—— (2005) *Fundamentals of Nursing*, 6th edn. Mosby, St Louis

—— (2008) *Fundamentals of Nursing*, 7th edn. Mosby, St Louis

Rosenberg IH, Sastre A (2002) *Nutrition and Aging*, 10th edn. Harcourt, Edinburgh

Saxelby C (2002) *Nutrition for Life*, 4th edn. Hardie Grant Books, Melbourne

University of New South Wales (2007) *High Rates of Malnutrition in the Elderly*. Online. Available: http://www.unsw.edu.au/news/pad/articles/2007/may/malnutrition.html [accessed 25 May 2008]

Wahlqvist ML (2002) *Australian and New Zealand Food and Nutrition*, 2nd edn. Unwin Pty Ltd, Sydney

Whitney EN, Rolfes SR (2002) *Understanding Nutrition*, 9th edn. Wadsworth Group, Belmont

Wiseman G (2002) *Nutrition and Health*. Taylor & Francis, New York

ONLINE RESOURCES

ABC Radio National: www.abc.net.au/rn

CSIRO nutrition information: www.csiro.au (search using 'nutrition')
Dietitians Association of Australia: www.daa.asn.au
Family Practice Notebook: www.fpnotebook.com/PHA44.htm
Food Standards Australia and New Zealand: www.foodstandards.gov.au
Foodwatch: www.foodwatch.com.au
Healthy Eating Club: www.healthyeatingclub.com
Health Insite: www.healthinsite.gov.au
Images of nursing feeding equipment: www.dinainternational.com/russian/hitex/web
Mayo Clinic: www.mayohealth.org
Micronix: www.micronix.com.au
Nasogastric tube placement. American Academy of Family Physicians: www.aafp.org/afp/20001115/tips/12.html
National Heart Foundation: www.heartfoundation.com.au
National Institutes of Health: www.nih.gov/
Nutrition and Food Sciences: www.nutritionandfoodsciences.org
Nutrition Australia: www.nutritionaustralia.org
Nutrition News Focus: www.nutritionnewsfocus.com
Queensland Diagnostic Imaging: www.qdixray.com.au/Procedures.htm
US Food and Nutrition Information Center, at the National Agricultural Library: www.nalusda.gov/fnic
US Food and Nutrition Information Center. Food pyramids: www.nal.usda.gov/fnic/Fpyr/pyramid.html

Chapter 32

URINARY ELIMINATION

OBJECTIVES

- Define the key terms/concepts
- Describe the transport mechanisms in the body related to the urinary system
- Explain homeostasis as related to the urinary system
- Name the parts of the urinary system and describe the structure and function of each part
- Identify the factors that affect urinary elimination, and associated problems
- Describe the different types of urinary incontinence and possible causes
- Describe the major manifestations of urinary system disorders
- State the diagnostic tests used to assess urinary system function
- Assist in planning and implementing nursing care for the client with a urinary system disorder

KEY TERMS/CONCEPTS

bladder
Bowman's capsule
cortex
glomerulus
kidney
medulla
micturition
nephron
tubules
ureter
urethra

CHAPTER FOCUS

The urinary system is responsible for maintaining homeostasis as well as eliminating some waste products of body metabolism. Many factors can affect voiding and result in alteration to this system. Nursing management of clients with urinary elimination disorders requires sensitivity and maintenance of client dignity as well as specific nursing skills.

LIVED EXPERIENCE

It is so embarrassing going to a urologist and having him examine me. The tests were even worse, as I had to have X-rays taken while I was passing urine. The nursing staff were sensitive and caring; one in particular, Joan, really helped me through what is still one of the worst experiences of my life.

Ray, age 56, after an intravenous pyelogram

THE URINARY SYSTEM

As a result of cellular metabolism, various waste products are produced. The urinary system plays a major role in the elimination of metabolic waste products and toxic substances and in regulating the rates of elimination of water and electrolytes from the body. By regulating the volume of the body fluid, the urinary system helps maintain blood pressure and the electrolyte content and pH of the blood. Because of this role, the kidneys are considered to perform one of the major homeostatic functions of the body. The urinary system (Figure 32.1) consists of the kidneys, which filter blood; the ureters, which transport urine to the bladder; and the bladder, which stores the urine until it is excreted through the urethra.

THE KIDNEYS

The kidneys are two bean-shaped organs situated behind the peritoneum on the posterior wall of the abdominal cavity, on either side of the vertebral column. The kidneys extend from about the twelfth thoracic vertebra to the third lumbar vertebra. The right kidney is situated a little lower than the left because of the space occupied by the liver.

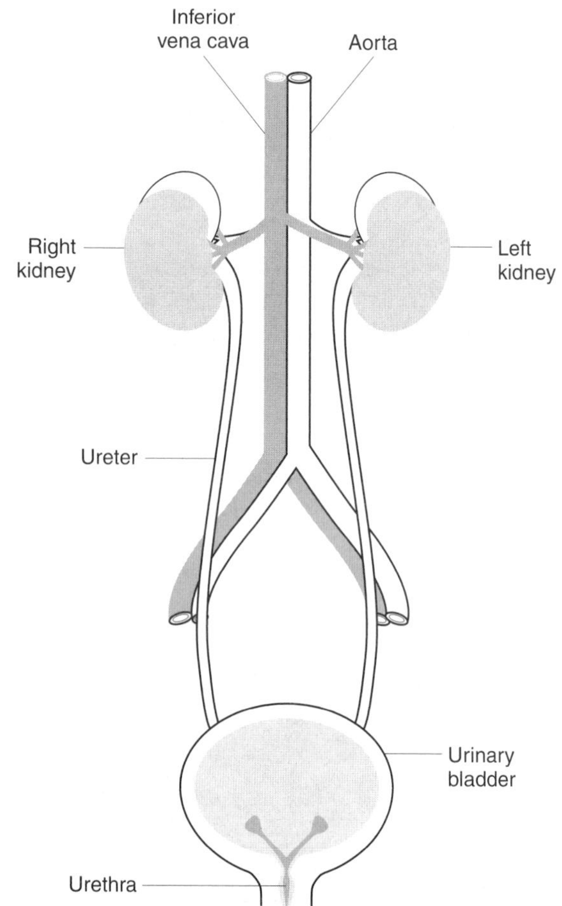

Figure 32.1 | The urinary system

GROSS STRUCTURE OF THE KIDNEY

A kidney (Figure 32.2) weighs 120–170 g, is 10–13 cm in length, 5–6 cm wide and 3–4 cm thick. The kidneys are protected and supported by renal fascia and by layers of perirenal fat. Three layers of tissue surround each kidney:

1. The fibrous renal capsule, covering the surface of the kidney
2. The adipose capsule, a layer of perirenal fat surrounding the renal capsule
3. The renal fascia, which surrounds and encloses the kidney and adipose capsule and anchors the kidney to the posterior abdominal wall.

The kidney consists of three general regions (Figure 32.2):

1. The cortex — the outer portion, lying directly beneath the renal capsule. This highly vascular area of tissue is reddish-brown in colour
2. The medulla — the inner portion, consisting of 8–18 triangular renal pyramids. It is purplish in colour. The apices of the renal pyramids open into the calyces. A calyx is a funnel-shaped extension of the renal pelvis
3. The pelvis — the inner portion formed by the dilated upper end of the ureter.

A deep indentation, the hilus, is present on the medial border of the kidney. It is from the hilus that the ureter emerges. The renal vein and the renal artery also pass through the hilus. The renal artery branches from the aorta to transport oxygenated blood to the kidney. The renal vein transports deoxygenated blood from the kidney to the inferior vena cava.

MICROSCOPIC STRUCTURE OF THE KIDNEY

The nephron

Each kidney contains at least 1 million nephrons, together with their collecting tubules or ducts. The nephron is the functional unit of the kidney. Each nephron (Figure 32.3)

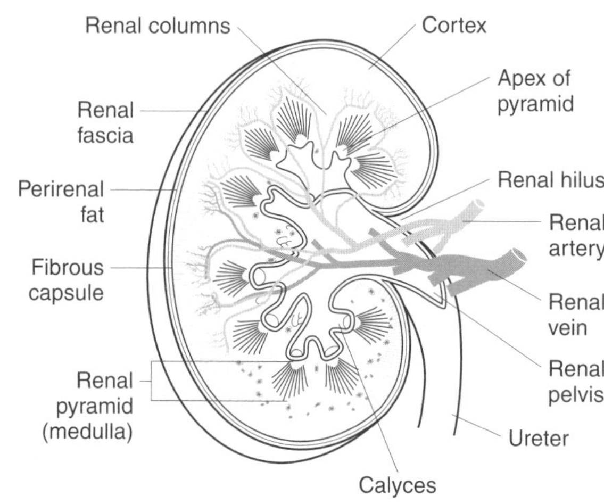

Figure 32.2 | Macroscopic structure of the kidney

is composed of a vascular and tubular system that allows for the formation of urine. The nephrons are located in the renal tissue, with most in the cortex and some extending deep into the medulla of the kidney. A nephron consists of several anatomically distinct regions:

- The glomerulus, located in the cortex and composed of a tuft of capillaries inserted into the horseshoe-shaped origin of the renal tube (the Bowman's capsule). The outer wall of the Bowman's capsule is composed of flattened squamous epithelium. The inner layer is made up of very specialised cells that form a semi-permeable membrane surrounding the glomerulus
- The proximal convoluted tubule — the first part of the renal tubule, situated in the cortex
- The loop of Henle, which consists of the straight portion of the proximal tubule, the straight part of the distal tubule, and the loop that joins them
- The distal convoluted tubule — the last portion of the renal tubule, which empties into a straight collecting tubule in the cortex
- The collecting tubule, which joins with other collecting tubules in the inner medulla of the kidney to eventually open into the calyces.

Division of the efferent vessels (the arterioles that carry blood away from the capillaries) forms a second set of capillaries. The veins that collect blood from these capillaries unite to eventually form the renal vein.

FUNCTION OF THE KIDNEYS

The functions of the kidneys are to maintain homeostasis by:

- Filtering the blood to maintain its normal composition, volume and pH
- Eliminating filtered wastes from the blood
- Regulating blood pressure.

In carrying out these functions the kidneys excrete urine.

Formation of urine

The formation of urine occurs in three phases: simple filtration, selective reabsorption, and secretion. Filtration occurs through the semi-permeable walls of the glomerulus and Bowman's capsule. Blood enters the glomerular capillaries under relatively high pressure and is forced into the lumen of the Bowman's capsule. Water and small molecules pass through the semi-permeable walls, while blood cells, plasma proteins, and other large molecules are unable to pass through healthy capillary walls. The resultant glomerular filtrate is thus plasma minus the plasma proteins.

The major factor assisting filtration is the difference between the blood pressure in the glomerulus and the pressure of filtrate in the glomerular capsule. A capillary hydrostatic pressure of about 70 mmHg builds up in the glomerulus because the calibre of the efferent arteriole is less than that of the afferent arteriole. The capillary pressure is opposed by the lower osmotic pressure of the blood and the lower filtrate hydrostatic pressure in the glomerular capsule. The amount of dilute filtrate formed in 24 hours is about 100–150 L. The amount actually excreted as urine in 24 hours is about 1–1.5 L, so most of the volume of the filtrate is reabsorbed.

Selective reabsorption occurs as the filtered fluid flows through the renal tubules. During this phase, substances such as glucose, amino acids, hormones, mineral salts, vitamins and most of the water are reabsorbed into the blood. Not reabsorbed are some of the water, substances in

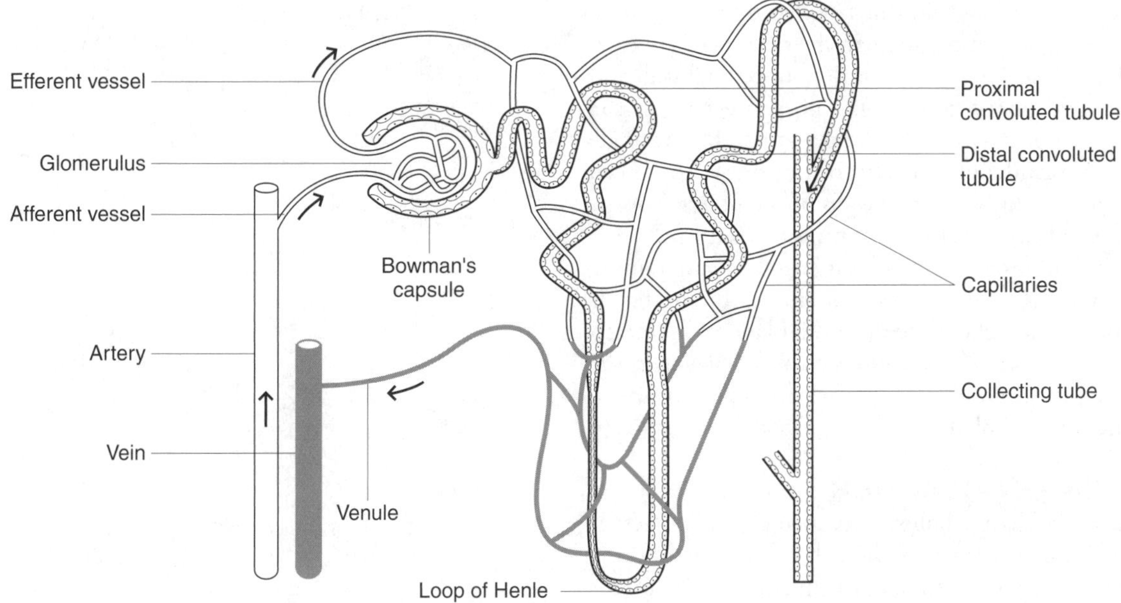

Figure 32.3 | The nephron

excess of body needs, and wastes, including drugs and toxic substances. Thus selective reabsorption helps to maintain fluid and electrolyte balance and blood pH.

Secretion is the process by which substances such as hydrogen and potassium ions move from the blood of the peritubular capillaries or from the tubule cells into the filtrate to be eliminated in urine. The fluid (urine) that flows from the collecting tubules contains substances not needed by the body. Urine flows into the pelvis of the kidneys for transport, via the ureters, to the urinary bladder.

Control of urine formation

The control of kidney function is both nervous and hormonal. Nervous control maintains the level of blood pressure required for filtration to occur. Hormonal control consists of:

- Adrenaline, secreted by the adrenal, or suprarenal, glands, which helps maintain the high level of blood pressure in the glomerulus
- Antidiuretic hormone (ADH), secreted by the pituitary gland, which controls the amount of water reabsorbed from the tubules
- Aldosterone, secreted by the suprarenal glands, which controls the tubules' reabsorption of mineral salts.

Composition of urine

Urine is a clear, amber-coloured slightly acidic fluid composed of 96% water, 2% urea and 2% mineral salts, uric acid and creatinine. Urea, uric acid and creatinine are waste products of protein metabolism. Mineral salts are excreted in the urine to maintain their normal level in the blood and to regulate the pH of the blood.

THE URETERS

The ureters are two narrow, thick-walled muscular tubes, 25–30 cm long, which originate in the renal pelvis of each kidney. They pass down the posterior abdominal wall and into the pelvic cavity to enter the posterior base of the bladder. The ureters enter the bladder at an oblique angle so that, as the bladder fills and contracts, urine is not forced back towards the kidneys. The walls of the ureters consist of an outer fibrous coat that is continuous with the renal capsule, a middle coat of involuntary muscle, and a lining of transitional epithelium. The function of the ureters is to carry urine from the kidneys to the bladder, by means of peristaltic action. The involuntary muscle layer in the walls of the ureters contract from 1–5 times per minute to force urine into the bladder.

THE URINARY BLADDER

The urinary bladder is a hollow muscular organ that acts as a reservoir for urine. It sits in the pelvic cavity behind the symphysis pubis. In the female it is in front of the uterus and in the male it sits in front of the rectum. The walls of the bladder consist of:

- A covering of peritoneum over the upper portion (the fundus)
- A layer of involuntary muscle
- A layer of connective tissue
- A lining of mucous membrane composed of transitional epithelium.

The trigone of the bladder is a triangle formed by the two ureteric orifices, where the ureters enter the bladder, and the urethral orifice, where the urethra leaves. Below the neck of the bladder lies the striated muscle that constitutes an external sphincter.

THE URETHRA

The urethra (Figure 32.4) is a muscular tube extending from the neck of the bladder to the external meatus. In the female the urethra is about 2.5–4 cm long and opens at the external urethral orifice in front of the vaginal opening. The external sphincter guards this opening. In the male, the urethra is about 15–20 cm long and opens at the tip of the penis. The male urethra has a double function: it forms a passage for urine as well as semen. It is guarded by an external sphincter immediately below the prostatic portion of the urethra. Near to the bladder, the urethra is lined with transitional epithelium that gives way to squamous epithelium. The function of the urethra is to provide a passage for urine from the bladder, out of the body.

MICTURITION

Micturition (or voiding) is the act of passing urine. Urine is carried down the ureters by peristaltic waves, each of which sends a spurt of urine into the bladder. While the normal capacity of the adult urinary bladder is about 450

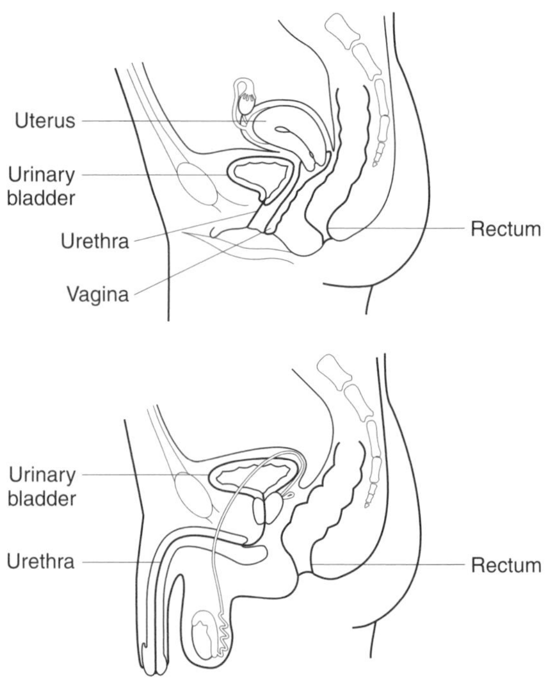

Figure 32.4 | Position of the male and female urethra

mL, the bladder is capable of expanding to hold larger amounts. The bladder fills slowly over a period of time and, when it holds about 300–500 mL, a desire to empty the bladder is experienced. A reflex initiated by impulses from stretch receptors in the bladder wall regulates the process of micturition. The sensory neurons transmit the impulses to the spinal cord, where they are relayed to the brain, which in turn stimulates parasympathetic neurons that innervate the bladder wall. When a client is ready to pass urine, these impulses cause the bladder muscles to contract, the urethral sphincters relax and urine is voided into the urethra and excreted. Urine is excreted in amounts of 1–2 L in 24 hours. Micturition is normally under voluntary control by about 2–3 years of age.

NURSING CARE AND MEETING ELIMINATION NEEDS

Metabolism produces wastes that must be eliminated regularly to maintain effective body function. Observation of urine and the client's ability to eliminate it provides the nurse with an objective assessment of the client's elimination status. As a result, appropriate nursing actions may be planned and implemented.

URINE COLLECTION

The nurse may be required to collect urine for observation or testing in the ward, or so that a specimen can be sent to the pathology laboratory for analysis. Key aspects related to the collection of urine include:

- Thorough washing and drying of the hands before and after and the wearing of gloves, as there is a risk of coming into contact with the urine
- The container in which the urine is collected must be clean, and in some instances sterile, to ensure collection of a specimen free from external contamination
- If testing or laboratory analysis is required, contamination of the container and urine must be prevented throughout the procedure
- Adequate information about the client and the specimen must be provided. The label on the specimen container must contain the client's name, identification number, the date and time of collection, and the method used to collect the specimen; for example, catheter specimen of urine. When a specimen is despatched for laboratory analysis, it must be accompanied by the medical officer's request form. The medical officer requests the collection of a specimen and indicates on the form which specific laboratory tests are to be performed
- Specimens must be sent to the laboratory as soon as possible after collection; if there is a delay in despatch, the specimen may require refrigeration
- Clients may be responsible for the collection of their own urine specimens, so the nurse should provide the information necessary to ensure that the collection is performed correctly.

Observation and urinalysis

If urine is to be collected for observation or testing in the ward, the client is requested to void into a clean bedpan or urinal (Figure 32.5). The urine should not be contaminated by faeces or menstrual blood, as a false assessment may result. The urine is transferred from the toilet utensil into a clean container in preparation for observation or testing. (For more detail regarding performing a urinalysis, see Chapter 22.)

Timed collection

All urine excreted during a timed collection, for example, during a 24-hour period, is collected and sent for laboratory analysis to measure the quantity of various substances present, such as specific hormones. A suggested method of collecting a 24-hour specimen is outlined in Table 22.1.

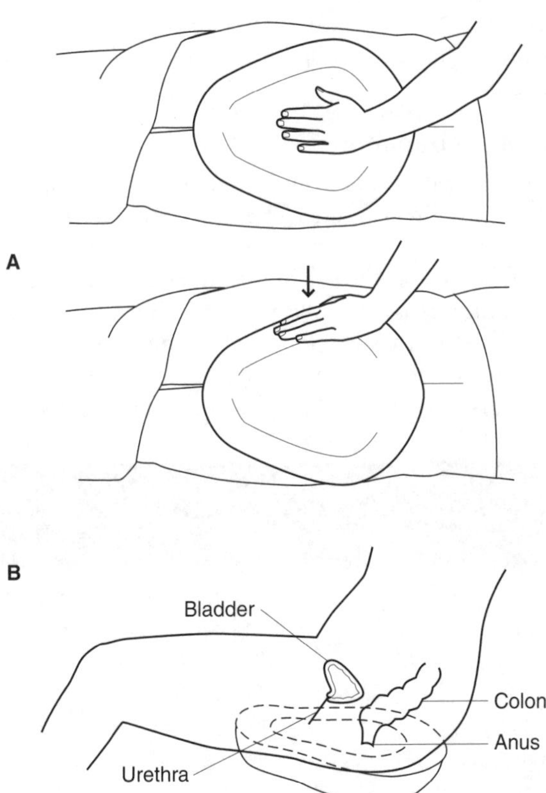

Figure 32.5 | Positioning a bedpan A: Another method of placing a bedpan is used when the client is unable to help. The client lies on one side and the bedpan is placed firmly against the buttocks B: The nurse pushes down on the bedpan and towards the client C: The client is positioned on the bedpan so that the urethra and anus are directly over the opening

Mid-stream specimen

This method of collection is used to obtain a sample of urine that is not contaminated by microorganisms from outside the urinary tract. The urine is sent to the laboratory to be tested for the presence of microorganisms and their sensitivity to antibiotics. The aim is to collect the middle portion of the stream of urine. A suggested method of collection is outlined in Table 22.2.

Using a collection bag

A urine collection bag may be used to obtain a specimen from a client who is unable to control the flow of urine, such as an infant or a client who is incontinent, unconscious or confused. A suggested method of collecting a sample of urine using a collection bag is outlined in Table 22.3.

Urine culture

A culture medium is sometimes used when the urine is to be tested for bacteria. Urine is first collected in a sterile container, then a slide containing culture medium is dipped into the urine. The culture slide is returned to its original container and despatched to the laboratory together with the urine in its separate sterile container. This method of collection may be necessary if there is a delay in despatch of the specimen and refrigeration is not practicable.

Catheter specimen

A catheter specimen of urine is obtained from a client who has an indwelling catheter. The insertion of a catheter for the sole purpose of obtaining a urine specimen is generally avoided because of the risk of introducing microorganisms into the urinary tract. Collecting a specimen from the end of the catheter that is connected to the drainage tubing should be avoided and the urine should be aspirated using a sterile syringe and needle through the sampling port (see Figure 22.1). The recommended method for obtaining a catheter specimen is outlined in Table 22.4.

Suprapubic bladder aspiration

This procedure is not commonly performed but, when necessary, it is performed by a medical officer, using sterile equipment and aseptic technique. It involves the insertion of a needle through the skin over the suprapubic area into the bladder. A quantity of urine is aspirated, placed in a sterile container and despatched to the laboratory. After this procedure the nurse should observe the puncture site for bleeding, and the urine for the presence of blood.

Straining urine

Stones, or calculi, are insoluble substances formed of mineral salts that may develop in the kidneys. They can range in size from microscopic, through resembling grains of sand or gravel, to several centimetres in diameter. If it is known or suspected that a client has developed renal calculi, careful observation of the urine is achieved by straining it to detect the passage of stones. Any stones collected are sent for laboratory examination, which reveals their exact composition and helps to identify their cause. The urine is strained by pouring it through a fine substance such as gauze or filter paper.

FACTORS AFFECTING THE URINARY SYSTEM

Problems associated with micturition may result from several factors, including a change of routine or environment, or as a consequence of certain disease states. Any alteration in a client's normal pattern of voiding (Table 32.1) must be recognised and reported immediately, so that appropriate actions can be planned and implemented.

Problems with urination include those outlined below.

TABLE 32.1 | ALTERATIONS IN URINARY ELIMINATION PATTERNS

Term	Definition
Anuria	The absence of urine production, or a urinary output < 100 mL/day (< 30 mL/hour)
Dribbling	Dribbling of urine from the urethra despite voluntary control of micturition. It may be at the end of micturition or continuous
Dysuria	Pain and burning on micturition, usually as a result of an infection or obstruction
Frequency	Voiding at frequent intervals, i.e. < 2-hourly
Haematuria	The presence of blood in the urine
Hesitancy	Difficulty starting micturition
Incontinence	The inability to control the passage of urine
Nocturia	Excessive or frequent urination at night
Oliguria	A decreased urine production resulting in an output < 500 mL/day
Polyuria	The excretion of an abnormally large volume of urine
Retention	The accumulation of urine in the bladder as a result of being unable to fully empty the bladder
Residual urine	The volume of urine remaining after voiding
Urgency	The feeling of needing to void immediately

ALTERED AMOUNTS

The term oliguria is used to describe decreased urine output of below 500 mL/day. This condition is caused by fluid and electrolyte imbalances, kidney dysfunction or urinary tract obstruction. Polyuria is the term used to describe the excretion of greatly increased amounts of urine, for example, over 2500 mL/day. It may occur as a result of a large fluid input, diuretic medications, or certain disease states such as diabetes insipidus.

SUPPRESSION OF URINE FORMATION

The term anuria refers to the cessation of urine excretion by the kidneys, or the production of less than 100 mL/day, and may result from kidney dysfunction or failure.

URINE RETENTION

When there is an accumulation of urine in the bladder and the client is unable to void, the condition is referred to as retention of urine. Retention of urine is commonly due to an obstruction of the bladder outlet or urethra, and it may also occur as a result of tension in the urethral sphincter, caused by anxiety or pain. Retention of urine with overflow occurs when the accumulation of urine in the bladder leads to stretching of the urethral orifice and, although small amounts of urine dribble away, the bladder remains full and distended.

INCONTINENCE OF URINE

Incontinence is the inability to control the excretion of urine and may result from a variety of local or generalised conditions that include:

- Sphincter incompetence; for example, as a result of urethral trauma, surgery to the bladder, or after childbirth
- Urinary tract infections (UTIs)
- Neurological lesions (refer to Clinical Interest Box 32.1)
- Bladder tumours or stones
- Impaired consciousness or awareness
- Medications that increase urinary output; for example, diuretics, or those that affect awareness
- Environmental causes such as difficult access to toilet facilities.

Incontinence of urine may be classified into six types:

1. Total incontinence, when the person experiences a constant involuntary loss of urine that is unpredictable and the client is unaware that it has occurred
2. Functional incontinence, when the person experiences an involuntary loss of urine that is unpredictable
3. Stress incontinence, when the person loses less than 50 mL of urine while sneezing, coughing, laughing, during exercise or other activities that result in increased intra-abdominal pressure
4. Urge incontinence, when the client experiences a strong sense of urgency to void, followed immediately by involuntary urination

CLINICAL INTEREST BOX 32.1
Incontinence and the client with dementia

Some individuals with dementia are occasionally incontinent. The nurse needs to consider that the individual may:

- Be embarrassed to ask for help
- No longer be able to express the need to go to the toilet
- Have trouble undressing to go to the toilet
- Be unable to find the toilet
- Be unable to recognise the toilet
- Not remember what to do
- Not want to go to the toilet in front of another person
- Not recognise the need to go to the toilet
- Have a urinary tract infection
- Have something obstructing the flow of urine from the bladder; for example, constipation, or enlarged prostate gland in men
- Be on medications that can reduce their sensitivity to the body's signals

(Alzheimer's Association Victoria)

5. Overflow incontinence, which is characterised by constant dribbling while the bladder remains full
6. Reflex incontinence — an involuntary loss of urine occurring when a specific bladder volume is reached. It may be predictable.

DYSURIA

Dysuria is the term used to describe painful micturition and is commonly due to a UTI or obstruction.

FREQUENCY OF MICTURITION

Frequency of micturition is when a client experiences the need to void more often than normal and commonly voids small amounts of urine each time. This condition is commonly associated with a UTI or may occur as a result of anxiety or stress.

Measures to induce micturition

When a client is experiencing difficulty in passing urine, the cause must be identified and treated. Difficulty in passing urine may result from an obstruction to the outflow of urine but may also be caused by other factors such as:

- Anxiety, stress, nervousness or embarrassment associated with the need to use toilet aids
- The need to remain in a supine position when using toilet aids
- The effects of medications, anaesthesia or the acute stress of surgery
- Pain, which can lead to tension in the muscles controlling the urethral opening.

Nursing actions that may be implemented to induce micturition include:

- Relieving pain: if a client is experiencing pain, the cause should be identified and treated. The nurse should report any complaints of pain immediately to the Registered Nurse (RN). Nursing actions to relieve

pain include ensuring that the client is positioned comfortably, checking any splints or dressings to detect whether they are causing the pain, and reporting to the RN for the administration of any prescribed analgesia
- Ensuring adequate privacy and sufficient time for the client to void. If possible, the client should be left alone to use the toilet aids (e.g. bedpan or urinal) as they are generally self-conscious about the need to eliminate in the presence of others. Ensure the client's safety and that the call bell is accessible
- Assisting the client to assume a natural voiding position: whenever possible the client should be permitted to use the toilet but, if this is contraindicated, an upright position may assist. Males may find it easier to pass urine if allowed to stand
- Helping the client to relax: unless contraindicated, a warm shower or bath may be beneficial. The RN should be consulted as to the advisability of pouring warm water over the genitalia of a female, as this action sometimes helps to stimulate micturition
- Stimulating the micturition response: this can often be achieved by providing the sound of running water (e.g. turning on a nearby tap)
- Encouraging the client to drink adequate amounts of fluids, unless this is contraindicated.

If these actions fail to induce micturition and the client is uncomfortable because of a distended bladder, it may be necessary to implement further actions, such as inserting a urinary catheter. This is ordered by a medical officer and performed by an RN.

CATHETERS

A catheter is a tube that is inserted into the bladder to drain urine. It is inserted through the urethra or, less commonly, through a small incision in the suprapubic area. A catheter may be inserted to empty the bladder then removed immediately, or it may be left in the bladder. A catheter that remains in the bladder may either be clamped and released at specified intervals, or connected to tubing and a bag to enable continuous drainage. A catheter that remains in the bladder is referred to as indwelling. A self-retaining catheter is used for this purpose. It has a small balloon that is filled with sterile water after the catheter is inserted, which stops the catheter falling out. Reasons for inserting a urinary catheter include to:
- Relieve retention of urine
- Closely monitor the urinary output
- Obtain a sterile specimen of urine
- Prevent skin maceration when a client is incontinent
- Remove residual urine when voiding does not completely empty the bladder
- Allow the drainage of urine and to keep the bladder empty during or after surgery on the abdominal, pelvic or perineal areas
- Facilitate bladder irrigation procedures.

Catheters are made from materials that cause minimal reaction when in contact with body tissues and are available in a variety of styles and sizes. Some of the materials from which catheters are made include: polyvinylchloride (PVC), which softens at body temperature and is commonly used for short-term purposes; silicone elastomer, which is a physiologically inert material causing few local reactions when in contact with body tissue and which can therefore remain in the bladder for long periods; and latex coated with silicone, which is not as inert as silicone, but may remain in the bladder for up to 10 days. Catheters are graded according to the French scale, and the larger the number the larger the lumen of the catheter. Sizes range from 1 to 30 French gauge (Fg), and the size is selected to suit the client's needs. It is important that a suitable size is selected to avoid leakage of urine around the catheter, or trauma to the urethra or bladder.

INSERTION OF A CATHETER

The procedure of catheter insertion is called catheterisation and is performed using sterile equipment and aseptic technique. As a catheter can cause trauma to the urethral or bladder mucosa and is a potential source of UTI, it is inserted only when absolutely necessary and only by an RN or a medical officer. Because the male urethra is longer and more curved than the female urethra and catheterisation is often more difficult, male clients are usually catheterised by a health worker skilled in this procedure. A suggested procedure for female catheterisation is outlined in Table 32.2. Nurses should be aware of their role and responsibilities regarding catheter insertion in the workplace. The basic requirements are:
- Sterile gloves
- Sterile catheters
- A sterile receiver for urine
- Sterile materials for cleansing the genital area
- Water-soluble lubricant
- Goggles
- Sterile forceps
- Sterile drapes.

If the catheter is to be indwelling, the following are also needed:
- Sterile water
- Sterile 5–10 mL syringe
- Drainage tubing and bag
- Holder for drainage bag
- Clamp
- Hypoallergenic tape.

In addition to preparing the equipment it is necessary to prepare the client by ensuring adequate lighting and privacy, placing the client in a supine position with legs extended, and promoting comfort during the procedure. The Enrolled Nurse (EN) may be asked to assist the RN or medical officer during the procedure.

Nursing care after the insertion of a catheter is similar

TABLE 32.2 | GUIDELINES FOR CATHETERISATION OF FEMALES*

Action	Rationale
Review and carry out the standard steps in Appendix 1	
Ensure adequate lighting	Visualisation of the urethral meatus is essential
Place the client in the dorsal position, with knees flexed and separated, and feet slightly apart on the bed	Provides a clear view of the urethral meatus
Ensure that the client is adequately draped	Reduces embarrassment
Place all the equipment in a convenient location	Facilitates easy access to it throughout the procedure
Wash and dry hands. Don gloves and goggles	Prevents cross-infection
Use sterile towels to create a sterile field around the genital area	Reduces risk of equipment becoming contaminated during the procedure
Cleanse genital area and urethral meatus, wiping from front to back	Reduces risk of introducing microorganisms from the genital/anal area into the urinary tract
Before inserting a self-retaining catheter, inflate and deflate the balloon	Necessary to check balloon for leakage before insertion
With forceps, hold the catheter about 7 cm from its tip	Assists in controlling the direction of the catheter
Dip tip of catheter into the water-based lubricant	Facilitates easier and more comfortable insertion
Place distal end of catheter into a sterile receptacle positioned between the client's legs	Urine will flow into the receptacle, not onto the bed
Keeping the client's labia separated, insert the catheter tip into the urethral orifice. Advance the catheter until 4–7 cm have been inserted	Length of catheter inserted must be in relation to the anatomical structure of the urethra. The average female urethra is about 3.8 cm long
If catheter is not to be left in, remove it gently when urine ceases to flow, or the required amount of urine has drained	Catheters are not left in any longer than necessary, and are removed gently to avoid discomfort
If a self-retaining catheter is being used, inflate the balloon, having first ensured that the catheter is draining adequately	Inflated balloon keeps the catheter in the bladder. Inadvertent inflation with the balloon in the urethra causes trauma and pain
Connect the indwelling catheter to the drainage bag and support the bag in a holder at the side of the bed. Alternatively, a clamp is placed on the end of the catheter	Urine flows from catheter, along the tubing and into the bag. Intermittent drainage may be prescribed
Attach the catheter to the client's inner thigh with hypoallergenic tape, and pass the catheter over the thigh	Prevents in–out movement of the catheter and prevents tension on the urethra
Position the tubing so that it is not obstructed by the client's weight or by tight bedclothes	Avoids blocking the flow of urine through the tubing
Remove excess lubricant from the client's genital area. Replace bedding and assist client into a comfortable position	Helps promote comfort
Remove and attend to the equipment in the appropriate manner. Wash and dry hands	Prevents cross-infection
Document the procedure, including the amount of water instilled into the balloon, and colour and characteristics of the urine	Appropriate care can be planned and implemented. When the catheter is to be removed, it is important that the water is first withdrawn and the balloon deflated to prevent trauma to the urethra

*This procedure is only performed by an RN or a medical officer

for both male and female clients and is planned and implemented to promote comfort, maintain the flow of urine and minimise the possibility of a UTI. The nurse needs to ascertain whether the catheter is to be clamped and released at specified intervals to provide intermittent drainage or if it is to be connected to a drainage bag for continuous drainage. If intermittent drainage has been prescribed, the end of the catheter is clamped. At specified intervals, for example, every 4 hours, the clamp is released to enable the urine that has accumulated in the bladder to drain. Aseptic technique should be used during this procedure to prevent the entry of microorganisms into the open catheter. An intermittent drainage regimen is commonly implemented before removal of an indwelling catheter, to promote and restore any lost bladder tone.

If continuous drainage has been prescribed, actions to promote free flow of urine and prevent stasis of urine include:

- Positioning the tubing so that it is not obstructed or kinked in any way
- Maintaining the tubing and drainage bag at a level below the client's bladder
- Ensuring that the client has a fluid input of at least 2000 mL daily, unless this is contraindicated.

To prevent ascending infection the catheter should be taped to the inner thigh to reduce any in–out movement. If continuous drainage is being used, the system should remain closed and sterile. If it is necessary to disconnect any part of the system, an aseptic technique must be used. To promote comfort and reduce the risk of ascending infection, the urethral meatus and catheter near the point of entry should be cleansed at least twice daily and whenever necessary, for example, after a bowel action. Cleansing should be performed by wiping in the direction away from the urethral meatus to avoid contaminating the urinary tract. An uncircumcised male's foreskin should be retracted before cleansing, and replaced after cleansing.

MAINTAINING AND SAMPLING FROM A CATHETER

The urine should be observed and the observations documented, for volume, colour, clarity, odour, and the presence of abnormalities such as blood, pus or sediment. Any deviations from normal must be reported immediately. Any inflammation of the urethral meatus, or pain or distension over the bladder area, should be reported immediately. The nurse should observe for signs that urine is bypassing or leaking around the catheter. This may be caused by bladder spasm, blockage of the catheter or tubing, or insertion of a catheter of incorrect size. If leakage occurs it should be reported and documented. To test the patency of a catheter or to remove clots or sediment, an RN may perform irrigation of the catheter or the bladder after review by a medical officer.

When a client has an indwelling catheter, it may be necessary to obtain a specimen of urine for laboratory analysis. A suggested technique for this procedure is described earlier in this chapter. Indwelling catheters are changed if contamination occurs or if any malfunction or obstruction cannot be corrected. If no complication occurs, the frequency with which a catheter is changed depends on the type being used, and ranges from about 10 days to 6 months.

When a catheter is being used to drain urine from an over-distended bladder, for example, during acute retention of urine, care is taken not to allow the urine to be drained too rapidly. Decompressing the bladder too quickly may result in bladder trauma or physiological shock; therefore, no more than 1000 mL should be released at any one time.

Urine meters (burettes) may be used in conjunction with drainage systems when precise measurements of urine output, such as hourly measurement, are required. A meter is commonly a rigid plastic container attached to the drainage system, which is calibrated to measure small volumes.

Disposable closed drainage sets consisting of tubing and a collection bag are commonly used. The collection bag is emptied at specified intervals or when it is almost full, and the tubing left in position until the entire set is changed or removed (Figure 32.6). The bag is emptied by releasing the valve at the bottom of the bag, using aseptic technique to avoid introducing infection.

Whenever the tubing or bag is changed or the catheter disconnected from the tubing, the sterility of the system must be maintained. To empty a urinary drainage bag the nurse requires a sterile jug and cover, alcohol swabs, goggles and disposable gloves. To change a urinary drainage bag the nurse will require the same equipment as for emptying, plus a receiver for used items, a clamp and a clean drainage bag. Key aspects related to emptying and changing collection bags are outlined in Table 32.3.

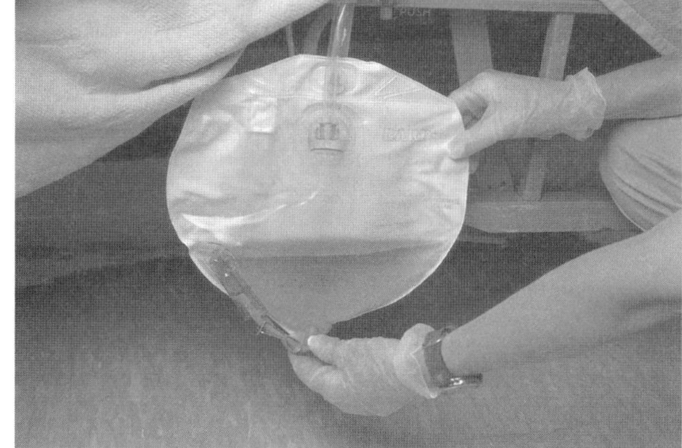

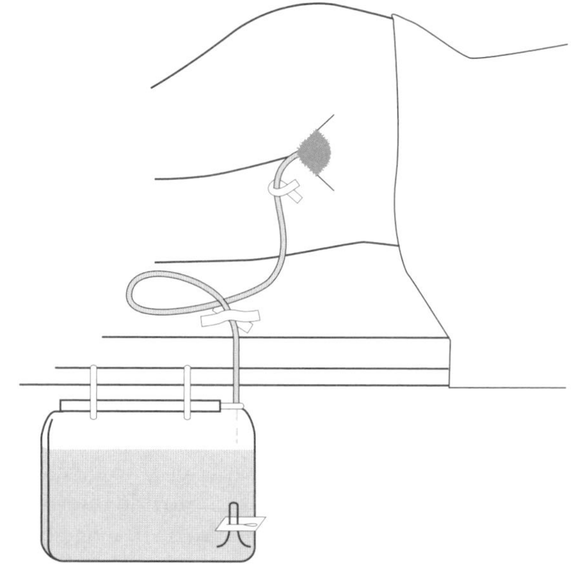

Figure 32.6 | Closed urinary drainage system *(deWit 2005; redrawn from Potter & Perry 2008)*

TABLE 32.3 | GUIDELINES FOR EMPTYING OR CHANGING COLLECTION BAGS

Action	Rationale
To empty a bag	
Review and carry out the standard steps in Appendix 1	
Swab the outlet valve on the collection bag with an alcohol swab	Reduces risk of introducing microorganisms
Place the jug below the valve and release valve	Allows urine to drain from the bag into the jug
When the bag is empty, tighten the valve	Prevents subsequent drainage of urine out of the bag
Swab the valve with an alcohol swab	Removes any traces of urine, and prevents cross-infection
Remove the jug, observe the urine and measure or test it if necessary	Assists in evaluating the client's urinary status
Empty and clean the jug, remove gloves, wash and dry hands	Prevents cross-infection
Report any deviations from normal and document accordingly	Appropriate care can be planned and implemented
To change a bag	
The first six steps are as for emptying a bag, above	
Swab the connection site where the system is to be disrupted	Reduces risk of introducing microorganisms
Clamp the catheter and remove the bag, and/or bag and tubing. Connect the catheter or tubing to the new bag	Prevents leakage of urine during the change
Swab the connection site with an alcohol swab	Removes traces of urine and prevents cross-infection
Release the clamp and ensure that the tubing and bag are positioned correctly	Allows urine to flow
Observe the urine and measure or test it if necessary	Assists in evaluating the client's urinary status
Remove the soiled articles and attend to them in the appropriate manner. Remove gloves, wash and dry hands	Prevents cross-infection
Report any deviations from normal and document accordingly	Appropriate care can be planned and implemented

BLADDER IRRIGATION

Bladder irrigation or washout may be performed to ensure patency of the catheter, to remove sediment or blood clots or to introduce an antibiotic or bacteriostatic agent. Bladder irrigation may be continuous or intermittent. Continuous irrigation may be necessary to flush out small blood clots that may form after prostate or bladder surgery and prevent urinary tract obstruction. During bladder irrigation, sterile equipment and aseptic technique are used to avoid introducing microorganisms. A triple lumen catheter is needed to perform bladder irrigation. One lumen is used to introduce the irrigating solution into the bladder, a second lumen allows the fluid to drain out, and the third lumen allows the instillation of fluid into the balloon that holds the catheter in the bladder.

For continuous irrigation, a container of irrigating solution is suspended on a stand and the tubing from the container attached to the catheter. Drainage tubing from the catheter is attached to a urine collection bag positioned below the level of the client's bladder. A clamp is used to regulate the rate at which the solution flows into the bladder. During irrigation the inflow and outflow tubing is checked to ensure the free flow of fluid. The outflowing fluid is checked for changes in appearance and presence of blood clots. Both the inflowing and outflowing fluid must be measured and documented and the collection bag emptied as necessary. The outflow volume should be greater than the inflow volume, allowing for urine production.

Intermittent irrigation involves the gentle introduction of small amounts of prescribed solution. Using a syringe, the solution is introduced into the distal end of the catheter. Small amounts, 30–50 mL for example, are introduced in succession and usually allowed to drain out by gravity. The technique is repeated until the prescribed amount of solution has been used, or until the return fluid is clear. The solution being introduced and returned is measured and documented, and the return fluid observed for changes in appearance or presence of blood clots.

REMOVAL OF A CATHETER

Depending on how long a catheter has been in position, the medical officer may prescribe bladder retraining before its removal. Bladder retraining involves clamping the catheter for specified periods, such as 2–4 hours, then releasing it to empty the bladder. This technique is repeated for several hours to help restore the bladder's muscle tone. Removing a catheter requires aseptic technique. Key aspects related to the procedure and after care include:

- Obtaining a specimen of urine for laboratory analysis if necessary, before the catheter is removed
- Ensuring that all water from the balloon is withdrawn before removing the catheter

- Gently withdrawing the catheter from the urethra, using aseptic technique
- Offering a bedpan or urinal immediately after the catheter is removed, as catheter removal often creates a desire to void
- Encouraging the intake of fluids to stimulate urine production, to dilute the urine and to help decrease any discomfort the client may experience on resuming voiding
- Observing and documenting urine output after the catheter is removed. If the client is voiding only small amounts, the bladder may not be emptying completely, and the medical officer should be informed
- Observing for and reporting any difficulty with voiding, incontinence, dribbling or bladder distension
- Documenting the date and time the catheter was removed and the client's response to the procedure.

ALTERATIONS IN URINARY SYSTEM FUNCTIONING

The kidneys are essential in the maintenance of homeostasis, as they regulate the rates of elimination of water and electrolytes from the body and contribute to the maintenance of a constant blood pH and blood pressure. The kidneys also eliminate metabolic waste products and toxic substances. Therefore, any dysfunction in the formation or excretion of urine can have major adverse effects on homeostasis.

PATHOLOGICAL INFLUENCES AND EFFECTS

Alterations in normal function of the urinary system can be classified as changes in kidney structure, fluid and electrolyte balance, elimination of waste substances, and alterations in the output of urine.

CHANGES IN KIDNEY STRUCTURE

Atrophy of the kidneys because of destruction of the renal tissue can occur in many chronic renal diseases. Alternatively, the kidneys can become enlarged because of blockage of the ureters, enlargement of the prostate gland or from invasion of the kidneys by neoplastic cells. If there is an obstruction lower down in the urinary tract, the ureters may become enlarged in diameter as they fill with urine that cannot pass the obstruction.

FLUID AND ELECTROLYTE IMBALANCE

If the kidneys are unable to concentrate the urine by regulating reabsorption, the loss of a large amount of dilute urine may result in fluid imbalance. If they fail to excrete sufficient water, an increase in the total circulating fluid volume impedes cardiovascular function. Failure of the kidneys to help control the balance of electrolytes in body fluids or to maintain normal osmolarity poses a major threat to homeostasis. Failure to excrete potassium will disrupt the conduction system of the heart, while failure to conserve sufficient potassium may result in altered cardiac muscle contraction. Renal disease may also result in abnormal retention or loss of sodium, calcium or phosphorus.

ELIMINATION OF WASTES

Normal metabolism produces an excess of acids. To compensate, the kidneys excrete acids and return bicarbonate to the plasma and extracellular fluid. An acid–base imbalance (metabolic acidosis) will result if this function is impaired; that is, if there is an increased amount of acid or a decreased amount of base in the body. The kidneys must also continually filter and excrete nitrogenous wastes derived from protein metabolism. Renal failure can result in an accumulation of urea, uric acid and creatinine in the blood, causing uraemia. The accumulation of uraemic toxins has adverse effects on several body systems, such as impaired neurological function.

URINE OUTPUT

Alterations in urine output may be temporary or long term. Urine output may be decreased, as in obstruction of the ureter or acute or chronic renal failure, or it may be increased, as during the diuretic stage of acute renal failure. The passage of urine along the urinary tract may be impeded by an obstruction, such as a tumour or calculus.

MAJOR MANIFESTATIONS OF URINARY SYSTEM DISORDERS

Disorders of the urinary system may produce signs and symptoms that vary according to the site and severity of the problem.

Pain

Pain is more common in acute, rather than chronic, disorders of the kidneys and urinary tract. Pain that originates from the kidneys is generally experienced as a dull ache in the lower back and may radiate to the lower abdominal area. Pain associated with renal colic is sudden and severe. It is felt in the lower back and may radiate to the groin area. Nausea and vomiting frequently accompany this type of pain.

Suprapubic pain may result from spasms or overdistension of the bladder, as in acute retention of urine. An infection of the lower urinary tract, such as cystitis, commonly causes pain and burning during and/or after voiding. Strangury is the term used to describe a burning pain that can occur during or after micturition. Discomfort, rather than pain, may occur if the bladder becomes abnormally distended.

Changes in voiding pattern

There may be an increase in the frequency of voiding, problems controlling the passage of urine, difficulty in initiating micturition, or a sense of urgency associated with the need to void. There may also be a tendency to nocturia.

Changes in output

Changes in the output of urine include voiding increased or decreased amounts, and cessation of the production or secretion of urine.

Changes in the urine

Abnormalities of the urine associated with urinary system disorders include changes in the normal colour, clarity or odour of urine. The urine may be bloodstained or dark amber, cloudy or smoky in appearance. Chronic renal disease can result in pale, almost colourless urine. A foul smelling 'fishy' odour is commonly present when there is a UTI (see Chapter 22).

Other manifestations

A client with a lower UTI commonly experiences pyrexia, malaise, nausea and vomiting, and pelvic and abdominal discomfort, whereas those with renal disease may experience hypertension, oedema, anorexia, nausea and vomiting, skin changes, and neurological symptoms such as headache or altered consciousness.

SPECIFIC DISORDERS OF THE URINARY SYSTEM

Disorders of the urinary system may be classified as congenital, infectious, immunological, degenerative, neoplastic, obstructive, traumatic, or those resulting from multiple causes.

Congenital disorders

Certain disorders may be present at birth, although the manifestations may not become evident for some time. Vesico-ureteric reflux is a mechanical problem that may be congenital or acquired. Abnormal backflow of urine from the bladder to the ureter(s) increases the hydrostatic pressure in the ureters and kidneys. Reflux into the kidneys causes damage to the renal parenchyma, and reflux nephropathy. In the congenital form the child is born with a short ureter, which often grows to normal size as the child develops and matures, so that the condition resolves. Acquired vesico-ureteric reflux may be caused by repeated UTIs, by inadequate functioning of the detrusor muscles in the bladder, or from a high pressure within the bladder as a result of an obstruction. Symptoms of the disorder generally appear only in the presence of a UTI and there may be no symptoms with chronic infection. The condition may not be diagnosed until signs of renal damage become evident.

Polycystic kidney disease is an inherited disorder characterised by grape-like clusters of fluid-filled cysts that enlarge the kidneys. There are two forms of this disorder; one affecting children and the other affecting adults. In its infantile form the disorder manifests as bilateral masses in the kidney areas, with symptoms of respiratory distress and cardiac failure. Adult polycystic disease is frequently asymptomatic until the client is about 40 years of age. Initial symptoms include hypertension, haematuria and low back pain. UTI is common and progression to renal failure is gradual.

Infectious disorders

Infection may occur in any part of the urinary tract, as urine provides an ideal medium for the growth of microorganisms. Most commonly they gain access to the urinary tract by ascending the urethra, although rarely they may descend from the kidneys to the lower urinary tract. Hospital-acquired UTIs are commonly related to the use of catheters, as repeated insertion or prolonged use of catheters increases the risk of infection.

Pyelonephritis is inflammation of the renal pelvis and may be an acute or chronic condition. Acute pyelonephritis results from bacterial infection of the kidneys, commonly as a consequence of a lower UTI. A client with acute pyelonephritis may experience severe pain or a continual dull ache in the kidney region, as well as pyrexia, nausea and vomiting and fatigue. Rigors may be present, and urination may be frequent and painful. The urine is generally cloudy, bloodstained and offensive in odour. Chronic pyelonephritis can result in the formation of renal scar tissue, which may in turn lead to chronic renal failure. This condition most commonly occurs in clients who experience recurrent acute pyelonephritis as a result of a urinary tract obstruction or vesico-ureteric reflux.

Cystitis is inflammation of the urinary bladder, and is usually the result of bacterial contamination. Causative organisms include *Escherichia coli*, *Proteus* spp, and *Pseudomonas pyocyaneus*. Cystitis is more common in females than in males because of the short length and proximity of the urethra to the bowel and vagina. Clients with cystitis experience a burning pain during micturition, which may be accompanied by frequency, urgency and bladder spasms. Incontinence of urine may occur. The urine is generally cloudy and offensive and may contain blood cells. Other features of the disorder include pyrexia, pain or discomfort in the bladder area, and fatigue.

Urethritis, inflammation of the urethra, may result from bacterial infection or traumatic irritation. Causative organisms are often of the type transmitted sexually, such as *Chlamydia trachomatis* and *Neisseria gonorrhoeae.* Symptoms of urethritis include dysuria and the presence of pus in the urine.

Immunological disorders

These disorders are caused by inflammation of the glomeruli. It is generally believed that the disorders are autoimmune in origin and that glomerular damage is the result of antigen–antibody complexes that circulate in the blood and bind to cells of the glomeruli. Acute glomerulonephritis results from an infection that has recently occurred elsewhere in the body, such as the respiratory tract. The common causative organism is the haemolytic streptococcus. The client generally experiences signs and symptoms of glomerulonephritis within 1–3 weeks after an infection. The most common manifestations are peripheral and periorbital oedema, decreased urine output, and hypertension. The urine contains red blood cells and protein and is smoky or dark in appearance.

In chronic glomerulonephritis there is progressive kidney damage, with a corresponding impairment of kidney function and retention of metabolic waste products. This condition is characterised by hypertension, oedema, high blood urea levels, and by the presence of protein and red and white blood cells in the urine. Early chronic renal failure causes nausea and vomiting, pruritus, fatigue and muscle cramps. As the disease progresses the client experiences severe headaches, dyspnoea, oedema, cardiac arrhythmias and disturbances of vision. Death from uraemia will occur if the condition is not treated by either dialysis or a renal transplant.

Nephrotic syndrome can occur in any condition that results in damage to the glomerular capillary membrane, such as glomerulonephritis, allowing loss of fluid into the interstitial spaces. The condition is characterised by marked proteinuria, hyperlipidaemia, and oedema primarily in dependent areas of the body. Periorbital oedema may be evident, particularly in the morning. Accompanying manifestations include lethargy, anorexia, depression, pallor and orthostatic hypotension.

Degenerative disorders

This group includes disorders in which there are degenerative changes in the renal structure or changes in the blood vessels that supply the kidneys. Degeneration occurs over a long period, and the client may not experience any symptoms until significant damage has occurred. Nephrosclerosis is necrosis of the renal arterioles, resulting from untreated or uncontrolled hypertension that impairs the blood supply of the kidneys. Renal damage occurs from a combination of fibrosis of the blood vessels walls and the resulting ischaemia. The client presents with high blood pressure, headaches, visual disturbances and altered neurological functioning. The urine contains protein and blood. If untreated, this condition can lead to renal and cardiac failure.

Analgesic nephropathy results from chronic ingestion of substances containing phenacetin. Aspirin–paracetamol combinations have also been found to cause similar renal tubule damage. The client complains of low back pain, haematuria and the symptoms of uraemia (nausea, vomiting, pruritus, muscle cramps). If end-stage renal failure develops, dialysis or kidney transplantation will be necessary.

Neoplastic disorders

Tumours that arise in the urinary system may be benign or malignant. Kidney tumours are generally malignant, and usually well advanced before haematuria, the first and most common sign, appears. Later features include pain as the tumour enlarges and presses on adjacent structures, nausea and vomiting, loss of weight, and metastatic symptoms such as bone pain. Wilms' tumour is a malignant tumour of the kidneys that occurs primarily in children. With suitable treatment, the prognosis is favourable.

Bladder tumours are generally malignant, and more common than kidney tumours. Most occur in men over age 50. Evidence shows that prolonged exposure to certain substances such as aniline dyes is associated with increased incidence of bladder cancer. A variety of other carcinogenic substances, such as artificial sweeteners, are linked to bladder cancer. The prime manifestation of a bladder tumour is intermittent haematuria.

Cancer of the prostate gland is a relatively common form of cancer and is thought to be a result of hormonal changes. As the tumour develops it causes the prostate gland to increase in size and causes difficulty in initiating micturition, a feeling that the bladder is not empty after voiding, and dribbling of urine after micturition. As obstruction increases, urination becomes more frequent, with nocturia, urgency and incontinence. Haematuria may be present due to rupture of dilated blood vessels at the neck of the bladder. Acute retention of urine may occur if the flow from the bladder is severely obstructed.

Calculi are stones that form in the kidneys and urinary tract. Most stones form in the kidneys and pass down into the ureters or bladder. They are usually composed of calcium salts or uric acid. Multiple small calculi may remain in the renal pelvis or pass down the ureter, while a staghorn calculus remains in the kidneys (Figure 32.7). Although the precise cause is unknown, predisposing factors in the formation of calculi include some medications, dehydration, metabolic factors, infection, prolonged immobility and urinary stasis.

The major symptom of calculi is pain, felt as a dull ache while the stone remains in the kidney (see Clinical Interest Box 32.2). If a stone passes into the ureter, the client may experience excruciating colicky pain that is frequently accompanied by nausea and vomiting. The pain results as the ureter goes into spasm in an attempt to move

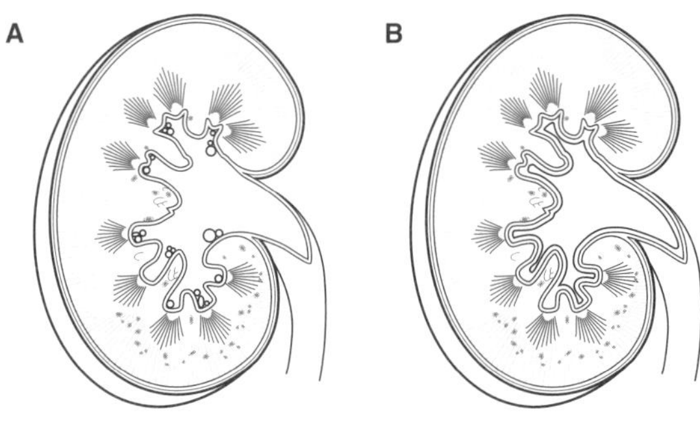

Figure 32.7 | Renal calculi A: Multiple small calculi B: A staghorn calculus

CLINICAL INTEREST BOX 32.2
Adapting procedure for a client with severe renal pain

Mr Allen has come to the emergency department at 2 a.m. complaining of severe colicky pain in the lumbar region, radiating down the left side of his abdomen to his groin. He states that the pain started about an hour ago and has gotten worse, and that he vomited once on the way to the hospital. His vital signs show a pulse rate of 96/min, respiratory rate of 24/min and temperature is normal, although his skin feels clammy and damp.

While waiting for the medical officer to attend, Sarah, Mr Allen's nurse, is keen to let him know that she cares and understands that he is suffering from severe pain, while still remaining professional. She also realises that the pain will be uppermost in Mr Allen's mind and that he will not be interested in small talk and so is only able to obtain an outline history. After the medical officer has been and has diagnosed a urinary calculus, Sarah gives pain relief as ordered. Mr Allen then relaxes somewhat and Sarah is able to take a more comprehensive history before admission to a ward.

the calculus out of the ureter by peristalsis. There may be haematuria, and small stones may be passed in the urine.

Obstructive disorders

Obstruction of the urinary tract may be caused by factors other than the presence of tumours and calculi. Benign prostatomegaly (enlargement of the prostate gland surrounding the male urethra) may compress the urethra and cause urinary obstruction. The cause of hypertrophy of the prostate gland is not fully understood but is probably related to hormonal mechanisms. It is more common in men over age 50.

Hydronephrosis, or dilation of the renal pelvis, may result from obstruction of the urinary tract. The build up of pressure behind the area of obstruction eventually results in damage to the kidneys, and renal dysfunction. Causes of hydronephrosis include prostatomegaly, urethral stricture, calculi, congenital abnormalities and neurogenic bladder. The client usually presents with dull lower back pain and tenderness, decreased urine flow, dysuria and haematuria. Infection or renal failure can occur if the problem is not corrected.

Traumatic disorders

Injuries to the kidney or urinary tract can have serious consequences. Because the kidney receives a large amount of blood from the abdominal aorta via the renal arteries, even a small laceration can cause massive haemorrhage. Injuries to the kidney include contusion, haematoma and laceration. The renal artery or renal vein may be ruptured. Symptoms include haematuria, back and abdominal pain, and symptoms of hypovolaemic shock if the injury is severe. Bladder trauma may be associated with pelvic fractures or result from a blunt or penetrating injury. Symptoms of bladder injury include haematuria, dysuria, decreased urinary output, suprapubic pain and tenderness. Scrotal or perineal swelling may occur if urine escapes from the damaged bladder into surrounding tissues.

Disorders of multiple cause

Various urinary system disorders have more than one cause. Acute renal failure is the sudden disruption of kidney function due to obstruction, reduced blood circulation or renal damage. The condition is characterised by oliguria, electrolyte imbalance and metabolic acidosis.

Acute renal failure generally consists of four phases: onset, oliguric, diuretic, and recovery. During the oliguric phase, urine output may be as little as 50–150 mL in 24 hours. At the same time the serum creatinine and blood urea nitrogen levels rise steadily. The diuretic phase is characterised by a urine output greater than 400 mL in 24 hours or as much as 3 L in 24 hours. During this phase, the risk of electrolyte imbalance remains high. Recovery of renal function may take from a few days to 12 months. During this phase the serum electrolyte levels return to normal.

Chronic renal failure is the gradual loss of functional nephrons and may be due to several causes, including chronic kidney infections, polycystic kidneys, renal vascular disease, hypertension and obstructive diseases such as calculi, nephrotoxic agents and diabetic nephropathy. The condition produces major changes in all body systems.

It consists of four phases: diminished renal reserve, renal insufficiency, renal failure, and end-stage renal disease. During the first phase, renal damage occurs but the client may be asymptomatic. With renal insufficiency the kidneys still function, but urinary concentration is impaired and blood urea levels are elevated. The renal failure stage produces uraemia, metabolic acidosis, electrolyte imbalance and impaired urine dilution. In the final end stage, renal function is severely impaired and most other body systems are affected. When renal function is impaired to such an extent that conservative treatment is no longer effective, dialysis therapy and/or kidney transplantation are necessary.

Neurogenic bladder causes the client to experience loss of perception of bladder fullness and loss of the desire to void. It may result from a variety of causes, including cerebral or spinal cord disorders and disorders of the peripheral nervous system. As a consequence, the bladder becomes distended, and overflow incontinence occurs. Because of incomplete emptying of the bladder, susceptibility to UTIs is increased.

Urinary incontinence, which may result from many causes, is characterised by the inability to control the elimination of urine.

DIAGNOSTIC TESTS

Certain tests may be performed to assist or confirm the diagnosis of urinary system disorders.

Urine tests

Urine may be obtained and tested for the presence of abnormal substances to provide information about renal and urinary functions. (Information on methods of collection and testing urine is provided in Chapter 22.)

Blood tests

Blood may be obtained and tested in the laboratory to assess renal function. The tests most often performed are:

- Serum creatinine measurements, which reflect the ability of the kidneys to excrete creatinine, the waste product of energy metabolism
- Blood urea nitrogen levels, which reflect the ability of the kidneys to excrete urea
- Uric acid levels, which may indicate renal dysfunction if elevated
- Measurement of haemoglobin and haematocrit levels, white blood cell counts, serum potassium and phosphorus levels.

Endoscopic examination

A cystoscopy allows visual examination of the bladder; urethroscopy allows visual examination of the urethra. Both endoscopic techniques may be performed at the same time (panendoscopy). A cystoscope is inserted into the bladder via the urethra to enable visualisation of the bladder wall and contents of the bladder. Ureteric catheters can be inserted via the endoscope, a biopsy obtained, and small tumours or stones may be removed.

Radiological investigations

Plain X-ray films may be taken to show the size, shape and position of the kidneys, or to show the presence of calculi in the urinary tract.

An intravenous pyelogram (IVP) involves the intravenous injection of a contrast medium, followed by a series of X-rays. Before this procedure it is necessary for the client to fast and have an empty bowel by the administration of an oral laxative, suppositories or enema. This prevents the presence of faeces in the bowel obstructing the radiologist's view of the urinary system. Well-functioning kidneys excrete the contrast medium rapidly, whereas impaired kidney function delays excretion. The IVP also provides information about the size and shape of the kidneys and ureters and the presence of calculi in the urinary tract. After any procedure involving the use of contrast medium, the nurse must observe the client for any adverse reactions such as numbness, tingling, or palpitations and report these to the RN or medical officer.

A retrograde pyelogram involves the insertion of catheters into the ureters through a cystoscope. Contrast medium is introduced through the ureteric catheters into the pelvis or the kidneys, and X-ray films are taken.

A cystourethrogram involves the introduction of contrast medium into the bladder through a urethral catheter. X-ray films are taken before, during and after micturition to show the outline of the bladder, the urethra and any backflow of urine into the ureters.

Renal angiography involves passing a special catheter into the femoral artery through a small incision in the groin. The catheter is passed into the aorta to the level of the renal arteries. Contrast medium is injected through the catheter to outline the renal arteries on X-ray film.

Urodynamics is the study of the hydrology and mechanics of the urinary bladder filling and emptying.

Computerised axial tomography (CAT) scan of the abdomen may be performed to identify kidney size or structural alterations within the urinary system. It may be done with or without contrast medium.

A renal scan demonstrates blood flow to the kidneys, following the intravenous administration of a small quantity of radioactive isotope. Pictures are taken at various intervals after injection of the isotope.

Abdominal ultrasound is a non-invasive technique whereby high frequency sound waves enable body organs to be examined on a computer screen.

Renal biopsy

A biopsy of kidney tissue may be taken for microscopic tissue examination. After injection of local anaesthetic a special biopsy needle is inserted through the skin to obtain a sample from the cortex of the kidney. After a renal biopsy the client must be monitored closely for haematuria, rapid weak pulse, pallor or low blood pressure, as these may indicate haemorrhage from the biopsy site.

CARE OF THE CLIENT WITH A DISORDER OF THE URINARY SYSTEM

Although specific nursing actions and medical management vary depending on the disorder, the main aims of care are to prevent and manage alterations in elimination, promote comfort, maintain skin integrity, and maintain fluid and nutritional status.

PREVENTING AND MANAGING ALTERED ELIMINATION OF URINE

Care includes assisting the patient with micturition, observation and collection of urine, maintenance of urinary continence, and care of the patient who requires internal or external urinary drainage apparatus. (See Clinical Interest Box 32.3 for a sample nursing plan for a client with urinary incontinence.)

PROMOTING COMFORT

A client with a urinary system disorder may experience discomfort or pain from a distended bladder, dysuria associated with a lower UTI, or severe pain caused by renal or ureteric calculi. The nursing care plan should be designed to provide for pain management that is appropriate for each client. Nursing measures should be implemented to assist

CLINICAL INTEREST BOX 32.3
Nursing care plan for a client with urinary incontinence

Assessment
Mr James has been admitted to your ward for investigation of urinary incontinence. His wife of 60 years has recently passed away and his GP has prescribed diazepam 5 mg before retiring at night to help relieve his anxiety. Since starting the medication, Mr James reports urge incontinence first thing in the morning. He is very embarrassed and distressed.

Nursing diagnosis
Urge urinary incontinence

Planning
Client outcomes
- Client will report relief from urge urinary incontinence or a decrease in incidence
- Client will maintain skin integrity

Nursing interventions and rationales
- Perform a complete urinalysis to determine underlying medical disorders
- Maintain a continence chart for at least 48 hours to establish continence pattern
- Review all medications in consultation with the medical officer to determine if any are thought to be contributing to the incontinence
- Teach pelvic floor exercises and distraction techniques to help prevent incontinent episodes
- Review client fluid intake and types of fluid consumed, as alcohol irritates the bladder and caffeine can cause urgency
- Teach the client the importance of skin integrity and the impact that incontinence can have on this
- Provide the client with information about the Continence Foundation of Australia to enable him to seek support after discharge if necessary

Evaluation
- Client reports urinary continence or reduced incidence of incontinence episodes
- Client reports that he performs pelvic floor exercises at least three times daily
- Client's fluid intake is at least 2 L per day and caffeine intake stops after 4 p.m.
- Client is clean and dry at all times and has good skin integrity
- Client understands the role and function of the Continence Foundation of Australia

comfort needs, and analgesics should be administered by an RN as prescribed. Other medications such as antibiotics and urinary antiseptics may be prescribed to help control the discomfort associated with infections, such as cystitis. Mild or severe generalised pruritus commonly accompanies uraemia and end-stage renal disease. Constant itching is distressing for clients, and the nurse should implement measures to relieve pruritus. Many clients are embarrassed so it is important that the nurse preserves dignity and privacy at all times.

MAINTAINING SKIN INTEGRITY

Several factors contribute to the loss of skin integrity in the client with a urinary system disorder:
- Pruritus accompanied by scratching
- Loss of urinary continence
- Oedema
- Dehydration
- Reduced mobility
- Altered sensation
- Decreased mental alertness.

These factors make the client susceptible to the development of decubitus ulcers. Measures that should be implemented to maintain skin integrity are described in Chapter 39 and include relief of pressure, provision of a well-balanced diet, adequate fluid intake (provided that the specific renal disorder does not contraindicate such a measure), and keeping the skin clean and free from moisture.

Maintaining nutritional and fluid status

Clients with impaired renal function are at risk of altered nutritional and fluid status. They may experience anorexia, nausea and vomiting, all of which can impair nutritional status. Dietary modifications and restrictions may be indicated for the client with impaired renal function. Commonly, salt, potassium and protein are restricted; client compliance is increased if the reasons for the dietary modifications are explained.

Excessive fluid loss may occur through the use of diuretics, in infectious processes, or through escape of fluid into the interstitial spaces as in nephrotic syndrome, whereas fluid retention occurs in some disorders such as renal failure. Maintenance of fluid balance may involve either an increased or restricted fluid input. The client is monitored by recording fluid input and output, daily weighing, and by observing for the signs and symptoms of dehydration or fluid retention (see Chapter 30).

ADDITIONAL NURSING ACTIVITIES

The nurse may be required to assist in the preparation of a client before specific diagnostic procedures and to monitor the condition afterwards. Catheterisation may be necessary to obtain a specimen of urine or to treat acute urinary retention. Nursing care of the client with a urinary catheter is provided earlier in this chapter.

Urinary diversion

A client whose bladder has been removed, for example, because of malignancy, will require urinary diversion. Various surgical techniques that divert the flow of urine are available (Figure 32.8):
- Ureterosigmoidostomy involves the implantation of the ureters into the sigmoid colon, resulting in urine being passed via the rectum
- Cutaneous ureterostomy involves bringing the ureters through the abdominal wall, with urine draining out through the stoma(s) into an ostomy appliance

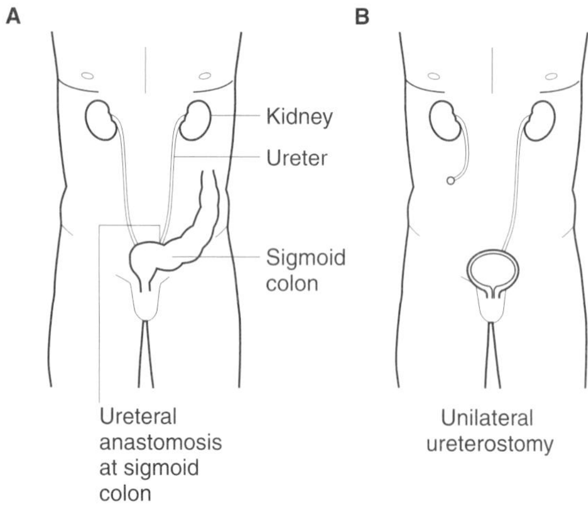

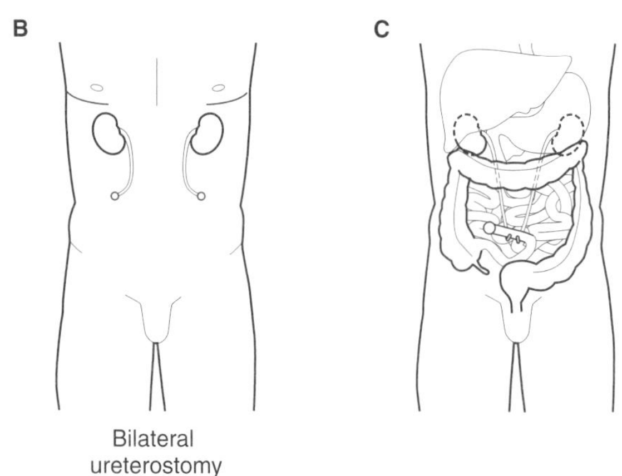

Figure 32.8 | Urinary diversion **A**: Ureterosigmoidostomy **B**: Cutaneous ureterostomy **C**: Ileal conduit

- Ileal conduit involves resection of part of the ileum. Both ureters are implanted into the proximal end of the ileal segment, and the distal end of the ileum is brought through the abdominal wall to form a stoma. The urine then drains out through the stoma into an ostomy appliance. This particular surgical technique is generally considered to be the most satisfactory if urinary diversion is required.

Care of the client with a urinary stoma is similar to the care required by a client who has a stoma created for the passage of faeces. The main aspects of care are the selection and management of ostomy appliances, care of the stoma and surrounding skin, and provision of psychological support.

Dialysis

When renal function is impaired to such an extent that conservative treatment is no longer effective, the client may be started on dialysis therapy. Dialysis combines the principles of diffusion, osmosis and filtration. It involves the transfer of solutes across a semi-permeable membrane, and the removal of waste products, excess salts and fluid from the blood. The method of dialysis is determined by the client's condition and may be performed by the client at home if the facilities are available. Home dialysis provides the client with greater independence.

There are three types of dialysis: peritoneal dialysis, continuous ambulatory peritoneal dialysis, and haemodialysis.

In peritoneal dialysis the client's peritoneum provides the semi-permeable membrane (Figure 32.9). The procedure may be performed on an intermittent or continuous basis. A catheter is placed in the abdominal cavity, and dialysate is instilled through the catheter. Dialysate may be an isotonic or hypertonic solution composed of water, electrolytes and dextrose. Through diffusion and osmosis, waste products together with excess electrolytes and fluid are transported from the blood into the dialysate. The dialysate is drained out by gravity before fresh dialysate is instilled. In intermittent dialysis each treatment takes about 9–12 hours, and is performed 3–4 times per week.

Continuous ambulatory peritoneal dialysis (CAPD) (Figure 32.10) enables the client to have greater mobility and independence. In this form of treatment the dialysate is run into the peritoneal cavity through a catheter and remains there for about 4 hours. The empty dialysis bag remains attached to the tubing and can be rolled up under the client's clothing. At the end of 4 hours the bag is unrolled, and the fluid is allowed to drain into it by gravity. After drainage, a fresh bag is connected and the procedure is repeated 3–5 times every day.

In haemodialysis the semi-permeable membrane is contained within a dialysis machine. Haemodialysis is performed an average of three times per week for a period of 4–6 hours. This method requires regular and convenient access to the client's blood circulation. Several systems are available that provide this access including an arterio-venous shunt (Figure 32.11a) or the creation of an arterio-venous fistula (Figure 32.11b). An arterio-venous shunt is an artificial passageway that allows blood to flow from an artery to a vein without going through a capillary network. An arterio-venous fistula, is created surgically to provide vascular access for haemodialysis. During haemodialysis, the client's blood is passed through the artificial kidney (haemodialysis machine) and then returned to the client's own circulation. The haemodialysis machine delivers the prescribed dialysate to the artificial kidney, which allows the removal of waste products and excess water and helps maintain or establish correct electrolyte levels and acid–base balance. The client's blood is anticoagulated during haemodialysis to prevent clotting in the tubing and machine. Heparin is used for this purpose and can be administered as a continuous infusion or intermittently. Although dialysis is a lifesaving treatment, it is nonetheless accompanied by risk. Table 32.4 lists the possible complications associated with either peritoneal dialysis or haemodialysis.

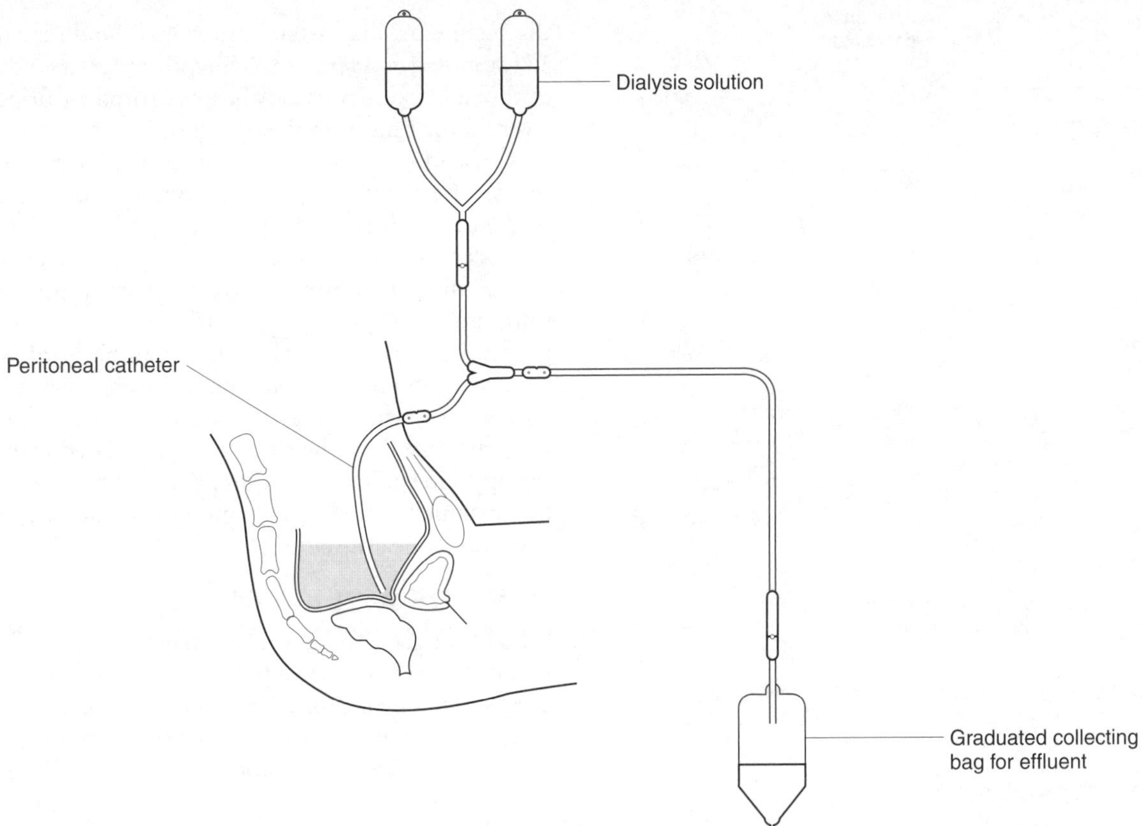

Figure 32.9 | Peritoneal dialysis *(Chilman & Thomas 1987)*

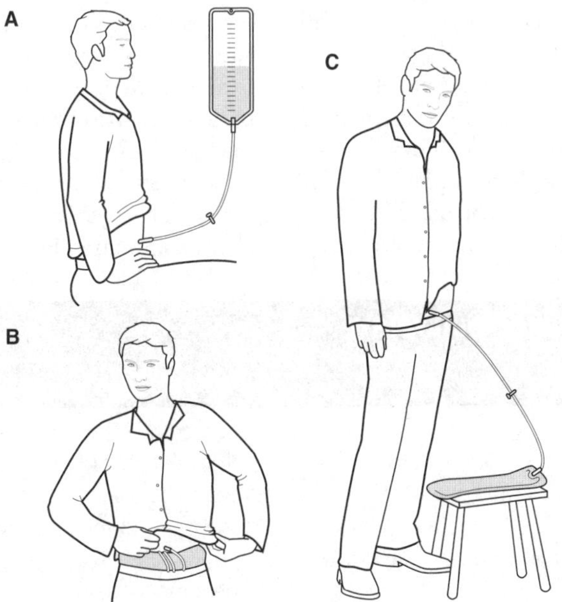

Figure 32.10 | Continuous ambulatory peritoneal dialysis (CAPD)

A: A bag of dialysate is attached to a tube in the client's abdomen so that the fluid flows into the peritoneal cavity

B: While the dialysate remains in the peritoneal cavity, the individual can roll up the bag, place it under their clothes and go about their normal activities

C: The bag is unrolled and suspended below the pelvis, which allows the dialysate to drain from the peritoneal cavity

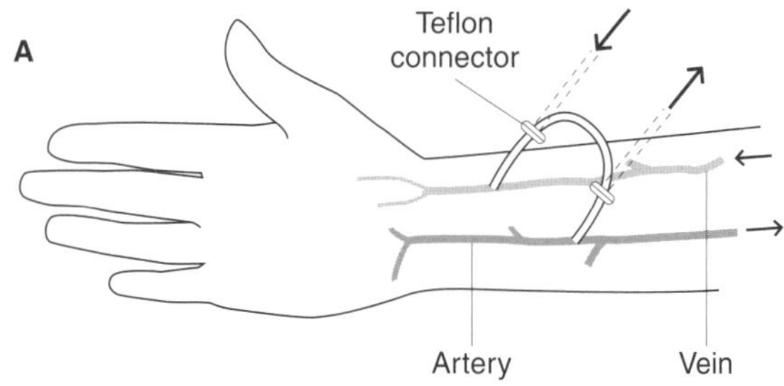

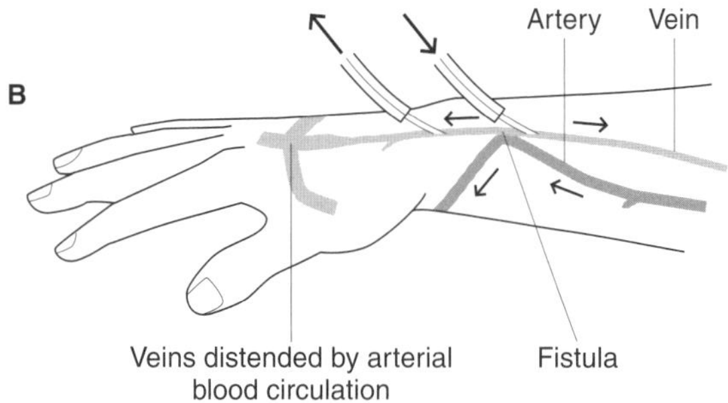

Figure 32.11 | **A**: Arterio-venous shunt **B**: Arterio-venous fistula *(Game et al 1989)*

Renal transplantation

As an alternative to long-term dialysis, the client with chronic renal failure may be assessed to determine suitability for a renal transplant. Unfortunately, the waiting list for potential recipients far exceeds the availability of donor kidneys. Transplant centres establish their own criteria and guidelines regarding recipient suitability and the procedures involved in obtaining donor kidneys. Renal transplant is a surgical procedure in which a donor kidney is transplanted into the recipient. The recipient's own kidneys may be either left or removed. The new kidney is placed in the left or right iliac fossa, outside the peritoneal cavity, and the renal vessels of the donor kidney are anastomosed to the recipient's iliac artery and vein. The donor ureter is anastomosed either to the recipient's ureter or bladder. The transplanted kidney usually begins to produce urine within a very short time after the operation.

Close monitoring of the client after surgery is essential to assess renal function and to detect early signs of rejection of the new kidney. To help prevent graft rejection, which may occur within 1–30 days or up to several years after the transplant, immunosuppressive drugs are administered. As immunosuppressive drugs increase the risk of infection, protective isolation techniques may be implemented. (Information on infection control is provided in Chapter 25.) A successful kidney transplant enables the client to lead a life free from the restrictions associated with dialysis therapy. However, immunosuppressive therapy will need to be continued as well as close monitoring of renal function and general health status.

CARE OF A CLIENT WITH INCONTINENCE OF URINE

Incontinence of urine is a relatively common problem that affects many people of all ages and both sexes. As a result there are now nurses who specialise in the management of incontinence. Continence advisors are also available to do a continence assessment of the client (see Clinical Interest Box 32.4 and Figure 32.12) and plan appropriate management to promote continence, and may use a variety of methods, such as a bladder chart (Figure 32.13) or continence assessment chart (Figure 32.14). The management of incontinence depends on identifying the cause and treating any underlying conditions. Nursing care of a client with incontinence requires understanding, patience and awareness of the need to preserve dignity and self-esteem.

A variety of products is available for managing incontinence. These have been designed to keep the incontinent client's skin and clothing dry, and it is important that the

TABLE 32.4 | COMPLICATIONS OF DIALYSIS

Peritoneal dialysis	Haemodialysis
Peritonitis	Haemorrhage, from heparinisation or from accidental disconnection of the apparatus
Obstructed catheter due to fibrin clot formation	Infection, at the insertion site or from contaminated equipment
Excessive protein loss	Thrombosis at the insertion site
Hyperglycaemia, if the dialysate contains high level of dextrose	Oedema of the hand or ischaemia of the fingers, as a result of the shunt or fistula
Candida or herpes zoster infections	Air embolism
Abdominal hernia or uterine prolapse, due to persistently raised intra-abdominal pressure	Hypotension from fluid and sodium removal
Psychological reactions to the therapy, e.g. anger or depression	Psychological reactions to the therapy (e.g. anger or depression)
Perforation of abdominal structures by the catheter	Hypothermia or hyperthermia as a result of a malfunctioning thermostat on the machine
	Hypertension (e.g. from fluid overload)

CLINICAL INTEREST BOX 32.4
Assessing incontinence

When assessing an individual with a continence problem, the nurse first needs to establish if there are any:

- Age-related changes
- Physical limitations
- Mental limitations
- Psychological problems
- Lifestyle factors
- Medications being taken
- Bladder-related medical problems

Secondly the client's environment needs to be assessed:

- Is the client close enough to the toilets?
- Is the height of the toilet appropriate?
- Are there physical barriers to the toilet?
- Are there enough toilets for the number of clients and residents?
- Can help be summoned if required?
- Do the staff respond quickly to the call bell?

client chooses the aids that are most suitable for them. The Continence Aids Assistance Scheme (CAAS) may be useful for some clients, as they assist not only with choice but also with cost. CAAS is an initiative of the Commonwealth Department of Health and Family Services. Choice depends on the type of incontinence (e.g. someone with mild stress incontinence would not need to wear a large pad), how much urine is lost, the ability of the person, the frequency of access to a toilet or changing facilities, and the cost.

Aids include disposable pads made of absorbent pulp and containing a powder that turns to gel when wet. They have a waterproof backing to prevent leakage and the more expensive brands have a special layer that keeps the skin dry. They come in a variety of shapes and sizes and manufacturers claim that the materials are biodegradable. Disposable bed and chair pads are also available to protect furniture. A range of reusable products is also available. These usually have an absorbent layer sandwiched between a stay-dry layer and a waterproof layer to prevent leaking. There are pants that are not absorbent but which hold a pad in place, as well as washable sheets that protect both the bed and the client.

Other aids are collection devices such as catheters, drainage bags and penile sheaths or condoms. Condoms are fitted over the penis and attached to a collection bag. Leg bags can be worn under normal clothing and provide the male incontinent client with greater freedom of mobility. As there are several styles of condom fittings and various methods of attaching them to the penis, the nurse should follow the manufacturers' directions regarding their use. Before any appliance is fitted, the penis must be cleaned and dried and observation made to ensure that the foreskin is not retracted (Table 32.5). The appliance is placed over the penis and secured in position. A special adhesive tape is commonly used and care must be taken to ensure that it is not applied too tightly. The tubing from the appliance is connected to either a bedside collection bag or a leg bag. The penis should be observed for oedema and discolouration; if this is detected, the appliance is removed immediately and reapplied more loosely. At least every 24 hours the appliance is removed and the penis cleaned and dried before reapplication. Use of such appliances may be discontinued if there are signs of skin excoriation, persistent oedema of the penis or UTI.

Commodes are also useful for people with incontinence, as well as toilet frames that can make getting on and off the toilet easier. Client clothing can be adapted if necessary to suit the client's needs and to facilitate easy access to any incontinence aids being used, such as use of velcro fastenings on pants. For photographs of different continence aids, see: www.health.qld.gov.au/mass/prescriber/products.asp.

KEY ASPECTS RELATED TO THE NURSING CARE OF A CLIENT WITH INCONTINENCE

- **Hygiene.** As constant moisture on the skin may lead to excoriation and the development of decubitus ulcers, it is essential that the skin is kept clean and dry. When the client is incontinent their skin should be washed with mild soap and water and gently dried. Particular attention is paid to the genital area, the groin and the crease between the buttocks. A protective cream may be applied to repel moisture and prevent excoriation.
- **Clothing.** Any wet clothing or bedclothes should be removed immediately and taken from the room to prevent offensive odours. The client should be provided with clean dry clothing.
- **Toilet facilities.** The client should be encouraged to void at regular intervals (e.g. every 2 hours). Ambulant people should have easy access to the toilet, and non-ambulant people should be provided with toilet utensils. Any request for use of toilet facilities should be responded to promptly.
- **Fluids.** Unless contraindicated, the client should be encouraged to drink at least 1500 mL daily, as an inadequate fluid input may further decrease the functional capacity of the bladder.
- **Attitude.** As a client is generally distressed and embarrassed by incontinence, the nurse should adopt a positive approach to continence management. The nurse should demonstrate discretion, tact and understanding to promote the client's dignity and self-esteem.
- **Incontinence aids.** As previously mentioned, a variety of aids is available to assist in the management of incontinence. These are used according to the client's needs.
- **Perineal exercises.** The client may be required to perform a regimen of isometric exercises designed to improve the retention of urine. These are called Kegel exercises (Clinical Interest Box 32.5) and consist of

Mount Henry Hospital **CONTINENCE SCREENING** WARD: ____________ DATE: ____________	LABEL
Relevant factors	**Information**
Presenting problem: urinary/faecal incontinence history, stress, urge, how long?	
Relevant diagnosis C.V.A.M.S. Dementia, Spina Bifida, Diabetes, Parkinson's Disease	
Gynaecological/urological history: Prostatectomy, multiple pregnancies, atrophic vagina/urethra	
Previous investigations: M.S.U. Ward, urinalysis, bladder scans, urodynamics, I.V.P. Sigmoidoscopy	
Psychosocial effects: Embarrassed, withdrawn, apathetic, denial, depression	
Self-awareness: Is resident aware of incontinence? Insight	
Communication: Ability to request toileting, familiar terms used, language difficulties	
Behavioural cues: Restless when wants to void/defecate, verbally agitated	
Coping strategies: Regular toileting, use of tissues/pads, fluid reduction	
Environmental: Location of toilet, raised seat commode, clothing — belts, buttons, stockings	
DOCUMENTATION AND ACCOUNTABILITY MANUAL	1–105

Figure 32.12 | Continence screening *(Aged Services Association, NSW)*

AGED SERVICES ASSOCIATION
NSW & ACT INC.

URINARY CONTINENCE ASSESSMENT

FACILITY:

Clinical Record No: ....
Surname: ....
Given Names: ....
D.O.B: .... Sex: ....
Room No: .... Doctor: ....
Pension No: ....
Medicare No: .... PHB No: ....

To be used if it has been established that the person has a problem or potential problem maintaining continence. Address all relevant questions, indicating if not applicable.
NOTE: Comments should include description of individual's needs or program required.

Q1. IS IT AN AGE RELATED CHANGE?

YES ❑ NO ❑ 1.1 Decreased Capacity? ....
YES ❑ NO ❑ 1.2 Decreased Warning Time? ....
YES ❑ NO ❑ 1.3 Increased Nocturnal Volume? ....

Q2 IS THERE A PHYSICAL LIMITATION?

YES ❑ NO ❑ 2.1 Pain? ....
YES ❑ NO ❑ 2.2 Posture? ....
YES ❑ NO ❑ 2.3 Able to rise from chair? ....
YES ❑ NO ❑ 2.4 Able to balance while attending clothes? ....
YES ❑ NO ❑ 2.5 Able to bend at the hips? ....
YES ❑ NO ❑ 2.6 Able to attend clothing? ....
YES ❑ NO ❑ 2.7 Able to attend own hygiene? ....
YES ❑ NO ❑ 2.8 Able to leave bathroom and return to where they wish to be? ....

Q3 IS THERE A MENTAL LIMITATION?

YES ❑ NO ❑ 3.1 Can the person recognise the urge to go? ....
YES ❑ NO ❑ 3.2 Can the person remember to go? ....
YES ❑ NO ❑ 3.3 Can the person find the way? ....
YES ❑ NO ❑ 3.4 Can the person remember what she/he is there for? ....
YES ❑ NO ❑ 3.5 Can the person recognise the toilet? ....

Q4 IS THERE A PSYCHOLOGICAL PROBLEM?
Consider Referral to GP/Specialist or Nurse Continence Advisor or other appropriate source.

YES ❑ NO ❑ 4.1 Lost Inhibitions? ....
YES ❑ NO ❑ 4.2 Lost Motivation? ....
YES ❑ NO ❑ 4.3 Denying the problem? ....
YES ❑ NO ❑ 4.4 Depression? ....
YES ❑ NO ❑ 4.5 Stress? ....
YES ❑ NO ❑ 4.6 Anxiety? ....

Figure 32.13 | Bladder chart

St Joseph's Private Hospital

CONTINENCE ASSESSMENT

Client name ______________________________

Address ______________________________

____

Unit Record No: ____________________

Medical Officer: ____________________

Directions for use

1. Complete the chart over a full 3-day period
2. Make an entry on every occasion the client passes urine, either in the toilet/commode or when has an episode of incontinence
3. Document clearly according to the following indicators:
   DRY = no urine passed on checking underwear/pad/bed
   DAMP = underwear or pad is damp but outer clothing is not affected (not damp)
   WET = incontinent to the extent that outer clothing is wet or pad is soaked
   SATURATED = outer clothing is extremely wet/urine has leaked through onto furniture/floor

Date and time commenced: ____________________

Date and time to complete: ____________________

Date	Time	Dry Damp Wet Saturated	Continent in toilet/commode Volume voided (note with ** if approximated)	Fluid intake type and amount	Comments	Signature

Figure 32.14 | Continence assessment chart

TABLE 32.5 | GUIDELINES FOR APPLYING A CONDOM CATHETER

A condom catheter is used for a male client who is incontinent but can void on his own

Action	Rationale
Review and carry out the steps in Appendix 1	
Assess the need for and the client's willingness to use a condom catheter	If the client is unwilling, he may detach the condom catheter
Assess the condition of the skin on the penis	Urine incontinence places the skin at risk for breakdown
Collect equipment: condom catheter; disposable gloves, adherent tape, basin, warm water, soap, washcloth, towel, urine collection bag with drainage tubing or leg bag and straps	Promotes work efficiency
Explain the procedure to the client and maintain privacy	Reduces anxiety
Place the client in a supine position and cover the upper torso with a blanket, then fold the sheet down so it covers the legs and can be lowered to expose the genitalia	Provides comfort and prevents unnecessary exposure
Prepare the urinary drainage bag for easy attachment to the condom catheter. Roll the wider tip of the condom sheath towards the narrower tip	Prepares the system for use
Wash hands and don disposable gloves	Prevents transfer of microorganisms
Wash and dry the penis and surrounding skin	Cleanses the skin before application of the condom device
Apply the double-sided elastic tape in a spiral fashion from the base of the penis downwards	Provides a surface on which the condom catheter can be attached without impeding circulation in the penis. Some condom catheters attach with a velcro strip over the sheath
Grasp the penis along the shaft. Hold the condom sheath at the tip of the penis and smoothly roll the sheath onto the penis, leaving 2.5–5 cm of space between the tip of the penis and the drainage tube of the condom sheath	Positions the condom catheter on the penis. Allows free passage of urine into the collecting tube and drainage bag
Position the penis downwards and connect the drainage tube to the collection bag	Allows urine to flow into the collection bag
Return bed to the low position and make the client comfortable; place call bell within reach	Provides comfort and security
Check the penis after 30 minutes and then every 2 hours to ensure catheter is not twisted	Ensures that the catheter is not too tight and impairing circulation; twisting of the catheter impedes urine flow
Remove gloves and wash hands	Reduces risk of transfer of microorganisms
Document the date, condition of the genital area, size and type of catheter applied, type of drainage collection attached to the catheter, amount, colour and character of urine obtained in bag, and the client's tolerance of the procedure	Documents the use of condom catheter

(adapted from deWit 2005)

a series of voluntary contractions of the muscles of the pelvic floor and perineum. The nurse may be required to instruct and supervise the client in the performance of these exercises.

- **Medication.** The nurse should be aware of the various medications that may be prescribed in the management of incontinence, and their side effects; for example, antibiotics to treat a UTI.
- **Surgical intervention.** This is sometimes indicated in the treatment of incontinence; for example, an operation may be performed to elevate the bladder into an improved anatomical position.
- **Retraining regimens.** Planned bladder-retraining regimens are commonly implemented to promote continence or to modify incontinence. Before a regimen starts, complete assessment of the client is necessary to provide accurate information about the incontinent episodes. The recording of every episode of incontinence and the time of occurrence is made for 24–48 hours. A regimen is then started, according to the client's usual toileting pattern, whereby the client is encouraged to void at specified intervals; for example, 2 hourly, day and night. Documentation is continued and the schedule is adjusted as necessary. If the client remains continent in between the 2-hourly toileting, the intervals may be increased to 3- and then 4-hourly. Consistency and a client-centred approach are essential for success.

CLINICAL INTEREST BOX 32.5
Pelvic muscle (Kegel) exercises

Exercise program for making pelvic floor muscles stronger:

- Check with a continence adviser or physiotherapist to ensure that exercises are being performed correctly
- Find the right muscles: when passing urine, stop the flow mid-stream. Then relax and finish passing urine. The muscles you tighten and pull upwards to stop the flow of urine are the pelvic floor muscles. Tighten the muscles around the anus by imagining that you are trying to stop passing wind.
- Test your muscle strength: women — place one or two clean fingers in the vagina and tighten the pelvic floor muscles; men — press one finger on the area between the anus and scrotum; when the pelvic floor muscles are tightened, this area will move up and away from the finger.
- To do the exercise, squeeze the muscle identified and hold for a count of 10 seconds. Relax for a count of 10 seconds. It may take 2 weeks to be able to hold for 10 seconds.
- Do the exercise three times a day: 15 in the morning, 15 in the afternoon and 20 at night. Or for 10 minutes three times a day. Try to work up to 25 repetitions at one time. It will take about 2 weeks to notice a difference. Within a month of regular exercise, there should be a decrease in instances of incontinence.

(adapted from deWit 2005)

CLINICAL INTEREST BOX 32.6
Nursing diagnoses in urinary problems

- Body image disturbance
- Incontinence, stress
- Incontinence, urge
- Incontinence, urinary, functional
- Pain
- Self-care deficit, toileting
- Skin integrity impaired
- Urinary elimination, altered
- Urinary retention

- Some clients — for example, those who have a neurogenic bladder as a result of a neurological dysfunction — may be educated to perform intermittent self-catheterisation, or Credé's manoeuvre. Credé's manoeuvre involves applying manual pressure over the lower abdomen to promote complete emptying of the bladder.
- Urinary incontinence is a major but largely hidden problem in Australian society. Fortunately, recognition of the needs and problems of clients who experience incontinence is increasing. Remember that incontinence is sometimes treatable and always manageable. Clinical Interest Box 32.6 lists possible nursing diagnoses for a client with altered urinary elimination.

SUMMARY

The urinary system is essential for homeostasis. It is the means by which the body rids itself of a variety of metabolic wastes and maintains fluid and electrolyte balance. The urinary system consists of the kidneys, the ureters, the urinary bladder and the urethra. The kidneys filter the blood to maintain its normal composition, volume and pH. In carrying out this function, the kidneys secrete urine.

Urine forms by the processes of filtration, selective reabsorption and secretion. Urine is composed of water, urea, mineral salts, uric acid and creatinine. When the kidneys form urine it passes down the ureters by peristaltic action, to the bladder. It is then stored in the bladder until micturition is initiated and it is excreted from the body through the urethra. Micturition is initiated when the bladder walls are stretched, usually when the bladder holds about 300 mL of urine. Urine is a waste product of metabolism, and regular elimination is necessary for the maintenance of normal body function. Elimination of urine is affected by various factors ranging from the intake of food and fluids to the changes that occur as a result of certain disease states.

As part of the assessment of a client's elimination status, urine is observed and, if necessary, tested in the ward or sent to the laboratory for analysis. The nurse must ensure that specimens are collected and tested correctly so that accurate results are obtained.

Problems associated with the elimination of urine may occur, and the implementation of certain nursing actions may be necessary to assist the client to meet elimination needs. All procedures must be thoroughly understood so that the desired effects are achieved and safety and comfort are promoted.

Normal functioning of the urinary system may be impaired as a result of changes in kidney structure, changes in the ability of the kidneys to secrete and excrete urine, or alterations in the passage of urine through the urinary tract. The major problems associated with urinary system disorders are pain, changes in voiding pattern or urine output, and changes in the urine. Disorders of the urinary system can be classified as those that are congenital, resulting from multiple causes, infectious, immunological, degenerative, neoplastic, obstructive or traumatic in origin.

Diagnostic tests used to assess urinary system function include: laboratory analysis of urine, blood and tissue; radiological examination; and endoscopy.

Care of the client with a urinary system disorder includes preventing and managing altered elimination of urine, promoting comfort, maintaining skin integrity, and maintaining nutritional and fluid status. Nursing activities include observation and collection of urine and assisting with the care of a client who requires intervention to eliminate urine.

Dialysis and renal transplant are two forms of therapy that may be indicated for a client with specific end-stage renal dysfunction.

REVIEW EXERCISES

1. Describe the structure and function of each part of the urinary system.
2. Describe normal urine and voiding.
3. Identify the factors that affect urinary elimination.
4. Outline the different types of urinary incontinence.
5. Describe at least three different aids used for incontinence.
6. Describe the major manifestations of urinary system disorders.
7. List at least six diagnostic tests that may be performed to determine urinary function.

CRITICAL THINKING EXERCISES

1. Mr Fitzgibbon has brought his 87-year-old wife to the clinic where you are working for a check-up. Mrs Fitzgibbon has Alzheimer's-type dementia and has associated total incontinence. While waiting for the doctor, you are checking Mrs Fitzgibbon's weight and her husband tells you that she has become excoriated around the genital area.
   (a) What do you think has caused this?
   (b) What advice would you give to Mr Fitzgibbon?
   (c) What organisation can you refer them to?
2. Mr Larouche has had a prostatectomy and you are caring for him postoperatively. He has an indwelling catheter attached to a drainage bag. The urine has been slightly bloodstained. When you go to check Mr Larouche's vital signs he complains of a sense of fullness in the lower abdominal region. You note that his lower abdomen is distended and that his catheter has not drained any urine since you emptied the drainage bag 6 hours ago despite the fact that he has been drinking extra fluids as ordered.
   (a) What is the likely cause of the abdominal distension?
   (b) What could be done to relieve it?
   (c) Whose role is this?

REFERENCES AND FURTHER READING

Ackley BJ, Ladwig GB (2002) *Nursing Diagnosis Handbook — a Guide to Planning Care*, 5th edn. Mosby, St Louis

Ankner GM (2007) *Case Studies in Medical–Surgical Nursing*. Thomson Delmar Learning, Clifton Park, NY

—— (2008). *Medical–Surgical Nursing*. Thomson Delmar Learning, Clifton Park, NY

Chilman AM, Thomas M (1987) *Understanding Nursing Care*, 3rd edn. Churchill Livingstone, Edinburgh

Commonwealth Department of Health and Ageing. *Types of Continence Products*. Australian Government Publishing Service, Canberra

Crisp J, Taylor C (eds) (2005) *Potter & Perry's Fundamentals of Nursing*, 2nd edn. Elsevier Australia, Sydney

deWit SC (2005) *Fundamental Concepts and Skills for Nursing*, 2nd edn. WB Saunders, Philadelphia

Game C, Anderson R, Kidd J (eds) (1989) *Medical Surgical Nursing: a care text*. Churchill Livingstone, Melbourne

Moore KH (2001) The cost of urinary incontinence. *Medical Journal of Australia*, 174: 436–7

Potter PA, Perry AG (2008) *Fundamentals of Nursing*, 7th edn. Mosby, St Louis

Stamoulos P, Bakalis S (2005) *Renal and Urinary System and Electrolyte Balance*. Hodder Arnold, London

Thibodeau GA (2008) *Structure and Function of the Body*. Mosby, St. Louis

Tortora GJ, Grabowski SR (2000) *Principles of Anatomy and Physiology*, 9th edn. John Wiley & Sons Inc, New York

ONLINE RESOURCES

Australian Government of Health and Ageing. Continence Aids Assistance Scheme: www.health.gov.au/acc/continence/caas.htm

Continence Foundation of Australia: www.contfound.org.au. Got to go? … Again? email: anne@contfound.org.au

Queensland Health, continence resources: http://www.health.qld.gov.au/mass/resourcescont.asp

The National Public Toilet Map: www.toiletmap.gov.au

Chapter 33
BOWEL ELIMINATION

OBJECTIVES

- Define the key terms/concepts
- Describe the anatomical position and structure of the digestive system
- Describe the physiological functions of the various areas of the digestive system
- List the four functions of the large intestine
- Explain how the presence of bile influences the colour of faeces
- List six functions of the liver
- Describe normal faeces and the defecation process
- Identify the factors that affect bowel elimination
- Apply appropriate principles when implementing nursing actions to assist the individual to meet their bowel elimination needs
- Perform procedures described in this chapter, accurately and safely, including the observation, collection and testing of faeces, and assisting clients with bowel elimination
- Briefly describe the specific disorders of the digestive system
- Describe the diagnostic tests that may be performed to assess digestive system function
- Employ critical thinking to provide care for clients with alterations in bowel elimination

KEY TERMS/CONCEPTS

colon
colostomy
constipation
defecation
diarrhoea
endoscopy
enema
faeces
flatulence
haemorrhoids
hepatitis
ileostomy
impaction
incontinence
peristalsis
peritoneum
stoma
stomatitis
suppository

CHAPTER FOCUS

The digestive process enables consumed food and fluids to be broken down into nutrients and electrolytes that can be absorbed by the body for cell energy and function. This process produces waste products that must be eliminated regularly. Healthy bowel function is maintained by routine elimination habits, a nutritional diet with the recommended amount of fibre and fluid intake, and daily mild exercise to stimulate colonic motility. The variety of factors that can affect normal bowel elimination are explored in this chapter. Observation of the individual's ability to eliminate faeces, together with observation of the faeces, provides the nurse with an objective assessment of the client's bowel elimination status. As a result, appropriate nursing actions may be planned and implemented to assist the individual to meet their bowel elimination needs.

LIVED EXPERIENCE

I was raised by my mother, who gave me laxatives — chemical laxatives are harsh and irritating to the bowel and should never be used. They provide only temporary relief and add to the problem. I have learnt that diet and exercise and drinking adequate water prevents constipation.

Lucy, 63, retired teacher

THE DIGESTIVE TRACT

Every cell in the body requires energy to carry out its normal functions. Cellular energy is produced when nutrients in food are broken down and absorbed. Solid wastes that accumulate during the digestive process must be eliminated. The digestive system is the means by which food is ingested, digested and eliminated. In the digestive tract, food is digested to its elemental components — nutrients, fluid and electrolytes. The digested elements are absorbed into the bloodstream for transport to all body cells, and the solid wastes that accumulate during digestion are excreted from the body.

ANATOMY

The digestive tract is a muscular tube about 9–10 metres in length, which extends from the mouth to the anus (Figure 33.1). The structure of the alimentary canal is similar for most of its length and consists of an outer covering, middle layers of involuntary muscle and connective tissue, and an inner mucous membrane lining (Figure 33.2).

The outer covering of the alimentary canal consists of fibrous tissue (the serosa) or, in the abdomen, peritoneum. The *peritoneum* is a double-layer serous membrane that secretes serous fluid to prevent friction between the abdominal organs. The inner layer is called the visceral serous membrane and the outer layer the parietal serous membrane. The two layers of the peritoneum are kept proximate and separated by peritoneal fluid. The peritoneum forms a lining for the abdominal cavity (parietal layer) and a covering for most of the abdominal organs (visceral layer).

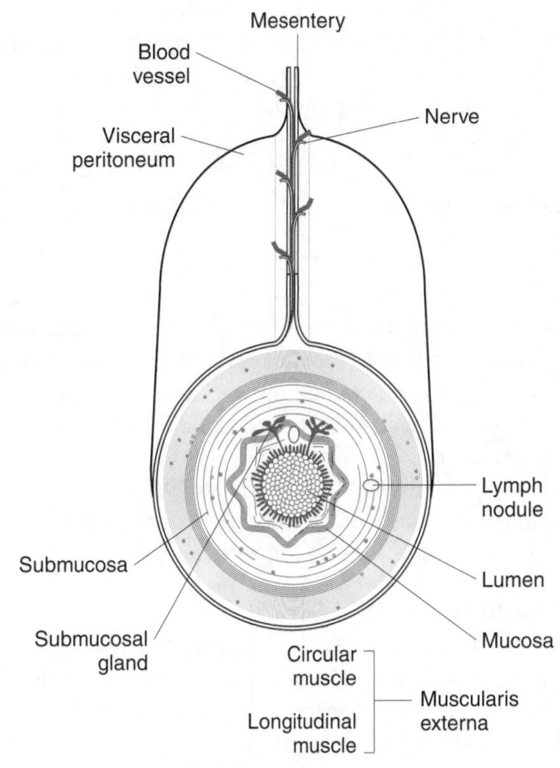

Figure 33.2 | Structure of the alimentary canal

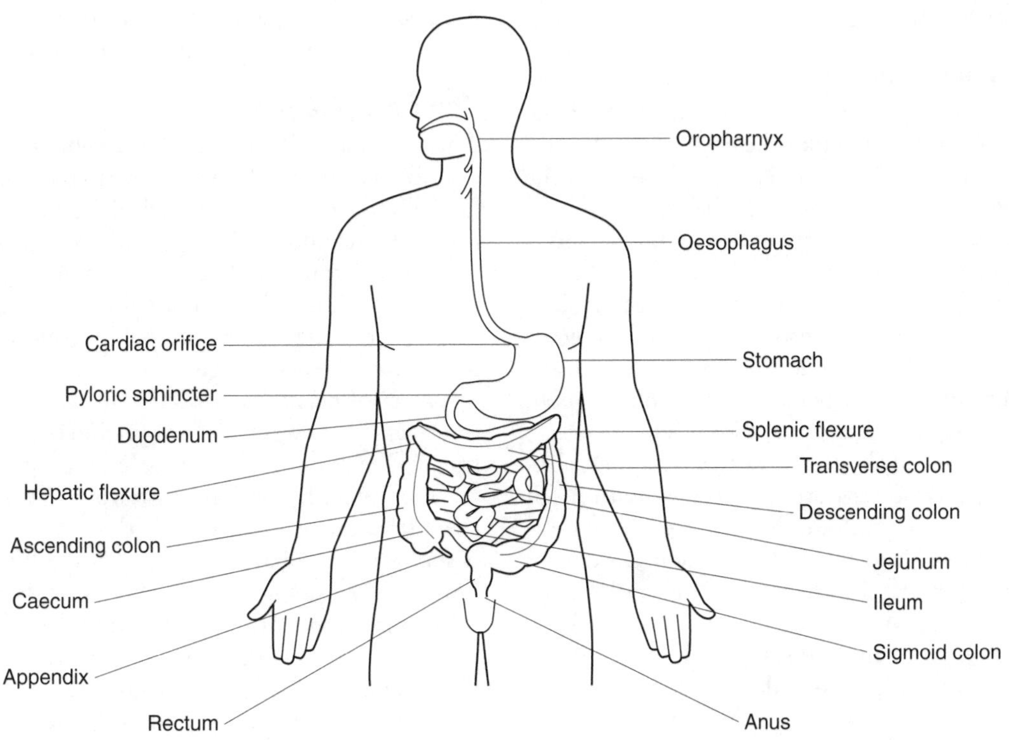

Figure 33.1 | The parts of the alimentary canal

The mesentery, which is formed by the peritoneum, covers the intestines and attaches them to the posterior abdominal wall. Ligaments are formed by folds of peritoneum to attach some organs to each other or to the abdominal wall. The greater omentum is attached to the lower border of the stomach and hangs down like an apron and loops up to be attached to the transverse colon. The lesser omentum extends from the lower border of the liver to the lesser curvature of the stomach.

The middle layer of the digestive tract contains smooth involuntary muscle with both circular and longitudinal fibres.

The innermost layer of the digestive tract is composed of connective tissue (the submucosa), which contains many large blood and lymph vessels, and an inner lining of mucous membrane (the mucosa), which secretes mucus into the digestive tract. The mucosa also contains a small amount of loose connective tissue and a thin layer of smooth muscle.

The organs that make up the digestive tract are the mouth, the oropharynx, the oesophagus, the stomach, the small intestine and the large intestine.

The mouth

The mouth, or oral cavity, has boundaries of muscle and bone and is lined by mucous membrane. The lips protect its anterior opening, the cheeks form the lateral walls, the hard palate forms its anterior roof, and the soft palate forms its posterior roof. The uvula is a finger-like muscular projection hanging down from the midline of the soft palate. It helps prevent the entry of food and fluids into the nasal cavities.

Components of the mouth

The mouth contains the tongue and the teeth. The tongue is a muscular organ that occupies the floor of the mouth. It is attached to the hyoid bone and also to the floor of the mouth by folds of mucous membrane called the frenulum. The tongue consists of a mass of voluntary muscle and is covered by squamous epithelium. On the upper surface of the tongue there are many small projections called papillae, which contain tastebuds, the sensory endings of the nerve that perceives taste. The tongue is a very mobile organ which is important in the chewing (mastication) of food, assists in swallowing and is essential for speech.

The teeth are embedded in the maxillae and the mandible. All teeth have the same basic structural organisation but differ in shape and size. Each tooth has one or more roots embedded in the maxilla or mandible, a portion (the crown) above the gum, and a neck, which joins the root and the crown and which is surrounded by the gum. Each tooth is made up of an ivory-like substance called dentine; a central pulp cavity containing blood and lymphatic vessels, nerves and connective tissue; and a thin layer of enamel covering the crown. In children there are 20 deciduous (milk) teeth, consisting of 10 in each jaw; in adults there are 16 permanent teeth in each jaw. The teeth are named according to their shape and function. In each jaw there are four incisors, used for biting; two canines, used for tearing; four premolars, used for crushing; and six molars, used for grinding. A wisdom tooth is the third molar tooth and it is the last tooth to erupt. Wisdom teeth usually erupt from age 18 to 25.

The salivary glands, of which there are three pairs, pour their secretions into the mouth. The salivary glands are:

1. The parotid glands, each of which lies below the ear and between the mandible and the sternocleidomastoid muscle. Each parotid duct opens through a papilla on the cheek opposite the crown of the second upper molar
2. The submandibular glands, each of which lies beneath the mandible. Each duct opens on either the left or right side of the frenulum of the tongue
3. The sublingual glands, situated beneath the mucous membrane on the floor of the mouth.

The salivary glands are accessory digestive organs.

The oropharynx

The oropharynx is the muscular canal forming the passage between the oral cavity and the major parts of the alimentary canal. Lined by mucous membrane, it is a tube about 13 cm long and is continuous with the nasopharynx above and the oesophagus below.

Functions of the oropharynx

Through the act of swallowing, masticated food formed into a bolus is pushed into the oesophagus by the muscles of the pharynx. Together with the other two sections of the pharynx, it forms part of the respiratory tract.

The oesophagus

The oesophagus is a muscular tube about 20–25 cm long, extending from the pharynx above to the stomach below. It lies behind the larynx and trachea, in the midline through the neck and thorax, and passes through the diaphragm to join the stomach. The oesophagus has an outer layer of fibrous tissue, a layer of involuntary muscle, a layer of connective tissue, and a lining of mucous membrane. The function of the oesophagus is to carry food to the stomach by means of peristaltic action.

Peristalsis is a wave-like progression of alternate contraction and relaxation of the muscle fibres of the oesophagus or intestines, by which contents are propelled along the alimentary canal. At rest, the opening between the oesophagus and pharynx (oesophageal sphincter) is closed. During swallowing the muscles contract and cause the sphincter to open, thereby allowing the bolus of food to pass down into the oesophagus. A wave of contraction in the circular muscle layer then propels the bolus down to the stomach. The bottom end of the oesophagus acts as a functional sphincter, which is normally in a state of tonic contraction. As the peristaltic wave approaches the sphincter,

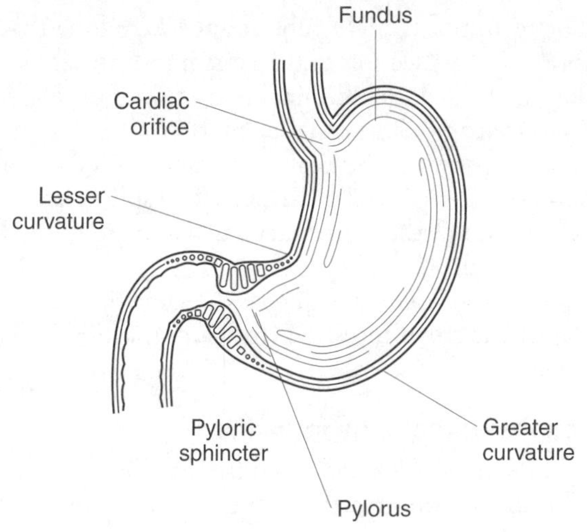

Figure 33.3 | The stomach

the muscle relaxes and allows food to enter the stomach. The sphincter then closes again and prevents regurgitation of gastric contents back into the oesophagus.

The stomach

The stomach is a hollow muscular organ that lies primarily in the upper left quadrant of the abdomen, beneath the diaphragm (Figure 33.3). It is commonly described as being 'J shaped', but the size and shape of the stomach varies according to its contents. The stomach is divided into four areas: the fundus (the upper portion); the cardia, where the oesophagus joins the stomach; the body, or main part of the stomach; and the pylorus (the narrowed lower portion).

The 'curvatures' of the stomach are the lesser curvature, which is the medial border; and the greater curvature, which is the lateral border.

The opening of the oesophagus into the stomach is called the cardiac orifice, and is surrounded by a functional sphincter called the cardiac sphincter. The pyloric orifice is the opening between the stomach and the small intestine and is surrounded by the pyloric sphincter, which consists of a thickened layer of circular muscle and is normally partly open. Peristaltic waves in the stomach push some of the gastric contents through the orifice and into the duodenum. The orifice then closes.

The stomach wall consists of four layers:

1. The serosa, an outer covering of peritoneum
2. The muscular layer, consisting of longitudinal and circular muscles and an additional oblique layer of muscle on the inside
3. The submucosa, a layer of connective tissue that contains many large blood and lymph vessels
4. The mucosa, which is a lining of mucous membrane arranged in folds, which flatten out as the stomach distends. The lining consists of a single layer of epithelial cells, which continually secrete pH-neutral mucus onto the surface. The mucosa is covered by small depressions, which contain the openings of the gastric glands that secrete gastric juice.

Functions of the stomach

The stomach acts as a temporary reservoir for food, allowing the digestive enzymes time to act, breaks up the food into a liquid state by rhythmic muscular contraction of its walls, and produces gastric juice, which contains:

- Hydrochloric acid, which is released in response to the hormone gastrin, and activates pepsins, provides an optimal pH for pepsin activity, and destroys bacteria
- Intrinsic factor, which is vital for the absorption of vitamin B12 from the diet, which is needed for the development of erythrocytes
- Mucus, which is secreted by the surface cells of the stomach mucosa and forms a lining that protects the mucosal cells from the gastric contents
- Gastric enzymes (pepsinogens), which are inactive until exposed to hydrochloric acid, when the active pepsins are released. Pepsins act as a catalyst in the chemical breakdown of protein, forming polypeptides and free amino acids
- Water.

The small intestine

The small intestine is a coiled muscular tube about 5–6 metres in length, extending from the pyloric end of the stomach to the large intestine. The small intestine is divided into several anatomically recognisable areas: the duodenum — the proximal section, which is the widest section and is about 20 cm long and curved; the jejunum, which is the middle section and is about 2.5 metres long; and the ileum, which is the distal section and is about 4 metres in length.

Covering the mucosa are very fine projections called villi (Figure 33.4). Intestinal glands in the mucous membrane secrete an intestinal juice containing enzymes to complete

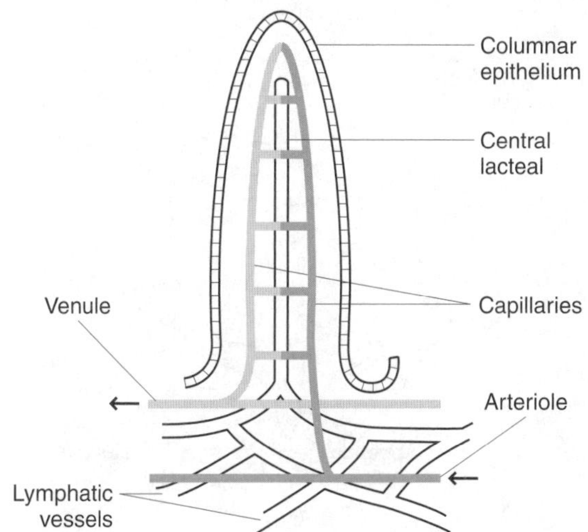

Figure 33.4 | A villus

the digestion of food. Solitary and aggregated patches of lymphatic tissue (Peyer's patches) are also found in the mucosa of the intestinal wall, especially in the lower ileum. An opening in the duodenum (ampulla of Vater) allows for the entry of the common bile duct, carrying bile from the liver, and the pancreatic duct, carrying pancreatic juice. At the junction of the ileum and the caecum of the large intestine is the ileo-caecal valve, which prevents a backward flow of contents from the large to the small intestine.

Functions of the small intestine

The functions of the small intestine are the secretion of intestinal juice, completion of chemical digestion of food, and absorption of digested food through the villi.

The large intestine

The large intestine is a muscular tube about 1.5 m in length and 6 cm in diameter, and extends from the end of the ileum to the anus (Figure 33.5). Lying in the abdominal and pelvic cavities, the large intestine may be divided into regions that are distinguished by their anatomical structure and position:

- The caecum, a blind-ended sac about 6 cm long and 7.5 cm in diameter, leads into the ascending colon and has the appendix attached
- The ascending colon, which is about 15 cm long and passes up the right side of the abdominal cavity to the lower surface of the liver
- The transverse colon, which is about 50 cm long and crosses the upper abdomen from right to left then curves in the vicinity of the spleen
- The descending colon, which is about 25 cm long and passes down the left side of the abdomen to the left iliac region
- The sigmoid colon, which is variable in length and is the S-shaped continuation of the descending colon and lies in the pelvic cavity

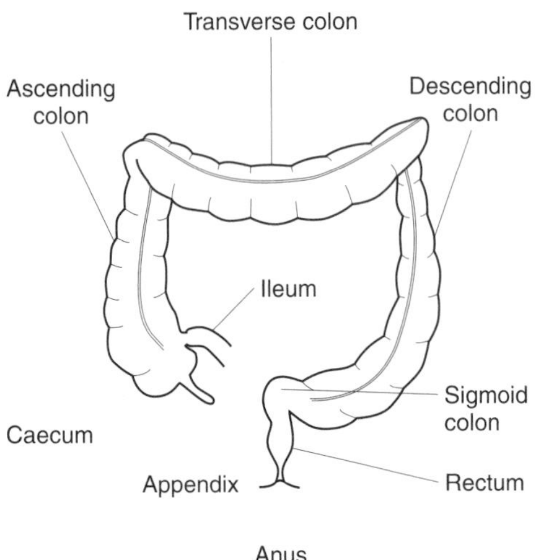

Figure 33.5 | The large intestine

- The rectum, a straight tube about 12 cm long that forms the last section of the large intestine
- The anal canal, the terminal part of the rectum, about 4 cm in length. The canal opens on to the external skin at the anus. The anal canal contains the internal and the external anal sphincters. The sphincters seal off the end of the alimentary canal and are normally constricted.

The wall of the large intestine has the same basic structure as that of the small intestine (the serosa, muscular layer, submucosa and mucosa).

Functions of the large intestine

The four functions of the large intestine are:

1. The absorption of large amounts of water and some mineral salts
2. Production of microorganisms (mainly bacteria) that are necessary for the normal functioning of lymphatic tissue in the large intestine and thus, resistance to infection. These bacteria also synthesise vitamins B and K
3. Transformation of the intestinal contents into semi-solid faeces, and storage of faeces until they are excreted
4. Secretion of mucus to lubricate faeces.

THE ACCESSORY DIGESTIVE ORGANS

The accessory organs secrete enzymes into the alimentary canal, secretions (enzymes) that are actively involved in the process of digestion. An enzyme is a substance, usually protein in nature, that initiates and accelerates a chemical reaction. The accessory organs are the salivary glands, the pancreas, the liver and the biliary tract.

The salivary glands

There are three pairs of salivary glands that secrete saliva into the mouth. The anatomical position of each pair is described above. Saliva is a watery fluid containing ions, mucin and the digestive enzyme salivary amylase. Salivation is largely initiated by sensory stimulation, including the presence of food in the mouth, and by taste and smell. Salivation may also be induced by the presence of irritating substances in the stomach or small intestine. Saliva has the following functions:

- Moistens and softens food
- Contains mucin, which acts as a lubricant to aid swallowing
- Moistens the mouth
- Has an antibacterial activity
- Enables molecules to dissolve on the surface of the tongue and stimulate the tastebuds
- Contains the enzyme salivary beta-amylase, which begins the chemical digestion of starch.

The pancreas

The pancreas is a soft gland, lying across the abdominal cavity behind the stomach. It is divided into a head, which fits into the curve of the duodenum; a central portion, or body; and a tail, which extends out to the spleen. The pancreatic duct runs centrally through the length of the pancreas, while smaller ducts carry the pancreatic juice secreted by the pancreas into the central duct. The pancreatic duct joins the common bile duct from the liver, to enter the duodenum (Figure 33.6).

The bulk of the tissue in the pancreas is composed of exocrine cells, which produce pancreatic juice. The pancreas secretes about 1200 mL of pancreatic juice daily. Pancreatic juice is a watery alkaline fluid rich in digestive enzymes. The enzymes and their actions are summarised in Table 33.1. The overall function of pancreatic juice is the digestion of nutrients. Scattered among the exocrine tissue are groups of hormone-secreting cells, the islets of Langerhans. The function of the islets of Langerhans is described in Chapter 41 on endocrine health, as these cells belong to the endocrine system.

Digestive function of the pancreas

Table 33.1 provides a summary of chemical digestion.

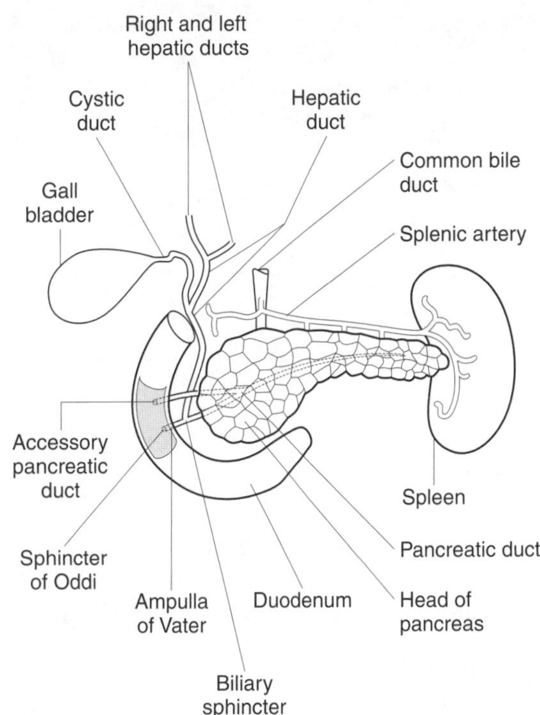

Figure 33.6 | The pancreas and neighbouring structures

The liver

The liver is an organ situated in the upper part of the abdominal cavity, immediately beneath the diaphragm. The greater part of the liver lies in the right upper abdomen but the organ extends across to the left upper abdomen (Figure 33.7). The liver is divided into two parts, a large right lobe and a much smaller left lobe. Like the alimentary canal, the liver is almost entirely covered by a layer of peritoneum. Beneath this is a fibrous capsule, which is continuous with areolar connective tissue situated within the liver. The areolar tissue forms a tree-like structure, which carries branches of the hepatic artery, hepatic portal vein, bile ducts and lymphatic vessels. These vessels enter and leave the liver through the porta hepatis, a short transverse fissure on the inferior surface of the liver.

The hepatic artery carries oxygenated blood to the liver. The portal vein carries deoxygenated blood, rich in nutrients from the small intestine, to the liver. Three hepatic veins carry deoxygenated blood from the liver to the inferior vena cava. The right and left hepatic ducts carry bile, secreted by the liver, to the common hepatic duct. The latter combines with the cystic duct from the gall bladder to form the common bile duct, which drains into the duodenum. The biliary tract, which transports bile from

TABLE 33.1 | SUMMARY OF CHEMICAL DIGESTION

Secretion	Daily volume (mL)	Enzyme	Substrate	Result
Saliva	1000–1500	Salivary amylase	Starch	Dextrins, maltose
Gastric juice	2000	Pepsin	Protein	Polypeptides and a few free amino acids
Bile	700	—	Fat	Facilitates action of lipase to emulsify fats
Pancreatic juice	1200	Lipase Amylase Maltase Trypsin	Triglycerides Starch Maltose Proteins	Fatty acids and monoglycerides Maltose Glucose Peptides and amino acids
Intestinal juice	2000	Peptidases Amylase Maltase Lactase, sucrose Lipase Enterokinase	Peptides Starch Maltose Disaccharides Glycerides	Amino acids Maltose Glucose Monosaccharides Fatty acids, glycerol and trypsin Activates pancreatic trypsinogen

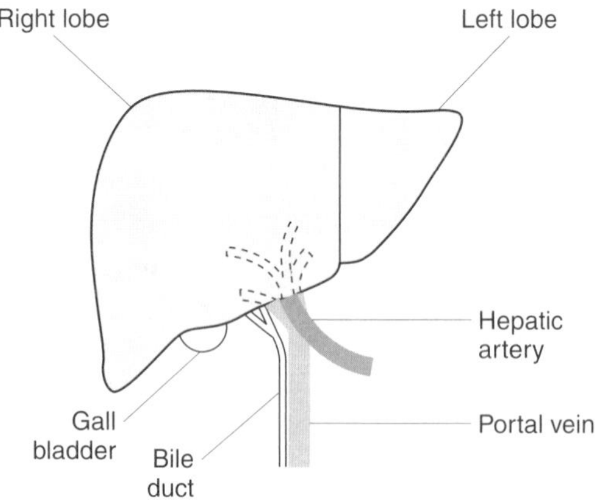

Figure 33.7 | The liver

the liver to the duodenum, consists of the left and right hepatic ducts, the common hepatic duct, the cystic duct, the gall bladder and the common bile duct (Figure 33.8).

The gall bladder

The gall bladder is a small muscular sac that lies on the inferior surface beneath the right lobe of the liver.

Functions of the liver and gall bladder include:

- Secretion of bile, a watery fluid containing a variety of organic and inorganic substances, but no enzymes. As much as a litre of bile may be secreted by the liver per day, and stored in the gall bladder before its release into the duodenum. Bile contains bile salts and bile pigments. Bile salts are derived from cholesterol and are able to break down (emulsify) fat droplets entering the small intestine from the stomach. Bile pigments, such as bilirubin and biliverdin, are derived from haemoglobin, in particular the erythrocytes removed from circulation. Bile has the following functions:
  - — provides the alkaline medium required by the enzymes in the small intestine
  - — emulsifies fats in preparation for the action of enzymes
  - — stimulates peristalsis in the intestine
  - — colours and deodorises faeces
  - — helps in the absorption of fats and vitamin K from the small intestine
- Bile not needed immediately travels from the common hepatic duct into the cystic duct and passes into the gall bladder for storage. When bile is required in the duodenum, the gall bladder contracts and forces bile through the cystic duct into the common bile duct to enter the duodenum
- Preparation of nutrients. The liver converts any glucose not needed immediately into glycogen for storage. It converts excess protein to glucose to be used as an energy source, and changes the nitrogenous part of excess protein to urea, which is excreted. The liver also converts fats into a form that can be used by the tissues
- Production of plasma proteins (albumin, globulin, fibrinogen, prothrombin, heparin) and vitamin A
- Storage of glycogen, iron and vitamins A, B-group and D
- Destruction of erythrocytes and toxic substances such as alcohol, poisons and drugs
- Production of a considerable amount of heat, as a result of the many activities of the liver.

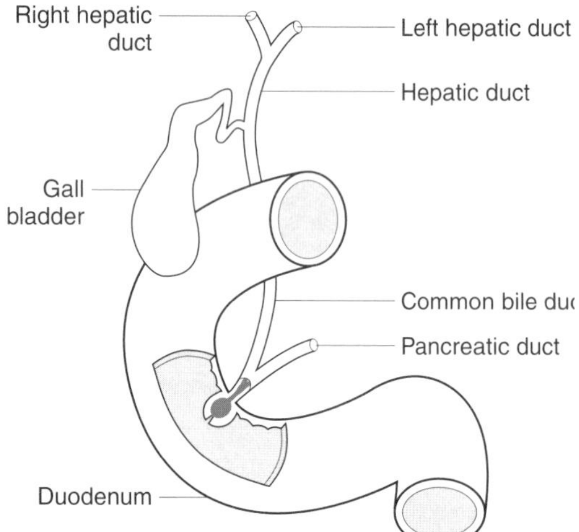

Figure 33.8 | The biliary tract

PHYSIOLOGY OF DIGESTION

DIGESTION OF FOOD

During the process of digestion, food is reduced to its simplest chemical form so that it can be absorbed into the bloodstream and used by the tissues. Digestion occurs through both mechanical and chemical actions. Mechanical action involves the physical process of liquefying the food, mixing it with digestive juices and moving it through the alimentary canal. Chemical action occurs when the digestive juices mix with the food, resulting in complex chemical substances being split into simple substances.

Digestion in the mouth

In the mouth food is broken down physically by the process of chewing (mastication), and mixed with saliva to bring about the formation of a moist ball, or bolus. Chewing softens the food so that it passes more easily through the alimentary canal. The presence of food in the mouth, together with its taste and smell, stimulates the secretion of saliva, gastric and pancreatic juices and bile (by means of parasympathetic pathways). The enzyme salivary beta-amylase in saliva begins to digest starches.

After the food has been formed into a bolus it is passed through the pharynx and down the oesophagus into the stomach by the act of swallowing. Swallowing is a complex reflex regulated by a 'swallowing centre' in the medulla oblongata of the brain. Swallowing is initiated when the tongue muscles push the bolus upwards and backwards into the oropharynx. The soft palate is elevated and comes into contact with the posterior wall of the pharynx, thereby closing off the nasopharynx. The larynx is pulled upwards and forwards, and the bolus pushes the epiglottis back over the glottis to prevent food from entering the respiratory tract. The oesophageal sphincter opens and the bolus enters the oesophagus.

Peristaltic waves carry the bolus through the oesophagus, and the cardiac sphincter relaxes to allow food and fluids to enter the stomach. The cardiac sphincter contracts to close the cardiac orifice at the end of each wave of contraction of the oesophagus, then relaxes to open the orifice when the next wave of contraction begins.

Digestion in the stomach

The stomach stores the food and later releases it at a rate that is optimal for digestion. Food is mixed with gastric juice, thereby changing its consistency so that it will be more easily transported along the alimentary canal. The food is exposed to enzymes (pepsins) which begin the digestion of proteins, and the gastric juice converts ferric iron (Fe^{3+}) to ferrous iron (Fe^{2+}). When the stomach muscles are stretched by swallowed food, peristaltic contractions are stimulated, which results in a churning movement. When the food is mixed with gastric juice it develops a pasty consistency and becomes known as chyme. The rate of emptying of the stomach depends on the:

- Consistency of the chyme
- Degree of opening of the pyloric orifice
- Force of the peristaltic contractions
- Type of food in the stomach (fats tend to delay emptying, while carbohydrates are usually emptied quickly).

The average time for the stomach to empty after a meal is 4–6 hours. When the food has been well mixed in the stomach, peristalsis begins in the lower half of the stomach and forces the chyme through the pyloric sphincter. Because this sphincter is only partially opened, only small amounts of chyme enter it at one time. When the duodenum is filled with chyme a nervous reflex (the enterogastric reflex) occurs, which inhibits the vagus nerves from stimulating the stomach muscles, and slows the emptying of the stomach. This mechanism ensures that food does not enter the small intestine too rapidly, to enable its digestion.

Digestion in the small intestine

After it leaves the stomach, chyme is mixed with intestinal secretions as well as with bile and pancreatic juice. Digestion is completed and the products are absorbed through the villi of the intestinal wall. The wall of the small intestine is capable of several different types of movement:

- Peristalsis, which ensures an onward movement of the contents of the intestine
- Segmentation, which ensures mixing of the intestinal contents. Segmentation contractions occur regularly, causing the chyme to be broken up into segments
- Pendulum movements, which are small contractions that sweep forwards and then backwards to cause more effective mixing of the intestinal contents (Figure 33.9).

ABSORPTION OF DIGESTED FOOD

Absorption is the passage of the end-products of digestion through the villi into the bloodstream. Although absorption mainly occurs in the villi in the small intestine, some absorption takes place in the stomach and large intestine. Neighbouring segments of the intestine alternately contract and relax, moving food along the digestive tract. Small, lipid-soluble substances such as alcohol, water, glucose and drugs such as salicylic acid (aspirin) are able to diffuse through cell membranes and can therefore be absorbed in the stomach. Absorption of water and digested nutrients occurs all along the length of the small intestine.

Most substances, for example, amino acids and monosaccharides, are absorbed through the villi walls by the process of active transport, and enter the capillaries in the villi to be transported in the blood to the liver via the portal vein. The exception is lipids (fats), which are absorbed passively by the process of diffusion. Lipids enter central

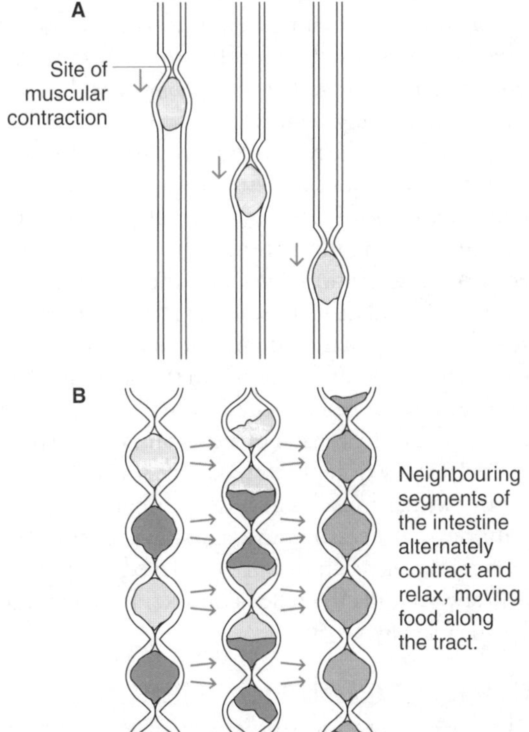

Figure 33.9 | Movements of the small intestine
A: Peristalsis: food moves along the digestive tract, as neighbouring segments of the intestine contract and relax in turn. B: Segmentation: single segments contract and relax alternately. Because there are inactive segments between the active ones, the food mixes but does not move along the tract

lacteals in the villi to be transported in the lymph. Lymphatic vessels empty their contents into the thoracic duct, which then drains the lymph into the blood at the subclavian vein. The proximal colon is the main site for the absorption of certain substances from chyme, including mineral salts and water. Vitamins B and K are synthesised by bacteria in the colon and absorbed into the bloodstream.

EXCRETION

Chyme enters the caecum through the ileo-caecal valve, which is normally closed but opens briefly to allow a small amount of chyme through with each peristaltic wave. Movement of chyme through the large intestine is a slow process. Various types of movement occur in the colon, including peristalsis, segmentation, and mass movements. Mass movements are brought about as a result of distension of the stomach or duodenum by ingested food. This sudden movement of colonic contents can push large amounts of faeces into the rectum and initiate the desire to defecate.

FAECAL MATTER AND DEFECATION

The faeces consists of a semi-solid brown mass. Even though absorption of water takes place in the large intestine, water still remains and makes up 60–70% of the weight of faeces. The remainder consists of fibre, indigestible cellular plant and animal matter, dead and live microbes, digestive enzymes, epithelial cells from the walls of the gastrointestinal tract together with the mucus they secrete, fatty acids and bile pigments.

Most of the time the rectum is empty of faeces; however, when a mass movement forces faeces into the rectum the desire to defecate is initiated. Faeces collect in the sigmoid colon before entering the rectum. As the faecal mass enters the rectum the defecation reflex and the desire to defecate are initiated. Impulses from sensory neurons in the rectal wall travel to the spinal cord, and peristalsis is stimulated in the descending colon, rectum and the anal canal. When the peristaltic wave reaches the internal anal sphincter it relaxes. Voluntary relaxation of the external anal sphincter enables the faeces to be excreted. Voluntary contraction of the abdominal muscles and deep inhalation raise the intra-abdominal pressure and assist evacuation. If it is not convenient, defecation can be delayed temporarily, as within a few seconds the reflex contractions cease and the rectal walls relax.

MEETING ELIMINATION NEEDS

The client's elimination status is assessed by obtaining information about elimination practices and by observing bowel actions. The nurse should enquire about the client's usual pattern of defecation and whether they have experienced any recent alterations to this pattern. Information should also be obtained about the client's usual fluid and dietary intake so that, whenever possible, it can be maintained or improved to facilitate normal elimination. The nurse should identify early signs of any problems associated with elimination so that appropriate care can be implemented to assist the client to meet their elimination needs. The nurse should also be aware of the numerous factors that affect bowel elimination:

- Age: developmental changes affect bowel elimination throughout life. As the body develops and changes, so do the size of the small and large intestines, amount of secretions and rate of peristalsis. Infants have developing digestive tracts, so complex foods are poorly digested, peristalsis is rapid and control of the bowel is not coordinated by the neuromuscular system until 2–3 years of age. During adolescence, the rate of gastric secretions increases. With ageing the rate of peristalsis is reduced. The slowing of nerve impulses delays the sensation to defecate and can lead to constipation
- Personal habits: privacy is considered to be important by most people when defecating, as the odours are linked to embarrassment. The urge to defecate can be suppressed if there is a lack of privacy, and this can lead to distension and constipation
- Diet: regular daily food intake helps maintain a regular peristalsis of the colon. Variety in the amount of dietary intake and types of foods can directly influence the bowel routine. For example, spicy foods may irritate the gastric and intestinal lining. A high-fibre diet increases the movement of food through the intestines. Fibre softens and adds weight to stools and increases bowel frequency. Fresh fruits and vegetables are rich sources of fibre
- Fluid intake: an inadequate fluid intake can result in hardening of the stool contents and discomfort when defecation occurs. The recommended fluid intake for adults is 1400–2000 mL/day. This may be contraindicated in clients with cardiac and renal disorders
- Physical activity: physical activity promotes peristalsis, while inactivity reduces motility of the bowel. It is recommended that all individuals perform regular mild exercise to promote regular bowel elimination
- Infection: the infection process can directly affect the protective lining of the gastrointestinal tract. Gastric and duodenal ulcers are known to be caused largely by the *Helicobacter pylori* bacterium
- Position: the normal defecation process has been addressed earlier in this chapter. Any interference from the usual body position (e.g. due to surgery) can lead to difficulty defecating
- Pain: pain on defecation may be due to the presence of lesions such as haemorrhoids or anal fissures. Tenesmus is the term used to describe persistent ineffectual spasms of the rectum accompanied by the desire to empty the bowel, and may be associated with disorders such as inflammatory bowel disease
- Psychological state: the psychological state of a person influences the motility and secretions of the

gastrointestinal tract. If a person is angry, anxious or stressed, the secretions and motility of the bowel are increased and can lead to diarrhoea. Alternatively, a person who is depressed will have reduced secretions and motility of the bowel, which could lead to constipation
- Pregnancy: as the fetus develops in size through pregnancy, the pressure it exerts on the bowel is increased, impeding the movement of faecal matter through the bowel
- Medication: laxatives are used to soften the stool to ease the discomfort in defecating. Excessive or chronic use of laxatives leads to reduced bowel muscle tone and less responsiveness to the normal stimulation of defecation. Narcotic medication will slow peristalsis. Anticholinergic medication inhibits gastric acid secretion and motility. Antibiotic medication affects normal bowel flora levels, leading to bowel irritability and increased motility. Non-steroidal anti-inflammatory medication also causes gastrointestinal irritation. Non-enteric-coated aspirin directly affects the protective lining of the gastrointestinal tract and, if taken daily, can predispose a client to gastritis and ulceration
- Surgery and anaesthetics: anaesthetics stop bowel peristalsis. Direct and prolonged surgery and nerve damage to the bowel can lead to a prolonged period of reduced peristalsis
- Diagnostic procedures: before procedures such as endoscopy, barium swallow or enema, the client is required to fast. These procedures will affect bowel routine.

PROMOTING A BOWEL ELIMINATION PROGRAM

A program to promote bowel elimination is an important part of the nursing care plan for a client. The goal of a bowel management program is to assist the client to evacuate the bowel comfortably and completely at a determined time without laxative support, by promoting privacy, regular mild exercise, high-fibre foods and an adequate fluid intake. The client's overall lifestyle becomes healthier, and general wellness and outlook improve.

EXAMINING FAECES

To detect and identify abnormalities, faeces are examined by observation (Table 33.2), by chemical testing in the workplace or by analysis in the laboratory. Laboratory analysis of faeces provides information about the condition and functioning of the digestive system. Testing the faeces for abnormalities involves analysing the specimen for the presence of blood, parasites and/or their ova, bile, fat, pathogenic microorganisms or pancreatic enzymes. Clinical Interest Box 33.1 provides information on the collection of a faecal specimen.

COMMON PROBLEMS ASSOCIATED WITH ELIMINATION OF FAECES

Constipation

Constipation is the infrequent passage of dry hard stools and is often the result of some deficiency in the three elements necessary for normal bowel activity: dietary fibre, adequate fluid input and sufficient physical activity. Other causes include disregarding the urge to defecate, chronic use of laxatives or certain disease states. When constipation occurs, the individual often strains to produce hard dry stools, and

TABLE 33.2 | ABNORMALITIES OF FAECES DETECTED BY OBSERVATION

Observation	Deviation from normal	Possible cause
Colour	Grey, pale or clay coloured	Absence of bile due to disorders of the liver or gall bladder, or obstruction of the common bile duct
	Dark and tar-like (melaena)	Presence of digested blood due to bleeding in the upper digestive tract
	Containing blood	Bleeding from the lower colon, rectum or anus
	Black	Medications containing iron supplements
	Green	Gastrointestinal infections
Consistency	Hard and dry	Insufficient fluid or fibre
		Medications that reduce motility of the intestines
		Prolonged inactivity
	Loose and watery	Reaction to certain foods or fluids, medications that increase the motility of the intestines, or gastrointestinal infections
Foreign substances	Pus or mucus	Infection or irritation of the intestines
	Undigested food substances	Inflammatory disease or malabsorption states
	Worms	Helminth infestation
Odour	Foul smelling	Specific disease processes

CLINICAL INTEREST BOX 33.1
Collecting a faecal specimen

The nurse may be required to collect faeces for observation or testing in the ward, or so that a specimen can be sent to the laboratory for analysis. Key aspects related to the collection of faeces include:
- Thorough washing and drying of the hands before and after collection, and wearing disposable gloves to prevent cross-infection
- The container in which the faeces are collected must be clean, and in some instances sterile, to ensure a specimen free from external contamination
- Contamination of the container and faeces must be prevented throughout the procedure
- Adequate information about the client and the specimen must be provided. Specimen containers are labelled with the client's name and registration number, time and date of collection, and type of specimen. If the specimen is to be sent to the laboratory for analysis, it must be accompanied by relevant documentation (e.g. the medical officer's request form)
- Specimens must be sent to the laboratory as soon as possible after collection. Most tests require the provision of a fresh specimen, and this is of particular importance when the faeces are to be tested for the presence of parasites such as amoebae. A warm specimen facilitates the isolation of such organisms
- The client may be responsible for collecting their own faecal specimen; if so, the nurse should provide the client with the information necessary to ensure that the collection is performed correctly.

straining may aggravate pre-existing rectal conditions such as haemorrhoids. Constipation is often accompanied by abdominal distension and discomfort, nausea, headache and diminished appetite. Natural measures to prevent constipation include:
- Sufficient dietary fibre: foods such as wholegrain cereals, fruit and vegetables contribute bulk and induce peristalsis
- Adequate fluid input: at least 1500 mL/day is necessary to help keep the intestinal contents in a semi-solid state for easier passage and excretion
- Responding to the desire to empty the bowel as soon as practicable
- Maintaining a regular time for bowel movement
- Incorporating sufficient exercise into the daily routine
- Relaxing and assuming a natural position when having a bowel action. Some people find the use of a small footstool to promote thigh flexion helpful
- Avoiding undue anxiety about bowel habits. While some people have a bowel action every day, it is quite normal for others to have a 2–3 day interval between bowel actions.

Other measures to assist elimination from the bowel may be necessary, including:
- Laxatives: substances taken orally that promote evacuation of the bowel by increasing bulk, softening the faeces or lubricating the walls of the colon
- Suppositories: small solid masses, medically ordered and inserted into the rectum to promote the evacuation of faeces
- Enemas: the introduction of fluid through the anus into the lower colon to promote the evacuation of faeces.

Impaction

If the faeces remain in the rectum for a long time, a large hardened mass develops that is difficult to expel. Impacted faeces is the term used to describe this condition.

Flatulence

Excessive formation of gas in the stomach and intestines is called flatulence. If the gas is not expelled, the intestines become distended and the person may experience abdominal discomfort and swelling. Flatus is the term used for gas in the intestine that is expelled through the anus. Flatulence may result from swallowed air, the consumption of gas-forming food or liquid, or bacterial action within the intestines.

Diarrhoea

Diarrhoea is the discharge of frequent, loose unformed stools resulting from the rapid passage of contents through the intestines. The person with diarrhoea may be exhausted from frequent defecation and the presence of accompanying abdominal distension and pain. If diarrhoea is prolonged, the absorption of nutrients and fluids is impaired and the person begins to show signs of fluid and electrolyte loss. Diarrhoea is a symptom of various conditions, including:
- Irritation or inflammation of the gastrointestinal tract; for example, due to pathogenic infection, highly spiced foods, or medications that increase intestinal motility
- Disorders of digestion or absorption
- Disorders that affect secretion and function of bile or pancreatic juice, such as in obstructive jaundice
- Emotional states such as anxiety or stress.

Diarrhoea should be assessed in terms of the frequency of defecation and the characteristics of the faeces. The cause of diarrhoea must be investigated and treated. Key aspects related to the care of a client with diarrhoea include:
- Reducing intestinal peristalsis: dietary management of an adult client involves the withholding of food until the diarrhoea diminishes, then the gradual resumption of food. Foods low in fibre may be provided initially to reduce stimulation of the intestines
- Administering any prescribed medications: anti-diarrhoeal medications such as codeine phosphate may be prescribed, as may antispasmodic preparations, to reduce abdominal cramps and pains
- Maintaining fluid input to replace lost fluids and to

prevent dehydration. Oral fluids are given if tolerated, or fluids may be administered intravenously. Input and output should be observed and documented as part of the client's fluid balance assessment
- Ensuring that the client has adequate privacy whenever toilet facilities are being used, and that used toilet utensils are removed from the room immediately
- Ensuring that the client's hygiene needs are met: after each bowel action the anal area and buttocks should be cleansed with a mild soap and thoroughly dried. A protective cream may be applied to reduce discomfort, and the area should be observed for signs of excoriation
- When using a bedpan or commode chair, the client may be embarrassed by the odours associated with diarrhoea, so measures to eliminate odours should be taken. Any soiled linen should be changed and removed from the room immediately. The room should be well ventilated, and room deodorants may be used with discretion
- Implementing isolation precautions if the diarrhoea is due to a pathogenic infection, to prevent cross-infection.

Faecal incontinence

Faecal incontinence is the inability to control the excretion of faeces, and may occur as a result of lesions in the brain or spinal cord, impaired consciousness or awareness, or various other factors. The principles of management of a client with faecal incontinence are similar to those for the management of urinary incontinence. The cause must be identified and treated, the person's hygiene needs attended to, and measures taken to maintain dignity and self-esteem. Clinical Interest Box 33.2 provides further facts on faecal incontinence.

Artificial openings into the intestine

As a result of certain disorders such as obstruction or tumours in the bowel, the passage of faeces through the rectum and anus may not be possible. In these instances, the surgical creation of an artificial opening from the colon to the surface of the abdomen may become necessary. For the latest information and research findings on this subject, see the Australian Council of Stoma Associations website at (www.australianstoma.org.au).

CLINICAL INTEREST BOX 33.2
Facts on faecal incontinence

- Faecal incontinence affects as many as one in 100 people. It is more common as you get older, but a lot of younger people are also affected (Department of Health and Ageing 2002)
- Incontinence is NOT a 'normal' part of ageing or the 'natural' aftermath of giving birth
- The National Continence Helpline (1800 33 00 66) is a free call information and referral telephone service for people with incontinence and their carers.

NURSING INTERVENTIONS

Clients with bowel elimination disorders may require various forms of nursing intervention.

SUPPOSITORIES

Suppositories may be ordered and inserted into the rectum to promote the evacuation of faeces or to facilitate rectal administration of a drug. The required equipment consists of:
- Prescribed suppository/suppositories
- Disposable gloves
- Water-soluble lubricant
- Receptacle for used articles
- Appropriate toilet facilities (e.g. bedpan, toilet paper)
- Soap, face washer and towel (for hands).

Suppositories prescribed to promote a bowel action are composed of various substances, such as glycerine. Evacuant suppositories act by softening and lubricating the faeces to facilitate easier passage and excretion, or by increasing peristalsis through the irritation of intestinal sensory nerve endings. The nurse must be aware of the different types of suppositories available and work within the scope of practice regarding the checking and administration of drugs. Types of medications that may be administered rectally by suppository include those that relieve nausea, relieve bronchospasm during an asthma attack, or provide anti-inflammatory action to minimise gastric irritation. Table 33.3 outlines the procedure for inserting a rectal suppository.

ENEMAS

Giving an enema is introducing a solution into the rectum and sigmoid colon. Most commonly it is ordered and administered to promote the evacuation of faeces and alleviate constipation, to administer a drug rectally, to prepare a bowel for diagnostic procedures or surgery, or to begin a bowel training program. When a solution or medication is introduced and retained it is referred to as a retention enema. When a solution is administered to promote evacuation of the bowel, it is referred to as an evacuant enema. An evacuant enema acts by distending the bowel and stimulating the nerves in the rectal wall, thus promoting peristalsis. An evacuant enema may be administered to relieve constipation or to empty the lower colon before examination, radiological investigation or surgery. Before administration, the nurse should ascertain the type and purpose of the enema that has been prescribed.

Enema solutions may be commercially prepared and packaged in disposable sets, or prepared in the ward immediately before administration. Substances used include a solution of enema soap and water, emollients such as olive or mineral oil, and hypertonic solutions. The quantities administered are in the range 5–1200 mL,

TABLE 33.3 | GUIDELINES FOR INSERTING A RECTAL SUPPOSITORY

Action	Rationale
Review and carry out standard steps in Appendix 1	
Explain the procedure	Reduces anxiety
Assemble the equipment and follow the nursing policies related to checking medications	The correct type, size and quantity must be administered
Ensure adequate privacy	Reduces embarrassment
Place the individual in a left lateral position	Anatomical site of the lower colon means that this position is the most effective for the introduction and retention of suppositories
Ensure that the person is adequately covered, with only the buttocks exposed	Promotes warmth and comfort
Wash and dry hands and put on disposable gloves	Prevents cross-infection
Lubricate finger of glove and suppository	Facilitates insertion of suppository
Gently insert the suppository by directing it with the finger, through the anus about 3.5 cm into the rectum	Suppository must pass the internal anal sphincter and come in contact with rectal mucosa
During insertion, encourage the client to take deep breaths through the mouth	Helps relax the anal sphincters
Encourage the client to retain the suppository for the correct length of time. A suppository administered to cause a bowel action should be retained for at least 20 minutes	Client must be aware of whether the suppository is to be retained to allow any medication to be dissipated, or whether to expect a bowel action. Suppositories to promote a bowel action must be retained long enough to be effective
Ensure that the client has easy access to toilet facilities and the signal device	Reduces anxiety related to accidental expulsion of the suppository or faeces
Dispose of used equipment appropriately; wash and dry hands	Prevents cross-infection
If a bowel action results, the faeces are observed and the observations reported and documented	Helps in assessing the effectiveness of the treatment and detects any abnormalities
Attend to the client's hygiene and position	Helps promote comfort
Report and document the procedure	Appropriate care may be planned and implemented

depending on the substance used and the age of the client. A suggested method of administering a non-disposable enema is outlined in Table 33.4. Disposable or re-useable equipment may be used to administer the solution, with a basic set consisting of:

- A container of solution
- Funnel
- Length of tubing with a clamp
- Rectal catheter
- Water-soluble lubricant
- Lotion thermometer
- Disposable gloves
- Extra equipment as listed in the organisation's policy and procedure manual.

Enemas may produce dizziness or faintness, excessive irritation of the mucosa, electrolyte imbalance, or cardiac arrhythmias from the vasovagal reflex.

TREATING IMPACTED FAECES

The term faecal impaction refers to the presence of a large, hard dry mass of faeces in the lower colon. When the condition occurs it is a result of prolonged constipation, poor bowel habits, inactivity, dehydration, use of constipation-inducing drugs or incomplete bowel cleansing after a barium swallow or enema. If measures to promote a bowel action, such as a suppository or enema, are ineffectual, surgical removal of the mass may be prescribed under an anaesthetic.

DISORDERS OF THE DIGESTIVE SYSTEM

SPECIFIC DISORDERS

Stomatitis

Stomatitis is a term that refers to inflammation of the mouth. It may be a primary condition or a symptom of another disease. Inflammation may affect the lips, tongue, gums, mucous membranes or palate. Stomatitis is characterised by pain, bleeding, swelling, ulceration and halitosis and can be managed with good oral hygiene and treating underlying disorders that are contributing to the condition, such as vitamin deficiencies.

Parotitis

Parotitis is inflammation of the parotid glands, which may be related to poor oral hygiene, dryness of the mouth, or

TABLE 33.4 | GUIDELINES FOR ADMINISTERING A DISPOSABLE ENEMA

Action	Rationale
Review and carry out steps in Appendix 1	
Check the medical officer's order. Explain the enema procedure to the client	Ensures that a medical order has been written. Informs the client
Collect all equipment: disposable enema, bedpan, bedside commode, underpad/bluey, water soluble lubricant, disposable gloves, paper towel and toilet tissue. Ensure that there is a bedpan or bedside commode by the bed	Facilitates access during procedure
If possible, place the client onto left side and drape with a blanket or sheet. Place the underpad/bluey under the buttocks. Ensure privacy	Solution travels up the colon more easily when the client is lying on the left side. The underpad/bluey protects the bedsheets from moisture or soiling
Wash and dry hands and put on disposable gloves	Prevents cross-infection
Apply lubricant to the tip of the disposable enema. Gently insert the tip into the anal opening, about 10 cm in an adult. Gently squeeze the container and roll it up from the bottom as the contents enter the bowel. Squeeze as much of the fluid into the rectum as possible. Remove the tip slowly and hold the buttocks together	Slow instillation of an enema achieves the best result. The client should retain the solution for about 20 minutes to 2 hours so that it will soften the stool
Assist the client onto the bedpan or bedside commode. If the client uses the toilet, request to see the result before flushing. If a bedpan is used, raise the head of the bed to a sitting position, if this is not contraindicated. Place call bell and toilet paper within reach	Provides an opportunity to observe the characteristics of the stool expelled
When the bowel contents have been expelled, assist the client in cleaning the anal area, observe the results of the enema, noting the colour, amount and consistency of the stool. Remove and clean the bedpan or bedside commode	Results of the enema are judged by the stool expelled
Restore the client's area, lower the bed, replace the side rails (if being used) and place the call bell within reach	Provides safety
Document the date, time, type of enema and amount of fluid instilled. Describe the result and how the client tolerated the procedure	Appropriate care can be planned and implemented

infection. Infectious parotitis (mumps) is an acute viral disease. Parotitis may also result from a calculus in the parotid gland. Symptoms of parotitis include tenderness and swelling of the gland, and pain associated with the ingestion of food or sour fluids.

Gastritis

Gastritis is inflammation of the gastric mucosa and may be acute or chronic. Acute gastritis is associated with irritation of the mucosa related to the ingestion of irritating foods, alcohol, caffeine or certain medications. Acute gastritis may also be caused by food poisoning, microorganisms or psychological stress. Chronic gastritis is commonly associated with an underlying disorder such as peptic ulcer, chronic alcohol abuse or malignancy. Many people with chronic gastritis have no symptoms, while others experience anorexia, a feeling of fullness, eructation (burping) and vague epigastric pain. The same symptoms appear in acute gastritis, and the individual may also experience abdominal cramps, nausea, vomiting and diarrhoea. Haemorrhage may occur, presenting as haematemesis (vomited blood), occult blood in the faeces or melaena.

Gastroenteritis

Gastroenteritis is inflammation of the stomach and intestines. It is an acute disorder characterised by diarrhoea, nausea, vomiting and abdominal cramps. Gastroenteritis has many causes, including the ingestion of bacteria, amoebae, parasites, viruses, toxins or food allergens, and drug reactions. The symptoms vary according to the cause, the extent to which the digestive tract is involved, and the age of the individual. Infants and aged and debilitated clients are more vulnerable to the rapid loss of fluid and electrolytes that occurs with the condition.

Hiatus hernia

A hiatus (diaphragmatic) hernia is the herniation of the stomach through the diaphragm into the thoracic cavity. The incidence of hiatus hernia increases with age and is more common in females. It may be the result of muscular weakening or diaphragmatic abnormalities, or may occur when the intra-abdominal pressure is raised, for example, by pregnancy, obesity, malignancy, trauma or persistent coughing or sneezing. There may be no symptoms, or the individual may experience reflux, regurgitation, heartburn, eructation and flatulence, a feeling of fullness after eating, and some chest discomfort. Chest discomfort or pain commonly occurs after meals and is frequently aggravated when the person lies flat.

Haemorrhage

Gastrointestinal haemorrhage may occur as a result of a variety of disorders. Common causes of bleeding from the upper digestive tract are peptic ulcer disease, oesophageal varices, malignancy and erosive gastritis. Causes of bleeding from the lower digestive tract include haemorrhoids, fissures, inflammatory bowel disease, polyps, diverticular disease and malignancy. Gastrointestinal bleeding is sometimes associated with disorders of the blood, such as leukaemia. Upper gastro-intestinal haemorrhage may be accompanied by haematemesis, melaena or occult blood in the faeces. Haemorrhage from the lower intestinal tract may present as bright-red blood excreted through the anus, or as occult blood present in the faeces. If blood loss is severe, the signs and symptoms of hypovolaemic shock will be evident.

Peptic ulcer

Peptic ulcer disease encompasses gastric ulcer, duodenal ulcer and stress ulcer. Peptic ulceration is related to erosion of the gastric or duodenal mucosa by acidic digestive juices. In severe or chronic cases, erosion may penetrate the muscle tissue and serosa. This allows acidic juices to enter the abdominal cavity. Although a precise cause has not been determined, factors that have been implicated in gastric ulcer development are smoking and certain medications which render the mucosa susceptible to damage.

A duodenal ulcer results from excessive gastric acid secretion, possibly due to an overactive vagus nerve. Factors that appear to be related to duodenal ulcer development are the ingestion of caffeine, alcohol, certain medications, and smoking. A stress ulcer may affect either the stomach or the duodenum, and occurs in a high percentage of people who have experienced severe trauma, shock, burns or infection.

The manifestations of an ulcer vary according to the site and whether it is a chronic or acute condition. The individual with chronic ulcer disease may experience burning epigastric pain, which may be aggravated by stress or fatigue. The pain of a gastric ulcer tends to occur sooner after eating than does the pain of a duodenal ulcer. Eating or taking an antacid tends to relieve the symptoms of a duodenal ulcer.

Complications of peptic ulcer disease include perforation, haemorrhage, intestinal obstruction and peritonitis. If gastrointestinal bleeding occurs it may be manifested by haematemesis and melaena and, if severe, by signs of hypovolaemic shock.

Cholecystitis

Cholecystitis is acute or chronic inflammation of the gall bladder and is commonly associated with impaction of a gall stone in the cystic duct. The gall bladder becomes dilated and filled with bile, pus and blood. Cholelithiasis is the term used to describe the presence of stones or calculi in the gall bladder. Choledocholithiasis is the presence of gallstones in the common bile duct. Major manifestations of cholecystitis are intense pain and tenderness in the right upper abdominal quadrant, nausea and vomiting. If a stone obstructs the common bile duct, jaundice may be evident.

Hepatitis

Hepatitis, which is inflammation of the liver, may be viral or non-viral in origin. Viral hepatitis is classified as infection with hepatitis A virus (HAV), hepatitis B (HBV) or hepatitis C (HCV). Hepatitis A is an infectious disorder that is generally spread via the faecal–oral route, for example, through the ingestion of contaminated food. The individual may have few symptoms or may experience headaches, fatigue, anorexia, pyrexia, dark urine, pale faeces, liver enlargement, jaundice and pruritus.

Hepatitis B (serum hepatitis) is generally transmitted parenterally by contact with infected blood. The virus may also be spread via contact with body secretions such as saliva, vaginal secretions, menstrual blood and semen. The virus may also be transmitted from an infected mother to her baby, during passage through the birth canal or via breast milk. The incidence of hepatitis B is higher in people who receive blood or blood products, use or share contaminated needles or engage in unprotected sexual practices. A person may be a carrier of HBV but experience no symptoms of the disease. Manifestations of HBV are similar to those of HAV but in a more severe form. The infection may persist for a long time, resulting in chronic liver failure and cirrhosis.

Hepatitis C (originally termed non-A–non-B hepatitis) is more common in people who have received numerous blood transfusions. The manifestations may be symptomless or similar to those of hepatitis B.

Non-viral hepatitis generally results from exposure to certain chemicals which, when ingested or inhaled, cause necrosis of hepatitic cells. Manifestations of the disorder are similar to those of viral hepatitis.

Diverticular disease

Diverticular disease (diverticulosis) is the presence of bulging pouches (diverticula) in the intestinal mucosa. Faecal matter becomes trapped in the pouches and the resulting inflammation is called diverticulitis. High intraluminal pressure on areas of weakness in the intestinal wall, and a lack of dietary fibre, are considered to be contributing factors. Diverticulitis causes mild to severe abdominal pain, some nausea, and altered bowel habits. In severe cases, the diverticula can rupture, producing abscesses or peritonitis.

Irritable bowel syndrome

Irritable bowel syndrome (IBS) is a relatively common disorder. The condition is thought to result from food intolerance, psychological distress, or in the presence of increased gastrin levels. The individual experiences alternating bouts of diarrhoea and constipation, which may be accompanied by abdominal distension or pain. The faeces usually contain excessive amounts of mucus.

Intestinal hernia

An intestinal hernia is the protrusion of part of the intestine through the abdominal wall. Various types of hernias are named according to their location: umbilical, inguinal, and femoral. A ventral, or incisional, hernia occurs at the site of an abdominal incision. An intestinal hernia may occur as a result of factors that increase intra-abdominal pressure or cause weakening of the abdominal wall, such as obesity, constipation or pregnancy. The hernia appears as a lump in the affected area and tends to disappear when the person is supine. The swelling increases in size when a standing position is assumed, or during exertion. The major complication of a hernia is strangulation, when the blood flow to the protruding loop of bowel may be so obstructed that necrosis occurs.

Haemorrhoids

Haemorrhoids are distended veins in the anal area, and can be internal or external. Internal haemorrhoids remain within the anal area, while external haemorrhoids prolapse through the anal canal. Haemorrhoids commonly result from increased pressure in the anal area related to constipation, straining to defecate, obesity, pregnancy and prolonged sitting or standing. The individual commonly experiences pain in, and bleeding from, the anus, particularly during defecation. Pruritus of the anal area may occur in the presence of external haemorrhoids. Thrombosis of external haemorrhoids produces sudden anal pain, and the appearance of a palpable firm lump protruding from the anus.

Anal fissure

An anal fissure is a crack in the lining of the anus and, like haemorrhoids, is associated with increased pressure in the anal area. Sudden occurrence is characterised by a tearing or burning pain during or immediately after defecation, and by the appearance of a few drops of blood. An anal fissure may heal spontaneously or it may partially heal and recur. A chronic fissure produces scar tissue, which may impede normal defecation.

Rectal prolapse

Rectal prolapse is the protrusion of one or more layers of the mucous membrane of the rectum through the anus. Prolapse may be partial, or complete with displacement of the anal sphincter and rectum. Rectal prolapse is associated with increased intra-abdominal pressure from straining to defecate or malignancy, for example. It may also result from weak rectal sphincters or muscles. Protrusion of tissue from the rectum is evident, and the individual may experience a sensation of rectal fullness, bleeding and pain due to ulceration of the exposed tissues.

INFLAMMATORY AND INFECTIOUS DISORDERS

Inflammatory and/or infectious disorders of the digestive system may be related to internal or external irritation or to the proliferation of pathogenic microorganisms.

Appendicitis

Appendicitis is inflammation of the appendix and may occur as a single attack or as repeated episodes. The condition commonly results from an obstruction of the lumen of the appendix, for example, by a faecal mass, or as a result of inflammation and oedema due to a viral infection. The obstruction causes inflammation, which can lead to infection, necrosis and perforation. If the appendix perforates, the contents spill into the abdominal cavity, causing peritonitis. Commonly, the manifestations of appendicitis are anorexia, nausea, vomiting and diffuse abdominal pain. The pain eventually localises at McBurney's point in the right lower quadrant of the abdomen. Pyrexia and leukocytosis are generally present.

Peritonitis

Peritonitis is inflammation of the peritoneum and may be associated with many conditions. Causes of peritonitis include a perforated peptic ulcer, appendix or diverticulum; abdominal trauma; or as a complication of abdominal surgery. The peritoneum becomes inflamed and oedematous, which generally results in decreased intestinal motility and intestinal obstruction. The onset of peritonitis may be acute, or slow and progressive. The inflammatory process causes accumulation of fluid in the abdominal cavity, leading to abdominal distension and rigidity, severe pain, nausea and vomiting. As a result of loss of fluid and electrolytes into the abdominal cavity, the individual displays signs of hypovolaemic shock. Abdominal distension results in upward displacement of the diaphragm and, typically, the individual's ventilations become shallow.

Inflammatory bowel disease

Inflammatory bowel disease is the term generally used to describe ulcerative colitis and Crohn's disease, both of which are chronic and recurrent disorders. Although the precise cause of inflammatory bowel disease is unknown, factors that have been implicated include a familial tendency, infection, autoimmune reactions and psychological stress.

Ulcerative colitis primarily affects the superficial mucosal layers of large areas of the colon. The inflammation associated with the disorder destroys tissue, causing ulceration and necrosis. Symptoms may be intermittent or continuous and include abdominal pain and diarrhoea. The faeces are generally watery and may contain blood and mucus. Complications of ulcerative colitis include haemorrhage, formation of abscesses or fistulas, and bowel obstruction.

Crohn's disease (regional enteritis) affects all layers of the ileum and/or the colon. Sometimes the regional lymph nodes and the mesentery are also involved. Symptoms vary according to the site and extent of the lesions and, in acute episodes, the individual experiences lower right abdominal pain and cramps, flatulence, diarrhoea, nausea and vomiting, and pyrexia. The faeces may contain large quantities of blood and mucus. Complications of Crohn's disease are similar to those of ulcerative colitis. Chronic or prolonged episodes of inflammatory bowel disease lead to nutritional imbalances and marked weight loss.

Clinical Interest Box 33.3 provides current statistics on Crohn's disease and ulcerative colitis.

Pilonidal cyst

A pilonidal cyst forms in reaction to ingrown hair, and develops in the upper section of the cleft between the buttocks. A pilonidal cyst is more common in people who have heavy hair growth in that area. The condition is exacerbated by friction, warmth and moisture. Generally, a pilonidal cyst causes no problems unless it becomes infected, resulting in local pain, tenderness and swelling. There may be several openings from the cyst to the skin (pilonidal sinus or fistula), which discharge purulent material.

NEOPLASTIC AND OBSTRUCTIVE DISORDERS

Neoplasms of the digestive system may be benign or malignant. Obstruction of part of the digestive tract, such as the small intestine, may occur as an acute or chronic disorder.

Polyps — projections of the mucosal surface of an organ — may develop in the stomach or intestine. Polyps may be benign or malignant and the most common form is adenoma. An adenomatous polyp may begin in the benign form and later undergo malignant changes. Polyps may be asymptomatic or they may cause diarrhoea, haemorrhage, or the manifestations of intestinal obstruction. Familial colonic polyposis is a hereditary disorder characterised by numerous polyps, and has a high association with colonic malignancy.

Cancer may develop in the mouth, oesophagus, stomach, intestines, rectum, liver or pancreas. Dietary factors have been implicated as one cause of gastric cancer. Dietary factors, particularly a lack of dietary fibre, are considered to be related to carcinogenic changes in the intestines and rectum. Clinical Interest Box 33.4 provides current facts on bowel cancer in Australia. The manifestations of cancer of the digestive system vary according to the site. Bowel cancer can develop with few, if any, early warning symptoms. Symptoms of bowel cancer can include:

- Bleeding from the anus or any sign of blood after a bowel motion
- A recent and persistent change in bowel habit; for example, looser bowel motions, severe constipation and/or needing to go to the toilet more than usual
- Unexplained tiredness (a symptom of anaemia)
- Abdominal pain, especially of recent onset.

Intestinal obstruction may occur as an acute or a chronic condition. When an obstruction occurs, the passage of intestinal contents is inhibited. Part of the small or large intestine may become partially or totally obstructed. Obstruction of the small intestine is more common and may be due to adhesions or a strangulated hernia. The small intestine may also be obstructed by foreign objects or compression of the bowel wall from stenosis. In this condition, the motility of the small intestine is decreased or absent. Obstruction of the large intestine is related to diverticulitis, cancer and volvulus (twisting of the colon).

Manifestations of intestinal obstruction appear when fluids, gas and ingested substances accumulate proximal to the site of obstruction. The individual generally experiences abdominal pain, distension and vomiting; and is usually unable to pass flatus or faeces. If the obstruction is at the distal end of the intestine, vomiting may occur, and the vomitus has a faecal odour caused by bacterial overgrowth in the intestinal tract. The individual commonly exhibits the manifestations of fluid and electrolyte imbalance because of progressive dehydration and plasma loss. Complications

CLINICAL INTEREST BOX 33.3
Australian Crohn's and Colitis Association

The Australian Crohn's and Colitis Association (www.acca.net.au) is a voluntary non-profit organisation committed to providing and implementing services to assist members' needs. They estimate that over 23 000 Australians have irritable bowel disease, over 10 000 have Crohn's disease and over 13 000 have ulcerative colitis.

CLINICAL INTEREST BOX 33.4
Bowel cancer

According to the Australian Department of Health and Ageing 2002, in Australia the lifetime risk of developing bowel cancer before age 75 is about one in 17 for men and one in 26 for women. This is one of the highest rates of bowel cancer in the world, and results in about 11 300 new cases and 4600 deaths from bowel cancer a year.

Because of these findings, a bowel-screening pilot program is in progress. Screening involves testing for bowel cancer in people who do not have any obvious symptoms of the disease. The aim is to find the cancer early when it is easier to treat and cure. Regular screening is important because bowel cancer can develop without any early warning symptoms. While no cancer is completely preventable, it is believed that eating a healthy diet and exercising regularly could prevent 66–75% of bowel cancer cases.

of intestinal obstruction include peritonitis, ischaemia and necrosis of the bowel.

TRAUMATIC DISORDERS

Trauma to parts of the digestive system may be related to injury or to irritation, such as the ingestion of a corrosive substance. Abdominal trauma may be localised or it may involve more than one abdominal structure. When a part of the digestive system is damaged the processes of digestion, absorption and elimination may be impaired. As a consequence, alterations in nutritional, electrolyte and fluid status occur. Depending on the type and extent of injury, the manifestations include external bruising, abdominal distension, pain, altered bowel sounds and haemorrhage, either internal and concealed, or presenting as haematemesis and/or melaena. Complications of trauma to the digestive system include haemorrhage, shock, infection, peritonitis and obstruction.

DIAGNOSTIC TESTS

Certain tests may be performed to assist or confirm the diagnosis of digestive system disorders.

Laboratory tests

Specimens that may be obtained from the client for laboratory analysis include blood, faeces, gastric or peritoneal fluid, urine, and samples of tissue:

- The blood may be tested to determine haemoglobin level, haematocrit, leucocyte count, serum electrolytes, bilirubin levels, glucose levels or pancreatic enzyme levels
- The faeces may be tested to identify bleeding disorders, biliary obstruction, infections and disorders of digestion or absorption
- Gastric fluid analysis involves examination of gastric secretions, and may be performed by examining a specimen of vomitus or by testing a sample of the gastric contents aspirated via a nasogastric tube
- Peritoneal fluid analysis assesses a sample of peritoneal fluid obtained by abdominal paracentesis. The test may be performed when bleeding or infection is suspected by a medical officer. Abdominal paracentesis involves the insertion of a trocar and cannula through the abdominal wall to aspirate a quantity of peritoneal fluid
- The urine may be tested to detect the presence of any abnormal substance (e.g. bilirubin) which may be excreted in the urine as a result of a digestive system disorder
- Biopsy: specimens of tissue may be obtained during endoscopic examinations or surgery. The specimens are examined microscopically for changes in cellular structure, to confirm diagnosis or to determine the cause of a disease (e.g. malignancy).

Radiological examination

Several different types of radiological investigation may be performed:

- Plain X-rays may be taken to aid in the diagnosis of abdominal masses, bowel obstruction, trauma to abdominal organs, and ascites
- Fluoroscopy (visualisation with motion) involves use of a contrast agent (e.g. barium sulphate) which can be visualised as it passes through and outlines structures in the digestive tract. Fluoroscopic examination of the digestive tract includes barium swallow, barium meal and barium enema
- For a barium swallow or barium meal the individual drinks the contrast medium. Its progress is observed on a fluorescent screen, and X-ray films are taken as the substance moves through the upper digestive tract. To visualise the lower digestive tract, a barium enema is administered. The contrast medium is instilled into the colon by means of a rectal tube, then the progress of the substance is observed on a fluorescent screen and X-ray films are taken
- Computerised tomography (CT) scanning involves the direction of a narrow X-ray beam at parts of the body, from various angles. Contrast medium is often administered intravenously to enhance visualisation. A computer reconstructs the information as a three-dimensional image on a screen
- Ultrasound involves the use of soundwaves to visualise body structures. A transducer is passed over the area, such as the abdomen, and receives echoes, which are bounced off body structures. The echoes are converted into electrical impulses, which may be viewed on a screen or photographed
- Endoscopy is the visual examination of part of the digestive tract using a flexible fibre-optic endoscope. The endoscope also provides a channel for the introduction of instruments for the purpose of obtaining a sample of tissue for microscopic examination. The various forms of endoscopy derive their names from the part of the body being examined:
  - — oesophagoscopy (the oesophagus)
  - — gastroscopy (the stomach)
  - — duodenoscopy (the duodenum)
  - — proctoscopy (the anus and rectum)
  - — sigmoidoscopy (the sigmoid colon)
  - — colonoscopy (the colon).

CARE OF THE INDIVIDUAL WITH A DIGESTIVE SYSTEM DISORDER

Although specific nursing actions and medical management vary depending on the disorder, the main aims of care are to:

- Prevent and manage alterations in elimination
- Promote comfort

CLINICAL INTEREST BOX 33.5
Nursing diagnoses relating to bowel problems

- Bowel incontinence
- Constipation
- Constipation, colonic
- Constipation, perceived
- Diarrhoea
- Skin integrity, impaired

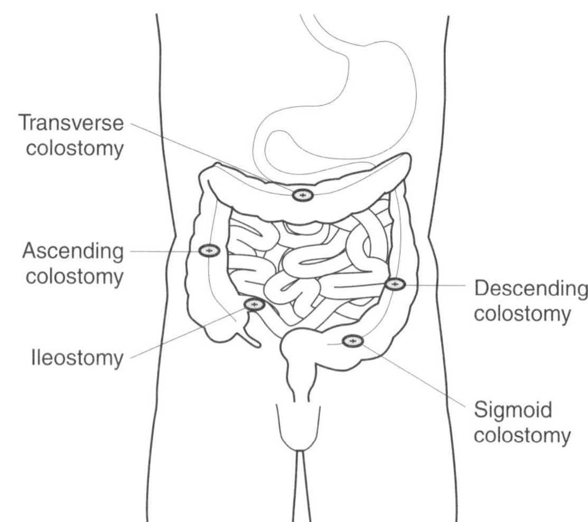

Figure 33.10 | Stoma sites

- Maintain skin and mucous membrane integrity
- Maintain nutritional and fluid status.

Specific nursing activities include implementing measures to assist elimination from the bowel, observing and collecting excreta, and care of an individual with a stoma. Examples of nursing diagnosis relevant to bowel problems can be located in Clinical Interest Box 33.5.

CARE OF CLIENT WITH A STOMA

Specific disorders of the digestive tract may require surgical treatment involving the creation of an artificial opening on the abdominal wall. Part of the intestine is brought through this opening to form a stoma. A *colostomy* involves the creation of an artificial opening into a section of the colon, which is brought out through an opening in the abdomen. An *ileostomy* involves the creation of an artificial opening into part of the ileum, usually the terminal ileum, also brought out through an opening in the abdomen. As a result of both surgical procedures, faecal elimination occurs through the stoma, which may be created as a temporary or a permanent measure.

A temporary colostomy is created to divert faecal contents, for example, to allow healing of an incision in the distal colon or rectum. A permanent colostomy is indicated principally in colorectal cancer after a partial or total colectomy has been performed. A temporary ileostomy is created to rest the bowel, as in ulcerative colitis. A permanent ileostomy may be formed after total colectomy in the management of Crohn's disease or ulcerative colitis. The site is selected according to which part of the bowel is affected and with consideration of the client's physique, clothing, occupation and any other factors that may influence the client's ability to successfully manage the care of the stoma.

In many health care institutions a stoma therapist liaises with the client and surgeon to select the most appropriate site. The site of the stoma (Figure 33.10) will determine the consistency of the faecal matter excreted through it. The closer the stoma is to the small intestine, the more liquid the faeces will be. Faeces excreted through an ileostomy are liquid to paste-like, whereas faeces excreted through a sigmoid colostomy are semi-formed to solid. Figure 33.11 illustrates the types of colostomy or ileostomy that may be created.

Care of the client with a stoma includes the selection and management of appliances (Figure 33.12), care of the stoma and surrounding skin, colostomy irrigation, meeting nutritional needs and providing psychological support. Table 33.5 outlines the procedure for changing an ostomy appliance. A stoma therapist may be available to assist in the preparation of the client and their significant others before the operation and also plays a major role in providing support and education after the operation.

A dietitian can help a client with a colostomy choose a balanced diet. It may be desirable to eliminate some foods; for example, foods that cause excessive gas and odour are often avoided. These foods include members of the cabbage

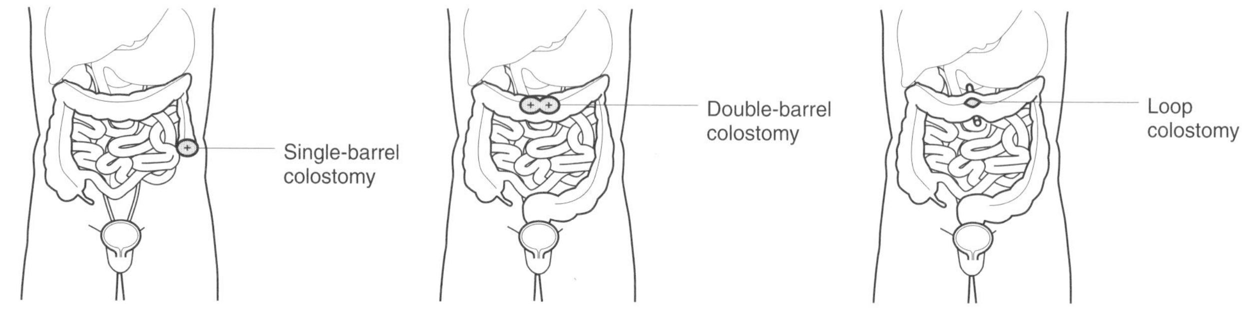

Figure 33.11 | Types of ostomy

TABLE 33.5 | GUIDELINES FOR CHANGING AN OSTOMY APPLIANCE

Action	Rationale
Review and carry out standard steps in Appendix 1	
Explain the procedure to the client and provide privacy	Reduces anxiety and embarrassment
Place the equipment in a convenient location	Facilitates performance of the procedure in an organised manner
Wash and dry hands and put on gloves	Prevents contamination
Remove the old appliance gently and place it in a plastic bag. Remove the skin barrier (e.g. pectin wafer) if necessary	Avoids damage to surrounding skin surface
Wipe the stoma and surrounding skin, using swabs and warm water. Pat dry	Cleanses the skin of mucus and faecal drainage
Inspect the stoma and surrounding skin. The stoma should be pink or red, and free from excoriation	Deviations from normal must be reported immediately so that appropriate care can be planned
Apply the skin barrier to the surrounding skin	Protects the skin
Remove the adhesive backing and place the new appliance over the stoma. Ensure that it is secured firmly in position with no gaps exposing the skin around the base of the stoma	Prevents leakage of faeces
Assist the client into a comfortable position and attend to their needs	Promotes comfort
Remove the equipment and attend to it in the appropriate manner. Wash and dry hands	Prevents odour and cross-contamination
Document and report the procedure	Appropriate care can be planned and implemented

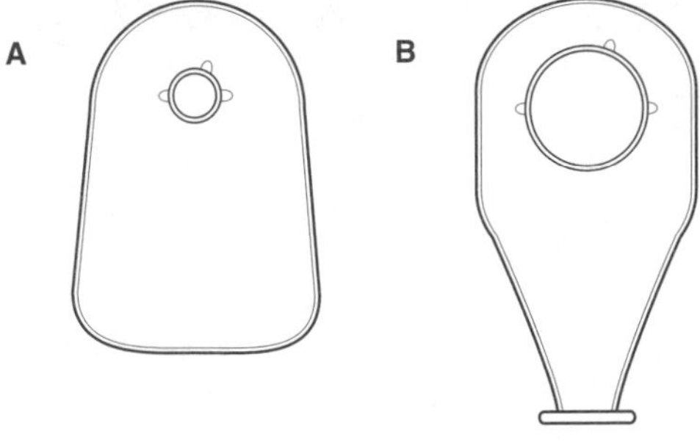

Figure 33.12 | Ostomy appliances. **A**: Non-drainable stoma bag. **B**: Drainable stoma bag

family, beans, eggs, fish and nuts. Foods or fluids such as fruits, soda, coffee, carbonated beverages or high-fibre items may cause diarrhoea. Foods with hard-to-digest kernels, such as popcorn, may need to be avoided as well. Non-irritating foods can be substituted for those that must be restricted.

SUMMARY

The functions of the digestive system are to ingest and digest foods so that nutrients can be absorbed into the bloodstream, and to eliminate wastes from the body. Normal functioning may be impaired as a result of alterations in swallowing, secretory function, motility, digestion, absorption or elimination. Disorders of the digestive system can be classified as those occurring from multiple causes, from inflammation or infection, as a result of neoplasms, obstruction, or as a result of injury. Diagnostic tests used to assess digestive system function include laboratory analysis of body fluids, excretions or tissue; radiological examinations; and endoscopy. Care of the client with a digestive system disorder includes preventing and managing altered elimination, promoting comfort, maintaining skin and mucous membrane integrity, and maintaining nutritional and fluid status.

Nursing activities include care of the client who has a gastric tube, implementing measures to assist bowel elimination, observing and collecting excreta, and assisting with artificial feeding. A client with a specific disorder of the digestive tract may require the surgical creation of a stoma, through which faeces are excreted.

REVIEW EXERCISES

1. Describe the physiological functions of the various areas of the digestive system.
2. List the four functions of the large intestine.
3. List six functions of the liver.
4. Describe normal faeces and the defecation process.
5. Identify the factors that affect bowel elimination.
6. Briefly describe the specific disorders of the digestive system outlined in this chapter.

CRITICAL THINKING EXERCISES

1. Lucy, 28, has been diagnosed with IBS. What are the classic symptoms affiliated with IBS? What client education points can you cover with Lucy to assist her in managing IBS?

2. Mark, 40, is admitted for a colonoscopy because of a family history of bowel cancer and intermittent presence of blood in his bowel actions. What education can you provide Mark about this procedure?
3. Veronica, 78, is admitted with severe constipation. While interviewing Veronica she states that she has managed her constipation in the past with laxatives, and that she restricts her fluid intake because she suffers with urinary incontinence. She has not been as mobile since her left knee replacement 1 month ago. What key changes can you suggest to Veronica to maintain a regular bowel elimination program?
4. An elderly client is admitted with a history of 3 days of diarrhoea. What are the possible causes of diarrhoea? What is your primary concern for this client? What key information should be charted regarding the bowel actions?

REFERENCES AND FURTHER READING

Anderson DM (chief lexicographer) (2002) *Mosby's Medical, Nursing and Allied Health Dictionary*, 6th edn. Mosby, St Louis

Ankner GM (2007) *Case studies in Medical–Surgical Nursing*. Thomson Delmar Learning, Clifton Park, NY

—— (2008) *Medical–Surgical Nursing*. Thomson Delmar Learning, Clifton Park, NY

Blackwell J (2001) Clinical practice guidelines: management of chronic hepatitis C. *Journal of the American Academy of Nurse Practitioners*, 13(10): 440

Briggs J (2000) Identification and management of dysphagia in children with neurological impairment. *Best Practice — Evidence Based Practice Information Sheets for Health Professionals*, 4(3): 1–6

—— (2000) Identification and nursing management of dysphagia in adults with neurological impairment. *Best Practice — Evidence Based Practice Information Sheets for Health Professionals,* 4(2): 1–6

—— (2000) The impact of preoperative hair removal on surgical site infection. *Best Practice — Evidence Based Practice Information Sheets for Health Professionals*, 7(2): 1–6

Crisp J, Taylor C (eds) (2005) *Potter & Perry's Fundamentals of Nursing*, 2nd edn. Elsevier Australia, Sydney

Department of Health and Ageing (2002) *Faecal Incontinence*. Online. Available: http://www.health.gov.au/internet/wcms/Publishing.nsf/Content/continence-info-faecal.htm [accessed 25 May 2008]

Keshay S (2004) *The Gastrointestinal System at a Glance*. Blackwell Science, Malden, MA

Thibodeau GA (2008) *Structure and Function of the Body*. Mosby, St Louis

ONLINE RESOURCES

Australian Council of Stoma Associations: www.australianstoma.org.au

Australian Crohn's and Colitis Association: www.acca.net.au

Australian Government Department of Health and Ageing: www.health.gov.au

Australian Prescription Products Guide: www.appco.com.au/appguide/home.asp

Health Insite: www.healthinsite.gov.au

Joanna Briggs Information sheets: www.joannabriggs.edu.au

Chapter 34
REST AND SLEEP

OBJECTIVES

- Define the key terms/concepts
- Describe the importance of rest and sleep to the wellbeing of the individual
- Outline and describe the phases of the sleep cycle
- State the factors that may interfere with the process of rest and sleep
- Describe the supportive nursing measures that may be implemented to promote the individual's need for rest and sleep
- Demonstrate an awareness that a number of sleep disorders exist and that some are potentially life-threatening

KEY TERMS/CONCEPTS

central sleep apnoea
continuous positive airway pressure (CPAP)
narcolepsy
non-rapid eye-movement sleep (NREM)
obstructive sleep apnoea (OSA)
rapid eye-movement sleep (REM)
rest
sleep
sleep cycle
sleep disorder
sleep disturbance

CHAPTER FOCUS

Sleep is a specific state of consciousness that occurs on a cyclic basis. It is a period of rest and recuperation for the body and the brain. The amount of sleep an individual may require depends on age, lifestyle, personality, environment and state of health. The need for sleep usually becomes less as we age.

An important nursing responsibility is implementing measures that will promote physical and emotional comfort and thereby assist the individual to receive sufficient rest and sleep. Discomfort that affects sleep can result from stimuli of physical or psychosocial origin. When possible the nurse should implement measures to prevent the development of, or relieve, discomfort, so that effective sleep can be achieved. Without sufficient and appropriate rest and sleep, all other activities of daily living may be affected. Most people complain of 'trouble sleeping' at some stage in their lives, although this is usually a temporary problem.

This chapter addresses promotion of the clients' physical and psychological comfort and wellbeing by providing sufficient rest and sleep. The need for comfort is closely associated with the ability to achieve adequate rest and sleep. The nurse should be aware of the measures necessary to ensure that comfort needs are met. Rest and relaxation can occur only when there is freedom from physical discomfort and emotional tension, and clients are more likely to sleep well if normal sleeping habits are maintained.

LIVED EXPERIENCE

How are people expected to sleep well in hospital? During my recent stay after surgery I was woken continually for observations, medications and by noise — phones ringing, buzzers sounding, nurses talking loudly, noisy equipment, lights and an uncomfortable bed! What with this, and a confused elderly gentleman entering my room and trying to get into bed with me, I was glad to go home in order to sleep!

Olivia, 57, a private hospital client

PHYSIOLOGY OF SLEEP

Sleep is a basic physiological need that is necessary for survival. It can be defined as a period of reduced consciousness, diminished muscular activity and depressed metabolism. Sleep provides the greatest degree of rest, with all body systems functioning at a reduced level. Although sleep is a state of reduced consciousness, certain stimuli, for example, a sudden loud noise, will usually rouse the person.

There are large individual variations in the optimal amount of sleep required, with about 7 hours a night being the average required for an adult. The quality of sleep is equally as important as the quantity of sleep achieved. Sleep patterns change throughout the life cycle and the quantity of sleep diminishes from about 20 hours a day in infancy to about 8 hours a day in adolescence, to perhaps as little as 4 hours in older adulthood. As a person ages, the amount of time spent sleeping at night is usually decreased from earlier in life. Many older adults will wake more often during the night, and report an inability to return to sleep after rousing. They may then report 'napping' more often during the day.

There are several theories about the purpose of sleep, with the most commonly accepted concept being that sleep promotes the growth and repair of body cells. It appears that the level of circulating hormones, such as growth hormone and those secreted by the adrenal glands, vary during sleep. The alteration in the amount of these hormones circulating during sleep is considered to facilitate cell growth and repair. Sleep is also a time that allows for conservation of energy, prevention of fatigue, and provision of organ respite. It is therefore of particular importance that the person who is ill or hospitalised has the opportunity to benefit from the restorative nature of sleep. People who suffer from chronic illness or chronic pain syndrome that disturbs effective sleep may spend much time in bed but not wake feeling rested or restored.

SLEEP REGULATION

Sleep involves a sequence of physiological states maintained by central nervous system activity that is associated with changes in the peripheral nervous, endocrine, cardiovascular, respiratory and muscular systems (Crisp & Taylor 2005). In current theory, sleep is thought to be an active inhibitory process. The control and regulation of sleep may depend on the interrelationship between two cerebral mechanisms that intermittently activate and suppress the brain's higher centres to control sleep and wakefulness. One mechanism causes wakefulness, while the other causes sleep (Crisp & Taylor 2005). The reticular activating system (RAS) is located in the upper brainstem. It is believed to contain special cells that maintain alertness and wakefulness. The RAS receives visual, auditory, pain and tactile sensory stimuli (Crisp & Taylor 2005). Sleep may be produced by the release of serotonin from specialised cells in the raphe sleep system of the pons and medulla. This area of the brain is also called the bulbar synchronising region (BSR). As people try to fall asleep, they close their eyes and assume relaxed positions. Stimuli to the RAS decline and, if the room is dark and quiet, activation of the RAS further declines. At some point the BSR takes over, causing sleep (Crisp & Taylor 2005).

Stages of sleep

Sleep is described as being of two major types, non-rapid eye-movement sleep (NREM), and rapid eye-movement sleep (REM). Normally a period of sleep consists of about 4–6 cycles, each lasting around 100 minutes. It is generally recognised that each sleep cycle consists of five stages. The first four stages are stages of NREM sleep, while the fifth stage is REM sleep. The five stages of sleep are:

- Stage 1: this stage is characterised by general relaxation and drowsiness and is the transitional stage between wakefulness and sleep. During this stage, which lasts about 15 minutes, the person can still be woken by any slight stimulus (e.g. the sound of a dog barking in the distance)
- Stage 2: during this stage, muscle relaxation intensifies, brain activity decreases and body functions are slowing down. During this stage, which usually lasts 10–20 minutes, the person can still be woken easily but there is greater relaxation than in stage 1
- Stage 3: this stage occurs about 30 minutes after the person goes to sleep. During this stage the person is not usually roused by familiar noises. There is complete relaxation in which most body systems slow down. Some effects are that the pulse rate is reduced, gastrointestinal function decreases and muscles are relaxed
- Stage 4: during this stage the person is in a deep sleep, is difficult to rouse, the body is relaxed and body functions are markedly decreased. This stage is also known as slow-wave sleep (little brainwave activity occurs), and is associated with physical repair and restoration
- Stage 5: this is a period of light sleep during which most dreaming is thought to occur, and the eyes move rapidly back and forth (REM). If awakened during this stage, the person may recall vivid dreams. It is possible to reach this stage of sleep within 90 minutes of sleep initiation. REM sleep is thought to be necessary for mental restoration and adaptation to stress. The act of dreaming, while not fully understood, is considered by some as necessary for the promotion of psychological integration. Dreams can be described as a sequence of thoughts, images and emotions that pass through the mind during the REM stage of sleep.

It is thought that to achieve high-quality restorative sleep most people complete several sleep cycles. With each successive cycle, stages 1 and 2 are normally not re-entered, and so continuing sleep tends to fluctuate between stages

3 and 4, with lengthening periods of REM sleep. Infants spend a greater proportion of time in REM sleep than do adults, with about 40% of total sleep time being REM sleep. With adults, about 20% of total sleep time is REM sleep. If the person wakes fully on occasions during sleep, the sleep cycle needs to restart at stage 1, and so total time spent in deep sleep may be lessened. The length of lighter stages of sleep (especially stage 1) is often increased in older people and stages 3 and 4 often decrease. This is why many older adults often report feeling less rested even after being observed to have slept soundly.

During a 24-hour period there is a cycle of physiological functions that tend to be highest during the early evening and lowest during the early morning. Examples of these functions are metabolic rate, heart and ventilation rates and body temperature. A pattern based on this 24-hour cycle is referred to as a circadian rhythm (or body clock), in which certain actions such as eating and sleeping are repeated regularly. It appears that the 24-hour cycle of light and dark is the pattern to which humans synchronise their body rhythms, and this is an important factor in the cycle of sleeping and waking. This pattern of synchronisation is highly individualised, allowing variation — some people are distinctly described as 'morning people', while others fit well into the 'night-owl' category. Any disruption to a person's circadian rhythm can cause discomfort, and manifest in a disturbed sleep pattern.

One example of the consequences of disrupted circadian rhythm is the state known as 'jet lag'. This condition occurs when a person's circadian rhythm is disrupted by travel across several time zones in a relatively short time, and is characterised by fatigue, insomnia and sluggish physical and mental function. Clients who are being nursed in intensive care units (ICUs) may experience the same phenomenon. Intensive care units may be brightly lit during the night as well as during the day. Without a regular pattern of light and dark, together with perhaps disturbing sights and sounds, a client in an ICU may experience disruption to this normal 24-hour rhythm. A person who engages in shift work may experience symptoms similar to jet lag, as the body adapts to changes in the 24-hour biological clock. Working on night shift removes sleeping from the normal night-time activities and renders it out of order with the body's time.

Any interruptions to sleep may cause interference with a person's ability to carry out their usual activities. A person who experiences a sleep-pattern disturbance may exhibit changes in behaviour and performance. A person may show signs of increased irritability, lack of energy and fatigue. Sleep-pattern disturbances include difficulty in falling asleep, periods of wakefulness during the night, waking earlier than usual, and not feeling rested after sleep. Some people experience nightmares or sleepwalking. A nightmare is a dream that arouses feelings of intense fear or extreme anxiety and usually wakes the sleeper. Sleepwalking is a state that culminates in walking about, but the individual has no recollection of the episode. Other sleep disorders include sleep apnoea and narcolepsy. A person who develops a sleep disorder may require referral to a sleep disorders centre for investigation.

DREAMS

Although dreams occur during both NREM and REM sleep, the dreams of REM sleep are more vivid and elaborate and are believed to be important to the consolidation of long-term memory. REM dreams may progress in content throughout the night from dreams about current events to emotional dreams of childhood or the past (Crisp & Taylor 2005).

Most people dream about immediate concerns such as an argument with a partner or worries over work. Another theory suggests that dreams erase certain fantasies or nonsensical memories. Since most dreams are forgotten, many people have little dream recall and do not believe they dream at all. To remember a dream, a person must consciously think about it on waking. People who recall dreams vividly usually wake just after a period of REM sleep (Crisp & Taylor 2005).

SLEEP DISORDERS

If a sleep disturbance persists despite the implementation of a good pre-sleep routine and lifestyle changes, advice may be sought from a medical officer. In the longer term a person may be referred to a sleep physician and may then undergo specific investigation in a sleep disorders unit, which is usually attached to an acute-care hospital or facility. Treating sleep disorders is a specialised branch of medicine and nursing.

An individual may undergo polysomnography (sleep studies). This involves being admitted overnight and sleep patterns being monitored. A specialised nurse or technician obtains a thorough sleep history from the client, which includes information of both past and current sleep problems. Specific information is collected in relation to sleep, including the time of settling, time of waking and number of times sleep is broken. Other data may include information on physical illnesses, medications and diet, any aids or techniques that the person is currently using to achieve sleep, and an environmental assessment. Polysomnography involves attaching monitoring leads to multiple areas of the body. While the person sleeps, brainwave activity, muscular activity, heart rate and oxygen saturations are monitored and recorded. Data collected are analysed to observe the person's stages of sleep and sleep patterns, to detect any sleep abnormalities.

INSOMNIA

People commonly complain about insomnia — trouble either falling asleep or staying asleep. Most people experience insomnia transiently, often in relation to one or a number of the above factors (illness, stress, change in sleeping environment). Usual sleeping habits usually return once the acute event or causative factor is over or eliminated. In the short term, having less sleep than normal usually causes no harm. Teaching individuals about the factors influencing sleep may help in improving sleep quality. Often lifestyle and environmental conditions are able to be easily modified, such as reducing alcohol and caffeine intake before bed, not napping through the day and use of stress-modifying techniques.

Chronic insomnia is usually termed as that lasting for a month or longer. It may be the result of an underlying medical, behavioural or psychiatric problem. Depression can often cause insomnia. Chronic insomnia usually requires investigation as to its cause, and treatment other than simple lifestyle and environmental modifications.

SNORING

Snoring is defined as breathing during sleep accompanied by harsh sounds and is caused by any obstruction of the air passages at the back of the mouth and nose. Poor muscle tone, excessive tissue or deformities such as a deviated septum may cause snoring. Obstructed airways due to colds or allergies can also cause snoring. Snoring can also be a symptom of sleep apnoea. The mild snorer should exercise to develop good muscle tone and lose weight if needed (deWit 2005).

OBSTRUCTIVE SLEEP APNOEA (OSA)

This occurs when a person's airway collapses during sleep. Breathing stops for a variable period until the brain registers a lack of breathing and sends a message to the sleeper. The sleeper rouses slightly, often snorting and gasping, but continues to sleep. Often the individual is not aware that they are rousing, but deep sleep is not maintained. This pattern may repeat itself many times during the night, leaving the person sleep-deprived and fatigued.

Obstructive sleep apnoea (OSA) is a serious and potentially life-threatening condition. The episodes of apnoea during sleep may cause various organ systems to function abnormally and possibly contribute to many disorders such as hypertension, heart attack and stroke. It also commonly leads to excessive daytime sleepiness and poor concentration and potentially increases the risk of having a road accident. Obesity is one of the contributing factors to OSA.

Treatment options may begin with lifestyle changes, if these are indicated, such as weight loss and a decrease in alcohol intake. Referral may be made to an ear, nose and throat (ENT) surgeon to assess whether airway obstruction could be caused by other mechanical factors. A dental splint may be utilised in mild cases of OSA to hold the jaw in a forced-forward position and thus keep the airway open. Moderate to severe sleep apnoea usually requires the long-term use of a nasal continuous positive airway pressure (CPAP) device. This is a mask worn while sleeping. It keeps the back of the throat open by forcing air through the nose, thereby preventing snoring and airway collapse. Clients require education and support to adapt to the use of a CPAP device but, in the long term, OSA can be controlled, and effective restorative sleep restored.

CENTRAL SLEEP APNOEA

Central sleep apnoea occurs when the brain fails to send a signal to the chest and diaphragm to keep breathing. There is no obstruction in the throat but, because of a disorganised breathing control, there is no effort made to breathe. When the signal does come through, breathing is quietly resumed, without the snorts and jerks associated with obstructive apnoea. The condition is usually also managed with CPAP therapy, at low-pressure. 'Mixed sleep apnoea' is a combination of obstructive and central apnoea.

NARCOLEPSY

Narcolepsy is a sleep disorder characterised by persistent and excessive daytime sleepiness. Uncontrollable brief episodes of sleep occur during hours of wakefulness. This is thought to be caused by an abnormality in the wake–sleep area of the brain. It often occurs in people in their teens or early 20s. There is no cure, but narcolepsy may be managed with medication (i.e. amphetamines), changes in lifestyle, counselling and support. Narcolepsy is usually diagnosed by conducting a daytime sleep study, used to measure the individual's tendency to fall asleep.

SLEEP DEPRIVATION

Many clients experience sleep deprivation as a result of hospitalisation (see Clinical Interest Box 34.1). This involves decreases in the amount, quality and consistency of sleep. When sleep becomes interrupted or fragmented, changes in the normal sequence of sleep stages occurs, and cycles cannot be completed. Gradually a cumulative sleep deprivation occurs. Individuals may experience a variety of physiological and psychological symptoms. The severity of symptoms is often related to the duration of sleep deprivation. The most effective treatment for sleep deprivation is elimination or correction of factors that disrupt sleep.

CLINICAL INTEREST BOX 34.1
Sleep deprivation

Physiological Symptoms	Psychological Symptoms
Ptosis, blurred vision	Confusion and disorientation
Fine motor clumsiness	Increased sensitivity to pain
Decreased reflexes	Irritable, withdrawn, apathetic
Slowed response time	Agitation
Decreased reasoning and judgment	Hyperactivity
Decreased auditory and visual alertness	Decreased motivation
Cardiac arrhythmias	Excessive sleepiness

(Potter & Perry 2008)

PARASOMNIAS

The parasomnias are sleep problems that are more common in children than in adults. Sudden infant death syndrome (SIDS) is thought to be related to apnoea, hypoxia and cardiac arrhythmias caused by abnormalities in the autonomic nervous system that are manifested during sleep. It is recommended that infants be placed in the supine position during sleep. Parasomnias that occur among older children include sleepwalking (somnambulism), nightmares, bed-wetting (nocturnal enuresis), and tooth grinding (bruxism). Specific treatment for these disorders varies. However, in all cases it is important to support the individual and maintain their safety (Crisp & Taylor 2005).

FACTORS LEADING TO SLEEP DISTURBANCES

A variety of factors may affect the quantity and quality of sleep. These factors are often transient, but the individual may seek advice about a sleeping problem. It is vital that the nurse is aware of such factors. Any physical illness that causes pain, difficulty breathing (even simple nasal congestion from a common cold), or requires the person to assume an awkward position (e.g. traction or a plaster cast), may compromise the ability to sleep. Nocturia, or getting up to urinate during the night, may disrupt the sleep cycle, as may other physical disorders, such as hyperthyroidism and cardiac dysrhythmias. Eating food such as a spicy or heavy meal late at night may also have an adverse effect on the ability to sleep.

Drugs and other substances, especially those containing caffeine, may adversely influence the ability to sleep. Prescribed medications used in the treatment of diseases or disorders not related to sleep can act alone or in combination and produce effects that may seriously disrupt sleep. The increased use of medications, commonly in the older adult, and the potential for altered pharmacokinetics (due to delayed elimination of medication) may result in interactions that induce insomnia or cause over-sedation. It is important for the nurse to consider the effects of the prescribed medications that a client is taking, if there is an otherwise unexplained problem with sleep (see Clinical Interest Box 34.2).

Alcohol and stimulants affect sleep patterns. Excessive alcohol disrupts REM sleep, although it may hasten the onset of sleep, and people often experience nightmares. Caffeine-containing beverages act as stimulants of the central nervous system, which can then interfere with sleep (Kozier et al 2000). Smoking affects sleep patterns. Nicotine has a stimulating effect on the body, and smokers often have more difficulty falling asleep than non-smokers. By not smoking after the evening meal, the individual usually sleeps better (Kozier et al 2000).

Lifestyle factors, including a person's daily routine, may influence sleep patterns. Any alteration in routine, such as engaging in late-night social activities or changing work times or mealtimes can disrupt sleep. Emotional stress, such as anxiety, depression or worry over personal problems and situations may cause difficulty sleeping. Often the difficulty sleeping is compounded by frustration, when sleep does not happen. The environment — particularly the person's home sleeping environment — may also cause wakefulness. Sleeping with a restless or snoring bed partner will usually alter the partner's ability to achieve sound sleep. Also, the

CLINICAL INTEREST BOX 34.2
Effects of medications on sleep

Hypnotics
Interfere with reaching deeper sleep stages
Provide only temporary (1 week) increase in quantity of sleep
Eventually cause 'hangover' during day; excess drowsiness, confusion, decreased energy
Sometimes worsens sleep apnoea in older adults

Antidepressants and Stimulants
Suppress REM sleep
Decrease total sleep time

Alcohol
Speeds onset of sleep
Reduces REM sleep
Awakens person during night and causes difficulty returning to sleep

Caffeine
Prevents person from falling asleep
Causes person to awaken during night
Interferes with REM sleep

Diuretics
Nighttime awakenings caused by nocturia

Beta-Adrenergic Blockers
Cause nightmares
Cause insomnia
Cause awakening from sleep

Benzodiazepines
Alter REM sleep
Increase sleep time
Increase daytime sleepiness

Narcotics
Suppress REM sleep
Cause increased daytime drowsiness

Anticonvulsants
Decrease REM sleep time
Causes daytime drowsiness

REM, Rapid eye movement.
(Potter & Perry 2008)

effects of light, noise, temperature and comfort also affect sleep patterns in the home environment.

The many stressors associated with daily living, and particularly with illness, may have a detrimental affect on a person's ability to rest and sleep, and further impact on their general wellbeing. Some people may find various relaxation techniques helpful. For many people, physical exercise is an effective method of relieving stress, but as this is not always practical, relaxation techniques may be used instead.

Exercise and fatigue can affect sleep patterns. A person who is relatively fatigued usually achieves a restful sleep. Exercising 2 hours or more before bedtime allows the body to cool down and maintains a state of fatigue that promotes relaxation (Crisp & Taylor 2005). Good eating habits are important for proper health and sleep. Eating a large, heavy and/or spicy meal at night may result in indigestion that interferes with sleep. Weight gain or loss influences sleep patterns. When a person gains weight, sleep periods become longer, with fewer interruptions. Weight loss can cause short and fragmented sleep (Crisp & Taylor 2005).

ASSESSING SLEEP PATTERNS

When assessing a client's status in relation to comfort, rest and sleep, the nurse should obtain information about usual sleeping behaviour, such as the time the person normally goes to sleep, the quality of sleep and the time of waking up (see Clinical Interest Box 34.3). It is helpful to know whether they have a bedtime routine, for example, if they normally have a hot drink before bedtime, and if they require medication to help them sleep. The nurse should also ascertain whether there is currently any discomfort that may disturb rest and sleep, such as nausea, difficulty breathing or pain associated with present illness. The information obtained, together with observation of the client, provides the nurse with a foundation on which to plan and implement nursing actions to promote comfort, rest and sleep (see Clinical Interest Box 34.4). When possible the person's usual bedtime routine should be maintained, and the immediate environment arranged so that it is conducive to comfort, rest and sleep.

SLEEP-PROMOTION MEASURES

During the night the nurse continues to observe clients and perform procedures or treatments as necessary. Clients should be disturbed as little as possible and, if woken and they experience difficulty resettling, measures such as a change of position, adjustment to the bedding or a warm drink may help with resuming sleep. The Registered Nurse (RN) must be notified if a client does not resettle after these supportive measures have been implemented. The nurse on night duty must ensure that the individual's comfort and safety are promoted. Continuity of care is essential and, as there are usually fewer staff working at night, the nurse's observational skills are vital in detecting any change in an individual's condition or comfort. The nurse is also in a position to observe any specific problem related to sleep, such as not settling, excessive restlessness, excessive snoring or airway obstruction.

Sleep is influenced by a variety of factors that may be described as physical, psychological or environmental. Effective sleep may be facilitated by a range of natural measures, which include:

- Sleep in a room that is quiet, darkened, at a comfortable temperature (coolness or warmth) and which has sufficient fresh air or ventilation
- Engage in physical exercise during the day to promote rest at night, and go to bed when tired
- Spend some time relaxing and unwinding before going to bed. Sleep may also be more easily achieved if the person is able to resolve any problems before going to bed
- Resisting stimulants such as tea, coffee or cocoa immediately before going to bed. People may find it easier to sleep if they avoid going to bed feeling hungry or overfull
- Adopt a pre-sleep routine, e.g., similar time each night, warm bath or shower, warm drink and some peaceful music or relaxing reading. For children, this may include quiet time and perhaps story reading, as well as settling with a familiar object, such as a doll or soft toy.

The need for comfort is closely related to the need for sufficient rest and sleep. Rest depends on relaxation and to be relaxed a person must be physically comfortable and

CLINICAL INTEREST BOX 34.3
Questions to determine a client's usual sleep pattern

- What time do you usually go to sleep?
- How quickly do you fall asleep?
- What is the average number of hours you sleep during the night?
- How many times do you wake at night?
- When do you usually wake in the morning?
- Do you rise once you wake or do you stay in bed?

CLINICAL INTEREST BOX 34.4
Components of a sleep history

- Description of client's sleep problem
- Usual sleep pattern before the sleep problem
- Recent changes in sleep pattern
- Bedtime routines and sleeping environment
- Use of sleep and other prescription medications and over-the-counter drugs
- Pattern of dietary intake and amount of substances that influence sleep
- Symptoms experienced during waking hours
- Physical illness
- Recent life events
- Current emotional and mental status

(adapted from Potter & Perry 2008)

free from emotional tension. Rest and relaxation do not necessarily mean inactivity; for example, a person who has a sedentary occupation may find the physical exercise of a brisk walk relaxing. People confined to bed may find it more relaxing if they are reading or watching television rather than lying in bed with nothing to do.

A person may find it difficult to rest in a hospital environment because of physical discomfort, stress, constant activity levels by nursing staff, or disturbing sights and smells that may occur with illness and hospitalisation. A person may be subjected to bright lights or disruptive noises (see Clinical Interest Box 34.5), and effective rest may be disturbed by the constant attention of members of the health care team. Anxiety related to illness, and its consequences, may prevent relaxation and interrupt sleep. Being in hospital involves a variety of potential stressors; the nurse should therefore implement measures to provide as stress free an environment as possible.

A person may experience difficulty in maintaining the usual sleep pattern because of illness or hospitalisation. Clients should be encouraged to maintain the usual pre-sleep routine. Nursing care should be planned so that repeated disturbance to clients is avoided. Emotional tension may be reduced by providing clients with adequate information before any treatment or procedure starts. To provide opportunities for questions to be asked and answered, the nurse should promote a climate that is conducive to communication by spending time with the client and their significant others. Unnecessary noise should be eliminated and clients told the reasons for unavoidable noises.

Some regulations regarding visiting times may be necessary to avoid overtiring a hospitalised person. Many health care agencies have specified times during the day that are regarded as rest periods. Throughout these periods, visitors to, and activities in, the ward are kept to a minimum to provide a quiet relaxed environment. During rest periods, clients should be encouraged to try to sleep or to engage in some relaxing non-stressful activity. To facilitate rest and relaxation, the client's physical comfort should be promoted, as it is difficult to rest in the presence of discomfort such as pain, a full bladder or an uncomfortable position (see Clinical Interest Boxes 34.6 and 34.7).

CLINICAL INTEREST BOX 34.5
Control of noise in the hospital

- Close doors to clients' room when possible.
- Keep doors to work areas on unit closed when in use.
- Reduce volume of nearby telephone and paging equipment.
- Wear rubber-soled shoes. Avoid clogs.
- Turn off bedside oxygen and other equipment that is not in use.
- Turn down alarms and beeps on bedside monitoring equipment.
- Turn off room TV and radio unless client prefers soft music.
- Avoid abrupt loud noise such as flushing a toilet or moving a bed.
- Keep necessary conversations at low levels, particularly at night.
- Conduct conversations and reports in a private area away from client rooms.

(Potter & Perry 2008)

MEETING SLEEP NEEDS

In hospital, the nurse should assist a person in preparation for sleep, by ensuring that the following key physiological and psychological needs are met.

Hygiene needs

When required the client should be assisted to meet all hygiene needs, such as washing face and hands and cleaning teeth. An ambulant client may like to have a warm shower or bath before settling to sleep. A non-ambulant client may require repositioning and turning.

Nutritional and fluid needs

A warm drink and snack could be offered to the client, unless this is contraindicated. A client may prefer a non-stimulating milk-based drink rather than tea or coffee, which can have a stimulating effect. A client permitted oral fluids should also be provided with fluid that can be consumed during the night if desired.

CLINICAL INTEREST BOX 34.6
Promoting Safe Sleeping

The SIDS and Kids Safe Sleeping program teaches parents how to create a safe sleeping environment for babies and young children.

1 Put baby on the back to sleep from birth
2 Sleep baby with head and face uncovered
3 Avoid exposing babies to cigarette smoke before birth and after
4 Sleep baby in a safe cot and in a safe environment
5 Sleep baby in its own cot or bassinette in the same room as the parents for the first 6–12 months.

(Sids and Kids 2007)

CLINICAL INTEREST BOX 34.7
Promoting sleep in adult clients

- Administer any analgesics or sedatives about 30 minutes before bedtime
- Encourage clients to wear loose-fitting nightwear
- Remove any irritants against the client's skin, such as moist or wrinkled sheets or drainage tubing
- Position and support body parts to protect pressure areas and aid muscle relaxation
- Administer necessary hygiene measures
- Keep linen clean and dry
- Encourage the client to void before going to sleep
- Provide a quiet environment

(Kozier et al 2000)

Elimination needs

Clients should be provided with toilet facilities before settling for sleep. The nurse may need to assist an ambulant person to the toilet or provide a non-ambulant person with the appropriate toilet utensil. Urinary drainage equipment should be checked, and the collection bag emptied if necessary.

Comfort needs

Preparing the client's room includes ensuring that there is adequate ventilation and warmth and that lighting is reduced to a minimum. The client's signal device and any other items that may be required during the night need to be placed within easy reach. Nursing measures include ensuring that the client is positioned comfortably and that the bedclothes and pillows are arranged to meet individual needs. The bottom sheets should be free of wrinkles or creases, and supplementary items such as a sheepskin or bed cradle may be used to enhance comfort. Whenever possible, treatments and procedures are completed before clients settle for sleep. For example, any splints or dressings should be checked and, if necessary, adjusted or changed.

Protection and safety needs

Measures need to be taken to promote the individual's safety during sleep. If a person is restless or confused, the use of bed rails may be indicated. Appropriate consent and documentation should accompany this action when undertaken. It is usually appropriate to adjust the height of the bed to its lowest level. As an alternative safety measure, 'hi-low' beds, which can be situated at floor level, and use of a concave mattress may be appropriate for a client who is disoriented and inclined to get out of bed and wander.

Adequate lighting should be provided, perhaps via a night light, particularly if the individual needs to get out of bed during the night. The individual should be monitored regularly throughout the night, to assess condition, ensuring that any equipment such as intravenous infusion apparatus is functioning appropriately.

Pain-avoidance needs

It is the role of the Enrolled Nurse (EN) to notify the RN if a client is experiencing pain or any other distressing symptoms, such as a troublesome cough, which may affect adequate rest and sleep. Any acute or chronic pain should be assessed and managed, either by non-pharmacological or pharmacological means (see Chapter 28).

Psychological needs

If a client is anxious or worried the nurse should try to ascertain the reason and provide appropriate support. For example, a person may be concerned about some aspect of treatment, such as forthcoming surgery, and providing them with further information may help to alleviate some of their anxiety. Reassurance that a nurse will be available to respond to needs may also be helpful.

Pharmacological measures

In the short term, and particularly while hospitalised, a client may be prescribed medication by a medical officer to promote sleep, for example, a sedative. Natural measures to promote settling should be undertaken first but, if trouble getting to sleep persists, sedation may be considered by the medical team to be appropriate. After a sedative medication has been administered, the client should be encouraged to relax and allow it to take effect. The response to, and effects of, such medication must be noted. When the client has settled for sleep, it is best that all activity, noise and light be reduced to a minimum.

Stress reductions

A range of techniques is available for reducing stress and promoting relaxation, all of which aim to help the individual control reactions to stress. To promote relaxation so that the need for rest and sleep may be met, the teaching of a constructive method of coping with stress may be indicated. Relaxation techniques should initially be learned in a quiet restful environment and, with practice, may then be used in most situations to reduce stress. To practise these techniques, the client should be lying or sitting comfortably, with the limbs relaxed, the eyes closed, and with sensory stimulation reduced to a minimum.

Yoga and meditation

Yoga and meditation are forms of relaxation that are helpful to many people and, while neither is difficult, they should be taught by people with expertise in these methods.

Relaxation breathing

This technique consists of controlled breathing, performed while the client assumes a comfortable position. The person is encouraged to concentrate on their breathing, and may find it helpful to visualise each breath as providing muscles with energy-giving oxygen. The person is encouraged to take a deep breath, hold it briefly, then exhale slowly. With each exhalation the person is encouraged to say 'relax' and, as the technique is repeated, should feel progressively more relaxed.

Progressive muscular relaxation

The theory behind this technique is that a relaxed body leads to a relaxed mind. The technique consists of consciously tensing and relaxing the major muscles of the body in sequence. The client is encouraged to tense one or a group of muscles, feel the tension, then slowly ease the tension by relaxing the muscles. As the technique is repeated, there should be an awareness of the sensation of relaxation in the muscles.

Visual imagery

This technique involves encouraging the client to imagine a restful and pleasant scene. By imagining the scene, together with the associated sounds and smells, it is possible to become quite relaxed.

Touch and massage

It is generally considered that the sense of touch is as important a contact with reality as the senses of sight and sound. Massage is a method of communication without words, and can induce a feeling of physical and mental relaxation. There are many types of massage and, while most are relatively easy to learn, instructors with experience should teach the basic techniques. Muscles contract and become tense in stressful situations, and massage can be an effective method of promoting muscle relaxation. Some of the key aspects of massage are:

- Providing a quiet private environment free from harsh lighting
- Providing warmth. The room, the person receiving the massage and any oils being used should be comfortably warm
- The person who is giving the massage should have short fingernails and clean warm hands
- Verbal communication should be limited, and the recipient encouraged to concentrate on the sensation of physical contact
- The person giving the massage should convey, in their touch, an impression of confidence and ability. Remembering that the recipient is a person with dignity will influence the quality of touch
- After the massage the recipient should be encouraged to remain resting, quiet and relaxed.

Although a massage can be beneficial, some people may not feel comfortable about being massaged. Also, a client's physical condition may contraindicate the use of massage. In the right situation, however, massage, particularly of the neck and back, can be very relaxing and promote rest.

Clinical Interest Box 34.8 outlines some ways in which sleep and rest can be promoted at home. Clinical Interest Box 34.9 lists the possible nursing diagnoses for a client with sleep disturbances.

SUMMARY

Comfort is necessary for relaxation, rest and sleep. A person's ability to achieve comfort and relax, and therefore to receive sufficient rest and sleep, may be disrupted during illness or hospitalisation. Measures that can be implemented to promote rest may include certain techniques that facilitate relaxation. Sleep can also be promoted by allowing the hospitalised individual to maintain their normal pre-sleep routine, and by ensuring that the person's safety and comfort are promoted during the night, as at any other time. Sleep behaviours and patterns can be assessed by the nurse, and simple measures to promote effective sleep may be taught and implemented. Assisting clients to meet their needs for comfort, rest and sleep is essential in the promotion of individual physical and psychological wellbeing.

CLINICAL INTEREST BOX 34.8
Promoting rest and sleep at home

Sleep pattern

- Establish a regular bedtime and waking time for all days of the week. Eliminate lengthy naps during the day. Limit them to only 30 minutes a day
- Exercise adequately during the day. Avoid physical exertion 2 hours before bedtime
- Avoid dealing with work or family problems before bedtime
- Establish a regular routine before sleep, e.g., reading, listening to music, etc
- When unable to sleep, pursue a relaxing activity until you feel drowsy
- If having trouble falling asleep, get up until you feel sleepy
- Use the bed mainly for sleep

Environment

- Ensure appropriate lighting, temperature and environment
- Keep noise to a minimum

Diet

- Avoid heavy meals 3 hours before bedtime
- Avoid alcohol- and caffeine-containing foods and beverages at least 4 hours before bedtime
- Decrease fluid intake 2–4 hours before sleep
- If a bedtime snack is necessary consume only light snacks or a milk drink

Medications

- Use sleeping medications only as a last resort
- Take analgesics 30 minutes before bedtime to relieve aches and pains
- Consult with a health care provider about adjusting other medications that may cause insomnia

(Kozier et al 2000)

CLINICAL INTEREST BOX 34.9
Nursing diagnoses related to sleep disturbances

- Anxiety
- Breathing pattern ineffective
- Confusion, acute
- Coping, ineffective, family
- Coping, ineffective, individual
- Fatigue
- Sensory perception alteration
- Sleep-pattern disturbance: insomnia, sleep apnoea

(Potter & Perry 2008)

REVIEW EXERCISES

1. What is the importance of rest and sleep to a person's wellbeing?
2. What are the phases of the sleep cycle?
3. What factors may interfere with the process of rest and sleep?
4. Describe the supportive nursing measures that may be implemented to promote the individual's need for rest and sleep.

CRITICAL THINKING EXERCISES

1. Mrs Smith, aged 50, is a client on your surgical ward who has recently undergone knee surgery. You are on night shift, and find her awake at 1 a.m. While she has no specific complaints, she tells you that she has been having trouble sleeping since her surgery 4 days ago. Develop a nursing care plan for Mrs Smith to promote effective sleep during this current period of hospitalisation.
2. Mr Brown is a middle-aged factory worker who works permanent evening shift, which finishes at 11 p.m. After work he eats his main meal of the day and drinks at least six cans of beer. He normally goes to bed at 1 a.m. and sleeps in short periods, for about 6 hours. He gets up at least once to urinate. He relaxes by watching television in bed. As a nurse, what would you assess about Mr Brown's sleep habits and history? What could you recommend to him to improve his sleep patterns?

REFERENCES AND FURTHER READING

Akerstedt T, Fredlund P, Gillberg M, Jannson B (2002) Sleep disturbances, work stress and work hours: a cross sectional study. *Journal of Psychosomatic Research*, 53 (3): 741–8

Ambrogetti A, Hensley M & Ols L (2006) *Sleep Disorders: a Clinical Textbook*. Quay Books, London

Anon. Coping with CPAP Treatment. [Patient information brochure] ResMed Limited, NSW

Bryant B, Knights K, Salerno E (2003) *Pharmacology for Health Professionals*. Harcourt Australia, Sydney

Crisp J, Taylor C (eds) (2005) *Potter & Perry's Fundamentals of Nursing*, 2nd edn. Elsevier Australia, Sydney

deWit S (2005) *Fundamental Concepts and Skills for Nursing*, 2nd edn. WB Saunders, Philadelphia

Kozier B, Erb G, Berman AJ, Burke K (2000) *Fundamentals of Nursing: Concepts, Process, and Practice*, 6th edn. Prentice-Hall Inc, Upper Saddle River, NJ

Marieb E (2006) *Human Anatomy and Physiology*, 6th edn. Benjamin Cummings, San Francisco

Parmeggiana PL, Velluti RA (2005) *The Physiologic Nature of Sleep*. Imperial College Press, Hackensack, NJ

Potter PA, Perry AG (2001) *Fundamentals of Nursing*, 5th edn. Mosby, St Louis

—— (2005) *Fundamentals of Nursing*, 6th edn. Mosby, St Louis

—— (2008) *Fundamentals of Nursing*, 7th edn. Mosby, St Louis

Sharp T (2001) *The Good Sleep Guide*. Penguin Books, Sydney

Sids and Kids (2007) *Fact Sheet: Safe Sleeping*. Online. Available: http://www.sidsandkids.org/documents/FAQOctober2007_2__000.pdf [accessed 25 May 2008]

ONLINE RESOURCES

Sids and Kids: www.sidsandkids.org

Chapter 35

PAIN MANAGEMENT

OBJECTIVES

- Define the key terms/concepts
- Describe the physiological processes whereby pain sensations are received, transmitted and interpreted
- State the factors influencing an individual's perception of, and reaction to, pain
- Describe pain assessment methods, including the differences required in approach with an individual suffering chronic pain
- Describe various methods of pain management, including both non-pharmacological and pharmacological approaches
- Apply appropriate principles in planning and implementing nursing actions to prevent and to alleviate an individual's pain

KEY TERMS/CONCEPTS

acute pain
analgesic
chronic pain
endorphins
epidural infusion
gate-control theory
pain
pain tolerance
patient-controlled analgesia (PCA)
threshold
transcutaneous electrical nerve stimulation (TENS)

CHAPTER FOCUS

Pain is both an unpleasant physical sensation and a social and emotional experience. Each episode of pain is a unique personal event. It is a universal human experience occurring across the life span, but, because no one can fully appreciate the pain of another person, pain is always a subjective experience.

Pain may be mild or severe, acute or chronic. Pain is difficult to define, as it is an individual experience with varying levels of intensity, and it may be physical, psychological or emotional in origin. Pain is often described as being a sensation of distress or suffering caused by a particular stimulus. A definition of pain that has been widely accepted and used by many nurses is that of McCaffery, a highly recognised pain care specialist (McCaffery & Pasero 1999). Her definition encompasses the idea that 'pain is what the person says it is, and exists when he [sic] says it does'. Pain is increasingly being considered a condition rather than a symptom, and ideas about pain and its management are constantly changing.

Assessment and management of an individual's pain may pose a significant challenge for the health care team. Supportive nursing care for a person in pain can play a huge part in this challenge.

LIVED EXPERIENCE

I'd like to, just once, wake up in the morning and know that today there would be no discomfort or pain. I spend a few hours each morning just trying to get 'ready' for the day — I use warm water, heat packs, medication, magnets . . . anything to try and help achieve some comfort. The end of the day often isn't much better than the start, but hopefully for a couple of hours in the middle of the day, I'm reasonably functional. I try other alternative treatments too; acupuncture seems to help a little, but some days, it all seems too hard, and the whole of my being is affected by my pain.

Rebecca, 41, with chronic pain syndrome

PHYSIOLOGY OF PAIN

Pain is one of the most common causes of discomfort, and pain avoidance is viewed by Maslow (in Crisp & Taylor 2005) as a first priority physiological need. Pain avoidance appears to be an instinctive reaction to harmful factors in the environment; for example, a newborn will draw away from a painful stimulus. Throughout the life cycle, people will avoid painful stimuli or take actions to withdraw from such stimuli. The ability to relieve or to control pain depends on an understanding of how it occurs and how it is controlled by the brain. The physical experience of pain can be divided into four distinct phases: the stimulus which causes the pain, the transfer of pain, the perception of pain and the reaction to pain.

When pain receptors are stimulated they send electrical impulses along special pathways to the spinal cord. These pathways may be seen as being similar to a two-lane road, one lane with large diameter fibres for fast message transmission ('A' fibres), and one lane with smaller diameter fibres for slower message transmission ('C' fibres). 'A' fibres have the most insulation, and carry information that reflects throbbing and pricking types of pain. Slow pathways ('C' fibres) have less insulation, and carry impulses that represent burning pain. Pain receptors in the skin and other tissues are free nerve endings, some of which are the peripheral terminations of small diameter 'C' fibres, while others are the slightly larger diameter 'A' fibres. When histamine and other naturally occurring chemical substances are released as a result of tissue damage, pain sensations travel along the nerve fibres. Regardless of the type of pain, and whether travelling slowly or quickly, pain impulses are transmitted to the dorsal root ganglia of the spinal cord, where they synapse with certain neurons in the posterior horns of the grey matter. Pain sensations are then transmitted to various areas of the brain by synapses at the thalamus, where they are perceived and interpreted (Figure 35.1).

Pain causes both reflex motor reactions and psychic reactions. Some of the reflex actions occur directly from the spinal cord, where small neurons in the grey matter transmit an impulse straight from the skin to the muscles, without brain involvement. For example, a painful stimulus to the hand, such as extreme heat, initiates reflex contraction of the flexor muscles that cause withdrawal of the arm from the heat source.

Although the complex mechanisms of the physiology and psychology of pain are not understood completely, there are several theories of pain. The gate-control theory of pain (Melzack & Wall 1965) suggests that neural mechanisms in the dorsal horns of the spinal cord can act like a gate. This theory suggests that activity in the large diameter nerve fibres can close the gate and block pain impulses, resulting in a decrease or elimination of pain sensation. Therefore, according to this theory, it is possible to block pain impulses travelling to the brain by stimulating the large 'A' nerve fibres and 'closing the gate'. This theory may help to explain the reason why cutaneous stimulation (rubbing a sore spot) or acupuncture can relieve pain, as in acupuncture, stimulation of non-painful nerve fibres can 'confuse' messages and suppress pain signals.

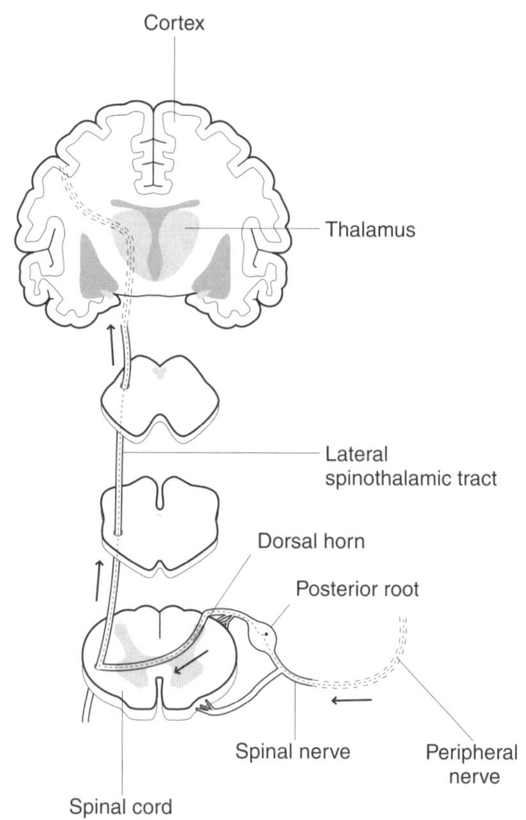

Figure 35.1 | The pathway of pain

It is acknowledged that pain can be inhibited along the course of transmission and that endorphins play a complex role in closing the gate to pain. Endorphins are naturally occurring substances with opioid qualities, which combine with the same receptors as morphine and other narcotics, producing the same effect (i.e. analgesia). They act as neurotransmitters that mediate the transmission of pain information. As a result of pain or stress, an impulse from the brain may trigger the release of endorphins from pain-inhibiting neurons in the dorsal horn, which block transmission of the pain impulse before it reaches the brain. Various studies have shown that plasma endorphin levels increase in states of stress, and also that acupuncture and transcutaneous electrical nerve stimulation (TENS [discussed later in this chapter]) increase endorphin release. Therefore, although incompletely understood, it is known that the body has some internal mechanisms that help to control pain and its perception.

CAUSES OF PAIN

Pain is often a useful protective signal, as it can be a warning of actual or impending tissue damage. The sensation of pain can also warn the individual of emotional or stress-related problems, such as a headache caused by tension or anxiety. Pain can result from many sources or stimuli, including mechanical trauma, chemical irritants, extremes of temperature, ischaemia and psychological factors.

Ischaemia

Ischaemia (decreased blood supply to an area or body part) causes cell damage or destruction with the subsequent release of irritating chemical substances that stimulate the pain nerve endings.

Chemical irritation

Stimulation of sensory nerve endings by irritant chemicals from an external source, such as acid, or by chemical substances released by damaged cells (histamine) will cause pain. Substances may leak from an organ into the peritoneal cavity and stimulate large areas of pain fibres causing severe pain; for example, gastric juice may escape as a result of a perforated gastric ulcer.

Mechanical trauma

Pain may result when body tissues are stretched; for example, distension of a hollow organ such as the stomach or bladder. When tissues are contracted, as in muscle spasm, pain occurs as a result of local ischaemia, stretched nerve endings and from an accumulation of metabolic wastes. Prolonged pressure on tissues causes local ischaemia and pressure on nerve endings and, consequently, pain. Physical force, such as a hard blow to the tissues results in initial pressure on the nerve endings and subsequent irritation from substances released by the damaged cells.

Extremes of temperature

Extremes of heat or cold (thermal trauma) may damage tissues and cause pain. Burns or scalds damage nerve endings, and frostbite causes local blood vessel constriction and ischaemia.

Psychological factors

Pain may be experienced in the absence of any physiological cause, or as a result of the physical manifestations of psychological disorders, such as abdominal cramp or headache resulting from stress or anxiety. Emotional distress causes increased muscle tension that can lead to aches and pains in a variety of areas, such as neck or back pain.

TYPES OF PAIN

Acute pain is usually of rapid onset and varies in intensity and length of time it lasts. It is often perceived as an incident of high severity. In most cases it is self-limiting, and has a predictable management and end. It is often able to be precisely located and described. Acute pain, if mild, may require no specific intervention, and more severe acute pain can usually be managed successfully. Acute pain may result from injury, infection, or after surgical intervention. When tissue damage is the cause, pain declines as the tissues heal.

Chronic pain is considered to be pain that has lasted for at least 6 months and is an ongoing experience that fails to resolve naturally or does not respond well to intervention. It is often no longer considered to be pain that warns of impending danger or tissue damage. Chronic pain is constant or intermittent and the individual often has difficulty localising it. The pain from arthritis may be regarded as chronic pain. An individual who experiences unrelieved pain for an extended period often feels trapped and helpless. The client's anxiety increases and they become preoccupied with their pain and state of health. Sleep disturbances and fatigue may be experienced and irritability, aggression, or withdrawal and depression may result.

Superficial (cutaneous) pain originates in the skin or mucous membranes, as a result of stimulation of nerve receptors in those areas. Because there are large numbers of sensory nerve endings on the surface of the body, a person is usually able to localise and describe surface pain accurately.

Deep (visceral) pain originates in internal body structures as a result of stimulation of receptors in those areas. As there are fewer sensory nerve endings in the viscera than in skin or mucous membranes, it is more difficult to localise and describe visceral pain. Localised damage to the viscera rarely causes severe pain, whereas widespread damage causing diffuse stimulation of the nerve ending produces extreme pain. For example, occlusion of the blood supply to a large section of the intestine stimulates many diffuse fibres and can result in severe pain.

Visceral pain may be felt at a site far removed from the affected area, through the mechanism known as referred pain. Referred pain is felt in a part of the body away from the pain's point of origin; for example, pain in the left shoulder and arm associated with myocardial infarction. In this instance, sensory neurons that transmit signals from the skin enter the same area of the spinal cord as do nerve fibres from the myocardium. The neurons carry pain signals from both areas to the brain and, because cutaneous pain is more common than visceral pain, the brain interprets the pain as originating in the skin. Figure 35.2 illustrates the common sites of referred pain in a female, but it can be noted that the sites are the same in both females and males.

Phantom pain is a sensation of pain felt in a body part that has been removed, such as when the lower leg has been amputated. Although the nerves supplying the amputated part have been severed, the remaining neurons may continue to send impulses as before, and the brain still interprets the impulses as if that part were still there.

Intractable pain refers to pain that is severe and constant or unrelenting, and which is unrelieved by usual pain management measures. For example, the extreme and constant pain often associated with cancer may not be relieved by strong analgesics alone, and the individual may also require non-drug therapy such as surgery to block the nerve fibres conducting the pain impulses.

Total pain, the experience of a person with an ongoing pain syndrome, is derived from several sources. The term

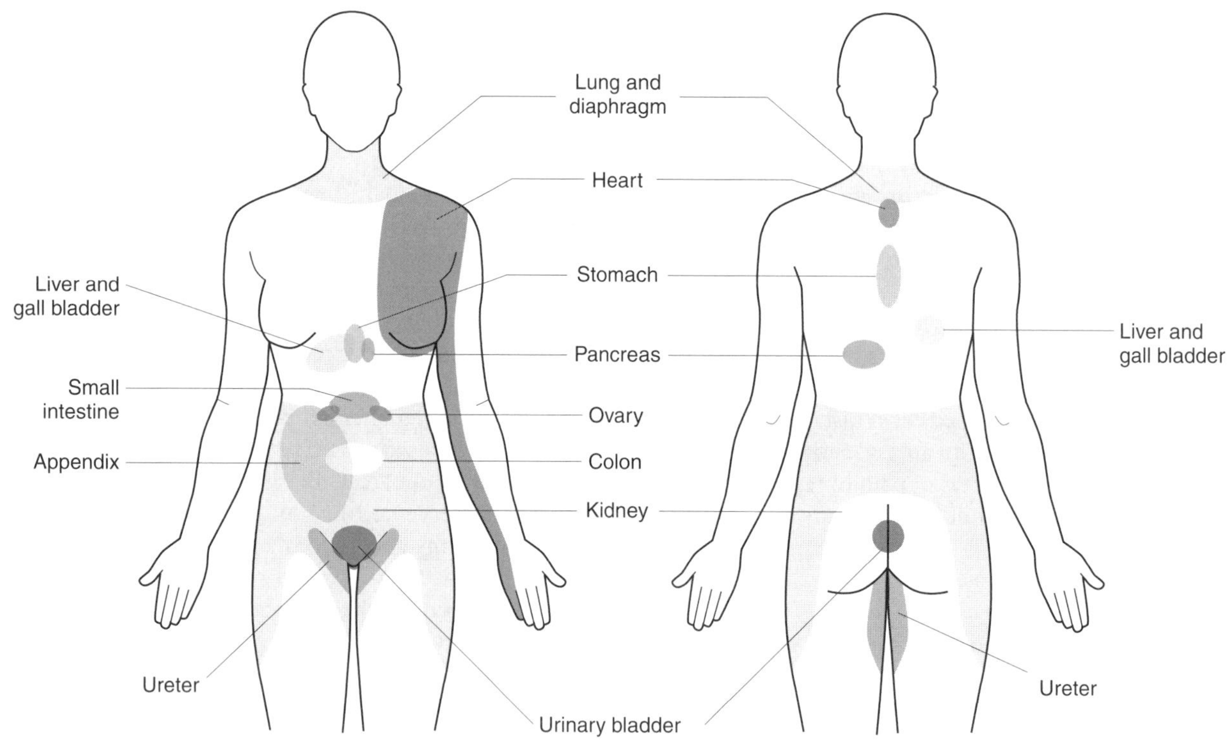

Figure 35.2 | Referred pain sites: cutaneous areas to which pain from certain viscera are referred

'total pain' has been devised to address the complexity of pain as both a somatic and a psychological experience. It has been well documented that a person's pain threshold can be lowered by psychological factors such as fear, depression and isolation, with the result that the pain experience is increased.

PERCEPTION OF PAIN

The perception of pain is individual and is therefore different for each person. In addition, a person may perceive pain differently at different times. Clinical Interest Box 35.1 provides some common biases and misconceptions about pain. The pain threshold is the point at which a stimulus, such as pressure, activates pain receptors and produces a sensation of pain. Four identifiable levels of pain threshold have been described:

1. Sensation threshold: the lowest stimulus level at which an individual perceives sensation (e.g. tingling)
2. Pain perception threshold: the lowest stimulus level at which the individual states that the continuing stimulation is painful
3. Pain tolerance: the lowest level at which the individual withdraws from the stimulation or asks to have it stopped
4. Encouraged pain tolerance: this is the same as pain tolerance, but the individual is encouraged to tolerate higher levels of stimulation.

Because the perception of pain is individual, some will experience pain much earlier than others. Studies have shown that all individuals have a similar sensation threshold but that the ways in which they react to pain vary greatly.

CLINICAL INTEREST BOX 35.1
Common biases and misconceptions about pain

The following statements are false:

- Substance abusers and alcoholics overreact to discomforts
- Clients with minor illnesses have less pain than those with severe physical alteration
- Administering analgesics regularly will lead to drug addiction
- The amount of tissue damage in an injury can accurately indicate pain intensity
- Health care personnel are the best authorities on the nature of a client's pain
- Psychogenic pain is not real
- Chronic pain is psychological
- Clients should expect to have pain in a hospital
- Clients who cannot speak do not feel pain.

(Potter & Perry 2008)

FACTORS INFLUENCING PAIN

The ways in which different people react to pain may vary tremendously and many factors may be involved. Behavioural manifestations of pain vary according to both the individual and to factors in the environment.

Age

As infants and young children lack the ability to express themselves verbally, their pain, or the degree of pain they experience, may not be recognised or appreciated. Many misconceptions exist in relation to pain in infants, including that infants do not feel pain or are incapable of expressing pain. In addition to the physiological changes, behavioural cues, such as facial activity (including brow bulge, eye squeeze and open lips), crying behaviour and gross motor activity may indicate pain in the infant. Additionally, many children are taught from an early age that they are expected to be brave and that 'only babies cry'. As a result, a child who is experiencing pain may endeavour to hide it. Conversely, a child may invent or exaggerate pain as a method of gaining attention.

When older children or adolescents experience pain they may think of it in terms of how it will affect their activities and the attainment of goals. As a result of misunderstanding about their body and illness, young clients sometimes harbour distressing fantasies about the significance of pain. Consequently, both anxiety and pain are increased.

The ability to tolerate pain generally seems to increase with age, and this may be partly due to expectations about what constitutes 'adult' behaviour. Many myths also exist, however, in relation to pain experienced by older adults, particularly those with cognitive impairment. This has resulted in an underestimation and management of pain in people with disorders such as Alzheimer's disease. Clinical Interest Box 35.2 provides more information about pain management in clients with Alzheimer's disease. Common misconceptions include that pain is a natural consequence of growing old, that pain perception decreases with age, and that, if the older adult does not report pain, they do not have pain.

Gender

Many males have been conditioned by society to be strong and brave. Some people consider that any display of emotion by a male, such as crying, is a sign of weakness. As a result of society's expectations of acceptable behaviour, a male may internalise or suppress expressions of pain.

CLINICAL INTEREST BOX 35.2
Pain management in clients with Alzheimer's disease

No evidence exists that cognitively impaired older adults experience less pain or that their reports of pain are less valid than those people with intact cognitive function. It is probable that clients with dementia and progressive deficits of cognition, particularly those in long-term care facilities, suffer significant unrelieved pain and discomfort. Assessing pain in these clients is challenging but possible. The best approach is to accept the client's report of pain and treat the pain as it would be treated in a person with intact cognitive function.
(Potter & Perry 2008)

Culture

Cultural values, attitudes and feelings contribute to the way people react to pain. Some people have a matter-of-fact attitude to pain, with little outward expression of their suffering, while others are more expressive and seek immediate pain relief. Most Western cultures place strong values on the ability to bear pain with silent fortitude, so that external behaviours may not reveal the intensity of pain. People from Latin cultures are permitted to display their suffering openly, such as by crying or moaning, as a socially accepted response to pain. It must also be appreciated, however, that there are enormous differences within every culture and that not every person from a specific culture will react in the same manner. Clinical Interest Box 35.3 provides an example of a cultural experience of pain.

Emotional state

A person who is emotionally or physically exhausted often has a reduced capacity to tolerate pain. Individual resistance to, and control over, reactions to pain may be lessened. This is often a cyclic phenomenon — continual pain results in anxiety, and anxiety and fear exacerbate pain.

Previous pain

Previous episodes of severe pain often cause great apprehension, and individuals can suffer greatly if they anticipate recurrent severe pain. Anxiety may be increased if the previous experience of severe pain was poorly managed. Previous pain experience may at times be useful as a form of comparison, when assessing a subsequent pain episode. Overall, the amount of previous pain experiences a person has had may influence their current response to an episode.

Self-image

A person's self-perception can influence a reaction to pain. For example, a person who has a low self-esteem may try to bear pain stoically to be regarded highly by others. Conversely, another person with a poor self-image and feelings of worthlessness may tolerate pain poorly in an attempt to gain attention and recognition. A pain episode may be interpreted by some people as being punished for something.

Time of day

Night, with accompanying darkness and reduced sensory input, often increases a person's sensation of pain. Fear

CLINICAL INTEREST BOX 35.3
A cultural experience of pain

Certain religious groups, for example, Muslims, may believe that it is God's will for them to experience pain. Some clients may be unwilling to accept medication in case it clouds or impairs their senses. Buddhists, for example, may prefer to use meditation techniques to help relieve their pain.
(Heath 1995)

and anxiety may be increased and, as a result, so too is the sensation of pain. The latter part of the day may also be when the person is fatigued physically and emotionally.

Environment

There is a relationship between anxiety and pain, and environmental factors can either contribute to or reduce anxiety levels. The environment can act as an anxiety-provoking stressor, for example, if it is ugly, if there is an atmosphere of tension or if there is a lack of privacy. Privacy allows a person uninhibited expression of pain, such as crying or moaning. The continued presence of other people, as in a shared ward, results in a sense of loss of privacy. This may be a cause of anxiety and a contributing factor in the perception of, and reaction to, pain.

It is therefore important to recognise the many factors that influence pain reactions and to appreciate that each pain experience is unique and personal. Anyone caring for a client experiencing pain should not judge the appropriateness of that person's reaction to pain, and must be sensitive to individual needs.

Although behavioural reactions to pain are individual, the physiological manifestations that occur with an acute episode of pain can be observed in all people. When acute pain occurs the autonomic response is activated, so that:

- Heart rate increases
- Blood pressure rises
- Breathing often becomes rapid and shallow
- Muscles tense
- Blood flow to the hands and feet is constricted, and they become cold
- The skin becomes pale and sweaty
- Nausea and vomiting may occur.

These physiological changes are often less observable in a person with chronic pain. Over time the changes are unable to be sustained, and the individual with chronic pain may exhibit a general appearance of not being in pain. To these clients, their pain is present and it is real.

ASSESSING PAIN

In addition to observing a client for the physiological and behavioural manifestations of pain, the nurse should ask questions that enable the client to describe the pain in their own words. A nurse should never ignore a client's statement that they are in pain, and should remember that 'pain is what the person says it is'. A client can usually sense if the nurse does not believe that they are experiencing pain, and this can increase a sense of helplessness. As a consequence, the client may compensate by under-reporting pain or by anxiously over-reporting. Either reaction aggravates the circle of mistrust–anxiety–more pain. When assessing a client's pain, the nurse should make certain of obtaining sufficient and appropriate information by observation and questioning.

Location

A client may be able to locate a painful area specifically, by describing it or by pointing to the body area involved, such as the tip of the thumb on the left hand, or they may describe the painful area more generally, for example, all over the abdomen. Pain that radiates from its point of origin should also be noted.

Time of occurrence

Information should be obtained regarding the onset of pain; for example, whether it was sudden or gradual. The client should also be asked if the pain increases or decreases at specific times of the day or night; that is, if there is rhythmic variation or pattern in the pain. For example, a client who has arthritis aggravated by inactivity may experience severe joint pain on waking, but the pain may become less severe throughout the day.

Duration

It is important to establish how long the pain lasts; for example, whether it is continuous or intermittent.

Precipitating factors

Certain physical activities or psychological factors may precipitate pain. For example, chest pain may occur after physical exercise, or abdominal pain may occur after eating. A change of posture may aggravate or relieve pain, and factors such as anxiety or fear may also precipitate pain. It is important to establish factors that aggravate the pain as well as those that modify or bring about pain relief.

Impact on activities

Assessment should include whether or not the pain interferes with lifestyle or the performing of any activities of daily living; for example, does it affect the ability to eat, move freely or sleep? Are roles and relationships being affected in a significant way by the pain that is being experienced?

Character, or type

This is the way the pain is described by the person who is experiencing it, and it is important for the nurse to report and record the client's own words. Some of the terms that may be used to describe the type and quality of pain are gripping, knife-like, burning, prickling, tingling, dull, aching, cramping, gnawing, constricting, throbbing, vice-like, crushing, stabbing and shooting.

Intensity

The severity of pain is not always evident from a person's reaction, especially with a chronic pain problem, and must therefore be assessed as the client's own perception. Several measurement tools, or pain scales (Figure 35.3), have been designed to assist a client to describe the intensity of pain. Health care institutions may devise their own measurement tool, or may use a standard tool. One method of assessment is a linear scale from 1–10, on which the

A

Numerical

1	2	3	4	5	6	7	8	9	10

No pain — Severe pain

B

Description

No pain	Mild pain	Moderate pain	Severe pain	Unbearable pain

C

Visual analogue

No pain — Unbearable pain

Figure 35.3 | Scales for measuring pain intensity in adults. The individual identifies a point on the scale that corresponds to their perception of the severity of the pain

client indicates the intensity of their pain, with 0–1 being no pain at all, and 10 representing severe and intense pain. A similar scale using 'smiley faces' may be used for children (Figure 35.4).

This type of measurement device facilitates both assessment and management of pain in many cases. However, the use of pain-scale assessment tools makes the assumptions that the client has a past experience of pain, that they can understand the scale and verbalise, and that they are not cognitively impaired. With elderly clients, issues such as poor memory, depression and sensory impairment may also make pain assessment difficult. The Abbey Pain Scale (Figure 35.5) is a measurement of pain in people with dementia who cannot verbalise.

Associated signs or symptoms

The painful area, as described by the client, should be observed for signs of distension or oedema, discolouration (such as bruising or inflammation), change in skin temperature, and any loss of function or mobility. The nurse should also ascertain whether there are any accompanying signs, such as nausea with abdominal pain, cyanosis with chest pain, or skin pallor and sweating.

Posture and facial expression

The client's posture and facial expression may indicate that pain is being experienced. A certain position may be assumed to minimise the pain; for example, a client may lie on their side with the knees drawn to relieve abdominal pain. Severe pain may cause a client to lie rigidly, as any movement may increase the pain. It is important to consider that an older child or adult client's facial expression is not always a reliable guide to the presence or severity of pain, as facial expressions are varied and may be misleading. A client experiencing acute pain may grimace and look anxious, whereas a client with chronic pain may show few signs of distress, and suffering may be masked by a brave or exhausted facial expression. Pain assessment in the elderly, especially with impaired cognition, may rely heavily on the observation of behavioural changes, such as increased confusion or agitation, tenseness, fidgeting or even withdrawal or aggression.

Vital signs

The client's temperature, pulse, respirations and blood pressure should be measured when pain is first experienced. The results should be documented, and repeated measurements made to detect any alterations. Any abnormal result or significant variation should be reported immediately.

Signs of emotional tension

The client should be observed for signs of increased emotional tension, such as irritability, anxiety, depression, aggression, exhaustion or sleeplessness. When a client experiences pain or a change in the nature of pain already present, the nurse should monitor and assess by questions and by making the observations as described. This assessment is then documented and reported appropriately. Clinical

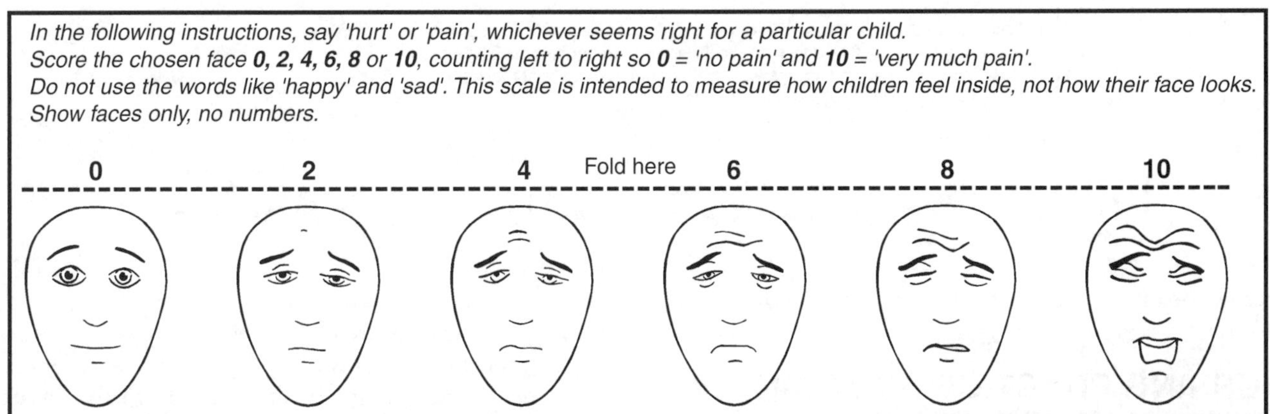

Figure 35.4 | Faces Pain Scale — Revised *(Hicks, von Baeyer, Spafford, van Korlaar, Goodenough: Pain (2001); 93(2): 173-83. Used with permission from IASP®. See www.painsourcebook.ca for instructions on use of the scale)*

Place identification label here

Name: ....
DOB: ....
Room No: ....

ABBEY PAIN SCALE

For measurement of pain in people with dementia who cannot verbalise

How to use scale: While observing the resident, score questions 1 to 6.

Name of person completing the scale:...
Date: .... Time: .... Designation:...................................
Latest pain relief given was .... at .... hrs.

Q1 Vocalisation **Q1** ☐
(e.g. whimpering, groaning, crying)

Absent 0 Mild 1 Moderate 2 Severe 3

Q2 Facial expression **Q2** ☐
(e.g. looking tense, frowning, grimacing, looking frightened)

Absent 0 Mild 1 Moderate 2 Severe 3

Q3 Change in body language **Q3** ☐
(e.g. fidgeting, rocking, guarding part of body, withdrawn)

Absent 0 Mild 1 Moderate 2 Severe 3

Q4 Behavioural change **Q4** ☐
(e.g. increased confusion, refusing to eat, alteration in usual patterns)

Absent 0 Mild 1 Moderate 2 Severe 3

Q5 Physiological change **Q5** ☐
(e.g. temperature, pulse or blood pressure outside normal limits, perspiring, flushing or pallor)

Absent 0 Mild 1 Moderate 2 Severe 3

Q6 Physical changes **Q6** ☐
(e.g. skin tears, pressure areas, arthritis, contractures, previous injuries)

Absent 0 Mild 1 Moderate 2 Severe 3

Add scores for 1–6 and record here **Total Pain Score** ☐

Now tick the box that matches the Total Pain Score

0–2 No pain	3–7 Mild	8–13 Moderate	14+ Severe

Finally tick the box which matches the type of pain

Chronic	Acute	Acute on Chronic

Abbey, J; Do Bellis, A; Piller, N; Esterman, A; Giles, I; Parker, D and Lowcay, B.
Funded by the JH & JD Gunn M Medical Research Foundation 1998–2002
(This document may be reproduced with this acknowledgement retained)
Taken from: www.health.gov.au/acc/reports/download/

Figure 35.5 | The Abbey Pain Scale *(Abbey J, Do Bellis A, Piller N, Esterman A, Giles I, Parker D, Lowcay B. Funded by the JH & JD Gunn Medical Research Foundation 1998–2002. [This document may be reproduced with this acknowledgement retained.] Taken from: www.health.gov.au/acc/reports/download/)*

Interest Box 35.4 outlines some behavioural indicators of the effects of pain.

NURSING PRACTICE AND PAIN AVOIDANCE NEEDS

The nurse is in a position to make a major contribution to the prevention and alleviation of a client's pain. As described previously, pain is a subjective experience, and not easy to measure objectively. Therefore the nurse has an important responsibility to observe the client for visible evidence of pain, listen carefully to the client's description of pain, and implement measures that prevent pain.

It is important for the nurse to remember that pain

CLINICAL INTEREST BOX 35.4
Behavioural indicators of effects of pain

Vocalisations
- Moaning
- Crying
- Screaming
- Gasping
- Grunting

Facial expressions
- Grimace
- Clenched teeth
- Wrinkled forehead
- Tightly closed or widely opened eyes or mouth
- Lip biting
- Tightened jaw

Body movement
- Restlessness
- Immobilisation
- Muscle tension
- Increased hand and finger movements
- Pacing activities
- Protective movement of body parts

Social interaction
- Avoidance of conversation and of social contacts
- Focus only on activities for pain relief
- Reduced attention span

(Heath 1995)

is not a single entity but is rather the consequence of a conflict between the stimulus and the whole individual. The nurse has a responsibility to the client, firstly not to cause or allow the experience of unnecessary pain; and secondly, if pain is experienced, to do all that is possible to relieve the pain and suffering. The nurse also has a responsibility to monitor and report the client's response to, and the efficacy of, any prescribed pain management.

From a medical point of view, the management of pain includes treating the underlying disease to remove or diminish the cause; treating any other symptoms such as nausea or constipation that may increase the perception of pain; and using non-pharmacological and pharmacological therapy. Specific nursing interventions as described later in this chapter, include minimising the stimulus that is causing or contributing to the pain, alleviating pain with supportive nursing intervention, and assisting the client to cope with pain. It must be considered that even the simple provision of information and explanation may have a powerful effect in assisting people to feel in control of their pain-management situation.

NON-PHARMACOLOGICAL THERAPY

Pain management and control may be achieved by a variety of supportive measures other than medication. Non-drug approaches to pain management may include the use of heat or cold, massage and psychological methods.

Application of heat or cold

Heat applied to the skin causes dilation of the local blood vessels and, as a result, may improve the blood supply to an area, relax muscles and relieve spasm, promote healing and relieve pain. Cold applications may also be used to relieve swelling and pain. Cold has a numbing effect that helps to reduce pain in a body part.

Massage

Massage involves the manipulation of soft tissue and can increase circulation, reduce muscle tension, relax the individual and relieve pain. Cutaneous stimulation often acts to alter the client's conscious awareness of pain. Aromatherapy and massage using essential oils may also be of benefit in some situations. Soothing touch and gentle rocking motion to promote contact, warmth and closeness may help to relax an infant in pain.

Psychological methods

Various techniques may be used to promote general relaxation of the client, and therefore reduce anxiety and relieve pain. Music and art may be used as a sensory distraction or as a soothing method of reducing stress. Other methods of distraction may be helpful to lessen the individual's awareness of painful stimuli, such as encouragement of concentration on slow, deep, rhythmic breathing exercises, or even guided imagery, singing, praying or tapping. Several other methods of non-pharmacological pain management may be prescribed or undertaken. While it is not the role of the nurse to implement these, they may form part of the overall treatment plan, so an awareness of them is required.

Acupuncture

This technique, which is a form of traditional Chinese medicine, involves the insertion of fine needles into the skin at selected points on the body. Acupuncture may be used to manage both acute and chronic pain, and there are several theories about how it relieves pain. Some authorities believe that acupuncture achieves analgesia by stimulating the release of endorphins, while others believe that it stimulates the large diameter nerve fibres that effectively close the gate and block pain impulses (gate-control mechanism).

Transcutaneous electrical nerve stimulation (TENS)

A specific technique of peripheral nerve stimulation, TENS involves the application of electrodes to trigger points on the skin (Figure 35.6). The electrodes are activated by a battery-powered device to produce a tingling or vibrating sensation in the painful area. The impulses block the transmission of pain impulses to the brain. TENS may be indicated for many people, especially those with joint or bone pain. It is normally well tolerated, although skin irritation is sometimes experienced. It should not be used

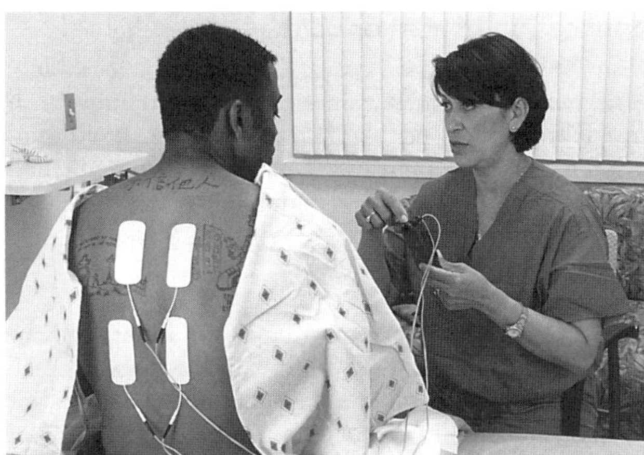

Figure 35.6 | A transcutaneous electrical nerve stimulation (TENS) device *(Lewis et al 2008: 144)*

for patients with cardiac pacemakers, as it can interfere with pacemaker function.

Hypnosis

Hypnotic analgesia may be achieved when a person enters a state of self-induced relaxation and concentration. During hypnosis, cognitive thinking is bypassed, allowing the individual to become more susceptible to suggestion. The individual enters a passive trance-like state, which is induced by a trained hypnotist, who may use the repetition of words and gestures. Susceptibility to hypnosis varies from person to person.

Biofeedback

Biofeedback is a method that assists a person to become aware of, and subsequently to control, certain autonomic physiological responses, such as blood pressure, muscle tension and heart rate. Through concentration, and with the aid of instruments, the individual can learn to control and modify these processes, which are normally involuntary. The technique of biofeedback is more effective when accompanied by other relaxation techniques.

Placebo therapy

Placebo therapy involves the administration of inactive substances (such as lactose pills or sterile water), and may be effective for certain people in certain situations. It is thought that placebos relieve pain or other symptoms by causing the body to release endorphins, combined with an expectation that the treatment will be effective. The use of placebos involves a degree of recipient deception and poses many ethical and moral problems. Its use in mainstream pain management should generally be limited.

Pain clinics

People who experience chronic pain may be helped by attending a multidisciplinary pain clinic. Pain clinics commonly attempt to reduce use of pain medication, help clients resume normal activities and restore a positive self-image. Management includes a thorough physical and psychological examination before a program is designed for the individual. Approaches to pain management in a pain clinic include psychological counselling, acupuncture, TENS or any of the other methods of pain relief. The individual is taught alternative ways of carrying out the activities of daily living so that associated pain is minimised.

PHARMACOLOGICAL THERAPY

Medications prescribed by a medical officer to relieve pain may be either local or systemic, analgesic or co-analgesic. The nurse's role in relation to medication administration involves assessment and monitoring of individual client responses to therapeutic treatments ordered. When medications have been prescribed, it may be within the nurse's scope of practice to administer them.

Nerve block

Peripheral nerve transmission of pain can be interrupted temporarily by the injection of a local anaesthetic, or permanently by injecting a sclerosing agent into the nerve root area. As the latter method can result in destruction of tissue adjacent to the injected area, other pain-relieving methods are usually preferred, with this being an option in cases when other pain-relieving methods have been unsuccessful.

Counter-irritants

Counter-irritants, such as mentholated ointments and heat rubs, applied locally to the skin, can produce an inflammatory response, thereby relieving congestion in underlying tissues and reducing pain from the original source.

Radiotherapy and/or chemotherapy

The pain associated with malignant disease may be relieved by radiation, which shrinks a tumour that is actively causing compression in an area. Chemotherapy (also considered as pharmacological therapy) may sometimes control pain if the tumour is sensitive to the medications used.

Analgesic

Analgesic or pain-relieving medications may be mild, for example, non-narcotics such as acetylsalicylic acid (aspirin) or paracetamol, or strong, for example, narcotics such as morphine or pethidine. Analgesics may be administered via a number of routes, including orally, by injection or infusion (intramuscularly, subcutaneously, intravenously or into the epidural space), or in some instances they may be applied topically (via creams or patches onto the skin). The type, dosage and route of analgesic medications given will be prescribed by the medical officer according to the client's needs. Good pain control, especially in post-operative and chronic pain situations, is achieved by administering appropriate amounts of the most effective medication at regular intervals, thus avoiding the experience of peaks and troughs of pain. In some cases analgesia is ordered on a 'prn' (as required) basis, which may be appropriate for intermittent episodes of pain. Clinical Interest Box 35.5 provides a caution related to pain and the older adult.

Analgesics are frequently given intravenously for severe pain, either as a bolus dose (a concentrated dose given in a short period of time) or, preferably, as an infusion, which has the advantage of avoiding repeated injections and establishes a constant blood level of analgesic drug, thus avoiding considerable pain between doses.

Patient-controlled analgesia (PCA) is another method using intravenous opioids and a programmable pump. A dose of drug is delivered each time the client pushes a button, within limitations set by the physician. This allows the client to choose how often and when to receive the medication, and often enables them to establish a greater sense of control over pain management.

Epidural analgesia is an alternative method of pain control that uses a fine catheter inserted into the epidural space of the spine, again connected to a programmable pump. This method of pain relief is effective in controlling pain while allowing the client to remain alert. It is frequently used in obstetrics, postoperative clients and sometimes in clients with cancer. The primary responsibilities for caring for clients with either narcotic or epidural infusions lie with the Registered Nurse (RN). However, response to medications and evaluation of pain control measures are within the scope of practice of all nurses. Clinical Interest Box 35.6 outlines nursing measures for a client with an epidural infusion.

CLINICAL INTEREST BOX 35.5
Pain and the older adult

Because of the normal changes of ageing, the older adult may respond differently to analgesics than a younger client. The older adult should be monitored closely for side effects and toxicity.
(deWit 2005)

Co-analgesic medications, while not true analgesics in the pharmacological sense, act to augment pain relief, either alone or in combination with analgesics. Examples of medications that may be used as co-analgesics are corticosteroids and non-steroidal anti-inflammatory drugs, both of which may act to decrease inflammation and oedema. The use of anti-anxiety drugs or drugs producing muscle relaxation may also be incorporated into a treatment plan. Sometimes a dose of co-analgesic medication together with an analgesic can produce greater pain relief than a higher dose of an analgesic alone.

NURSING CARE OF A CLIENT EXPERIENCING PAIN

The nurse has a responsibility to try to eliminate or minimise the stimulus that is causing pain. The nurse also observes the client who is experiencing pain, reports and documents their observations and implements nursing measures to alleviate pain. Continued assessment and monitoring of the client is necessary to evaluate the effectiveness of any prescribed therapy. Particular attention must be paid to clients who cannot clearly articulate their needs or feelings, such as infants and small children and those with cognitive or communicative impairment. Pain management, both of non-pharmacological and pharmacological nature, must still be addressed in these situations, and responses evaluated. The nurse also plays an important role in supporting the client's significant others, who are usually distressed by the pain experience of their loved one,

CLINICAL INTEREST BOX 35.6
Nursing care for clients with epidural infusions

Goal	Actions
Prevent catheter displacement	Secure catheter (if not connected to implanted reservoir) carefully to outside skin.
Maintain catheter function	Check external dressing around catheter site for dampness or discharge. (Leak of cerebrospinal fluid may develop.)
	Use transparent dressing to secure catheter and to aid inspection.
	Inspect catheter for breaks.
Prevent infection	Use strict aseptic technique when caring for catheter (see Chapter 34).
	Do not routinely change dressing over site.
	Change infusion tubing every 24 hours.
Monitor for respiratory depression	Monitor vital signs, especially respirations, per policy.
	Use pulse oximetry and apnoea monitoring.
Prevent undesirable complications	Assess for pruritus (itching) and nausea and vomiting.
	Administer antiemetics as ordered.
Maintain urinary and bowel function	Monitor intake and output.
	Assess for bladder and bowel distention.
	Assess for discomfort, frequency and urgency.

(Potter & Perry 2008)

particularly when the pain is chronic or is a result of terminal illness.

The importance of clear and effective communication between the nurse and the client and significant others cannot be over emphasised. A positive relationship facilitates effective communication, which can affect the client's response to pain and pain relief. The client should be encouraged to express feelings openly, in an atmosphere of trust. The nurse should learn to listen actively to the client, so that not only the verbal interactions are heard but any nonverbal cues are also detected and acted on. For example, clients may deny pain or state that they are not experiencing much pain, but the body language and tone of voice may indicate otherwise. To promote peace of mind and to reduce anxiety, clients should be provided with information about their illness, including expected pain and its management. Clients should be aware that they have a right to pain relief and that varied pain-relieving measures are available. It is important to prevent or reduce the cycle of pain–stress–anxiety–pain. A variety of nursing measures, some very simple, may help to minimise or alleviate pain.

Changing position

At times pain can result from, or be increased by, an uncomfortable posture. The client should be assisted into a more comfortable position, with appropriate pillows arranged for support. The addition of a sheepskin underneath the back and buttocks may enhance comfort, and the bedclothes should be arranged to meet individual needs. It is important to ensure that the client's body is in alignment, and the placement of a pillow under a painful limb may further enhance comfort. Correct positioning should ensure that there is no undue stress on incisions, and no tension applied to any tubing present (surgical drain tube or urinary catheter).

Meeting general comfort needs

The nurse should ensure that all basic comfort needs are provided for; for example, discomfort and pain can result from a distended bladder. The client may feel more comfortable if the face and hands are washed, hair brushed and teeth cleaned. If not contraindicated, a drink of the client's choice should be offered. A warm drink in the evening may help to promote settling and sleep. Comfort needs for an infant in pain may include containment (swaddling) to increase feelings of security, and the pacifying effect of non-nutritive sucking.

Gentle handling

When the client is being assisted to move, the nurse should ensure that any movements are made gently. Pain is usually increased on movement, so clients should be permitted and assisted to move at their own pace. As the client moves, the nurse should ensure that painful areas are supported. An incision can be supported during movement; the client or the nurse may place a hand over the incision to 'splint' it, or hugging a pillow may provide support on movement.

Promoting rest and sleep

Pain is very tiring, and fatigue increases reactions to pain; therefore the nurse should ensure that the client receives adequate and effective rest and sleep. Measures should be implemented during the day, as well as during the night, to facilitate rest; for example, the blinds may be drawn, and all care planned so that repeated interruptions and visits to the client are avoided. Relaxation reduces anxiety, can enhance the effect of pain relief and facilitates sleep. The client can be taught and encouraged to practise one of several relaxation techniques, as described earlier. If appropriate, and with client consent, gentle massaging of the neck and back may relieve tension and facilitate relaxation.

Checking dressings and splints

Any dressing, bandage or splint should be checked at regular intervals and, within medical orders, changed or adjusted if necessary. A poorly positioned dressing can irritate a wound, a bandage may be too tight, or an inappropriately applied or positioned splint may cause pressure and pain.

Adapting the environment

The nurse should consider the client's immediate surroundings and adapt them according to individual needs. While some clients experiencing pain may prefer to rest in a darkened room, others may prefer that their room is bright and cheerful. A client may choose to attempt to distract themself from their pain by watching television or listening to music, or may prefer to lie quietly. The presence of fresh flowers in the room may be a source of pleasure or irritation, and some clients may find it comforting if there are appropriate paintings on the wall. The nurse should ensure adequate privacy and appropriate ventilation and heating, while adapting the environment to meet individual needs.

Implementing prescribed therapy

The nurse may be responsible for being with the client during therapy, or may be involved in its implementation. Whenever therapy is prescribed, the nurse should implement measures to promote the client's comfort and safety. The nurse should also monitor the client to assess the efficacy of prescribed therapy, and report and document all observations. Clinical Interest Box 35.7 lists the possible nursing diagnoses when caring for a client with pain.

SUMMARY

Pain, which is often a protective signal of actual or impending tissue damage, is both an unpleasant physical sensation and an emotional experience. Each episode of pain is unique and subjective and it is important for the nurse to appreciate that 'pain is what the patient says it is'. Pain may be mild or severe, acute or chronic, physical or psychological.

CLINICAL INTEREST BOX 35.7
Nursing diagnoses relating to pain

- Anxiety
- Hopelessness
- Mobility, impaired physical
- Pain
- Pain, chronic
- Self-care deficit
- Sexual dysfunction
- Sleep pattern disturbance

Pain receptors transmit impulses along nerve fibres to the brain, where the impulses are perceived and interpreted. The body has some internal mechanisms that may be activated to help control pain and its perception, such as the gate-control mechanism and the endorphin system.

The perception of pain varies with the individual, therefore some people will experience pain much sooner and more intensely than others. Many factors influence an individual's reaction to pain, including age, gender, culture, emotional state, history of pain, self-image, the time of day and the environment. Although each individual's behavioural reaction to pain is different, the physiological responses to acute pain are the same.

The nurse has a responsibility to assess a client's pain in terms of site, time it occurs, duration, precipitating factors, type, intensity, associated signs and symptoms, body posture, vital signs and emotional manifestations.

The management of pain includes non-pharmacological and pharmacological therapy, and depends on each client's individual needs. The nurse has a responsibility to eliminate or reduce painful stimuli and to plan and implement supportive nursing measures to help alleviate pain or to assist the client to manage their pain.

REVIEW EXERCISES

1. What are the physiological processes whereby pain sensations are received, transmitted and interpreted?
2. What are the factors influencing an individual's perception of, and reaction to, pain?
3. State the pain assessment methods, including the differences required in approach, with a person suffering chronic pain.
4. Describe various methods of pain management, including both non-pharmacological and pharmacological approaches.

CRITICAL THINKING EXERCISES

1. Mrs Jones is 65 and, up until admission to hospital, has lived alone. She has had rheumatoid arthritis for the past 25 years, resulting in severely deformed hands. She is unable to walk without assistance and is no longer managing at home, despite full community services. Chronic pain is a major issue for her — she states that 'the pain is there most of the time but gets worse when I move suddenly'. What is the nursing role in assessment and planning of care in relation to the management of Mrs Jones' pain?
2. It has been observed that pain in certain groups, especially children and the elderly, is not always well managed, and that these groups may be among the most under-treated for pain. Why do you think that this may occur? What can the nurse do to improve this situation?

REFERENCES AND FURTHER READING

Bryant B, Knights K, Salerno E (2003) *Pharmacology for Health Professionals*. Elsevier Australia, Sydney

Clayton BD, Stock YN, Harroun RD (2007) *Basic Pharmacology for Nurses*. Mosby Elsevier, St Louis

Crisp J, Taylor C (eds) (2005) *Potter and Perry's Fundamentals of Nursing*, 2nd edn. Elsevier Australia, Sydney

deWit S (2005) *Fundamental Concepts and Skills for Nursing*, 2nd edn. WB Saunders, Philadelphia

Heath HBM (1995) *Potter and Perry's Foundations in Nursing Theory and Practice*. Mosby, London.

Helmrich S, Yates P, Nash R et al (2001) Factors influencing nurse's decisions to use non-pharmacological therapies to manage patient's pain. *Australian Journal of Advanced Nursing*, 19(1): 29–35

Hicks, von Baeyer, Spafford, van Korlaar, Goodenough. The Face Pain Scale — revised: toward a common metric in pediatric pain measurement. *Pain* (2001); 93(2): 173–83. See www.painsourcebook.ca

Karch M (2008) *Focus on Nursing Pharmacology*. Lippincott Williams & Wilkins, Philadelphia

Kozier B, Erb G, Berman AJ, Burke K (2000) *Fundamentals of Nursing: Concepts, Process and Practice*, 6th edn. Prentice-Hall Inc, Upper Saddle River, NJ

Lewis S, Heitkemper M, Dirksen S (2008) *Medical–Surgical Nursing*, 7th edn. Mosby, St Louis

Marieb E (2006) *Human Anatomy and Physiology*, 6th edn. Benjamin Cummings, San Francisco

Max EE (2007) *Complimentary Therapies for Pain Management: an Evidenced Based Approach*. Elsevier/Mosby, Boston, MA

McCaffery M, Pasero C (1999) *Pain Clinical Manual*, 2nd edn. St Louis, Mosby

McClean W, Higginbotham N (2002) Prevalence of pain among nursing home residents in rural NSW. *Medical Journal of Australia*, 177(1): 17–20

Melzack R, Wall P (1965) Pain mechanisms: a new theory. *Science Journal (ISC)*, 171–9

Potter PA, Perry AG (2008) *Fundamentals of Nursing*, 7th edn. Mosby, St Louis

Waldman SD (2007) *Pain management*. Saunders, Philadelphia

ONLINE RESOURCES

Pain assessment tools: www.health.gov.au/acc/reports/download/assesstls3b.pdf

Chapter 36

MOVEMENT AND EXERCISE

OBJECTIVES

- Define the key terms/concepts
- Describe and implement the principles of good posture and body mechanics
- Describe the role of the musculoskeletal system in the regulation of movement
- Describe how joints are involved in movement
- State differences between isotonic, isometric and isokinetic exercise
- Describe and define range of movement (ROM)
- Identify and demonstrate joint movements involved in ROM exercises
- Define obesity and describe how variables such as family values and diet influence adult obesity
- Describe how older adults may benefit from exercise
- Identify and describe the complications associated with immobility, and implement appropriate preventive measures
- State the influences and effects associated with disorders of the musculoskeletal system
- Describe the major manifestations of musculoskeletal system disorders
- Briefly describe the specific disorders of the musculoskeletal system outlined in this chapter
- State the diagnostic tests that may be used to assess musculoskeletal function
- Assess clients for impaired mobility and activity intolerance
- Assist in planning and implementing nursing care for a client with a musculoskeletal disorder
- According to specified role and function, perform the nursing activities described in this chapter, safely and accurately

KEY TERMS/CONCEPTS

active and passive exercise
arthrography
benign tumours
body mechanics
contractures and ankylosis
dangling, gait and crutch walking
deep vein thrombosis (DVT)
diplopia and ptosis
haematopoiesis
hypostatic pneumonia
isotonic/isometric/isokinetic exercises
metastatic bone tumours
muscle atrophy
obesity and overweight
orthostatic hypotension
osteoclasts and osteoblasts
osteogenic sarcoma
osteomyelitis
plantar flexion (footdrop)
PRICE: prevention, rest, ice, compression and elevation
pursed-lip breathing
range of movement (ROM)
rheumatoid factor
tendinitis
wellbeing

CHAPTER FOCUS

Regular exercise is one of the keys to wellbeing and can add quality years to one's life, as well as prevent disease. Encouraging regular activity is both a challenge and an opportunity for nurses who are in a unique position to support clients making lifestyle changes that improve health. Even limited amounts of movement and exercise have the potential to prevent many complications of immobilisation. By focusing on the remaining abilities of a person, however small, nurses can often prevent problems.

The human body is ideally suited to movement, and regular exercise promotes health, feelings of wellbeing and prevents illness throughout the lifespan. Exercise is made possible by the musculoskeletal, nervous and cardiovascular systems that work together to make movement possible. Information on the function of the cardiovascular and nervous systems is provided in Chapters 38 and 41.

Sustained regular exercise stimulates the body and mind and there are numerous benefits such as maintenance of cardiopulmonary efficiency, increased muscle tone and strength, joint mobility, sound sleep as well as a decrease in boredom and stress. Regular exercise can affect blood cholesterol levels by increasing high-density lipoproteins (the 'good' cholesterol). Goldberg and Elliot (2000) suggest that the risk of developing diabetes decreases in those who are active, regardless of body weight, which is thought to be a factor in the development of this disease. Current information suggests that obesity and being overweight can cause serious health problems, but moderate regular exercise can control weight.

Stress and illness deplete the body of energy. Even though carrying out any type of exercise is often the last thing people want to do, regular exercise is energising and can allow a person to better cope with life's daily stresses. Strenuous exercise, however, can result in injury and fatigue and should be undertaken with caution and under medical supervision. People of all ages gain real health benefits from activities such as walking, which is easy to do every day and need not be strenuous or difficult, just regular; for example, walking three to four times per week briskly would be sufficient. Even if a person does not end up very lean, exercise is beneficial and many of the health problems once thought to be a part of ageing can be prevented with regular exercise.

LIVED EXPERIENCE

I am in my late 40s now, but 20 years ago I wanted to enhance my appearance, lose weight as well as gain fitness. So I decided to take up walking, and I soon discovered that there were many benefits and, as well as improving my appearance, I gained muscle tone, felt stronger and had higher energy levels. I also found I was sleeping better and woke up ready for the day and better able to deal with the daily stresses at work or home. Now I really think that exercise will always be an essential part of my life and I can't imagine not exercising and hope to be active well into my 80s!

Angela, age 48

THE MUSCULOSKELETAL SYSTEM

The musculoskeletal system is composed of many structures that work together to produce movement and provide support and protection for organs. About 600 voluntary or skeletal muscles form the flesh of the body. Skeletal muscle is attached to bone and classified by the kind of movement it makes; for example, flexors allow joints to bend or flex, while abductors allow shortening so that joints are straightened or abducted (moved away from the body). Muscle tissue is capable of contraction and relaxation, after stimulation by a motor nerve. Muscle develops under several influences such as exercise, nutrition, gender and genetic predisposition, which accounts for variations in muscle size and strength between individuals. When muscle contracts it pulls on a bone or bones and produces movement at a joint, where two bones meet. As joints are weak points in the skeleton, synovial fluid, cartilage, ligaments and tendons add protection. See Clinical Interest Box 36.1 for facts on muscle coordination.

The skeleton (Figure 36.1) gives the body shape, protection, stores minerals, forms blood cells (haematopoiesis) and allows movement. Normally there are over 200 separate bones and supportive ligaments, as well as fibrous bands of tissue called tendons, which connect muscle to bone. The human skeleton is separated into the axial and appendicular skeleton. Axial skeleton bones form the head and trunk, all others belong to the appendicular skeleton, or bones of the extremities.

Bone is composed of different tissue and classified by location and shape, such as long, short, flat, irregular or sesamoid, such as the patella, or kneecap. Long bones in the arm and leg differ from short bones in the wrist and ankle, and flat bones that form the shoulder blade are different again from irregular shaped bones such as the

CLINICAL INTEREST BOX 36.1
Muscle coordination and facial expressions

The muscular system plays a vital role in maintaining correct body posture by means of good muscle tone and coordinated activity. Most skeletal muscles work in pairs or groups, with one pair or group antagonising the action of another pair or group to achieve controlled movement. For example, during elbow flexion, the triceps muscle relaxes to allow the forearm to be pulled up when the biceps muscle contracts. Extension of the arm is made possible by the relaxation of the biceps, as the triceps contracts and pulls on the arm. The erect position of the trunk is maintained as a result of coordination of groups of muscles.

A good example of muscle coordination is our facial expressions, which come about as a result of many tiny complex facial muscles working together to allow an incredible range of expressions. However, unlike other muscles, they are actually attached to the skin, so that people can change expression with a slight muscle movement. For instance when you smile your upper lip muscle (levator labii superioris) lifts your top lip, at the same time your cheek and jaw muscles pull the mouth up and out so that you look happy. However, when you frown, the forehead muscle furrows the brow, eye-socket muscles narrow the eyes, while the lower lip muscle (depressor labii inferioris) pulls the lower lip down and you appear angry or upset.

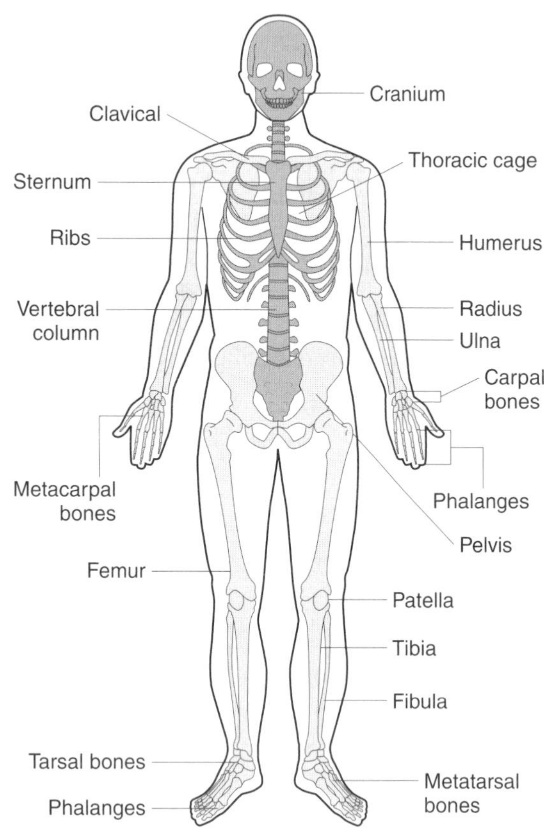

Figure 36.1 | The skeleton, anterior view
The axial skeleton appears a darker grey than the appendicular skeleton *(Wilson & Waugh 1996)*

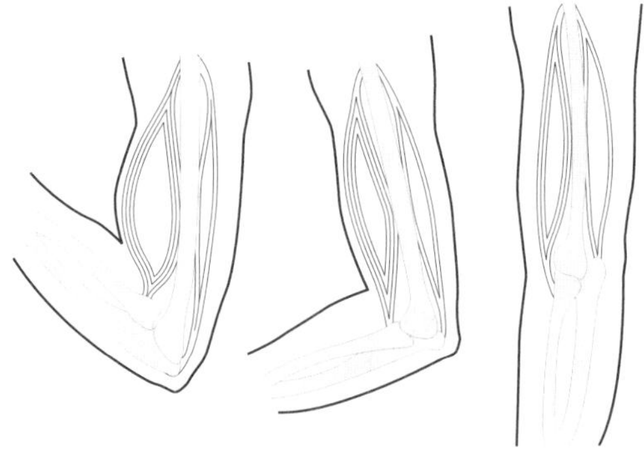

Figure 36.2 | Arm muscles showing contraction and relaxation

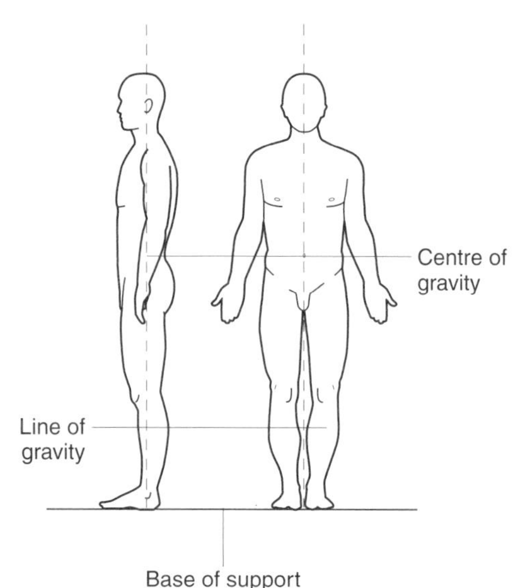

Figure 36.3 | Body mechanics: correct standing posture

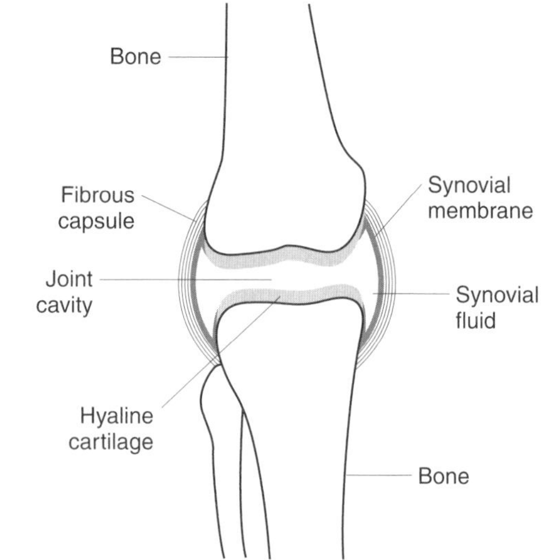

Figure 36.4 | Synovial or freely movable joint

jaw and vertebrae. Bone begins as cartilage that eventually hardens to form bone. Bone remodelling (the creation and destruction of bone) is a lifelong process and performed by bone-forming cells called osteoblasts, and bone-absorbing cells called osteoclasts. Normal bone growth depends on a healthy diet, as well as other hormonal factors (e.g. oestrogen affects bone formation) and physical factors. Despite the rigidity of the skeleton, humans are capable of moving and bending in almost any direction and this flexibility is largely due to the skeleton's many movable joints (Figure 36.2).

BODY POSTURE AND MECHANICS

Fatigue, muscle strain and injury can result from improper use or positioning of the body during activity or rest. Good posture is achieved when all parts of the body are in correct body alignment, and is important when sitting, lying, standing or moving. Normal spinal curves should be maintained and the joints should be supported in their normal positions. Good posture (Figure 36.3) and alignment reduces strain on all muscles and joints (Figure 36.4) and enables internal organs to function without interference; for example, full lung expansion is facilitated. Body mechanics is the term used to describe the physical coordination of all parts of the body to promote correct posture and balanced effective movement. The practice of correct body mechanics results in less fatigue and reduces the risk of muscle and joint injury.

ATTITUDES, VALUES AND FEARS TOWARDS EXERCISE

Children learn the value of regular exercise if they are brought up in an environment in which exercise is seen in a positive way and both parents and children discover ways to incorporate exercise into their daily routine. Later on, these children are more likely to continue to exercise into their old age. On the other hand, sedentary parents may send the message to their children that exercise is too much trouble and not worth the effort. Thus early familial attitudes towards exercise can form lifetime patterns of behaviour. Personal values about one's appearance (e.g. it is better to be slim or build up muscle to produce a 'good' body) can motivate both young and older adults to exercise regularly. Nurses need to dispel fears and anxiety about exercise and activity that many people may have because of chronic conditions or lack of information about the benefits of exercise, and respond appropriately to clients' questions. (See Clinical Interest Boxes 36.2 and 36.3.)

THE OLDER ADULT AND EXERCISE

According to the National Health and Medical Research Council (NHMRC) in Australia, up to half of the functional decline associated with ageing is the result of disuse and can be reversed by exercise. Exercise improves cardiopulmonary fitness, ability to stretch and balance and endurance. Benefits of regular exercise are particularly important for older adults, as being fit makes it easier to perform daily activities and improves recovery after illness as well as minimising the risk of future ill-health. Light exercise is beneficial and, as long as individuals ease into exercise, especially if they have led sedentary lives, there is nothing to stop older adults from starting a regular exercise program. However, it is wise that they consult with their medical officer first. (See Clinical Interest Box 36.4.)

OVERWEIGHT AND OBESITY

In Australia in 2001, 30% of adult males and 36% of adult females aged 45–74 considered themselves to be overweight. The prevalence of obesity (those with a body mass index [BMI] greater than 30) in Australians has risen from one in 14 in 1980, to one in seven in 1989, and one in five by 1995. Based on current trends, by 2025 it could be one in three. It is known that being severely overweight puts a load on the heart and increases the risk of high blood pressure and diabetes, but what was not known until fairly recently is just how many years of life are lost if a person is obese. In the late 1990s American researchers asked that simple question of tens of thousands of Americans and the results were compelling, with reports of females with BMIs over 30 (especially if about 20 years old) losing 5–8 years, and obese men up to 12 years. These data are easily transferable to Australia. (See Chapter 31 for further information on BMI.)

Childhood obesity is of particular concern because the evidence shows that one in three obese children will become obese adults, increasing their vulnerability to weight related diseases. Overweight and obesity in children and adolescents is generally caused by lack of physical activity, unhealthy eating patterns, or a combination of the two, with genetics and lifestyle both important determinants of a child's weight. Nurses need to be aware that inactivity is a health risk and that obesity is a serious health risk, not just a cosmetic issue, and that obese people risk losing many productive years of their lives. Clinical Interest Box 36.5 provides an outline of some self-care behaviours and exercises.

CLINICAL INTEREST BOX 36.2
Positive physical and psychological effects of regular exercise

- Increases muscle strength and balance
- Decreases blood pressure
- Prevents constipation by maintaining muscle tone in the digestive tract
- Increases bone density and prevents osteoporosis
- Stimulates the nervous system, resulting in improved coordination
- Improves sense of control over one's life
- Improves body image

CLINICAL INTEREST BOX 36.3
Walking to control or lose weight

Walking can promote weight loss and control. A brisk 30-minute walk burns about 200 calories, a slow 30-minute walk about 100 calories. By parking further from work or a shopping centre 3–4 times a week, a person can make up the 30 minutes by walking to and from their destination.

CLINICAL INTEREST BOX 36.4
The older adult and exercise

'But people of our age just don't do that sort of thing!'

Seventy-two-year-old Dorothy protested when her friend Mary suggested she join the gentle exercise class at the local gym. 'I've already had one fall — what if it makes me fall over again?' 'But Dorothy', Mary said, 'the good thing about gentle exercise is that it makes your bones stronger and less likely to break — gentle exercise can make a big difference.'

The New South Wales Health Department (2000) suggests that being active helps keep muscles strong, improves balance and can prevent falls in the elderly. However, if you do fall, stronger muscles mean faster reactions so that you can grab hold of something or put your hands out to save yourself.

(www.mhcs.health.nsw.gov.au/health-public-affairs/mhcs/pdfs/5920/BHC-5920-ENG.pdf)

CLINICAL INTEREST BOX 36.5
Self-care behaviours and exercise

- Make the most of opportunities for exercise — use stairs, park a kilometre away from work or walk to work once or twice a week, walk faster and use lunchtimes for exercise
- Choose an enjoyable physical activity
- Plan 3–4 exercise activities per week
- Before starting exercise sessions, ensure medical clearance if in a high-risk group
- Alternate different types of exercise to keep interest up; for example, Pilates followed by weight-training sessions then walking or bike riding
- Invite a friend to walk or join a health club or gym
- Build up exercise sessions to avoid over-exertion

TYPES OF EXERCISE

ISOTONIC, ISOMETRIC AND ISOKINETIC EXERCISE

Isotonic exercise involves muscle shortening and active contraction and relaxation of muscles and occurs with movement, such as carrying out activities of daily living, independent range-of-movement (ROM) exercises, swimming, walking, running, cycling or jogging. Examples of isotonic bed exercises are pushing or pulling against a stationary object, using a trapeze to lift the body off the bed, lifting the buttocks off the bed by pushing with the hands against the mattress and pushing the body to a sitting position (Kozier et al 2000).

Isometric exercise involves muscle contraction without shortening, so that there is minimum movement, for example, asking an immobilised client to contract and relax their quadriceps or gastrocnemius (calf) muscle without moving the leg. Nurses encourage both types when caring for clients. Two examples of isometric exercise are:

- Quadriceps: the client assumes a supine recumbent position. Instruct the client to press the back of the knee against the mattress while trying to lift the heel of the foot from the bed. Hold for 8 seconds, relax completely and repeat as tolerated. This exercise strengthens and maintains larger muscles of the thigh that will enable the client to ambulate and get out of a chair
- Hand muscles: instruct the client to grip a tennis, squash or sponge ball with the entire hand 5–10 times, then dig each fingertip, one at a time, into the ball 5–10 times each. This exercise strengthens the grip to hold onto crutches or a walker more efficiently (Crisp & Taylor 2005).

When isotonic exercises are not possible, isometric exercises are encouraged. Clients are taught to contract the muscle for the count of 10, then relax it. This exercise should be repeated about 10 times every 3–4 hours while awake. Benefits of isotonic and isometric exercise include increase in muscle tone, mass and strength, improved joint mobility, increased circulation and osteoblastic activity. However, when a nurse performs passive range-of-movement (ROM) exercises, in which the client's muscles do not exert effort, some of the potential benefits are reduced in favour of improved joint mobility and circulation. Isokinetic exercise involves muscle contraction with resistance; for example, rehabilitative exercises for knee and elbow injuries. In this case, isokinetic devices are used to take muscles and joints through a complete ROM without stopping, with resistance at each point.

Mechanical devices are available for specific joints, which place these joints through continuous passive ROM (CPM). These CPM machines are used postoperatively to place joints through a selective repetitive ROM. The CPM can be set to certain degrees of joint mobility, with increasing joint mobility or flexion as the required outcome (Crisp & Taylor 2005).

JOINT MOBILITY

RANGE-OF-MOVEMENT (ROM) EXERCISES

Joints are capable of a wide range of movement (Table 36.1). ROM or motion exercises are either active, when the clients are able to move the joints themselves, or passive, when the nurse moves clients' joints within the normal ROM, noting joint flexibility and/or limitations of movement. ROM exercises are illustrated in Figure 36.5. Joints that are not moved regularly can develop contractures (shortening of a muscle and eventually ligaments and tendons and eventual loss of function). The following 11 terms are associated with joint movement:

1. Abduction: movement away from the midline of the body
2. Adduction: movement towards the midline of the body
3. Flexion: bending
4. Extension: straightening
5. Hyperextension: extension beyond the normal ROM; that is, bending the head back towards the spine
6. Rotation: turning around a fixed axis. Internal rotation is turning inwards, and external rotation is turning outwards
7. Circumduction: circular movement
8. Pronation: turning downwards
9. Supination: turning upwards
10. Inversion: turning a part in towards the body
11. Eversion: turning a part out away from the body.

The frequency with which ROM exercises are performed depends on the client's condition and medical and nursing management, but they are commonly performed at least twice daily. However, it is important not to overtire the client. ROM exercises may be performed independently or with assistance. Using appropriate movements, all joints are exercised in a logical sequence. Exercise routines

TABLE 36.1 | JOINT MOVEMENTS

Type of movement	Joints where movement occurs
Flexion	Shoulder, hip, knee, elbow
Extension	Wrist, interphalangeal joints
Abduction	Shoulder, hip, joints between
Adduction	Metacarpals, wrist and phalanges, or metatarsals and phalanges
Rotation	Shoulder, radius and ulna joints, hip, the joint between the atlas and axis
Circumduction	Shoulder
Pronation or turning the palm downwards. Supination or turning the palm upwards	Radius and ulna joints

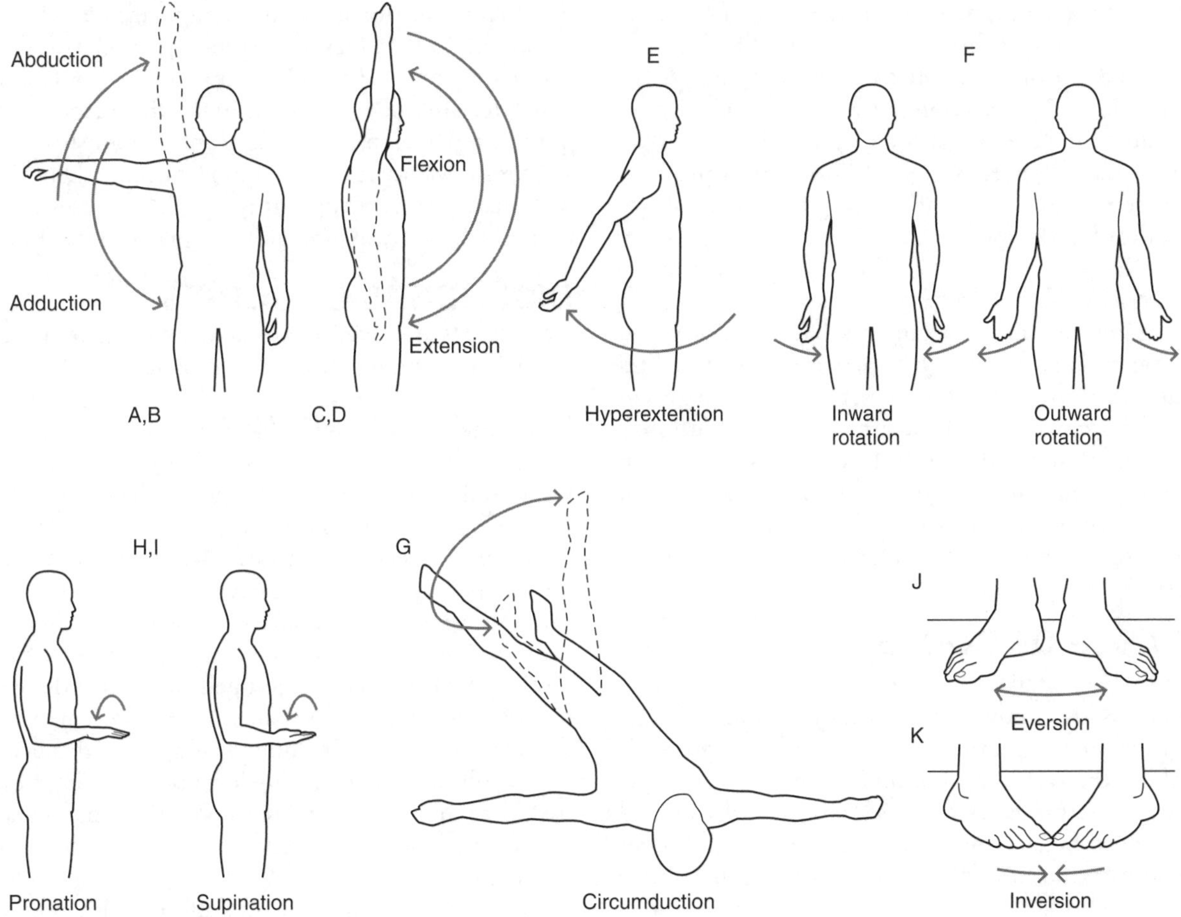

Figure 36.5 | Range-of-movement joint movements

are normally individually designed and the intensity and frequency depend upon the client's general condition, level of fitness and capabilities.

GAIT

Gait is the term used to describe the manner of walking and, while varying from one person to another, there is normally a certain rhythm to a person's walk. Gait abnormalities may occur when there is a disorder of the musculoskeletal or nervous system; for example, unilateral hip dislocation produces a distinct 'waddle' with each step. A staggering, or ataxic, gait may be caused by a lesion in the brain or spinal cord, and a 'scissors' gait is one in which the legs cross each other in progression. An abnormal gait may also result from pain or discomfort due to a lesion on the foot, such as a corn, or from ill-fitting and uncomfortable shoes.

DISEASES OF MUSCLES

MYASTHENIA GRAVIS

This condition affects females more than males, usually occurs between age 20 and 40, and is an autoimmune disease of unknown origin. Defective muscle stimulation is caused by the development of antibodies that damage receptors in the neuromuscular junction, blocking impulses to muscle fibres. Progressive and extensive muscle weakness occurs, with the eyelids affected first by drooping (ptosis), and clients sometimes complaining of diplopia or double vision, owing to extraocular muscle weakness. The neck and limb muscles are affected next, with remissions and relapses precipitated by extreme exercise, infections, emotional disturbances and pregnancy.

MYOPATHIES AND PROGRESSIVE MUSCULAR DYSTROPHIES

Progressive muscular dystrophies are an inherited group of diseases in which there is progressive degeneration of groups of muscles. The major differences between these types of conditions are age of onset, rate of progression and groups of muscles involved. For example, the Duchenne type is gender-linked and presents at about age 5, while myotonic dystrophy usually begins in adulthood. Both progress without remission, and death occurs from respiratory failure or cardiac disease.

CRUSH SYNDROME

Sustained pressure on limbs causes ischaemia resulting in muscle necrosis or death. When pressure is released and circulation restored, necrotic products enter the blood and the filtration system of the renal system. Death may result from acute renal failure. Infection is a common complication and may cause gas gangrene (necrosis of soft tissue accompanied by gas bubbles; it can occur after surgery or trauma and is caused by infection with anaerobic organisms).

DISEASES OF BONES

OSTEOPOROSIS

Osteoporosis is a condition in which the amount of bone tissue is reduced because the rate of bone deposition lags behind the rate of resorption. It may be progressive, temporary or permanent. Cancellous bone is usually affected before compact bone. Osteoporosis may be localised or occur throughout the skeleton. Bones are brittle and susceptible to fracture. The factors that contribute to excessive bone loss include diminished oestrogen levels, immobility, lack of exercise, nutritional deficiencies and certain endocrine disorders. Manifestations include low back pain, kyphosis (rounded back) and spontaneous or pathological fractures resulting from minor injury.

RICKETS

Rickets occurs in children, and osteomalacia in adults after ossification is complete, and both are caused by vitamin D deficiencies. Vitamin D is formed in the skin by the action of sunlight. In vitamin D deficiency, bones become soft, bowed and prone to fractures. Paget's disease is found in people over age 40, is of unknown origin and characterised by hyperactivity of osteoblasts and osteoclasts; that is, rapid turnover of bone tissue. Bones are soft, thick and enlarged and may 'bow'. Usually the pelvis, long bones, lumbar vertebrae and skull are affected.

TUMOURS OF BONE

Tumours of the bone may be benign, primary malignant or metastatic. Benign tumours may be single or multiple, or of several types. The most common benign form is giant-cell tumour, which is composed of multinucleate giant cells or osteoclasts. Clients complain of pain and tenderness, with localised swelling. Osteogenic sarcoma is the most common primary malignant bone tumour. The areas most often affected are the ends of long bones, especially the distal femur or proximal tibia, and metastases may occur, commonly in the lungs. Bone tumours are characterised by the gradual onset of pain in a limb, or the sudden onset of pain after a minor injury to the limb, where a localised mass or swelling develops, as well as a limp. Fatigue is a common symptom. Metastatic bone tumours occur when cells of a malignant primary tumour in another part of the body enter the blood or lymph and are spread to the bone.

DISORDERS OF JOINTS

The tissues involved in diseases of synovial joints are synovial membrane, cartilage and bone.

RHEUMATOID ARTHRITIS

Rheumatoid arthritis is a systemic disease characterised by chronic inflammation of the synovial joint linings, with periods of remission and exacerbation. Joints most commonly affected are those of the wrists, hands and feet. Rheumatoid arthritis results in muscle atrophy, osteoporosis and anaemia, as well as cardiovascular and pulmonary symptoms. The cause is unknown but the disease involves release of antigen–antibody (rheumatoid factor) complexes into the joints. More common in females, signs and symptoms include swelling and stiffness of the joints, followed by marked deformities resulting from soft tissue weakness and joint destruction. Rheumatoid nodules may be present over the extensor surfaces of the elbows or Achilles tendons.

Juvenile rheumatoid arthritis affects children under the age of 16. As for adult rheumatoid arthritis, the cause is unknown and, when acute, is characterised by pyrexia and arthralgia. Arthritis can be self-managed with the correct diagnosis by professionals, regular and appropriate exercise, pain relief and a well-balanced diet to maintain an ideal body weight. Infectious arthritis is inflammation of a joint that results from microorganisms that invade the synovial membrane. Symptoms include severe pain, inflammation and swelling of the affected joint, accompanied by systemic signs and symptoms of infection.

ANKYLOSING SPONDYLITIS

Ankylosing spondylitis is a chronic inflammatory disease that primarily affects the axial skeleton (spine and adjacent soft tissue) and has characteristics similar to those of rheumatoid arthritis, but the rheumatoid factor is absent. The cause is unknown but heredity, immune responses and infection are suspected. Signs and symptoms include gradual onset of back pain, decreased spinal mobility, peripheral arthritis and, in advanced stages, kyphosis (hunched back).

OSTEOARTHRITIS AND GOUT

Osteoarthritis is a degenerative non-infectious disease that causes pain and restricted movement of affected joints. Cartilage in the joints becomes thinner and eventually the two bones come into contact and begin to degenerate, followed by inflammation and effusion. Thought to be caused by excessive use, it usually develops in late middle age and affects large weight-bearing joints (hips, knees and cervical and lower lumbar spine).

Gout is a condition characterised by joint inflammation due to deposits of sodium urate crystals in joints and tendons. Causes include a metabolic defect responsible for increased serum uric acid production and impaired excretion of uric acid by kidneys. Use of alcohol and diuretics may precipitate attacks. The large toe is commonly affected and becomes tender, inflamed and very painful. It occurs in males more often than females.

MUSCULOSKELETAL INFECTIONS AND INFLAMMATORY DISORDERS

Tendinitis is painful inflammation of tendons and of tendon–muscle attachments to bone, which commonly affects the shoulder rotator cuff, hip, Achilles tendon or hamstring muscle. Bursitis is inflammation of the synovial membrane lining a bursa, and usually occurs in the subdeltoid, olecranon, trochanteric, calcaneal or prepatellar bursae. The cause of tendinitis and bursitis is overuse of a particular muscle group, which can eventually damage a tendon or bursa. Tendinitis can also result from other musculoskeletal disorders such as rheumatoid arthritis, whereas bursitis can result from calcium deposits in bursae, or infection. Signs and symptoms include pain, swelling and limited movement.

Occupational overuse syndrome (also known as repetitive strain injury [RSI]) is a collective term for a range of conditions that are mainly work related and characterised by discomfort or persistent pain in muscles and tendons. The syndrome results when activities performed on a repetitive basis cause gradual injury to specific muscles and tendons.

Osteomyelitis is a pyogenic (pus-forming) infection involving bone, bone marrow, and surrounding soft tissues, and may be acute or chronic, with resultant bone destruction. Acute osteomyelitis is characterised by rapid onset of severe pain in the involved bone, with local heat, swelling and inflammation as well as pyrexia, tachycardia, nausea and malaise. Chronic osteomyelitis is characterised by slight pyrexia, pain and persistent drainage of purulent material from a sinus tract.

COMMON SIGNS AND SYMPTOMS OF MUSCULOSKELETAL DISORDERS

Pain and nerve (sensory) changes

Pain is a common symptom of musculoskeletal disorders, as a result of trauma, inflammation or degeneration. Clients describe the pain as mild, aching, severe or throbbing, and it may be localised or generalised, depending on the specific disorder. Pain may increase with movement, be exacerbated by changes in external temperature, and relieved by rest. It may be worse at certain times; for example, joint discomfort from degenerative disease is often worse in the evenings. Numbness, tingling and lack of sensation are other sensory changes. Swelling from injury or tumours causes pressure on nerves, resulting in loss of sensation.

Swelling, deformity and impaired mobility

Swelling of an affected area may be the result of the formation of inflammatory exudate in response to injury from physical trauma, chemicals or infection. Swelling will also occur when blood is lost from the circulation into surrounding tissues (haematoma); for example, after a fracture. A joint may become swollen if there is an increase in the amount of synovial fluid or if blood or purulent discharge is present in the joint capsule. Deformity may be the result of growths, fractures, dislocations, abnormal curvature of the spine, or contractures. The effects of a deformity include changes in range of joint motion, posture and gait. Mobility may be impaired to such an extent that the client is unable to move without pain or unable to carry out activities of daily living, or it may only restrict mobility at certain times, such as after activity or related to certain positions.

Sprains, strains and fractures

A sprain is an injury to a ligament, caused when a joint is forced beyond its normal ROM. A ligament may be stretched or torn and local bleeding and bruising present with restricted movement. A strain is an injury to a muscle and/or a tendon, resulting from excessive physical effort. Both sprains and strains cause pain and swelling, but strains may cause muscle spasm as well. A fracture is a broken bone, often with nearby soft tissue, blood vessel and nerve damage, and is most commonly caused by injury to the bone. A stress fracture occurs when a bone is subjected to repeated or prolonged stress such as jogging. A pathological fracture may occur in weakened bone as a result of osteoporosis. Fractures are classified as open or closed, simple or complicated. Open (or compound) fractures are those in which the bone breaks through the skin, while closed fractures are those where the skin is intact. In a simple fracture only the bone is involved, while in complicated fractures nearby blood vessels, nerves or organs are affected.

Table 36.2 lists the various types of fractures, according to the way in which the bone has broken. Signs and symptoms vary but mostly there is pain, swelling, involuntary and painful muscle spasm, bruising, obvious deformity, abnormal mobility and loss of function. Crepitus (grating caused by bone fragments rubbing together) may be heard or felt. Shock may occur as a result of haemorrhage or extensive damage.

A neurovascular assessment is performed for every client who has experienced a fracture, whether treated with a cast or traction. It should be performed every hour for the first 24 hours and, if the cast is dry, then every 4–8 hours. Check the health facility's protocol. The assessment includes inspection of:

- Skin: inspect area distal to the injury; palpate skin temperature with the back of the hand and compare with the opposite extremity or site
- Movement: have the client move the area distal to the injury, or move it passively — there should be no discomfort
- Sensation: enquire about feelings of numbness or tingling; check sensation with a paper clip and compare bilaterally — sensation should be the same
- Pulses: palpate pulses distal to the injury; compare bilaterally
- Capillary refill: check this in the nail beds distal to the injury. Capillary refill should occur within 3 seconds and within 5 seconds in the older adult
- Pain: enquire about the degree, location, nature and frequency of pain, noting any increase in intensity or change in the type of pain (deWit 2005).

The cast should be inspected for rough edges, cracking, moisture, signs of bleeding or drainage from under the cast, and odour emanating through the cast (refer to Table 36.3).

Dislocation refers to complete displacement, and subluxation to partial displacement, of a joint's articulating surfaces; both damage surrounding soft tissue structures. Joint effusion is the accumulation of synovial fluid in a joint and occurs if blood vessels in the synovium are damaged. Joint effusions may result from severe sprains, dislocations or fractures. Signs and symptoms of dislocation and effusion include severe pain, limited movement, joint deformity and swelling. (Chapter 48 covers the first aid care of sprains, fractures and bandaging.)

Lower back pain

Lower back pain is a common symptom that has a variety of causes, including poor posture, injury, inflammatory conditions, obesity, metabolic bone disorders, degenerative processes and intervertebral disc disease. Discomfort or pain may be mild, severe, continuous or intermittent and aggravated by certain movements or posture, and may radiate into the buttocks or down the back of the legs. People with lower back pain should not sit for more than 30 minutes at any one time, and frequent stretching (thrusting the hips forward while the upper body leans back) are recommended. Most lower back pain can be safely and effectively treated after an examination by an orthopaedic surgeon and a prescribed period of activity modification and medication to relieve the pain and diminish the inflammation. Although a brief period of rest may be helpful, most studies show that light activity speeds healing and recovery. It may not be necessary to discontinue all activities, including work. Instead, people may adjust their activity under the guidance of medical officers or physiotherapists.

When the initial pain has eased, a rehabilitation program may be suggested to increase muscle strength in the lower back and abdominal muscles, as well as stretching exercises to increase flexibility. If overweight, weight loss is recommended, as this may decrease the chance of recurrence of lower back pain. The best long-term treatment is an active prevention program of maintaining optimal physical condition. This can be achieved by regular exercise, as well as practising proper lifting techniques and assuming good posture.

When is surgery needed?

Whether acute or chronic, lower back pain can almost always be treated without surgery. The most common reason for

TABLE 36.2 | TYPES OF FRACTURES

Type	Description
Greenstick	The fracture is incomplete and does not extend through the bone. The bone bends, and splits or cracks on one side
Transverse	The fracture line is straight across the bone
Oblique	The fracture line is at an angle across the bone
Spiral	The fracture line coils around the bone. This type of fracture generally results from twisting of the limb
Impacted	The fragments of broken bone are pushed (telescoped) into each other
Comminuted	The bone is broken into a number of fragments
Depressed	The broken edges are pushed below the level of the rest of the bone. This type of injury may occur when the skull is fractured
Avulsion	A fragment of bone, connected to a ligament, breaks off from the rest of the bone
Intracapsular	The fracture is within the joint capsule
Extracapsular	The fracture is close to a joint, but is outside the joint capsule

TABLE 36.3 | PROCEDURE FOR INITIAL CARE OF THE PATIENT IN A CAST

Review and carry out standard steps in Appendix 1

Action	Rationale
Validate the medical orders in the patient record	Ensures correct procedure is about to take place
Explain the procedure to the client	Reduces anxiety and gains client's consent and cooperation
Critically think through your assessment data and problem solving, e.g. provide privacy, comfort measures, pain relief	Evaluating each aspect and its relationship to other data will help identify specific problems and modifications of the procedure that may be needed for the individual
Identify the type of cast and its purpose Inspect the bed for type of mattress support	Ensures patient comfort
Critically think through your data, carefully evaluating each aspect and its relationship to other data	Identify specific problems and modifications of the procedure needed for this client
Planning	
Determine individualised patient outcomes in relationship to the cast. Include the following: (a) Patient expresses comfort (b) Cast is supported (c) Patient engages in activity to prevent complications of the cast and of immobility (d) Neurovascular status in extremity remains stable (e) Skin at the edges of the cast remains free of breakdown (f) There are no signs or symptoms of infection or complications of immobility (g) Identify any transfer device or assistance that will be needed to move patient into bed	Knowledge of the equipment required and procedures needed to be performed is essential to be able to choose the correct equipment required for your client Performing a baseline examination allows the nurse to evaluate accurately
Wash or disinfect your hands	Prevents cross infection and contamination
Conduct neurovascular checks immediately and then every hour while the cast is in the drying stage: 1. Circulation checks: (a) Check skin temperature of the toes or fingers of the extremity. (b) Check the colour of the nails and the colour of the extremity. (c) Check for capillary filling by pressing on tissues 2. Motion checks: (a) Ask patient to move fingers or toes 3. Sensation checks: (a) Ask whether patient can feel pressure when you press on the nails of the fingers or toes (b) Ask about pain (c) Ask about abnormal sensations (paraesthesia) such as numbness or tingling Monitor the amount, colour, and odour of any drainage that appears on the outside of the cast. Mark boundaries of the drainage area so that increases in size can be identified Elevate the extremity with the cast if possible Change patient's position during the drying process	The limb is assessed distal to the injury or site of surgery to determine if the trauma/surgery has interfered with vascular or neurovascular function Comparing the affected limb with the unaffected limb gives a basis for determining what is normal for the client Compartment syndrome can be identified by performing neurovascular observations and early detection can prevent nerve and muscle damage or even necrosis, which may result in amputation Provides a baseline that can be used to determine increase in bleeding Minimises swelling Ensures the pressure on the cast is not in one spot
Teach the patient how to prevent complications through activity. (a) Encourage the patient to turn after cast is completely dry. (b) Give instructions in performing isometric exercises including gluteal settings and quadricep settings if the patient is on continuous bed rest	Prevents pressure sores Isometric exercises involve muscle contraction without shortening, so that there is minimum movement. Isometric exercises increase muscle tone, mass and strength and increase circulation
Wash or disinfect your hands	Prevents cross infection and contamination

(Continued)

TABLE 36.3 | PROCEDURE FOR INITIAL CARE OF THE PATIENT IN A CAST—cont'd

Action	Rationale
Evaluation	
Evaluate in relation to the previously identified outcomes: (a) Patient expresses comfort. (b) Cast is supported to prevent strain on muscles and joints (c) Patient engages in activity to prevent complications of the cast and of immobility (d) Neurovascular status in extremity remains stable (e) Skin at the edges of the cast remains free of breakdown (f) There are no signs or symptoms of infection or the complications of immobility	Evaluation ensures you are leaving the client pain free, comfortable and safe
Documentation	
Document the evaluation of status including specific findings relating to circulation, motion and sensation	These observations are most often entered on a neurovascular observation chart Neurovascular status should be recorded in client's progress notes at least once per shift Any deterioration in neurovascular status is noted in the progress notes and the client's doctor informed Also record any relevant psychological data

surgery on the lower back is to remove the pressure from a 'slipped disc' (prolapsed disc) when it causes nerve and leg pain and has not responded to other treatments. Some arthritic conditions of the spine, when severe, can cause pressure and nerve irritation and can often be improved with surgical treatment.

DIAGNOSTIC TESTS

Tests assist or confirm the diagnosis of musculoskeletal disorders. Plain X-ray films may detect bone or joint abnormalities. An arthrogram is an X-ray of a joint after injection of radio-opaque dye into the joint. Arthrography outlines soft tissue (i.e. the meniscus) which is not usually visualised by plain X-ray. Bone scans provide imaging of the skeleton after intravenous injection of a radioactive isotope that collects in bone tissue at sites where there is increased activity (i.e. at the site of a tumour) and lesions can be detected earlier. Arthroscopy, the visual examination of a joint with a fibre-optic endoscope, is mostly performed on the knee to remove loose fragments, view suspected damage or obtain a biopsy. Biopsies may be performed on bone, muscle or synovial membrane. Synovial fluid may be aspirated (arthrocentesis) and analysed to detect infection or inflammation, while blood is tested for enzymes, antibodies and antigens, calcium, phosphorus and uric acid levels, as well as erythrocyte sedimentation rate.

CARE OF THE INDIVIDUAL WITH A MUSCULOSKELETAL DISORDER

While medical management and nursing care will depend on the specific disorder, the main aims of care are to:

- Promote rest and relieve pain
- Prevent complications of inactivity and promote movement when possible
- Maintain skin integrity
- Maintain or improve nutritional status
- Prevent psychosocial problems
- Promote rehabilitation.

HEALING OF BONES

Bone fractures can take weeks or months to heal, and healing occurs in stages. The first stage is the formation of a haematoma between the two ends of the bones. This is followed by inflammation and accumulation of white cells to phagocytose the haematoma (about 5 days). Lastly, the development of granulation tissue and new blood vessels is followed by the development of a callus (calcified osteoblasts) and shaping of new bone by osteoclasts, which remove excess callus (Figure 36.6). Factors that delay healing are infection, fat emboli (from the medullary canal) that lodge in the lungs, splinters of dead bone not removed by phagocytosis, ischaemia (the neck of femur is vulnerable, as it has a poor blood supply), continued mobility and age of the client.

PROMOTING REST

Rest helps minimise pain and swelling, promotes healing of injured tissues, relieves muscle spasms and prevents further tissue destruction in inflammatory conditions. Rest may be classified as general, when the individual is confined to bed (e.g. if several joints are inflamed) or local, when a specific body part is immobilised, such as a limb in a splint or cast (see Table 36.3 Caring for a client with a cast).

General care during the rest phase involves:

- Providing a suitable bed with a firm mattress, pillows and sheepskins to promote comfort
- Meeting basic needs; that is, helping those who are immobilised with activities of daily living

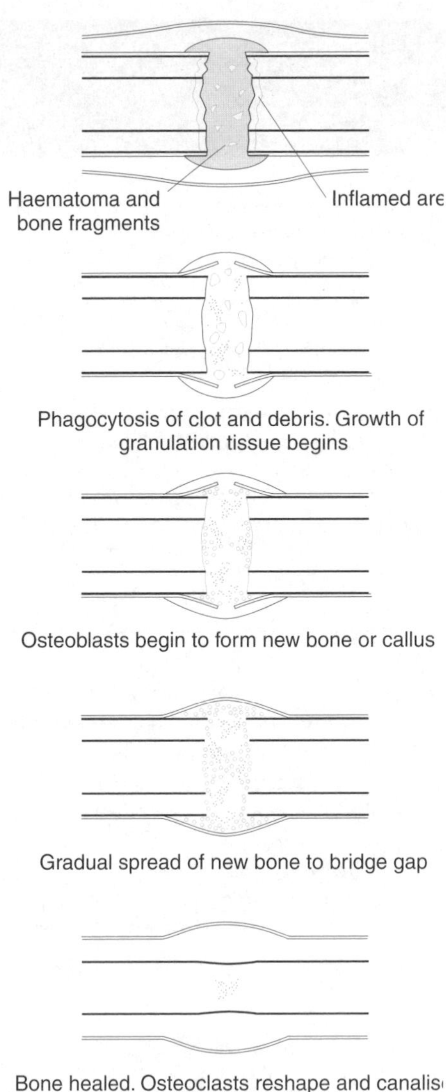

Figure 36.6 | Stages in bone healing *(Wilson & Waugh 1996)*

- Preventing complications associated with immobility
- Maintaining correct posture and body alignment.

TRACTION

Traction reduces and immobilises fractures. A steady pull from two directions keeps the bone in place. Traction is also used for muscle spasms, to correct or prevent deformities, and to relieve pressure on a nerve. Weights, ropes and pulleys are used to create the pull required to stabilise the limb. Traction can be applied to the neck, arms, legs or pelvis. Skin traction is applied to the skin. Tape, a boot or a splint is used. Weights are attached to the device. Skeletal traction is applied directly to the bone with wires or pins are inserted through the bone. Weights are attached to the device (see Table 36.4).

MAINTAINING SKIN INTEGRITY

Clients who are immobilised for prolonged periods are at high risk of developing pressure sores or decubitus ulcers. Skin must be maintained in good condition and protected from irritation, friction and prolonged pressure. (General care of the skin and prevention of pressure sores are described in Chapter 37.)

PROPER POSITIONING TECHNIQUES

Clients with musculoskeletal disorders who are immobilised require help from nurses to ensure proper body alignment and comfort. Aids to comfort in bed, such as pillows, foot boards, trochanter rolls, trapeze bars, sandbags and slippery-type sheets for ease of movement in bed, are all useful to ensure that an immobilised client is comfortable. (Various positions and proper positioning are discussed in Chapter 27.)

MAINTAINING OR IMPROVING NUTRITIONAL STATUS

Nutrition for clients with a musculoskeletal disorder includes a well-balanced diet and maintenance of recommended body weight. The diet should contain adequate amounts of protein, calcium and vitamin D to promote healing and maintenance of the musculoskeletal system. Adequate fibre and fluids aid elimination. If overweight, a weight-reduction diet is recommended to prevent stress on inflamed or diseased joints.

RELIEVING PAIN

While the general approaches to pain management described in Chapter 35 are relevant to clients with musculoskeletal disorders, specific measures may also be indicated. Clients may experience acute or chronic pain, depending on the specific disorder, and general measures to promote comfort and minimise pain should be implemented; that is, changing position, massage, handling a painful limb gently, and rest. If not contraindicated, elevating the limb may relieve discomfort and pain. Specific measures include checking to ensure that splints, casts or dressings are not too tight or rubbing against the skin. Hot or cold packs or treatments may be used to provide relief and increase ROM. Heat is sometimes used in chronic joint disorders, as it relaxes muscles, relieves stiffness and provides analgesia, and is often applied before exercise and massage. Applying a cold pack to a limb or area is useful for acute pain or acutely inflamed joints. When these treatments are used, caution is necessary to prevent tissue damage. (Information on heat and cold applications is provided in Chapter 35.) Analgesia may be prescribed and administered in accordance with nursing regulations and the institution's policy.

PREVENTING PSYCHOSOCIAL PROBLEMS

Management of a musculoskeletal disorder may require a person to be confined to bed, and possibly hospital, for

TABLE 36.4 | PROCEDURE FOR CARING FOR THE PATIENT IN SKELETAL TRACTION OR WITH AN EXTERNAL FIXATION DEVICE

Action	Rationale
Review and carry out the standard steps in Appendix 1	
Review the doctor's order: type of traction or external fixation device, the weight, activity and the position of the bed	Ensures correct type of traction and weight is applied
Assess the patient returning to the unit from surgery for signs of general discomfort or pain	Provides a baseline and gives an indication whether the traction is correctly applied
Critically think through your data, carefully evaluating each aspect and its relationship to other data	Identifying specific problems and modifying the procedure if needed for this individual
Determine individualised desired patient outcomes in relationship to skeletal traction or an external fixation device. Include the following: (a) Patient expresses comfort (b) *For traction*: ropes, pulleys, and weights correctly placed *For external fixation*: all components in place without pressure (c) Pin sites are clean without signs of infection	Early detection of signs or symptoms of adverse outcomes, such as pain, burning, complications of immobility, skin breakdown, pin site infection or changes in circulation, motion and sensation of the affected body part can prevent major complications and prolonged hospitalisation for the client
Implementation	
Gather the equipment needed for the traction or external fixation device and obtain assistance if needed	Ensures all equipment is at client's bedside to maximise efficiency, reduce apprehension on the client's part and increase the confidence in the nurse
Wash or disinfect your hands	Prevents cross infection and contamination of tubing
Raise the bed to an appropriate working position based on your height	Prevents injury to the nurse and complies with occupational health and safety guidelines
Inspect the devices: (a) *For skeletal traction,* all ropes and pulleys should be in proper alignment, correct weights should be attached and ropes should be hanging freely (b) *For an external fixation device,* all components should be free of pressure and the extremity supported	Inspecting all operative sites including pin or tong insertions for excessive bleeding or drainage and providing pin site care maintains skin integrity and decreases the risk of infection
Check circulation, motion and sensation (CMS) of the affected extremity as a baseline: (a) *Circulation:* assess by checking peripheral pulses, colour, capillary refill and temperature of the extremity (b) *Motion:* assess by having the patient move fingers or toes on the affected extremity (c) *Sensation:* assess by asking the patient about pain, tingling, numbness or other sensations in the extremity	Observing neurovascular observations provides an assessment of the client's circulatory system distal to fracture or skeletal traction. This ensures any early deficits with circulation are noticed early and interventions to prevent ischaemia can be taken
Place call signal, all personal possessions and items needed for self-care within easy reach of patient	Allows client to maintain independence
Teach patient methods for moving in bed and any appropriate exercises	Encourages the client to move (as required) minimising the risk of pressure sores and problems associated with immobility
Evaluation	
Evaluate (a) Client expresses comfort (b) *For traction:* ropes, pulleys, and weights are correctly placed *For external fixation:* all components in place without pressure (c) Pin sites are clean without signs of infection (d) There are no signs or symptoms of adverse outcomes, such as pain, burning, complications of immobility, skin breakdown, pin site infection or changes in circulation, motion and sensation of the affected body part	Evaluation ensures you are leaving the client pain free, comfortable and safe

TABLE 36.4 | PROCEDURE FOR CARING FOR THE PATIENT IN SKELETAL TRACTION OR WITH AN EXTERNAL FIXATION DEVICE—cont'd

Action	Rationale
Documentation	
Document the following on the appropriate form: (a) Patient comfort and tolerance of the procedure (b) Type of traction and weight applied or location of the external fixation device (c) Neurovascular status (circulation, motion and sensation) and any observations or concerns	Documentation increases the communication between health care professionals and complies with legal requirements for reporting change

an extended time, and often leads to boredom, frustration or depression. To prevent such problems, clients are encouraged to express their feelings and are allowed to participate in making decisions about their care. Active involvement in all aspects of care and self-care techniques are taught, as this allows clients to take responsibility for some of their care and can help to reduce problems associated with dependence and immobilisation. Regular programs of activity developed with the client and other allied health professionals need to be incorporated into the nursing care plan.

PROMOTING REMOBILISATION AND REHABILITATION

As the musculoskeletal system is crucial to activity, a routine of exercise and rehabilitation is developed and implemented. A planned exercise program is generally developed by the physiotherapist, but the nurse is required to encourage and supervise regular exercise. Programs contain exercises designed to prevent muscle atrophy or joint contracture and to prepare for ambulation. Range-of-movement exercises are important during this time. A program of gradated, non-weight-bearing exercises is started, designed to regain or increase muscle tone, build muscle strength and promote joint mobility. When clients are able to bear weight on the affected limb, the exercise program is aimed at restoring as much mobility as possible. The overall aim of rehabilitation is independence in activities of living, and requires a multidisciplinary team approach consisting of nurses, medical officers, physiotherapists and occupational therapists. Depending on specific needs, a social worker and splint-maker may be involved. (Information on rehabilitation is provided in Chapter 46.) Preparation for discharge includes informing clients of the need to continue any exercise program, on the use of splints or braces, about limits of physical activity and the importance of attending any future appointments or ongoing rehabilitation programs.

GENERAL TREATMENT FOR EXERCISE-RELATED INJURIES

Exercise can be the cause of injuries that are mostly orthopaedic in nature and caused by irritation of bones, tendons and ligaments and/or muscle tissue. Injury may be as a result of weight-bearing stress or collision. Nurses can teach clients the acronym PRICE: prevention, rest, ice, compression and elevation, and advise of the need for a medical officer to diagnose the injury. Generally, further injury can be avoided by resting the affected limb.

NURSING PRACTICE IN MEETING MOVEMENT AND EXERCISE NEEDS

To plan and implement appropriate nursing actions, a client's ability to mobilise should be assessed. By observation and obtaining factual information, nurses are able to plan and implement measures to meet each client's movement and exercise needs. When admitting clients, nurses obtain information about usual movement and exercise habits and whether assistance is required to mobilise. It is important to note whether a client experiences problems that limit independent movement, such as a painful hip or knee, and whether an aid, such as a walking stick, is required. Nurses observe and document posture and gait, strength and tone, ROM and other factors such as dyspnoea at rest or on exertion, which may limit exercise.

It is important to identify potential problems that may affect a client's ability to exercise. Impaired mobility may result from a decrease in the individual's strength; presence of pain or discomfort; impaired cognition or perception, such as dementia, severe anxiety or depression; impaired neuromuscular or skeletal function; or as a result of imposed restrictions such as bed rest. Being in hospital is likely to alter a person's normal movement and exercise routine and, although there is often a degree of restriction in activities, clients able to ambulate should be encouraged to do so, while those who are immobilised may require assistance to move. Nurses promote safety and comfort while encouraging, when possible, a return to independent function.

When planning care to meet a client's need for movement and exercise the nurse must consider factors such as:

- Maintaining and promoting normal mobility
- Assisting those with restricted mobility
- Providing and assisting with use of equipment to aid mobility
- Preventing and alleviating discomfort associated with reduced mobility.

A sample nursing care plan is shown in Table 36.5.

AMBULATION AFTER PROLONGED IMMOBILISATION

'Dangling' before ambulating

Ambulating, or walking, is encouraged and facilitated to prevent the complications associated with even short-term but especially long periods of immobility. Certain clients may need to relearn how to walk; for example, after a cerebrovascular accident or leg surgery, clients may need the assistance of aids such as a walking stick, crutches or walking frame. After an extended period of immobility, nurses need to instruct clients to mobilise progressively. Bedridden clients who are able to raise each leg 4–6 cm straight up from the bed usually possess enough strength to walk, provided that they are mentally alert.

Nurses begin re-educating muscle groups by first allowing the client to sit on the edge of the bed for 1–2 minutes with their feet on the floor, a technique called dangling. Clients then progress to standing, then walk a few steps, gradually increasing the distance. Blood pressure can drop dramatically and the client could faint if they were to stand up suddenly. Dangling for a few minutes helps prevent hypotension and dizziness when a previously immobilised client stands for the first time. If a client complains of dizziness or suddenly looks pale when they are standing, quickly return the person to bed or the nearest chair. Clients' rates of progress will depend upon their general condition, nursing and medical management and previous levels of fitness. Preparing a person to restart mobilisation involves both psychological and physical factors, and nurses need to provide encouragement, reassurance and physical support as necessary.

When the nurse assists a client who has a one-sided weakness, or hemiplegia, it is important to decide which walking aid or technique has been recommended. Although the method used to assist is individualised, most clients require assistance and support on the affected side. When assisting a person to walk it is helpful if they remain close to a railed wall and able to rest on a chair before beginning the return walk. If an ambulant client has an intravenous infusion, urinary or wound-drainage bag, the nurse ensures that therapy or drainage is not affected, by checking tubing or drainage bags in case they have become dislodged after exercise. When planning to assist a client to ambulate, the following needs to be considered:

TABLE 36.5 | A NURSING CARE PLAN FOR AN OLDER CLIENT

Assessment	
Mrs J is a 75-year-old lady in an aged-care facility who does not do much walking or exercise because of a fear of falling and because of her belief that even small amounts of exercise may not be beneficial. She is able to walk about 10 metres but quickly tires, complaining of fatigue, and lacks energy for activities of daily living. Baseline assessment includes height 163 cm, weight 68 kg, blood pressure 160/100 mmHg, pulse 90 bpm at rest	
Nursing diagnosis	
Activity intolerance related to generalised weakness and sedentary lifestyle	
Planning	
Goals	**Expected outcomes**
Client's activity tolerance will improve	Client will discuss effects of exercise on activities of daily living
Client will develop plan of exercise incorporating isotonic and isometric exercises	Client will perform and record regular exercise 3–4 times per week
Client's cardiopulmonary response will improve	Client will be able to walk 20 metres to exercise and perform activities of daily living without fatigue
Interventions	**Rationale**
Exercise promotion — educate client regarding benefits of exercise	Exercise energises and can prevent injury
Develop a plan of exercise with client that gradually develops fitness, increasing walking distance 5 m each walk	Exercise should be performed every 48 hours
Encourage client to document exercise	Keeping a diary or log increases compliance
Monitor activity to prevent over-exertion	Client is unlikely to continue with program if too strenuous
Evaluation	
Observe client's ability to perform increased level of exercise Ask client about improved performance of activities of daily living and feelings of wellbeing. Review client's exercise log/records	

- Height
- General condition
- Physical disability
- Mental attitude
- Confidence
- Environment
- Whether assistance from other health professionals or walking aids is required.

Well-fitting footwear should always be worn (non-slip soles) and potential hazards eliminated, such as obstacles or liquids on floors. Clients should not be allowed to walk barefoot or with just socks or slippery footwear (e.g. women with nylon hose) on the feet. Clients are encouraged to walk at their own pace and, if they become distressed or complain of pain, faintness, giddiness or undue fatigue, should be seated and the nurse should remain with the client and call for assistance.

WALKING AIDS

Walking aids broaden the base of support and increase stability. The type of aid used depends on the client's condition, amount of support required and type of disability. Clients are commonly instructed in the use of walking aids by a physiotherapist; however, it is important for nurses to know the principles involved, to reinforce instructions and safe use of walking aids. Walking aids that may be required on a temporary or permanent basis include crutches, walking sticks and walking frames. Callipers, leg braces or splints may be used to provide extra support for a weak leg, to prevent or correct deformities, or prevent joint movement. It is important that a leg brace is applied correctly, as a poorly fitting brace is ineffective and may cause pressure and discomfort.

Crutches

Crutches enable a person to ambulate by taking the weight of the body off one or both legs. Successful use of crutches requires balance and upper body strength. Selection of crutches and particular type of gait depends on individual needs, but must be appropriate to be safe and effective. Clinical Interest Box 36.6 provides information on how to teach clients about crutch safety. The two types commonly used are the underarm and forearm crutches.

Underarm crutches are often used by clients with a sprain or leg cast, while forearm crutches are more commonly used by those with a through gait, as in paraplegia. Underarm crutches must be measured so that the person's weight is carried on their wrists and palms and not on the axillae. The axilla bar should be 4–5 cm below the axilla, and the hand bar positioned to permit 15–30 degree flexion of the elbow at rest (Figure 36.7). Forearm crutches must also allow 15–30 degree flexion of the elbow at rest. Before crutches are used they should be assessed for safety, ensuring that all screws and bolts are tightened and rubber tips are in good repair. It is important to ascertain the amount of

CLINICAL INTEREST BOX 36.6
Teaching clients about crutch safety

Objective
- Client will state and demonstrate safe crutch walking

Teaching strategies
- Teach client with axillary crutches about the dangers of pressure on the axillae, which occurs when leaning on the crutches to support body weight
- Explain why client must use crutches that were measured for him or her
- Show client how to routinely inspect crutch tips. Rubber tips should be securely attached to the crutches. When tips are worn, they should be replaced. Rubber crutch tips increase surface friction and help prevent slipping
- Explain that the crutch tips should remain dry. Water decreases surface friction and increases the risk of slipping
- Show client how to dry the crutch tips if they become wet; client may use paper or cloth towels
- Show client how to inspect the structure of the crutches. Cracks in a wooden crutch decrease its ability to support weight. Bends in aluminium crutches can alter body alignment
- Provide client with a list of medical supply companies in the community for obtaining repairs, new rubber tips, handgrips and crutch pads
- Instruct client to have spare crutches and tips readily available

Evaluation
- Client states and demonstrates principles of crutch safety

(Potter & Perry 2008)

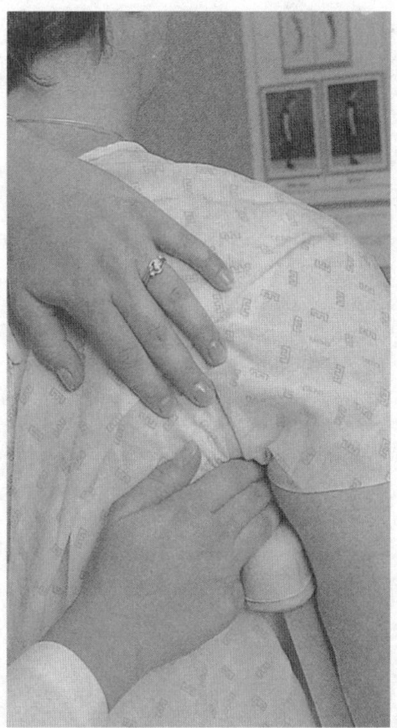

Figure 36.7 | Verifying correct distance between crutch pads and axilla *(Potter & Perry 2008)*

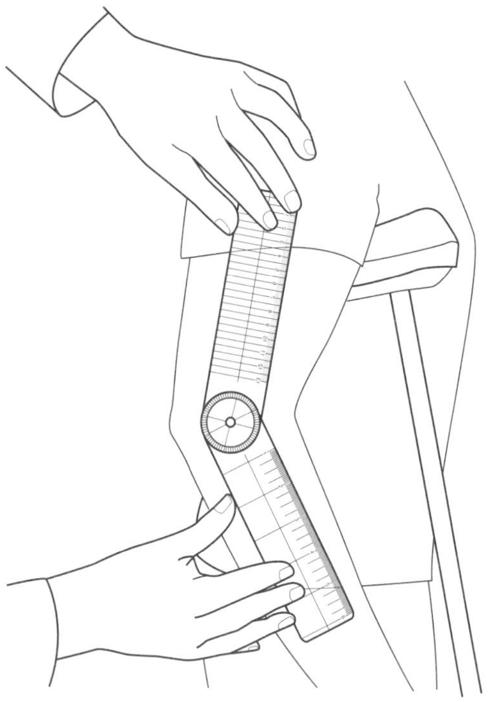

Figure 36.8 | Using the goniometer to verify correct degree of elbow flexion for crutch use

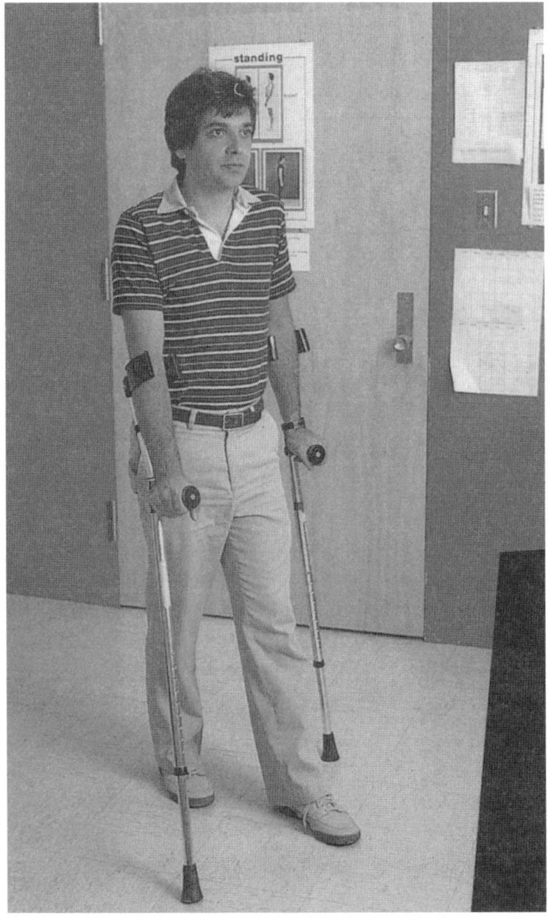

Figure 36.9 | Double adjustable forearm crutch *(Potter & Perry 2005)*

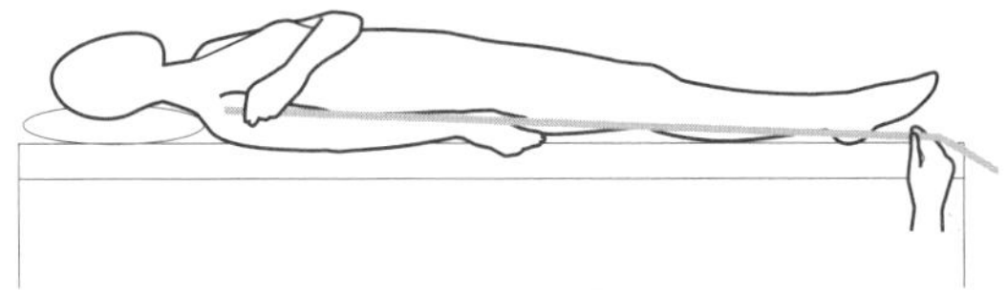

Figure 36.10 | Measuring crutch length

weight bearing allowed on the affected leg(s); that is, partial or none (Figures 36.8–36.10).

Crutch-walking gaits

Clients are instructed in one of several gaits, according to need. The most common is the three-point gait, in which weight is borne on the unaffected leg, and the crutches moved forward first, followed by the unaffected leg, then the affected leg follows in a swinging movement because it is raised from the ground. This gait is used when a person is unable to bear weight on one leg (Figure 36.11). The two-point and four-point gaits are used when both feet can bear some weight; that is, partial weight bearing. The two-point gait requires the individual to advance one crutch and the opposite leg together, followed by the other crutch and

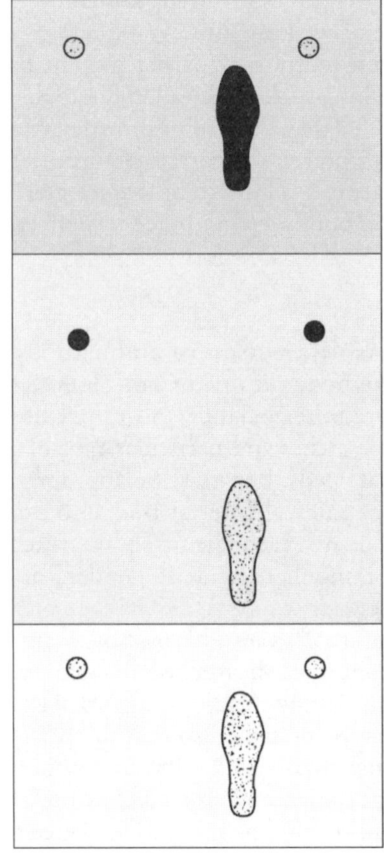

Figure 36.11 | Three-point gait, with weight borne on the unaffected leg. Solid foot and crutch tips show weight bearing in each phase (read from bottom to top) *(Potter & Perry 2008)*

leg. The four-point gait requires greater coordination but provides more stability, as there are always three points on the floor as each leg is moved alternately with the opposite crutch (Figures 36.12 and 36.13).

The swing-through gait is used when a person has no use of the lower body (i.e. in paraplegia), and both crutches are advanced simultaneously. The person swings both legs either parallel with or beyond the crutches, the pelvis moving first, followed by the shoulders and head in order to maintain balance.

When rising from a chair the individual is taught to hold both crutches in one hand, with the tips resting firmly on the floor, and to push up with their free hand, using the crutches for support. To sit down, the process is reversed — the person supports themselves with the crutches in one hand, holds the arm of the chair with a free hand, and lowers into the chair (Figure 36.14). To use stairs, the three-point gait is easiest, so that when going up stairs a person leads with the unaffected leg, follows with both crutches then the affected leg. When going down stairs a person leads with the crutches and affected leg, followed by the unaffected leg (Figures 36.15 and 36.16).

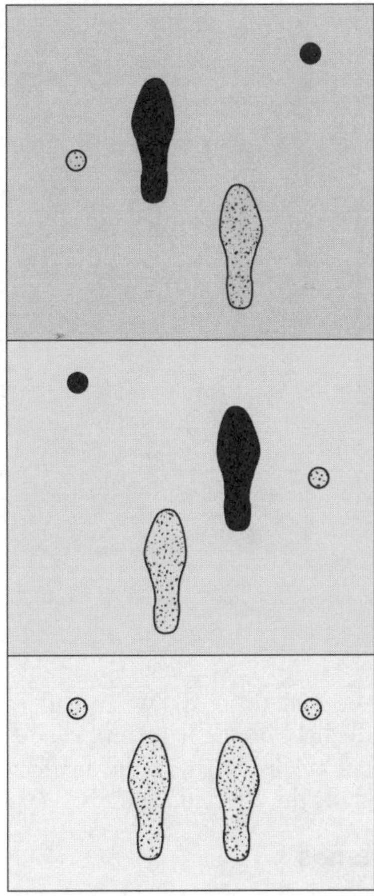

Figure 36.12 | Two-point gait, with weight borne partially on each foot, and each crutch advancing with the opposite leg. Solid areas indicate leg and crutch tips bearing weight (read from bottom to top) *(Potter & Perry 2008)*

Sticks

A walking stick may be used for people with one-sided weakness or injury, occasional loss of balance, or to reduce weight bearing on a hip or knee, as well as to provide balance and support for walking, reducing fatigue and strain on weight-bearing joints. Walking sticks should extend from the individual's greater trochanter to the floor, and be fitted with a rubber tip to prevent slippage. Sticks are available

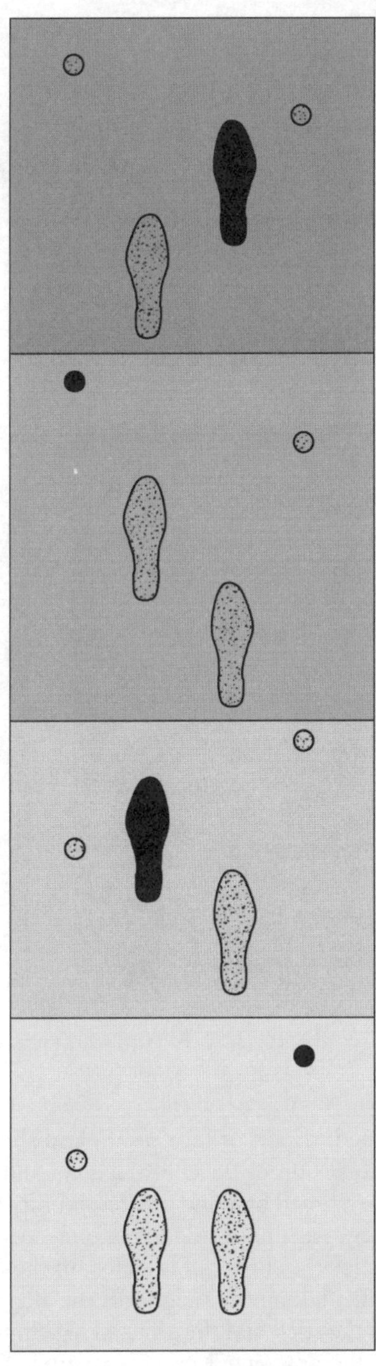

Figure 36.13 | Four-point alternating gait. Solid feet and crutch tips show foot and crutch tip moved in each of the four phases (read from bottom to top) *(Potter & Perry 2008)*

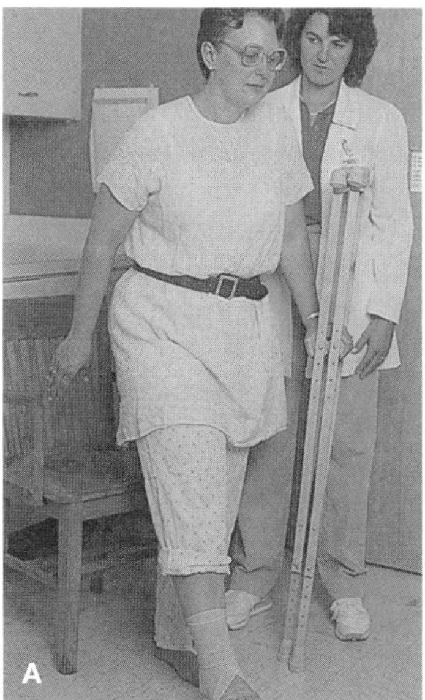

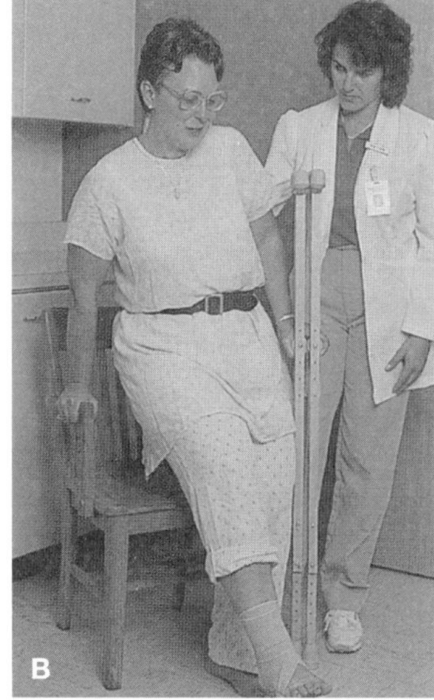

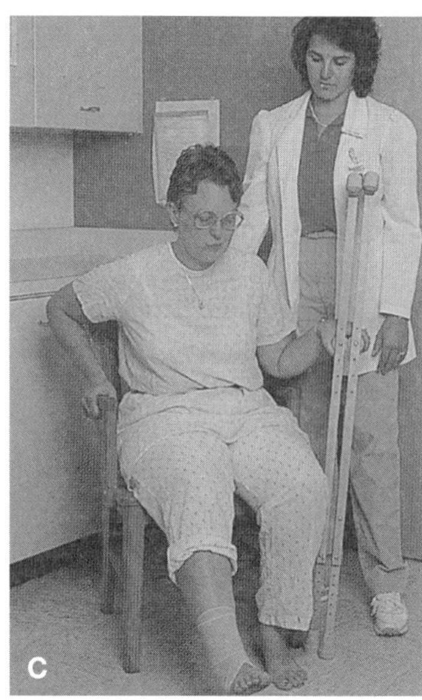

Figure 36.14 | Sitting in a chair. **A**: Both crutches are held by one hand; client transfers weight to crutches and unaffected leg. **B**: Client grasps arm of chair with free hand and begins to lower herself into chair. **C**: Client completely lowers herself into chair *(Potter & Perry 2008)*

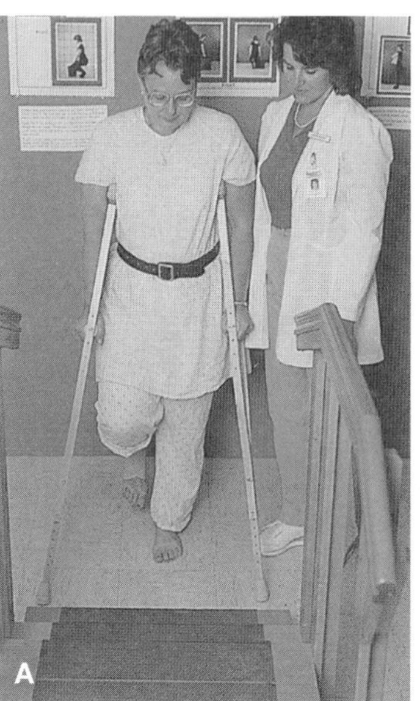

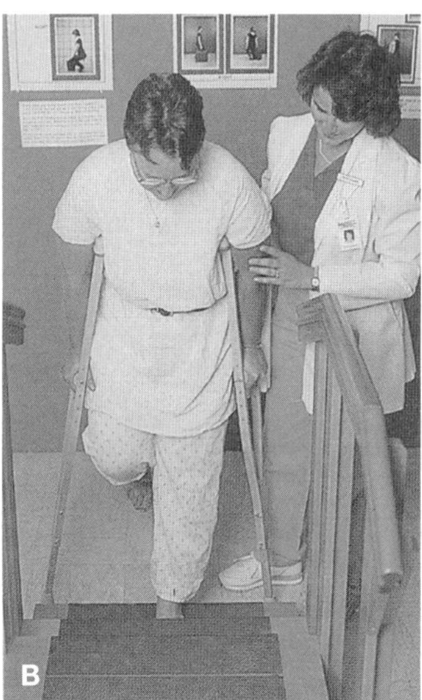

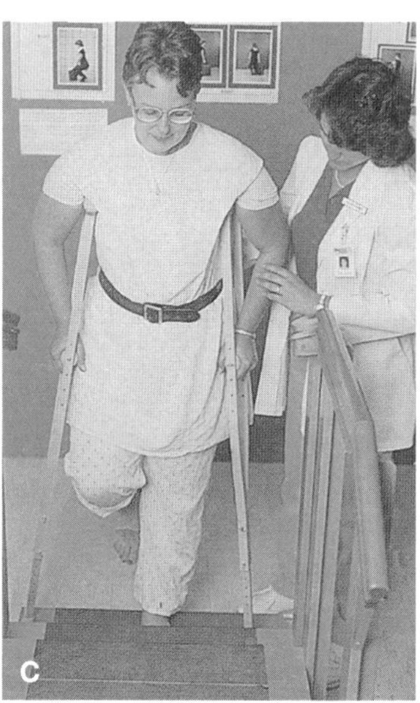

Figure 36.15 | Ascending stairs. **A**: Weight is placed on crutch **B**: Weight is transferred from crutches to unaffected leg on stairs **C**: Crutches are aligned with unaffected leg on stairs *(Potter & Perry 2008)*

as single-tipped, tripod or four point, and should permit 15–30 degree flexion of the elbow. Three- and four-point sticks provide a broad base and greater stability and may be used by a client with poor balance or one-sided weakness.

To use a stick the client holds it close to the body on the unaffected side; taking the weight off the affected leg, the client moves the stick and the affected leg simultaneously, followed by the unaffected leg. Sometimes the three- or four-pronged stick (Figure 36.17) is held on the affected side. Clients are encouraged to keep the stride of each leg, and the timing of each step, equal. While a client is learning to use the stick, the nurse stands behind them to support them if they become unsteady. When going up stairs the stick should be held in one hand and clients encouraged to hold the stair rail, leading with the unaffected leg; when going down stairs the affected leg leads.

Walking frames

Walking frames consist of a metal frame with hand grips, four legs, and one open side (Figure 36.18). A frame may be used by an older adult, as it provides greater support and sense of security than a stick and is useful for those with an unsteady gait, or when partial weight bearing is recommended. The height is selected to allow 15–30

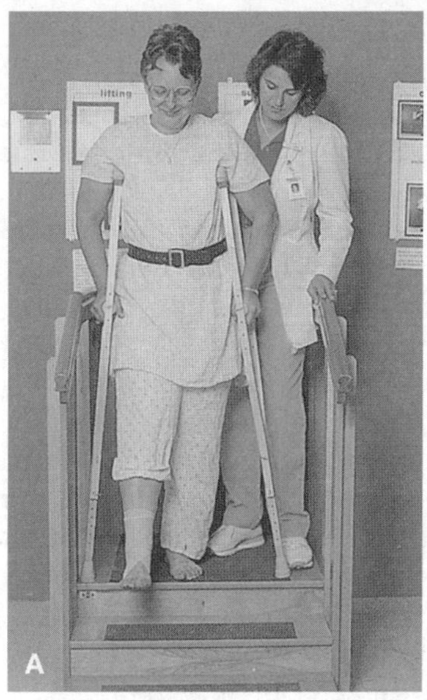
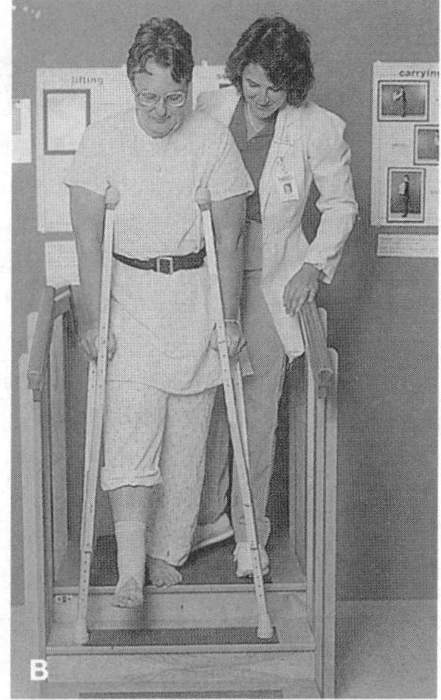
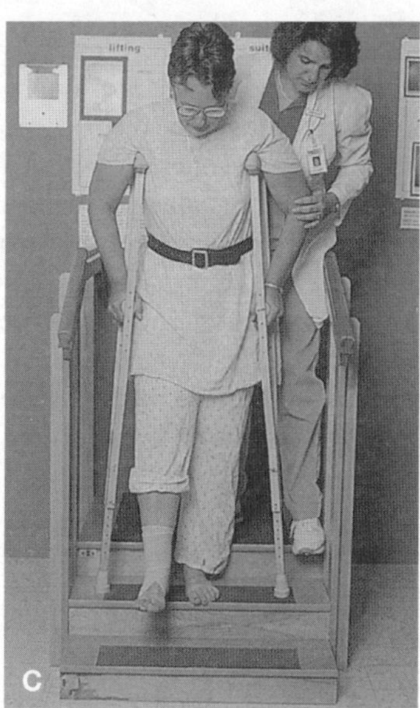

Figure 36.16 | Descending stairs. **A**: Body weight is on unaffected leg **B**: Body weight is transferred to crutches **C**. Unaffected leg is aligned on stairs with crutches *(Potter & Perry 2008)*

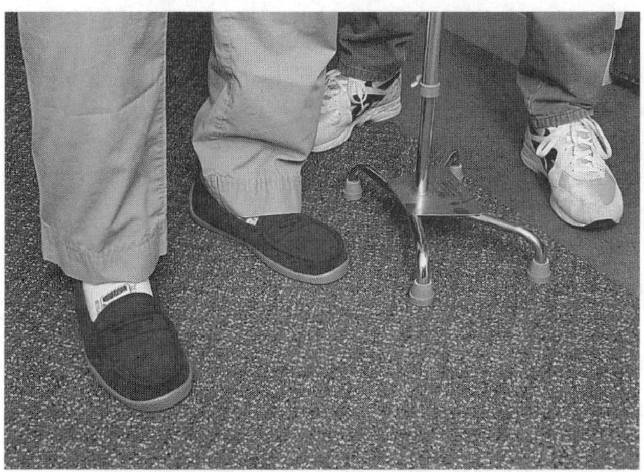

Figure 36.17 | Quad, or four-point stick *(Potter & Perry 2008)*

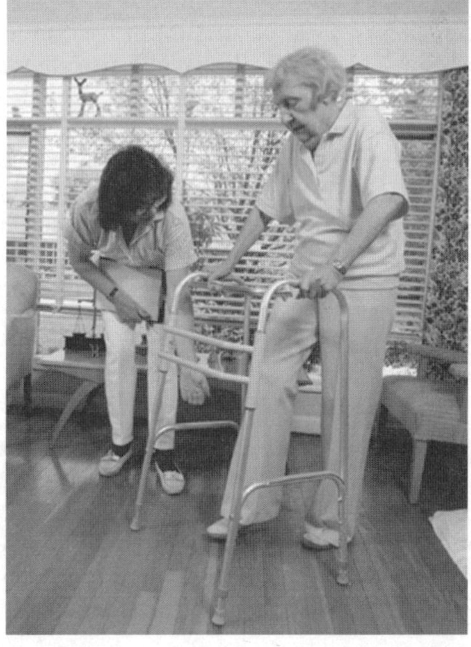

Figure 36.18 | Client using a walking frame *(Potter & Perry 2008)*

degree flexion of the elbows when the hand grips are held. Attachments such as baskets and trays are available to meet specific needs and to promote greater independence. To safely rise from a chair, the frame is placed in front of the client, who then inches forward in the seat of the chair and, with both feet firmly on the ground, and both hands on the arms of the chair, pushes with their arms to stand and, when standing, grasps the frame. Commonly, the client picks the frame up and moves it 15–20 cm forward, then moves one foot, followed by the other, up to the frame. If a client has a one-sided weakness, the affected leg is moved first.

When clients are learning to use a frame, the nurse stands behind them to support the hips and encourage the client to stand upright and look straight ahead. To sit down, the person stands with the back of their knees against the front of the chair, then reaches behind to securely grip the armrests, bending their arms to lower themselves into the chair. When a walking aid is used, the person is assisted until they are confident in the use of the aid and when unassisted use is decided by their medical officer, physiotherapist or nurse, in consultation with other health professionals.

COMPLICATIONS ASSOCIATED WITH REDUCED MOBILITY

The body works more efficiently when people are active, so when a client is confined to bed or immobilised, each system is affected in a negative way. Depending on age, health status, and length and degree of immobility, inactivity can cause both short- and long-term complications. Disuse of muscles leads to degeneration and subsequent loss of function and it is important that clients receive some form of exercise to prevent muscle atrophy. Atrophy begins almost as soon as muscles are immobilised. Clients also experience a limitation in their endurance, which makes activities of daily living difficult. Restoring muscle strength and tone in clients who have been immobilised for any length of time is a slow process. Systemic effects of immobility include:

- Pressure sores or decubitus ulcers
- Contractures
- Cardiovascular and pulmonary stasis
- Urinary stasis
- Constipation
- Depression, anxiety or boredom.

PRESSURE SORES OR DECUBITUS ULCERS

Pressure sores result from localised damage to the skin and underlying tissue caused by pressure, shear or friction (for bedridden clients, shear or amount of friction increases as their head is elevated). Pressure, especially on bony prominences, results in poor circulation, so that the area is deprived of essential nutrients and oxygen, and cellular death may occur. Any client with a mobility or activity deficit should be subject to a pressure-sore risk assessment. Pressure sores remain a significant problem in hospitals and residential care settings despite being largely preventable. (See Chapter 37 for factors that affect skin integrity.)

EFFECTS ON THE MUSCULOSKELETAL SYSTEM

Effects of immobility upon the musculoskeletal system are quickly evident after even short periods of inactivity. People who attempt to walk after several days of bed rest are surprised at how weak their leg muscles have become. Immobilisation and the resultant disuse of muscles leads to atrophy, decreased size, strength and tone of muscles, decreased joint mobility and bone demineralisation.

Contractures and ankylosis

Contractures are abnormal conditions of a joint, characterised by flexion and fixation, caused by atrophy and shortening of muscle fibres. Ankylosis is joint consolidation and immobilisation. Contractures may result from improper support or positioning of a joint, or as a result of inadequate joint movement. For example, if a joint is allowed to remain in one position for an extended length of time, the muscle fibres that normally provide movement shorten to accommodate that position, and lose the ability to contract and relax. Weight-bearing activity stimulates bone formation and balance; however, during immobilisation, bone formation slows, while breakdown of bone increases. With the subsequent loss of bone calcium, phosphorus and matrix, disuse osteoporosis results, and the brittle demineralised bones fracture easily.

For prevention, encourage physical activity and isometric or isotonic active ROM exercises while the client is in correct body alignment. An immobilised person may need direction as well as assistance when they perform ROM exercises. Pressure-relieving devices, such as a bed cradle, may prevent the bedclothes pressing down and forcing joints into abnormal positions.

Footdrop

Footdrop is another term for plantar flexion, which is caused by damage to the nerve supply of the muscle responsible for dorsiflexion of the foot. If a client's feet are allowed to assume plantar flexion for long periods they become fixed in that position so that, when the client attempts to stand or walk, they will be unable to place their heels on the floor and walk normally (Figure 36.19).

Prevention includes using a foot board or firm pillow in the bed to maintain the feet in proper alignment, or dorsiflexion, as if in a standing position (if not contraindicated); that is, at a 90 degree angle. Devices and techniques to keep pressure off the feet should be used, such as a bed cradle or foot pleat in the upper bedclothes. The person's feet should be exercised through their ROM, either actively or passively. If footdrop occurs, management includes use of an orthopaedic brace, intensive physiotherapy or surgical intervention.

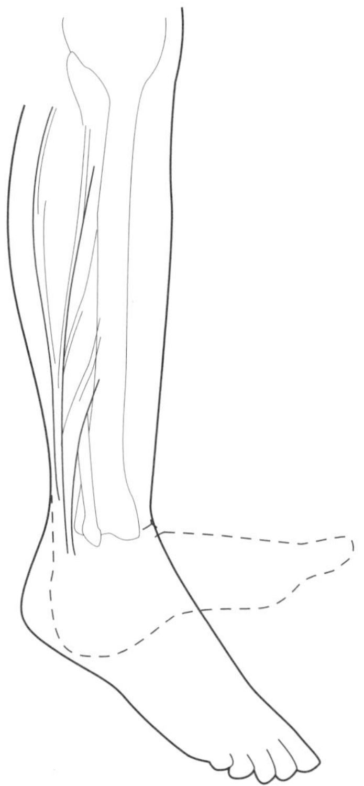

Figure 36.19 | Footdrop. The ankle is fixed in plantar flexion. Normally the ankle is able to flex (dotted line), which eases walking

EFFECTS ON THE CARDIOVASCULAR AND PULMONARY SYSTEMS

The primary negative effects of immobility on the cardiovascular system are increased cardiac workload; orthostatic, or postural, hypotension; and venous thrombosis. An increase in the workload on the heart is probably due to less resistance by blood vessels and changes in blood distribution. Heart rate increases and cardiac output falls after prolonged rest. A significant drop in blood pressure on standing (25 mmHg systolic and 10 mmHg diastolic) is termed orthostatic, or postural, hypotension and is due to a decrease in neurovascular reflexes and muscle tone. In addition, stasis of blood may precipitate clot formation due to a lack of muscular activity that would normally help move blood towards the heart. Serum calcium levels increase as calcium exits bone and enters the bloodstream, which influences clot formation. If a clot or thrombus detaches from the vessel wall and is transported in the bloodstream, it is called an embolus. Emboli that lodge in the pulmonary artery tree are referred to as pulmonary emboli. Depending on the size of the embolus, consequences may be serious.

Prevention of deep vein thrombosis (DVT)

Prevention of pulmonary embolus includes exercises to stimulate venous blood circulation in the legs. Active or passive 2-hourly exercises should be performed and consist of rotating the ankles, dorsiflexion and plantar flexion of the feet, flexing and extending the knees, and raising and lowering each leg. Clients are advised not to cross their legs while lying in bed or sitting. Prolonged pressure on the backs of the legs should be avoided by careful positioning and repositioning. Upper bedclothes should remain loose to allow movement of the legs.

Anti-embolic elastic stockings may be prescribed to facilitate venous return from the lower extremities, prevent venous stasis and venous thrombosis, and reduce peripheral oedema. The stockings expose the toes but cover the foot and extend up the leg to the knee or groin (Figures 36.20 and 36.21). They give firm support to superficial veins in the leg, maintaining adequate venous pressure and reducing the incidence of thrombi. The client's leg(s) are measured to ensure correct fit, then the stockings applied by rolling them slowly from the foot up the leg. Firm even pressure is essential, and the toes are exposed to check that they remain warm and pink and blood supply is not impeded by the stockings. Table 36.6 presents guidelines for applying anti-embolic stockings. For clients requiring surgery, additional preventive measures may include antithrombotic agents pre- and post-operatively (i.e. anticoagulants).

PREVENTION OF POSTURAL OR ORTHOSTATIC HYPOTENSION

Prevention involves the gradual reintroduction of ambulation and allowing clients time to adjust to changes such as going from a lying to a sitting or standing position (see dangling technique, earlier in this chapter).

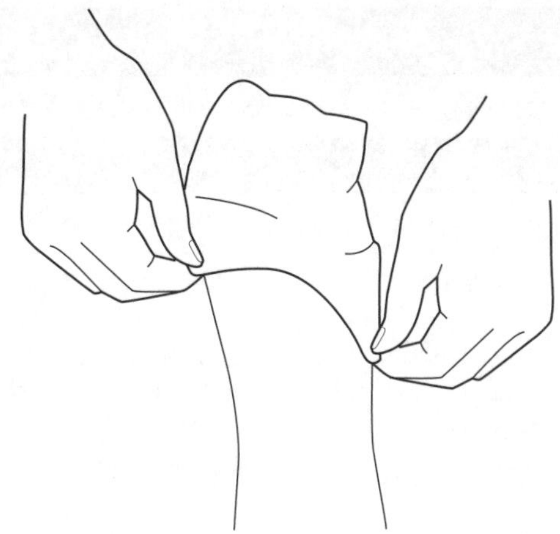

Figure 36.20 | Applying the inverted stocking over the toes

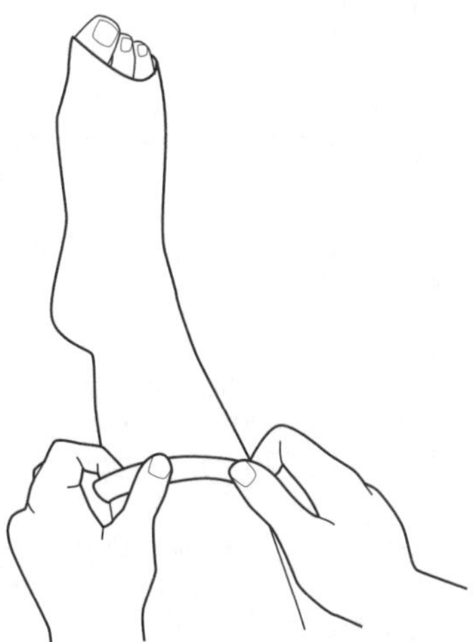

Figure 36.21 | Pulling the stocking snugly over the leg

MANAGEMENT OF PULMONARY EMBOLUS

Management of emboli in the pulmonary system includes administration of oxygen, analgesia and anticoagulant therapy. When immobilised, a person's pulmonary system declines in function, and effects are related to a decrease in the rate and depth of breathing and effort, as well as an increase in bronchial secretions. Lung expansion decreases and breathing deeply is inhibited. In addition, secretions pool in the bronchial tract, which predisposes clients to respiratory tract congestion and infection. Hypostatic pneumonia may result and the risk increases when a person is dehydrated or is given medication that causes respiratory depression, such as morphine.

Atelectasis, or collapse of the lung, may occur and inhibits gaseous exchange at the alveoli. This results in hypoxaemia secondary to hypostatic pneumonia, resulting in an acid–base imbalance. Signs and symptoms of lung congestion include a cough and production of sputum, rattling, distressed or painful breathing, and increased body temperature.

TABLE 36.6 | APPLYING ANTI-EMBOLIC STOCKINGS

Equipment required: tape measure, anti-embolism stockings and talcum powder

Action	Rationale
Review and carry out the standard steps in Appendix 1	
Check the orders for the type of stocking to be applied	Stockings come in three sizes: knee high, thigh high and full length
Measure the client's leg length and circumference of both legs. Compare the measurements to the size chart to obtain stockings of correct size	Ensures that the stockings will fit properly
Apply stockings in the morning if possible, before the client rises	In sitting and standing positions the veins can become distended so that oedema occurs. The stockings should be applied before this happens
Assist the client to a lying position. Ensure that the client's legs are clean and dry and apply a light coating of talcum powder to each leg	This eases application of stockings
Place your hand in one stocking and turn it inside out, down to the heel	Makes it easier to slip the stocking onto the foot without discomfort to the client
Stretch open the stocking at the heel and fit it over the client's foot (Figure 36.20)	Stocking must fit smoothly without wrinkles that might damage the skin's surface
Grasp the top of the stocking and fit it over the ankle and calf (Figure 36.21)	If knee-high stockings are being used, do not pull over the knee or fold the top of the stocking down. The stockings must be the correct length, or they can impair circulation or damage the skin's surface
If thigh-high, fit the top of the stockings over the knee and thigh. Smooth the entire surface to eliminate any wrinkles. Instruct the client not to cross the legs or ankles when sitting in a bed or chair	Leg crossing causes pressure points that can impair venous return
Remove the stockings for 30 minutes every 8 hours	Allows for inspection of the skin and legs for any oedema and peripheral pulses, skin colour and temperature
Document the size, type and application of the stockings	Verifies that the ordered stockings are in place and supports changes for the stockings
Special considerations:	
• Stockings should be washed when soiled. Obtain a second pair for use while stockings are drying. To wash, use mild soap and warm water. Hang to dry	• Stockings should not be off the client for more than 30 minutes at any one time
(adapted from deWit 2005)	

Prevention of pulmonary stasis

Preventing this problem includes nursing clients sitting up when possible and encouraging coughing and deep breathing. Deep breathing exercises are performed with the person in a sitting position. The nurse places one hand on the chest and the other on the abdomen just below the ribs. The client is instructed to inhale slowly and deeply, pushing the abdomen out to promote optimal distribution of air to the alveoli, then breathe out through pursed lips while contracting their abdomen, which forces air out of the lungs. 'Pursed-lip breathing' improves oxygen diffusion, encourages a slow deep-breathing pattern, and puts positive back-pressure on the airways so that they stay open longer and expel greater amounts of stale air. Abdominal contraction pushes the diaphragm upwards, exerts pressure on the lungs and helps to empty them. After several breaths, clients are encouraged to cough up sputum.

Additional chest physiotherapy such as postural drainage and chest percussion and vibration may be added. Fluids should be increased (provided there are no contraindications) to help liquefy secretions and facilitate coughing up secretions or phlegm. Oxygen therapy may be necessary, and medications such as antibiotics may be prescribed if infection is present. Analgesia is offered before chest physiotherapy begins. Nebulisation using normal saline can loosen secretions for ease of expectoration.

URINARY STASIS

Immobility can lead to retention of urine, urinary tract infection or renal calculi. Difficulty in using the pan or bottle in bed can result in incomplete bladder emptying and stasis of urine. Immobility reduces the amount of circulating lactic acid, which leads to alkaline urine (i.e. high urinary pH values) and, together with excess blood calcium (which is excreted by the kidneys), may result in kidney stones.

Prevention of urinary stasis

To prevent stasis of urine, nurses promote an adequate intake of fluids (unless contraindicated), and ensure that clients understand the importance of not postponing urination and of the need to empty the bladder completely.

Management of urinary stasis

Management depends on the cause and includes increasing fluids and treating any infection. (Information on elimination of urine and disorders affecting the urinary system is provided in Chapter 32.)

CONSTIPATION

Constipation may occur as a result of decreased intestinal peristalsis due to reduced mobility or as a result of difficulty in using the bedpan in bed. Preventing and managing constipation includes promoting adequate fluids, exercise and fibre, as well as the appropriate aperient or suppository when required. Clients are encouraged to maintain as normal a routine as possible to promote normal bowel function. (Information on bowel elimination is provided in Chapter 33.)

PSYCHOLOGICAL EFFECTS

Psychological stress, anxiety, depression or boredom can occur when a client is immobilised. Loss of independence occurs when clients have to rely on other people or aids to carry out activities of daily living. It interferes with all aspects of living, and people become bored by the lack of stimulation or variety. A change in the level of independence, and physical impairment or isolation from family and friends, result in feelings of depression, and people may also be anxious and feel worthless, irritable, apathetic and restless. Nurses need to try to improve clients' self-esteem.

Clients are encouraged to participate in decisions regarding care, which allows some control over their life. Changes of environment may be beneficial; for example, some time spent in the day room or outside, reading, using the radio, TV or telephones may prevent boredom. Clients are encouraged to pursue hobbies or studies, or the occupational therapy department may be able to provide alternative activities. A social worker may assist with any problems about finance or the home situation. Flexible visiting hours are important, as well as communication with clients showing concern, respect and empathy, active listening and providing information about care and treatment. It is important that clients are allowed to express their emotions.

CLINICAL INTEREST BOX 36.7
Nursing Diagnoses pertaining to immobility

- Impaired mobility and improper body mechanics
- Activity intolerance
- Body image disturbance
- Coping, ineffective individual
- Gaseous exchange, impaired
- Injury, risk for
- Mobility, impaired physical
- Nutrition, altered
- Pain
- Skin integrity, impaired

See Clinical Interest Box 36.7 for nursing diagnoses pertaining to immobility.

SUMMARY

Movement and exercise are necessary to maintain cardiopulmonary efficiency, muscle strength and tone, and joint mobility. Some form of movement and exercise is advisable for health and wellbeing, as it stimulates the mind, enhances awareness and improves the psychological state. The practice of good body posture and body mechanics reduces muscle fatigue and prevents injury and is important whether lying, sitting, standing or moving. During exercise the joints should move through their full ROM.

A client's ability to exercise should be assessed in order to plan and implement nursing measures to meet their needs. Some clients will be able to move and ambulate independently, while others require assistance. Any technique or aid used to assist a person to move should be one that promotes safety and comfort. Immobility presents challenges for nurses, who can often prevent serious complications by implementing simple measures for movement and exercise. Nurses have a duty of care to identify clients at risk of developing complications while immobilised, and to promote movement and exercise in those who are capable, encouraging independence.

Knowledge of the musculoskeletal system gives the nurse insight into how the body functions during exercise and movement and the way in which exercise can improve health and wellbeing. Pathological changes in the musculoskeletal system can result from inflammation, infection, degeneration, nutritional influences, neoplasms or trauma. Major manifestations include pain, sensory changes, swelling, deformity and impaired mobility. Disorders of the musculoskeletal system may be classified as congenital, degenerative, infectious or inflammatory, immunological, metabolic, neoplastic, traumatic or from multiple causes.

Care of clients with musculoskeletal disorders includes promoting rest, preventing complications of immobility, maintaining skin integrity and nutritional status, relieving pain, preventing psychosocial problems, remobilisation, regaining independence and rehabilitation. Nurses need to be aware of correct positioning of clients who are immobilised, as comfort and correct body alignment are important aspects of care. The general objectives of fracture management are reduction, immobilisation and restoration of function. Exercise has many physical and psychological benefits that greatly enhance wellbeing. Healthy attitudes towards regular exercise can mean a population that ages well and values exercise to prevent disease and illness.

REVIEW EXERCISES

1. What are the principles of good posture and body mechanics?
2. What is the difference between isotonic, isometric and isokinetic exercise?
3. Define range of movement (ROM).
4. Describe how older adults may benefit from exercise.
5. What are the complications associated with immobility?
6. Describe the major manifestations of musculoskeletal system disorders.

CRITICAL THINKING EXERCISE

Mary, 70, recently reported a sudden pain in her lower back when bending down to pick up something. She also says that she has had backache for years, gradually worsening around her trunk, as well as an inability to move as she used to. What precautions would you take when moving Mary? Describe the type of exercise that would be best in Mary's situation and suggest how she can build strong bones.

REFERENCES AND FURTHER READING

Ankner, GM (2007) *Case studies in Medical–Surgical Nursing*. Thomson Delmar Learning, Clifton Park, NY

—— (2008) *Medical–Surgical Nursing*. Thomson Delmar Learning, Clifton Park, NY

Crisp J, Taylor C (eds) (2005) *Potter & Perry's Fundamentals of Nursing*, 2nd edn. Elsevier Australia, Sydney

deWit SC (2005) *Fundamental Concepts and Skills for Nursing*, 2nd edn WB Saunders, Philadelphia

Goldberg I, Elliot DL (2000) *The Healing Power of Exercise: Your Guide to Preventing and Treating Diabetes, Depression, Heart Disease, High Blood Pressure, Arthritis and More*. John Wiley & Sons, New York

Hopman-Rock M, Westhoff MH (2002) Development and Evaluation of Aging Well and Healthily: a Health-Education and Exercise Program for Community-Living Older Adults. *Journal of Aging And Physical Activity*, 10: 364–381

Kozier B, Erb G, Berman AJ, Burke K (2000) *Fundamentals of Nursing: Concepts, Process and Practice*, 6th edn. Prentice-Hall, Upper Saddle River, NJ

Marieb EN (2006) *Essentials of Human Anatomy & Physiology*. Pearson/Benjamin Cummings, San Francisco

Potter PA, Perry AG (2005) *Fundamentals of Nursing*, 6th edn. Mosby, St Louis

—— (2008) *Fundamentals of Nursing*, 7th edn. Mosby, St Louis

Skinner HB (2003) *Current Diagnosis & Treatment in Orthopedics*. Lange Medical Books, New York

Thibodeau GA, Patton KT (2003) *Structure and Function of the Body*, 12th edn. Mosby, St Louis

—— (2007) *Anatomy & Physiology*. Mosby, St Louis

Wilson KJW, Waugh A (1996) *Ross and Wilson's Anatomy and Physiology in Health and Illness*. Churchill Livingstone, London

ONLINE RESOURCES

Health Scout News (2003) *Can Exercise Lower your Blood Cholesterol?* www.health.yahoo.com/health/centers/cholesterol

NSW Government. Gentle exercise classes: www.mhcs.health.nsw.gov.au/health-public-affairs/mhcs/pdfs/5920/BHC-5920-ENG.pdf

NSW Health (2001) *Overweight and Obesity in Australian Children*: www.health.nsw.gov.au/obesity/adult/summit/summit.html

Walking and Health: www.health.yahoo.com/health/centers/fitness/_2146.html

Chapter 37

SKIN INTEGRITY AND WOUND CARE

OBJECTIVES

- Define the key terms/concepts
- Describe the structure of the skin
- Describe the functions of the skin
- Identify the risk factors for loss of skin integrity
- Discuss the wound-healing process
- Describe the different wound-healing intentions
- Describe the classifications of wound types
- Identify the principles of wound management
- Describe the differences between acute and chronic wounds
- Describe the procedures related to care of surgical wounds
- Describe the care required to prevent and manage decubitus ulcers/pressure sores
- Discuss the differences between arterial and venous leg ulcers
- Describe the care required to prevent and manage skin tears
- Describe the management of loss of skin integrity related to burns
- Describe the major manifestations of skin disorders
- Complete an assessment for an individual with impaired skin integrity
- List the nursing diagnoses associated with impaired skin integrity
- Assist in planning and implementing nursing care for the individual with a loss of skin integrity
- List appropriate nursing interventions for the individual with impaired skin integrity

KEY TERMS/CONCEPTS

burns
modern wound-management principles
normal wound-healing process
pressure sores
risk factors
skin disorders
skin structure and function
skin tears
wound assessment
wound stages

CHAPTER FOCUS

The skin has several functions, which are largely concerned with protection of the body against infection, physical trauma and ultraviolet radiation. Any disorder that disrupts normal skin function will affect the efficiency with which it carries out its functions, and may place the physiological integrity of the individual at risk. The effects that disorders of the skin have on the individual range from being minor and temporary, to major and life threatening. Some serious skin disorders such as burns affect the individual to the extent that self-concept and body image are severely impaired. Wound management is a major role of the nurse. It is important that all nurses have a good knowledge of normal wound healing and the variances that can occur with ageing and disease processes. There is an abundance of literature on wound management and a vast array of wound-care products. The aim of this chapter is to assist the nurse unravel some of the confusion.

LIVED EXPERIENCE

After I had open heart surgery, I was very concerned about the scars on my chest. I thought I would never be able to wear a low-cut blouse again. But the nurses explained to me that with the new dressings available today the wound will heal very well and the scar will become less noticeable over time.

Joy, 56, heart surgery client

THE INTEGUMENTARY SYSTEM

The integumentary system consists of the skin and its appendages; the hair, nails, sweat and sebaceous glands. The skin (or integument) is the largest organ of the body, covering about 7500 cm^2 of surface area in an average adult (Figure 37.1). It is a protective barrier to the outside world, plays a vital role in homeostasis, and also provides a major means of communication through touch and sensation. The appendages of the skin — hair, nails and glands — arise from the epidermis but are present in the dermis.

STRUCTURE OF THE SKIN

The skin is comprised of two basic layers: the epidermis and dermis. Under the dermis is a layer of adipose tissue called subcutaneous tissue. While this layer is not considered to be part of the skin, subcutaneous tissue does protect and insulate the deeper tissues.

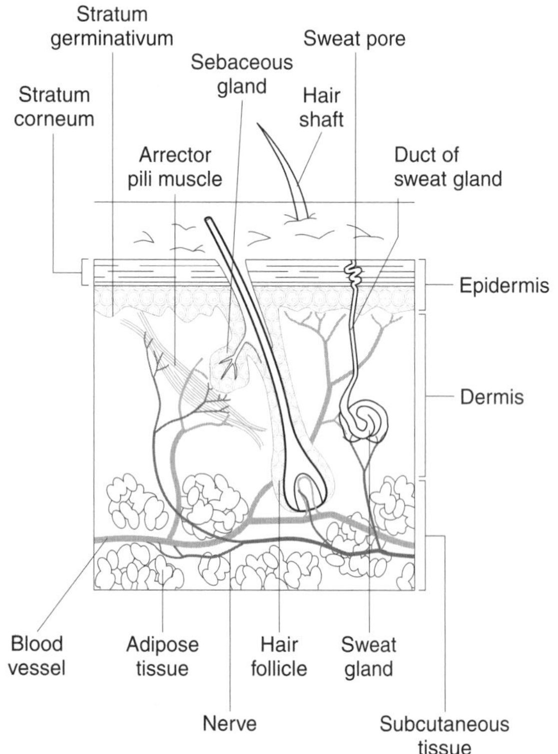

Figure 37.1 | Structure of the skin

The epidermis

The epidermis is the thin outermost layer and is composed of epithelial cells arranged in layers of stratified epithelium. The number of layers varies according to the amount of wear and tear experienced; for example, there are many more layers on the soles of the feet and the palms of the hands than there are between the toes and the fingers.

The epidermis is divided into two layers. The horny layer (stratum corneum) is the uppermost layer, and consists of about 30 layers of dead, flattened keratinised cells. These keratinocytes contain a waterproof hard protein substance called keratin. Keratin's waterproofing properties protect the body and prevent escape of fluid from the deeper tissues. Keratin is also responsible for the formation of hair and nails. The germinative layer (stratum germinativum) is the deeper layer of the epidermis. It is here that new cells are constantly being formed and pushed upwards to replace cells that die and are rubbed off. Millions of new cells are produced daily and are pushed up away from the source of nutrition, to become part of the outermost layer.

Melanocytes are present in the germinative layer. Their function is to produce a brown pigment called melanin. Melanin gives colour to the skin and protects the body against the damaging effects of ultraviolet rays in sunlight. Brown-toned skin results when large amounts of melanin are produced, whereas light-toned skin results when the body produces less melanin.

The epidermis does not contain any blood vessels, but receives its essential substances from fluid that comes from the blood supply to the dermis. As cells are pushed towards the surface, away from the source of nutrition, they die and are eventually rubbed off. Thousands of dead epithelial cells are flaked off every day, which means that they are deposited on clothing and on every surface touched. They become part of the dust in a room, serve as food for mites, and harbour microorganisms. A person sheds about 0.5 kg of dead cells per year, much of which goes down the bathroom drain.

The patterns of lines and ridges in the epidermis are due to projections in the dermis called papillae. On the fingertips these patterns are the fingerprints, which are different in every individual. For this reason, fingerprints are useful for purposes of identification. Nails are formed from the stratum corneum and are composed of modified epithelium.

The dermis

The dermis consists of white fibrous tissue containing many elastic fibres. Elasticity of the skin is essential to allow for changes in the size of a part of the body without tearing, such as the abdominal area during pregnancy. In old age the fibres become less elastic, causing wrinkles and folds to appear in the skin. The following structures are contained in the dermis.

Network of blood vessels

The blood vessels transport blood containing oxygen and nutrients to the dermis and transport blood containing wastes such as carbon dioxide away from the dermis. The blood vessels also play a role in regulating body temperature. If the body temperature is elevated the dermal capillaries become engorged with blood, which allows loss of body heat from the skin surface through radiation. If the environmental temperature is low, blood vessels in the skin constrict, conserving body heat by reducing radiation from the body.

Nerve endings

The dermis has a rich nerve supply consisting of several types of nerve endings. Each type of nerve ending reacts to a different stimulus, such as pain, touch, pressure and temperature. Impulses are transmitted from the nerve endings to the brain for interpretation.

Hair follicles and hairs

Hairs grow from hair follicles, which are deep pouch-like cavities in the skin. Although hair follicles are present in most areas of the skin, they are not found on the palms of the hands or the soles of the feet. Hair is composed of modified epithelium and grows from roots deep in the follicles. The part of a hair projecting above the epidermis is called the shaft. Hair colour reflects the amount of pigment, generally melanin, in the epidermis. Hair is a protection from the elements and from trauma; for example, the scalp hair and eyebrows are barriers against sunlight, and the nasal hairs filter inhaled air.

Hair growth is influenced by the sex hormones oestrogen and testosterone. An excessive growth of hair is called hirsutism. Like other cells that compose the skin, the hair cells also become keratinised. The hair that we brush, blow dry and curl is a collection of dead keratinised cells. Hair colour is genetically controlled and is determined by the type and amount of melanin. The absence of melanin produces white hair. Grey hair is due to a mixture of pigmented and non-pigmented hairs. Red hair is due to a modified type of melanin that contains iron. Hair is important cosmetically. Hair loss can be very distressing for some people. The most common type of hair loss is male-pattern baldness. It is a hereditary condition characterised by a gradual loss of hair with ageing.

Arrector pili muscles

These are minute involuntary muscles, with one end attached to a hair follicle and the other end to the dermis. When these muscles contract, for example, during fear or exposure to cold, the follicles and hairs become erect. Contraction of the muscles also causes some elevation of the skin around the hairs, giving rise to the 'goose pimple' appearance. The contraction of the arrector pili muscles increases heat production. This response is called shivering.

Sebaceous glands

Sebaceous glands are small glands, most of which open into hair follicles. The glands produce sebum, which is an oily substance and a lubricant that keeps the skin soft and moist and prevents the hair from becoming brittle. Combined with sweat, sebum forms a moist, oily acidic film that is mildly antibacterial. During periods of increased hormonal activity, such as adolescence, sebaceous glands become very active and the skin becomes oilier.

Sweat glands

Sweat glands, which are widely distributed, are either eccrine or apocrine. Eccrine glands are present all over the body and produce a clear perspiration. Apocrine glands are found mainly in the axillary and genital areas, and secrete sweat that has a strong characteristic odour. Sweat glands are coiled in appearance, with a straight duct that releases sweat onto the surface of the skin through an opening called a pore.

Sweat glands play a part in regulating body temperature. They excrete large amounts of sweat when the external, or body, temperature is high. When sweat evaporates off the skin's surface it carries large amounts of body heat with it. Sweat consists of water that contains sodium chloride, phosphates, urea, ammonia and other waste products. Under normal circumstances, the amount of sweat secreted by an individual is about 700 mL/day. Under some conditions, such as strenuous physical exertion or pyrexia, the amount can be increased to as much as 1500 mL/day. Much of the water lost through the skin evaporates immediately, so it is not noticeable and is called insensible perspiration. Sweat that makes the skin damp and is noticeable is called sensible perspiration.

FUNCTIONS OF THE SKIN

The major functions in which the skin and its appendages play a role are protection, thermoregulation, metabolism and sensory perception.

Protection

The skin is the first line of defence against the external environment. It provides a barrier to a variety of harmful agents, such as microorganisms, radiant energy and chemical substances. The skin acts as a barrier to harmful agents only as long as it remains intact. The waterproof quality of the outer layer prevents excess water absorption and abnormal loss of body fluids. The skin contains nerve endings that are sensitive to painful stimuli. The nerve endings transmit impulses to the brain that alert the individual that damage is occurring.

Thermoregulation

The skin plays a major role in the maintenance of constant body temperature. Blood conducts heat from internal structures to the skin for dissipation. The skin dissipates excess body heat by radiation, conduction, convection and evaporative cooling. Body temperature is controlled by the hypothalamus, which is the heat-regulating centre in the brain. This centre is sensitive to the temperature of the blood passing through it and also receives sensory stimuli from nerve endings in the skin that react to heat and cold (thermoreceptors). The hypothalamus in turn relays impulses requiring vasodilation and activation of the sweat glands (for cooling), or vasoconstriction and inhibition of sweat glands (for heat retention). Thus, the hypothalamus acts like a thermostat that initiates heat-losing activities when the body temperature begins to rise, and heat-retaining activities when the body temperature starts to fall.

Metabolism

The skin assists in the regulation of fluid and electrolyte balance by eliminating water and small amounts of sodium chloride through the sweat glands. Sweat consists of 99.4% water, 0.2% salts, and 0.4% urea and other wastes. In the presence of sunlight or ultraviolet radiation, the skin begins the process of forming vitamin D (calciferol), a substance required for absorbing calcium and phosphates from food.

Sensory perception

Through perception of a painful stimuli, the skin causes an avoidance reaction, while other receptors perceive sensations of pressure and touch. The skin is therefore an agent of communication between the outside environment and the body, as the activity of sensory nerve endings informs the individual of what is happening outside the body.

Factors that affect skin integrity

Many risk factors can affect the integrity of the skin, including:

- Immobility and inactivity
- Restlessness
- Sedation
- Neurological factors, such as paraplegia, quadriplegia and multiple sclerosis
- Poor nutrition and hydration status
- Systemic and local circulation and oxygenation
- Presence or absence of excessive moisture
- Vascular conditions such as peripheral vascular disease
- Age-related factors
- Obesity
- Exposure to pressure, friction, shearing forces or burns
- Exposure to chemicals
- Diseases such as diabetes mellitus
- Immunological suppression as a result of systemic conditions or medications
- Trauma from falls, accidents or burns
- Surgical intervention
- Inappropriate or ill-fitting prostheses and footwear
- Infection
- Skin disorders, e.g., genetic factors, idiopathic causes, hypersensitivity rashes.

WOUND HEALING

Wound healing is a dynamic and complex process and consists of four stages: haemostasis, the inflammation stage, the reconstruction phase and the maturation phase. The process of wound healing begins at the moment of injury and can continue for some years.

HAEMOSTASIS

The first stage of wound healing is haemostasis, which has three components, vasoconstriction, platelet response and the biochemical response. Vasoconstriction is when the bleeding in the wound is arrested by spasm in the arteries, arterioles and capillaries.

The platelet response is commonly described as the formation of the platelet plug. When platelets come into contact with parts of a damaged blood vessel, such as collagen or endothelium, their characteristics change. They become larger and irregular in shape and stick to the collagen fibres in the wall of the vessels and to each other. The platelets release various chemicals — serotonin, prostaglandins, phospholipids and adenosine diphosphate (ADP)—which attract more platelets, which stick to the original platelets and form the plug. This platelet plug is very effective in preventing blood loss in a small vessel.

The biochemical component is the formation of a blood clot through the processes of the intrinsic and extrinsic clotting pathways, clot retraction and fibrinolysis. This is a complex process involving different clotting factors that are released from the damaged tissue. A clot is developed and retraction of the wound takes place.

The next stage of the healing process is termed tissue repair. This stage also has three phases — inflammation, reconstruction and maturation — which overlap each other and have varying time intervals.

THE INFLAMMATION PHASE

This phase begins the moment that injury is incurred. The capillaries contract and thrombose to facilitate haemostasis. Vasodilation of the surrounding tissues occurs in response to the release of histamine and other vasoactive chemicals. This process causes increased blood flow to the surrounding tissue, which produces erythema, swelling, heat and discomfort, such as throbbing. A variety of white blood cells called polymorphonuclear leucocytes arrives at the site of the wound as a defence response and is involved in the immune response to fight infection. Polymorphs, macrophages and their associated growth factors produce various local and systemic effects. This phase continues for about 3 days.

THE RECONSTRUCTION PHASE

This is a time of cleaning and temporary replacement of tissue. The polymorphs kill bacteria, and the phagocytic macrophages digest the dead bacteria and debris to clean up the wound. Dermal repair is necessary if the wound is one of full thickness. New blood capillaries are developed (angiogenesis) and granulation tissue, which consists largely of collagen, is laid down. Epithelial cells migrate over the granulation tissue from the surrounding wound edges, hair follicles, sweat or sebaceous glands in the wound. These cells are very fragile. When the wound is covered the epithelium begins to thicken to 4–5 layers, forming the epidermis. Wound contraction then occurs, reducing the overall size of the wound. This phase can continue for 2–24 days.

THE MATURATION PHASE

This is commonly known as the remodelling phase. The matrix of collagen cells is reorganised and strengthened. This phase can continue for about 24 days to 1 year. The wound is still at risk during this phase and should be protected.

HEALING INTENTIONS

When the wound has minimal tissue loss and the edges can be brought together by sutures or clips, as in a surgical wound, the wound is said to heal by primary intention, or first intention. Granulation tissue is not obvious. Healing by secondary intention occurs when wound edges cannot be brought together, as with a gaping wound. Granulation tissue fills in the wound until re-epithelialisation takes place and a large scar results. Third intention, or delayed primary intention, healing occurs when wound closure is delayed for a few days, so that an infected or contaminated wound can be debrided (dirt, foreign objects, damaged tissue and cellular debris are removed from a wound or burn to prevent infection and promote wound healing). Closure of contaminated wounds is usually delayed until all layers of wound tissue show no signs of infection, usually within 4–10 days. At other times some wounds need surgical intervention such as the application of skin grafts or flaps to speed the healing process and reduce the risk of infection. Clinical Interest Box 37.1 provides details on skin grafts.

CLINICAL INTEREST BOX 37.1
Skin grafts

Skin grafts speed up the healing process and reduce the risk of infection. Grafts may be partial or full thickness. Skin grafts are classified as:

- Autograft: a surgical relocation of skin to the wound from another site of the body. A second wound results and is known as the donor site
- Allograft: a donor graft of skin between allogenic individuals, such as from one person to another
- Xenograft: a donor graft of tissue transplanted between different species, such as tissue of porcine origin transplanted to a human being
- Cultured: the cultivation of epidermis from a small amount of epithelial cells taken from the donor or recipient's body and cultivated under laboratory conditions to form epidermis, before being transplanted back to the individual.

FACTORS THAT AFFECT WOUND HEALING

Factors that affect wound healing include:

- Wound infection
- Allowing the wound to dry out and form a scab (wound hydration)
- Allowing maceration of the wound to occur (exudate management)
- Inappropriate dressings
- Temperature variances
- Not treating the underlying cause
- Keloid formation
- Foreign bodies
- Friction, shearing forces and pressure
- Age
- Underlying disease
- Vascularity
- Obesity
- Disorders of sensation and movement
- Drugs
- Psychological state
- Nutritional status
- Radiation therapy.

TYPES OF WOUNDS

SEPTIC AND ASEPTIC WOUNDS

Clean wound

These wounds are made under aseptic conditions such as surgery, and heal by primary intention. These wounds generally do not require drainage.

Clean-contaminated wound

This is a wound made under aseptic conditions, but involving a body cavity that normally harbours microorganisms, such as the gastrointestinal, respiratory or urinary tract.

Contaminated wound

This term applies to a wound in which microorganisms are likely to be present, and includes open, traumatic and accidental wounds and surgical wounds in which a break in asepsis occurred.

Dirty wound

This term applies to traumatic wounds that are generally more than 4 hours old. Purulent discharge is evident. The wounds involve perforation of viscera and spillage of contents.

Infected wound

Wounds that show signs of early infection are red, swollen, hot and painful. If not treated appropriately, cellulitis develops and may lead to conditions such as lymphangitis, lymphadenitis, bacteraemia, septicaemia and possibly even death.

ACUTE AND CHRONIC WOUNDS

Acute wounds

Acute wounds in early stages are frequently not colonised with bacteria, but infection can become a complication. Although infection cannot always be prevented, care should be taken to minimise transmission by thorough aseptic technique when attending to the wound. Examples of acute wounds are those made by surgical incision or traumatic injury. An example of a surgical wound is a skin flap (refer to Clinical Interest Box 37.2).

Chronic wounds

Chronic wounds are rarely sterile. Microbial colonisation is usually present, predisposing the wound to infection. Clinical infection depends on the virulence of the bacteria and the resistance of the host. Clinical Interest Box 37.3 provides the differences between inflammatory response and infection. An example of a chronic wound is a venous leg ulcer.

Wounds can be described according to the amount of damage done to the tissues:

- Superficial: wounds affecting the epidermis
- Partial thickness: wounds affecting the epidermis and the dermis
- Full thickness: wounds that have affected the epidermis, dermis and the subcutaneous tissue; the muscle, tendon and bone may also be involved.

CLASSIFICATION OF WOUNDS BY STAGES

Stage I

Observable pressure-related alteration(s) of intact skin, whose indicators, as compared to the adjacent or opposite area on the body, may include changes in skin temperature (warmth or coolness), tissue consistency (firm or boggy feel) and/or sensation (pain, itching).

Stage II

Partial-thickness skin loss involving the epidermis and/or dermis. The ulcer is superficial and presents clinically as an abrasion, blister or shallow crater.

Stage III

Full-thickness skin loss involving damage or necrosis of subcutaneous tissue that may extend down to, but not through, underlying fascia. The ulcer presents clinically as a deep crater with or without undermining of adjacent tissue.

Stage IV

Full-thickness skin loss with extensive destruction, tissue necrosis or damage to muscle, bone or supporting structures (e.g. tendons or joint capsules) (Australian Wound Management Association 2001; Cuddigan, Ayello & Sussman 2002).

CLASSIFICATION OF WOUNDS BY COLOUR

Wounds may be classified by colour, as follows:

- Black: necrotic tissue can be dry or moist
- Yellow: usually moist sloughy wound
- Green: moist, sloughy; can be indicative of infection. Usually accompanied by pain, heat, swelling, redness and exudating pus

CLINICAL INTEREST BOX 37.2
Skin flaps

A flap is a surgical relocation of tissue from one part of the body to another part to reconstruct a primary defect. This creates a secondary defect that will require skin grafting or primary closure.

Types of flaps

Skin, or cutaneous, flaps are grafts of tissue consisting of skin and superficial fascia. Composite tissue flaps are described according to the type of tissue they are composed of; for example, fasciocutaneous flap.

Flaps can be classified as free and pedicle. A free flap is the relocation of skin and subcutaneous tissue as a complete segment, with an anastomosis of the segment's blood supply to vessels at the affected site. A pedicle flap is the surgical transfer of skin and subcutaneous tissue to another body site. Blood supply to the flap is maintained via a vascular pedicle attached to the body donor site.

CLINICAL INTEREST BOX 37.3
Recognising the differences between inflammatory response and infection

Inflammation	Infection
Localised redness	Erythema (spreading redness)
Pain	Increasing local wound pain
Heat	Change in the appearance of the wound tissue
Swelling	Increase in the amount of wound exudate
	Purulent or very foul smelling exudate
	Induration (hardness of the surrounding tissue)

- Red: healthy granulating wound
- Pink: epithelialising wound, usually has a translucent appearance.

PATHOPHYSIOLOGICAL INFLUENCES/EFFECTS AND MAJOR MANIFESTATIONS OF SKIN DISORDERS

PATHOPHYSIOLOGICAL INFLUENCES AND EFFECTS

The major factors that affect normal structure and functions of the skin can generally be classified into six categories:

1. Genetic factors
2. Idiopathic causes
3. Hypersensitivity
4. Trauma
5. Neoplasia
6. Infections and infestations.

Genetic factors

Genetic factors determine skin colour and the amount and distribution of hair. Congenital skin disorders include birthmarks, hypopigmentation (albinism) and a condition called ichthyosis, which involves excessive scaling or thickening of the outermost skin layer. Heredity also plays a role in predisposition to the development of acne and atopic dermatitis.

Idiopathic causes

Many skin disorders have no one known cause, for example, vitiligo and psoriasis. Other skin disorders may be associated with emotional or physical stress but there does not seem to be any one identifiable cause.

Hypersensitivity

Some individuals have a tendency to react adversely to contact with various substances, for example, when a substance is inhaled, ingested or comes in contact with the skin. Some allergic reactions are manifested in alterations in the skin; for example, reddening and itching of the skin may be side effects of certain medications.

Trauma

Damage to the skin can result from exposure to extremes of temperature, from prolonged pressure on the skin or from physical injuries resulting in lacerations, punctures or abrasions.

Neoplasia

Any abnormal growth of new tissue, whether benign or malignant, is called a neoplasm. Examples include calluses, which can develop on the toes from friction and chronic pressure, or keloid scarring, which can result after injury to the skin. Benign or malignant neoplasms may develop from any type of cell in the skin, but the melanocytes and keratinocytes are the cells most frequently involved. A mole (naevus) is a common type of benign skin tumour. Some benign epithelial cell lesions may develop into malignant neoplasms.

Infections and infestations

If the skin is broken and pathogenic microorganisms gain entry, infection may result.

Primary skin infections are commonly caused by bacteria, fungi and viruses. Secondary skin infections may occur in conditions such as stasis dermatitis, in which impaired circulation damages skin cells of the lower limbs.

Systemic infections, such as measles, chickenpox and some sexually transmitted diseases, also result in manifestations on the skin. Skin infestations occur when parasites such as lice or mites invade and subsist on the skin.

MAJOR MANIFESTATIONS OF SKIN DISORDERS

Various structural and functional changes accompany skin disorders.

Pruritus

Pruritus (itching) is one of the more common and distressing symptoms of a skin disorder. Pruritus is thought to result from a disruption in the skin nerve endings. Scratching to relieve pruritus can result in tissue damage and infection, thereby causing further discomfort.

Lesions

Depending on the type of skin disorder, one or a variety of lesions may be present. Observation of the patient includes assessing any lesions to determine their shape, size and distribution. Table 37.1 lists and describes the various types of skin lesions. Some types of lesions may discharge fluid, which is referred to as exudate.

Alterations in sensation

In addition to pruritus, the individual may experience other abnormal skin sensations such as numbness, tingling, burning or pain.

Alterations in skin colour

Disorders of the skin may be accompanied by darkened areas of skin (hyperpigmentation), patches of pale skin (hypopigmentation) or inflammation. Burned skin may be reddened, blanched or charred, depending on the extent of the burn. Cold injuries can result in red areas, as in chilblains, or in extreme pallor, as in frostbite.

Alterations in skin temperature

In certain skin disorders such as bacterial infection the skin may feel hot to touch, whereas in other conditions such as frostbite the skin is cool to touch.

TABLE 37.1 | SKIN LESIONS

Term	Description	Examples
Bulla	Elevated, filled with clear fluid. Similar to a vesicle, but larger	Pemphigus vulgaris, drug eruptions, partial thickness burns
Comedo	A plug of secretion contained in a follicle	Acne
Crust	A superficial mass caused by dried exudate	Impetigo, eczema
Cyst	Encapsulated mass in the dermis or subcutaneous layer. May be raised or flat, and contain fluid or solid material	Sebaceous cyst
Erosion	Moist, red, depressed break in the epidermis. Follows rupture of a vesicle or bulla	Chickenpox
Excoriation	Superficial break in the skin	Scratches, abrasions
Fissure	Deep, linear, red crack or break exposing the dermis	Tinea pedis
Macule	Small circumscribed discolouration, e.g., red, white, tan or brown	Freckle, rubella, scarlet fever
Nodule	Circumscribed, elevated area — usually 1–2 cm in diameter	Ganglion, acne
Papule	Circumscribed, elevated, firm palpable area	Mole, wart, pimple
Plaque	Elevated, rough flat-topped areas	Psoriasis, seborrhoeic warts
Pustule	A vesicle or bulla containing pus	Acne, furuncle, folliculitis, impetigo
Scale	Mass of exfoliated epidermis	Dandruff, psoriasis
Scar (cicatrix)	Ranges from a thin line to thick, irregular fibrous tissue. May be white, pink or red	Healed surgical incision or wound
Tumour	Elevated, solid formation	Lipoma, melanoma, fibroma
Ulcer	Depressed circumscribed area involving loss of the epidermis, exposing the dermis, and may involve subcutaneous tissue	Decubitus ulcer, stasis ulcer
Vesicle	Circumscribed, elevated superficial area filled with clear fluid	Blister, herpes simplex infection, contact dermatitis
Weal	Transitory, elevated irregularly-shaped swelling of the epidermis	Urticaria, insect bites

Alterations in texture

Abnormalities of texture, for example, roughness or hardness, may result from the presence of certain types of lesions such as scabs or papules. Scaling may occur, or the skin may be thick, wrinkled, or atrophied. Some skin disorders may result in areas of oedema; for example, injuries from heat or cold.

Presence of an odour

Certain skin disorders, particularly those that are accompanied by oozing lesions, may give rise to an offensive odour.

Systemic manifestations

Certain skin disorders, such as acute contact dermatitis or carbuncles, may be accompanied by systemic effects such as fatigue, nausea, headaches and an elevated body temperature.

SPECIFIC DISORDERS OF THE SKIN

GENETIC DISORDERS

Genetic disorders are those that are present at birth, become evident soon after birth, or those that may be passed on to the next generation.

Acne vulgaris is a chronic inflammatory condition involving the sebaceous glands and the pilosebaceous follicles, particularly of the face. A blackhead forms and blocks the opening of a sebaceous gland, which becomes infected. Later, a pustule forms. This condition is most often present in adolescents and young adults. Familial tendencies are thought to contribute to the cause or exacerbation of acne. Other causative factors include endocrine imbalances, use of oral contraceptives, hormone therapy, emotional stress and lack of personal hygiene.

Ichthyosis is any one of several inherited conditions in which the skin is dry, hyperkeratotic and fissured, resembling fish scales. It usually appears at, or shortly after, birth. Ichthyosis vulgaris is the most common type and the least severe.

IDIOPATHIC DISORDERS

Idiopathic disorders are those in which no definite cause can be identified.

Psoriasis is a chronic skin disorder characterised by red patches covered by thick, dry, silvery scales. The lesions may be present on any part of the body but are more common on the extensor surfaces of the elbows and knees and on the scalp. Psoriasis can be exacerbated by trauma, infection, stress and the use of specific systemic medications.

Pityriasis rosea is thought to be caused by a virus, and

is characterised by a scaling, pink macular rash that spreads over the trunk and other parts of the body. The condition is self-limiting and usually disappears within 4–6 weeks.

Vitiligo is a benign disorder consisting of irregular patches of skin totally lacking in pigment.

Seborrhoeic dermatitis is a chronic inflammatory condition characterised by dry or moist, red scaly eruptions. Common sites are the scalp, eyelids, face and trunk. The scales have a greasy feel and yellow crusts. Cradle cap is one form of seborrhoeic dermatitis.

HYPERSENSITIVITY DISORDERS

These disorders result from an immediate or delayed reaction after exposure to a certain substance.

Contact dermatitis is caused by an irritant substance that comes into direct contact with the skin, such as detergents, hair dye, metals, preservatives, perfumes or specific fabrics. The resultant inflammation and skin rash may be mild or severe, depending on the individual's response. Chronic exposure to an irritant may result in the skin becoming reddened, scaly or cracked.

Atopic dermatitis usually occurs when there is a history of asthma and/or hay fever. The condition is characterised by pruritus, redness of the skin, papules and thickening of the skin. Common sites are the face and neck, behind the knees and in the cubital fossae, and on the back of the hands.

Urticaria is a pruritic skin eruption characterised by transient weals with well-defined red margins and pale centres. Urticaria (hives) is most frequently caused by foods, insect bites and inhalants. Specific types of urticaria are associated with systemic diseases. Pruritus associated with urticaria is frequently intense and is commonly accompanied by stinging, numbness or prickling sensations. Urticaria may also be a manifestation of an adverse reaction to a drug, and the skin lesions may appear almost immediately or several days after the drug has been absorbed. Drugs responsible for such adverse reaction include acetylsalicylic acid, penicillin and codeine.

Pemphigus vulgaris is an uncommon disorder of the skin and mucous membranes, characterised by the formation of large bullae containing clear fluid. The disorder is thought to result from an autoimmune response, and may be fatal if untreated. The bullae erupt, ooze and bleed readily, and death is often due to a secondary bacterial infection or loss of blood protein.

TRAUMA

A traumatic injury, which involves damage to the skin, may be due to direct force, penetration or extremes of temperature.

Erythrocyanosis (chilblains) is redness and swelling of the skin as a result of excessive exposure to cold. Burning, itching, blistering and ulceration may occur; the areas most commonly affected are the toes, fingers, nose and ears.

Frostbite is the traumatic effect of extreme cold on the skin and subcutaneous tissues, characterised by pallor of the exposed areas, such as the nose, ears, fingers and toes. Vasoconstriction and damage to blood vessels impair local circulation, resulting in oedema, anoxia and necrosis.

Immersion (trench) foot is a condition of the skin on the feet that develops from continued exposure to wetness and coldness, such as prolonged immersion in cold water. The feet appear pale, cold and swollen, and the individual experiences tingling followed by loss of sensation.

Burns are injuries to the body tissues caused by heat, electricity or chemicals. Thermal burns include injuries caused by flame, steam or hot liquids. Electrical burns result from contact with an electrical current, and chemical burns most often result from contact with caustic substances. A burn may be minor or major, and the degree of local effects and systemic consequences depend on many factors, including the severity of the burn and the age of the individual. (Further information on burns and the care of clients with burns is provided later in this chapter.)

NEOPLASIA

A keloid is a benign overgrowth of fibrous tissue at the site of a wound to the skin. The new tissue is elevated, thickened and reddened. Most keloids flatten and become less noticeable over a period of years. Keloids are more likely to develop if a wound has been infected or if the edges of a wound have been poorly aligned during healing.

Sebaceous cysts are one type of epithelial cyst and consist of a capsule containing a soft yellow–white material. These benign cysts are elevated and firm and range in size from about 0.2–5.0 cm.

A lipoma is a common benign tumour composed of adipose tissue, which is generally encapsulated in the subcutaneous layer of the skin. Lipomas vary in size and most frequently occur on the neck, back, thighs or forearms.

Neurofibromatosis is a congenital condition characterised by numerous neurofibromas of the skin and nerves, by café-au-lait spots on the skin and in some cases by abnormalities of the muscles, bones and internal organs. Many large, pedunculated soft-tissue tumours may develop.

Basal cell carcinoma is a malignant lesion characterised by a shallow ulcer surrounded by a raised well-defined edge. Basal cell carcinomas may also be referred to as rodent ulcers. The most common site is the face, particularly the nose, eyelids and cheeks. Basal cell carcinomas usually occur in people aged over 40 and, as metastasis is rare, the prognosis is favourable.

Squamous cell carcinoma is a malignant lesion characterised by a firm, elevated painless nodule. The most common sites are areas of the body most often exposed to ultraviolet rays. Squamous cell carcinoma is most frequently seen in men over age 55 and, as metastasis is probable, this neoplasm has a higher mortality rate than does basal cell carcinoma.

A melanoma is a malignant tumour that arises from melanocytes. The incidence of melanoma seems to be related to prolonged exposure to the sun, particularly by fair-skinned people. Because metastatic dissemination is relatively common, the mortality rate is high. In its premalignant stage, a melanoma appears as a flat, irregularly pigmented macule. Colour changes appear as the melanoma becomes malignant and invasive, with the colour ranging from red, brown and blue to black. Melanoma can occur on any part of the body but most frequently occurs in areas of the skin exposed to sunlight. There are many types of melanoma and, because of its invasive nature, the nodular type is the most serious. Australians have the highest rate of malignant melanoma in the world, and the incidence is particularly high in Queensland and the tropics.

INFECTIONS AND INFESTATIONS

Because the surface of the body is constantly exposed to large numbers of pathogenic microorganisms, the skin is a potential area for infection. In addition, dermatological problems are often the result of infestation by parasites. Many factors increase a person's vulnerability to a skin infection, including ill-health, poor standard of hygiene or a break in the continuity of the skin. Bacterial skin infections include carbuncles, erysipelas, folliculitis, furuncles (boils), impetigo and paronychia.

A carbuncle is a cluster of staphylococcal abscesses or boils containing purulent matter. Eventually, pus discharges to the skin surface through numerous openings.

Erysipelas is an acute streptococcal inflammatory infection involving subcutaneous tissue. The skin of the affected area is bright red and oedematous, with a sharply defined border. The area may develop vesicles and the individual commonly experiences pain and an elevated body temperature.

Folliculitis is a common infection of the hair follicles, caused by staphylococci. Superficial or deep pustules are evident, and the most common site is the face.

A furuncle (boil) is an infection caused by either staphylococci or streptococci. A furuncle starts as a painful, hard, deep follicular abscess, and the overlying skin is hot to touch. The area becomes soft and opens to discharge a core of tissue and pus.

Impetigo is an acute contagious disorder of the superficial layers of the skin, caused by either staphylococci or streptococci. The condition begins as local erythema and progresses to pruritic vesicles, which ooze, with the exudate from the lesion forming a yellow-coloured crust. Lesions usually form on the face and spread locally.

Paronychia is a painful inflammatory infection of the tissue around the nails.

Viral skin infections include herpes simplex and herpes zoster infections, and verrucae.

Herpes simplex virus (HSV) has an affinity for the skin and usually produces small irritating or painful fluid-filled blisters on the skin and mucous membranes. HSV-1 infections tend to occur in the facial area, particularly around the mouth and nose, whereas HSV-2 infections are usually limited to the genital region. The blisters erupt and thin yellow crusts form as the lesions begin to heal.

Acute infection with herpes zoster, or varicella-zoster virus (V-ZV), is characterised by the development of very painful vesicular skin eruptions that follow the underlying route of cranial or spinal nerves inflamed by the virus. After about 1 week the vesicles develop crusts, and the condition may last several weeks. The pain may last for much longer.

A verruca (wart) is caused by the human papilloma virus, and presents as a firm skin lesion with a rough surface. Different types of verrucae include those that commonly affect the hands, fingers or knees; and those that affect the genito-anal region.

Fungal skin infections include candidiasis and tinea. Candidiasis is any infection caused by a species of *Candida*, usually *Candida albicans*, characterised by pruritus, a white exudate, peeling and easy bleeding. Oral or vaginal thrush are common topical manifestations of candidiasis, as are red eroded patches in the genito-anal region.

Tinea (ringworm) is a group of fungal skin diseases caused by dermatophytes of several kinds. It is characterised by itching, scaling and painful lesions. Types of tinea include tinea capitis, affecting the scalp, tinea pedis, affecting the feet, and tinea corporis, affecting non-hairy smooth skin on the body.

Infestations of the skin by parasites include scabies and pediculosis. Scabies is a condition caused by a mite, *Sarcoptes scabiei*, and characterised by a papular rash, intense pruritus and excoriation of the skin from scratching. The sites most commonly affected are the thin-skinned areas between the fingers, flexor surfaces of the wrists and the inner aspect of the thigh. The mite burrows into the outer layers of the skin, where the female lays eggs. Small, thread-like red streaks appear where the mite has burrowed into the skin.

Pediculosis is infestation by blood-sucking lice, which causes intense pruritus, often resulting in excoriation from scratching. Different varieties of pediculi affect the hair on the scalp, the body or the pubic area. The lice can be seen with the naked eye, and their eggs (nits) can be seen as small pear-shaped bodies attached to the hairs.

DIAGNOSTIC TESTS

To diagnose specific disorders of the skin a variety of tests may be performed.

Direct examination

A lesion may be examined using a magnifying lens, or a Wood's lamp may be used to determine the presence of fungal infections. Fungal infections such as ringworm show a characteristic fluorescence under black light.

Skin biopsy

The medical officer obtains a sample of skin or part of a lesion for pathological examination. Certain lesions may be surgically excised to provide sufficient tissue for histological diagnosis.

Microscopic examination

Specimens for microscopic examination may be obtained by gently scraping the scales or crusts of lesions. Exudate from oozing lesions may also be obtained for microscopic examination.

Skin testing

Skin testing may be performed to determine which substance or substances cause a hypersensitive reaction. Patch testing provides a means for assessing contact sensitivity. One or more suspected allergens are placed on a hairless part of the body. The test site is later examined for a visible reaction.

CARE OF THE INDIVIDUAL WITH A SKIN DISORDER

Although nursing care is planned to meet the individual's needs, according to their specific skin disorder, the nursing care of a person with any dermatosis generally involves the following aspects.

RELIEF OF PRURITUS

Itching, which can be a source of considerable distress, is a feature of many skin disorders. The natural response to pruritus is to scratch, and scratching can cause further discomfort and may lead to tissue damage and infection. While medical therapy is aimed at resolving the problem responsible for the pruritus, certain nursing measures can be employed to provide some relief:

- As heat tends to aggravate itching, the room should be maintained at a moderate and comfortable temperature. The bedclothes and personal clothing should be light, loose and cool
- Soothing tepid baths may be helpful in alleviating the itching
- Diversions that are of interest to the individual, such as reading or watching television, may be helpful.

TOPICAL APPLICATIONS

The application of local soothing preparations or topical medications may be prescribed. The most common mediums used to apply medications to the skin are creams, lotions, ointments and pastes, or powders. Medications that are mixed with the appropriate medium for topical application include: anti-inflammatory drugs such as corticosteroids, antipruritic agents such as tar or corticosteroids, antiseptics such as phenol, and antibiotics such as neomycin. Specific substances to be added to the bath water may also be prescribed. For example, oatmeal, bath oils or coal-tar preparations may be prescribed when large areas of the body surface are affected. The nurse must ensure that the bath water is at a comfortable temperature and should be aware that many skin disorders result in changes in sensory perception, so it is essential that the water is not too hot.

Whenever topical applications have been prescribed, the nurse must know the level of responsibilities and the regulations regarding administration of medications in the health care facility and geographical area in which they work. Each type of topical medication requires proper application, and the nurse must know the amount to use, whether gloves are required during application, and the signs of any adverse effects of the medication. The five rights of administration of medication (right person, right medication, right time, right dose, right route) are just as relevant for topical applications as they are for systemic medications.

In addition to topical applications, systemic medications may be prescribed, such as analgesics to relieve pain, antibiotics to combat infection, or mild sedatives to promote adequate rest.

Dressings may be prescribed as part of the local treatment of skin disorders. Moist dressings may be used in the management of acute inflammatory skin disorders. Any solution that is used to soak the dressing should be warmed to body temperature. Occlusive dressings may be applied over a topical medication, to promote penetration of the drug into the epidermis.

MAINTENANCE OF FLUID AND NUTRITIONAL BALANCE

Fluid and electrolyte balance may be disrupted because of loss of fluid in exudate from skin lesions. It is important to ensure that adequate fluid replacement is provided to compensate for any abnormal fluid loss.

A diet that is rich in protein may be prescribed to replenish losses and to promote healing. It is important to ascertain whether the individual is allergic to any specific foods, as skin disorders can be caused or aggravated by food allergies. Any known allergens must be eliminated from the diet.

PREVENTING INFECTION

Any disruption to the integrity of the skin increases the risk of infection, so measures such as the following should be implemented to protect the skin:

- After bathing or showering, the skin should be gently patted dry. Brisk rubbing could cause damage to already tender skin
- The nails should be kept short and clean to prevent damage from scratching, and the person should be encouraged to resist scratching. It is important to explain that scratching increases the risk of skin trauma and infection. In some instances, e.g., with a young child or a disoriented person, mittens may be placed over the hands to reduce skin damage by scratching

- All dressings and applications of topical substances must be performed aseptically
- If the skin disorder is contagious, isolation precautions may be implemented to prevent the spread of infection to others.

PROVIDING PSYCHOLOGICAL SUPPORT

A severe skin disorder may cause distress and embarrassment to the person who has it. They may be self-conscious about their appearance, and their body image may be severely impaired. If the person feels that other people will avoid contact because of their unsightly appearance, they may experience anxiety or depression, both of which may be exacerbated if the disorder is likely to result in permanent disfigurement. To assist the client with a skin disorder, the nurse should be careful not to demonstrate any distaste or repugnance. It is important that the client and their significant others are kept well informed about the disorder and its likely outcome. The client should be given the opportunity to express their emotions and fears, such as the fear of disfigurement or alienation from their loved ones.

PRESSURE SORES (DECUBITUS ULCERS)

Pressure sores result from ischaemic hypoxia of the tissues, owing to prolonged pressure on the area. As a result of impaired blood circulation the area is deprived of essential nutrients and oxygen, and cellular death occurs. Pressure sores are also referred to as decubitus ulcers, trophic ulcers, stasis ulcers, ischaemic ulcers and bedsores. The major factors likely to interrupt local capillary blood supply are pressure and shearing forces; however these can be exacerbated by a variety of other factors. One, or a combination, of these factors increases the risk of pressure sores. Predisposing factors can be classed as either intrinsic or extrinsic.

INTRINSIC FACTORS

Intrinsic factors are characteristics specific to an individual's condition.

Nutritional status

Inadequate nutrition prevents efficient cellular growth and repair, and renders the tissues more vulnerable to damage. A poorly nourished person will usually have less protection over the bony prominences and be more vulnerable to the effects of prolonged pressure. Clinical Interest Box 37.4 addresses the correlation between vitamin C and wound healing.

Body type

As the sites of maximum skin compression are located over bony prominences, a thin person is more at risk. Conversely, an obese person may be at risk due to shearing forces and added pressure caused by body weight pressing on the skin.

CLINICAL INTEREST BOX 37.4
Vitamin C and healing

Question: Why is vitamin C essential in the diet, especially in the reconstruction phase of the healing process?

Answer: Because the fibroblasts require an acidic environment to manufacture collagen.

Mobility

Limited mobility restricts the movements a person usually makes to redistribute pressure on weight-bearing areas.

Neurological factors

Reduced sensitivity to pressure or pain may occur in certain disease states, such as spinal cord injury, paralysis, multiple sclerosis or diabetes mellitus. Transmission of impulses from receptors in the skin or to the muscles may be impaired, so that the person does not receive the 'message' to move. Sometimes, although a message is transmitted, the person is unable to move independently.

Vascular factors

Reduced local tissue perfusion may result from certain disease states, such as arteriosclerosis, cardiac failure or diabetes mellitus. As reduced local tissue oxygenation and nutrition are the primary cause of pressure sores, people with vascular perfusion abnormalities are at risk.

Incontinence

Incontinence of urine or faeces may result in skin excoriation or maceration. Abrasions are more likely to form from friction between the skin and the surface under the person, making shearing forces more severe.

EXTRINSIC FACTORS

Extrinsic factors are those derived from the individual's environment.

Pressure

The greater the pressure on the skin, the more the tissues are distorted. Pressure on the skin over bony prominences can distort the blood vessels to such an extent that the blood flow is interrupted. Pressure can also occlude lymphatic vessels, and the consequent accumulation of toxic substances can contribute to cell damage. The areas of the body where bony prominences are covered by a thin layer of tissue are those most likely to develop pressure sores. However, pressure sores can develop on other body areas if they are subjected to prolonged or excessive pressure (Figure 37.2).

Shearing forces and friction

When pressure is applied at an angle, the layers of the skin move over one another, causing distortion of the tissue. The forces involved (shearing forces) distort and occlude the dermal capillaries, resulting in tissue necrosis and the

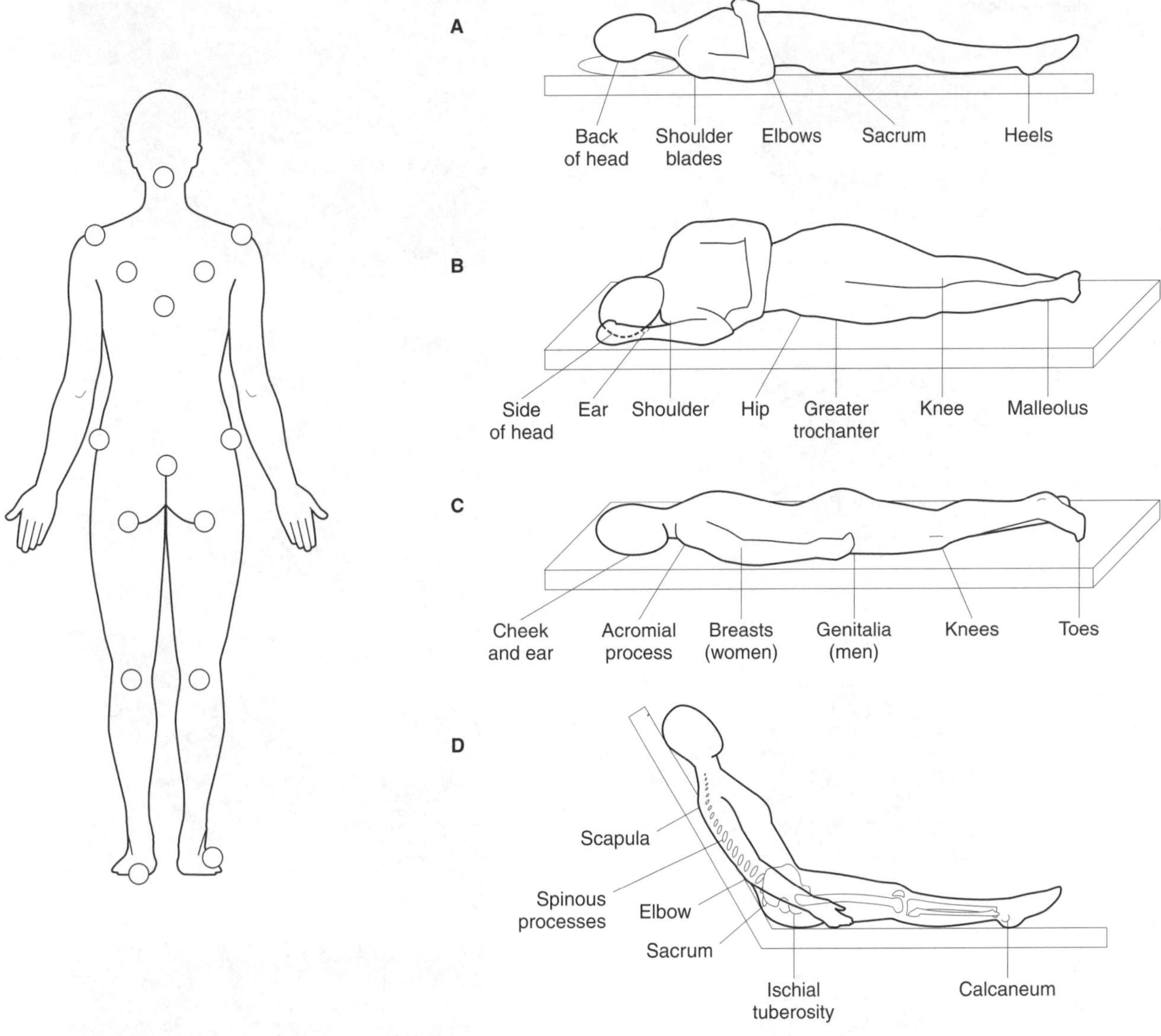

Figure 37.2 | Pressure area sites
A: In the supine position **B**: In the lateral position **C**: In the prone position **D**: In the sitting position

development of a pressure sore. Friction between the skin and another surface, such as a sheet, also results in tissue distortion due to shearing forces. Friction immobilises the epidermis while the deeper layers move, and is an important factor in a client whose skin is fragile.

Loss of skin integrity

Any skin damage increases the risk of pressure sores. Actions such as excessive washing with soap, prolonged exposure to moisture, or rubbing can damage the skin's integrity.

DEVELOPMENT OF A PRESSURE SORE

Pressure sores commonly develop through four stages, unless measures are taken early to relieve pressure and increase local tissue perfusion (Figure 37.3):

- Stage one: the skin is red and does not return to normal colour with relief of pressure. The area may also be oedematous and the person may experience tenderness or a sensation of burning
- Stage two: the skin blisters, peels or cracks
- Stage three: the full thickness of skin is damaged. Subcutaneous tissue damage can also occur, and commonly a serous or bloodstained discharge is evident. A slough forms and appears as a black area, which is composed of dead tissue. Microorganisms invade and multiply rapidly
- Stage four: a deep ulcer is formed as the full thickness of skin and subcutaneous tissue is destroyed. Structures such as fascia, muscle, connective tissue or bone underlying the ulcer are exposed and may be damaged. If any signs or symptoms of a developing decubitus ulcer are observed, the nurse in charge must be notified immediately.

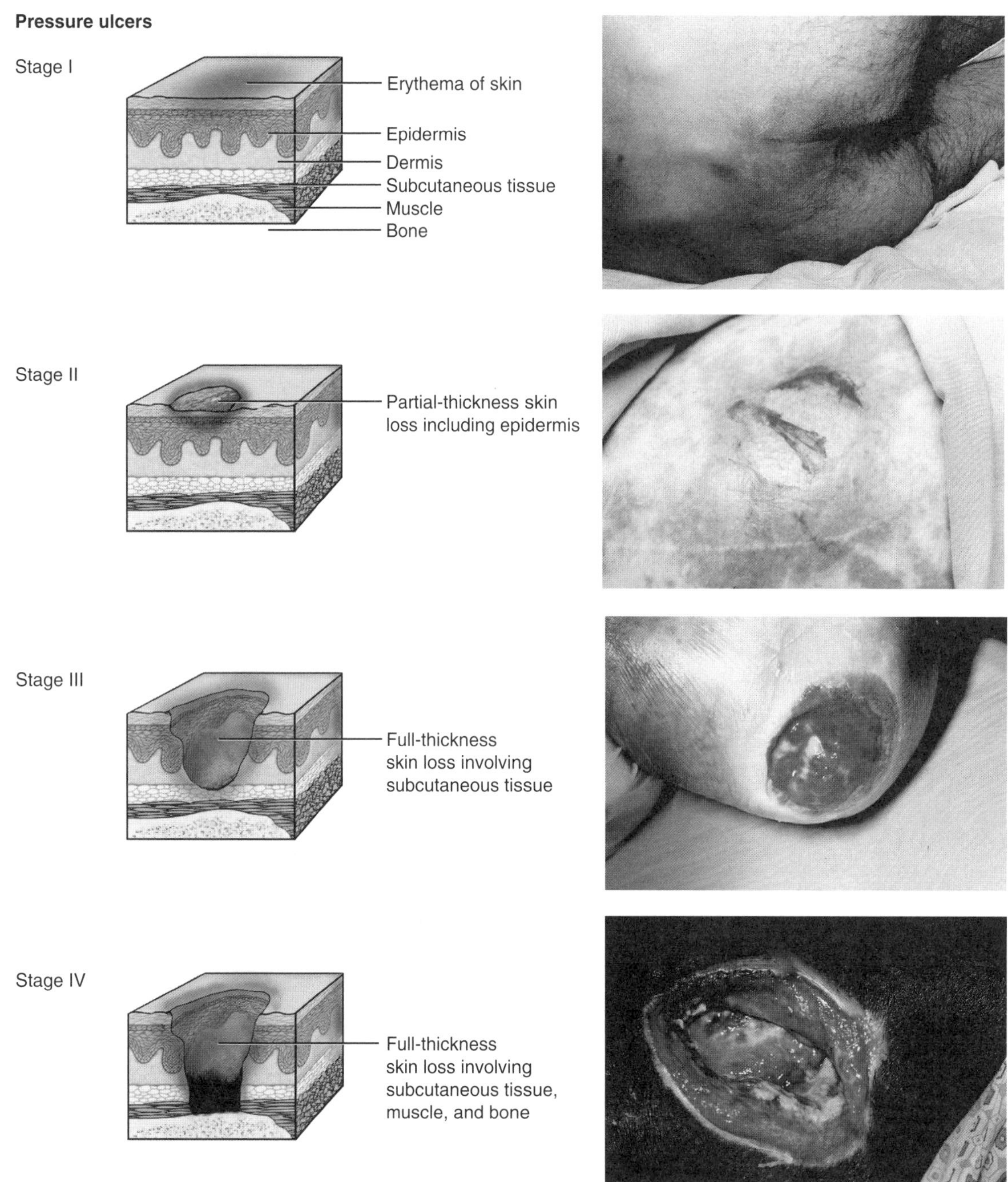

Figure 37.3 | The four stages of pressure ulcers *(deWit 2005)*

PREVENTING PRESSURE SORES

It is important to identify clients at risk of decubitus ulcers, and many assessment systems have been designed to aid identification. Health care facilities may devise their own risk assessment tool or may use an established one, such as the Norton scale (Table 37.2) or the Braden scale (Table 37.3).

An assessment tool is used as a guide to facilitate the implementation of a rational preventive regimen. Thermography may also be used as a screening technique to detect incipient or actual pressure damage. Skin pressure may be measured using a specific gauge such as the Denne pressure gauge, to estimate the pressure on a site.

Pressure sores form in a few hours but may take many months to heal; preventing them is therefore of prime importance. Ensuring good blood supply to pressure areas is critical because poor blood supply is the primary cause of pressure sores and because, if a pressure sore occurs, poor blood supply delays tissue healing, which depends on a good blood supply bringing antibodies and leucocytes to combat infection, as well as nutrients and oxygen for regeneration of tissues.

Research has shown a direct correlation between malnutrition and the development of pressure sores. A well-balanced diet is necessary to maintain the health of tissues and to prevent tissue breakdown. An adequate fluid intake is important to prevent skin dryness. If a person's appetite is poor, high-protein fluids and added vitamins may be prescribed. If a person is unable to tolerate oral food or fluids, an alternative method of meeting nutritional needs, such as gastric tube or intravenous (IV) feeding, may be necessary.

Maintaining skin integrity

It is important to keep the skin clean, dry, supple and intact. The skin is washed as necessary, using a non-irritating soap sparingly to avoid causing dryness. Dry skin may require the application of an oil or cream. Thorough drying, following

TABLE 37.2 | THE NORTON SCALE FOR ASSESSING RISK OF PRESSURE SORES

Name	Date	Physical condition		Mental condition		Activity		Mobility		Incontinent		TOTAL SCORE
		Good	4	Alert	4	Ambulant	4	Full	4	Not	4	
		Fair	3	Apathetic	3	Walk/help	3	Slightly limited	3	Occasional	3	
		Poor	2	Confused	2	Chair bound	2	Very limited	2	Usually/urine	2	
		Very bad	1	Stupor	1	Bed	1	Immobile	1	Doubly	1	

(modified from the Centre For Policy on Ageing: London, England 1962)

TABLE 37.3 | THE BRADEN SCALE FOR ASSESSING RISK OF PRESSURE SORES

Patient's name______		Evaluator's name______		Date of assessment
Sensory perception Ability to respond meaningfully to pressure-related discomfort	1. *Completely limited* Unresponsive (does not moan, flinch or grasp) to painful stimuli due to diminished level of consciousness or sedation OR Limited ability to feel pain over most of body surface	2. *Very limited* Responds only to painful stimuli. Cannot communicate discomfort except by moaning or restlessness OR Has a sensory impairment which limits the ability to feel pain or discomfort over half of body	3. *Slightly limited* Responds to verbal commands, but cannot always communicate discomfort or need to be turned OR Has some sensory impairment that limits ability to feel pain or discomfort in one or two extremities	4. *No impairment* Responds to verbal commands. Has no sensory deficit that would limit ability to feel or voice pain or discomfort.
Moisture Degree to which skin is exposed to moisture	1. *Constantly moist* Skin is kept moist almost constantly by perspiration, urine, etc. Dampness is detected every time patient is moved or turned	2. *Very moist* Skin is often, but not always, moist. Sheets must be changed at least once a shift	3. *Occasionally moist* Skin is occasionally moist, requiring an extra sheet change approximately once a day	4. *Rarely moist* Skin is usually dry, sheets require changing only at routine intervals
Activity Degree of physical activity	1. *Bedfast* Confined to bed	2. *Chairfast* Ability to walk severely limited or non-existent. Cannot bear own weight and/or must be assisted into chair or wheelchair	3. *Walks occasionally* Walks occasionally during day, but for very short distances, with or without assistance. Spends majority of each shift in bed or chair	4. *Walks frequently* Walks outside the room at least twice a day and inside room at least once every 2 hours during waking hours

(Continued)

TABLE 37.3 | THE BRADEN SCALE FOR ASSESSING RISK OF PRESSURE SORES—cont'd

Mobility Ability to change and control body position	1. *Completely immobile* Does not make even slight changes in body or extremity position without assistance	2. *Very limited* Makes occasional slight changes in body or extremity position but unable to make frequent or significant changes independently	3. *Slightly limited* Makes frequent though slight changes in body or extremity position independently	4. *No limitations* Makes major and frequent changes in position without assistance
Nutrition Usual food intake pattern	1. *Very poor* Never eats a complete meal. Rarely eats more than one-third of any food offered. Eats 2 servings or less of protein (meat or dairy products) per day. Takes fluids poorly. Does not take a liquid dietary supplement OR Is NBM and/or maintained on clear liquids or IVs for more than 5 days	2. *Probably inadequate* Rarely eats a complete meal and generally eats only about half of any food offered. Protein intake includes only 3 servings of meat or dairy products per day. Occasionally will take a dietary supplement OR Receives less than optimum amount of liquid diet or tube feeding	3. *Adequate* Eats over half of most meals. Eats a total of 4 servings of protein (meat, dairy products) each day. Occasionally will refuse a meal, but will usually take a supplement if offered OR Is on a tube feeding or total parenteral nutrition regimen that probably meets most of nutritional needs	4. *Excellent* Eats most of every meal. Never refuses a meal. Usually eats a total of 4 or more servings of meat and dairy products. Occasionally eats between meals. Does not require supplementation
Friction and shear	1. *Problem* Requires moderate to maximum assistance in moving. Complete lifting without sliding against sheets is impossible. Frequently slides down in bed or chair, requiring frequent repositioning with maximum assistance. Spasticity, contractures or agitation leads to almost constant friction	2. *Potential problem* Moves feebly or requires minimum assistance. During a move skin probably slides to some extent against sheets, chair, restraints or other devices. Maintains relatively good position in chair or bed most of the time but occasionally slides down	3. *No apparent problem* Moves in bed and in chair independently and has sufficient muscle strength to lift up completely during move. Maintains good position in bed or chair at all times	
				TOTAL SCORE

(Crisp & Taylor 2005, courtesy Barbara Braden and Nancy Bergstrom)

a bath, for example, is necessary to prevent skin excoriation or maceration. Particular attention should be paid to skin folds and creases, such as under the breasts, between the buttocks, and in the groin. Careful handling prevents damage to the skin, and there should be the appropriate number of staff, or a lifting device, to minimise the risk of injury to the skin when moving a client.

Incontinence should be managed appropriately, and devices used to protect the skin from constant moisture. After each incontinent episode the skin is washed, dried carefully, and may be protected by the application of a barrier cream. Wet or soiled bed linen or clothing must be removed immediately.

The presence of any skin breaks should be reported immediately to the nurse in charge so that early treatment can be implemented.

Preventing pressure

Prolonged periods of pressure should be avoided, the aim being to prevent occlusion of the blood vessels that may lead to a disruption of the blood supply. Repositioning clients at regular intervals, such as every 2 hours, is an effective way of preventing prolonged pressure on any area. Several repositioning schedules have been designed to assist nurses in implementing a regular position change regimen. The Lowthian 24-hour turning clock (Figure 37.4) is one such design, and should be accompanied by documentation that records implementation of the schedule.

Special beds, such as a net suspension bed, may be used to relieve pressure and to facilitate position change. An overhead hand grip may be used by a client to lift up and relieve pressure from the buttocks and sacral area. Pressure-relieving devices such as sheepskin, ripple or

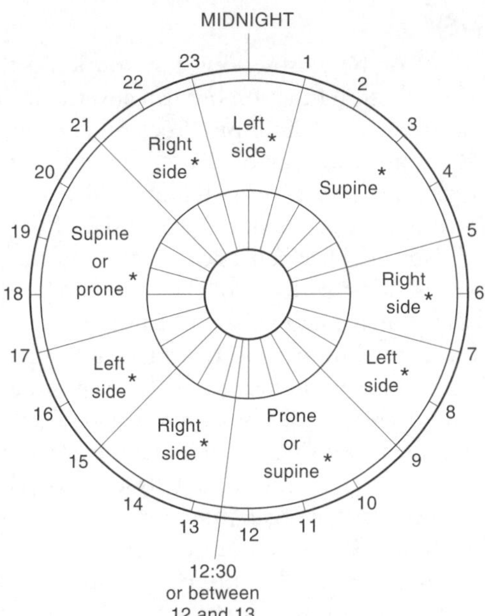

Figure 37.4 | Lowthian turning clock *(reproduced with permission of Peter Lowthian, Senior Nurse (Research), Royal National Orthopaedic Hospital, Stanmore. Modified from original illustration by Peter Lowthian)*

egg-crate mattresses may be used to reduce pressure or to distribute the person's weight evenly. For maximal effect, a sheepskin should be placed so that it is in direct contact with the skin. Cushions or pads containing gel, foam or water may be placed on seats; for example, of a wheelchair. The person sitting in a chair is encouraged to lift up from the seat frequently, to relieve pressure and facilitate tissue perfusion in the buttocks and sacral area. The person is assisted in this action if unable to lift independently. All splints, plasters, braces and bandages should be checked regularly and adjusted if necessary to relieve pressure.

Relieving shearing forces

Shearing may be prevented by careful positioning and lifting techniques, so that sliding in any direction is avoided. Pillows should be arranged for adequate support, and a foot board or firm pillow at the feet may assist the person to maintain a sitting position (foot boards are contraindicated with clients who have had strokes, as they increase tone and contribute to clonus). The person must be lifted carefully to avoid dragging the skin along any surface, and surfaces such as sheets must be kept smooth.

MANAGEMENT OF A PRESSURE SORE

If a pressure sore develops despite preventive measures, early detection and management increases the likelihood of successful treatment. Management aims to remove pressure from the area, treat any predisposing factors and promote healing of the decubitus ulcer. The client must be positioned so that the ulcerated area is free from all pressure. Management of the ulcer should follow the principles of general wound management to promote healing. Controversy exists over pressure-sore management, and many forms of treatment have been implemented, with varying degrees of success. Applications or techniques for which no scientifically based explanation can be provided should be avoided. Instead, nurses should refer to the results from current clinical research to select products or techniques that have been demonstrated as being beneficial.

Whatever treatment is prescribed, healing is promoted by relief of pressure, a diet containing adequate nutrients and fluid, removal of predisposing causes, and maintenance of a good blood supply to the area. If infection has developed, systemic antibiotic therapy may be prescribed.

SKIN TEARS

The older adult is susceptible to skin tears because of the complex ageing process, which leaves skin fragile. The epidermis begins to atrophy and there is a loss of elasticity. Manual handling, knocks on wheelchairs and generally minor accidents can result in a skin tear. Prevention strategies such as padding sharp edges of coffee tables and wheelchairs, care with removal of tapes and dressings, extremely careful manual handling and the use of padding to protect vulnerable areas of the body all need to be considered. Skin tears are one of the most common injuries in frail older adults. Thorough assessment of the risk factors and prevention protocols can assist in preventing this type of injury.

Treatment of skin tears depends on the amount of tissue damage and/or loss. Moist wound-management principles are still appropriate for this type of wound. Preventing infection is important, especially if the wound is on the lower extremity of a client with diabetes or peripheral vascular disease.

LEG ULCERS

Leg ulcers are costly and debilitating. Chronic leg ulceration is a common and often recurrent condition in the elderly population and is disruptive to lifestyle and comfort of the individual. Non-compliance with treatment of venous leg ulcers is a common problem, which leads to a failure to heal and recurrence. However, there are different types of leg ulcers and it is important to differentiate between them so that the correct management strategies can be followed.

TYPES OF LEG ULCERS

Leg ulcers are classified according to the vasculature involved:

- Arterial, involving arteries and arterioles
- Venous, involving veins and venules
- Mixed arterial–venous, involving arteries, arterioles, veins and venules
- Lymphatic, involving the lymphatic drainage system.

CLINICAL INTEREST BOX 37.5
The cost of leg ulcers

It is estimated that approximately one per cent of the Australian population suffers from chronic leg ulceration. The most common cause is poor blood circulation. Other causes or exacerbating factors include relentless pressure (bed sores), poorly managed diabetes, high cholesterol, smoking, dietary problems and poor arterial circulation. Older people are at greater risk (Department Human Services, Victoria 2004). It is estimated that chronic wounds, such as venous leg ulcers, cost the Australian community in excess of $500 million per annum.

Clinical Interest Box 37.5 looks at the burden that venous ulcers place upon the Australian community.

Arterial leg ulcers

These ulcers are usually located between toes or at the tip of the toes, over phalangeal heads and above the lateral malleolus, over the metatarsal heads or on the side of the sole of the foot. Arterial ulcers have a well-demarcated edge and a deep pale wound base. The ulcer is exceedingly painful and the person often needs to hang their leg down in a dependent position when in bed. The person's leg takes on a hairless, thin, shiny, dry skin appearance. The toenails are thickened and often brittle. The leg is pale when elevated and cool to touch. The pedal pulses are often diminished or absent and neuropathy may be present. Predisposing factors for arterial leg ulcers are arteriosclerosis, advanced age, diabetes mellitus, hypertension and smoking.

The management of arterial leg ulcers is very different from the management of venous leg ulcers:

- Consultation with a vascular surgeon is recommended at an early stage
- Treatment of the underlying disease is important
- Angiography or angioplasty may be required
- Chemical sympathectomy may be required
- Bypass surgery or amputation may be required
- Compression bandaging is contraindicated.

Venous leg ulcers

Venous ulcers usually occupy the lower one-third of the leg in the pretibial area and anterior to the medial malleolus. The ulcers have uneven edges and a ruddy granulation tissue and appear to be superficial compared with the arterial ulcer. There is moderate to no pain. Discomfort is relieved by elevation of the leg. Venous ulcers are often accompanied by oedema, with fluid leaking out and macerating the surrounding skin. Pruritus and scale formation occurs. The leg can take on a reddish–brown pigmentation, oedema is present and the leg can be quite firm. There is usually evidence of old healed ulcers, tortuous superficial veins, and the limb may be warm to touch. Foot and leg pulses are present. The predisposing factors for venous leg ulcers are a history of deep venous thrombosis (DVT), valvular incompetence in the perforating veins and obesity.

BURNS

Burns are one of the most serious skin injuries, as they not only disrupt physical function but can also result in severe emotional trauma for the injured person and significant others. Burn injuries may be caused by dry heat, moist heat, chemicals, electricity or radiation. When a hot object comes in contact with the skin, the transfer of heat causes structural damage. Heat causes coagulation of the protein in tissue cells, and the depth of the burn is related to the amount of thermal energy dissipated in the skin.

After a thermal injury, intravascular fluid is lost as the capillaries become more permeable. As the intravascular fluid volume decreases, the venous return and cardiac output fall. The clinical signs of 'shock' become apparent, and tissue hypoxia threatens internal organs such as the kidneys. Other changes occur in organ function, in electrolyte levels and in metabolic function. Subsequently, complications of major burns can involve any body system because all systems are stressed during the injury and during healing. (See Chapter 48 for the first aid care of burns.)

CLASSIFICATION OF BURNS

A burn is described as superficial, partial thickness or full thickness.

Superficial burns

In superficial burns the basal layer of the epithelium remains intact and the skin is dry, red and oedematous. The area is painful because cutaneous nerve endings are injured. Superficial burns generally heal within 1 week in a healthy person, often without treatment.

Partial-thickness burns

In partial-thickness burns there is damage to the epidermis and to the superficial dermis. As the dermis contains blood vessels, any injured vessels exude serum, thus raising the epidermis to form blisters. The skin is painful and red and, if a blister bursts, the area beneath is pink, swollen and wet. When the superficial dermis has been injured, the raw area is resurfaced with epithelium growing from the undamaged walls of the sweat glands and hair follicles. Deeper partial-thickness burns result in diminished sensation, as the dermal nerve endings are destroyed. Blood vessels are destroyed and so there is less leakage of serum from them. Re-epithelialisation becomes slower when more skin structures, such as hair follicles, are destroyed. Deep partial-thickness burns can heal over time but may be skin grafted to speed recovery, reduce the risk of infection and minimise scarring.

Full-thickness burns

In full-thickness burns, all layers of the skin are destroyed and the injury may extend to underlying fat, muscle and bone. The area is painless because cutaneous nerve endings have been destroyed. The appearance of the area can vary and may be white, waxy, tan-coloured, red or charred.

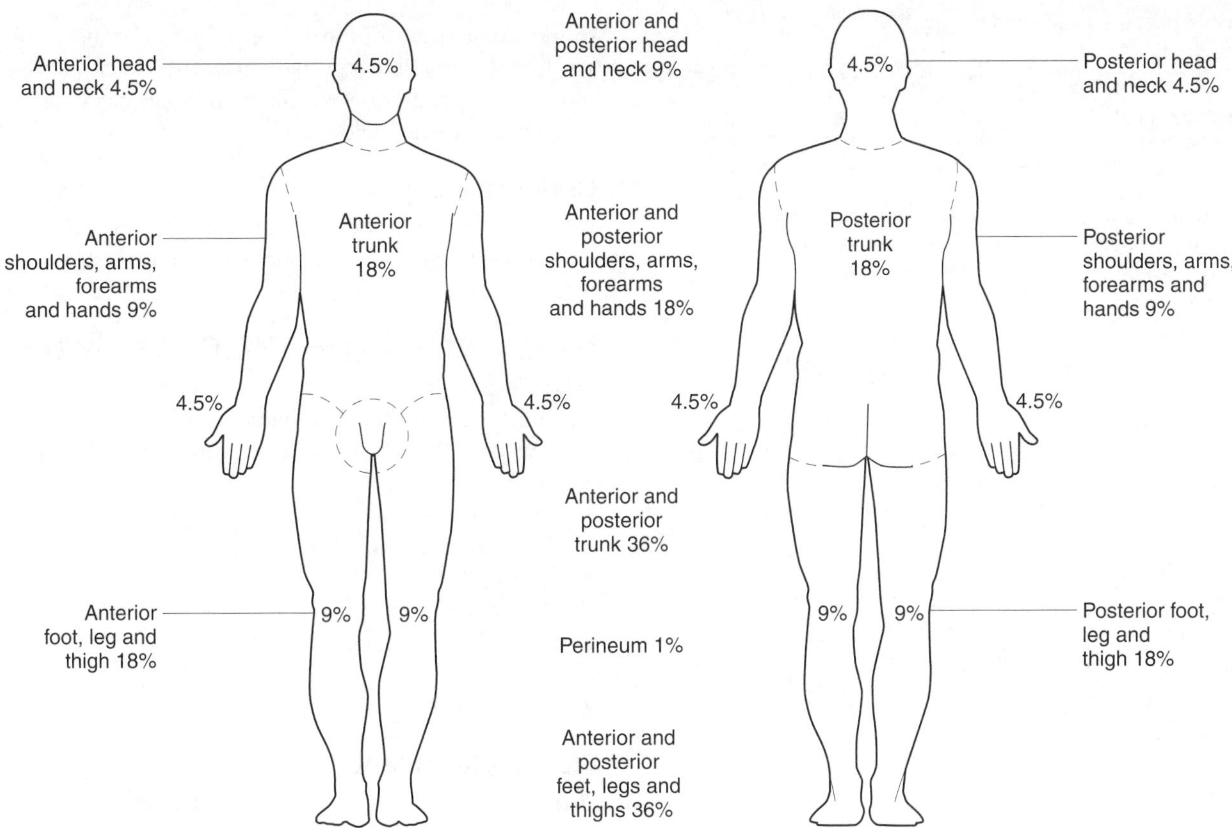

Figure 37.5 | Assessing burn surface area: rule of nines (adults)

The area is dry and feels hard. Because all parts of the skin are destroyed, healing is only possible by epithelial proliferation from the wound edges. Skin grafting is commonly performed, unless the burn is very small.

ASSESSING BURN SIZE

The severity of a burn depends more on the surface area than on the depth of tissue involved. The greater the area involved, the greater the amount of fluid lost from the body, and the greater the degree of shock that ensues. To assess the size of a burn accurately, a chart is used on which the size is expressed as a percentage of the total body surface. The two methods generally used to calculate burn size are the 'rule of nines' (Figure 37.5) and the Lund–Browder method (Figure 37.6). The Lund–Browder method is the more accurate, as it allows for changes in body proportion with age. The numbers on each body portion on the chart indicate the percentage of body surface for that part. Both types of chart provide a rapid and accurate means of determining the extent of the burn.

COMPLICATIONS OF BURNS

After a severe burn, all body systems are involved in an attempt to maintain homeostasis. Complications are relatively common and can involve any body system.

Shock

Shock is due to loss of fluid from the circulation. The greatest loss of fluid occurs at the site of the burn, but loss also occurs throughout the body. Substances such as kinins, released by the body in response to the injury, increase capillary permeability, allowing serum to escape into the tissues. This loss of serum causes reduced blood volume (hypovolaemia), which may lead to severe shock. As a result of hypovolaemia, cardiac output decreases, blood pressure falls, and acute renal failure and death may follow.

Infection

Infection may occur if microorganisms gain entry through areas where the skin has been damaged or destroyed. Although a burn wound is usually sterile initially, the area provides an ideal culture medium for a wide range of microorganisms. Necrotic tissue, oedema, and transudate all provide a nutrient medium for bacteria. The individual's resistance to infection is reduced by factors such as shock, anaemia and electrolyte imbalance.

Septicaemia

Septicaemia occurs when there is bacterial invasion of the tissues and bloodstream, and is a major cause of death in severely burned individuals. Septic shock is a form of shock that occurs in septicaemia, when endotoxins are released from bacteria in the bloodstream. The endotoxins cause

Percentage of areas affected by growth

	0	1	5	10	15	Adult age
A = half the head	9.5	8.5	6.5	5.5	4.5	3.5
B = half of one thigh	2.75	3.25	4	4.25	4.5	4.75
C = half of one leg	2.5	2.5	2.75	3	3.25	3.5

To estimate the total of the body surface area burned, the percentages assigned to the burned sections are added. The total is then an estimate of the burn size.

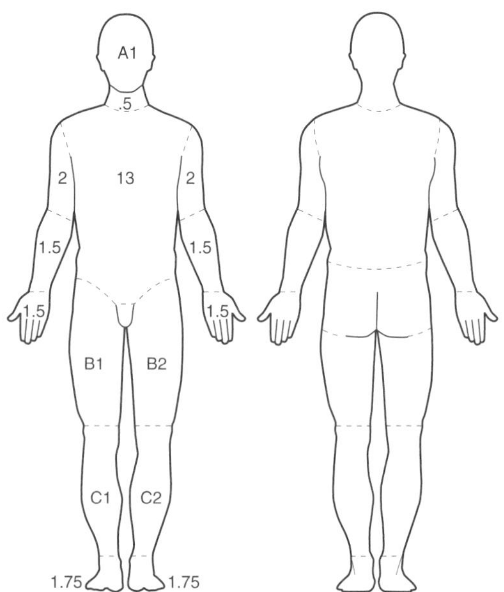

Figure 37.6 | Assessing burn surface area: Lund–Browder method

decreased vascular resistance, resulting in a drastic fall in blood pressure. Pyrexia, tachycardia, rapid ventilations, confusion and coma may also occur.

Pulmonary problems

Pulmonary damage can occur from smoke, chemical inhalation or carbon monoxide intoxication. In the acute period, pulmonary oedema may develop, and later pulmonary complications include pneumonia and respiratory distress syndrome.

Scarring and contractures

Scarring and contractures may occur after healing has taken place. Within weeks, hypertrophic scarring results in red, itchy raised scars, which are hard to the touch. The shrinkage of these scars may cause contracture across joints and can lead to severe disfigurement and disability unless treated. The amount of scarring depends upon the severity of the burn, the area affected, the age of the individual and the effectiveness of treatment.

Psychological effects

A person who has been severely burned is likely to experience depression, anxiety and difficulty in adjusting to the consequences of injury. The person's significant others are likely to experience similar emotions. If a child has been burned, the parents are also likely to experience severe guilt feelings about the incident.

Curling's ulcer

A Curling's ulcer is a duodenal ulcer that may develop in a person with severe burns. It is thought to be the result of stress.

MANAGEMENT OF THE CLIENT WITH BURNS

The management of an individual with burns will depend on a range of factors, but the basic aspects of care are:

- Fluid replacement
- Prevention of infection
- Adequate nutrition
- Pain relief
- Promotion of mobility
- Psychological support
- Promotion of healing
- Preparation for discharge.

Fluid replacement

If the burned area is not too great (e.g. less than 15% in an adult, less than 10% in a child), the body generally compensates adequately for the fluid loss, and only the provision of extra oral fluids is indicated. In more extensive or severe burns, fluid loss is a major cause of shock, so fluid replacement is of prime importance. The medical officer calculates the volume of fluid replacement required then prescribes the type of fluid and method of administration. Intravenous fluids are commonly prescribed and, in extensive full-thickness burns, blood transfusion may be required to compensate for a reduction in erythrocyte numbers. Large volumes of intravenous fluids containing replacement electrolytes may be necessary, and individual fluid requirements are continually calculated and adjusted according to need.

Monitoring techniques that may be performed to assess fluid requirements include:

- Insertion of a urinary catheter to enable hourly monitoring of urine output. Fluid replacement aims at maintaining a urine output of 30–50 mL/hour in an adult
- Blood tests. Frequent (e.g. hourly) haematocrit measurements act as a guide to fluid deficit and therefore enable fluid requirements to be calculated. Electrolyte levels are also commonly measured
- Weighing. If the person's condition permits, they may be weighed daily, as measurement of body weight provides an accurate method of assessing fluid status.

Prevention of infection

As stated previously, the burn wound provides an ideal culture medium for a range of microorganisms. Preventing infection is directed at preventing contamination of the wound and preventing invasion of the tissues and bloodstream. A special burns unit may be available where the air is filtered, the client is received into a bed prepared with sterile linen, and isolation techniques are used to protect against infection. When a special unit is not available, the client is generally nursed in a single room using protective isolation techniques. (Protective isolation techniques are described in Chapter 25.) Methods of preventing infection include:

- Aseptic dressing techniques
- Topical antiseptic applications in dressings
- Use of sterile linen on the bed
- Wound excision and skin grafting
- Systemic antibiotic therapy
- Enhancing natural defences, e.g., by providing a high protein/kilojoule diet and treating any anaemia.

Providing adequate nutrition

In addition to the loss of erythrocytes and protein-rich serum, the hypermetabolic response of the body to a burn rapidly depletes stores of energy. The individual must be provided with adequate carbohydrates, protein, fats, minerals, vitamins and fluid. Energy and protein requirements are generally assessed using a formula, and oral dietary intake is often augmented by nasogastric feeding or parenteral therapy to meet these requirements. Accurate monitoring of tolerance to the diet enables continual assessment of nutritional requirements.

Relieving pain

In most superficial burn injuries pain can be severe, but in deeper burn injuries the nerve endings are destroyed, thus pain is not generally experienced initially. Pain management is complex, because the perception of pain has physical and psychological origins. Analgesic medications are commonly administered together with anxiolytic medications. Nursing measures also include explanation and assurance to the client to reduce fear, and careful positioning may be beneficial. The nurse has a responsibility to observe the client continually and to be directed by the client on the level of analgesia required. (Further information on pain management is provided in Chapter 35.)

Promoting mobility

Because of the nature of the injury, and its management, a person with burns may experience prolonged periods of immobility. Thus, the individual is subject to the complications of immobility, such as venous thrombosis, pneumonia, decubitus ulcers and contractures. (See Chapter 36 for measures to manage problems associated with immobility.) Regular and careful position changes are essential. Clients must be positioned for comfort and repositioned frequently to prevent decubitus ulcers and contractures. Splints and other devices may be used to improve positioning and to prevent contractures. The client's limbs should be correctly positioned to decrease joint flexion.

Physiotherapy is essential for a person who is immobile, and involves chest physiotherapy and range of motion (ROM) exercises. ROM exercises may be performed actively or passively, and the degree of motion should be recorded to document progress. Ambulation is started as soon as possible and the nurse may be required to assist. If skin grafting has been performed, the client will be required to increase ambulation slowly, as too rapid ambulation may destroy new grafts. The client may be placed in a bath of warm water, for example, before having dressings renewed, as the warmth and buoyancy of the water may enable them to move more freely with less pain.

Providing psychological support

As this type of injury can have devastating emotional impact on the individual and their significant others, psychological support is an extremely important aspect of care. After the injury, the person will experience various emotions such as fear of death, fear of disability and fear of disfigurement. Feelings of despair, anger, frustration, depression and guilt may all be experienced at any time after the burn.

Communication between team members caring for the client is important to achieve adequate support for both them and their significant others. The nurse can help to provide support by:

- Developing a trusting relationship and by being available to listen. The nurse should encourage the client to talk through feelings and fears
- Providing information about all the procedures and equipment in a way that can be understood. Fear will be reduced if information is provided to the client and significant others in a way that facilitates understanding of the injury, the treatment and the prognosis. People who are experiencing stress often have difficulty in remembering, so information should be repeated whenever necessary
- Assisting the client to adapt gradually to body changes, and by being supportive when the client views the injury, particularly for the first time
- Supporting the client's coping mechanisms for as long as necessary. The nurse should understand that any expressions of anger, aggression or intolerance are not being directed at the nurse personally. Rather, it is the person's way of reacting to the injury and its consequences
- Involving the client in all aspects of care as much as possible, to promote independence and self-esteem.

Promoting healing of the injury

Care of the burned area varies according to the site and severity of the injury. The aims of wound care are to prevent infection and promote healing with minimal scarring. Two or more methods of burn care may be used simultaneously, and methods may change during the course of healing.

The open method of treatment involves the application of antimicrobial creams without the use of dressings. The burns are left exposed to the air to allow the exuding serum to dry and form a protective crust, which prevents further fluid loss and the entry of microorganisms. A topical antibacterial agent, such as silver sulphadiazine, is usually applied to the area. The cream is applied with a sterile gloved hand and, as the heat of the room and of the client's skin melts the cream, it must be applied frequently. The individual may be nursed on a special type of bed frame that allows ventilation, and a bed cradle is used to keep the bedclothes away from the burned areas. The open method of treatment eliminates the need for dressings, and the antibacterial agent reduces the incidence of infection. As there is rapid heat loss from the burned areas, keeping the person warm may be a problem. The individual is generally nursed in a room that is warm enough to maintain normal body temperature. Clinical Interest Box 37.6 provides a sample nursing care plan for a client with a burn injury.

The closed method of treatment involves the application of a dressing, which may be impregnated with petroleum jelly, paraffin or an antibacterial agent. The dressings are held in position with bandages and may remain in place for up to 72 hours before being changed. The outer layers of absorbent padding that cover the dressing are reinforced if serum seeps through. Dressing changes are performed with strict aseptic precautions. The client is given an analgesic before the dressing change or may be given a general anaesthetic before the procedure is performed. After the dressings have been removed, the wounds are cleansed. Warm saline baths may be used to help clean the burn, remove dead tissue and to loosen adherent dressings.

The frequency with which the dressings are changed depends on many factors, and may range from 3–4 times a day, to daily, to once in 2–3 days.

Surgical management

Surgical management of burns involves the initial cleaning and debridement before the open or closed method of treatment is used. Other surgical procedures are skin grafting and escharotomy.

Skin grafting

Skin grafting promotes healing, prevents infection and prevents the contraction of scars. It is performed as early as possible in the treatment of some partial-thickness burns and in the treatment of all full-thickness burns. Split skin grafting involves the removal of sheets of the epidermis and part of the dermis from a donor site, and placing them over the burned surface. In extensive burns the sheets of skin can be 'meshed' by machine to give them a net-like appearance. By stretching the net, the skin graft can cover a greater area. A full-thickness graft includes the epidermis and the entire dermal layer, and is generally used when full-thickness skin loss has occurred.

Skin from a source other than the client's own body

CLINICAL INTEREST BOX 37.6
Nursing care plan for a client with a BURN INJURY

Nursing diagnosis

One of the many nursing diagnoses that needs to be considered by the nurse is disturbance in self-concept related to changes in appearance associated with tissue loss and scarring, alterations in motor and sensory function, dependence on others to meet basic needs, changes in usual lifestyle and roles and inability to participate in usual sexual activities.

Short-term and long-term goals

- The client will demonstrate beginning adaptation to changes in appearance, body functioning, lifestyle and roles, evidenced by the verbalisation of feelings of self-worth and sexual adequacy.
- The client will maintain relationships with significant others and have an active participation in activities of daily living.
- The client will take an active interest in personal appearance, have a willingness to participate in social activities and begin to plan a lifestyle to meet the restrictions imposed by the burn injury.

Actions and rationale

- The nurse will determine the meaning of the effects of the burn injury to the client by encouraging them to verbalise feelings and noting the non-verbal responses to the changes experienced.
- The nurse will assist the client to identify strengths and qualities that have a positive effect on self-concept.
- The nurse will implement measures to assist the client to cope with the effects of the burn injury by:
  - — reinforcing the reason for wound-care procedures
  - — not encouraging the use of a mirror until the client is ready
  - — arranging for a visit by another burns client who has successfully adjusted to a similar burn injury
  - — reducing pain
  - — reducing fear and anxiety, reassuring the client regarding nightmares if they occur and reinforcing that these will gradually stop
  - — including the client in all aspects of planning care and allowing choices when possible to increase the client's control
  - — providing diversional activities according to the client's interests
  - — clarifying misconceptions about future limitations on activity and sexual function
  - — encouraging family and significant others to allow the client to do self-care as much as possible, as this assists in building self-esteem
  - — assisting the client to be well informed, and communicating with all members of the multidisciplinary team
  - — monitoring the client for signs and symptoms of depression and referring them to the appropriate discipline for assistance.

may be used as a temporary cover for large burned areas, to decrease fluid loss. The donor site is generally covered with a non-adherent dressing and layers of dressing material to absorb blood and serum that ooze from the wound. A new technique has been developed in which sections of the individual's unburned skin are grown in the laboratory, and later used to graft onto their burned areas.

To promote successful transplantation, the graft must be immobilised to prevent displacement. Immobilisation is achieved by one of several methods, such as suturing, and the graft area is covered for protection. Successful 'take' of the graft depends on many factors, including absence of infection in the area, prevention or elimination of haematomas or seromas, and adequate blood circulation.

Escharotomy

Eschar is a dry crust caused by contraction of burned skin. Its development frequently causes increased tissue pressure, which may impair circulation and lead to ischaemia. An escharotomy is a surgical procedure in which longitudinal incisions are made through the eschar to relieve pressure on the underlying tissues. As the eschar does not contain nerve endings the procedure is painless, but it does result in open wounds, which provide a portal for infection.

Contractures and keloids

Contractures and keloid formation after healing are always a possibility and it is important that preventive measures are implemented. Pressure placed over the healing wounds is generally successful in reducing keloid formation, and constant pressure applied during scar maturation retards the development of keloid. Tailored elastic garments (Jobst suits), which are fitted exactly over any burned body part, apply pressure to prevent and correct post-burn hypertrophic scarring and contractures. Pressure garments may be required for between 6 months and 2 years after healing.

PREPARATION FOR DISCHARGE

Before discharge from hospital, it is important that the client understands that the healed burned and grafted skin is tender and will break down more easily than normal skin. The client is informed that these areas are very vulnerable to extremes of temperature, irritant substances and physical trauma. As part of discharge preparation the nurse should advise the client, or the parents of the young child, to:

- Avoid sunlight on the burned areas for at least 12 months. Burned and grafted skin tans unevenly and unpredictably, and burns easily. The incidence of skin cancer in burned skin is quite high
- Use only non-irritant soaps and cosmetics on the burn areas
- Exercise care if engaging in activities such as sports in which there is the possibility that the burned areas may be bumped or damaged
- Wear clothing made from soft fabrics that will not irritate the healed burned or grafted areas
- Continue with prescribed management of the areas. Management may include the continual wearing of a tailored elastic garment, or application of a cream to the areas. The person may also be required to follow a planned program of exercises designed to improve mobility
- Seek appropriate help, such as psychological counselling, if there is difficulty in adapting to a changed physical appearance.

WOUND MANAGEMENT

Wound assessment is very important. The nurse must make a holistic assessment of the person and consider factors such as the present and past history, age, underlying disease, nutritional status, psychological status, medication, mobility and activity, vascularity, and other therapies or treatments that are taking place. The nurse must identify the cause of the wound, type of wound, location, measurements, stage of the wound, whether the wound is acute or chronic, what interventions have already been tried and whether infection is present. Clinical Interest Box 37.7 outlines the principles of wound management.

WOUND MANAGEMENT PRINCIPLES

Wound management employs the principles of moist wound healing; that is, to keep the wound floor moist enough to facilitate the movement of cells across the floor of the wound. Research suggests that moist wounds granulate 40% faster than dry wounds. The benefits of moist wound healing are reported to be:

- Thermoregulation
- Less pain
- Less infection
- Less injury and damage to cells on removal of the dressing
- More efficient autolytic debridement of necrotic tissue
- Less risk of transmission of microorganisms
- Fewer dressing changes and therefore less disturbance of the wound, resulting in reduced costs in dressing consumables and reduced workload for care staff
- The client's lifestyle is interrupted less and, with most dressings, the client can continue to shower as usual.

WOUND DRESSINGS

Wound dressings may be classified into four main types:

1. Wound-hydration products

CLINICAL INTEREST BOX 37.7
Principles of wound management

- Assess or define aetiology
- Control factors affecting healing, e.g., smoking, nutrition
- Select an appropriate wound dressing
- Plan for maintenance of wound healing
- Evaluate and review

2. Moisture-retentive dressings
3. Exudate-management products
4. Compression dressings.

Wound-hydration products

Wound-hydration products rehydrate the wound. These dressing products are composed of water, bound together by cross-linked polymers. They can be used as cavity fillers in wounds with light exudate. These dressings are usually in the form of a gel.

Moisture-retentive dressings

Moisture-retentive dressings keep the wound bed moist, allowing cells to migrate across the surface of the wound with ease. These dressings are used on light-to-moderately exudating wounds. They are composed of hydrophilic particles (cellulose) and come in various thicknesses, shapes and sizes. These dressings aid the process of natural autolysis and stimulate regranulation and re-epithelialisation. They retain moisture and are the ideal secondary dressing to support wound hydration. They can be left in position for several days, they do not adhere to the wound, they allow the passage of oxygen to the wound and are impermeable to microorganisms and water. The dressings are usually of such a nature that visual inspection can be made of the wound healing. These semi-permeable film dressings are comfortable for the client and alleviate pain because they protect exposed cutaneous nerve endings.

Exudate-management products

Exudate-management products absorb exudate from the wound surface. These dressings are the calcium alginates, which are composed of polysaccharides derived from seaweed; polyurethane foam dressings; hydrofibre dressings, which are made from pure cellulose (hydrocolloids) pectin and gelatine; and the combination dressings, which marry the technologies of hydrocolloids and the absorption capacity of diaper technology.

Compression dressings

Compression dressings aid in oedema control by maintaining various pressures. There are lightweight compression bandages and high-compression bandages. Zinc paste bandages also come into this category — both those with and those without antibacterial properties. Dressing changes depend on the health care facility's protocol and the type of dressing used. Many of the manufacturing companies that produce wound dressings will assist in the education of how to use their products and provide after-hours information services. Clinical Interest Box 37.8 outlines the basic factors to consider when selecting a dressing, while Clinical Interest Box 37.9 discusses the selection of dressings and Clinical Interest Box 37.10 addresses a myth about wound management.

CLINICAL INTEREST BOX 37.8 Factors to consider when selecting a dressing

- Wound type: superficial, full thickness, cavity
- Wound description: granulating, epithelialising, necrotic, sloughy
- Wound characteristics: dry, moist, heavily exuding, malodorous, excessively painful, difficult to dress, bleeds easily
- Bacterial profile: sterile, colonised, infected, infected and potential source of cross-infection

CLINICAL INTEREST BOX 37.9 The right dressing for the right wound type

Modern wound dressings improve healing time, reduce pain, reduce the time required to dress the wound and require less frequent changes. If used appropriately, they can be very cost effective. The answer is using the most appropriate dressing for the wound. Match the action of the dressing to the aim of the treatment, as follows:

Wound type

Black wound (hard, dehydrated, black, necrotic)
Yellow wound (soft, yellow, creamy slough)
Green wound (infected)
Red wound (moist, red granulation)
Pink wound (evidence of epithelial growth on surface)

Aim of treatment

Rehydrate, debride, promote granulation tissue
Debride slough, promote granulation, absorb excess exudate
Treat infection with systemic antibiotics, absorb excess exudate, debride slough
Retain moisture, promote and protect granulation tissue and epithelialisation, absorb excess exudate
Retain moisture, promote and protect epithelialisation

Examples of dressings that can be used

Hydrogels, TenderWet
Hydrogels, alginates, hydroactive dressings, Cadexomer Iodine,TenderWet, hydrocolloids, foams
Hydrogels, alginates, silver-impregnated dressings, TenderWet, foams, Cadexomer Iodine
Foams, alginates, hydroactive dressings, hydrocolloids, hydrogels
Hydrocolloids (thin), non-adherent dressings, polyurethane films

SURGICAL WOUNDS

Care of a surgical wound is directed towards promoting healing and preventing infection. In the immediate post-operative period, assessing for haemorrhage is a major responsibility of the nurse. Both the dressing and the bed linen under the client should be checked for signs of haemorrhage. Any increase in blood staining on the dressing or an increase of blood in a drainage tube or bottle must be reported immediately to the nurse in charge. Strict asepsis is necessary when caring for surgical wounds, and the nurse must follow the individual health care facility's protocol.

CLINICAL INTEREST BOX 37.10
Myths in wound management

Myth: Patients with wounds should not let the wound come into contact with shower water.

Truth: Showering postoperative wounds does not increase infection or slow the healing process and promotes a sense of wellbeing and health associated with cleanliness. Showering of chronic wounds and ulcers may be undertaken with caution. Tap water should not be used if declared unsuitable for drinking.
(The Joanna Briggs Institute 2003)

Adequate oxygenation of the tissues is promoted by deep breathing and coughing exercises, and early ambulation to promote full lung expansion will enhance oxygenation of the blood. Adequate circulation of blood to the area should be promoted to transport all the substances required for healing and combating infection. Adequate blood volume can be maintained by ensuring sufficient fluid intake, and circulation can be stimulated by exercises and mobility.

Movement of the area should be restricted in the early stages of healing. If strain is placed on a wound, the newly formed granulation tissue may tear. The wound area should be stabilised, rested and supported.

Surgical wound management

To provide the conditions necessary for healing, the wound must be free of dead or infected tissue, protected against external agents, which may delay healing, and provided with a moist environment, which is conducive to healing.

Controversy exists about many aspects of wound care, such as the type of dressing applied, frequency of dressing changes, cleansing procedures and solutions used. Most health care facilities develop their own protocols and procedures for wound management and it is the nurse's responsibility to know these procedures and be aware of the protocols and regulations relating to wound care. Clinical Interest Box 37.11 provides interesting reading on which solution to use.

CLINICAL INTEREST BOX 37.11
Are antiseptics cytotoxic? True or false?

Research has shown that antiseptics once commonly used in hospitals for wound management actually damage important cells such as macrophages.

True: Professor George Rodeheaver challenged health care workers to put into their eye the substances that they put onto their patient's wounds (Thomas, Rodeheaver & Bartolucci 1997). His research showed that cells such as macrophages and fibroblasts were damaged by chemicals such as povidine iodine and hydrogen peroxide in vitro. This research and subsequent following research has changed wound-management practices markedly.

Changing a surgical wound dressing

If a dressing is to be changed, sterile equipment and aseptic techniques are used to prevent cross-infection. To prevent the spread of airborne microorganisms, activities in the room should be reduced to a minimum, windows and doors should be closed and conversation should be limited while the equipment and wound are exposed to the air. A suggested technique for performing a dressing change is outlined in Table 37.4. The equipment required includes:

- A sterile dressing pack that consists of:
  - — cotton wool swabs
  - — dressing(s)
  - — dressing towels
  - — bowl(s) for cleansing solution
  - — dressing forceps
- Prescribed skin-cleansing lotion
- Sterile disposable gloves
- Receptacle for waste
- Scissors
- Hypoallergenic tape or bandage
- Sterile syringe if required.

DRAINAGE TUBES

At the time of operation, the surgeon may place a drain tube through a separate 'stab' incision near the principal wound. A drain promotes healing by providing an exit for blood, serum and debris that may otherwise accumulate and result in postoperative swelling, pain or infection. The type of drain inserted depends on the site and extent of the wound; a drain may be freestanding or attached to a drainage bag, intermittent suction or to a self-contained disposable drainage system that supplies its own suction.

When a free drainage is inserted, a sterile safety pin is usually passed through the tubing just above skin level to prevent the drain from slipping into the incision. A gauze dressing is placed between the pin and the skin. Alternatively, the drain may be secured in position by one or two sutures. An absorbent dressing may be placed over the drain to collect exudate, or a pouch or bag may be applied to the surrounding skin for drainage collection. A closed-wound drain consists of tubing connected to a vacuum unit. Using aseptic technique, the container is emptied as necessary. Vacuum in the container is re-established each time the container is emptied. The unit is always positioned below wound level to promote drainage by gravity. The exit drain site may be protected by an absorbent or occlusive dressing.

The length of time a drain remains in position depends on several factors, such as the amount of drainage required. Before its removal, a drain may be rotated and shortened daily to prevent the body tissues becoming adhered to it and also to promote healing. A suggested technique for rotating and shortening a drain tube is outlined in Table 37.5.

The nurse is required to perform this procedure only if it is within the scope of practice and if institutional policy permits. As this action may be quite painful, administration

TABLE 37.4 | GUIDELINES FOR DRESSING A WOUND

Action	Rationale
Review and carry out the steps in Appendix 1	
Explain the procedure	Reduces anxiety
Inspect the dressing	To determine dressing requirements
Ensure privacy and assist the client to assume an appropriate position, ensuring that only the wound area is exposed	Promotes comfort and facilitates performance of the procedure
Ensure adequate lighting	Facilitates observation of the wound
Wash and dry hands thoroughly	Prevents cross-infection
Assemble the required equipment, using aseptic technique	Prevents contamination of sterile items
Place the equipment in a convenient location near the bedside	Facilitates performance of the procedure
Wash and dry hands thoroughly, don gloves if required	Prevents cross-infection
Use forceps to remove any dressing from the wound and place it in the waste receptacle	Prevents cross-infection
Position dressing towels around the wound	Creates a sterile field
Observe the wound for union, signs of infection, exudate, inflammation and healing	Evaluates condition of the wound, and stage of healing
Cleanse the wound in accordance with the practices of the health care facility, medical officer's orders or as directed by the nurse in charge. Clean from a clean area towards a less clean area	Avoids transferring wound exudate and normal flora from the surrounding skin into the wound, and thus prevents wound contamination
Using forceps, apply a clean dressing over the wound and secure it in position. Or, if ordered, the wound may be left exposed to the air	Protects the wound from infection and irritation, e.g., from clothing
Remove gloves and towels and place them in an appropriate receptacle	Prevents cross-infection
Assist the individual to reassume a comfortable position	Promotes comfort
Remove and attend to the equipment appropriately. Wash and dry hands	Prevents cross-infection
Report and document the procedure	Appropriate care can be planned and implemented

TABLE 37.5 | GUIDELINES FOR SHORTENING A DRAIN TUBE

Action	Rationale
Review and carry out the steps in Appendix 1	
Follow the steps described in the guidelines for dressing a wound, up to and including cleaning the wound	The stab wound is cleansed to remove exudate, thus preventing contamination
Using the stitch cutter, remove any suture securing the tube in the wound	Enables the tube to be rotated, if necessary, and shortened
If the tube is round, gently rotate it	Rotation of the tube frees any adherent granulation tissue
Withdraw the tube the prescribed length, e.g., 1.25 cm	Tube must only be shortened the prescribed length, to allow the wound to heal from within
Secure tube with sterile safety pin below level of planned cut	Prevents tube from slipping into the wound
Cut off excess tube	Prevents it pressing on the wound
Place and secure a clean dressing or pouch over the tube	Protects the skin from irritation from wound drainage
A gauze dressing is generally placed between the pin and the skin, and another dressing or pouch placed over the tube	Protects the skin from irritation
Remove and discard gloves and towels	Prevents cross-infection
Assist the client to reassume a comfortable position	Promotes comfort
Remove and attend to the equipment appropriately. Wash and dry hands	Prevents cross-infection
Report and document the procedure	Appropriate care can be planned and implemented

of a prescribed analgesic by a Registered Nurse (RN) 30 minutes before the procedure is usually necessary. The equipment required includes:

- A sterile tray containing sterile:
  - — cotton wool swabs
  - — bowl for cleansing solution
  - — dressing
  - — safety pin
  - — gloves
  - — scissors
- Artery forceps (if required)
- Sterile stitch cutter if necessary
- Receptacle for waste
- Hypoallergenic tape.

Removal of a drain tube requires similar technique to that for dressing a wound and shortening a drain tube (see Tables 37.4 and 37.5). Any retaining suture is removed and the tube is withdrawn steadily and gently to minimise discomfort. If the tube is attached to a suction device, the nurse must ascertain whether suction is to be discontinued before removal of the tube. Generally, suction is discontinued to avoid damaging the tissues as the tube is being withdrawn. Check the health care facility's protocol.

SUTURES AND CLIPS

When surgery has been completed, the wound edges are approximated and held together by sutures, clips or staples. Generally a single line of sutures or clips is sufficient for closure. In some instances, tension sutures are also required to ensure closure and to provide additional support for the wound. Suturing methods include intermittent and continuous. With intermittent (interrupted) suturing the surgeon ties each individual suture. Continuous suturing is a series of sutures with only two knots: one at the beginning and one at the end of the suture line. The manner in which the suture crosses and penetrates the skin determines the method of removal. Figure 37.7 illustrates two methods of achieving skin closure.

When healing has progressed well, sutures, clips and staples are removed, usually within 7–10 days after insertion. The wound is checked for union of the edges before sutures or clips are removed. Sometimes alternate sutures or clips are removed one day, and the remainder are removed the following day. The most important principle in suture removal is never to pull the visible portion of a suture through underlying tissue, as pulling the exposed portion of the suture through tissues may lead to infection. The nurse may be required to perform this procedure if it is within the specified role and function, and if institutional policy permits. Sutures are generally removed using a disposable sterile stitch cutter, and staples or clips are removed using a sterile staple extractor. Figure 37.8 illustrates the technique of staple removal. A suggested technique for removing sutures or staples is outlined in Table 37.6. The equipment required includes:

- A sterile stitch cutter or staple extractor
- Sterile swabs and solution to cleanse the incision
- Sterile gloves
- Receptacle for waste
- Adhesive butterfly strips or paper tapes if required.

SUMMARY

The integumentary system consists of the skin and its appendages — the hair, nails, sweat and sebaceous glands. The skin is the largest organ of the body and is composed of two layers. The epidermis is the thin outermost layer composed of epithelial cells, many of which are keratinocytes. Keratin has waterproofing qualities and is also responsible for the formation of hair and nails. Melanin, which is produced by cells in the deeper layer of the epidermis, gives colour to the skin and protects the body against the damaging effects of ultraviolet rays in sunlight. The dermis, or deeper layer of the skin, contains blood vessels, nerve endings, hair follicles and hairs, arrector pili muscles, sebaceous glands and sweat

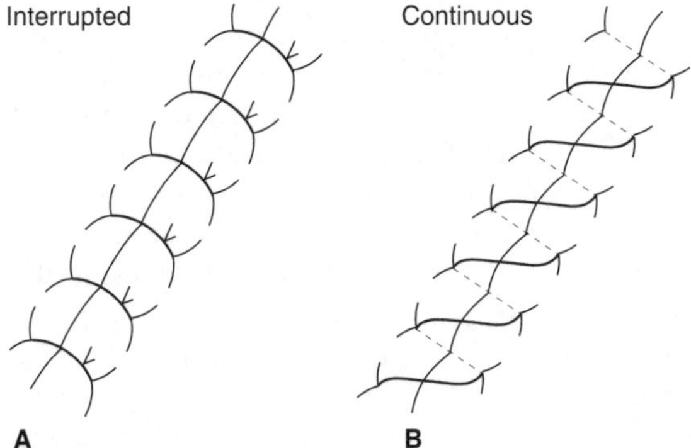

Figure 37.7 | Suturing techniques

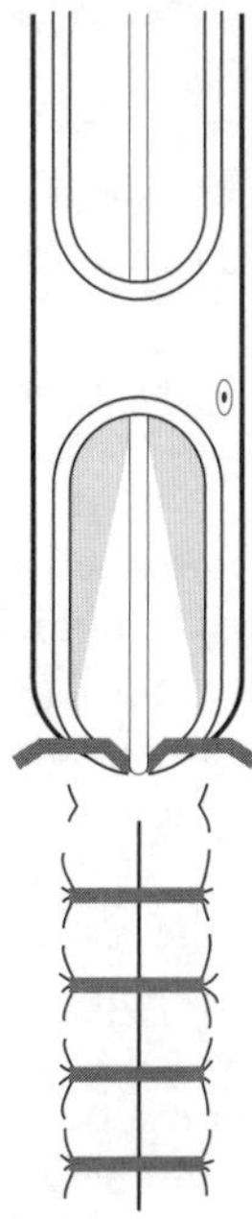

Figure 37.8 | Removing a staple

TABLE 37.6 | GUIDELINES FOR REMOVAL OF SUTURES AND STAPLES

Action	Rationale
Review and carry out the steps in Appendix 1	
Explain the procedure	Reduces anxiety
Ensure adequate lighting, and place the equipment in a convenient location	Facilitates performance of the procedure
Assist the individual into a suitable position, and ensure privacy	Promotes comfort and reduces embarrassment
Wash and dry hands thoroughly	Prevents cross-infection
Remove any dressing, and swab the suture line	Removes any exudate and dried blood, thus reducing the risk of infection
Removal of each intermittent suture involves: • Using forceps to grasp the knot and gently raise it off the skin • Cutting the suture as close to the skin as possible, away from the knot • Pulling the cut suture up and out of the skin, ensuring that the exposed portion of the suture is not pulled through the tissues	Avoids risk of pulling exposed suture through the tissues, which prevents infection
Removal of a continuous suture involves: • Using forceps to grasp the first knot and gently raise it off the skin • Cutting the first suture on the side opposite the knot • Cutting the same side of the next suture in line • Lifting the first suture out in the direction of the knot • Repeating the process down the suture line, using forceps to hold each suture where you would grasp the knot if the suture were intermittent	Minimises discomfort and ensures that the sutures are removed in the correct direction
To remove staples, position the extractor's lower jaws beneath the span of the first staple	The extractor re-forms the shape of the staple and pulls the prongs out of the intradermal tissue
Squeeze the handles until they are completely closed then lift the staple away from the skin. Remove alternate staples at first. Repeat the process for each staple	To ensure that the incision has healed before removing all staples
Wipe the incision line gently with swabs and solution	Prevents infection, and irritation from clothing
Apply a light dressing if necessary	Provides additional support, and promotes union of the wound edges if healing is not complete
If necessary, apply butterfly strips or tapes across the incision	To keep the edges of the incision closed
Assist the individual to reassume a comfortable position	Promotes comfort
Remove and attend to equipment appropriately	Prevents cross-infection
Wash and dry hands	Prevents cross-infection
Report and document the procedure	Appropriate care can be planned and implemented

glands. Nails and hair protect certain areas of the body, for example, nails protect the tips of toes and fingers, while hair protects areas such as the scalp. The major functions of the skin are protection, thermoregulation, sensory perception, excretion, immunity, synthesis of vitamin D, and to act as a blood reservoir.

Surgical wounds are the result of intervention by the surgeon and can range from an uncomplicated suture line to a more complex wound requiring drainage tubes or skin grafts. A surgical wound must be treated with strict aseptic technique and the nurse must be cognisant of the individual health organisation protocols.

Pressure ulcers result from ischaemic hypoxia of the tissues due to prolonged pressure in an area of the body, usually over a bony prominence. Both intrinsic and extrinsic predisposing factors contribute to the development of a pressure ulcer. Pressure ulcers can be classified as stages 1–4, depending upon the amount of tissue damage. Risk assessment and preventive strategies that are employed by the nurse play an important role in ensuring that the incidence of pressure ulcers, which are largely predictable and preventable, is kept to a minimum. The nurse engages the multidisciplinary team to assist in the prevention of pressure ulcers within the vulnerable client population such as the elderly and frail.

Skin tears are a traumatic injury that can occur especially

to the frail elderly population. Preventive strategies paying particular attention to the environment and equipment used for caring for this vulnerable age group are important.

Leg ulcers are a costly and debilitating disorder and the nurse must be able to differentiate between the different types to employ the correct wound management method. The use of compression bandaging, which can be quite effective in the management of venous leg ulcers, is contraindicated and dangerous for the management of arterial leg ulcers.

Burns may be caused by dry heat, moist heat, chemicals, electricity or radiation. A burn is described as superficial, partial thickness or full thickness, depending on the depth of tissue involved. The size of the burn is estimated by using either the Lund–Browder method or the rule of nines. Complications are common after a burn and include shock, infection, scarring and contracture and adverse psychological effects. Medical and nursing management of a client with burns will vary according to the severity of the injury. The care of the individual generally involves fluid and electrolyte replacement, prevention of infection, provision of adequate nutrition, relief of pain, promoting mobility, providing psychological support and promoting healing of the injury.

The effects that disorders of the skin have on the individual range from being minor and temporary, to major and life threatening. Some serious skin disorders affect the individual to the extent that self-concept and body image are severely impaired. Disorders of the skin may have a single cause or may result from several interrelated factors, while for some disorders the cause is unknown. Tests used to diagnose skin disorders include direct examination, biopsy, microscopic examination and skin testing. Clinical Interest Box 37.12 addresses nursing diagnoses in wound management.

In all skin integrity deficits the psychological support for the individual is of major importance. Pain management and nutritional support are also vital. The correct method of wound care is essential and must be given with a clear understanding of the normal healing processes and the effect that certain pathologies have on those processes.

The website of the Australian Wound Management Association (www.awma.com.au) is a recommended resource for nurses wanting to enhance their knowledge further, as it provides up-to-date information, links to other wound associations throughout the world and future wound management conferences. Membership of the Australian Wound Management Association entitles the member to receive a copy of the journal *Primary Intention*.

CLINICAL INTEREST BOX 37.12
Nursing diagnoses in wound management

- Infection, risk for
- Nutrition, altered: less than body requirements
- Pain
- Physical mobility impaired
- Self-esteem disturbance
- Skin integrity impaired
- Skin integrity, impaired, risk for
- Tissue perfusion, altered

(Crisp & Taylor 2005)

REVIEW EXERCISES

1. What are the risk factors for loss of skin integrity?
2. Describe the wound-healing process.
3. What are the principles of wound management?
4. What care is required to prevent and manage pressure sores (decubitus ulcers)?
5. What are the major manifestations of skin disorders?

CRITICAL THINKING EXERCISES

1. Cathy, 77, is admitted to the acute-care hospital for a right total knee replacement. She has been fairly immobile for some time because of deterioration in her right knee. Cathy also has diabetes mellitus and is obese. Cathy's postoperative recovery is marked by pain and subsequent wound infection. She experiences a pressure ulcer to her right heel. What measures could have been taken to prevent Cathy from developing a pressure ulcer?
2. What discharge instructions would you give a client about assessing for signs of wound infection?

REFERENCES AND FURTHER READING

Australian Wound Management Association Inc (2001) *Clinical Practice Guidelines*, 1st edn. Cambridge Publishing, WA

—— *Standards for Wound Management*, 1st edn. Cambridge Publishing, WA

Bale S, Jones V (2006) *Wound Care Nursing: a Patient-Centred Approach*. Mosby Elsevier, Edinburgh

Brandeis GH, Berlowitz DR, Katz P (2001) Are pressure ulcers preventable? A survey of experts. *Advances in Skin & Wound Care: The Journal for Prevention and Healing*, 14(5) Sept/Oct, 244–8

Carville K (2001) *Wound Care Manual*, 4th edn. Perth Silver Chain Nursing Association, Perth WA

Coloplast Wound Care. We've Got It Covered Wound Chart. Coloplast Pty Ltd, Vic

Crisp J, Taylor C (eds) (2005) *Potter & Perry's Fundamentals of Nursing*, 2nd edn. Elsevier Australia, Sydney

Cuddigan J, Ayello EA, Sussman C (eds) (2002) *National Pressure Ulcer Advisory Panel. Pressure Ulcers in America: Prevalence, Incidence, and Implications for the future*. NPUAP, Reston, VA

Department Human Services, Victoria (2004) *Leg Ulcers*. Online. Available: http://www.horizonscanning.gov.au/internet/horizon/publishing.nsf/Content/8E7F31F58B3AEC50CA25714F0004A65C/$File/v7_4.pdf [accessed 28 May 2008]

deWit S (2005) *Fundamental Concepts and Skills for Nursing*, 2nd edn. WB Saunders, Philadelphia

Herlihy B, Maebus NK (2003) *The Human Body in Health and Illness*, 2nd edn. Elsevier Science, St Louis

Hess CT (2008) *Skin & Wound Care*. Lippincott Williams & Wilkins, Philadelphia

Marieb EN (2006) *Essentials of Human Anatomy & Physiology*. Pearson/Benjamin Cummings, San Francisco

Martin R (2001) Early identification and management of infected wounds. *Woundcare Network Issue* 7, ArtiFact Pty Ltd

Ovington LG (2001) Wound care products: how to choose. Advances in Skin & Wound Care. *The Journal for Prevention and Healing*, Sept/Oct

The Joanna Briggs Institute (2003) Solutions, techniques and pressure for wound cleansing. Best practice. *Evidence Based Practice Information Sheets for Health Professionals* 7(1): 5

Thomas DR, Rodeheaver GT, Bartolucci AA (1997) Pressure ulcer scale for healing: derivation and validation of the PUSH tool. The PUSH task force. *Adv Wound Care*, 10(5): 96–101

White W (2001) Skin tears: a descriptive study of the opinions, clinical practice and knowledge base of RNs caring for the aged in high care residential facilities. *Primary Intention*, 9(4), Nov, p. 138

Chapter 38
OXYGENATION

OBJECTIVES

- Define the key terms/concepts
- Describe the structure of the respiratory system
- State the functions of the respiratory system
- Describe the position of the heart and the function of the circulatory system
- State the factors that affect respiratory function
- Describe the major manifestations of respiratory system disorders
- Briefly describe the specific disorders of the cardiac and respiratory systems outlined in this chapter
- Describe the major manifestations of circulatory system disorders
- Assist in planning and implementing nursing care for the client with a cardiac and respiratory system disorder
- Apply relevant principles in the planning and implementation of nursing actions to assist the client receiving oxygen therapy

KEY TERMS/CONCEPTS

acid–base
airway
alveolar
artery
bradypnoea
cardiovascular
diffusion
endotracheal
erythrocytes
expiration
gaseous exchange
hypercapnia
hypocapnia
hypoventilation
hypoxaemia
hypoxia
inhalation
intercostal
interstitial
leucocyte
lymph
perfusion
respiration
tachypnoea
thrombocyte
tracheostomy

CHAPTER FOCUS

The role of the cardiac and respiratory systems is to supply the body's oxygen demands. Cardiopulmonary physiology involves delivery of oxygenated blood from the lungs to the left side of the heart and thence to the tissues, and deoxygenated blood from the tissues to the right side of the heart and thence to the pulmonary circulation for re-oxygenation. Blood is oxygenated through ventilation, perfusion and transport of respiratory gases.

The overall function of the cardiovascular system, which includes the lymphatic system, is to move blood around the body. Blood is circulated by the heart through blood vessels to transport oxygen, nutrients and other substances to the cells and to transport wastes away from the cells. Blood also assists in protecting the body against infection and distributing heat evenly throughout the body, and prevents its own loss by means of a built-in clotting mechanism. The respiratory system provides the body with the ability to absorb oxygen and excrete carbon dioxide and other waste products from the body. The two systems work in conjunction to maintain homeostasis.

Every cell in the body requires a constant supply of nutrients and oxygen, and every cell must rid itself of waste products. The cardiovascular, lymphatic and respiratory systems are the means by which these activities are achieved. The overall function of the circulatory system is transportation of substances to and from the cells.

The respiratory system is the means by which oxygen from the atmosphere is delivered to the bloodstream and carbon dioxide is diffused out from the bloodstream. This is achieved through the capillary alveoli membrane in the lungs. Ventilation is the method of delivering air into and out of the lungs. Respiration, which is the intake and use of oxygen and the elimination of carbon dioxide to the atmosphere, is achieved by the respiratory system and the cardiovascular system.

An adequate supply of blood is necessary for the normal function of every cell. Cells temporarily deprived of blood or oxygen will not function normally, and continued disruption of blood supply causes irreversible damage or cell death. Any disorder that interferes with the distribution or delivery of blood to tissues or the uptake or excretion of gases in respiration is a potential harm to body cells and may have permanent effects on a part, or all, of the body. The most common complication of a respiratory disorder is carbon dioxide retention. This can be a result of alveolar hypoventilation, or a cardiovascular disorder altering the ventilation or the perfusion of the lungs and other tissues.

Homeostasis depends on the ability of the heart to adequately circulate the required volume of blood and oxygen to the tissues. One of the most important aspects of nursing care is the maintenance or restoration of a clear airway, which includes measures directed at removing secretions by the use of suction via the nasal, oropharyngeal or endotracheal routes or by tracheostomy. Education is essential to promote exercise, which maintains optimal circulation of blood, and deep breathing and coughing exercises are encouraged to minimise the retention of secretions and secondary infections. Circulation can be assisted by changes in diet, fluid, exercise, medications and positioning. The patency of airways can be assisted by the use of humidification, nebulisation and physiotherapy using isotonic or hypotonic solutions or certain medications.

Although disorders of the cardiovascular and the respiratory system are common in most communities, the incidence of cardiac and respiratory disease is controlled to some extent by: legislation to minimise airborne irritants; immunisation programs; and health education regarding risks such as bad diet, smoking, hypertension and environmental pollution.

LIVED EXPERIENCE

My dad had a pulmonary embolism, which caused him to collapse 4 days after an appendectomy. The day before it happened, I can remember he was complaining of pain in his leg, and they were actually taking him down to the X-ray department when he collapsed. Now, 18 years later, dad is on warfarin to keep his blood from clotting and has to wear antiembolic stockings. He has clots all up his right leg, which then leads to lymphoedema and, occasionally, leg ulcers. Dad is also often breathless — just doing little things — and he easily becomes puffed out. Mum and I were concerned about this, then dad's doctor showed us an X-ray of dad's lungs. It looked like his lungs had bullet holes in them — from the embolism. This explained the breathlessness.

Gabrielle, daughter and Registered Nurse

STRUCTURE OF THE RESPIRATORY SYSTEM

The function of the respiratory system (Figure 38.1) is to deliver oxygen from the atmosphere to the bloodstream and to deliver carbon dioxide from the bloodstream to the atmosphere. The structures that make up the respiratory tract constitute the means by which this exchange of gases occurs. The respiratory system consists of cavities and conducting airways that begin at the nasal and oral cavity and end at the alveoli, the functional unit of the respiratory system. The larger airways are composed of cartilage and smooth muscle that maintain their patency, and are gradually replaced with smooth muscle in the terminal airways, which allow alterations in airway diameter and ventilation. The two lungs are located in the thoracic cavity, encased by a double membrane known as the pleura, and are separated by the mediastinal cavity that contains the heart and great vessels. The thoracic cavity has ribs that aid in ventilation and protect the lungs from damage. The diaphragm and the internal and external intercostal regions are composed of skeletal muscle and constitute the main muscles of ventilation; other muscles are used when required for more forceful inhalation or expiration.

NASAL CAVITIES

The nose is a bony cartilaginous structure divided into a right and left nasal cavity by the nasal septum. The anterior portion of the septum is cartilage and the posterior portion is bone, formed by the vomer and part of the ethmoid bone. Inside each nostril (nares) is a vestibule lined by skin containing sebaceous and sweat glands and coarse hairs that act as filters. Apart from the vestibules, all other areas of the nasal cavity are lined by mucous membrane. In most of the cavity the membrane is covered by ciliated epithelium with many 'goblet' cells. Mucous cells are also present in the underlying connective tissue. The nose consists of these chambers, with specific structures and cells that have the following functions:

- Hairs and cilia line the nasal cavities and filter foreign particles and pathogens from the inhaled air
- Mucus secreted by the mucosa traps substances in inhaled air, and the cilia move particles of mucus towards the pharynx to be swallowed or expectorated
- Inhaled air is warmed and moistened as it passes over the mucosa. The three nasal turbinate bones in each cavity cause air flow to become turbulent, which enhances contact of air with the mucosa
- Sensory organ for the sense of smell (olfaction).

THE PHARYNX

The pharynx is a muscular tube about 12 cm long, lying in front of the cervical vertebrae and behind the nose, mouth and larynx. It is lined with mucous membrane and has three sections:

1. The nasopharynx, which is continuous with the nasal cavity above and with the oropharynx below. Its functions include:
   — warming and moistening inhaled air

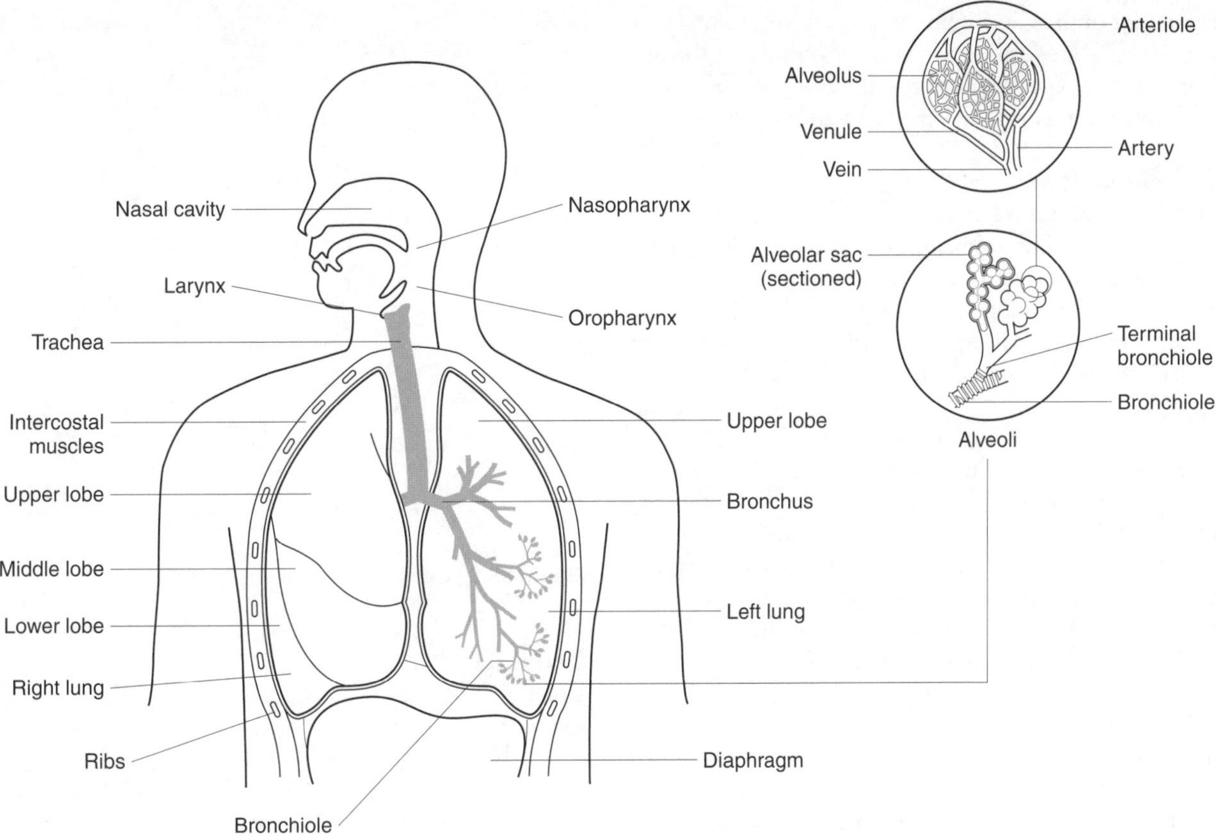

Figure 38.1 | The respiratory tract

— protection from infection, by patches of lymphoid tissue such as the adenoids

— equalisation of pressure in the middle ear with the atmospheric pressure by allowing air to travel along the eustachian tubes to the middle ear

2. The oropharynx, the section that lies behind the mouth and is separated from the cavity of the mouth by two folds of mucous membrane (the fauces). Between these folds lie the oral tonsils, which are patches of lymphoid tissue involved in the immune system. The oropharynx provides a common passage for air, food and fluids. The uvula is a muscular projection of the soft palate in the middle of the arch formed by the fauces, and prevents the entry of food and fluid into the nasal cavity
3. The laryngopharynx, which is the section that opens into both the larynx and the oesophagus. It contains the epiglottis (see next section).

THE LARYNX

The larynx is situated in the upper region of the neck and extends from the pharynx above to the trachea below. It is composed of pieces of cartilage connected by membranes and provides a passageway for air between the pharynx and trachea. As air passes through, it is further moistened, warmed and filtered. The main cartilages that form the larynx are:

- The thyroid cartilage, which is the largest and forms a prominence known as the 'Adam's apple'
- The epiglottis, a leaf-shaped cartilage attached to the upper part of the thyroid cartilage. During swallowing, the larynx rises and the epiglottis covers its opening, directing food and fluid into the oesophagus and preventing its entry into the trachea and subsequent aspiration into the lungs
- The cricoid cartilage, which lies below the thyroid cartilage, and is shaped like a wide banded ring.

The larynx is lined with mucous membrane, which becomes ciliated in the lower part. In the upper part, two folds of membrane containing embedded fibrous and elastic tissue form the vocal cords. The vocal cords extend from the anterior wall to the posterior wall of the larynx to form the glottis, or voice box, which produce sounds. The nerve supply to the larynx is from the laryngeal and recurrent laryngeal nerves, which are branches of the vagus nerve.

Voice production

The vocal cords are apart during normal breathing. Contraction of muscles attached to the cords brings them closer together, and expired air is used to cause vibration of the cords. The brain, tongue, lips, nasal cavity and facial muscles all help to convert the resultant sounds into speech. The pitch of the voice depends on the length and tightness of the cords, and the air sinuses in the skull bones influence the resonance of the voice. The vowels and consonants that make up speech are formed by various positions of the lips and tongue. Speaking requires coordination of the larynx, mouth, lips, tongue, throat, lungs and abdomen.

THE TRACHEA

The trachea is about 12 cm long and lies in front of the oesophagus, extending from the larynx to the mid-thorax, where it divides into a right and a left bronchus. The trachea consists of 15–20 C-shaped rings of cartilage joined by involuntary muscle and fibrous tissue. Posteriorly the trachea lacks cartilage and is replaced with smooth muscle to enable the oesophagus to expand, while the cartilages maintain the patency of the airway. It thus provides a permanently open passageway for air travelling to and from the lungs. The trachea is lined with ciliated epithelium containing mucus-secreting goblet cells. The cilia sweep the mucus, cell debris and any foreign particles that enter the trachea up into the pharynx to be swallowed or expectorated. Air travelling through the trachea is further warmed and moistened to prevent drying and damage to tissues.

BRONCHI

At about the middle of the thorax, the trachea divides to form the right and left bronchus. The bronchi enter the lungs; the right bronchus dividing into three, and the left bronchus dividing into two branches. There are three lobes in the right lung and two lobes in the left lung, therefore one branch of each bronchus enters each lobe. The left bronchus is longer than the right because of the position of the heart. Smooth involuntary muscles surround the airways to allow for alteration in airway diameter.

BRONCHIOLES

Bronchioles are the smallest branches of the bronchi, and their walls consist of involuntary muscle with elastic fibrous tissue, allowing for expansion and constriction. They divide to form terminal bronchioles that give rise to microscopic alveolar ducts, which terminate in clusters of air sacs called alveoli.

ALVEOLI

Alveoli are microscopic air sacs in the lungs. Their walls are composed of one layer of type I, simple squamous epithelial cells, and type II cells that produce surfactant that maintain alveolar expansion by reducing surface tension. Macrophages are present and their role is to phagocytose cell debris and pathogens. The alveoli form a surface area of about 70 m^2 for semi-permeable membrane diffusion of gases. The alveoli are surrounded by networks of capillaries, arising from the pulmonary arteries and their tributaries. The function of alveoli is the interchange of oxygen and carbon dioxide between the air in the alveoli and the blood in the capillaries (Figure 38.2).

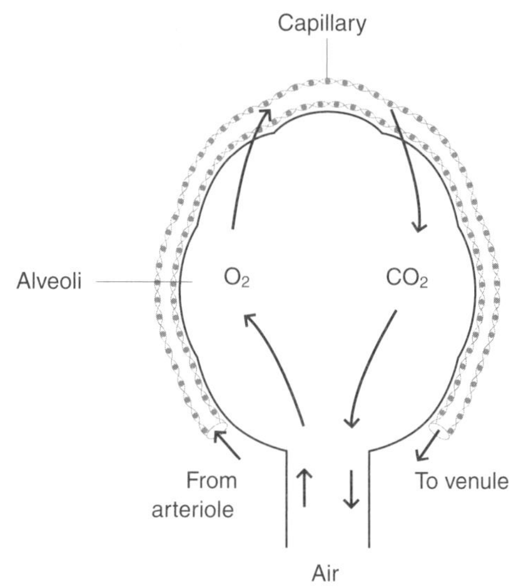

Figure 38.2 | Exchange of gases in the alveoli

LUNGS

The two lungs lie in the thoracic cavity on either side of the mediastinum. The mediastinal cavity contains the heart, major blood vessels and the oesophagus. The lungs are light and spongy and consist of the bronchioles, alveoli and blood vessels and are supported by areolar tissue. There is also a great deal of elastic tissue to enable the lungs to expand and recoil freely during respiration. The base of each lung rests on the diaphragm and the apex of each extends to just above each clavicle. The right lung has three lobes and is shorter and wider than the left lung, which has two lobes (Figure 38.1). Each lobe is made up of lobules, each with its own blood, nerve and lymph supply. On the medial side of each lung is a depression called the hilus, through which the bronchi, lymphatic vessels and blood vessels enter and exit.

PLEURA

The pleura (Figure 38.3) comprise a double layer of serous membrane, consisting of the visceral pleura, which adheres to the surface of the lungs, and the parietal pleura, which lines the thoracic cavity and covers the superior surface of the diaphragm. The pleura secrete a thin film of serous fluid, maintained at about 50 mL, which lies between the two layers and prevents friction between the surfaces. The pressure within the pleura is 2 mmHg below atmospheric pressure to prevent lung collapse.

MUSCLES OF VENTILATION

The main muscles responsible for ventilation are the diaphragm and internal and external intercostal muscles. During difficult or forced breathing, accessory muscles are used, such as the muscles of the neck, thorax (e.g. sterno-cleidomastoid, anterior serrate, scalene) and abdominal muscles, including the rectus abdominus and transverse abdominus.

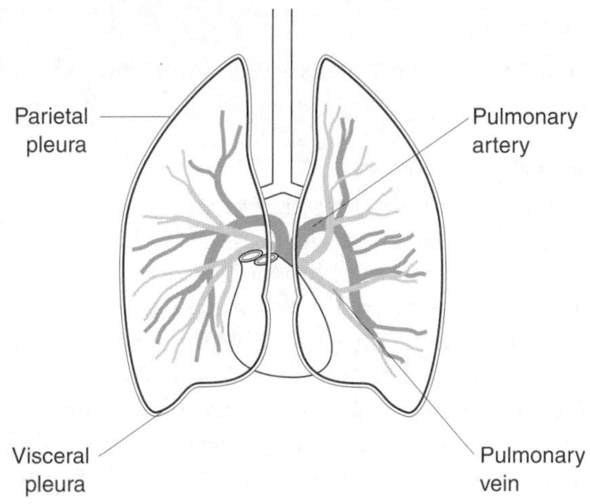

Figure 38.3 | The lungs and pleura

SCIENTIFIC PRINCIPLES RELATED TO THE RESPIRATORY SYSTEM

Air is moved into and out of the lung by alterations in pressures in different areas in relation to the atmosphere. An understanding of pressure relationships and laws concerning gases will assist in the understanding of ventilation and respiration discussed later in this chapter.

PRESSURE

Pressure may be defined as force (or stress) per unit area applied to a surface. The concept of pressure, or force, applies equally to solids, liquids and gases. Described below are some of the principles and concepts relating to pressure that are relevant to nursing.

ATMOSPHERIC PRESSURE

Atmospheric pressure arises by virtue of the weight of the air above the earth. Atmospheric pressure decreases as altitude increases because of the reduced amount of air above. Even at a particular altitude, atmospheric pressure is not constant, but varies according to atmospheric conditions. The total pressure exerted by the atmosphere is about 6.8 kg per 25 mm^2 of surface area at sea level. The atmosphere consists principally of nitrogen (N_2) 79.03%, oxygen (O_2) 20.93%, and carbon dioxide (CO_2) 0.0004%, which totals 99.9604%. Other gases such as carbon monoxide (CO) are present in minute quantities. Oxygen, a colourless and odourless gas, is essential in sustaining most forms of life.

Water vapour and gases in the atmosphere have weight and, at sea level, exert a pressure defined as 1 atmosphere of pressure ('atmospheric pressure') equivalent to 760 mmHg. The terms negative and positive pressure are used to compare a pressure to normal atmospheric pressure at sea level. Any pressure above normal atmospheric pressure is regarded as a positive pressure, and any pressure below normal atmospheric pressure is regarded as a negative pressure.

The following three laws of physics define the characteristics of gases:

1. Pascal's principle, which states that a confined liquid transmits pressure, applied to it from an external force, equally in all directions
2. Boyle's law, which states that the volume of a given mass of gas is inversely proportional to the pressure to which it is subjected, provided that the temperature remains constant
3. Charles' law, which states that the volume of a given mass of gas is directly proportional to its absolute temperature, provided that the pressure remains constant; for example, as the temperature of a gas is increased (at constant pressure) the gas expands.

The combined effects of atmospheric pressure and the application of the gas laws above provide the basis for the operation of many common devices, and also of the lungs. Boyle's law refers to pressure differentials and is able to be applied to the process of breathing. By changing the volume of the thoracic cavity, the air pressure in the lungs can be made lower or higher than atmospheric pressure, leading to inhalation or exhalation, respectively.

REGULATION OF VENTILATION

SENSORY MECHANISMS OF THE RESPIRATORY SYSTEM

Every cell in the human body requires oxygen for normal metabolism and must excrete the metabolic waste product, carbon dioxide. To maintain homeostasis, cells in different locations of the body react to changes in oxygen and CO_2 levels. Sensory cells include chemoreceptors, pressorreceptors and baroreceptors.

CHEMORECEPTORS

Chemoreceptors are specialised cells located centrally in the upper medulla of the brainstem and peripherally in bodies located in the carotid and aortic arteries. They respond to slight increases in arterial or cerebrospinal fluid CO_2 pressure (P_{CO2}) and acidity (an increased concentration of hydrogen [H^+] ions). Regulation of ventilation depends mainly on the level of CO_2 in the blood. A slight increase in CO_2 concentration stimulates chemoreceptors to increase the respiratory rate and depth until the excess CO_2 is eliminated. Conversely, a decreased CO_2 level slows the ventilatory rate. Oxygen levels are normally sensed by the carotid bodies, which are sensitive to a fall in oxygen concentration of less than 50%. Stimulation of the carotid receptors increases the respiratory rate, the exception being clients with chronic hypercapnia such as emphysema.

PRESSORRECEPTORS

Pressorreceptors, or mechanoreceptors, are stretch receptors present in lung tissue and within the thoracic wall. The bronchioles and alveoli also have stretch receptors that respond to extreme over-inflation as well as extreme deflation.

When over-inflation occurs, impulses are transmitted from the stretch receptors to the medulla by the vagus nerve, the expiratory centre is activated and exhalation occurs. When extreme deflation occurs impulses from the lungs activate the inspiratory centre, and inhalation occurs.

BARORECEPTORS

Baroreceptors are cells sensitive to blood pressure, and which normally monitor changes in blood pressure. When blood pressure increases, impulses are sent to the respiratory centres to cause a decrease in respiratory rate. Rate, depth and rhythm of respirations are further affected by reflex responses, chemical signals and voluntary control; for example, during actions such as swallowing, impulses from gustatory centres are conveyed to the respiratory centre, and breathing stops temporarily.

Any abnormal mechanical disturbance, such as the presence of chemical substances such as cigarette smoke, causes excitement of the lung irritant receptors, which induces hyperventilation and a reflex bronchoconstriction. Information from other parts of the body may also be received by the respiratory centres; for example, a rise in body temperature initiates an increase in the rate of ventilation, while a sudden cooling of the body induces a sudden inhalation followed by hyperventilation.

THE RESPIRATORY CENTRES

Respiration is controlled both voluntarily and involuntarily. The automatic control of breathing is regulated by three respiratory centres, known as the medullary centre, located in the medulla oblongata, the apneustic centre in the pons, and the pneumotaxic centre in the upper pons of the brainstem. These centres receive stimuli from sensory cells described above, and from each other. Their function is to control the rate, rhythm and depth of ventilation. Impulses travel from the respiratory centres along separate nerves that exit the spinal cord at different levels to separately innervate and control the diaphragm and internal and external intercostal muscles. Impulses are also transmitted to the other centres and cause stimulation of the respiratory muscles via the phrenic nerves, to stimulate the diaphragm to contract, and the intercostal nerves, which stimulate the intercostal muscles.

VENTILATION AND RESPIRATION

Respiration is the term used to describe an interchange of gases. The main purpose of respiration is to supply the body with oxygen and dispose of carbon dioxide. The four processes involved are:

1. Ventilation: movement of air containing different gases into the respiratory tract
2. External respiration: exchange of oxygen and CO_2 between the blood and the alveoli (Figure 38.2)
3. Internal respiration: exchange of oxygen and CO_2 between the bloodstream and the tissues
4. Cellular respiration: exchange of gases by cells.

Ventilation

Ventilation has two phases: inhalation and exhalation (Figure 38.4).

Inhalation

During inhalation the diaphragm contracts and flattens, enlarging the thoracic cavity lengthwise, particularly in males. In females normal inhalations occur primarily by contraction of the external intercostal muscles, which raise the ribs and sternum, thus increasing the size of the thoracic cavity from side to side and front to back. As the chest wall moves up and outward, the parietal pleura moves with it and, because of the 2 mmHg negative pressure within the pleura, the visceral pleura follows the parietal pleura. This causes stretching of the lungs, which expand to fill the enlarged thorax, and air is pushed into the respiratory passages.

Exhalation

Exhalation is normally a more passive process than inhalation except in exercise and respiratory conditions in which active expiration occurs via internal intercostal and accessory muscles. During exhalation the diaphragm relaxes

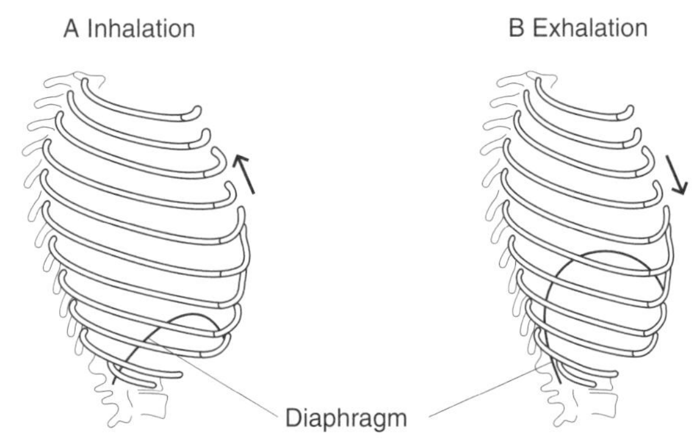

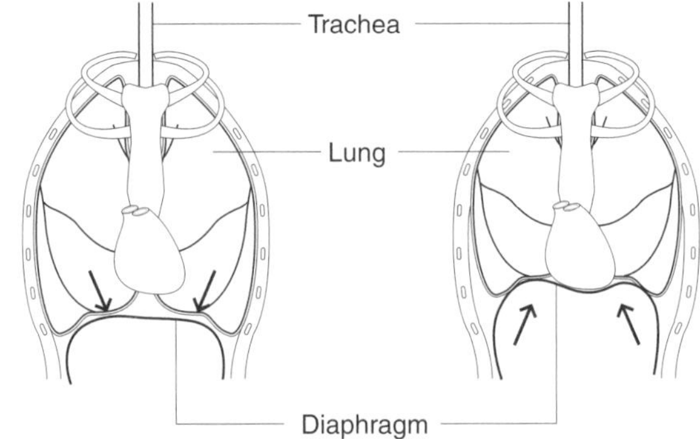

Figure 38.4 | Rib cage and diaphragm positions during breathing
A: At the end of normal inhalation: chest expanded (top left) and diaphragm depressed (bottom left)
B: At the end of a normal exhalation: chest depressed (top right) and diaphragm elevated (bottom right)

thus decreasing the size of the thoracic cavity. The external intercostal muscles also relax, allowing the ribs and sternum to return to their former position, further decreasing the size of the thoracic cavity. The elastic tissue of the lungs allows for recoil, further forcing air out of the respiratory passages.

Respiration

External respiration

External respiration is the exchange of gases between air in the alveoli, and the blood travelling through the capillaries surrounding the alveoli. Branches of the pulmonary artery bring deoxygenated blood to the capillaries surrounding each alveolus. During gas exchange, gases normally diffuse through the semi-permeable walls of the alveoli and capillaries to the area of lowest concentration of each gas, as each gas diffuses independently of other gases, until the pressure is equal on both sides. Thus, oxygen moves from an area of higher concentration in the alveoli to an area of lower concentration in the blood capillaries, while CO_2 moves from an area of a higher concentration in blood capillaries to an area of lower concentration in the alveolar air. Pulmonary venules then collect the blood rich in oxygen from the capillaries and unite to form the two pulmonary veins which leave each lung to enter the left atrium of the heart. Table 38.1 illustrates the concentration and movement of gases in the alveoli and capillary blood. Table 38.2 illustrates the approximate composition of inspired and expired air.

Internal respiration

Internal respiration is the exchange of gases between the bloodstream and the tissues (Figure 38.5). During this exchange, the gases diffuse through the semi-permeable walls of the capillaries to equalise the concentration of gases on both sides. Oxygen moves from the blood into the tissues, down a concentration gradient, to replenish oxygen used in cellular metabolism. Carbon dioxide moves from the tissues into the blood, down a concentration gradient, to rid the tissues of waste produced by cellular metabolism. Table 38.3 illustrates the concentration and movement of gases in the tissues and capillary blood.

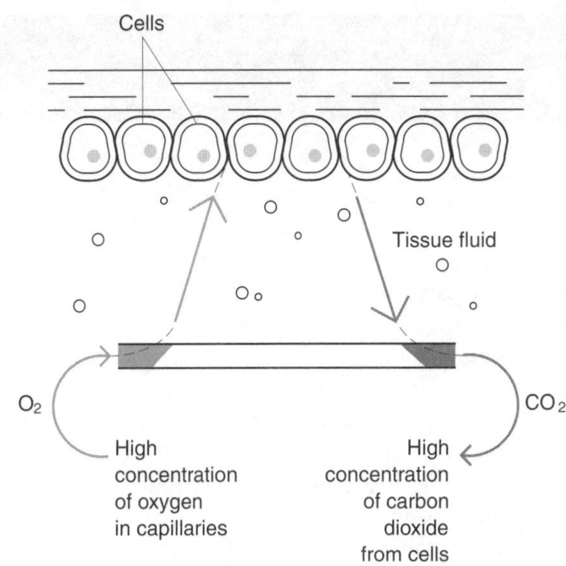

Figure 40.5 | Internal respiration

Cellular respiration

The gases that diffuse from the interstitial tissue into cells are used by the cells for metabolism. The metabolism of nutrients uses oxygen and produces CO_2, which diffuses from cells into the interstitial tissue. This level of respiration is termed cellular respiration.

FACTORS NECESSARY FOR VENTILATION AND RESPIRATION

The passage of oxygen from the atmosphere to the alveoli in the lungs, and the passage of carbon dioxide from the alveoli to the atmosphere, requires an unobstructed airway.

TABLE 38.1 | CONCENTRATION AND MOVEMENT OF GASES IN THE ALVEOLI AND CAPILLARY BLOOD

Gas	Concentration in alveoli	Movement	Concentration in blood
Oxygen	100 mmHg	—	38 mmHg
Carbon dioxide	38 mmHg	—	46 mmHg

TABLE 38.2 | COMPOSITION OF INHALED AND EXHALED AIR (APPROXIMATE)

Substance	Inhaled air	Exhaled air
Nitrogen	78.62%	74.5%
Oxygen	20.84%	15.7%
Carbon dioxide	0.04%	3.6%
Water vapour	0.50%	6.2%
Total	100.0%	100.0%

TABLE 38.3 | INTERNAL RESPIRATION

Gas	Concentration in tissues	Movement	Concentration in blood
Oxygen	Low		High
Carbon dioxide	High		Low

In addition, the process of respiration requires:

- Adequate oxygen in the atmosphere
- A patent functioning respiratory tract
- Functioning thoracic muscles and nerves to control the thoracic cage and diaphragm
- Capillaries in close proximity to the cells to allow the exchange of gases
- A functioning cardiovascular system that contains adequate amounts of plasma and normal erythrocytes and haemoglobin to transport the gases.

STRUCTURE OF THE CARDIOVASCULAR SYSTEM

The structures that make up the cardiovascular system are the:

- Heart, which acts as a pump to circulate the blood through the body
- Blood, which carries essential substances to cells and carries wastes away from cells
- Blood vessels, which contain and transport the blood throughout the body
- Lymphatic system, which transports tissue fluid containing electrolytes, proteins and some waste products, recognises and destroys pathogens before they reach the bloodstream, and delivers nutrients from the digestive tract into the cardiovascular system.

BLOOD

Blood, which is classed as a connective tissue, constitutes about one-twelfth of the weight of the body. It is a viscous substance composed of a fluid portion (plasma) and formed elements (cells and cell fragments). Depending on the weight of the individual, the average total volume of blood is about 5–6 L. Blood varies in colour, from bright red when it has a high oxygen content, to dark red when the oxygen content is low. Arterial blood normally has a pH range of 7.35 to 7.45.

Functions of blood

Blood has the following functions:

- Transporting oxygen, nutrients, water and ions to all tissue cells
- Removing waste materials to excretory organs
- Transporting hormones to cells
- Supplying materials from which cells and glands make their secretions
- Protecting the body against infection by means of the leucocytes and antibodies
- Regulation of body temperature by distributing heat evenly throughout the body
- Preventing loss of body fluid and blood cells by means of its clotting mechanism.

Constituents of blood

Plasma and formed elements make up the components of blood. Plasma, the fluid part of blood, is a straw-coloured watery fluid in which blood cells are suspended. Plasma forms about 55% of the blood volume and contains:

- Water: about 90–92% of the plasma is composed of water, which is important in the maintenance of all body fluids and in the production of secretions
- Proteins: albumin, globulin, fibrinogen, prothrombin and heparin are some of the proteins found in plasma. The liver normally produces proteins, with the exception of serum globulin, which is derived from lymphocytes. Plasma proteins have several important functions: they assist in retaining water in the plasma and interstitial tissue; factors such as prothrombin and fibrinogen are essential for blood clotting; proteins such as heparin help to prevent abnormal clotting of blood in the blood vessels
- Mineral salts: the main mineral salts found in blood plasma are sodium chloride, iodine, potassium, phosphorus, calcium, iron, magnesium and copper. Mineral salts are necessary for the regulation of cellular functioning and electropotentials, and maintenance of the blood pH
- Nutrients: those found in blood plasma are numerous and include amino acids, glucose, fatty acids, glycerol and vitamins. They have been reduced to their simplest form by the digestive processes and absorbed from the alimentary tract into the blood and lymph for circulation to the cells
- Waste products resulting from fat and protein metabolism, including urea, uric acid and creatinine
- Gases, including oxygen, nitrogen and carbon dioxide. Oxygen and nitrogen enter the bloodstream after inhalation of air, and carbon dioxide is an end product of oxidation in the cells
- Hormones: chemical substances secreted directly into the bloodstream by endocrine glands and carried to the areas of the body where they are required to stimulate activity
- Antibodies and antitoxins: complex protein substances produced by the body in response to an invasion by a foreign protein (antigen). They are part of the body's defence mechanism

- Enzymes, produced by the body, which initiate or accelerate chemical reactions.

Blood group types

Human blood is grouped into four classifications based on immune reactivity. The groups are O, A, B, AB. The Rhesus factor (either negative or positive) is also determined. Eighty-five percent of the population has Rh antibodies on the surface of the red blood cell (that is RH positive). Generally speaking the blood of any one group is incompatible with the blood group of another. Therefore blood transfusions should be an exact match to the client's blood group and Rh factor. When blood transfusions occur with mismatched blood a haemolytic reaction can occur (refer to Table 38.4 Preparing and monitoring a client undergoing a blood transfusion) (Tollefson 2004).

BLOOD CELLS

The blood cells and fragments are suspended in the plasma and are called formed elements. The three types of blood cells or fragments of cells are erythrocytes, leucocytes and thrombocytes.

Erythrocytes (red cells) are biconcave non-nucleated discs measuring about 7 microns in diameter. In adults, erythrocytes are produced in the red bone marrow of cancellous bone tissue, where they pass through several stages of development. They begin as large nucleated cells but when mature (after they have produced haemoglobin) they lose the nucleus and are liberated into the circulation. Haemoglobin is a complex protein composed of four different 'haem' chains, each containing a central atom of iron and a globulin protein. It has a strong affinity for both oxygen and carbon monoxide and gives the blood its colour. The normal haemoglobin level is about 14–16 g/100 mL of blood.

The number of erythrocytes is about 5 000 000/mm^3 of blood, and their average life span is 100–120 days. As their nucleus is absent, they are unable to repair damage and become worn out in circulation, and are destroyed in the spleen and liver. The haemoglobin is split; its iron is stored by the liver for future use, and the pigment is used by the liver in the production of bile. The primary function of erythrocytes is to carry oxygen. In the lungs, oxygen combines with haemoglobin to form oxyhaemoglobin, making the blood bright red in colour. As blood circulates through the tissues, the oxygen is released, forming deoxyhaemoglobin, and the blood becomes dark red in colour.

Leucocytes (white cells) measure about 10 microns in diameter. They differ from erythrocytes in that they are larger, possess a nucleus and are less numerous. They also have the power of independent movement, known as diapedis, or emigration, which erythrocytes do not possess. There are two main types of leucocytes: granulocytes and agranular leucocytes. Granulocytes contain granules of enzymes and are classified as neutrophils, basophils or eosinophils. Neutrophils are the most numerous of the leucocytes and are important to the body in defence against bacteria, as they have the ability to engulf phagocytose and digest them. Neutrophils also play an important part in the inflammatory response. Injured tissues, and other leucocytes, secrete substances that stimulate the bone marrow to release increased numbers of neutrophils. Basophils release substances in infected tissue that are toxic to many microorganisms. They also play a part in the allergic response and act to limit the inflammatory response. Eosinophils are also involved in phagocytosis, as they ingest antigen–antibody complexes and parasites. They also play a role in clot retraction.

Agranular leucocytes lack granules of enzymes and are classified as monocytes or lymphocytes. Monocytes have the ability to move into the tissues, where they become macrophages and are capable of phagocytosis. They also secrete a variety of substances involved in the body's defence, and play a role in the immune response. Lymphocytes are either T lymphocytes or B lymphocytes, both of which divide when stimulated by antigens. T lymphocytes are responsible for cellular immunity, and adhere to cells identified as foreign to the body. They secrete cytotoxic substances that kill the foreign cells. B lymphocytes are involved in humoral immunity, as they produce antibodies and are also responsible for immunoglobulin production. While the life span for granular leucocytes is only about 21 days, lymphocytes may survive for up to 100 days.

The total number of leucocytes is about 8000–10 000/mm^3 of blood, but this number increases considerably (leucocytosis) when there is any infection in the body. The life span of a leucocyte is variable and depends to some extent on the degree of activity.

Thrombocytes (platelets) are colourless microscopic fragments of the megakaryocyte cell. Measuring about 3 microns in diameter, they do not possess a nucleus. Thrombocytes are produced in the red bone marrow, which is present in cancellous bone tissue. The number of thrombocytes is about 250 000–300 000/mm^3 of blood, and the average life span of a thrombocyte is 5–9 days. The function of thrombocytes is to play a major role in the clotting of blood to reduce blood loss when a vessel wall is injured. The process involves many substances (clotting factors) which are produced by the liver and circulate in the plasma, as well as some substances released by the platelets and injured tissues. Normally a blood clot will form within 2–6 minutes after a blood vessel wall has been damaged.

The mechanism of clotting (haemostasis) involves three phases: vasoconstriction, formation of a temporary platelet plug and formation of a clot. When a small vessel becomes damaged:

- Local vasoconstriction occurs, which reduces blood flow and therefore blood loss
- The vessel wall becomes 'sticky' and platelets adhere to the damaged area
- The platelets release serotonin and adenosine

TABLE 38.4 | PREPARING AND MONITORING A CLIENT UNDERGOING A BLOOD TRANSFUSION

Review and carry out the steps in Appendix 1

Action	Rationale
Check medical orders to ascertain type, frequency and amount of fluid to be administered, and time prepared	Ensures correct quantities are given to client
Explain procedure to client	Reduced anxiety/apprehension and gains client's trust and cooperation
Measure and record blood pressure and vital signs	Provides a baseline of the client's haemodynamic health status
Prepare equipment	
Wash and dry hands	Prevents cross infection and contamination of blood and tubing
Don appropriate equipment and clothing as per infection control guidelines	Minimises risk of cross infection
Gather equipment including: • Sphygmomanometer (aneroid or mercury) • Stethoscope • Blood or blood product • Client's blood order sheet	Ensures all equipment is at client's bedside to maximise efficiency, reduce apprehension on the client's part and increase the confidence in the nurse
Establish an IV infusion with normal saline	IV access is established by a doctor or accredited Registered Nurse (RN). Normal saline is the solution used during a blood transfusion because it is compatible with blood and does not cause red blood cell lysis
Identify the client and the blood product according to policy Two nurses check the: • Client's armband • Blood order sheet • Information on the blood product • Expiry date	Group and type of blood product matches on the order and the product
The blood transfusion must be initiated within 15 minutes of arrival to the ward	Minimises risk of bacterial infection
Initiate the blood transfusion • Gently invert the blood product several times • Wearing gloves, close clamp on saline infusion and attach blood product to the short tubing on the administrating set • Tip the blood and gently squeeze to fill the filter • Place blood on IV stand and open the clamp, squeeze the drip chamber and release it until blood begins to flow	Ensures cells and plasma are mixed Stops the back flow of blood from mixing with the saline Filling the filter prevents air from entering the system Ensures no air bubbles enter the giving set
Initiate the transfusion slowly	Most reactions occur within the first 10 minutes. Beginning the transfusion slowly reduces the amount of blood for the system to react against reducing the severity of the reaction
Monitor the client	Vital signs are taken as per facility guidelines. Most are generally taken every 15 minutes for the first hour of the infusion then hourly for the remainder of the infusion
Observe for reactions such as: • Fever, chills, headache, malaise	Signs of a febrile reaction. Slow infusion rate
Observe for reactions such as: • Flushing of the skin, urticaria, wheezing, itchy rash	Signs of an allergic reaction. Stop infusion, flush with normal saline Notify doctor, give IV corticosteroids as ordered Restart the transfusion with a new blood product
Observe for reactions such as: • Restlessness, anxiety, chest pain, tachypnoea, tachycardia, nausea, shock, haematuria	Signs of a haemolytic reaction Stop transfusion, start new giving set with normal saline Commence oxygen therapy Notify doctor, give adrenaline and IV corticosteroids as ordered
Complete the transfusion	Ensures client receives the entire transfusion

TABLE 38.4 | PREPARING AND MONITORING A CLIENT UNDERGOING A BLOOD TRANSFUSION—cont'd

Action	Rationale
Dispose of the blood unit as per facility guidelines	Some facilities require all blood units (including the giving set) to be returned to blood bank and kept for 24 hours in case of a delayed reaction
Monitor client	Clients can have a delayed reaction to the blood product for up to 24 hours Vital signs are often recorded hourly for 4 hours then 4 hourly for 24 hours
Report and document the procedure and any complications	Most blood products have a peel off identification tag that is identical to the blood unit ID number, grouping and Rh factor so that errors in transcription are avoided. This tab should be removed and placed in the client's progress notes

diphosphate (ADP), which attract other thrombocytes, leading to the formation of a temporary platelet plug

- The temporary platelet plug is converted into a clot by the deposition of fibrin, which is formed from fibrinogen. The conversion of fibrinogen to fibrin involves a 'cascade' of reactions that requires a number of plasma factors (numbered I to XIII). A series of reactions culminate in the conversion of prothrombin to thrombin, which converts fibrinogen to fibrin. This conversion requires the presence of platelets, Factor V, Factor X and calcium ions. Vitamin K is also necessary for the conversion of Factors VII, IX and X
- The fibrin forms a meshwork of fibres that traps the erythrocytes and form the basis of a clot
- The clot plugs the injured blood vessel, drawing the edges together.

The clotting mechanism is a complex one that will not occur if any of the necessary elements are reduced, defective or missing.

BLOOD VESSELS

Blood is circulated throughout the body within vessels that form a closed continuous system (Figure 38.6). The walls of blood vessels have three layers: an outer coat of fibrous tissue, a thick middle layer of involuntary muscle with elastic fibrous tissue and an inner lining of endothelium to form a smooth surface for contact with blood (Figure 38.7). Blood vessels include the arteries, veins and capillaries (Figure 38.8).

Arteries

Arteries carry blood away from the heart (efferent). All arteries carry oxygenated (bright red) blood, with the exception of the two pulmonary arteries which carry deoxygenated (dark red) blood from the heart to the lungs. Arteries vary in size, and large arteries divide to form smaller arteries. Further division, or branching, occurs to form the smallest arteries, called arterioles, which divide into

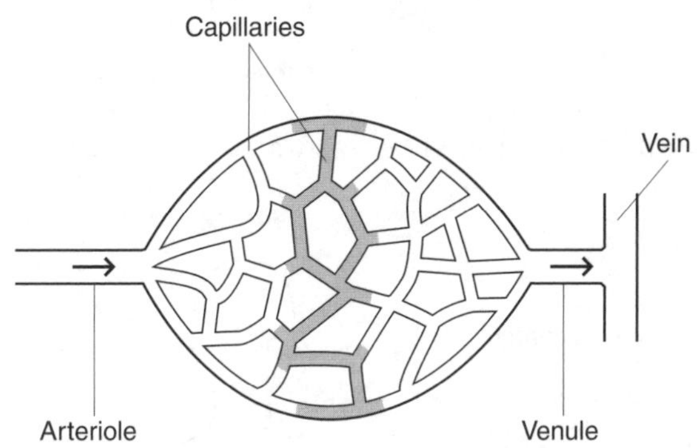

Figure 38.6 | Circulation of blood through the tissues

capillaries. Arteries and arterioles have the same tissue structure that allows them to stretch and recoil as the heart pumps the blood into them.

Veins

Veins carry blood towards the heart (afferent). All veins carry deoxygenated (dark red) blood, with the exception of the four pulmonary veins, which carry oxygenated blood from the lungs to the heart. Veins vary in size, and large veins divide to form smaller veins. The smallest veins are called venules, which divide into capillaries. Venules carry deoxygenated blood away from the capillary beds and unite to form veins. The walls of veins are composed of the same three layers as those of arteries, but the walls are thinner and have less elastic and muscular tissue. Veins join up until the two largest veins are formed — the superior and inferior vena cavae. These two veins empty their contents into the right atrium of the heart.

The larger veins possess pocket-like valves on their inner surfaces. These valves aid the unidirectional flow of blood towards the heart, and prevent a backward flow of blood. Skeletal muscle activity also helps venous return. As the muscles surrounding the veins contract and relax, the blood is 'milked' through the veins towards the heart.

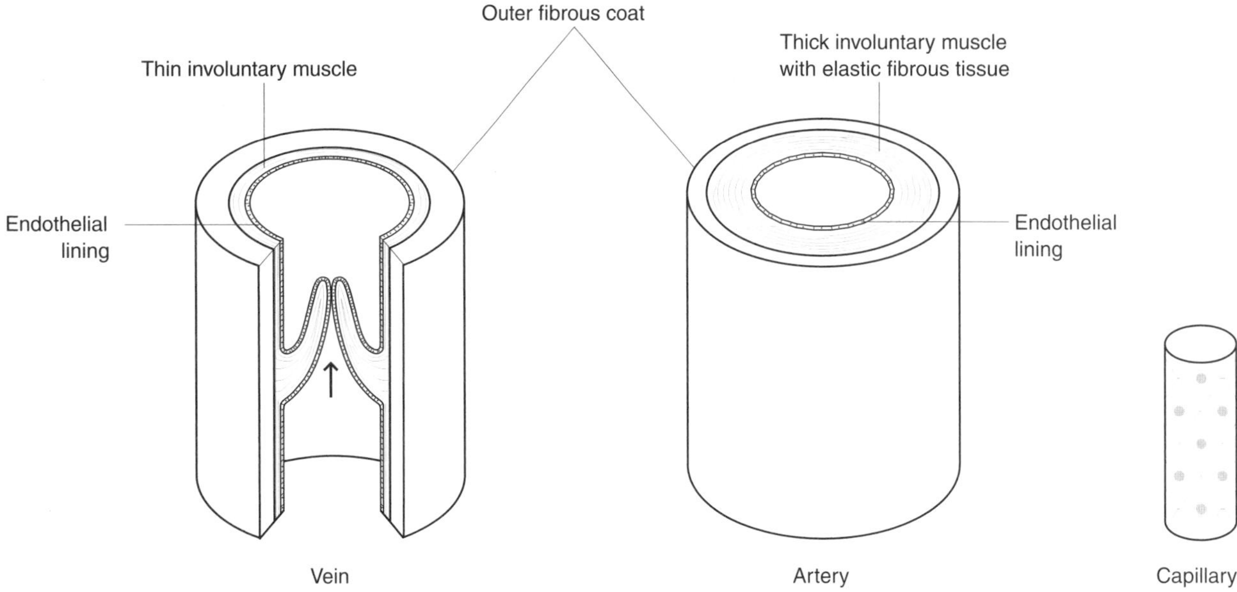

Figure 38.7 | Structure of blood vessels

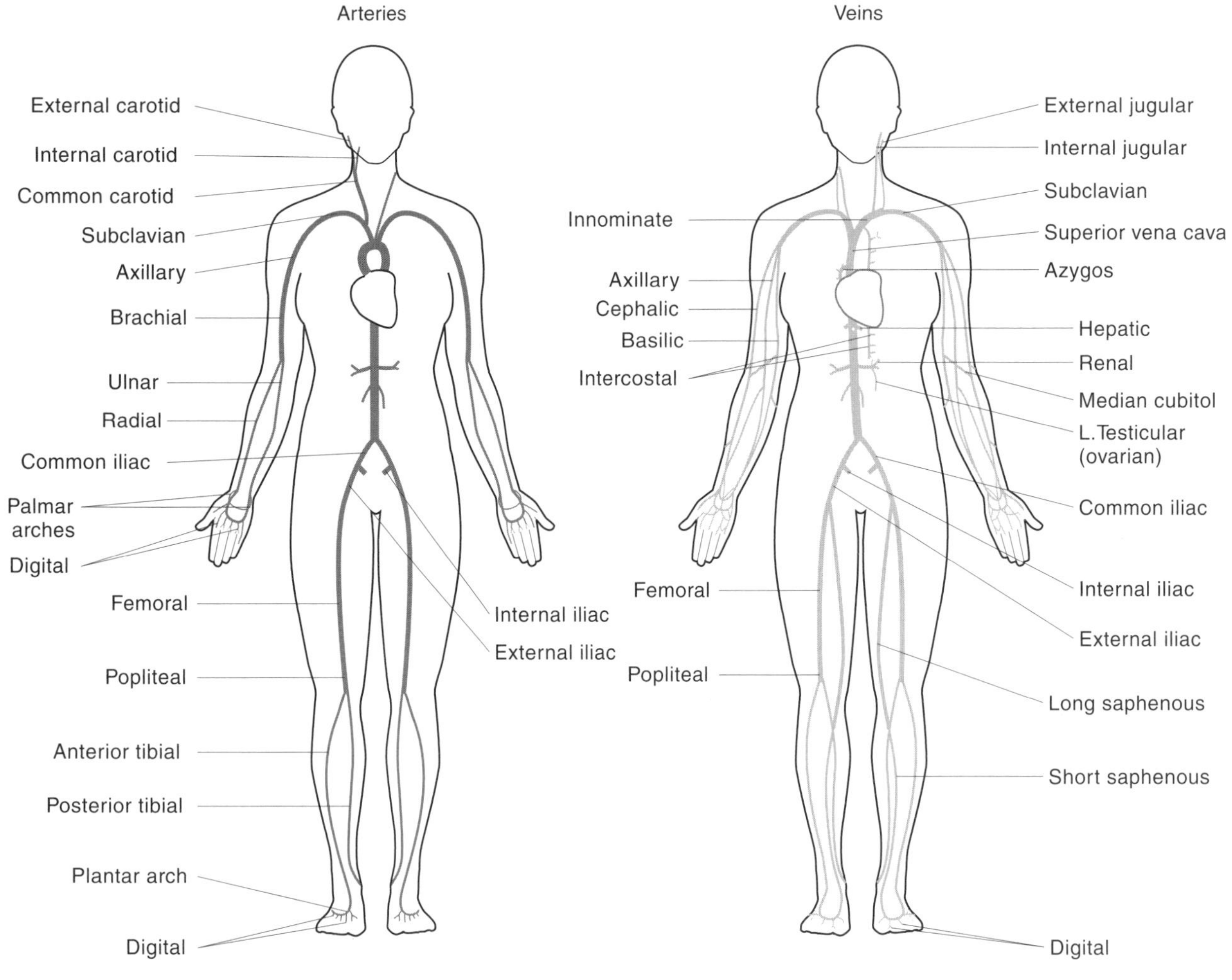

Figure 38.8 | Major arteries and veins of the systemic circulation

Capillaries

Capillaries are microscopic vessels about 5–7 microns in diameter and are composed of a single layer of endothelium, with little surrounding connective tissue. They form closed networks through all tissues and are structurally adapted for their role in the rapid diffusion of substances between the plasma and interstitial fluid. This allows water, oxygen, nutrients and other essential substances to pass rapidly from the blood to the tissue cells, and waste products from the tissue cells pass through the capillary walls to the blood.

THE HEART

The heart is a hollow, conical muscular organ situated obliquely in the thoracic cavity between the lungs and behind the sternum. One third of the heart lies to the right, and two thirds lie to the left of the median plane. Its base is uppermost and points towards the right shoulder, and its apex is below, pointing to the left. The adult heart is about 12 cm × 8 cm × 6 cm, and weighs about 300 g.

Structure of the heart

The heart is divided into a right, and a left side by a muscular partition called the septum. Each side is further divided into an upper receiving chamber, the atrium, and a lower distributing chamber, the ventricle (Figure 38.9). The walls of the heart consist of the pericardium, myocardium and endocardium:

- The pericardium is the outer coat, consisting of two layers of serous membrane. The pericardium secretes a small amount of serous fluid to moisten the surfaces in contact with each other, so that the heart can beat with minimal friction
- The myocardium is the middle muscular layer consisting of cardiac muscle, which is a highly specialised type of muscle tissue present only in the heart. It is of varying thickness, being thicker in both ventricles than in the atria, and thicker in the left ventricle than in the right
- Endocardium is the innermost lining of the heart, and provides a smooth surface for the flow of blood. Folds of endocardium help to form the valves of the heart.

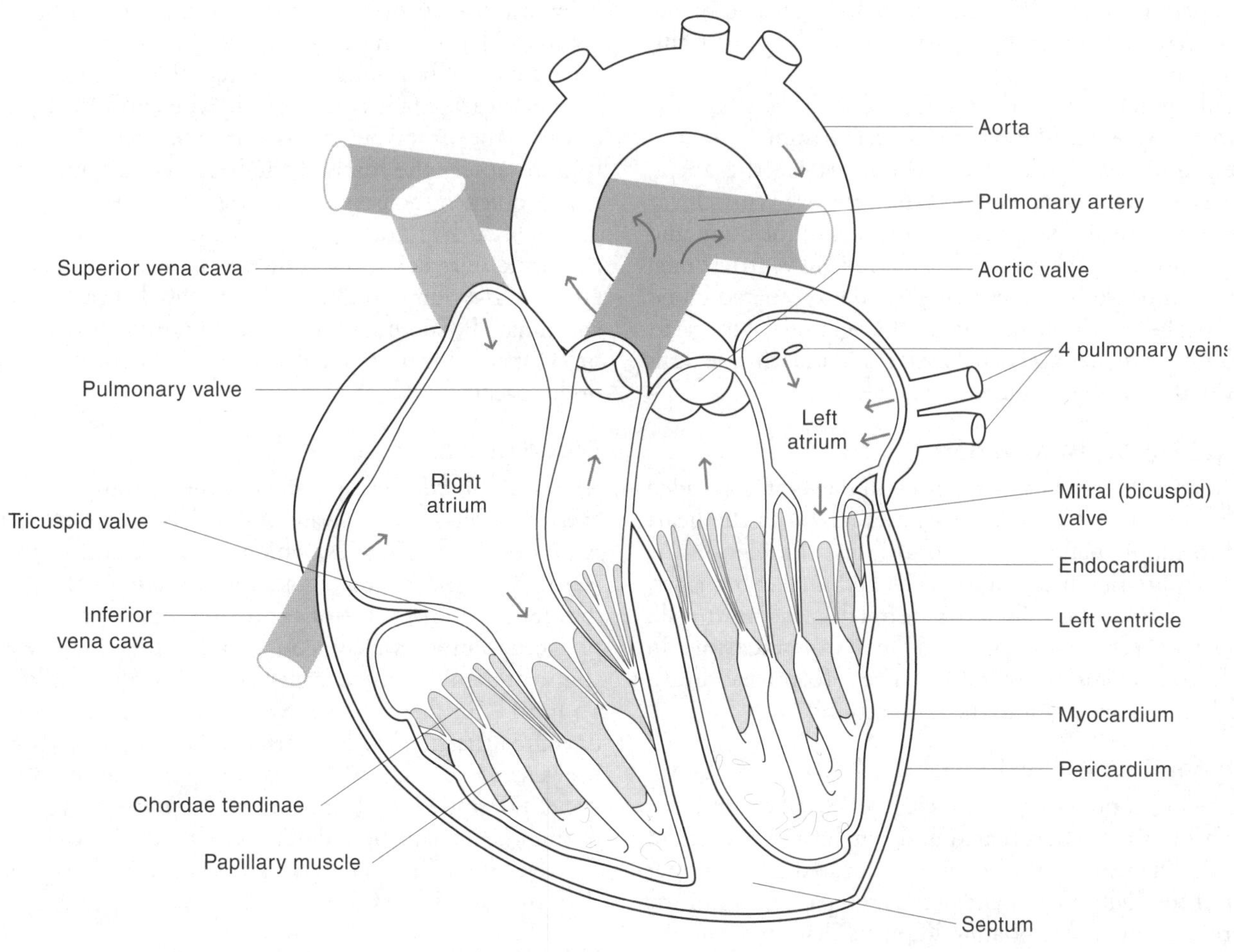

Figure 38.9 | Structure of the heart

Valves of the heart

Heart valves consist of flaps of fibrous tissue covered by endocardium, which allow blood to flow in one direction only, thus preventing a backward flow. The valves are the:

- Bicuspid (or mitral) valve, between the left atrium and left ventricle
- Tricuspid valve, between the right atrium and right ventricle
- Aortic valve, between the left ventricle and the aorta
- Pulmonary valve, between the right ventricle and the pulmonary artery.

Fine cords of tendons (chordae tendinae) are attached from the mitral and tricuspid valves to small projections from the muscle walls of the ventricles called papillary muscles. Contraction of the papillary muscles closes the valves, preventing blood from escaping back into the atria.

Blood vessels

Several blood vessels either enter or leave the heart. The blood vessels that enter the heart are the:

- Inferior vena cava, which carries deoxygenated blood collected from the lower part of the body to the right atrium
- Superior vena cava, which carries deoxygenated blood collected from the upper part of the body to the right atrium
- Four pulmonary veins, two from each lung, which carry oxygenated blood into the left atrium.

The blood vessels that leave the heart are the aorta, which carries oxygenated blood from the left ventricle for distribution to all the systems and tissues of the body, and the pulmonary artery, which leaves the right ventricle then divides into two branches that carry deoxygenated blood from the heart to each lung. Thus, the right side of the heart deals only with deoxygenated blood, and the left side deals only with oxygenated blood.

Blood supply to the heart

As the aorta leaves the heart it gives off two branches called the coronary arteries. These arteries pass into the heart wall to supply mainly the myocardium with blood. The coronary arteries divide into smaller and smaller branches, until networks of capillaries are formed in the heart wall. Venules collect the deoxygenated blood from the tissues in the heart wall and unite to form a vein (coronary sinus), which opens directly into the right atrium.

The conducting system of the heart

The heart's conducting system (Figure 38.10) ensures that it contracts in a coordinated and synchronised series of events. The sinoatrial (SA) node is located in the upper part of the right atrium and acts as the pacemaker of the heart, continuously initiating impulses that innervate the rest of the heart. The atrioventricular (AV) node lies in the lower part of the interatrial septum of the heart. The AV node is connected to the bundle of His and is the only natural pathway for the impulse to travel from the atria to the ventricles. The bundle of His divides into the right and left bundle branches, which in turn divide off into tiny fibres termed Purkinje fibres. These fibres rapidly conduct the impulse throughout the myocardium from the apex to the base.

Functions of the heart

The function of the heart is to act as a pump: it pumps deoxygenated blood to the lungs to excrete carbon dioxide and pick up oxygen, and pumps oxygenated blood to all other parts of the body.

The cardiac cycle is the series of pressure changes, valve actions and electrical potentials that bring about the movement of blood through the heart during one complete heart beat. The cardiac cycle takes about 0.8 of a second and consists of two phases, systole (the contraction phase) and diastole (the relaxation phase). During systole, both atria contract at the same time, emptying their contents into the ventricles. The two ventricles then contract simultaneously, forcing their contents into the aorta and pulmonary artery. Diastole follows after each contraction of the heart.

Cardiac output is the volume of blood pumped out by each ventricle during 1 minute. It is the product of the volume of blood pumped at each beat (stroke volume) and the number of beats during 1 minute (heart rate).

The heartbeat is controlled by the cardioregulatory centre in the central nervous system. The vagus nerve slows it and reduces the force of the beat, while sympathetic nerves quicken the beat and increase its force.

Each cardiac muscle cell is capable of spontaneous, rhythmic self-excitation known as autorhythmia. To be effective as a pump, the action of the whole heart must be coordinated. Coordination of the rhythmic movements is brought about by the specialised cells of the sinoatrial (SA) node (pacemaker).

Blood pressure

The term blood pressure refers to the pressure, or force, exerted by blood on the walls of the blood vessels. Pressure is highest in the arteries, which receive blood from the ventricles of the heart at about 120 mmHg. As the vessels divide, their cross-sectional area increases, causing the pressure to progressively reduce so that there is only very slight pressure in the capillaries (about 35 mmHg and 15 mmHg in the venules). Systolic blood pressure is the pressure registered in a large artery as blood is forced out of the ventricle during the contracting period of the cardiac cycle. Diastolic blood pressure is the pressure registered during the relaxing period of the cardiac cycle, when there is no ejection of blood into the arteries. It is therefore lower than the systolic pressure.

CIRCULATION OF BLOOD

Deoxygenated blood from all body regions is transported via the veins to the superior and inferior vena cavae, which enter

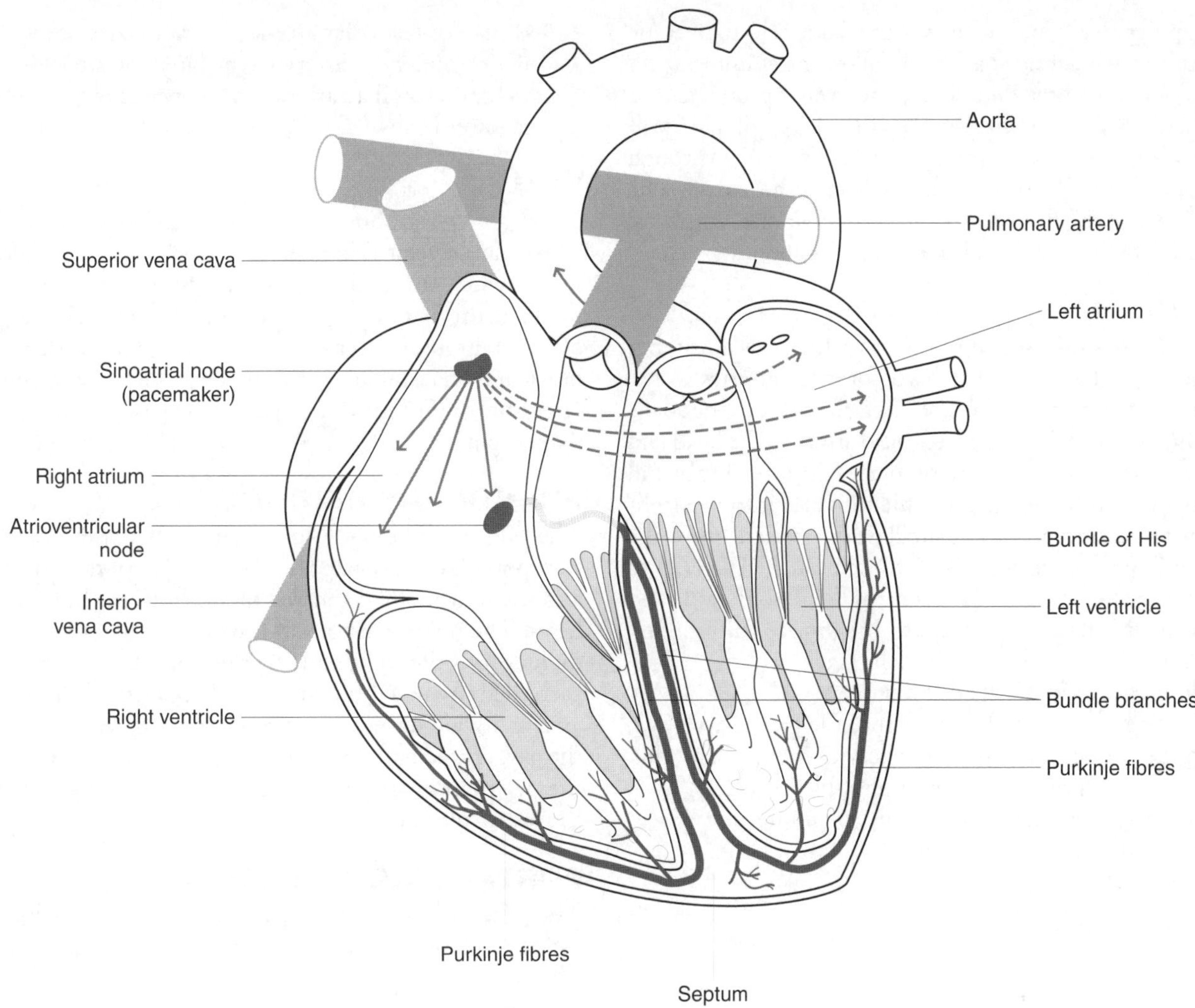

Figure 38.10 | The conduction system of the heart

the right atrium. The coronary sinus drains venous blood from the myocardium into the right atrium. At first, blood flows passively into the right ventricle as the tricuspid valve is open, then contraction of the right atrium (atrial systole) occurs to empty its entire contents. After the tricuspid valve closes, the right ventricle contracts (ventricular systole), and blood is ejected through the pulmonary valve into the pulmonary artery.

The pulmonary artery divides into the right pulmonary artery, which carries deoxygenated blood to the right lung and the left pulmonary artery, which carries deoxygenated blood to the left lung. In the lungs, oxygen is exchanged for carbon dioxide from the blood, and the oxygenated blood returns to the left atrium via four pulmonary veins. The left atrium contracts and blood passes through the mitral (bicuspid) valve into the left ventricle. After the mitral valve closes, the left ventricle contracts and blood is ejected into the aorta via the aortic valve. The aorta branches off to supply all areas of the body with oxygenated blood.

Blood is thus in constant circulation around the body, and the system of circulation can be divided into three parts:

1. Systemic circulation
2. Pulmonary circulation
3. Portal circulation.

THE SYSTEMIC CIRCULATION

The systemic circulation is the distribution of oxygenated blood to all tissues, and the return of deoxygenated blood from all tissues to the heart. When the left ventricle contracts it forces blood into the aorta under pressure. The elastic walls of the aorta distend to receive the blood. When the left ventricle relaxes the walls of the aorta recoil and, with the aortic valve closed, the blood is driven onwards through the aorta. Branches from the aorta also distend and recoil as the blood travels through them, and this wave of distension and recoil is felt as the pulse wherever a superficial artery crosses a hard structure such as a bone.

Arterioles supply networks of capillaries with oxygenated blood, and the hydrostatic pressure behind the blood causes water and other essential substances to be pushed through the capillary walls and wash over the tissue cells to become part of the tissue fluid. Tissue cells allow certain substances they require to enter, and excrete their waste products into the tissue fluid. The pressure within the capillaries will allow only a small amount of the fluid to return through the capillary and venule wall, back into the blood. The remainder of the fluid reaches the blood via the lymphatic system, which is discussed later in this chapter.

Arteries

The aorta has four sections, each of which has a number of branches (Figure 38.11). Two coronary arteries to the heart wall branch from the ascending aorta. From the aortic arch branch the left common carotid artery to the head and neck; the left subclavian artery to the left upper limb; and the right innominate artery, which divides into the right common carotid and right subclavian arteries. From the descending thoracic aorta branch the bronchial arteries to the lungs; the oesophageal artery to the oesophagus; and 10 pairs of intercostal arteries to the intercostal muscles. From the abdominal aorta, branch the:

- Phrenic arteries to the diaphragm
- Coeliac trunk, which divides into the gastric artery to the stomach, the hepatic artery to the liver and the splenic artery to the pancreas and spleen
- Superior mesentric artery to the small intestine
- Renal arteries to the kidneys
- Ovarian or testicular arteries to the ovaries or testes
- Inferior mesentric artery to the large intestine
- Two common iliac arteries to the pelvic organs and the lower limbs.

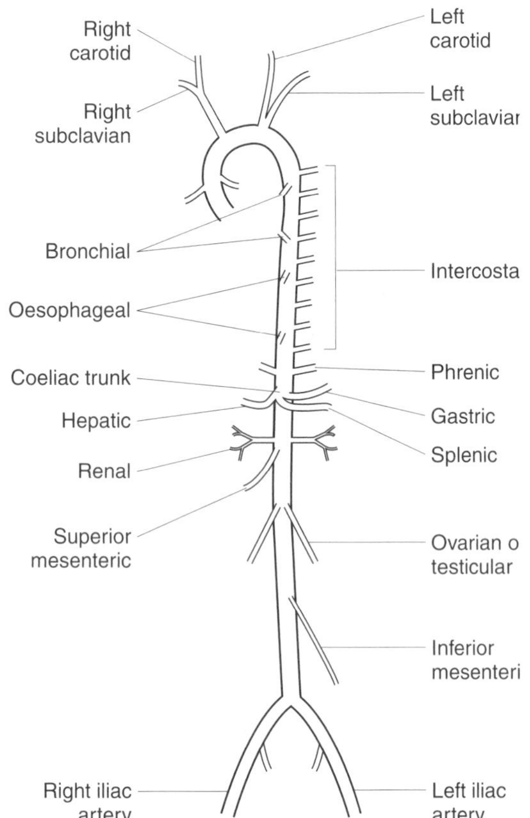

Figure 38.11 | The aorta and its branches

Veins

There are two groups of veins: superficial veins, some of which can be seen as bluish lines under the skin; and deep veins, which run beside arteries and often have the same name as the arteries. Veins rely on the squeezing action of skeletal muscles to assist in pushing blood towards the heart, and on respiratory movements, which have a milking effect on the inferior vena cava as it passes through the diaphragm.

PULMONARY CIRCULATION

The pulmonary circulation (Figure 38.12) involves the transport of deoxygenated blood from the heart to the lungs and the return of oxygenated blood from the lungs to the heart. The pulmonary artery leaves the right ventricle and divides into the right and left pulmonary arteries, which carry deoxygenated blood to the lungs. In the lungs, the arteries divide until capillaries are formed. Venules collect the oxygenated blood from the capillaries and unite to form the two pulmonary veins, which leave each lung and enter the left atrium of the heart.

PORTAL CIRCULATION

The portal circulation (Figure 38.13) is responsible for carrying blood that is deoxygenated but rich in digested

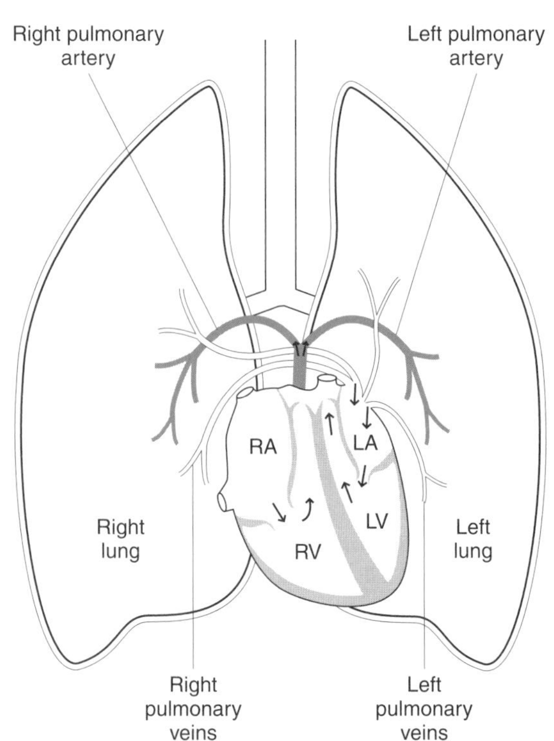

Figure 38.12 | Pulmonary circulation

nutrients, from some of the abdominal organs to the liver.

The splenic, gastric, inferior and superior mesenteric veins unite to form a large vein called the portal vein, which enters the liver. The liver converts the nutrients brought by the blood into a form to be either used by tissues throughout the body, or stored for future use. The liver thus receives blood from two sources: the hepatic artery, which supplies it with oxygenated blood; and the portal vein, carrying deoxygenated blood rich in nutrients. When the oxygen has been extracted from the former and the nutrients from the latter have been processed, the blood leaves via the three hepatic veins.

STRUCTURE OF THE LYMPHATIC SYSTEM

The lymphatic system (Figure 38.14) is closely connected with the circulation of blood and consists of an additional set of vessels through which some of the tissue fluid passes before reaching the large veins and entering the blood. This system consists of lymphatic capillaries, lymphatic vessels, lymphatic nodes and lymphatic ducts. The fluid in the system is called lymph.

The lymphatics serve an important function in preventing oedema, as the tiny vessels collect fluid and proteins from the interstitial spaces and promote their return to the blood circulation. They also collect the larger digested fat particles from the digestive system and empty them into the circulation. In addition, the lymphatics play a key role in the body's defence against microorganisms. They collect microorganisms in the interstitial spaces and carry them to the lymph nodes, where the lymphocytes (and macrophages) remove them from the lymph.

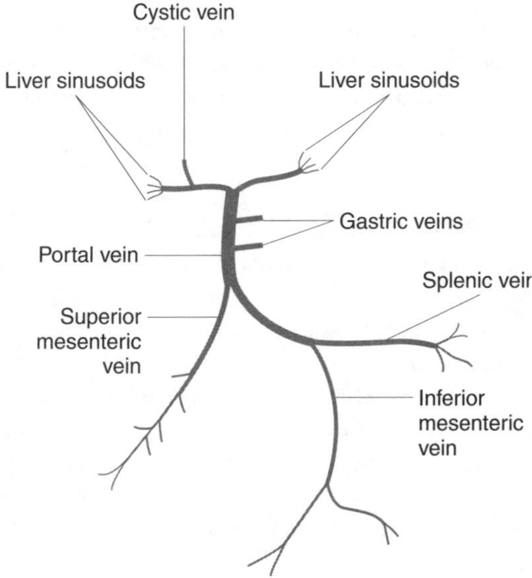

Figure 38.13 | Portal circulation

LYMPH

When fluid leaks out of the capillaries from the cardiovascular system it accumulates in the tissue spaces. When this fluid is drained from the tissues and collected by the lymphatic system, it is called lymph and has a composition similar to the blood plasma. Lymph is normally a colourless fluid, although lymph absorbed from the intestines is saturated with fats and is milky in colour. Lymph travels slowly through the lymphatic system — total lymph flow is about 2–4 L/day.

LYMPHATIC CAPILLARIES

Lymphatic capillaries are similar in size and structure to blood capillaries. They unite to form larger lymphatic vessels similar in structure to veins and, like veins, they have valves to prevent a backward flow of lymph. All lymphatic vessels pass through one or more lymph nodes. Afferent lymphatic vessels carry lymph to a node. Efferent lymphatic vessels carry lymph away from the node and empty it into the lymphatic ducts.

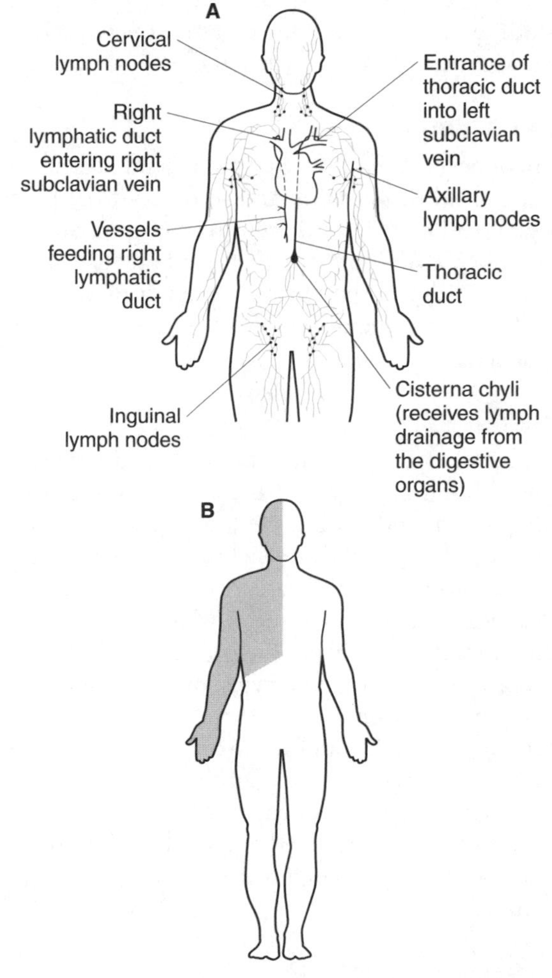

Figure 38.14 | The lymphatic system
A: The distribution of lymphatic vessels and nodes
B: Areas drained by the right lymphatic duct (shaded) and the thoracic duct (unshaded)

LYMPH NODES

Lymph nodes are found mainly in groups in many parts of the body, such as the neck, thorax, abdomen, groin and the limbs. Lymphatic nodes vary in size and consist of lymphatic tissue. The functions of lymphatic nodes are to filter and destroy bacteria from the lymph passing through the node; to produce lymphocytes, which are added to the lymph; and to produce antibodies and antitoxins.

OTHER AREAS CONTAINING LYMPHATIC TISSUE

In addition to the nodes already described, lymphatic tissue is found in several other anatomical structures, including the tonsils in the oropharynx, adenoids in the nasopharynx, the appendix attached to the intestines, the thymus gland in the thorax, Peyer's patches in the small intestine, and the spleen in the abdomen.

Tonsils

The tonsils form part of a protective ring of tissue at the entrance to the respiratory and digestive tracts. Lymphatic vessels leave the tonsils and enter the cervical nodes.

Thymus gland

The thymus gland is a soft grey-pink gland present in the thorax behind the sternum and in front of the heart. It is large in infants and children, reaching its maximum size at puberty. After puberty this gland gradually shrinks, until in adulthood there is only a small piece of tissue left. The thymus gland functions in the production of lymphocytes.

Spleen

The spleen is a purplish half-moon-shaped organ in the left hypochondriac region of the abdomen. It lies below the diaphragm and behind the lower ribs and is mainly composed of lymphoid tissue enclosed in a fibrous capsule. The functions of the spleen are to:

- Produce lymphocytes, some of which enter the bloodstream to carry out their phagocytic action
- Destroy worn-out erythrocytes, producing bile pigments and iron
- Produce antibodies and antitoxins
- Provide a storage area for erythrocytes needed in emergency situations (if haemorrhage occurs, the spleen vessels contract and empty blood into the circulation in an attempt to restore normal blood volume).

LYMPHATIC DUCTS

The two lymphatic ducts receive the lymph from lymphatic vessels and empty it into the bloodstream via the subclavian vein (Figure 38.14). They are the thoracic duct and the right lymphatic duct.

Thoracic duct

The thoracic duct, the larger of the two lymphatic ducts, begins in the abdominal cavity at lumbar level as a dilated sac called the cisterna chyli. The duct passes upwards through the aortic opening behind the diaphragm into the thorax, where it empties its contents into the left subclavian vein so that the lymph rejoins the bloodstream. Lymphatic vessels from all parts of the body below the diaphragm, and the left side of the body above the diaphragm, empty their contents into the thoracic duct.

Right lymphatic duct

The right lymphatic duct is very small (about 1 cm long) and lies in the root of the neck. It receives lymph from the right side of the head and neck, the right side of the thorax and the right upper limb. The right lymphatic duct empties its contents into the right subclavian vein.

FACTORS AFFECTING RESPIRATORY FUNCTION

OXYGEN CONCENTRATION

Oxygen makes up 20.93% of the air, which is normally sufficient to meet the needs of the body. A decrease in this amount of oxygen can cause problems. Two instances in which the available oxygen may be deficient are:

- High altitude: the total pressure of all gases in the air decreases as altitude increases. As the total pressure decreases, the oxygen pressure decreases proportionately, and the individual will experience difficulty in maintaining adequate tissue oxygenation (hypoxia). Acclimatising is a homeostatic response where initially the ventilatory rate is increased in an attempt to supply the body with sufficient oxygen, then later the bone marrow is stimulated to increase erythrocyte production (polycythaemia) to carry more oxygen
- Presence of noxious gases: some noxious gases such as carbon monoxide have a higher affinity for haemoglobin than does oxygen, which is displaced by them, causing a reduction in oxygen availability to tissues.

REGULATING MECHANISMS

Any factor that interferes with the respiratory centres in the brainstem or the nerves that transmit messages to and from them may cause ventilatory difficulties. Respiratory depression can be caused by increased intracranial pressure such as cerebral oedema, due to conditions such as hypercapnia, cerebral bleeds, meningitis, encephalitis, hydrocephalus, tumours, hypoalbuminaemia and keto-acidosis. Clinical Interest Box 38.1 discusses the effect pyrexia has on oxygen regulation mechanisms. Other factors include certain medications such as analgesics (e.g. morphine), and various anticonvulsant drugs (e.g. clonazepam). Ventilation increases when the pH of the

CLINICAL INTEREST BOX 38.1
OXYGEN REQUIREMENTS AND PYREXIA

Many respiratory conditions cause pyrexia. Historically clients have been treated with antipyretics or other methods to cool their skin, such as tepid sponges, fans and removing clothing. Pyrexia is the body's homeostatic mechanism for providing a hostile environment for pathogens and for increasing the immune response. Clients normally feel hot to touch on the 'up' state of the fever but state that they feel cold, and may shiver, while the 'down' state normally is the reverse.

Cooling a client's skin may actually increase the pyrexial state, as the body shivers to keep warm. Medical treatment of pyrexia is increasingly aimed at allowing the body's immune system to maintain the pyrexia, without nursing or medical interference, drugs or other care. The pyrexia is still investigated and the cause treated, and antipyretics administered if a client's other symptoms or past history (e.g. febrile convulsion) deem it safer or their discomfort may be alleviated by antipyretics.

Most at risk of pyrexial complication are some clients with congenital or chronic respiratory or cardiac conditions in which they have a diminished 'reserve', or ability for their bodies to supply the extra 10% of oxygen needed per 1°C of body temperature increase. In these clients not only are antipyretics commonly used but also supplemental oxygen is administered while the pyrexial state exists.

blood is lowered (a respiratory response to rid the body of the excess acid) whereas ventilation decreases when the pH increases (to retain acid). (See respiratory alkalosis and acidosis, later in this chapter.)

EXCHANGE OF GASES DURING VENTILATION AND RESPIRATION

The efficiency of ventilation and respiration can be affected by any factor that interferes with the patency of the respiratory tract or the actions of the ventilatory muscles. For example, an accumulation of secretions may result from respiratory conditions such as asthma, bronchitis or a reduced cough reflex. Ventilations may also be reduced by factors that affect the actions of the ventilatory muscles, such as brainstem or spinal cord injury or motor neuron diseases such as multiple sclerosis or Guillain–Barré syndrome. These conditions can restrict the movements of the diaphragm and/or intercostal muscles. Chest expansion and ventilation can also be affected by deformities of the chest wall or skeleton, such as scoliosis, flail chest (multiple rib fractures causing instability in part of the chest wall and paradoxical breathing movements — the part of the lung underlying the injured area contracts on inspiration and bulges on expiration) and pectus excavatum (a skeletal abnormality of the chest that is characterised by a depressed sternum).

DIFFUSION OF OXYGEN AND CO_2

Any dysfunction of the lungs that affects the alveolar capillary membrane thickness or causes a reduction in their surface area will affect respiratory function. Conditions such as pulmonary oedema, alveolitis, pneumonia or chronic obstructive airways disease may reduce the diffusion of oxygen and CO_2. Information on these and other respiratory disorders is provided later in this chapter.

TRANSPORT OF OXYGEN AND CO_2 TO AND FROM THE CELLS

Any condition affecting the efficiency of the heart, blood vessels or blood can interfere with the transportation of oxygen to the cells or CO_2 away from the cells. Such conditions include congestive cardiac failure, atherosclerosis, carbon monoxide poisoning and anaemia. Information on these and other cardiovascular disorders is provided later in this chapter.

INFLUENCES ON THE RATE, DEPTH AND RHYTHM OF BREATHING

Several factors influence the characteristics of breathing, such as pyrexia and physical activity. Oxygen requirements are greatest during exertion and least during sleep. The rate and depth of ventilations vary in response to the body's production of CO_2; for example, during strenuous exercise the volume of air drawn into the lungs with each breath may be increased from a normal tidal volume of 500 mL to as much as 3800 mL. Changes in mood, emotion and pain may also affect the rate, depth and rhythm of ventilation; for example, the ventilation rate is commonly increased during fear, anxiety or apprehension. Chronic irritation by inhaled irritants such as smoke or dust can also affect breathing and cause short-term effects such as coughing and shortness of breath, or long-term effects such as severe dyspnoea resulting from emphysema.

ADDITIONAL FACTORS

Numerous other factors can modify the rate and depth of ventilation, for example, involuntary and reflex mechanisms such as exercise, pain, hiccupping, sneezing, sighing and emotions, and conscious voluntary actions such as voluntary breath-holding, inhalation and exhalation. Clinical Interest Box 38.2 discusses the alteration to respirations in the older adult. Other factors that affect functioning include:

- Digestive system disorders and diminished appetite, potentiating an alteration in nutritional status
- Changes in renal function, which can affect erythropoietin production
- Osteoporosis
- Circulatory disorders.

These may all combine to affect blood cell production, with subsequent anaemias. In clients who are more sedentary such combinations of factors and subsequent alveolar hypoventilation increase the risk of primary or secondary infections. To avoid the complications of ageing, all clients can be educated to:

- Improve their nutritional status, including nutrients

CLINICAL INTEREST BOX 38.2
Respirations and the older client

Involutional changes that can occur with increasing age include; loss of elasticity of the lung tissue, costal cartilage calcification, kyphosis, weakening and loss of skeletal muscle fibre, reduction in cilia numbers and beating speed, and thickening of alveolar membranes. These factors and many more diminish the respiratory system's ventilatory capacity and the ability to excrete CO_2 and absorb oxygen, increasing the resting respiratory rate from the adult rate of about 20/min to 25/min for an older client.

and supplementation of additional sources of vitamins as required
- Increase their fluid intake, as permitted
- Perform routine breathing exercises
- Maintain their weight-bearing ability
- Increase their exercise and mobilisation.

RESPIRATORY PATHOPHYSIOLOGICAL INFLUENCES AND EFFECTS

Respiratory symptoms result from one or a combination of inadequate pulmonary ventilation, abnormalities of diffusion through the pulmonary membrane, or inadequate transport of oxygen from the lungs to the tissues.

INADEQUATE VENTILATION (HYPOVENTILATION)

Hypoventilation and alveolar hypoventilation is a reduction in the ventilation of the alveoli. The causes are many and varied and include airway obstruction by oedema, inhaled foreign bodies, retained secretions (mucus, casts), polyps, tumours, bronchospasm, emphysema, neuromuscular or skeletal abnormalities and central nervous system disorders. Hypoventilation occurs when the volume of air entering the alveoli is not adequate for the metabolic needs of the body. The reduction in ventilation causes an increase in the partial pressure of CO_2 in arterial blood (Pa_{CO_2}), termed hypercapnia, and may also cause hypoxaemia, a decrease in the partial pressure of oxygen in arterial blood (Pa_{O_2}).

IMPAIRED DIFFUSION

Diffusion is the process by which oxygen and CO_2 molecules are transported between the alveoli and the capillary network. Diffusion abnormalities can interfere with the passage of oxygen into the blood. Such diffusion abnormalities can result from: a thickening of the alveoli capillary walls, for example, in pulmonary oedema; a reduced amount of functioning lung tissue, such as in emphysema; or fibrosis of the alveolar walls, as seen in alveolitis and pneumonitis.

IMPAIRED PERFUSION

Not only is an adequate intake of oxygen by ventilation essential, but for oxygenation of the body tissues to occur, adequate perfusion of lung tissue with blood is essential. Any condition that decreases the circulation of blood to lung tissue may lead to ventilation–perfusion mismatches (V/Q principle) and hypoxaemia. Such conditions include decreased blood volume, pulmonary embolism, cardiac disorders and chronic obstructive pulmonary disease.

In addition to abnormalities of the lungs or respiratory structures, dysfunction of other body systems can adversely affect respiratory function. For example, a disease process that affects the nervous system may adversely affect respirations. When the spinal cord is damaged, the nervous system may greatly impair respiratory function. Cardiovascular dysfunction can affect respiratory function; for example, right-sided heart failure may affect the volume of pulmonary blood circulation. A deformity of the skeletal system, such as scoliosis, may restrict movement of the thoracic cage and thus alter respiratory function. Inadequate lung expansion can also occur after abdominal surgery, as pain in the operation site may inhibit deep breathing and coughing. Not only can abnormalities of other body systems adversely affect the respiratory system, but respiratory abnormalities generally affect all other body systems.

MAJOR CLINICAL MANIFESTATIONS OF RESPIRATORY DISORDERS

The signs and symptoms manifested by a client with a respiratory disorder vary with the location and severity of the disorder. The following are some common clinical features of respiratory disease.

CHEST PAIN

Disorders of the respiratory system such as pleurisy can result in chest pain. During ventilation, friction occurs between the inflamed pleura. Chest pain may be localised or may be experienced only when the client breathes deeply, and can vary from a continuous aching pain to a stabbing knife-like pain. Pain associated with respiratory disorders may be retrosternal, lateral or posterior and is exacerbated by deep inhalation.

COUGH

A cough is a common symptom of many respiratory disorders and may result from irritation or from retained secretions that obstruct some part of the airway. If sputum is swallowed, expectorated or the cough sounds moist, it is described as productive. A non-productive, or dry, cough is one that sounds dry or irritating and no sputum is expectorated or swallowed. Sputum is the result of excessive mucus production and may result from inflammation, infection or congestion.

Haemoptysis (the coughing or expectoration of blood) may occur in some lung diseases. Blood-streaked sputum frequently occurs in some respiratory tract conditions, such as infections (e.g. bronchitis, tuberculosis), pulmonary oedema or bronchogenic carcinoma. The expectoration of bright red or frothy blood indicates a more serious disorder, such as pulmonary embolism or lung abscess.

Voice changes, ranging from hoarseness to aphonia (no speech), may result from numerous causes, including viral upper respiratory tract infections (e.g. laryngitis), vocal cord polyps and laryngeal tumour. Unilateral or bilateral vocal cord paralysis may also result from congenital defects, intubation or other damage to the recurrent nerve, for example after thyroid or cardiac surgery.

Dyspnoea (difficult or laboured breathing) may result from disorders affecting either the upper or the lower respiratory tract or surrounding structures. Disorders of the upper respiratory tract that may cause dyspnoea include obstruction of the airway by inflammation, a tumour or foreign body. Disorders of the lower respiratory tract that cause dyspnoea include airway inflammations or infections, asthma, pneumonia, pneumonitis, carcinoma of the lung and chronic obstructive pulmonary disease. Any disorder affecting the thorax, such as trauma to the chest wall, commonly causes dyspnoea. Laboured breathing may be accompanied by nasal flaring, the use of the neck and accessory chest muscles and increased ventilation rate.

CHANGES IN BREATHING PATTERNS AND SOUNDS

Any disorder that affects the respiratory system may produce changes in the pattern of breathing. Examples include tachypnoea (increased respiratory rate), bradypnoea (decreased respiratory rate) and airway obstruction; for example, due to emphysema, which can result in prolonged forceful expiration and pursed-lip breathing. Certain disorders also result in abnormal breathing sounds, such as wheezing or 'grunting' ventilations. Information on abnormal breathing sounds is provided later in this chapter.

HYPOXIA

Hypoxia is a deficiency of oxygen in the tissues and may be due to lung disorders that prevent adequate supplies of oxygen from reaching the blood (hypoxaemia). Hypoxia may also be due to hypoventilation, anaemia or impaired tissue utilisation of oxygen. The initial manifestations of hypoxia include tachycardia, tachypnoea, breathlessness, pallor, lethargy or agitation, followed by increasing confusion and deepening cyanosis.

THORACIC ABNORMALITIES

Chronic respiratory system disorders may alter chest configuration; for example, a 'barrel chest' is characteristic of chronic obstructive conditions such as cystic fibrosis and emphysema. Abnormal curvatures of the spine, such as severe scoliosis, and congenital chest deformities such as pigeon chest (Figure 38.15) and pectus excavatum 'funnel chest' (Figure 38.16) may also affect pulmonary ventilation. Asymmetrical chest expansion can result from conditions such as flail chest, haemothorax, pneumothorax, retained secretions or inhaled foreign bodies causing atelectasis.

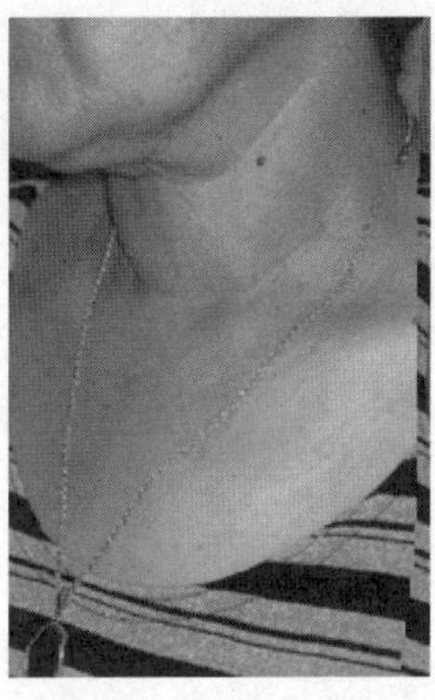

Figure 38.15 | Pigeon chest *(Lemmi & Lemmi 2000)*

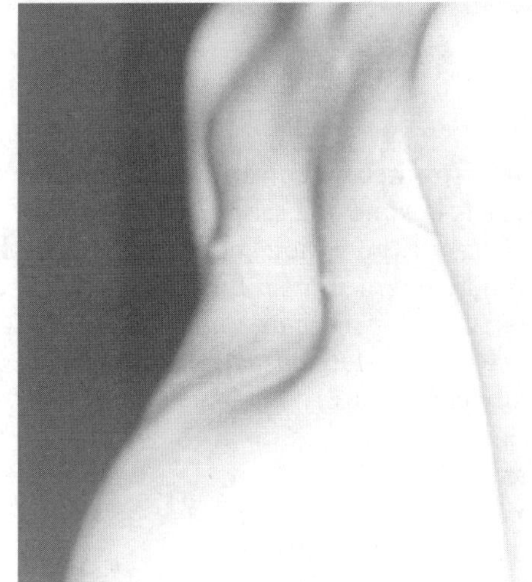

Figure 38.16 | Funnel chest *(Zitelli & Davis 1997)*

OTHER MANIFESTATIONS

Depending on the type and severity of the disorder, other manifestations may be evident. For example, infections of the respiratory tract generally result in pyrexia, headaches, aching muscles and lethargy. Difficulty in swallowing (dysphagia) may be present in disorders such as pharyngitis and tonsillitis. In certain chronic disorders of the respiratory system, clubbing of the fingers may be evident (Figure 38.17). The distal portions of the fingers are abnormally enlarged by anastamosis of blood vessels in response to peripheral hypoxaemia. The nails have an increased curvature and the angle of the nail bed increases to over 85 degrees.

SPECIFIC DISORDERS OF THE RESPIRATORY SYSTEM

DISORDERS OF MULTIPLE CAUSE

Certain disorders of the respiratory system have more than one cause and may be related to structural or functional

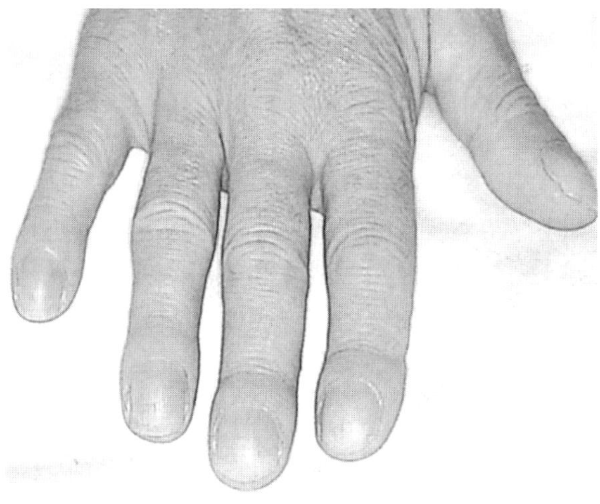

Figure 38.17 | Clubbing of the fingers *(Earis & Pearson 1995)*

changes, environmental conditions or a combination of factors. It is beyond the scope of this text to provide in-depth detail of the various conditions related to the respiratory system. For more information you are advised to refer to an anatomy and physiology or pathophysiology text, such as Marieb (2006). Listed below are some examples of respiratory conditions:

- Rhinitis
- Pleurisy
- Epistaxis
- Sarcoidosis
- Pneumoconioses
- Laryngeal oedema
- Adult respiratory distress syndrome.

INFECTIOUS DISORDERS

Infectious disorders can be classed as upper or lower respiratory tract infections. Infections of the upper respiratory tract are caused by bacteria or viruses, while a variety of microorganisms can cause lower respiratory tract infections. For more information you are advised to refer to an anatomy and physiology or pathophysiology text, such as Marieb (2006). Clinical Interest Box 38.3 looks at a viral infection, sudden acute respiratory syndrome (SARS). Listed below are some examples of respiratory conditions:

- Sinusitis
- Influenza
- Pharyngitis
- Tonsillitis
- Quinsy
- Laryngitis
- Epiglottitis
- Acute bronchitis
- Pneumonia
- Pertussis
- Croup
- Tuberculosis
- Empyema.

CLINICAL INTEREST BOX 38.3
Sudden acute respiratory syndrome (SARS)

Sudden acute respiratory syndrome (SARS) first appeared in the southern Chinese province of Guangdong in 2002 and by 2003 had been classified as an epidemic by the World Health Organization. Symptoms of SARS, which is believed to be spread mainly through droplet infection, include pyrexia, rigors, cough, headache, aches and pains and dyspnoea. These same symptoms are common for many other respiratory infections, making the positive diagnosis difficult.

The number of deaths to June 2003 was about 800 people worldwide, and the number of people infected, about 8500, since 2002. In 2002 and 2003 about 14% of those infected died from SARS, usually 5–6 weeks after becoming ill.

The virus was found to be a coronavirus, and the genome was sequenced in April 2003 by the US Centers for Disease Control and Prevention. After relaxation of SARS infection-control measures in Canada, a further outbreak occurred, due probably to transmission by an unrecognised SARS carrier, and affected five clients in a rehabilitation hospital. As a result, infection-control departments worldwide have introduced the most stringent infection-control policies for medical and paramedical workers seen to date, to limit the spread of SARS.

OBSTRUCTIVE DISORDERS

Obstructive disorders are lung diseases that cause a persistent obstruction of bronchial air flow. Airway obstruction can also be due to the inhalation of a foreign body, or one or both bronchi may become obstructed by a benign or malignant tumour. Some of the more common types of airways obstruction are grouped under the heading of chronic obstructive pulmonary disease (COPD) or chronic obstructive airways disease (COAD). Common forms of COAD include asthma, emphysema, bronchiectasis and chronic bronchitis. Asthma and emphysema will be discussed briefly here, however for more information you are advised to refer to an anatomy and physiology or pathophysiology text, such as Marieb (2006).

Asthma

Asthma is a disease manifested by difficulty in breathing caused by generalised narrowing of the airways. Asthma is characterised by recurring episodes of paroxysmal dyspnoea, wheezing on expiration, coughing and tenacious, mucoid bronchial secretions. A person having an asthma attack commonly experiences anxiety, diaphoresis, tachycardia and elevated blood pressure. The increased effort of breathing can cause extreme fatigue.

Episodes of asthma may be precipitated by inhalation or ingestion of allergens or pollutants, infection, or it may be exercise induced or occur in response to changes in air temperature or emotional stress. The severity and duration of asthma attacks vary; treatment may control the attack

CLINICAL INTEREST BOX 38.4
Childhood asthma

The incidence of children suffering from asthma has increased. Studies comparing the incidence of asthma in city-living and farming communities found that children living in a 'clean environment' were more at risk of asthma. They cited that the difference may be due to the 'obsession'-like trend towards a germ-free house and environment. They indicated that children in farming communities had more exposure to pathogens, which stimulated their immune system. However, a significant proportion of asthma in children in the 1–5-year-old age bracket is due to pathogens.

A study done on wheezing-associated respiratory infections reported that the identified pathogens were, in order of occurrence: respiratory syncytial virus (RSV), parainfluenza virus (PIV-1 and PIV-2) and influenza virus A and B. Children in the 6–15-year age bracket were affected more by *Mycoplasma pneumoniae*, influenza virus A and B and rhinovirus. Lower respiratory infections such as those mentioned above accounted for up to 30% of visits to the local medical officer in the first year of life, later dropping to 5% by age 9.

Commonly, city living exposes children to larger class sizes, crèches, child care centres and places of interest, all of which increase the contact with other people and pathogens.

rapidly, or the symptoms can become increasingly severe and prolonged.

A severe and prolonged asthma attack that resists treatment is referred to as status asthmaticus (indicated by a Pa_{CO_2} of over 50%, or extreme exhaustion). Unless treatment reverses the condition, the client may develop respiratory failure. Clinical Interest Box 38.4 provides an overview of the current incidence of childhood asthma.

Emphysema

Emphysema (pulmonary) is a chronically progressive disease characterised by over-distension and destruction of alveolar walls, resulting in a loss of lung elasticity and surface area for diffusion. The predisposing causes are the same as those for chronic bronchitis, with cigarette smoking being the major factor. Initially the peripheral bronchioles become inflamed and the subsequent narrowing of the airways traps air in the alveoli. As the disease progresses the alveolar walls become over-inflated and rupture. Because of loss of lung elasticity the terminal bronchioles tend to collapse prematurely during exhalation, making expulsion of air from the lungs more difficult.

Symptoms of chronic emphysema include shortness of breath, dyspnoea, cyanosis and cough. Individuals will commonly exhale through pursed lips to prolong expiration and reduce the tendency of the airways to collapse. As the disease becomes more severe, they may use their accessory muscles to breathe. The anteroposterior width of the chest usually increases because of expansion of the chest wall and loss of lung elasticity, giving the chest a barrel-shaped appearance. Distension of the neck veins may be present, as may clubbing of the fingers. In advanced emphysema, the person fights for every breath of air.

NEOPLASTIC DISORDERS

Benign or malignant neoplasms may affect the upper or lower respiratory tract. Tumours can affect the normal functioning of the respiratory tract and, if malignant, can cause extensive tissue damage by infiltration. The signs and symptoms of neoplastic disease vary depending on the location and extent of the lesion.

Nasal polyps are masses of hypertrophied mucosa that commonly form in response to recurrent swelling of the nasal mucosa. Obstruction of the nasal passages develops gradually as the benign polyps multiply and enlarge. The client experiences difficulty in breathing through the nose, and the voice may have a nasal quality.

Laryngeal polyps are growths that arise from the mucous membrane of the vocal cords. The major symptom is hoarseness. Laryngeal polyps are usually benign but they may become malignant.

Laryngeal carcinoma is a malignant neoplasm arising from or around the vocal cords. Persistent hoarseness is the major symptom, and heavy cigarette smoking is believed to be a major causative factor. If the lesion is large, dysphagia may be present.

Lung cancer commonly affects a bronchus. It arises from the bronchial epithelium and rapidly invades lung tissue, causing parts of the lung to collapse. It may spread through the lymphatic network and bloodstream to form metastases in other parts of the body, such as the liver, bones or brain. The incidence of lung cancer is related to several factors, the most important being the inhalation of cigarette smoke. Other factors include exposure to atmospheric pollution and occupational pollutants.

Unfortunately, the physical manifestations of lung cancer do not generally appear until the disease is well advanced. Symptoms include persistent cough, dyspnoea, purulent or blood-streaked sputum, chest pain and repeated attacks of bronchitis or pneumonia. Sometimes the initial symptoms are associated with organs that are the sites of metastasis, such as the liver, bones or brain. Cancer of the lung may also occur secondary to a primary malignant tumour elsewhere in the body, as a result of metastasis.

TRAUMATIC DISORDERS

Injury to part of the respiratory tract can result from a variety of causes.

Laryngotracheal trauma

Laryngotracheal trauma can be minor and cause hoarseness and some dysphagia, or it may be severe, as a result of laryngeal or cricoid fracture. In a severe injury, oedema of the larynx may occur and be accompanied by signs of respiratory distress.

Flail chest

Flail chest occurs when multiple rib fractures result in 'floating' of a segment of the rib cage. As a consequence there may be instability in part of the chest wall and paradoxical breathing. Paradoxical breathing is characterised by the injured chest wall collapsing in during inhalation, and moving out during exhalation. The lung underlying the injury contracts on inhalation and bulges on exhalation. If uncorrected, ventilation is impaired, which may lead to hypoxia and respiratory failure. Manifestations of a flail chest are paradoxical motion of the chest wall during breathing, severe pain, dyspnoea, tachycardia and cyanosis.

Pneumothorax

Pneumothorax is a collection of air in the pleural space causing the lung on the side of the injury to collapse. A pneumothorax may be open or closed. In an open pneumothorax, an injury creates an opening in the chest wall, allowing air to flow into the pleural cavity. In a closed, or spontaneous, pneumothorax, the chest wall is intact and air enters the pleural space from an opening on the surface of the lung.

Depending on the severity, a pneumothorax may cause severe dyspnoea, hypoxaemia, tachypnoea and associated pain, along with ipsilateral diminished chest expansion and breath sounds. There may be subcutaneous emphysema in the neck and upper chest, and a 'sucking' sound may be heard in the region of an open pneumothorax. Tracheal deviation to the contralateral side may be observed in severe cases in some clients.

Tension pneumothorax is a particularly severe form that occurs when air escapes into the pleural cavity. As a result, continuously increasing air pressure in the pleural cavity causes progressive collapse of the lung tissue. Emergency aspiration of air from the pleural cavity is necessary.

Haemothorax

Haemothorax is the accumulation of blood in the pleural space, usually as a result of trauma. Manifestations of haemothorax include dyspnoea and chest tightness, and may include signs of hypovolaemia if bleeding continues. If not treated, haemothorax can lead to shock from haemorrhage, and severe pain, or respiratory failure.

Haemopneumothorax is a collection of air and blood in the pleural cavity. Symptoms include those of both pneumothorax and haemothorax.

CARDIAC PATHOPHYSIOLOGICAL INFLUENCES AND EFFECTS

CHANGES IN CARDIAC FUNCTION

Cardiac failure occurs when the heart is unable to maintain an output of blood sufficient to meet the body's requirements and, as a result, the body tissues may become ischaemic.

Cardiac failure may result from mechanical failure due to disease of valves, obstruction to the blood flow, congenital heart disease, arteriosclerosis or hypertension. Cardiac failure can also occur as a consequence of a disease process, such as cardiomyopathy or myocardial infarction, or as the result of normal ageing. Consequently, the heart's ability to pump blood may be diminished.

When the heart fails to meet the requirements of the body, compensatory mechanisms occur in an attempt to improve cardiac output and to maintain the blood pressure. Compensatory responses include the sympathetic response, the renal response, and myocardial hypertrophy. The sympathetic response is stimulated by reduced cardiac output and results in increased heart rate, dilation of the coronary and cerebral arterioles, and constriction of the renal and skin arterioles. As a result, essential life functions are maintained. The renal response results in the secretion of substances that stimulate the production of aldosterone, causing vasoconstriction and retention of sodium and water. This response causes an increase in blood volume and peripheral resistance, which increases the workload of the heart.

Myocardial hypertrophy results from prolonged increase in myocardial wall tension and, while this initially maintains cardiac output, eventually cardiac output and tissue perfusion are decreased.

CHANGES IN THE BLOOD VESSELS

Disturbances in the ability of the arteries to stretch and recoil as blood is pumped from the heart, or changes in the ability of the veins to return the blood to the heart, result in ischaemia of the tissues. The ability of arteries to stretch and recoil may be affected by conditions such as arteriosclerosis, obstruction from inflammation or arterial spasms, or from excessive external pressure on an artery. When an artery is narrowed or constricted it is unable to transport sufficient blood to the area it supplies, resulting in ischaemia and possible tissue death (necrosis).

The ability of veins to return blood to the heart may be affected by impaired valves, a sedentary lifestyle, reduced skeletal muscle usage that normally assists venous flow, or from excessive external pressure on a vein. When blood flow through a vein is impeded, pooling of blood in the vein occurs. The hydrostatic pressure inside the vein increases and causes oedema in the surrounding tissues. Chronic venous insufficiency can result in thrombophlebitis, stasis cellulitis and stasis ulcers.

The formation of an embolus can cause obstruction of an artery or a vein. The most common embolus is a blood clot (thrombus), although an embolus can also consist of air or fat or foreign bodies. When the thrombus, or part of it, becomes dislodged from the vessel wall it travels in the bloodstream until it reaches a blood vessel that is too narrow for its passage. As a result, blood flow beyond that area is obstructed, and the ultimate consequence may be death of the tissues deprived of adequate oxygen and nutrition.

CHANGES IN THE BLOOD

Haemoglobin in the erythrocytes is responsible for transporting oxygen in the bloodstream. Any condition that affects the normal production or function of erythrocytes may decrease the supply of oxygen to the tissues. Conditions that may impede erythrocyte formation or their ability to carry oxygen include smoking, bone marrow aplasia, metabolic abnormalities, nutritional deficiencies, chronic or acute blood loss, drugs, living at high altitudes, flying, toxins, ionising radiation and genetic abnormalities. Tissue hypoxia results in a compensatory increased production of erythrocytes (polycythaemia), which causes the blood to become viscous and increases the risk of thrombi formation.

Leucocytes protect the body from infection through phagocytosis and the production of antibodies. Any disorder that decreases the production or maturation of leucocytes renders the client susceptible to overwhelming infection. Conditions that may impede leucocyte production or function include inadequate blood cell production, proliferation of immature leucocytes, viruses, drug reactions, radiation, nutritional deficiencies and bone marrow hypoplasia.

Thrombocytes are necessary for the clotting of blood. Any disorder that impairs thrombocyte production or function renders the client susceptible to bleeding. A decrease or increase in the formation of thrombocytes generally occurs in association with other disorders. Thrombocytopenia (decrease in thrombocyte number) is commonly due to viral infections but may be idiopathic or may result from bone marrow disease. It may also result from a condition that causes thrombocyte destruction, such as cirrhosis of the liver, or drug toxicity or continued bleeding. Thrombocythaemia (increase in thrombocyte number) is frequently idiopathic, but it may also accompany some disorders such as polycythaemia or chronic myeloid leukaemia.

CHANGES IN THE LYMPHATIC SYSTEM

The lymphatic system removes fluid and particles from the interstitial spaces, filters the lymph, and returns it to the circulation. Impaired lymphatic function may result from obstruction or inflammation of the lymphatic vessels or nodes, or from neoplastic disease. When lymphatic function is impaired, fluid accumulates in the interstitial spaces, and oedema results. As the function of lymphocytes is the key factor in immune responses, diseases of the lymphatic system, such as Hodgkin's disease, may seriously impair the immune processes. The client with immunodeficiency is vulnerable to infection and other pathological processes that would normally be inhibited by a healthy immune system.

MAJOR CLINICAL MANIFESTATIONS OF CIRCULATORY SYSTEM DISORDERS

The manifestations of disorders of the circulatory system vary depending on whether the disorder is one that affects the heart, the blood vessels, or the blood or blood-forming organs.

MANIFESTATIONS OF CARDIAC DISORDERS

Dyspnoea

Dyspnoea (difficult or laboured breathing) is the most common (and often the earliest) symptom of cardiac disease. Typically the dyspnoea occurs with exertion although, as cardiac disease progresses, the client may experience dyspnoea at rest. Paroxysmal nocturnal dyspnoea, which is associated with congestive cardiac failure, occurs during sleep; the client wakes suddenly with difficulty in breathing and a sensation of suffocation.

Chest pain

Chest pain (Table 38.5) may result from myocardial ischaemia or from pericarditis. Chest pain can also be caused by conditions not associated with cardiac disease, such as oesophagitis, reflux, pleurisy, musculoskeletal disorders, or stress and anxiety. Ischaemic pain is the result of a deficiency of blood to the myocardium, caused by a blocked or constricted coronary blood vessel. Angina (pectoris) is pain that results from diminished supply of oxygen to the heart, and is basically a reversible ischaemic process. Acute myocardial infarction represents the point when ischaemia becomes irreversible, blood flow to part of the heart is inadequate and unrelieved by rest, causing cardiac muscle necrosis.

Signs and symptoms that are textbook characteristics of angina or myocardial infarction, and any chest pain, should be suspected to be a myocardial infarction until proven otherwise. However, many myocardial infarctions may not follow the classic pattern of symptoms and as such may not be diagnosed and treated.

Palpitations

Palpitations are a sensation of fluttering in the chest or an awareness of the heart's action. The person may describe the heart's action as racing, pounding, stopping or skipping beats. Palpitations may be due to rhythm disturbances such as premature contractions (extra heartbeat), but they can also result from anxiety, stress, caffeine or nicotine, cough and cold medications and fatigue.

Cough

Cough may be associated with certain cardiovascular and most respiratory diseases. If cardiovascular disease is suspected it may be caused by an accumulation of fluid in

TABLE 38.5 | TYPICAL PATTERNS OF CARDIAC PAIN

Angina	Myocardial infarction
Gradual or sudden onset	Sudden onset
Episodic and temporary, usually lasting from 3–15 minutes	Lasts longer than 15 minutes
Substernal or anterior, not sharply localised. Radiates to back, neck, arms and jaw	Substernal, midline or anterior. Radiates to jaw, neck, back, shoulders, or one or both arms
Sensation of mild to moderate pressure. Described as lightness, squeezing or crushing	Persistent sensation of severe pressure. Described as crushing, heavy, vice-like, squeezing
Precipitated by exertion, stress, ingestion of food, exposure to cold	Not necessarily related to exertion or emotion, and may occur at rest
Accompanied by dyspnoea, diaphoresis, nausea, apprehension	Accompanied by nausea, vomiting, dyspnoea, apprehension, diaphoresis, a sensation of 'impending doom', pallor, cold clammy skin
Client keeps still to relieve the pain	Client moves about in search of a comfortable position
Relieved by rest and/or nitroglycerine	Not relieved by rest or nitroglycerine

the lungs (pulmonary oedema) often made worse at night or when lying in bed.

Fatigue

Fatigue frequently accompanies cardiac dysfunction and is related to inadequate cardiac output resulting in insufficient blood flow to the brain and skeletal tissues.

Cyanosis

Cyanosis (blue discolouration of the skin or mucous membranes) appears when haemoglobin oxygen saturation is greatly reduced below 92%. Central cyanosis is evident in all areas of the body, particularly in the lips, mucous membranes and nail beds, whereas peripheral cyanosis is evident mainly in the extremities.

Syncope

Syncope (transient loss of consciousness) may result when cardiac dysfunction causes an inadequate flow of blood to the brain. Sudden loss of consciousness due to heart block is known as Stokes–Adams syndrome. Heart block is defined as 'impairment of conduction in heart excitation; often applied specifically to atrioventricular heart block' (Hawley et al 2003: 200).

Oedema

Oedema (local or generalised accumulation of fluid in the tissues) may result from certain cardiac diseases. Peripheral or systemic oedema generally develops from right-sided cardiac failure and is first noticed in the lowest, or dependent, parts of the body, such as the legs, fingers, sacral area, periorbital area, in the abdomen (ascites) and intestines (causing constipation). As venous stasis increases, oedema increases. In left-sided cardiac failure fluid accumulates in the lungs (pulmonary oedema). In advanced cardiac failure total body oedema may develop. The severity of the oedema will depend on the degree to which venous return and/or cardiac output are reduced.

Pulse abnormalities

Pulse rate, volume or rhythm may be abnormal in the presence of cardiac dysfunction. Tachycardia may accompany cardiac failure, while heart block commonly results in bradycardia. A low cardiac output, and therefore a reduced pulse volume, is associated with cardiac failure and acute myocardial infarction. Certain cardiac disorders cause dysrhythmias accompanied by an irregular pulse.

MANIFESTATIONS OF PERIPHERAL BLOOD VESSEL DISORDERS

Intermittent claudication

Intermittent claudication is cramping pain in a muscle of the leg, brought on by exercise but relieved by rest. Commonly the pain is experienced in the calf muscle during walking and is thought to be due to accumulation of lactic acid in the tissues, rather than to ischaemia of the contracting muscle. Generally, it results from blockage of the superficial femoral artery; for example, due to atherosclerosis.

Rest pain

Rest pain is leg pain experienced even when resting and occurs when chronic arterial occlusive disease is advanced, or when a vessel is blocked by a thrombus or embolus. As a result, the blood supply to the surrounding tissues is diminished, causing ischaemic pain.

Pale cold extremities

Pale cold extremities indicate impaired blood flow to the limb. If an artery is suddenly occluded by a thrombus or embolus, there will be numbness and absence of distal pulses as well as coldness and pallor.

Altered peripheral pulses

Altered peripheral pulses may be present when arterial blood flow is impeded. Diminished or absent pulses suggest partial or total occlusion of an artery; for example, if the popliteal pulse is absent, the superficial femoral artery may be occluded.

Gangrene

Gangrene, which causes death of tissue, may occur as a result of chronic arterial insufficiency and is the consequence of severe and prolonged ischaemia. Gangrene first develops in the most distal parts of the lower limbs.

Leg ulcers

Leg ulcers or cellulitis may be present. Chronic occlusion of arterioles and small arteries results in ischaemia, skin breakdown and ulceration. Pooling of venous blood in the tissues of the extremities, for example, as a result of varicose veins, may lead to venous stasis ulcers. Aching or a feeling of fullness or heaviness in the legs is associated with venous insufficiency or valve incompetence. Homan's sign may be positive in the presence of thrombophlebitis. A positive Homan's sign is present when dorsiflexion of the foot (with the knee bent) produces pain in the calf. Tenderness, firmness and swelling in the calf are also suggestive of deep-vein thrombophlebitis.

MANIFESTATIONS OF BLOOD AND BLOOD-FORMING ORGAN DISORDERS

Bruising and bleeding

Bruising and bleeding may occur when there is abnormal thrombocyte production or function or reduced levels of clotting factors in the plasma. The appearance of any bruising or haemorrhagic spots in the absence of injury is suggestive of a blood disorder. Types of bruising and bleeding include:

- Purpura, haemorrhagic areas under the skin and in the mucous membranes. If the haemorrhages are small they are termed petechiae; larger purpuric areas are called bruises or ecchymoses
- Petechiae, red-brown pinpoint haemorrhages in the skin. Petechiae can occur over any part of the skin but are most common where pressure has been applied to a body part, seen in menigococcal meningitis and anthrax as well as common viral infections
- Ecchymoses are haemorrhagic spots larger than petechiae. They may be precipitated by an injury or may occur spontaneously
- Gastrointestinal bleeding, which appears as haematemesis and/or melaena and may occur in certain disorders of the blood such as thrombocytopenia, but may also occur as a result of liver failure, oesophageal varices, gastrointestinal ulcerations and drug therapies
- Menorrhagia, which may occur in haemorrhagic disorders as well as gynaecological disorders
- Haematuria, which may occur in haemorrhagic disorders as well as renal disorders
- Neurological changes (e.g. headaches, blurred vision, disorientation or altered consciousness), which may occur if there is bleeding within the central nervous system.

Changes in the skin may accompany disorders of the blood or blood-forming organs. Changes that may occur include pallor, rudor, jaundice, pruritus, thickened nails and ulcerations.

Fatigue

Fatigue or weakness are common manifestations of many haematological disorders, such as anaemia and leukaemia. A client with anaemia may also experience shortness of breath, particularly on exertion.

Enlarged lymph nodes

Enlarged lymph nodes may be present in disorders such as Hodgkin's disease or leukaemia. Pain may be experienced in many haematological disorders; for example, bleeding into a joint may result in joint pain, and bone pain can occur in leukaemia or lymphoma.

SPECIFIC DISORDERS OF THE CIRCULATORY SYSTEM

Disorders of the circulatory system may be congenital or due to multiple causes, pathogens or chemicals, or they may be drug related, neoplastic, obstructive, degenerative, or the result of trauma. It is beyond the scope of this text to provide in-depth detail of the various conditions related to the circulatory system. Listed below are some examples of circulatory system conditions. For more information you are advised to refer to an anatomy and physiology or pathophysiology text, such as Marieb (2006).

Congenital disorders

Congenital disorders are conditions which are 'present at and existing from the time of birth' (Hawley et al 2003: 105). These disorders include: ventricular septal defect; atrial septal defect; coarctation of the aorta; patent ductus arteriosus; Tetralogy of Fallot; transposition of the great vessels; thalassaemias (sickle-cell anaemia); and bleeding disorders (haemophilia A, haemophilia B, Von Willebrand's).

Disorders of multiple cause

It is beyond the scope of this text to provide in-depth detail of the various conditions related to the disorders of multiple causes and only a few of the most common conditions will be briefly discussed. For more information you are advised to refer to an anatomy and physiology or pathophysiology text, such as Marieb (2006).

Hypertension

High arterial blood pressure over 135/85 mmHg is generally classified as either primary ('essential') or secondary hypertension. Primary hypertension is the most common form and, while the cause is often unknown, many factors have been implicated as contributing to its development, including high sodium intake, obesity, diabetes, hypercholesterolaemia, genetic factors, alcohol, cigarette smoking and psychosocial factors.

Secondary hypertension is caused by either disease or certain medications. Diseases that result in secondary hypertension include those in which renal, vascular, endocrine or neurological mechanisms are involved, such as renal artery stenosis or intercranial lesions. Medications that may lead to secondary hypertension include oral contraceptives, corticosteroids and monoamine oxidase inhibitors.

Malignant hypertension is the term used to describe primary hypertension when there is a rapid rise of blood pressure to a very high level, such as 250/150 mmHg. It is accompanied by severe headache, visual disturbances and oliguria. If untreated, death may occur rapidly from cardiac or renal failure or cerebrovascular accident.

Hypertension is frequently asymptomatic until the client experiences a major problem such as cerebral haemorrhage, renal failure or myocardial infarction. Symptoms that may be due to hypertension include dizziness, chest pain, palpitations, epistaxis, headaches and brief episodes of memory loss (transient ischaemic attacks).

Coronary artery (ischaemic heart) disease

This is a disorder in which the arteries that supply blood to the heart muscle become diseased and fail to supply the heart with sufficient blood. Arteriosclerosis is the most common cause of coronary artery disease, causing disturbances of blood flow within the coronary arteries that gives rise to altered myocardial perfusion and disruption of the electrical cycle controlling heart rhythm. Atherosclerosis is one type of arteriosclerosis in which narrowing of the arteries occurs as a result of deposits of lipids in and around the smooth muscle, roughening of the endothelial lining, and loss of elasticity, with fibrosis and calcification. Eventually the artery becomes occluded, inelastic and incapable of dilating.

Although the precise cause of arteriosclerosis and coronary artery disease is unclear, there is general agreement that many factors contribute to its development, including genetic influences, gender (males are more commonly affected), hypertension, lack of exercise, cigarette smoking, stress, metabolic or endocrine disorders, obesity, diabetes mellitus, hypercholesterolaemia and dietary factors. The dietary factors that are considered to contribute to coronary artery disease are salt, saturated fats and lack of dietary fibre. Coronary artery disease may be asymptomatic until the client experiences angina or a myocardial infarction, which may result in sudden death.

Myocardial infarction

This is the death of part of the myocardium as a result of severe or total deprivation of its blood supply. Blood flow to the myocardium may be obstructed by arteriosclerosis or by thrombus formation within an atheromatous coronary artery. The most common site of infarction is the anterior surface of the left ventricle, resulting from occlusion of the left coronary artery. An infarction may affect some or all of the layers of the heart.

The major complications of a myocardial infarction are left ventricular failure, pericarditis and arrhythmias, which together account for a large percentage of deaths following myocardial infarction. It is generally recognised that the risk of death is greatest in the first few hours after myocardial infarction, with the risk decreasing after that time. Depression is common after recovery from the infarction and can result in non-compliance with treatment regimens and further infarctions.

A myocardial infarction may be asymptomatic (a silent myocardial infarction). More commonly it may manifest with pain in the centre of the chest, arms, neck, jaw or back lasting longer than five minutes, pallor, sweating, anxiety, shortness of breath, nausea or vomiting or sudden collapse.

Other disorders of multiple cause include: dysrhythmias, valvular heart disease, heart failure, cardiogenic shock, cardiac arrest, Raynaud's disease, disseminated intravascular coagulation, idiopathic thrombocytopenic purpura, agranulocytosis and Buerger's disease.

Anaemias

Anaemias are a group of disorders characterised by reduced oxygen-carrying capacity of the blood. Causes of anaemia are numerous and are related to the altered production or destruction of erythrocytes, and to blood loss. Anaemias can thus be classified as due to haemopoietic, haemolytic or haemorrhagic causes.

Aplastic anaemia is caused by injury or destruction of the haematopoietic cells in bone marrow, resulting in reduced or abnormal erythrocyte production. In this disorder the normal haematopoietic tissue is replaced by fatty bone marrow. Aplastic anaemia may be idiopathic or it may be caused by medications, toxic agents, radiation or immunological factors. Manifestations of aplastic anaemia are related to pancytopenia (abnormal depression of the cellular components of blood). They include pallor, tiredness, repeated infections and bleeding tendencies. Bleeding may present as petechiae, ecchymoses, haemorrhage from the mucous membranes, such as the gums, or gastrointestinal haemorrhage.

Pernicious anaemia is characterised by a metabolic defect involving the absence of intrinsic factor, which is secreted by the parietal cells of the gastric mucosa and is essential for vitamin B absorption in the terminal ileum. Pernicious anaemia is thought to result from an autosomal dominant defect. Other causes include gastric cancer, gastrectomy and malabsorption disorders involving the ileum. Manifestations of pernicious anaemia include pallor, tiredness, sore tongue, and numbness and tingling in the extremities. Because of vitamin B deficiency, demyelination of nerves and degeneration of nerve tissue occurs, producing neurological effects such as ataxia, altered vision, poor memory, depression and paralysis.

Iron-deficiency anaemia is characterised by small and pale erythrocytes because of reduced haemoglobin concentration. The two most common causes of iron-deficiency anaemia are chronic blood loss and an inadequate dietary intake of iron. Manifestations include pacophagia (craving for ice), pallor, chronic tiredness, tachycardia and shortness of breath on exertion.

Folate deficiency anaemia results from an inadequate dietary intake of folate, a disorder of the small intestine, where folate is absorbed, or from altered metabolism. Manifestations are similar to those associated with pernicious anaemia.

Acute blood-loss anaemia is a condition that results from sudden loss of erythrocytes and, consequently, depletion of haemoglobin and iron. Acute blood-loss anaemia may result from severe trauma, postoperative haemorrhage, invasive neoplasm, ruptured peptic ulcer, ruptured aneurysm or coagulation defects. Acute blood loss itself produces features associated with hypovolaemia and hypoxia, such as pallor, faintness, restlessness, anxiety, hypotension and a weak rapid pulse.

If anaemia is persistent and the client's haemoglobin levels decrease, the client may require a transfusion of blood. Table 38.4 provides information on preparing and monitoring clients undergoing a blood transfusion.

Neoplastic and obstructive disorders

Tumours may occur in any of the chambers of the heart and may affect one or all of the layers of the heart. Secondary metastatic tumours that infiltrate the heart are more common than primary cardiac tumours. Manifestations are related to which part of the heart is affected, and include signs of heart failure, dysrhythmias, angina, heart block and infarction. It is beyond the scope of this text to provide in-depth detail of the various conditions related to neoplastic and obstructive disorders and only a few of the most common conditions will be briefly discussed. For more information you are advised to refer to an anatomy and physiology or pathophysiology text, such as Marieb (2006).

Leukaemia

Leukaemia is a neoplastic disorder characterised by an accumulation and proliferation of abnormal cells in the bone marrow. Cells fail to develop and are unable to function normally, and the accumulation of leukaemic cells in the bone marrow prevents normal haematopoiesis. The precise cause of leukaemia is unknown but several factors have been implicated in its development including chromosome abnormality, exposure to radiation from power lines, viruses or chemicals, such as certain weed killers or insecticides. Leukaemia occurs either in acute forms, which involve the proliferation of immature cells, or in chronic forms which involve the proliferation of mature cells. The four most common forms of leukaemia are acute myeloid, chronic myeloid, acute lymphocytic and chronic lymphocytic.

Although manifestations of leukaemia vary according to the particular form of the disorder, there is a similarity in the signs and symptoms, which are related to the lack of normal haematopoiesis in the bone marrow. Bone marrow dysfunction results in:

- Anaemia, which may present as pallor, lethargy and shortness of breath
- Thrombocytopenia, which commonly manifests as petechiae, easy bruising, bleeding gums and haemorrhage (e.g. as occult haematuria)
- Leucopenia, which renders the client susceptible to recurrent infections. There is generally splenic enlargement, lymphadenopathy and bone pain.

Central nervous system involvement may be present in any of the leukaemias, giving rise to symptoms such as nausea and vomiting, irritability, headache and blurred vision.

Hodgkin's disease

Hodgkin's disease is a malignant disorder of the lymph node macrophages, characterised by painless and progressive enlargement of the lymph nodes, spleen and other lymphoid tissue. Untreated, Hodgkin's disease metastasises via the lymphatics to sites outside the lymphatic system. The precise cause of the disorder is unknown, but both genetic and environmental factors seem to be implicated in its development. Manifestations of Hodgkin's disease are painless enlargement of the lymph nodes, especially the cervical nodes, pruritus, night sweats, malaise and weight loss. Other symptoms depend on the degree and location of systemic involvement.

Other conditions related to neoplastic and obstructive disorders include: arteriosclerosis obliterans, acute arterial obstruction, thrombophlebitis, chronic venous insufficiency, Burkitt's lymphoma, multiple myeloma and malignant lymphomas.

Degenerative disorders

Cardiomyopathy

Cardiomyopathy results from extensive damage to the myocardial muscle fibres, causing hypertrophy of the entire heart, especially of the septum. Although the heart is enlarged, the ventricular chambers are small and are resistant to filling during diastole. Cardiomyopathy leads to congestive cardiac failure, arrhythmias and, frequently, sudden death.

The cause of most cardiomyopathies is unknown but the condition is thought to be genetically transmitted. Some forms of cardiomyopathy result from hypertension, congenital defects and myocardial destruction by toxic, infectious or metabolic agents. The most common manifestation of cardiomyopathy is dyspnoea, as a result of congestive cardiac failure. Angina, fatigue and syncope may occur because of inadequate cardiac output. As cardiac failure progresses, peripheral cyanosis, oedema, liver enlargement and jugular venous distension become evident.

Aortic aneurysm

Aortic aneurysm is a dilation of the wall of the aorta. There are several types of aneurysm:

- Saccular: an outpouching of one side of the arterial wall
- Fusiform: a spindle-shaped enlargement of the entire circumference of the artery
- Dissecting: a haemorrhagic separation between the medial and internal layers of the artery.

The most common cause of an aneurysm is arteriosclerosis, which weakens the aortic wall and gradually distends the lumen at the weakened area. Other causative factors include congenital defects, infection, hypertension and trauma.

Manifestations of an aortic aneurysm depend on its location, and may not develop until enlargement of the aneurysm exerts pressure on nearby structures. Depending on the location, an aortic aneurysm may manifest as dyspnoea; chest pain; dysphagia; dilated superficial veins on the chest, neck and arms; prominent abdominal pulsation; or dull abdominal or low back pain. A dissecting aneurysm may produce a sudden 'tearing' pain accompanied by pallor, shortness of breath, sweating and syncope. The main complication of an aortic aneurysm is rupture and, without immediate surgical intervention, the client may bleed to death.

Varicose veins

Varicose veins are dilated, tortuous branches of the saphenous veins. They result from incompetent valves, which cause a back-flow of venous blood. Varicose veins may result from congenital weakness of the valves, from injury or thrombophlebitis, or from conditions that produce venous stasis, such as pregnancy or occupations that necessitate standing for long periods. Superficial varicose veins may be unsightly but produce no symptoms. Deeper varicose veins may produce mild to severe leg symptoms, such as a feeling of heaviness, cramps, dull aching, and discomfort that increases with prolonged standing. Over time, dilation of the veins results in venous stasis, with oedema and changes in skin pigmentation. Visible and palpable protrusions frequently occur along the veins, resulting in disfigurement of the leg(s).

Infectious and inflammatory disorders

Pericarditis

Pericarditis (inflammation of the pericardium) may be an acute or chronic condition. Acute pericarditis may be accompanied by a purulent, serous or haemorrhagic exudate, which can produce further complications. Chronic pericarditis is characterised by fibrous pericardial thickening. As well as being caused by infection, pericarditis may result from trauma, radiation, neoplasms, cardiac surgery or myocardial infarction. The prime manifestation is chest pain that increases with deep inhalation, and decreases when the person sits up and leans forward. Other manifestations include dyspnoea and the signs of a systemic infection.

Myocarditis

Myocarditis (inflammation of the myocardium) may be an acute or chronic condition. Myocarditis may result from viral or bacterial infections, radiation, chemicals or metabolic disorders. Infective myocarditis usually causes non-specific symptoms that reflect a systemic infection. Myocarditis sometimes produces manifestations of severe congestive cardiac failure.

Endocarditis

Endocarditis (inflammation or infection of the endocardium) may result from invasion by microorganisms or from non-infective injury to the lining of the heart, or via intravenous (IV) cannulas, dental surgery or any other invasive procedure. Infective endocarditis involves the endocardium of the heart valves more frequently than the endocardium lining the heart chambers. The microorganisms stimulate the deposit of fibrin around them, producing vegetative growth on the endocardium.

Early manifestations are commonly non-specific, and the symptoms of acute endocarditis resemble those associated with influenza: pyrexia, sweats, anorexia, headaches and musculoskeletal aches. If a heart murmur develops, the pulse rate may be rapid and, if vegetations become dislodged, there may be manifestations of embolisation, producing the features of splenic, renal, cerebral, pulmonary or peripheral vascular occlusion.

Rheumatic heart disease

This refers to the cardiac manifestations of rheumatic fever and includes pericarditis, myocarditis, endocarditis and chronic valvular disease. Rheumatic fever is associated with the type A beta-haemolytic streptococcus and is thought to be immunological in origin. It may be as long as 10 years after an attack of rheumatic fever before signs of heart valve disease become evident. The end result of the disease progression is stenosis of a heart valve, inability of the valve to close properly, or valve incompetence, which leads to regurgitation of blood through the valve during systole. Manifestations of rheumatic heart valve disease depend on the valve affected and on the degree of valve dysfunction. There may be signs of reduced cardiac output, pulmonary congestion, cardiac enlargement, heart failure and the presence of heart murmurs.

Lymphangitis

Lymphangitis is an acute or chronic inflammation of the lymphatic vessels, which generally results from a streptococcal infection of an extremity. The accompanying lymph node enlargement (lymphadenopathy) may be localised or generalised. Lymphangitis is characterised by red, warm tender streaks spreading up a limb from a focal point of infection. The regional lymph nodes become enlarged and tender, and the client experiences pyrexia and malaise.

DIAGNOSTIC TESTS

RESPIRATORY DIAGNOSTIC TESTS

Certain tests may be used to assist or confirm the diagnosis and severity of respiratory disorders.

Pulmonary function tests

These tests measure the functional ability of the lungs. Spirometry or plethysmography is used to assess the client's lung volume by measuring and recording the volume of inhaled and exhaled air. The values are then compared with the normal values against predicted values for a client of the same sex, weight, height and age. Table 38.6 lists types of pulmonary function tests and the normal expected values.

Polysomonography

This test is used to measure upper obstruction and pattern of respirations during sleep, using various pieces of equipment.

Chest X-ray

A chest X-ray is one of the most common procedures used to evaluate the lungs, and generally involves posterior, anterior and lateral views. Abnormal findings that may be evident on a chest X-ray include areas of density, presence of a mass or accumulation of fluid.

Lung scan

A lung scan may be performed by administering radioactive dye. The radioactive particles are distributed and trapped in the pulmonary capillary bed, and the lung scan produces a visual image of pulmonary blood flow. Conditions such as pulmonary oedema, lung cancer or COPD may cause abnormal perfusion.

Cultures

A specimen of secretions is obtained, for example, via a nose swab or nasopharyngeal aspirate or throat swab. Care must be taken to ensure that only the back of the throat is swabbed, which represents microorganisms in the respiratory tract. Samples are sent to the laboratory so that any microorganisms present can be identified. Sensitivity studies are then done to determine which drug is effective against the specific microorganism.

Sputum cytology

A specimen of sputum is obtained and sent to the laboratory, where it is examined to detect the presence of pus, pathogenic microorganisms or malignant cells.

Skin tests

A common skin test performed is the Mantoux test, used in the detection of tuberculosis (TB). A medical officer or Registered Nurse qualified in intradermal administration injects intradermally 0.1 mL of solution containing old tuberculin. A positive reaction may be defined as an area of redness or induration of at least 5 mm in diameter appearing within 48–72 hours. The greater the reaction size the greater the exposure to antibodies to the tubercle bacillus.

Bronchoscopy

Bronchoscopy involves the direct viewing of the trachea and bronchi by means of an instrument called a bronchoscope. A bronchoscopy is used in the diagnosis of respiratory tract disorders and may be used to remove foreign bodies or flush out secretions in the airways and to obtain a specimen of secretions or tissue for microscopic examination.

Thoracentesis

In this procedure the thoracic wall is punctured with a needle to obtain a specimen of pleural fluid for analysis. The procedure may also be performed to relieve pulmonary compression caused by a pleural effusion. A local anaesthetic is injected into the skin before the needle is inserted.

TABLE 38.6 | PULMONARY FUNCTION TESTS

Tests	Explanation	Normal value*
Tidal volume	Amount of air inhaled or exhaled during normal breathing	500 mL
Total lung capacity	Total volume of the lungs when maximally inflated	5800 mL
Vital capacity	Total volume of air that can be forcibly exhaled after a maximum inhalation	3000–6000 mL
Functional residual capacity	Amount of air remaining in the lungs after normal exhalation	2300 mL
Inspiratory capacity	Amount of air that can be inhaled after normal exhalation	3500 mL
Expiratory reserve volume	Amount of air that can be exhaled after normal exhalation	1200 mL
Forced expiratory volume (in one second [FEV_1])	Maximal amount of air that can be forcibly exhaled, in one second, after full inhalation	3000–5000 mL
Residual volume	Amount of air remaining in the lungs after a maximal forced exhalation	1200 mL

Arterial blood gas analysis

Blood gas analysis shows how well a client's lungs are delivering oxygen to the bloodstream and eliminating carbon dioxide. Blood is collected for analysis of pH, Pa_{CO_2}, Pa_{O_2}, bicarbonate and base levels.

Capillary acid–base balance

This analysis is performed by a fingerpick. Blood is collected in a glass capillary tube to analyse the acid–base balance and P_{CO_2}.

Other tests

Blood microscopy and culture or viral tests may also be carried out to detect and identify the source of bacterial or viral infections. Other diagnostic tests that may be performed include fluoroscopy, tomography, bronchography and pulmonary angiography.

CARDIOVASCULAR DIAGNOSTIC TESTS

Assessment of the client with a suspected circulatory system disorder, or evaluation of the progress of a disorder, requires that certain cardiovascular tests be performed.

Assessment of cardiac function

Electrocardiography (ECG)

Electrocardiography (ECG, Figure 38.18) provides a graphical record, or trace, that represents the heart's electrical action. Cellular activity of the cardiac muscle generates electrical impulses that flow through the heart. This electrical activity can be measured by a system of electrodes placed at specific points on the body surface (refer to Figure 38.10 The conduction system of the heart). The ECG displays the electrical activity as waveforms, which are named P, Q, R, S and T waves. The ECG recording illustrates the rate and rhythm of electrical conduction and cardiac contractions through the heart. Abnormalities indicate enlargement of the chambers, inflammation of the pericardium or damage to the myocardium. Exercise electrocardiography (stress test) measures the cardiovascular effects of controlled physical stress, such as treadmill walking. Ambulatory (Holter) electrocardiography records the heart's electrical activity for a specified time, for example, 24 hours, as the client performs their usual activities (see Table 38.7).

A

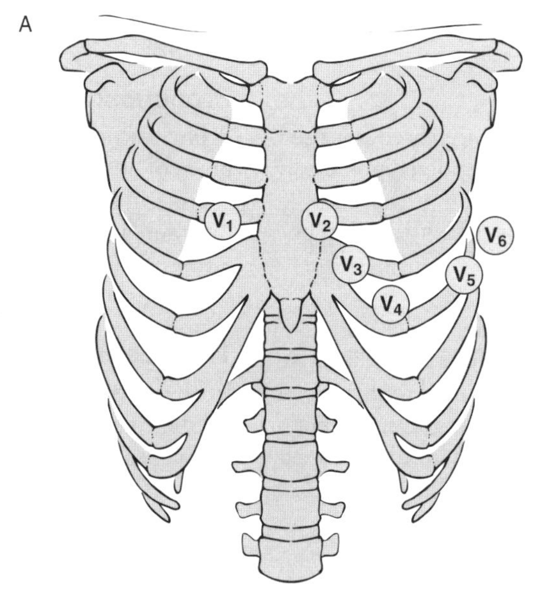

B(i)

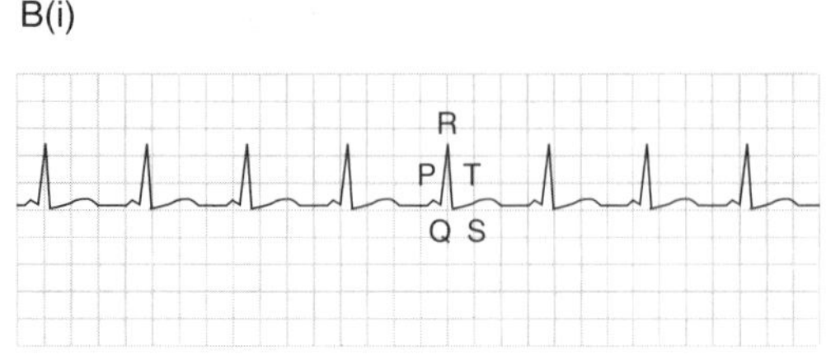

B(ii)

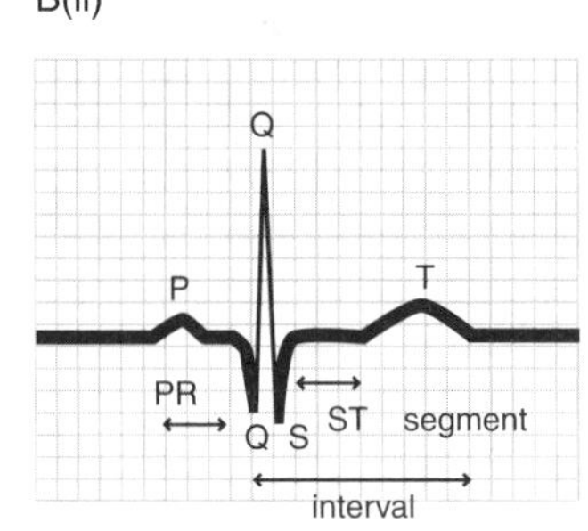

P wave = 0.04–0.08 sec
PR interval = 0.12–0.20 sec
QRS complex = 0.04–0.08 sec

Time: small squares = 0.04 sec
1 large square = 0.20 sec
5 large squares = 1.00 sec

Figure 38.18 | Electrocardiogram (ECG)
A: Placement of the chest leads *(Lewis et al 2004)*
B: A normal ECG (i) Regular sinus rhythm. (ii) Detail of an ECG

TABLE 38.7 | PERFORMING AN ECG

Review and carry out the steps in Appendix 1

Action	Rationale
Check medical orders to ascertain type, frequency and amount of fluid to be administered, and time prepared	Ensures correct quantities are given to client
Explain procedure to client	Reduced anxiety/apprehension and gains client's trust and cooperation
Prepare equipment	
Wash and dry hands	Prevents cross infection and contamination of blood and tubing
Don appropriate equipment and clothing as per infection control guidelines	Minimises risk of cross infection
Gather equipment including: • ECG machine • Electrodes • Gauze squares • Razor if necessary	Ensures all equipment is at client's bedside to maximise efficiency, reduce apprehension on the client's part and increases the confidence in the nurse
Assess client and prepare client	Ensure client is pain free, positioned in supine position, head supported Note: If client has breathing difficulties position in the semi-Fowler's position Loosen or remove clothing above the waist line Provision of privacy
Attach limb leads to clean, hair free sites on arms and legs	Area chosen should be over fleshy tissue not bony Skin needs to be clean to ensure the best conduction of electrical impulses Excess hair removed as it prevents adequate contact with the skin
Determine chest sites and attach electrodes to clean, dry hair free sites	Note: Care must be taken that the electrodes are accurately placed, since errors in diagnosis can occur if the electrodes are incorrectly placed. V1 — 4th intercostal space, right sternal border V2 — 4th intercostal space, left sternal border V3 — 5th intercostal space, left sternal border V4 — 5th intercostal space, left midclavicular line V5 — 5th intercostal space, left anterior axillary line V6 — 5th intercostal space, left midaxillary line
Attach lead wires to all electrodes	Attaching the electrodes to the leads ensures the electrical activity is conducted to the ECG machine
Set ECG paper speed, calibrate the machine according to manufacturer's instructions	Machines may be single channel or multi channel. Familiarity with the machine will increase accuracy of recording and decrease client and nurse stress
Record ECG and report to experienced Registered Nurse (RN)	Lack of experience and ability in interpreting an ECG recording might lead the student nurse to overlook changes that are significant
Removal of electrodes and conduction gel	Increases client comfort
Documentation	Includes inclusion of the actual recording—noting name, doctor, date and time and lead numbers. Some machines have the ability to program this information so that it is printed out on the ECG recording

Echocardiography

Echocardiography is a painless non-invasive test that directs ultra-high-frequency soundwaves through the chest wall into the heart, which then reflects those waves to a transducer and a recording device. As the sound transects the various heart structures, echoes are produced and recorded. Echocardiography evaluates cardiac structure and function and can reveal valve deformities, septal defects, cardiomyopathy and pericardial effusion.

Nuclear cardiology

Nuclear cardiology involves the use of radioactive tracers to evaluate myocardial blood flow and the status of myocardial cells. An IV injection, for example of the radioisotope thallium-201 or gallium, is administered to the client while they are exercising, and a scan performed to detect thallium uptake. Healthy myocardial tissue absorbs the radioisotope, but ischaemic or necrotic tissue does not.

Cardiac catheterisation

Cardiac catheterisation involves the insertion of a catheter into the right or left side of the heart to obtain information on cardiac pressures, cardiac output, oxygenation and heart valve function. The catheter is inserted through a vein in the arm or the groin and advanced into the vena cava; the passage of the catheter is observed on a fluorescent screen and X-ray films are taken. A contrast medium may be injected through the catheter and X-ray films taken (angiography). For coronary angiography, the catheter is advanced into the aortic arch and positioned into a coronary artery; a contrast medium is then injected to outline the coronary arteries as a series of X-ray films is taken.

Digital subtraction angiography

Digital subtraction angiography is less invasive than conventional angiography and involves injecting contrast dye into the venous system rather than directly into an artery. As the dye circulates through the heart and arterial system, a fluoroscopic image intensifier displays the vessels and focuses the image. A computer then converts the images into numbers. Several vessels can be evaluated with one injection of contrast dye.

Phonocardiography

Phonocardiography graphically records heart sounds produced as blood flows through the heart and great vessels. Microphones are placed on the chest, usually at the apex and base of the heart, and the sounds are picked up and converted into electrical impulses. The impulses are relayed to a recorder, which provides a graph of the heart sounds in wave form.

Central venous pressure

This test measures the functioning of the right atrium. A catheter, which is threaded through the subclavian or jugular vein into or near the right atrium, is connected to a manometer. This procedure enables accurate determination of right atrial blood pressure, which reflects right ventricular pressure. This test is also used to assess blood volume.

Intracardiac pressure monitoring

This test involves the insertion of a balloon-tipped flow-directed catheter, such as the Swan–Ganz catheter, into a large vein and then advancing it until it reaches the right atrium. Once the balloon is inflated, the flow of blood carries the catheter into the pulmonary artery. The procedure permits measurement of both pulmonary artery pressure (PAP) and pulmonary artery wedge pressure (PAWP). In addition, this procedure evaluates pulmonary vascular resistance and tissue oxygenation.

Blood tests

Blood tests may be performed to measure cardiac enzyme levels, which helps to assess myocardial function or cell death. Cardiac enzyme measurements help detect myocardial infarction, evaluate possible causes of chest pain and monitor the severity of myocardial ischaemia.

Assessment of peripheral blood vessels

Skin temperature studies

These may be performed to evaluate skin temperature of the extremities, which helps determine adequacy of blood circulation in arterial disease. Direct skin temperature readings are taken; in arterial disease the temperature in the extremities may be lower than in other body areas. The cold stimulation test may be used to demonstrate Raynaud's syndrome by recording temperature changes in the client's fingers before and after their submersion in ice water. Normally digital temperature returns to pre-test level within 15 minutes, but with Raynaud's syndrome return to pre-test level takes longer than 20 minutes.

Doppler ultrasonography

This involves the transmission of sound waves through the skin, which are reflected from moving blood cells in underlying blood vessels. This test evaluates blood flow in the major veins and arteries in the limbs, and helps to detect peripheral vascular aneurysms and deep vein thrombosis (DVT).

Arteriography

Arteriography (angiography) is the radiographic examination of one or more arteries after injection of a contrast medium into a major artery, usually the femoral artery. Arteriography can demonstrate blood flow status, collateral circulation, vascular anomaly and tumour and aneurysm formation.

Lower limb venography

This is the radiographic examination of a vein after an injection of contrast medium and is often used to assess the condition of the deep leg veins. Venography is the definitive test for DVT but may also be used to distinguish clot formation from other forms of venous obstruction or to locate a suitable vein for arterial bypass grafting.

Impedance plethysmography

This is a non-invasive test for measuring venous flow in the limbs and is helpful for detecting DVT. Electrodes are applied to the leg to measure changes in electrical resistance that result from blood volume variations.

Assessment of haematological status

For information on normal blood values, see Appendix 3.

Red blood cell (RBC) count

Red blood cell (RBC) (erythrocyte) count is the measurement of the number of erythrocytes found in a microlitre of blood. Together with haematocrit and haemoglobin determinations, this test is most often used to calculate mean corpuscular volume, mean corpuscular haemoglobin and mean corpuscular haemoglobin concentration.

Haematocrit

This is a blood test used to measure the percentage of a given volume of blood occupied by erythrocytes.

Erythrocyte indices

These involve examination of the size, weight and haemoglobin content of the average erythrocyte (mean corpuscular haemoglobin and mean corpuscular haemoglobin concentration).

Total haemoglobin

This test measures the grams of haemoglobin (Hb) in 100 mL of whole blood.

Stained red cell examination

This determines abnormalities in the size, shape or structure of erythrocytes.

Reticulocyte count

This measures the number of reticulocytes present in a sample of blood, which is then expressed as a percentage of the total RBC count. (Reticulocytes are immature erythrocytes.)

Erythrocyte sedimentation rate (ESR)

ESR measures the time required for erythrocytes, in a sample of whole blood, to settle to the bottom of a vertical tube.

Erythrocyte osmotic fragility

This measures red cell resistance to haemolysis when exposed to a hypotonic solution.

White blood cell (WBC) (leucocyte) count

WBC count is the measurement of the number of white cells found in a microlitre of whole blood. A differential WBC count determines the distribution and morphology of the various WBCs and provides more information about the immune system than the WBC count.

Coagulation

Coagulation function is measured by a wide variety of tests, including:

- Platelet count, which measures the number of circulating thrombocytes (platelets)
- Bleeding time, which measures the duration of bleeding after a standardised skin incision, commonly two small punctures made on the forearm
- Capillary fragility test, which measures the ability of capillaries to remain intact under increased intracapillary pressure. A blood pressure cuff is placed around the upper arm and inflated to midway between the systolic and diastolic pressures. After 5 minutes of sustained pressure, the number of petechiae on a selected area of the forearm are counted
- Clot retraction test, which estimates the quantity and quality of thrombocytes and fibrinogen
- Prothrombin time (PT), which measures the time required for a fibrin clot to form in a citrated plasma sample
- Partial thromboplastin time (PTT), which evaluates the entire coagulation system with the exception of Factors VII and XIII
- Factor VIII activity test, which measures the amount of Factor VIII in the blood and identifies a deficiency of that Factor (e.g. as in haemophilia).

Immunoglobulin studies

These evaluate the amount and types of immunoglobulins present.

Serum ferritin

Serum ferritin measurements evaluate the amount of iron stored in body tissues.

Total iron-binding capacity (TIBC)

TIBC measures the amount of available transferrin (a protein that binds with iron) in the blood.

Sickle-cell test

This detects the presence of haemoglobin S in suspected sickle-cell anaemia.

Gastric fluid analysis. This involves measuring the acidity of secretions in the stomach and is used in the diagnosis of pernicious anaemia.

Bone marrow examination

This provides information about the character, integrity and production of erythrocytes, leucocytes and thrombocytes in the marrow. Bone marrow can be removed by aspiration or needle biopsy. Aspiration of bone marrow involves the removal of a small amount, generally less than 5 mL. Biopsy, performed under local anaesthesia, is done when a larger amount of bone marrow is required. A needle is inserted through the skin and tissue, for example, over the iliac crest, until it reaches bone. The needle is then directed into the marrow cavity, and a sample of bone marrow is withdrawn.

Assessment of the lymphatic system

Lymphangiography is the radiographic examination of the lymphatic system after the injection of a contrast medium into a lymphatic vessel in each foot. X-ray films are taken to demonstrate the filling of the lymphatic vessels and, 24 hours later, to visualise the lymph nodes.

CARE OF THE CLIENT WITH A RESPIRATORY AND/OR CARDIAC SYSTEM DISORDER

Although specific nursing actions and medical management vary depending on the disorder, the main aims of care are to:

- Maintain airway patency
- Facilitate normal and effective breathing
- Promote efficient gas exchange
- Promote comfort and relieve pain
- Provide psychological support
- Maintain skin integrity
- Promote and maintain mobility
- Prevent infection
- Maintain fluid and nutritional status
- Administer prescribed medication
- Provide care, before, during and after a diagnostic test.

A client with a respiratory system disorder will commonly experience problems such as a change in breathing pattern and discomfort associated with breathing. Clients with cardiac disorders may experience multi-system problems associated with circulation, including pain or discomfort with exercise, difficulty breathing, palpitations and fatigue. Nursing activities include alleviating discomforts associated with exercise and breathing, administering oxygen, positioning, monitoring the client and their vital signs, and helping the client with cardiovascular and breathing exercises. As well as planning care to meet specific needs, nurses must also consider the client's other needs, such as nutrition, fluid intake, skin integrity, elimination and the need for comfort.

PROMOTING A CLEAR AIRWAY

One of the most important aspects of care is the maintenance or restoration of a clear airway, which includes measures directed at removing secretions. Commonly an inflammatory respiratory tract disorder results in the production of excessive secretions, made more tenacious by dehydration caused by tachypnoea, mouth breathing and pyrexia. The client may experience difficulty in maintaining a patent airway; some of the following steps may assist them in expectorating secretions.

Adequate hydration

Dehydration can make secretions more viscous and difficult to expectorate, so an adequate fluid input is important. Unless contraindicated, the client should be encouraged to drink at least 2–3 L a day. In certain conditions such as cardiac failure fluid may need to be restricted to 1500 mL or less. The nurse should assess fluid balance by measuring fluid input and output and by observing for signs of oedema. Weighing the client, for example, each day, is another way of assessing their fluid status. If they are unable to tolerate sufficient fluids orally because of dyspnoea, nausea and/or vomiting or the presence of an oxygen mask that can make drinking more difficult, alternative fluids may be administered by the IV route if necessary.

Maintaining nutritional status

Commonly a client with a cardiovascular disorder will be prescribed a diet that aims to reduce serum cholesterol and triglyceride levels. Sodium intake may also be reduced, for example, in the control and prevention of hypertension. If the client with either a respiratory or cardiovascular disorder is obese, a weight-reduction diet is generally prescribed. The diet generally should be low in total fat content, particularly saturated fats, and low in sodium. Kilojoules may be reduced to correct or prevent obesity, and alcohol should be restricted, as it can raise kilojoule intake and serum lipid levels. Beverages and foods containing caffeine should be restricted, as caffeine is a metabolic stimulant that can worsen tachycardia, hypoxaemia and dysrhythmias.

In specific blood disorders the client may be prescribed a diet high in one or more nutrients, for example, a diet high in iron is generally prescribed in the treatment of iron-deficiency anaemia. When a specific diet is prescribed the dietitian consults with the client to plan the diet and to ensure that they understand any dietary modifications or restrictions.

It is important that nurses are aware of the type of diet that has been prescribed and ensure that the client receives the correct tray at mealtimes. Nurses encourage the client to follow the diet and may need to assist at mealtimes, for example, if the client is unable to eat meals independently. (Information on assisting at mealtime is provided in Chapter 31.)

Cessation of smoking

If the client is a smoker, they should be encouraged to stop smoking. Cigarette smoke impairs function of the cilia, and smoking generally aggravates any existing respiratory and cardiac disorder.

Nebulisation and humidification

As well as drinking adequate fluid, additional fluid may be administered directly into the airways by means of humidifiers, inhalations or nebulisers. Nebulisation or humidification reduces the viscosity of secretions, facilitating easy expectoration. Physiotherapy may be used concurrently. (Information on the use of humidifiers and nebulisers is provided later in this chapter.)

Positioning

If a client with a respiratory condition experiences dyspnoea, they should be assisted into a more upright position. This facilitates alveolar expansion, as gravity allows more blood to perfuse the bases of the lung, improving the ventilation/perfusion (V/Q) ratio. Nurses should ensure that sufficient pillows are placed so that the client's back, neck, head and arms are well supported, or that the head of the bed is elevated.

Medication

Medications may be prescribed to reduce pain, loosen secretions, relieve bronchospasm, increase cilia beating speed, combat infection, increase or decrease coughing, relieve pulmonary oedema, alter blood pressure and cholesterol levels or correct dysrhythmias. Medications may be given by inhalation, orally, or by intramuscular or IV routes. The types of medications prescribed may include analgesics, decongestants, antihistamines, antibiotics, bronchodilators or expectorants.

Oronasopharyngeal suction

If coughing is ineffective in removing secretions, suction may be necessary. Oronasopharyngeal suction removes secretions from the pharynx by means of a suction catheter inserted through the mouth or nostril. This technique is used to maintain a patent airway and is indicated for a client who is unable to clear their airway effectively with coughing and expectoration. Table 38.8 outlines the guidelines for performing this procedure.

Chest physiotherapy

Chest physiotherapy assists the client to mobilise and eliminate secretions, re-expand airways and alveoli, and promote the efficient use of the muscles of ventilation. Chest physiotherapy includes postural drainage, chest percussion and vibration, coughing and deep-breathing exercises.

Postural drainage

Postural drainage (Figure 38.19) encourages pulmonary secretions to empty by gravity into the bronchioles, bronchi or trachea, so that they may be expectorated. The client with a respiratory disorder is assisted to assume positions that promote drainage from the affected parts of the lungs. Effectiveness of the technique largely depends on positioning that allows drainage by gravity. Postural drainage should be avoided immediately before or after meals, to prevent nausea and aspiration of food or vomitus.

Percussion and vibration

These techniques are employed to help loosen respiratory

TABLE 38.8 | GUIDELINES FOR ORONASOPHARYNGEAL SUCTION

Action	Rationale
Review and carry out the standard steps in Appendix 1	
Explain the procedure to the client and provide privacy	Reduces anxiety and embarrassment
If possible, position the client in a sitting position or with the neck extended	Promotes lung expansion and effective coughing. Facilitates catheter insertion
Wash and dry hands. Put on gloves	Prevents cross-infection
Attach collection bottle to the suction unit, attach connecting tubing, connector and catheter	Equipment must be assembled and checked for function before the procedure starts
Turn on the suction and dip the tip of the catheter into the water	Lubricates the catheter to facilitate insertion
With the suction off (e.g. by using the Y-connector), gently introduce the catheter into the mouth or nostril. If the oral route is used, the client's tongue may be depressed with a tongue depressor	Suction during insertion may damage the mucosa. Facilitates insertion of the suction catheter
Ensure that suction pressure is below 120 mmHg. Apply suction as the catheter is withdrawn, rotating the catheter as it is being withdrawn	Pressure above 120 mmHg may damage the mucosa. Rotating motion prevents tissue trauma and obtains maximal volume of secretions
Apply suction for a maximum of 8–10 seconds, or less in the young or critically unwell client, then remove from the airway. Allow the client time to rest between suctioning	Suctioning for longer than 10 seconds can cause tissue trauma and hypoxia
If secretions are tenacious, dip the tip of the catheter in water and apply suction. If a specimen is required for virology or bacterial studies, use of normal saline is recommended	Clears the lumen of catheter Normal saline prevents degradation of viruses or bacteria
Repeat the procedure, if necessary, until the mucous obstruction has been removed	Promotes a clear airway
After suctioning, instruct the client (if able) to take several slow deep breaths	Relieves hypoxia and promotes relaxation
Dip the catheter into the water and apply suction	Clears catheter and connecting tubing
Discard the catheter, water and gloves. Attend to the rest of the equipment. Wash and dry hands	Prevents cross-infection
Assist the client into a position of comfort	Promotes rest and relaxation
Wash and dry hands	Prevents cross-infection
Document and report the procedure, including observations of the aspirate	Appropriate care can be planned and implemented

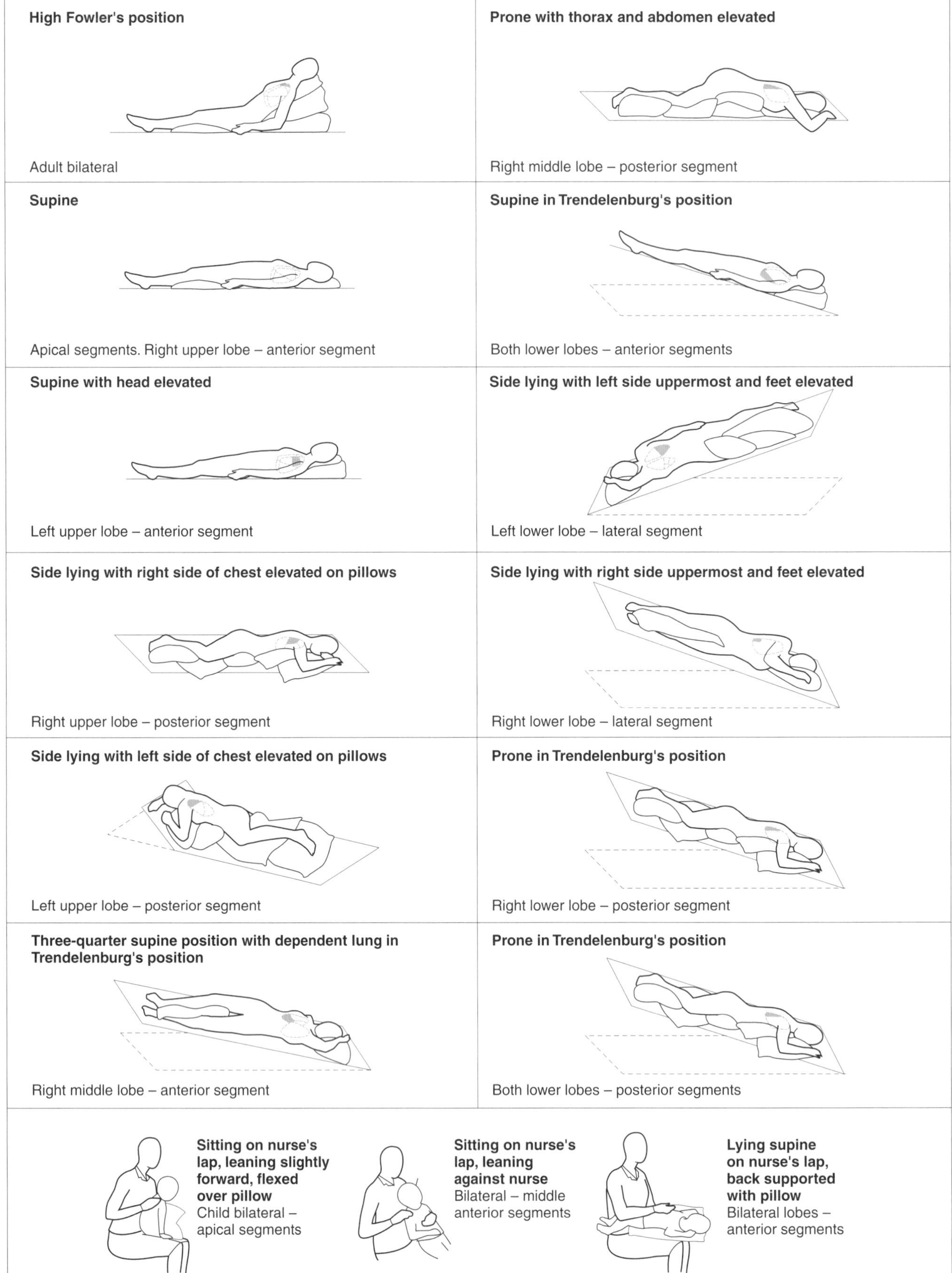

Figure 38.19 | Postural drainage *(redrawn from Potter & Perry 2008)*

secretions and are commonly used in conjunction with postural drainage. Percussion is performed by rhythmic tapping using cupped hands over the affected segments of the lungs. Care should be afforded to clients with osteoporosis, fractures or recent surgery. Vibration is performed by placing the hands over the affected area and shaking, so that the chest wall is vibrated while the client is forcibly exhaling. To ensure sufficient force is being used the client can be asked to vocalise and a vocal fremitus should be heard.

After postural drainage, percussion and vibration, the client should be asked to cough to remove the loosened secretions. This is performed by a physiotherapist. Oral hygiene should be attended to after the procedure because the expectorated secretions may have an offensive taste or odour.

PROMOTING COMFORT AND RELIEVING PAIN

In many disorders of the circulatory system the aim is to increase the client's activity progressively without pain. Comfort is promoted if the client is provided with a bed made to meet their specific needs.

The client may experience pain, for example, as a result of myocardial infarction or peripheral vascular dysfunction, so relief of pain is an important aspect in the promotion of comfort. In certain respiratory conditions such as pleurisy, severe pain may increase on inspiration. The presence of indwelling tubes, wires or cannulas all contribute to further discomfort. Pain-relieving measures such as the administration of adequate analgesic medication by the Registered Nurse (RN) are implemented so that the client is able to rest comfortably, sleep without discomfort and perform the activities of daily living without experiencing pain or significant side effects of the medication. The client is also advised on what precautions to take to avoid pain, which includes identifying any precipitating factors such as physical exertion or emotional stress. The incidence of pain can generally be reduced by careful planning of activity, modifying risk factors and use of prophylactic measures.

PROVIDING PSYCHOLOGICAL SUPPORT

Anxiety and fear are common responses to hospitalisation. A client who is experiencing a major respiratory or cardiovascular dysfunction, such as myocardial infarction, pneumonia or blood dyscrasias, often becomes extremely anxious, apprehensive and depressed about dyspnoea, pain, disability, loss of independence and dying. The client and their significant others may experience great concern about the alterations in lifestyle imposed by their disorder. Nurses provide psychological support by establishing and maintaining a trusting relationship with the client and their significant others and by encouraging them to express their feelings and concerns. They should be encouraged to discuss any lifestyle adjustments that may be necessary and they should be offered guidance on how to cope with change.

Stress and anxiety can be reduced if the client's symptoms, such as pain or dyspnoea, are alleviated, and the nurse should try to provide an environment that is as stress free as possible. The client should be provided with sufficient information about their illness, as knowledge helps to diminish anxiety and apprehension and assists them to develop effective coping skills. All procedures, treatments and monitoring techniques being implemented are explained so that the client understands the treatment. The client should be encouraged to participate in their care as much as possible and, when appropriate, to gradually assume responsibility for self-care to prevent loss of independence. The client should be informed about support groups and community resources such as rehabilitation classes, which may be helpful when they are discharged from hospital.

MAINTAINING SKIN INTEGRITY

A client with a respiratory, cardiac, peripheral vascular, blood or lymphatic disorder is at risk of impaired skin integrity. Decreased peripheral perfusion and oxygenation can result in skin breakdown. With poor arterial circulation the tissues lack adequate oxygen and nutrients and this can lead to cellulitis, ulcers, poor wound healing and necrosis. Maintenance of skin integrity includes:

- Assessing the skin for any signs of breakdown
- Keeping the skin clean and dry
- Protecting the extremities from exposure to extremes of temperature and from trauma
- Position changes to avoid prolonged pressure on the skin
- The use of accessories (e.g. a sheepskin) to reduce pressure, and promoting mobility.

Preventing skin breakdown includes keeping the feet clean and dry, avoiding rough drying movements, using creams or lotions that prevent drying and cracking, avoiding scratching itchy areas on the legs or feet, nail care provided by a podiatrist and protecting the feet with socks, slippers or well-fitting shoes.

PROMOTING AND MAINTAINING MOBILITY

Maintenance of mobility is necessary to prevent the complications of immobility, such as decubitus ulcers, venous stasis and pulmonary complications. Problems of immobility should be counteracted with position changes, range-of-motion (ROM) exercises and coughing and deep-breathing exercises. Ambulation of the client as soon as possible is important to prevent the complications of immobility.

In the initial stages of illness, such as immediately after myocardial infarction, the client's level of activity may be reduced to a minimum. As their tolerance increases, their level of physical activity gradually increases. The client should understand the importance of adequate physical exercise, which provides the necessary muscle contraction for movement of arterial blood and lymph to and from the peripheral areas of the body. Exercise or activity programs are generally implemented gradually, and the client is encouraged to rest after the exercise periods. As the client's condition improves, moderate exercise is encouraged as long as pain is not induced.

PREVENTING INFECTION

A client with any of the disorders mentioned previously may be susceptible to infection as a result of nosocomial infections, altered nutritional status, medications such as steroids, invasive procedures and changes in immune status. Measures to prevent infection must be implemented, such as good hand-washing techniques, and aseptic techniques for any procedure. Precautions must be taken to prevent damage to the skin or mucous membranes, as injured tissues create a portal for bacterial invasion. If the client's WBC count is low (leucopenia), it may be necessary to use protective isolation techniques to protect them against infection. The client must be monitored closely to detect the early manifestations of infection so that appropriate treatment can be prescribed.

PROMOTING EFFECTIVE BREATHING AND AERATION

In addition to the measures employed to promote a clear airway, other measures may be necessary to maintain adequate ventilation. Breathing exercises may be used by the client to promote and maintain optimal pulmonary ventilation, and oxygen may be prescribed to supplement that being obtained from the atmosphere.

Breathing exercises

When respiratory system disorders produce ineffective breathing patterns and inadequate ventilation, the client may be educated to perform deep-breathing exercises.

Deep breathing

Deep, or diaphragmatic, breathing uses the diaphragm and abdominal muscles to fully ventilate the lungs. The client should be assisted into a sitting position to promote optimal alveolar expansion. One hand is placed on the chest and the other hand is placed on the abdomen. If the client is breathing correctly the hand on the abdomen should rise with inhalation and fall with exhalation; the hand on the chest should remain still. The client is educated to inhale deeply and slowly, pushing the abdomen out, to promote optimal distribution of air to the alveoli. Clients may also be educated to exhale through pursed lips, while contracting their abdomen. Exhalation through pursed lips improves ventilation pressures and encourages a slow deep-breathing pattern. Abdominal contraction pushes the diaphragm upwards, exerts pressure on the lungs and helps to empty them.

Breathing exercises are performed according to the client's condition; for example, short sessions may be indicated if the client becomes fatigued easily. The duration and frequency with which deep-breathing exercises are performed vary; they may, for example, be performed for 1 minute, with gradual progression to a 10-minute exercise period four times daily.

Incentive spirometry

Incentive spirometry (Figure 38.20) uses a breathing device to encourage the client to achieve maximal ventilation. The device measures peak respiratory flow or respiratory volume, and induces the client to take a deep breath and hold it for several seconds. Incentive spirometry benefits the client, as it establishes alveolar hyperinflation for a longer time than is possible with a normal deep breath.

Oxygen therapy

A client with a respiratory system disorder may be prescribed supplemental oxygen to be administered intermittently or continuously. (See 'Meeting a client's need for oxygen' later in this chapter.)

PROMOTING EFFICIENT GAS EXCHANGE

Any disorder of the respiratory system may result in impaired gas exchange. Depending on the extent to which it interferes with ventilation and perfusion, hypercapnia, hypocapnia and/or hypoxaemia may develop. The aim of management of these conditions is to maintain adequate oxygenation and removal of carbon dioxide. In addition to the measures already described, which promote a clear airway and effective breathing, other measures may be necessary, including the insertion of an artificial airway and/or mechanical ventilation. (Information on both these

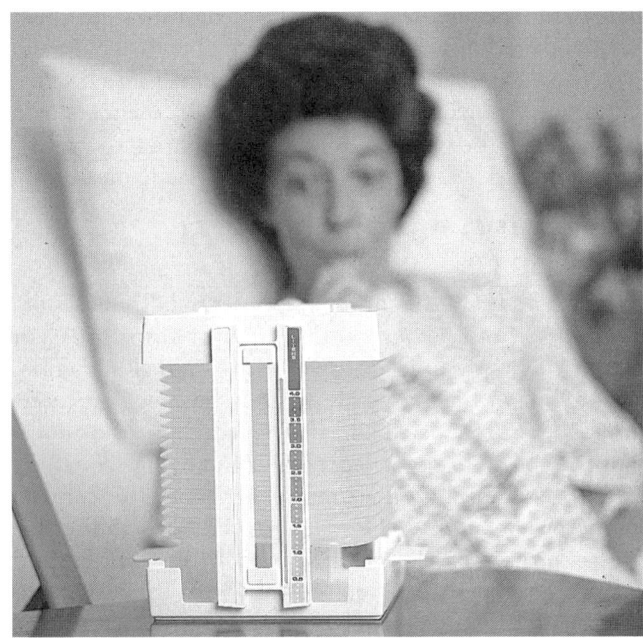

Figure 38.20 | Spirometry *(Potter & Perry 2008)*

TABLE 38.9 | IMPAIRED GAS EXCHANGE

Condition	Possible cause	Manifestations
Respiratory acidosis (hypercapnia)	Hypoventilation as a result of chronic obstructive pulmonary disease, pneumonia, drugs or trauma	Flushed warm skin, hypertension, tachycardia, headaches, drowsiness, confusion, irritability, coma
Respiratory alkalosis (hypocapnia)	Hyperventilation as a result of acute asthma, cerebral trauma or congestive cardiac failure	Diaphoresis, pallor, tachypnoea, tingling and numbness in the limbs, or around the mouth, carpopedal spasm (tetany) and convulsions
Hypoxia	Obstructive lung diseases, and restrictive lung diseases (e.g. chronic bronchitis, emphysema, sarcoidosis)	Pallor or cyanosis, tachypnoea, tachycardia, breathlessness, headaches, irritability, confusion

topics is provided later in this chapter.) The nurse must observe the client for the signs and symptoms of impaired gas exchange (Table 38.9).

NURSING ACTIVITIES

Specific nursing activities relevant to caring for a client with a respiratory system disorder include:

- Collecting specimens of sputum
- Obtaining nasal or throat swabs
- Administering oxygen
- Suction via the oral, nasal or tracheal routes
- Inhalation therapy.

Collecting sputum

Sputum is a mucous secretion produced by the mucous membranes that line the respiratory tract. Mucous secretion increases in response to inflammation, infection or congestion. Laboratory examination of sputum may be necessary to determine whether any microorganisms, blood or malignant cells are present. The nurse should observe the sputum, noting the amount, consistency, colour and presence of blood or odour. Sputum is normally clear in colour but may turn white if the client smokes or has a viral infection; yellow, rust-coloured, or green to dark-brown sputum may indicate the presence of an infection. It may be tinged with blood or contain streaks of blood that can suggest inflammations, dryness or infections or conditions such as pulmonary oedema or carcinoma. The consistency varies from watery to mucoid to tenacious. An Enrolled Nurse (EN) may only collect oral secretions via suctioning using a Yankauer-style suction unit.

When a specimen of sputum is required it is best collected early in the morning before any food or fluid is given, as this ensures that there is an accumulation of secretions to be obtained. To avoid the risk of cross-infection with airborne microorganisms the nurse should stand beside rather than in front of a client when collecting the sputum specimen. Sputum for laboratory testing should be free of saliva and food particles. A suggested procedure for collecting a specimen of sputum is outlined in Table 38.10.

Nasopharyngeal and throat swabs

Laboratory examination of secretions from the nasopharynx or throat may be necessary to determine the presence of pathogenic microorganisms. Collection of a specimen involves swabbing the inflamed tissues and collecting any

TABLE 38.10 | GUIDELINES FOR COLLECTION OF SPUTUM

Action	Rationale
Review and carry out standard steps in Appendix 1	
Explain the procedure to the client, ensuring that they understand it is sputum and not saliva that is required. Label the container appropriately	Reduces anxiety. Saliva will produce inaccurate test results
Wash and dry hands and don gloves	Prevents cross-infection
Assist the client to a sitting position	Facilitates coughing and expectoration
Instruct the client to cough and to expectorate into a sterile container	A sterile container ensures that the specimen is not contaminated
Place the lid on the labelled container, wipe the outside of the container, and wash and dry hands	Prevents cross-infection
Despatch the specimen, together with the request form, to the laboratory as soon as possible. Ensure that the container is clearly labelled with the relevant information	Proliferation of microorganisms occurs if the specimen is not despatched as soon as possible after collection. Avoids errors
Offer the client oral hygiene	Reduces bad taste or halitosis in mouth

exudate with a sterile cotton-wool-tipped swab. The nurse should refer to the health care institution's policy manual for information about the type of applicator, culture tube and transport medium to use. A suggested procedure for collecting a nasopharyngeal or throat swab is outlined in Table 38.11.

Oronasopharyngeal suction

Oronasopharyngeal suction may be required when secretions or foreign substances are causing an obstruction to the client's airway. Suction is indicated for the client who is unable to clear the airway effectively with coughing and expectoration, such as the severely debilitated or unconscious client. The removal of excess secretions and mucus from the airway aids breathing, promotes pulmonary gas exchange and prevents the accumulation of secretions that may cause secondary atelectasis or pneumonia. Suctioning is achieved by means of a catheter, which is introduced through the mouth or nose into the pharynx. A suggested procedure is outlined in Table 38.8. The basic equipment consists of:

- Wall suction or portable suction apparatus
- Collection bottle
- Connecting tubing
- Water suitable for flushing the catheter and tubing in a small container
- Sterile suction catheters
- Protective glasses
- Disposable gloves
- Tongue depressor.

Suction equipment is usually kept in readiness at the bedside if there is an indication that it may be needed frequently, as an emergency measure or as part of the health care institution's policies. In general the pressure is set at 80–120 mmHg for an adult (and considerably lower for a child), depending on the diameter of the catheter and the viscosity of the secretions. The medical officer will prescribe the level of suction to be used. If using the nasal route, suctioning should be alternated between the left and right nostrils to reduce trauma to the one nostril. It may also be necessary to lubricate the tip of the catheter with a sterile water-soluble lubricant before insertion into the nostril.

Inhalation therapy

Various forms of inhalation therapy may be prescribed for a client with a respiratory disorder, including humidified air or oxygen, and nebulised air or oxygen. These can be administered by aerosol devices, electric nebulisers and humidifiers or an intermittent positive-pressure ventilator.

Electrical humidifiers and nebulisers

Water vapour may be provided by means of a humidity cot, tent or via a mask or tube attached to the client. Various electrical devices such as the Concha Pak can provide both humidification and nebulisation, depending on the fitting used. The device has water fed by a sterile container to an electrically warmed core that heats up the fluid contained in it as it passes through a chamber. The warmed water

TABLE 38.11 | GUIDELINES FOR COLLECTING A NASOPHARYNGEAL OR THROAT SWAB

Action	Rationale
Review and carry out standard steps in Appendix 1	
Explain the procedure to the client. Inform them that they may experience the urge to sneeze or gag during the swabbing. Label the container appropriately	Reduces anxiety and promotes co-operation to minimise trauma
Assist the client, if possible, to a sitting position	Facilitates collection of the specimen
Wash and dry hands, and don gloves	Prevents cross-infection
If a nasopharyngeal swab is to be obtained, request the client to blow their nose	Clears the nasal passages
Request the client to tilt their head back	Facilitates collection of the specimen
To obtain a swab of the nasopharynx, gently pass the swab through the nostril until it reaches the posterior pharyngeal wall	Gentle insertion prevents tissue damage
Rotate, then withdraw the swab. To obtain a swab of the throat request the client to open their mouth, depress the tongue with a tongue depressor and use a torch to illuminate the throat	Facilitates access and visualisation
Ask the client to say 'ah'. Pass the swab over the tonsils, posterior pharyngeal wall and posterior edge of the soft palate	Raises the uvula to expose proper site of collection
Place the swab in the culture tube immediately and close the end of the tube. Wash and dry hands	Prevents cross-infection and contamination of the specimen
Despatch the specimen, together with the request form, to the laboratory as soon as possible. Ensure that the container is clearly labelled with the relevant information	Proliferation of microorganisms occurs if the specimen is not despatched and refrigerated as soon as possible after collection

vapour is delivered to the client via large bore corrugated tubing and the oxygen concentration can be regulated from room air to 100% oxygen by means of an oxygen venturitype diluter. The client inhales the vapour through a nebuliser-type mask.

Nebulisation provides a very visible mist of large water droplets that are delivered into the airways. Nebulisation is used to treat atelectasis and airway infections and to loosen and decrease the viscosity of secretions to facilitate expectoration. It can be delivered through a mask or tracheotomy tube. Humidification (Figure 38.21) provides water vapour in an almost invisible fine mist of small droplets that can travel further into the airways than by nebulisation by virtue of the droplet size and weight. Humidification is used to provide humidity to prevent stasis of mucus, tissue dehydration, and to reduce drying, inflammation and irritation of the air passages. These devices provide precise control of oxygen delivery and protection against cross-contamination by means of a sterile pre-filled container of solution, such as sterile water or normal saline.

Other similar devices are used in positive-pressure ventilators, such as Bird or Bennet ventilators, to deliver humidity or medication to a client on a ventilator or during intermittent positive-pressure breathing therapy. Nurses should know their role and responsibilities regarding inhalation therapy and administration of medications, and should be familiar with the health care facility's infection-control guidelines. The nurse should check the devices hourly for leaks, cracks and oxygen concentration. Bedding and clothing are changed as soon as they become damp. Care should also be taken to observe the skin surrounding the mask for signs of breakdown.

Mechanical and electrical nebulisers are used to deliver moisture or medication as a fine mist into the airways of clients with conditions such as asthma or emphysema. Bronchodilators are commonly prescribed

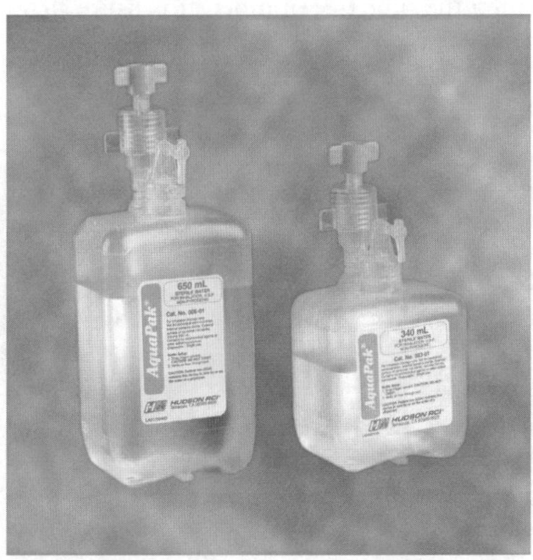

Figure 38.21 | A humidifier *(reproduced with permission from Hudson RCI)*

in the management of asthma. (Information on the use of hand-held inhalers is provided in Chapter 28.) The devices operate off mains or 12-volt power and are generally used by clients at home. Care must be taken to ensure that the device is placed on a stable surface, and regular maintenance of the filters is required.

Gas-driven nebulisers are used with compressed air or oxygen to deliver nebulised vapour or medication. The prescribed solution is inserted into the nebuliser, either alone or together with a prescribed amount of sterile water or saline, and one end of the oxygen tubing is attached to the nebuliser, which is directly connected to a nebuliser mask. The other end of the tubing is attached to an oxygen regulator and then to the pressurised gas source, which is turned on to check for proper misting. To produce particles of the correct size and to better ensure their arrival at the most distal airways, a flow rate of 10 L/min is generally required. The client is instructed to breathe deeply, slowly and evenly through the mouthpiece or mask and to hold their breath for 2–3 seconds at the end of inhalation to receive the full benefit of the medication. The client should be encouraged to cough and expectorate.

Steam inhalations are not generally used because of the risk of burns and the improved effectiveness in providing fluids by other means.

Mechanical ventilation

Mechanical ventilation is sometimes indicated for a client with a respiratory system disorder. Mechanical ventilation artificially assists or controls respiration and it is indicated to correct or prevent gas transport abnormalities. To maintain adequate pulmonary blood gas exchange, an endotracheal or tracheostomy tube is inserted (see below) and connected to the ventilator.

A variety of ventilators is available, which may be one of two main types: pressure controlled or volume controlled. With the pressure-controlled ventilator the gas is delivered to the lungs until a predetermined pressure is reached, then inspiration is terminated. With a volume-controlled ventilator a set volume of gas is delivered with each inspiration. The ventilation rate may be preset, controlled by the client, or may be a combination of both.

Care of a client receiving mechanical ventilation should be provided by nursing staff who are qualified and experienced to provide it. A client who requires mechanical ventilation is generally nursed in an ICU, as they require constant physical attention and emotional support.

THE CLIENT WITH AN ARTIFICIAL AIRWAY

The placement of an artificial airway is indicated to relieve obstruction, to facilitate suctioning of the lower respiratory tract, to prevent aspiration or to allow for mechanical ventilation. Artificial airways include the oropharyngeal airway, the endotracheal tube and the tracheostomy tube.

OROPHARYNGEAL AIRWAY

An oropharyngeal airway (Figure 38.22) is a curved rubber or plastic device inserted into the mouth to the posterior pharynx to establish or maintain a patent airway. The airway allows air to pass around and through the tube and facilitates oropharyngeal suctioning. It is used for the short term only, such as in the immediate post-anaesthetic period. If a client requires respiratory assistance for a longer period, an endotracheal or tracheostomy tube is generally used.

ENDOTRACHEAL TUBE

An endotracheal tube (Figure 38.23) is a flexible cuffed tube inserted via the mouth or nostril through the larynx into the trachea. Endotracheal intubation establishes and maintains a patent airway, prevents aspiration by sealing the trachea off from the digestive tract, facilitates the removal of tracheobronchial secretions and provides a means whereby optimal ventilation can be achieved. Endotracheal intubation may be required in an emergency or may be required for a short or long term.

The tube is inserted by a medical officer, who uses a laryngoscope to visualise the trachea and facilitate the passage of the tube. Most endotracheal tubes in adults have a cuff, which is inflated with air to provide a seal that prevents the leakage of air around the tube when the client is ventilated. Uncuffed tubes are generally used in infants and children unless there is excessive leakage of air past the tube. To avoid inadvertent removal or displacement of the tube, string and tape may be applied to secure the tube in position. Continuous expert care is required after endotracheal intubation to ensure airway patency and to prevent complications. A client who has been intubated is generally nursed in an ICU and receives constant physical attention and emotional support.

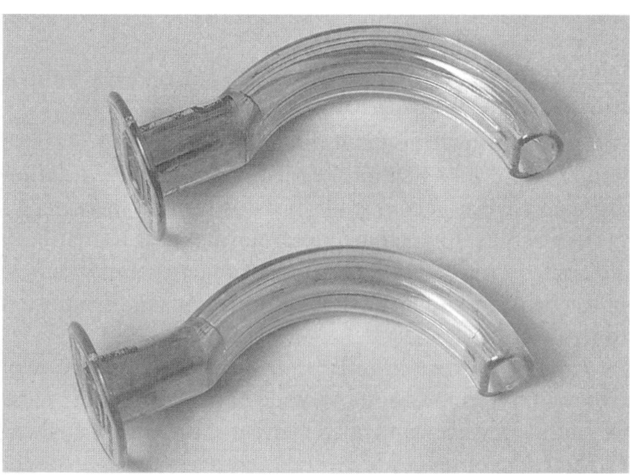

Figure 38.22 | Artificial oropharyngeal airway *(Potter & Perry 2008)*

TRACHEOSTOMY

A tracheostomy is a surgical creation of an external opening into the trachea, and may be performed as an emergency temporary measure or as a permanent measure. A tracheostomy tube may be inserted into the tracheostomy to provide a patent airway, prevent aspiration of secretions, allow removal of tracheobronchial secretions by suction and permit the use of a mechanical ventilation device. A tracheostomy tube (Figure 38.24) is a short curved tube fitted with a flange that assists in stabilising the tube. Tracheostomy tubes are available in a range of styles, materials and sizes, and some are fitted with an inflatable cuff.

CARE OF A CLIENT WITH AN ARTIFICIAL AIRWAY

The care of a client with an artificial airway — whether it has been inserted for a short or long term — involves many physical actions and the provision of emotional support. The main aspects of care include:

- Continued assessment of airway status
- Maintenance of correct cuff pressure to prevent tissue ischaemia and necrosis
- Continued monitoring for complications
- Keeping the tube free of mucus to ensure airway patency

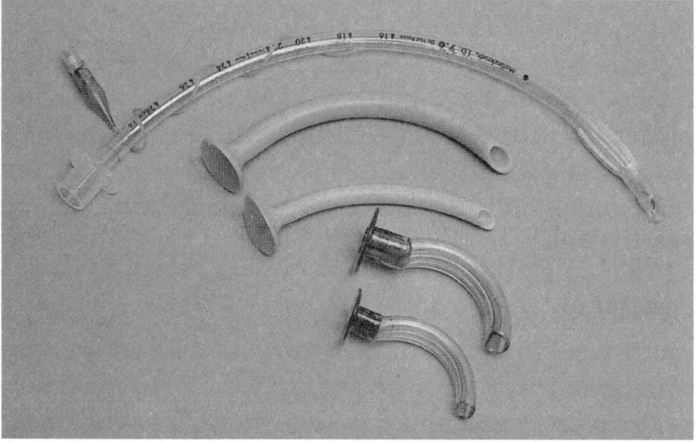

Figure 38.23 | An endotracheal tube (top) compared with nasal and oropharyngeal tubes *(deWit 2005)*

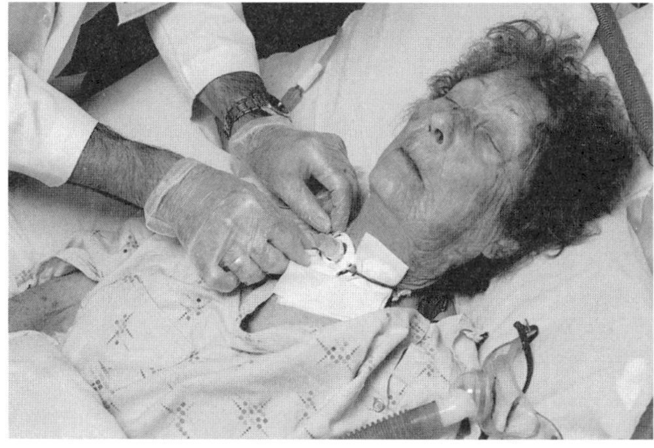

Figure 38.24 | A tracheostomy tube *(deWit 2005)*

- Preventing infection
- Providing psychological support.

Caring for a client with a tracheostomy

When caring for a client with a tracheostomy, the following should always be available at the bedside in case of accidental dislodgement or obstruction of the tube:

- Spare sterile tracheostomy tube or inner tube
- Tracheal dilator
- Scissors
- Syringe for a cuffed tube
- Oxygen and sterile 'Y' suction catheters.

A client with an artificial airway will be apprehensive about asphyxiation or choking, which can be further increased by an impaired ability to communicate their needs to others. The client's ability to effectively remove secretions by coughing may be grossly impaired. When unable to cough or expectorate secretions, suctioning must be performed. In the first few days after the insertion of a tracheostomy tube the procedure is uncomfortable and frightening, and the client must be provided with an explanation of the suctioning technique before it is performed. The nurse should be aware of their role in, and the regulations and the health care facility's, procedures and policies regarding tracheostomy suctioning. A suggested method of tracheostomy suctioning is outlined in Table 38.12.

The basic equipment for tracheostomy suctioning is:

- Sterile 'Y' suction catheters
- Wall or portable suction apparatus
- Connecting tubing
- Disposable gloves
- Container of sterile or tap water for clearing the catheter (depending on the institution's policy)
- Bag or container for contaminated catheters.

Care of the tracheostomy and tracheostomy tube (Table 38.13) is performed to minimise contamination and to decrease the possibility of obstruction by secretions. Tracheostomy care, which is performed using sterile equipment and aseptic technique to prevent infection, involves cleansing of the inner cannula and the area around the stoma. The frequency with which the care is provided may vary depending on the amount of secretions present, and may be as frequent as every ½ hour to 1 hour or may only be required once every 8 hours.

Some tracheostomy tubes have an inner replaceable tube that can be changed as part of routine daily care (e.g. 4-hourly to daily). It is essential that a spare inner

TABLE 38.12 | GUIDELINES FOR TRACHEOSTOMY SUCTIONING

Action	Rationale
Review and carry out standard steps in Appendix 1	
Explain the procedure and provide privacy. The client should be informed that suctioning may cause transient coughing or gagging	Reduces anxiety and embarrassment
Place the equipment within easy reach	Facilitates performance of the procedure in an organised manner
Remove any humidification (or ventilation) device	Allows access to the tracheostomy tube
Wash and dry hands and put on gloves	Prevents cross-infection
Attach the catheter to the suction tubing and set suction pressure to 80–120 mmHg	Pressure above 120 mmHg may damage the tracheal mucosa
Ask the client to cough and breathe slowly and deeply	Coughing helps loosen secretions, and deep breathing helps to minimise hypoxia
If necessary, or prescribed, the client's lungs are hyperoxygenated before aspiration	Helps to prevent hypoxia
Insert the catheter without suction into the tracheostomy tube	Prevents hypoxia and tracheal mucosa trauma
Apply suction and withdraw the catheter, rotating it gently. Suction for no longer than 10 seconds at a time. Allow the client to take 4–5 breaths between each aspiration. If secretions are thick, dip the catheter into sterile saline and apply suction	Rotating motion avoids tissue trauma Short-term suctioning limits the amount of oxygen removed and prevents hypoxia Helps to clear the lumen of the catheter
Report immediately if there is any difficulty in inserting the catheter into the tube	The tube may be partially blocked with secretions
When suctioning is completed, the client may need to be hyperoxygenated again. Replace any humidification device	Prevents hypoxia and promotes relaxation. Re-establishes delivery of humidity
Dispose of the gloves and suction catheter appropriately, wash and dry hands	Prevents cross-infection
Document and report on the procedure	Appropriate care can be planned and implemented

TABLE 38.13 | GUIDELINES FOR TRACHEAL STOMA CARE

Action	Rationale
Review and carry out the standard steps in Appendix 1	
Explain the procedure and provide privacy	Reduces anxiety and embarrassment
Open a sterile dressing pack and place any additional equipment within easy reach	Facilitates performance of the procedure in an organised manner
Wash and dry hands	Prevents cross-infection
Remove any humidification (or ventilation) device	Allows access to the tracheostomy tube
Suction the tracheostomy tube (refer to guidelines on suctioning)	Removes secretions from the airway
Remove and discard the tracheostomy dressing into a suitable waste receptacle	Correct disposal prevents cross-infection
For a newly formed stoma, use a sterile drape around the tracheostomy site	Provides a sterile field around the stoma
Put on sterile gloves	Prevents cross-infection
Cleanse the skin around the stoma and the flanges of the tube using gauze and appropriate solution. Take care not to let solution or strands of gauze enter the tube or stoma	Removes accumulated secretions and crusts. These may be aspirated into the lungs
Inspect the surrounding area and stoma site for inflammation or skin breakdown	Signs of impaired healing or infection require immediate attention
Apply a sterile tracheostomy dressing	Protects the stoma site
Replace the tracheostomy tapes if they are soiled or loose. Whenever possible, two people should be present to change the tapes	Tracheostomy tube must be secured in position. Soiled tapes predispose the client to infection. Prevents accidental dislodgement of the tube
Replace any humidification device	Re-establishes delivery of humidity
Remove gloves, dispose of the equipment appropriately, wash and dry hands	Prevents cross-infection
Assist the client into position and place the call bell within reach	Promotes comfort and relaxation
Document and report on the procedure	Appropriate care can be planned and implemented

tube is kept close at hand and replaced if the inner tube becomes blocked. The inner tube is cleaned using a suitable solution and dried and made accessible for future use. Many tracheostomy tubes are fitted with an inflatable cuff. Regular deflation of a cuffed tube is performed to prevent tracheal necrosis and stenosis. The frequency and length of time for cuff deflation varies depending on the type of tube used and the condition of the client.

To prevent the trachea or lower airways from drying and bleeding, a humidification connector 'Swedish nose' may be applied. It consists of a single or dual barrel that encloses the tube's orifice; humidity is provided by rolled absorptive paper filters pre-moistened with normal saline. If secretions are present on the outside of the suction catheter, additional sterile saline may be required to be instilled into the tracheostomy tube to loosen secretions and maintain the patency of the tracheostomy tube.

Communication is a significant problem and to alleviate anxiety and apprehension an alternative means of communication should be provided. A pad and pencil should be available, the client's call bell or buzzer must always be within easy reach and must be answered promptly. If unable to write, the client can be educated to use a series of gestures or sign language as an alternative method of communicating their needs. Alternatively, for clients with uncuffed tubes a speaking valve can be employed, or they can be educated how to cover the tube with their finger to occlude the airway on expiration and allow for limited communication. If the artificial airway is a temporary measure, the client should be informed that their voice will recover when the tube is removed. Before deflation, the tube and oronasopharynx are aspirated. When the cuff is inflated, only sufficient air is inserted to occlude the escape of air from around the sides of the tube.

The client should be provided with information about their progress and any procedures that are to be performed. They should be encouraged to participate in their own care as much as possible to reduce any sense of dependency, and the significant others should be involved in the care. The client may be discharged from hospital with a tracheostomy tube in situ. As soon as possible, they and the significant others are educated in self-care so that they feel comfortable and confident about caring for their tracheostomy. The client should be provided with information about relevant support groups such as tracheostomy associations that they may wish to contact.

Before the permanent removal of a tracheostomy tube the client will require sufficient information and emotional support, as they may feel that they will not be able to breathe without the tube. The tube may be removed when the client is able to maintain independent respiratory function, is able to breathe through the upper respiratory tract and has satisfactory protective reflexes such as the cough reflex.

To prepare the client for permanent removal of the tracheostomy tube a fenestrated tube may be inserted. This type of tube has an opening in the outer cannula that allows the client to breathe around as well as through the tube. Thus, they are able to adjust gradually to removal of the tube. Alternatively the tube may be occluded or 'corked' by an adhesive tape to determine the client's ability to cope without the tube. With uncuffed tubes this is routinely achieved to enhance communication by allowing the client to occlude the tube with their fingers while speaking. By covering the tube, they may be able to speak, breathe normally through the upper airway and expectorate secretions.

Before the tube is removed, suction is applied to remove tracheal and pharyngeal secretions. The cuff is then deflated and the tube removed. Generally a dry occlusive dressing is placed over the stoma and the client closely monitored for the first 24 hours. Healing and reduction in the tracheostomy can take 12 months or longer and care must be taken during this time to prevent aspiration and infections. After a period of time, when the client's airway is stable, the stoma can be surgically sutured together.

Complications of tracheostomy

The insertion of an artificial airway can result in several complications:

- Infection due to altered ciliary function or colonisation of the airway with bacteria
- Tracheal necrosis and stenosis due to excessive pressure on the trachea from the cuff
- Tracheo-oesophageal fistula
- Partial or complete airway obstruction (e.g. due to an accumulation of secretions in the tube)
- Subcutaneous emphysema
- Psychological effects, such as frustration at being unable to communicate as usual.

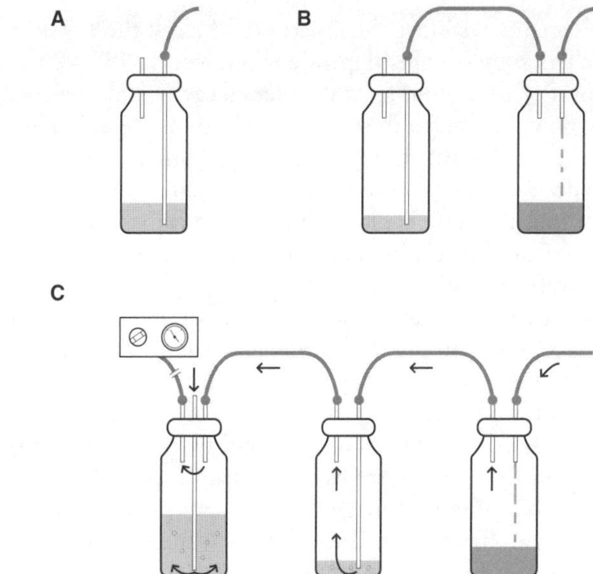

Figure 38.25 | Chest tube drainage **A**: One-bottle system **B**: Two-bottle system **C**: Three-bottle system with suction

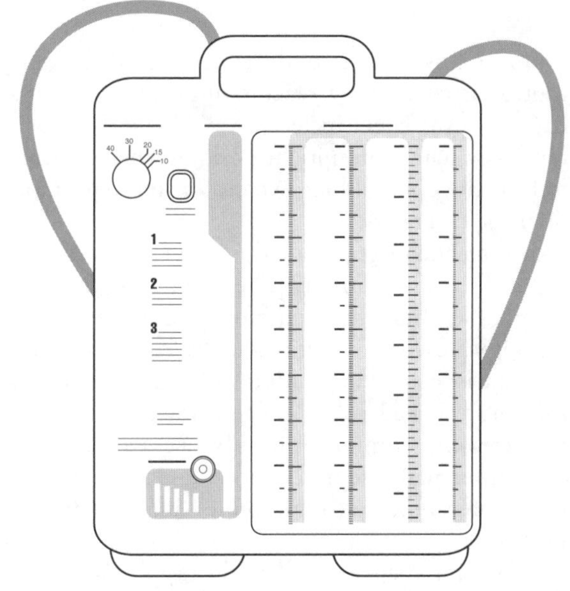

Figure 38.26 | Disposable, commercial chest-drainage system

THE CLIENT WITH THORACIC DRAINAGE TUBES

Insertion of chest drainage tubes (Figures 38.25 and 38.26) permits the drainage of air or fluid from the pleural space which, if not removed, alters intrapleural pressure and causes lung collapse. Ventilation is adversely affected by any disruption of the intrapleural pressure, which may be caused by surgery, trauma or pulmonary disease. Insertion of chest tubes drains the excess air or fluid and enables the lungs to function normally.

Chest drainage tubes may be inserted at the time of surgery while a client is anaesthetised, or they may be inserted using local anaesthetic. Because the procedure is painful, a conscious client is generally given analgesic medication about 30 minutes before tube insertion. The procedure is performed by a medical officer, using sterile equipment and aseptic technique. The insertion site is selected according to the client's condition, and one or more tubes may be inserted at the same time.

UNDERWATER SEAL DRAINAGE

After insertion the chest tube is connected to a drainage system that permits drainage out of the pleural space and prevents back-flow into that space. The tubing leads to a collection system positioned well below the level of the client's chest. This dependent position facilitates the removal of air or fluid from the pleural cavity and prevents back-flow. To prevent the entry of air into the pleural cavity the distal end of the tubing is submerged underwater. This provides a closed water-seal drainage system. The depth of water that the tube is placed under determines the water pressure used to create a seal, for example 5 cm, and is ordered by a medical officer.

Some commercially available systems of underwater seal drainage, for example the Pleurevac system, are available already assembled and are disposed of after use. Other types of thoracic drainage systems include the one-, two- or three-bottle systems. The one- and two-bottle systems are primarily gravity systems, which can be provided with suction to facilitate drainage. Such systems provide a water seal and can be connected to suction. A medical officer is required to order the application of suction, which is used to facilitate faster drainage of air or fluids. A low-flow suction regulator device is used to ensure that the suction provides a minimal bubbling effect.

CARE OF THE CLIENT WITH A CHEST DRAIN

The aim of closed-chest underwater seal drainage is to promote lung expansion by facilitating drainage of air and fluid. Care of the client includes:

- Nursing them in an upright position when possible, to facilitate optimal lung expansion and to promote drainage by gravity
- Providing adequate explanation and emotional support to reduce anxiety. The client may tend to restrict their breathing and movement for fear of dislodging the tube, so it is essential to explain that the tube is secured in position with tape and/or sutures
- Administering adequate analgesic medication to decrease discomfort. It may be necessary to administer analgesic medication 30–45 minutes before physiotherapy, to promote pain relief and relaxation
- Encouraging the client to breathe deeply and cough frequently (e.g. hourly, to help drain the pleural space and expand the lungs)
- Regularly assessing the client's respiratory status. The client should be observed for discomfort and any difficulty in breathing, and it is important to observe whether their chest is expanding symmetrically. The ventilations are assessed at regular intervals (e.g. hourly, for rate, rhythm and character)
- Maintaining the water seal and preventing air leakage, which is essential to prevent entry of air into the pleural space. The fluid level in the drainage bottle should be checked frequently (e.g. hourly) and sterile water added if necessary to ensure that the distal end of the water seal tube remains submerged at the ordered level
- Taking precautions to prevent separation of the connections, such as taping the joints and securing the tube to the client's clothing. Care must be taken to ensure that the underwater seal system remains below the client's chest to prevent fluid or air re-entering the pleural cavity, which can cause subsequent pneumothorax or empyema
- Securing the drainage system to the bed or placing it securely on the floor to protect it from toppling over and from accidental breakage. If the system is accidentally disconnected or broken, air will enter the pleural space and the lungs may collapse. It is general practice to have two chest clamps in plain view at the bedside for any client with a chest drain; in the event of disconnection, the two clamps are applied immediately to the chest tube, and assistance is summoned immediately.

  There is some controversy surrounding this emergency measure, as some authorities believe that clamping a chest tube could result in a tension pneumothorax. It is essential that the nurse be aware of the health care institution's measures to be taken should accidental disconnection of the system occur. If a chest tube is accidentally dislodged or falls out, the client is asked to exhale forcefully and the opening on the skin surface is sealed with an airtight dressing until the tube can be reinserted
- Maintaining patency of the drainage system, which is essential to facilitate expansion of the lung. The system must be checked hourly for loose connections and for fluctuation in the water-seal bottle. As the client inhales, the fluid should rise in the water-seal tube, and as they exhale the level should fall back (this is termed 'swinging')
- Ensuring that, if the system is connected to suction, the fluid line in the water-seal tube remains constant. During exhalation, bubbling is normally present in the water-seal bottle. Gently bubbling in a suction control bottle indicates that the correct level of suction has been achieved
- Observing the tubing for, and keeping it free from, kinks. Kinking of the tubing will obstruct the flow of air or fluid. To prevent kinking, or dependent loops of tubing, the tubing should be coiled flat on the bed and may be attached to the edge of the bed with tape and a safety pin. The tubing should fall in a straight line from the coil to the drainage bottle, to facilitate flow. The nurse should ensure that the client is able to move freely without pulling or lying on the tubing
- Double-clamping the chest tube near the site of insertion when it is necessary to replace a drainage system bottle. The bottle, and, if necessary, the connection tubing, is replaced and the clamps removed. The tubes should not be clamped for longer than 2 minutes, as a tension pneumothorax may result when air or fluid is prevented from escaping.

As a safety precaution, two nurses should be present whenever a drainage bottle or system is being replaced
- Protecting the insertion site by an occlusive dressing (e.g. Opsite). Using sterile equipment and aseptic techniques to prevent infection, the dressing is renewed in accordance with the health care institution's policy
- Assessing and documenting the colour, volume and type of drainage. Any alteration in the amount, colour or flow of drainage must be reported immediately. Sudden cessation of flow of drainage may indicate a malfunction of the system or disconnection of the tubing. A gradual reduction in flow may indicate occlusion by blood or proteins, that the tube position has moved in the pleural cavity or that the chest has reinflated.

Removal of a chest drain tube is performed by the medical officer. Generally the tube is clamped for up to 24 hours before removal, and a chest X-ray is performed immediately beforehand to determine lung expansion. If the client develops respiratory distress or a pneumothorax, the clamps are removed and the tube left in place. Analgesic medication is usually administered 30–45 minutes before tube removal. The tube is removed swiftly and immediately covered with an occlusive dressing to provide an airtight seal. In some cases the site is closed with purse string sutures that are tightened during removal.

One hour after the removal of the tube an X-ray is taken to ensure that there has been no ingress of air during or after the removal. The insertion site is checked regularly for sounds of air leakage and the client is observed for manifestations of pneumothorax, infection, subcutaneous emphysema and respiratory distress.

NURSING PRACTICE AND OXYGEN NEEDS

A client's respiratory status is assessed to ascertain whether they are receiving an adequate supply of oxygen and excreting sufficient carbon dioxide to meet their body's needs. Assessment is made by observing the client for signs and symptoms, identifying any deviations from normal and by assessing their ventilations. Assessing the respiratory status and identifying any actual or potential problems is assisted by obtaining information from the client regarding:

- Allergic reactions such as coughing, watery eyes, sneezing or shortness of breath that may occur as a result of exposure to allergens such as dust mites, pet hair or pollen
- Exposure to environmental air pollutants such as chemical wastes, smoke or dust
- Smoking habits
- Presence of a cough and the volume quality and quantity of sputum
- Chest pain.

The client should be observed for signs and symptoms of hypoxaemia, which is a diminished availability of oxygen to the body tissues. Hypoxaemia may result from disorders that limit the volume of air entering the lungs, or from obstructive lung diseases such as asthma and emphysema. The signs and symptoms of hypoxia and respiratory distress include:

- Cyanosis, which is a bluish discolouration of the skin and mucous membranes due to inadequate oxygenation, and can be either peripheral or central. Peripheral cyanosis results in local vasoconstriction and is usually visible in the nail beds and the lips. Central cyanosis is the result of more severe hypoxia and affects all body organs. It is most visible in highly vascular areas such as the lips, nail beds, tip of the nose, the external ear and the underside of the tongue. In people with naturally dark brown or black skin, cyanosis is most accurately detected by inspecting the mucosa inside the mouth
- Elevated blood pressure and pulse rate
- Shortness of breath (dyspnoea), fatigue and intolerance to exercise
- Abnormal respiratory rate, depth or rhythm
- Sighing, gasping, breath holding
- Flaring of the nares
- Use of accessory muscles during breathing (e.g. sub-sternal recession, tracheal tugging, shoulder shrugging and intercostal muscles during expiration)
- Apprehension, aggression, non-compliance or agitation
- Confusion or reduced level of consciousness
- Visible or excessive perspiration (diaphoresis).

A person with a chronic respiratory disorder should also be assessed for a barrel-shaped chest, which is an increase in the antero-posterior diameter of the chest wall, commonly associated with air trapping, as in atelectasis or chronic obstructive airways disease. Clients with chronic hypoxaemia may experience the same symptoms as above but may have clubbing of the fingers, where the angle of the nail bed increases to over 85°, caused by an increase in capillary numbers to supply poorly perfused tissue, with subsequent increase in size. (Assessment of ventilations is covered in Chapter 21.)

MEETING A CLIENT'S NEED FOR OXYGEN

Breathing is an automatic activity, but rate and depth can be changed voluntarily. Normally room air at normal atmospheric pressure, such as at sea level, provides sufficient oxygen to meet metabolic needs of the body. However, admission to hospital, or a respiratory condition, may affect a client's normal pattern of breathing. For example, if a person has an infection or is apprehensive or anxious, they may experience temporary breathing difficulties. In these instances measures to promote the return of normal breathing are performed. Nurses provide clients with adequate information to allay some of the anxiety relating

CLINICAL INTEREST BOX 38.5
Nursing diagnoses relating to disorders of oxygenation

- Activity intolerance
- Airway clearance, ineffective
- Anxiety
- Breathing pattern, ineffective
- Cardiac output, decreased
- Coping, ineffective individual
- Fear
- Gas exchange, impaired
- Health maintenance, altered
- Infection, risk for
- Knowledge deficit (specify)
- Tissue perfusion, altered (cardiopulmonary)
- Ventilation, inability to sustain spontaneous

(adapted from Potter & Perry 2008)

to their condition, investigations and hospitalisation. The nurse should also attempt to ensure that the room is ventilated adequately and at a comfortable temperature.

Clients who experience breathing difficulties due to a clinical condition may require assistance to meet any increase in either oxygen demands or carbon dioxide retention. Some methods include, for example, positioning in a more upright position, nebulisation, humidification, physiotherapy (which may include deep-breathing and coughing exercises), and mobilisation. Clients who suffer from an oxygen deficiency will commonly require administration of oxygen to supplement that being obtained from the atmosphere. Some nursing diagnoses relating to disorders of oxygenation are listed in Clinical Interest Box 38.5.

Administering oxygen

To prevent or reverse hypoxia and to improve tissue oxygenation, oxygen may be administered by nasal cannula (nasal prongs), nasal catheter, oxygen mask, headbox, cot or tent. Oxygen is a drug, so it is prescribed by a medical officer who determines the concentration, route and length of time that it is to be administered. To promote the safety and comfort of the client receiving oxygen therapy, the nurse should be aware of certain principles relevant to the administration of oxygen.

- Hypoxaemia can result from insufficient oxygen flow or delivery. Equipment and connections must be checked at regular intervals (e.g. hourly) to ensure that it is functioning properly. If signs or symptoms of hypoxaemia occur they must be reported immediately, as adjustment to the concentration being administered may be necessary, or alternative investigations or treatment implemented
- Although oxygen is not normally combustible, it does support combustion and it is essential to implement safety precautions to reduce the risk of fire. Smoking is prohibited in the vicinity, and measures are taken to prevent sparks, which may be given off by electrical or mechanical items. Inflammable substances such as oil or alcohol should not be used near or on the oxygen equipment
- Administration of any gas can dry and irritate mucous membranes; this is particularly so with nasal prongs. In some health care institutions the gas is humidified by passing it through a sterile water humidification system such as the Concha Pak before administration
- Oxygen is colourless and odourless, so accurate gauges on gas cylinders and oxygen concentrators are used to indicate the volume of oxygen remaining or rate of flow. An oxygen regulator limits the flow of the gas. Care must be taken to ensure that connections on the regulator are tight, otherwise a reduced volume or concentration will be administered
- Oxygen toxicity is a hazard with prolonged administration or concentrations over 50%. The client's capillary, venous or arterial blood gases are commonly measured during oxygen therapy and the concentration of oxygen or method of delivery can be adjusted. Damage and inflammation to airways, blood vessels and nervous tissue may result in acute respiratory distress syndrome (ARDS)
- Nosocomial infections can occur using oxygen therapy, particularly with the use of non-sterile oxygen bubble humidifiers. Masks, tubing, cannulae and catheters are for single client use and are discarded on discharge. Care must be taken to clean the mask or nebuliser regularly (e.g. every 8 hours).

The nurse must know how to check that the equipment is functioning correctly and that all connections are secure and do not leak. Cleaning and disposal of equipment is done as per the individual health care institution's infection-control guidelines.

Delivery of oxygen

Oxygen is piped to a wall outlet or, less commonly, is supplied via a portable cylinder or oxygen concentrator and may be delivered to the client via an oxygen regulator using one of several devices.

Nasal cannula

A nasal cannula (nasal prongs) is made from a soft plastic material and contains two short tubes that fit into the nostrils. It may be secured in position by an adjustable ring or strap around the back of the head (Figure 38.27) or taped onto the cheeks to prevent dislodgement. Because it does not enclose the nose or mouth, the cannula is comfortable and convenient for the person and there is less risk of aspiration of vomitus than a mask. The cannula is connected to the oxygen supply and the oxygen turned on at a low flow rate, with the flow checked before positioning it in the nares. The prongs are inserted following the natural curve of the nostrils, and the tubes are positioned over each ear and around the back of the head. The ring or strap is adjusted to maintain the position of the prongs, and care is taken to ensure that the strap is not too tight. An over-tight strap can cause pressure on the nostrils, the nose, the upper lip and cheeks. When the cannula has been positioned correctly, the flow of oxygen is adjusted to the prescribed rate. Minimum flow is 0.25 L/min to a maximum of 3 L/min. Higher volumes increase irritation and drying of the nasal mucosa. The oxygen concentration that the client receives is undeterminable and is reduced if the client mouth-breathes, eats or drinks.

Nasal catheter

An intranasal oxygen catheter (Figure 38.28) is made from a soft plastic material and contains a series of holes at the distal ends. The approximate length to be inserted is estimated by holding the catheter in a straight line from the tip of the client's nose to their earlobe, and marking the catheter with an indelible pen to ensure that the insertion length can always be seen. The tip of the catheter may be lubricated with sterile water or a water-soluble lubricant to facilitate insertion. Before insertion, the catheter is connected to the oxygen supply and the oxygen turned on at a low flow rate. As with nasal prongs, oxygen concentration varies with factors such as mouth-breathing. The catheter can induce gastric distension if forced into the stomach.

The catheter is gently inserted through one nostril into the nasopharynx to the pre-measured length. Using hypoallergenic tape, the catheter may be secured to the nose or cheek, avoiding traction on the nostril, which could cause skin breakdown. When the catheter has been positioned correctly, the flow of oxygen is adjusted to the prescribed rate. As it is an invasive device, the catheter may cause irritation of the mucosa, so it is usual to remove it after about 8 hours and insert a clean one into the other nostril. Rotating the site reduces the risks of mucous membrane irritation and skin breakdown at the tip of the nose.

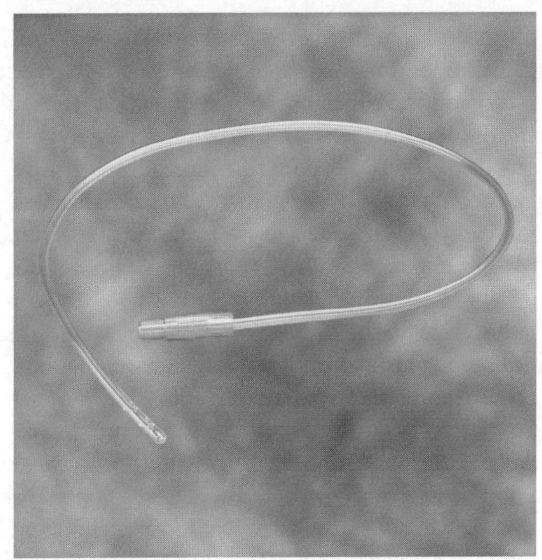

Figure 38.28 | Nasal catheter *(reproduced with permission of Hudson RCI)*

Face mask

Face masks (Figure 38.29) are available in several styles and sizes. They are made from a lightweight vinyl material and are designed to fit over the nose and mouth, secured in position by an elastic band around the head. As the mask covers both the nose and the mouth, it is confining and impedes activities such as eating, drinking and communication as well as potentiating the risk of aspiration of vomitus.

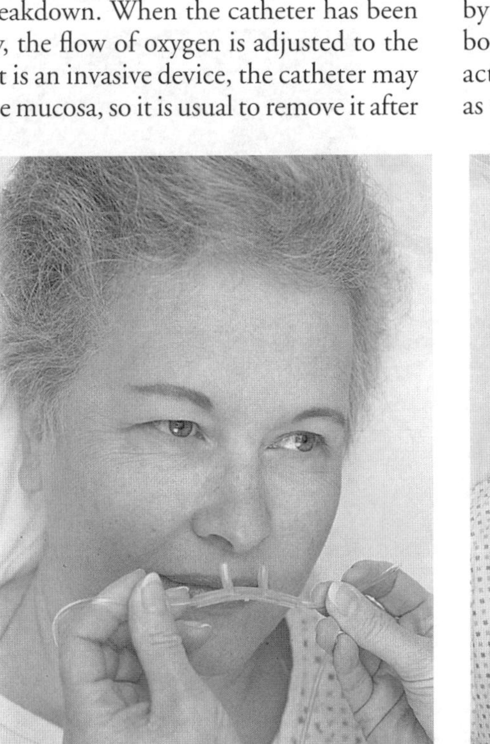

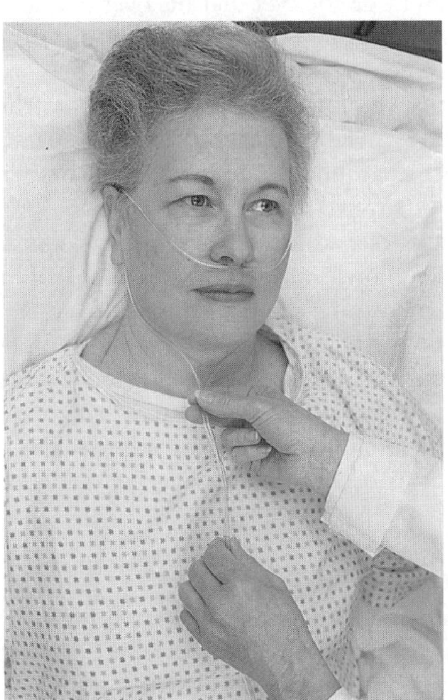

Figure 38.27 | Applying a nasal cannula *(Potter & Perry 2008)*

Minimum flow rates for masks is normally 4 L/min, as a lower flow rate is not adequate to clear the mask of exhaled carbon dioxide and can cause hypercapnia (CO_2 retention). Depending on the style, a mask can deliver oxygen from 28% at 4 L/min to 100% concentration at higher flow rates. A mask is commonly used when the client requires higher concentrations and more accurate amounts of oxygen, such as when the client is mouth-breathing, eating, talking or is able to breathe only through the mouth. Oxygen masks are recognisable by the presence of multiple small holes on the sides of the mask, as opposed to nebuliser masks, which have one large-diameter hole each side.

The style and size of mask is assessed by measuring from the chin to the top of the nose, and an appropriate size is selected. The mask is connected to the oxygen supply via a flexible plastic tube, and the oxygen turned on to check that there are no leaks at a low flow rate. The mask is placed over the nose, mouth and chin, and the elastic strap secured around the back of the head; some masks have pliable metal straps that can be used to mould the mask to the client's face shape. The strap is adjusted to ensure that the mask is firmly positioned but not uncomfortable, and the flow of oxygen adjusted to the prescribed rate. It is important that the mask fits closely but is not uncomfortable, and the nurse should ensure that there is no leakage of oxygen from the top of the mask. Leakage of oxygen from the top of the mask can flow across the eyes, causing dryness and irritation of the delicate tissues. Masks can create pressure areas on the skin and can be made more comfortable by applying self adhesive foam to the edges in contact with skin.

Head box

A head box may be used to deliver oxygen to an infant and consists of a transparent plastic box that fits over the head or shoulders. The infant can be observed easily, and high concentrations of oxygen can be administered.

The concentration of oxygen to be delivered to the client will be specified by the medical officer and depends on the delivery device used and the rate at which the oxygen flows. Oxygen can be delivered from concentrations of 21% to 100%, and the flow rate adjusted by oxygen regulators from 0.25 L/min (low flow) to 3 L/min (high flow). The flow rate is adjusted by turning the valve on the flow meter and observing the ball or dial that indicates the number of litres per minute at which the oxygen is flowing (Figure 38.30). Whenever oxygen is to be administered the nurse should refer to the directions that accompany the device, to ensure that the correct concentration of oxygen is delivered to the client.

MECHANICAL VENTILATION

In specific situations a client may require oxygen to be administered via a mechanical ventilator. These devices may use either positive or negative pressure.

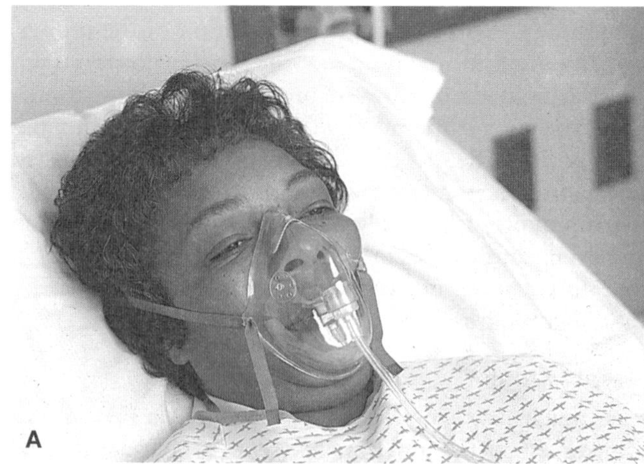
A

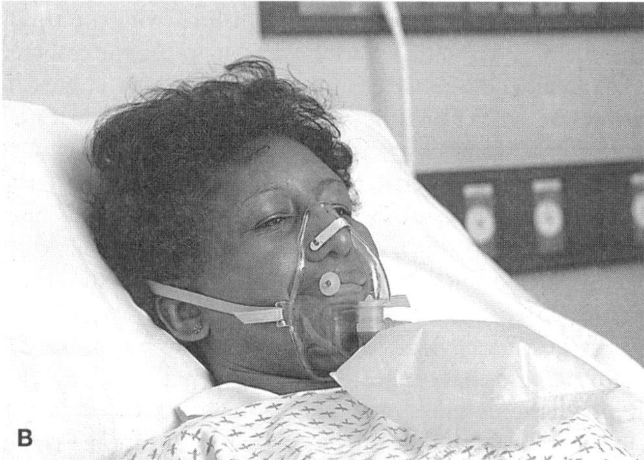
B

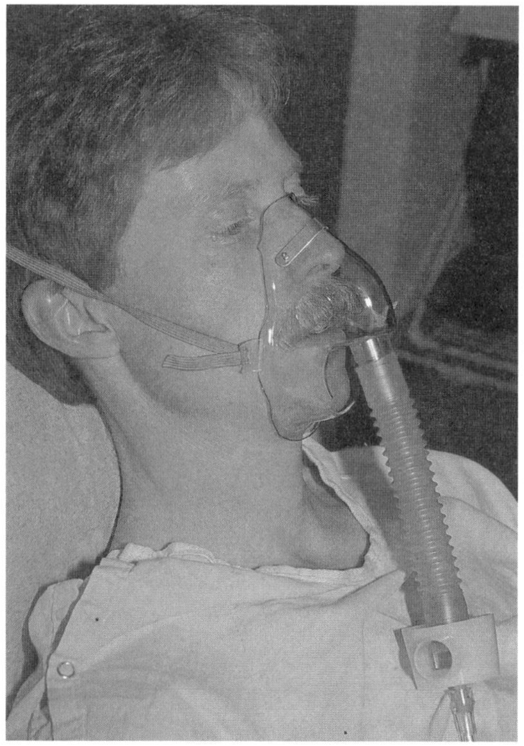
C

Figure 38.29 | **A**: Simple face mask **B**: Plastic face mask with reservoir bag **C**: Venturi mask *(Potter & Perry 2008)*

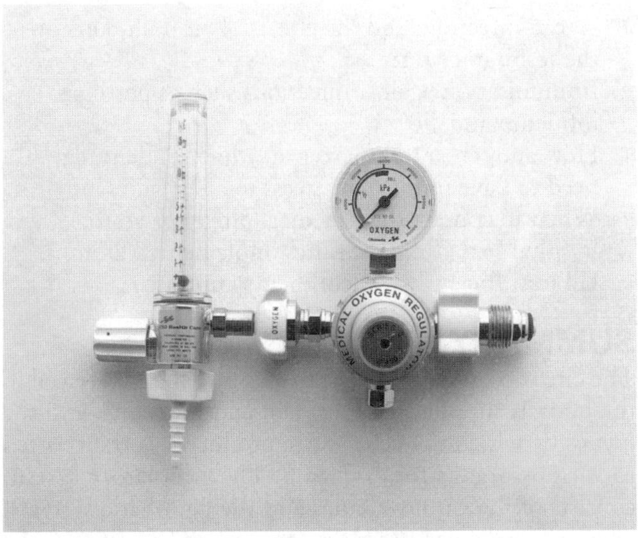

Figure 38.30 | Oxygen regulators *(BOC Gases Australia)*

Positive pressure

Intermittent positive-pressure ventilation (IPPV) devices push atmospheric or oxygen rich air into the client's airways to promote adequate lung expansion. Commonly, IPPV is performed via an endotracheal or tracheostomy tube and allows effective control of ventilation and oxygenation. The flow of air to the lungs is set at a predetermined pressure and, as the pressure is attained, the flow is stopped, pressure is released and the person exhales. Types of IPPV devices include:

- Positive end-expiratory pressure (PEEP): maintains a positive pressure in the lungs at the end of the client's respiratory cycle, by increasing pressure within airways
- Continuous positive airway pressure (CPAP) is a device that maintains a certain amount of pressure to maintain the patency of large and small airways and alveoli. CPAP devices are commonly used with a tight-fitting face mask or over a tracheostomy.

Negative pressure

Negative pressure chambers use a negative pressure to maintain inflation of the lung and can be used to administer high volumes of oxygen. Examples include the iron lung and barochamber.

KEY ASPECTS RELATED TO OXYGEN THERAPY

MEASURES TO PROMOTE THE COMFORT AND SAFETY OF THE CLIENT RECEIVING OXYGEN

- Constantly monitoring the equipment to ensure that it is functioning correctly. The nurse should check the flow rate and ensure that the prescribed concentration of oxygen is being delivered to the client. Connections on regulators, concentrators and humidifiers should be checked to ensure their tightness and that they are free of leaks. Measures should be taken to prevent the oxygen tubing becoming twisted, kinked or disconnected, to facilitate a free flow of oxygen to the client
- Prevention of infection. In the past, oxygen that was delivered by an oxygen mask, nasal cannula or nasal catheter was humidified to prevent drying of the mucous membranes. Normal practice in most health care agencies is to use only sterile methods of humidification and dispose of the equipment according to infection-control or manufacturer's guidelines to reduce the potential for nosocomial infections. Oxygen masks and cannulas provide sufficient atmospheric water to humidify the oxygen
- Reducing any anxiety that the client or their significant others experience related to the administration of oxygen. Some people may feel that the administration of oxygen is a sign that the client's condition is deteriorating, and clients using face masks may experience anxiety related to having both their nose and their mouth covered. The nurse should explain the purpose of the oxygen and the equipment that is being used. Some people may be educated to use the equipment independently and thus feel they have some control over the situation. Frequent visits to the client, prompt attention to their needs and efficient handling of the equipment will help to reduce their anxiety
- Informing the client of the importance of maintaining the delivery device in the correct position, as changing its position may alter the amount of oxygen being delivered
- Assisting the client to meet their hygiene needs. The skin under the tubing, elastic straps or mask should be kept dry to promote comfort and to reduce the risk of skin breakdown caused by humidity or perspiration. Both the client's face and face mask should be wiped dry at least every 2 hours, and the skin under the delivery device checked for signs of pressure or irritation. Oral and nasal hygiene needs should be met and a water-based cream or balm may be applied to the lips or nares to prevent dryness and discomfort
- Replacing the mask with a nasal cannula if necessary, while the client is eating or having their oral hygiene needs met
- Measuring the client's temperature by the tympanic or axillary route rather than the oral route, as placement of the thermometer in the mouth may cause further ventilatory distress
- Monitoring the client's condition constantly to assess the effectiveness of the treatment. The client should be observed for signs of hypoxia or oxygen toxicity.

Hypoxia may occur if the oxygen concentration is inadequate or if the equipment is not functioning properly. Oxygen toxicity is more likely to occur if the client is receiving high concentrations (e.g. over 50%), which can be detrimental to the central nervous system. Manifestations of oxygen toxicity include nausea, muscle twitching, dizziness, restlessness and irritability, convulsive seizures and coma. Prolonged administration of high concentrations of oxygen may also cause damage to the linings of the bronchi and alveoli, resulting in pulmonary congestion or collapse of lung tissue. Any indications of hypoxaemia, hypercapnia (CO_2 retention) or toxicity must be reported immediately, as the concentration of oxygen being administered may need to be adjusted. It should also be noted that people with chronic obstructive airways disease, such as emphysema, may have an 'oxygen drive', in which their respiratory rate is controlled by decreasing levels of oxygen, as opposed to the normal regulation of respiratory rate, which is due to an increasing CO_2 level. These clients are never prescribed high-flow oxygen, as it reduces their respiratory drive and rate and increases hypercapnia

- Observing the client closely after oxygen therapy has been discontinued, as the therapy may need to be resumed if signs of hypoxia become evident
- Handling the oxygen equipment. The equipment used to deliver oxygen to the person should be cared for in the manner specified in the health care institution's policy manual. Most of the delivery devices are disposable, which reduces the risk of cross-infection.

EDUCATION

Planning for a client's discharge from hospital is of particular importance if their respiratory disorder is chronic or recurrent. The client must be provided with sufficient information because, by understanding their condition and how to manage the symptoms, they will be better able to cope with chronic respiratory disease. The client should be encouraged to pursue as normal a lifestyle as possible and should be given information about:

- The importance of avoiding factors that may precipitate or exacerbate their condition, such as extremes of temperature, exposure to allergens or environmental irritants, fatigue or emotional stress
- The importance of avoiding close contact with clients who have a respiratory tract infection
- The importance of contacting their medical officer at the first sign of a respiratory tract infection
- The nature and correct use of any prescribed medications, nebulisers or aerosol therapy
- Public health education about smoking and its relationship to lung cancer and chronic obstructive pulmonary disease; the means of preventing droplet-spread infection; and the effects of air pollutants on the respiratory tract
- Immunisation against infections such as pertussis, influenza and TB
- How and when to use oxygen, which a client may need to have immediate access to at all times
- When to contact their medical officer or go to hospital (e.g. if the measures implemented at home fail to sufficiently control their symptoms).

SUMMARY

The circulatory system is the means by which every cell in the body is supplied with oxygen and nutrients, and the means by which the cells' waste products are transported to various organs for excretion. The circulatory system consists of the cardiovascular and the lymphatic systems. The cardiovascular system is composed of the blood, the blood vessels and the heart. The lymphatic system consists of lymph, lymphatic capillaries, vessels, nodes and ducts.

Blood is a viscous substance composed of a fluid (plasma) in which three types of formed elements are suspended — erythrocytes, leucocytes and platelets — each of which has specific functions. The overall functions of blood are to transport oxygen, nutrients and other substances to the cells, transport wastes away from the cells, protect the body against infection, distribute heat evenly throughout the body and prevent a loss of blood by means of a clotting mechanism. Blood is pumped by the heart into the major arteries, which then form increasingly smaller arteries and eventually arterioles. Arterioles are continuous, with a network of minute vessels called capillaries. Blood then enters small veins or venules, which join to form veins. The veins unite to form the major veins, which transport the blood back to the heart. Blood is in constant circulation around the body, either in the systemic, pulmonary or portal circulation. The lymphatic vessels pass through one or more nodes, the functions of which are to filter and destroy microorganisms and to produce lymphocytes, antibodies and antitoxins.

The heart is a hollow muscular organ situated in the thoracic cavity. It pumps deoxygenated blood to the lungs, and oxygenated blood to all parts of the body.

The act of breathing allows the passage of oxygen and carbon dioxide to and from the lungs, while the cardiovascular system transports these substances to and from the cells. Ventilation is controlled by centres in the brainstem that are sensitive to CO_2 level, while certain factors such as a client's clinical condition, disease, physical activity or emotions affect the rate, rhythm and depth of breathing. Diffusion is the process by which oxygen and CO_2 molecules are transported between the alveoli and the capillary network, and into and out of cells. Diffusion abnormalities can result from cardiac abnormalities such as cardiac failure causing pulmonary oedema, or respiratory disorders that cause a reduction in the amount of functioning lung tissue or fibrosis of the alveolar walls.

Respiratory dysfunction results from inadequate ventilation, from abnormalities of diffusion through the pulmonary membrane or inadequate transport from the lungs to the tissues. In addition to abnormalities of the lungs or respiratory structures, dysfunction of other body systems such as the cardiac system can adversely affect respiratory function, and vice versa. The major manifestations of respiratory system disorders are chest pain, cough, voice change, dyspnoea, altered ventilations, hypoxia and thoracic skeletal abnormalities. Disorders of the respiratory system can be classified as those occurring from multiple causes, from infection, as a result of neoplasms or obstruction or as a result of injury. Specific diagnostic tests used to assess function of the systems include full blood examinations, urea and electrolytes, ultrasound, pulmonary function tests, oximetry, chest X-ray, lung scan, blood gas analysis, cultures, sputum cytology, skin tests, bronchoscopy and thoracentesis.

Care of the client with a respiratory system disorder includes promoting a clear airway, promoting local hydration, proper positioning, administration of medications, oronasopharyngeal suction, chest physiotherapy and the administration of oxygen. The nurse may be required to obtain a specimen of sputum for laboratory examination, to obtain a nasal or throat swab or to administer inhalation therapy. A client with a specific disorder of the respiratory system may require the insertion of an artificial airway, and/or mechanical ventilation. The insertion of chest tubes may be necessary to promote the drainage of air or fluid from the pleural space. Care of clients with cardiac or lymphatic disorders include similar care to that of a respiratory client but may also include fluid restrictions, weighing and attention to chest or limb pain and skin integrity. Specific disorders of the circulatory system may require surgical intervention, which includes pacemaker implantation and heart or bone marrow transplantation.

Some clients require the administration of oxygen, which can be delivered using one of the various devices available. Whenever oxygen is being administered, the nurse must promote the client's safety and comfort as part of assisting them to meet their need for oxygen. Legislation exists to protect the client against environmental pollution. The aims are to ensure that clients in their place of work are not exposed to high levels of respiratory tract pollutants and irritants, and to control the processing, handling and sale of foods that may otherwise be responsible for the transmission of diseases.

The community health nurse, who plays a major role in illness prevention, health maintenance and health promotion, can make a significant contribution in reducing the incidence of cardiac and respiratory disease through the planning and implementation of community education programs.

REVIEW EXERCISES

1. Discuss the function of each of the cardiovascular, lymphatic and respiratory systems and how they interact together.
2. Explain the difference between ventilation, external ventilation and internal ventilation.
3. Discuss how a cardiac disorder may cause an effect on the respiratory system.
4. Explain the pathogenesis of oedema related to cardiac failure.
5. Explain three reasons why a person flying in an aircraft may develop a DVT or pulmonary embolus.
6. List four types of anaemia and outline the specific care for each.
7. Explain how carbon dioxide retention can occur and what the cardinal signs of hypercapnia are.
8. Discuss nursing care that can be employed to improve a client's tolerance to oxygen therapy.
9. List eight complications of oxygen therapy.
10. Discuss the safety procedures required when using oxygen therapy.
11. List all the different modes of oxygen administration.
12. Discuss the indications and contraindications for airway suctioning.
13. Explain the potential for harm when performing suction for each of the following: mouth, nose, pharynx, trachea and tracheostomy tube.
14. In what situations may oxygen therapy be required for a client.
15. Discuss why the use of oxygen can mask a client's underlying condition and status.

CRITICAL THINKING EXERCISES

1. A 36-year-old male professional cyclist is admitted to accident and emergency with a provisional diagnosis of spontaneous right-sided pneumothorax. What clinical features would you expect to see in this client? Describe what nursing procedures would be performed to alleviate the client's respiratory distress.
2. Mr Kirk, a 78-year-old chronic smoker diagnosed 30 years prior with emphysema, is a long-term client in your facility. During the previous 2 days his respiratory effort has increased, and his skin colour, previously pink, has now developed central and peripheral cyanosis that appears to be worsening. He has developed diaphoresis, his blood pressure has increased marginally and he is complaining of a headache. Describe the most appropriate oxygen delivery method and flow rate applicable in this situation and what complications may occur as a result of oxygen therapy.
3. Mrs Peters, 78, has cardiac failure from a 38-year history of chronic hypertension. She is prescribed one Lasix daily to promote diuresis but continues to drink more than her allowable daily limit, and her lower peripheries appear oedematous. She says she drinks because the 'Lasix makes her thirsty', and she cannot stop herself drinking. What nursing measures could you put in place to reduce her input and her thirst to prevent further oedema?

REFERENCES AND FURTHER READING

Crisp J, Taylor C (eds) (2005) *Potter & Perry's Fundamentals of Nursing*, 2nd edn. Elsevier Australia, Sydney

deWit SC (2005) *Fundamental Concepts and Skills for Nursing*, 2nd edn. WB Saunders, Philadelphia

Earis JE, Pearson MG (1995) Respiratory Medicine. *Times Mirror International Publishers*. London

Hargrave-Huttel RA (2001) *Medical Surgical Nursing*, 3rd edn. Lippincott, Philadelphia

Hawley R, King J, Weller BF (2003) *Australian Nurses' Dictionary*, 3rd edn. Baillière Tindall, Sydney

Jones I (2006) *Cardiac Care: an Introductory Text*. Whurr, Philadelphia; London

Kapit W, Meisami ME (2000) *The Physiology Coloring Book*, 2nd edn. Benjamin Cummings, San Francisco

Lemmi FO, Lemmi CAE (2000) *Physical Assessment Findings*. CD-ROM, WB Saunders, Philadelphia

Lewis SM, Heitkemper MM, Dirksen SR (2004) *Medical–Surgical Nursing. Assessment and Management of Clinical Problems*, 6th edn. Mosby, St Louis

Marieb EN (2006) *Human Anatomy and Physiology*, 6th edn. Benjamin Cummings Longman Inc, San Francisco

Nolan JD (2001) Prehospital and resuscitative airway care: should the gold standard be reassessed? *Current Opinion in Critical Care*, 7(6): 413–21

Peackock WFIV, Tiffany BR (2006) *Cardiac Emergencies*. McGraw-Hill Medical Publishing, New York

Potter PA, Perry AG (2005) *Fundamentals of Nursing*, 2nd edn. Mosby, St Louis

—— (2008) *Fundamentals of Nursing*, 7th edn. Mosby, St Louis

Santos C, Ferrer M, Roca J et al (2000) Pulmonary gas exchange response to oxygen breathing in acute lung injury. *American Journal of Respiratory and Critical Care Medicine*, 161: 26–31

Tollefson J (2004) *Clinical Motor Skills*, 2nd edn. Thomson, Southbank

Tortora GJ, Grabowski SR (2000) *Principles of Anatomy and Physiology*, 9th edn. Wiley & Sons, New York

Zitelli BJ, Davis HW (1997) *Atlas of Paediatric Physical Diagnosis*, 3rd edn. Mosby, St Louis

ONLINE RESOURCES

American Association for Respiratory Care: www.aarc.org (then type in client education tips in search box)

American Journal of Respiratory and Critical Care Medicine: http://ajrccm.atsjournals.org

American Lung Organisation: www.lungusa.org/diseases/oxygen_factsheet.html

Children's Virtual Hospital. Electric Airway: Upper Airway Problems in Children: www.vh.org/pediatric/provider/pediatrics/ElectricAirway/ElectricAirway.html

Development and Testing of Formal Protocols for Oxygen Prescribing (Article in the American Journal of Respiratory and Critical Care Medicine): http://ajrccm.atsjournals.org/cgi/content/full/163/4/942?maxtoshow=&HITS=30&hits=30&RESULTFORMAT=&titleabstract=oxygen&fulltext=oxygenation+oxygen+&searchid=1050095561893_6121&stored_search=&FIRSTINDEX=0&fdate=1/1/2001&journalcode=ajrccm

eMedicine: Altitude Illness — Pulmonary Syndromes: www.emedicine.com/emerg/topic795.htm

Oxygen Therapy: the First 150 Years: www.mtsinai.org/pulmonary/papers/ox-hist/ox-hist-intro.html

Pa_{O2}, Sa_{O2} and Oxygen Content: www.mtsinai.org/pulmonary/ABG/PO2.htm

Pleur-evac setup: www.nenhelp.com/pleurevac.htm

Pulmonary Physiology in Clinical Practice: www.mtsinai.org/pulmonary/books/physiology

The Four Most Important Equations in Clinical Practice: www.mtsinai.org/pulmonary/papers/eq/eqal.html

Chapter 39

ENDOCRINE HEALTH

OBJECTIVES

- Define the key terms/concepts
- Describe the position and structure of each endocrine gland
- Define the actions of the hormones secreted by each endocrine gland
- Explain the pathophysiological influences and effects associated with endocrine gland disorders
- Describe the disorders associated with each endocrine gland
- State the diagnostic tests that may be used when assessing endocrine function
- Assist in the planning and implementation of nursing care for the client with an endocrine disorder

KEY TERMS/CONCEPTS

acromegaly
Addison's disease
adrenal cortex
adrenal medulla
cretinism
Cushing's syndrome
diabetes insipidus
diabetes mellitus
dwarfism
gigantism
glands
goitre
hormones
pancreatic islets
parathyroids
pineal
pituitary
thymus
thyroid

CHAPTER FOCUS

The endocrine system is comprised of a number of small glands, some of which are structurally independent, while others are found within some organs. These glands secrete hormones, which aid in maintaining homeostasis in the body. Over- or under-production of these hormones can have widespread effects on the body because of the relation between the endocrine system and other systems in the body. An understanding of the function of these hormones gives health care professionals the ability to care for individuals with an endocrine disorder.

LIVED EXPERIENCE

I was dreaming that I was drinking an ice cold drink of water, it was great, so cool . . . then I woke up. Oh no, it's happening again! What is going on with me? I'm just so thirsty all the time. The teachers are getting really tired of me leaving the classroom heaps of times to go to the toilet. The thing is I'm not mucking around. I really do need to go. Plus, I'm so tired now, the thought of doing physical education at school freaks me out and there is no way I want to try out for the netball team, I'm just too tired. God, I'm scared, what if I'm sick? I'm at the fridge getting a cold drink. It's 4 am. I turn to go back to bed and there is mum . . . I just start crying.

Emma, age 14

I knew something was wrong with Emma, and had so many times thought it was just part of growing up — you know, hormonal changes and all that goes with an adolescent girl. I had discussed her continual thirst and tiredness with my friends and none of them seemed to have experienced the same problems with their girls. Now, this person who is a diabetes educator is trying to tell me Emma has diabetes! I don't believe it! She is my little girl, I feel as if my world is falling apart. I know I have to be strong for Emma but I faint at the sight of blood and the nurse is talking about injections and blood tests . . . I just don't understand — what have I done wrong?

Anne, Emma's mother

As a diabetes educator I am often faced with this situation when adolescents are diagnosed with type I diabetes. The experiences often involve parents feeling they have failed the child and done something wrong, and the child often feels as if their life is now virtually over. As these individuals are going to be dealing with diabetes now for life, an extensive education including family support is paramount to their continuing holistic health. That is where I come in.

Helen, RN, diabetes educator

STRUCTURE AND FUNCTION OF THE ENDOCRINE SYSTEM

ENDOCRINE GLANDS AND HORMONES

A hormone is a chemical substance secreted into the blood by an endocrine gland (Figure 39.1). The hormone is transported via the blood to areas of the body where it is needed to stimulate a specific cellular activity. Target organs are those that respond to a particular hormone. Some hormones can control other hormones by influencing their action, metabolism, synthesis and transport. A hormone can be described as a chemical regulator that integrates and coordinates cellular activities. Hormones are either steroids or proteins, and only target cells have the ability to respond to a specific hormone. After entering the blood, some hormones become bound to plasma proteins, while others are transported in an unbound state. Most hormones are continuously secreted at a rate determined by stimulation of the gland that releases them. Table 39.1 lists all the major hormones.

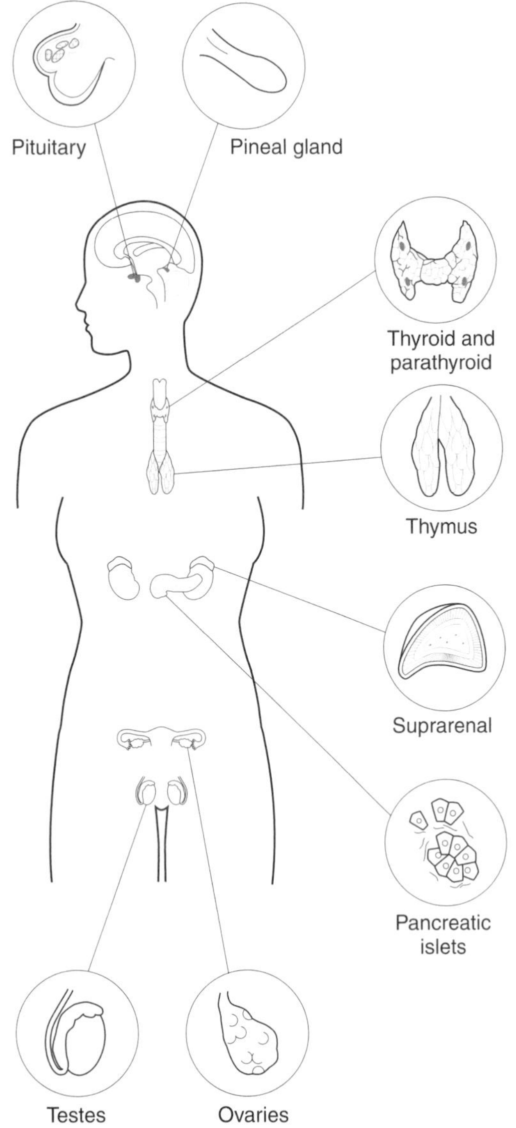

Figure 39.1 | The endocrine system

THE PITUITARY GLAND

The pituitary gland is about the size of a grape and is positioned at the base of the brain in a depression in the sphenoid bone. It lies just beneath the hypothalamus, to which it is connected by a stalk containing blood vessels and nervous tissue. It has two functional lobes: the anterior lobe comprised of glandular tissue, and the posterior lobe comprised of nervous tissue. Each lobe performs specific functions.

The anterior lobe produces:

- Growth hormone (GH), which is a metabolic hormone concerned with body growth, particularly skeletal muscles and long bones
- Thyrotrophic hormone (TH), also referred to as the thyroid-stimulating hormone (TSH), which is responsible for controlling the growth and activity of the thyroid gland
- Adrenocorticotrophic hormone (ACTH), which regulates the activity of the cortex of the suprarenal glands in hormone production
- Lactogenic hormone, also referred to as prolactin, which stimulates the mammary glands to secrete milk after the birth of a baby
- Gonadotrophic hormones, which control the development and functions of the ovaries and testes. These hormones are:
  - — follicle-stimulating hormone (FSH), which in the female stimulates the developing ovarian follicle to secrete oestrogen, and in the male stimulates the seminiferous tubules to produce sperm
  - — luteinising hormone (LH), which in the female is secreted after ovulation has occurred and stimulates the development of the corpus luteum in the ruptured follicle (the corpus luteum secretes progesterone), and in the male stimulates the testes to secrete testosterone (also known as interstitial-cell-stimulating hormone (ICSH).

The posterior lobe produces:

- Oxytocin, which has two functions:
  - — causing contraction of the uterine muscles during childbirth and lactation
  - — causing the ducts of the mammary glands to contract and expel breast milk.
- Antidiuretic hormone (ADH), which stimulates the kidney tubules to reabsorb water, resulting in decreased excretion of water in the urine.

DISORDERS OF THE PITUITARY GLAND

Hyperpituitarism

Hyper-function of the anterior pituitary gland commonly results from a tumour, which creates pressure on cerebral structures and causes neurological manifestations, such as severe headaches and visual disturbances, or excessive

TABLE 39.1 | THE MAJOR HORMONES

Endocrine gland	Hormone	Target	Effects
Pituitary (anterior lobe)	Growth hormone (GH)	Bones, muscles, organs	Promotes growth and metabolism
	Thyroid-stimulating hormone (TSH)	Thyroid gland	Regulates production of thyroid hormone
	Adrenocorticotrophic hormone (ACTH)	Adrenal cortex	Regulates secretion of cortisone, aldosterone and sex hormones
	Follicle-stimulating hormone (FSH)	Ovaries Seminiferous tubules	Regulates secretion of oestrogen Regulates production of sperm
	Luteinising hormone (LH)	Ovarian follicle	Formation of corpus luteum
	Interstitial-cell-stimulating hormone (ICSH)	Testes	Regulates production of testosterone
	Prolactin	Corpus luteum Breasts	Regulates secretion of progesterone Stimulates milk secretion
Pituitary (posterior lobe)	Oxytocin	Uterus Breasts	Stimulates uterine contractions Stimulates milk production
Thyroid	Antidiuretic hormone (ADH) Thyroxine Calcitonin	Tubules of kidneys Widespread Skeleton	Regulates reabsorption of water Increases metabolic rate, regulates growth Decreases plasma calcium levels
Parathyroids	Parathyroid hormone (PTH)	Bones Kidneys	Increases plasma calcium levels Regulates phosphorus excretion
Adrenals (cortex)	Glucocorticoids (e.g cortisone)	Widespread	Regulate metabolism of protein, fat and carbohydrate: • Promote gluconeogenesis • Mobilise amino acids • Promote lipolysis • Suppress inflammation • Effect on plasma glucose levels
	Mineralocorticoids (e.g. aldosterone)	Renal tubule	• Reabsorption of sodium • Excretion of potassium • Maintenance of fluid balance
	Sex hormones (e.g. androgens, oestrogens)	Gonads	Influence on development of secondary sexual characteristics and growth
Adrenals (medulla)	Epinephrine and norepinephrine	Widespread	• Vasoconstriction — increase in blood pressure • Gluconeogenesis • Response to stress • Stimulation of metabolism • Secretion of ACTH
Islets of Langerhans	Insulin	Widespread	• Decreases plasma glucose levels • Aids glucose transport into cells • Decrease in protein catabolism
	Glucagon	Liver Muscles Adipose cells	Increase in plasma glucose
Gonads (ovaries)	Oestrogen	Reproductive tissues	Development of secondary sexual characteristics Maturation of sexual organs Sexual functioning Development of mammary tissue
	Progesterone	Uterus Breasts	Maintenance of pregnancy, preparation of endometrium for implantation
Gonads (testes)	Testosterone	Widespread	• Development of secondary sexual characteristics • Maturation of sexual organs • Sexual functioning

(Continued)

TABLE 39.1 | THE MAJOR HORMONES—cont'd

Endocrine gland	Hormone	Target	Effects
Thymus	Thymosin	Immune system	Lymphocyte development
Pineal	Melatonin	Hypothalamus Midbrain Gonads	Regulating the gonads

secretion of pituitary hormones, with consequent increased stimulation of the target organs. It is a chronic progressive disorder marked by hormonal dysfunction and skeletal overgrowth, which can appear in two forms: gigantism and acromegaly.

Gigantism occurs in childhood and begins before epiphyseal closure. Children with gigantism may grow up to 15 cm a year, have slow sexual development and may have slow mental development. Gigantism is often the result of a tumour growing on the pituitary gland. Radiation therapy, surgical removal of the tumour and drug therapy may be used to decrease secretion of the growth hormone and slow down the excessive growth pattern. With this treatment, prognosis for the individual with gigantism is generally good.

Acromegaly occurs in adulthood and develops after epiphyseal closure. In acromegaly, over-secretion of growth hormone (GH) causes atrophy of skeletal muscle and formation of new bone and cartilage. The long bones are unable to grow in length, but the smaller bones of the hands, feet and face grow, giving the individual a characteristic appearance, with an enlarged lower jaw, bulging forehead and thickened ears and nose. The extremities become elongated and enlarged, resulting in large hands and feet. Thickening of the tongue may cause the voice to sound deep and hollow, associated with slurred speech. Acromegaly is a chronic disfiguring disease that often shortens life expectancy, as it may lead to respiratory, cerebrovascular and congestive heart diseases. Surgical intervention to remove the pituitary tumour often leads to hypopituitarism, and the tumours tend to recur.

Clients with anterior pituitary disorders require nursing interventions to assist them cope with the physical and emotional changes and also to prevent complications involving other organs.

Hypopituitarism

Hypofunction of the anterior pituitary gland can also result from a tumour in the gland, or it can be secondary to trauma of the hypothalamus. Other causes of hypofunction include disorders such as sarcoidosis, and infections such as tuberculosis or brucellosis. Hypopituitarism results in an absence or deficiency of growth hormone and gonadotrophin and is marked by growth retardation, which in children causes dwarfism and delay of puberty. It can present in three forms:

1. Frolich's syndrome, commonly caused by a tumour in the anterior pituitary gland and characterised by dwarfism, mental retardation, lack of sexual development and a reduction in all endocrine activity
2. Dwarfism, which results from hyposecretion of growth hormone and is characterised by proportionately small individuals who lack sexual development and may or may not suffer from mental retardation
3. Simmond's disease, due to atrophy of the anterior lobe of the pituitary gland, which is a rare disorder with widespread effects. Anorexia, atrophy of sexual organs, loss of weight, hypotension and anaemia are all clinical manifestations of this disorder.

Treatment of hypopituitarism involves hormone replacement of the needed hormones. Constant monitoring and adjusting of hormone levels is required to attain optimal results.

Diabetes insipidus

Damage to the posterior lobe of the pituitary gland can result in decreased or increased secretion of ADH. Diabetes insipidus is a rare condition caused by posterior lobe damage, and results from a deficiency of ADH. This results in the kidney tubules failing to reabsorb water. Without antidiuretic hormone, the individual has polyuria, passing vast quantities of dilute, colourless urine, up to 30 L in 24 hours. To compensate for the dehydration from the excessive fluid loss the individual experiences polydipsia (excessive thirst) and drinks large amounts of fluid. Treatment for people with diabetes insipidus involves medication such as vasopressin, which has a good prognosis. During the acute stage of this condition, clients need supportive care in relation to their polyuria and increased need for fluids.

Diagnostic tests

Pituitary function may be assessed by estimating the level of trophic hormones and by measuring the response to stimulation or suppression tests. The most common tests for evaluating anterior pituitary function are the serum growth hormone test and the insulin intolerance test. The insulin intolerance test, also called the growth hormone stimulation test, provides information about the secretion of growth hormone and ACTH. Investigations may also include X-ray or computerised tomography (CT) scan of the skull.

Testing posterior pituitary function includes the water-deprivation test, which is performed when the client's symptoms indicate diabetes insipidus. This test is based on the principle that withholding fluid for several hours stimulates secretion of ADH. In a person suspected of having diabetes insipidus, the urine may be tested to determine specific gravity. A low specific gravity is suggestive of diabetes insipidus.

THE THYROID GLAND

The thyroid gland lies in the neck just below the larynx. It consists of two lateral lobes positioned either side of the trachea. The lobes are joined together by a central mass called the isthmus, which lies anteriorly across the trachea. The thyroid gland is covered by a connective tissue capsule that forms trabeculae, which then pass inwards and divide the gland into lobes. The thyroid gland produces:

- Thyroxine (T4), which contains large quantities of iodine derived from the diet and stored in the thyroid gland. The function of thyroxine is to control the metabolic rate, thereby influencing:
  - — physical and mental development
  - — body temperature
  - — skin and hair health
- Calcitonin, also referred to as thyrocalcitonin, which decreases blood calcium levels by causing calcium to be deposited in the bones. In the kidneys, calcitonin promotes the excretion of phosphate and calcium, thus contributing to the regulation of blood calcium levels.

DISORDERS OF THE THYROID GLAND

Hyperthyroidism

Hyperthyroidism (also referred to as thyrotoxicosis) is hyper-functioning of the thyroid gland and may be caused by many factors, such as thyroiditis or an overproduction of thyroid stimulating hormone (TSH). An increase in the secretion of thyroid hormones affects the basal metabolic rate, as well as the functions of other body systems. The manifestations of hyper-functioning are generally related to increased metabolic processes. The condition can be caused by genetic or immunological factors, thyroid gland nodules or chronic inflammation of the thyroid gland.

Graves' disease

An autoimmune disorder, Graves' disease is a common hyperthyroid disease. Antibodies stimulate the thyroid gland, leading to glandular hypertrophy. Graves' disease more commonly affects young women. Symptoms include all the characteristics of hyperthyroidism — tachycardia, nervousness, hyperactivity and excitability. The individual will have a voracious appetite but loses weight and can be quite underweight. Diarrhoea is common, as peristaltic rate increases. Excessive sweating and extreme thirst are also common, because of the increased metabolic rate. One outstanding characteristic of Graves' disease is that of exophthalmos, or protrusion of the eyeballs, which is due to oedema in the tissues behind the eye, and does not resolve even when the hyperthyroidism is corrected. A serious complication of Graves' disease is thyroid storm (or crisis), which is discussed in Clinical Interest Box 39.1.

> **CLINICAL INTEREST BOX 39.1**
> **Thyroid storm, or thyroid crisis**
>
> This situation occurs in a person with advanced hyperthyroid disease. A thyroid crisis can be instigated by emotional stress, infection, trauma, cardiovascular disease or after thyroid surgery, and results from a sudden release of thyroid hormone into the bloodstream. This causes a sudden increase of the symptoms of hyperthyroidism and is considered a medical emergency, as the severe tachycardia, tachypnoea and increase in body temperature can be life-threatening.

Goitre

The thyroid gland can become enlarged, hyperactive or hypoactive as a result of pathophysiological changes. An enlarged thyroid gland may be the result of a simple goitre, thyroiditis or neoplasia. Goitre refers to any thyroid enlargement and may be associated with either over-secretion or under-secretion of thyroid hormones. Goitre can cause local problems by exerting pressure on the trachea, which may produce dysphagia or respiratory distress. Simple goitre (non-toxic goitre) is due to an iodine deficiency that causes a compensatory enlargement of the thyroid gland in an attempt to maintain thyroid hormone production. Endemic goitre occurs in regions away from coastal areas, where there is little iodine in the soil and water. The introduction of iodised salt has reduced the incidence in most Western countries. Exopthalmic goitre occurs in hyperthyroidism.

Management of hyperthyroidism involves assisting the individual and their family to manage the symptoms associated with hyperthyroidism until it is controlled with medication, or surgery if indicated. Surgical intervention may involve a subtotal thyroidectomy, which removes part of the thyroid gland, leaving enough gland to produce adequate thyroid hormone, or a total thyroidectomy may be performed if the gland is cancerous. A person who has had a total thyroidectomy requires long-term hormone replacement. The critical pathway in Table 39.2 outlines the nursing care of a client undergoing thyroidectomy surgery.

Hypothyroidism

Hypothyroidism is characterised by a decreased secretion of thyroid hormones. Hypothyroidism may be congenital or it may develop later in life. Cretinism is the congenital form of hypothyroidism and results from absence or underdevelopment of the thyroid gland or it may occur from severe maternal iodine deficiency during pregnancy.

TABLE 39.2 | CRITICAL PATHWAY THYROIDECTOMY

Expected length of stay — 3 days

	Day 1 preoperative	Operative day	Day 1 postoperative	Day 2 postoperative
Discharge planning	Assess discharge needs		Discuss wound care	Action if concerned
Psychosocial	Assess social situation	Reassurance	Assess emotional state	Reassurance Include family
Investigations	Assess emotional state Full ward test Electrocardiograph/chest X-ray Full blood examination Urea and electrolytes Thyroid function tests	Full ward test	Calcium	Calcium Thyroid function test
Observations	Baseline temperature, pulse, respiration, blood pressure and weight Oxygen saturation Assess facial nerve and Trousseau's sign	Postoperative observations Intravenous site and rate Wound Drain tubes	4/24 Observations Wound Drain tubes	Individual afebrile Wound clean No tetany evident
Assessments/ treatments	Consent form Preoperative check list	Facial nerve Trousseau's sign	Remove IVT and drain tube	
Diet/hydration/ elimination	Fast 6 hours preoperatively Chart bowel action	Nil orally Intravenous therapy and fluid balance chart Postoperative void	Commence light diet and fluids	Normal diet Normal elimination
Safety/mobility	Assess mobility Explain fire exit Call bell in reach Cot sides on bed	Rest in bed and pressure area care Thyroid tray Call bell in reach	Sit out of bed and gently ambulate	Limitations of activity
Hygiene	Shower pre-operation Remove make-up and jewellery	Postoperative sponge Mouth care	Shower	Individual able to shower independently
Medications	Ensure aspirin ceased Administer preoperative medications	Narcotic patient-controlled analgesia Routine medications	Analgesia Routine medications	Pain management Routine medications
Individual needs	Assess needs	Assess needs	Assess needs	Assess needs
Referrals	Surgical review	Surgical review		Surgical review Follow-up care
Education	Anaesthetic review Explain patient-controlled analgesia Explain signs and symptoms of tetany	Reinforce previous instruction		Wound care

The manifestations of cretinism are related to a marked depression of metabolic processes and progressive mental impairment. Typically the infant is overweight, lethargic, has dry thick skin, coarse features, a broad flat nose and protruding tongue and abdomen. If the disease goes unchecked, sexual organs fail to develop and muscle growth is retarded. Treatment is started as soon as diagnosis is made and involves lifelong thyroid hormone replacement therapy (HRT).

Myxoedema is acquired hypothyroidism and develops when the thyroid gland stops functioning effectively. Hypothyroidism can also result from surgical intervention used to correct hyperthyroidism. The most common natural cause of hypothyroidism is an autoimmune disorder, Hashimoto's disease. Symptoms of hypothyroidism are the opposite of those of hyperthyroidism. The individual is fatigued, drowsy, sensitive to cold temperatures, gains excessive weight, has thin nails and brittle hair, decreased pulse and respiratory rates and irregular menstruation. Hypothyroidism responds well to HRT and symptoms may disappear after a few months of treatment.

Diagnostic tests

A combination of tests is generally performed to evaluate thyroid function, including direct tests of thyroid function, tests that measure concentration and binding of the thyroid hormones and tests involving the use of scanning or imaging techniques. Blood tests are performed to measure serum hormone levels, which assist in the diagnosis of hyperthyroidism and hypothyroidism. Radioactive iodine tests, such as the radioactive iodine uptake test, evaluate thyroid function by measuring the amount of orally ingested iodine that accumulates in the thyroid gland after 2, 6 and 24 hours. Thyroid scanning is visualisation of the thyroid gland after administration of a radioisotope. Thyroid ultrasonography helps evaluate thyroid structure and differentiation between a cyst and a tumour on the thyroid gland.

THE PARATHYROID GLANDS

The parathyroids are four small glands embedded in the posterior surface of each lobe of the thyroid gland. The parathyroid glands produce parathyroid hormone (PTH), also referred to as parathormone, which is primarily responsible for the regulation of blood calcium and phosphate levels. Parathormone promotes the reabsorption of calcium into the blood after destruction of bone cells (osteoclasts) and inhibits the reabsorption of phosphate in the renal tubules.

DISORDERS OF THE PARATHYROID GLANDS

Hyperparathyroidism

Hyperparathyroidism involves hyper-functioning of the parathyroid glands resulting in an overproduction of PTH. This condition can be caused by hereditary factors, tumours or enlargement of the glands. Secondary hyper-functioning can be caused by renal disease, osteomalacia or rickets. Excessive parathormone production causes hypercalcaemia (excessive calcium in the blood). As the calcium is pulled from the bones, individuals with this condition display manifestations that are widespread and include symptoms such as backache, bone curvature and pathological fractures from bone weakness. Renal stones may develop because of the high calcium output in the urine. The digestive system increases absorption of calcium, causing abdominal pain, vomiting and constipation. Hypercalcaemia leads to hyperactivity of muscles, causing impaired neuromuscular coordination and cardiac arrhythmias.

Treatment of hyperparathyroidism is directed at the cause and often results in good prognosis for the client. Surgical removal of tumours or removal of the parathyroid glands may be necessary, leaving half of one parathyroid gland, which is all that is required to maintain normal parathormone levels. Other treatments include diuretic therapy to force increased excretion of calcium by the kidneys, and decreasing calcium intake in the diet.

Hypoparathyroidism

Hypoparathyroidism involves hypofunction of the parathyroid glands, resulting in a deficiency in PTH secretion. Causes include familial hypoparathyroidism, autoimmune disorders or surgical removal of parathyroid glands in an effort to treat hyperparathyroidism. Under-secretion of parathormone causes hypocalcaemia (low calcium levels in the blood), resulting in neuromuscular symptoms ranging from paraesthesia to tetany. Manifestations include anxiety, increased deep tendon reflexes and laryngeal spasm.

Tetany is a condition in which there is hyperexcitability of nerves and muscles because of low calcium blood levels. It begins with tingling in the fingertips, toes and around the mouth. The tingling increases and produces muscle tension and spasms, with consequent adduction of the thumbs, wrists, elbows and toes (carpopedal spasm). The tetany associated with hypoparathyroidism mainly affects the face and hands, causing uncontrolled contraction of these muscles. This should not be confused with lockjaw, which results from the infectious disease tetanus.

Treatment with calcium supplements and vitamin D, which controls absorption of calcium in the gastrointestinal tract, gives a good prognosis.

Diagnostic tests

Tests used to assess parathyroid function include estimation of serum calcium and serum phosphorus levels. A 24-hour urine collection may be performed to measure the total urine calcium. Hyperparathyroidism causes increased excretion of calcium in the urine, and hypoparathyroidism causes decreased excretion of calcium. Testing for hypocalcaemia and hypoparathyroidism involves checking for a positive Chvostek's sign (facial muscle spasm occurring when the facial nerve is tapped) and a positive Trousseau's sign (hand muscle spasm when pressure is applied to the nerves and vessels of the upper arm).

THE ADRENAL GLANDS

There are two adrenal glands located on top of each kidney. Each gland is surrounded by a capsule and contains an outer cortex and an inner medulla.

The adrenal cortex

The cortex, or outer portion, produces three major groups of steroid hormones, collectively called corticosteroids:

1. Glucocorticoids, which include cortisone, hydrocortisone and cortisol, are concerned with:
   — metabolism of protein, fat and carbohydrate
   — conversion of protein to glucose
   — storage of glycogen and its conversion to glucose
   — release of fat stored in adipose tissue for use as a fuel.

   When glucocorticoids have a high level in the blood, fats and proteins are broken down and converted to glucose. Hence, glucocorticoids are referred to as hyperglycaemic hormones
2. Mineralocorticoids, mostly aldosterone, which is concerned with the reabsorption of sodium ions and the elimination of potassium ions in the kidneys. Mineralocorticoids thus help regulate both water and electrolyte balance in the body fluids
3. Sex hormones — called androgens in males and oestrogens in females — are concerned with the development of secondary sexual characteristics and the functioning of the reproductive organs. Both male and female hormones are produced by the adrenal cortex, regardless of gender.

The adrenal medulla

The medulla, or inner portion of the adrenal glands, produces two similar hormones referred to as catecholamines: adrenaline (also referred to as epinephrine) and noradrenaline (also referred to as norepinephrine). When the medulla is stimulated by neurons of the sympathetic nervous system, the two hormones are released into the bloodstream. The physiological responses to the medullary hormones mimic those of the sympathetic nervous system:

- Dilation of coronary and skeletal muscle arteries
- Constriction of blood vessels in the skin and internal organs
- Increase in the rate and strength of the heartbeat
- Increase in blood pressure
- Dilation of the bronchial tubes
- Reduction of peristalsis in the digestive system
- Stimulation of the liver to release more glucose into the bloodstream
- Dilation of the pupils
- An increase in the metabolic rate.

Adrenaline prepares the body for fight or flight, and its secretion is increased when the body feels threatened or experiences strong emotions such as fear, anger or excitement, thereby helping the body cope with a stressful situation.

DISORDERS OF THE ADRENAL GLANDS

Hyperadrenalism

Hyper-functioning of the adrenal glands is usually confined to the cortex of the gland. Hyper-functioning of the cortex may be caused by neoplasia or hyperplasia, or it may be iatrogenic. A iatrogenic disorder is a condition caused by medical treatment or procedures. Iatrogenic diabetes mellitus is a form of diabetes that can develop from high doses of corticosteroids. Other factors resulting in hyper-functioning of the cortex include tumours or hyperplasia of the pituitary gland. Manifestations of hyper-functioning are generally related to an excess of glucocorticoids, mineralocorticoids and sex hormones. Three major disorders can result.

Cushing's syndrome

This condition may be caused by various factors, including hypersecretion of pituitary ACTH, steroid therapy or a tumour of the adrenal glands. Manifestations of this disorder are related to hyperglycaemia, abnormal distribution of lipids and protein wasting. Classic symptoms include obesity of the trunk with a pad of fat across the shoulders (buffalo hump), a moon face, striae on the breasts, abdomen and legs, muscle weakness, osteoporosis and skin fragility. Persistent hyperglycaemia may develop into diabetes mellitus. Hypertension is a common feature, which leads to atherosclerosis, ischaemic heart disease and nephrosclerosis. Surgical removal of the tumour or the adrenal cortex may correct this condition for the individual. Lifetime hormone therapy to replace the cortical hormones is then required. Clinical Interest Box 39.2 provides an overview of cortisone therapy.

Conn's syndrome

This condition is the result of hypersecretion of the mineralocorticoid aldosterone. Conn's syndrome leads to impaired reabsorption of sodium and water in the renal tubules. Manifestations of this disorder are hypertension, muscle weakness, polyuria, polydipsia, metabolic acidosis and neuromuscular dysfunction. This form of hyperadrenalism is often caused by a tumour on the adrenal cortex. Removal of the tumour usually gives a good prognosis.

Androgenital syndrome

Androgenital syndrome and adrenal virilism result from a hypersecretion of androgens. Excessive secretion of androgens causes pseudohermaphroditism, in which the gonads are those of one sex, but one or more contradictions exist in the secondary sexual characteristics. Female children are seen with excessive hair growth on the legs, chest and abdomen, an enlarged clitoris, a deepened voice and amenorrhoea. Male children experience precocious puberty

CLINICAL INTEREST BOX 39.2
Cortisone therapy

Cortisone is a therapy used to treat inflammatory conditions such as arthritis because of its anti-inflammatory properties. It does not cure the disease but gives individuals pain relief enabling them to continue their daily lives with as much normality as possible. However, Cushing's syndrome may develop in people receiving glucocorticoid steroids long term, so the nurse needs to monitor these clients for symptoms of Cushing's syndrome.

(premature sexual development) and gynaecomastia (breast development). Treatment of an adrenal cortex tumour is by surgical removal, and HRT is often indicated.

Hypoadrenalism

Hypofunctioning of the adrenal cortex may be caused by primary insufficiency, resulting in a condition known as Addison's disease. This is a rare condition thought to be due to an autoimmune reaction or an infective process such as tuberculosis. Up to 90% of the adrenal cortex can be destroyed before the symptoms become evident. The manifestations are related to a deficiency of the three types of adrenal cortical hormones. The lack of mineralocorticoids depletes sodium, which leads to diarrhoea, dehydration, weakness, weight loss and hypotension. The lack of glucocorticoids affects blood sugar levels, leading to hypoglycaemia. Increased ACTH level leads to brown pigmentation of the skin and mucous membranes, affecting the palms, elbows, scars, skin folds and areolae. Treatment includes corticosteroid therapy.

Disorders of the adrenal medulla

The medulla of the adrenal gland can be affected by neoplastic disorders. Neuroblastoma, which occurs primarily in children, is a malignant neoplasm that may metastasise to the lymph nodes, liver, lung and bone. Manifestations depend on the size of the tumour and the site of the metastasis.

Phaeochromocytoma is a generally benign tumour of the medulla or of the sympathetic chain, which causes oversecretion of adrenaline and noradrenaline. The resultant increase in sympathetic activity manifests as episodes of hypertension, tachycardia, chest pain, pallor, sweating, headaches, anxiety, tremor, nausea and vomiting and frequency of urination. These symptoms can cause life-threatening scenarios for the individual, so early diagnosis and treatment is imperative. Surgical removal of the tumour is often indicated as the treatment of choice.

Diagnostic tests

Both the cortex and the medulla of the adrenal glands secrete several hormones. Blood and urine tests are performed that enable measurement of the levels of these hormones. Blood tests determine the level of serum aldosterone, serum cortisol or serum catecholamines. These levels aid in the diagnosis of adrenal function; for example, serum cortisol levels are increased in Cushing's syndrome, while decreased serum cortisol levels are seen in Addison's disease. A 24-hour urine collection may be performed to estimate the total daily free cortisol, aldosterone or catecholamine levels. A CT scan or suprarenal venography may also be used to aid in the diagnosis of tumours.

THE GONADS

The female gonads are the ovaries, and the male gonads are the testes. The female and male gonads produce sex hormones identical to those produced by the adrenal cortex.

The ovaries are two small almond-shaped organs of the female reproductive system and lie in the pelvic cavity, either side of the uterus. The hormones produced by the ovaries are oestrogens and progesterone. Oestrogens influence development of the reproductive organs and the secondary sexual characteristics. Oestrogen also stimulates the lining of the uterus to thicken in preparation for a fertilised ovum to develop. Progesterone promotes the final thickening of the uterine lining and inhibits uterine contraction, enabling implantation of the fertilised ovum. Progesterone also inhibits ovulation during pregnancy and stimulates the mammary glands to produce milk.

The testes are two small organs of the male reproductive system, lying in a loose pouch of skin called the scrotum. The testes produce the hormone testosterone, which stimulates the development of male characteristics and the growth and function of the reproductive organs.

DISORDERS OF THE GONADS

Hypergonadism

Hypergonadism results from increased hormone production before puberty and leads to precocious sexual development in both sexes. In the male, the onset of puberty begins early, often before age 10. Signs include growth of facial and pubic hair and enlarged penis and testes. There may also be rapid growth of bones and muscle, leading to an early uniting of the epiphyses and a premature halt to long bone growth. Spermatogenesis also occurs, making the individual fertile. In the female, the onset of puberty can begin before age eight. Signs include the onset of menarche, appearance of pubic and underarm hair and breast enlargement. Ovarian development also enables pregnancy to occur.

Causes of hypergonadism are primarily unknown but some cases have been caused by ovarian tumours and testicular tumours. Treatment for both sexes involves removal or radiation of the tumours, and hormone therapy to suppress or counteract the effects of the sex hormone.

Hypogonadism

Hypogonadism results from decreased sex hormone production by the age of normal puberty. In the male, testes may fail to develop because of a pituitary disorder, resulting in the lack of development of male sexual characteristics. Testosterone therapy is an effective treatment for this condition. In the female, the secondary sexual characteristics do not develop because of the lack of oestrogen. Female children become abnormally tall because, without oestrogen, the long bones do not fuse normally. Oestrogen therapy is an effective treatment for this condition.

Diagnostic tests

Diagnosis of disorders of the gonads is based on a positive

clinical history and confirmed by blood tests showing elevated sex hormone levels.

THE THYMUS GLAND

The thymus gland is positioned in the upper thorax posterior to the sternum. It is large in infants and children, reaching its maximum size at puberty, then decreasing in size throughout adulthood. The thymus produces a hormone called thymosin, which promotes the growth of lymphoid tissue in the body and aids in the body's immune response. While dysfunction of the thymus gland is uncommon, a benign tumour of the gland is thought to be associated with myasthenia gravis. Congenital thymic hypoplasia causes deficient cellular immunity, making the individual more susceptible to infections.

THE PINEAL GLAND

The pineal gland is a small cone-shaped structure situated in the roof of the third ventricle of the brain. It begins to atrophy early in life and is replaced by fibrous tissue. The endocrine function of the pineal gland is unknown but it is believed to secrete the hormone melatonin, which appears to rise and fall during the course of the day and night and is believed to establish the body's day–night wake–sleep pattern. A rare neoplasm of the pineal gland (pinealoma) may either obstruct the flow of cerebrospinal fluid, causing hydrocephalus, or extend into the hypothalamus, causing precocious puberty.

PANCREATIC ISLETS

Formerly referred to as the Islets of Langerhans, these millions of pancreatic islets are small groups of cells scattered throughout the pancreas. They produce two hormones, insulin and glucagon, which both help to regulate blood glucose level.

Insulin and glucagon

Insulin is released into the blood when there is a high level of glucose present. The presence of some amino acids and fatty acids also increase insulin release. Insulin is released from the beta cells of the islets and increases the uptake of glucose into the cells and reduces the release of glucose from the liver, thereby decreasing the blood glucose level, hence having a hypoglycaemic effect. Insulin also promotes the conversion of glucose to fatty acids within the liver. Insulin acts generally to stimulate protein synthesis. Insulin is essential for the use of glucose by the cells of the body — without it, the cells would be unable to utilise glucose for energy.

Glucagon is released from the alpha cells of the pancreatic islets in response to a reduced blood glucose level. Its output is reduced in the presence of raised blood glucose and insulin; it thus acts as an antagonist of insulin. Glucagon raises blood glucose levels by stimulating the breakdown of glycogen in the liver and inhibiting glycogen synthesis.

DISORDERS OF THE PANCREATIC ISLETS

Diabetes mellitus

Diabetes mellitus is a disorder of glucose regulation characterised by abnormal metabolism of carbohydrate, protein and fat. A feature of the disorder is some degree of hyperglycaemia. Diabetes mellitus results from an insulin deficiency, or from the production of substances antagonistic to insulin, which cause it to be ineffective. It may be caused by hereditary factors, pancreatic disorders, or by disorders of other endocrine glands, such as the pituitary or adrenal glands. It is also thought to be autoimmune in origin. Gestational diabetes is one form of the disorder that appears only during pregnancy, and is characterised by impaired glucose tolerance. A woman who has had gestational diabetes runs a greater risk of developing diabetes mellitus later on in life. Diabetes mellitus is classified into two types: type 1, or insulin-dependent diabetes mellitus (IDDM); and type 2, or non-insulin-dependent diabetes mellitus (NIDDM). The diagnosis of diabetes mellitus is confirmed by the presence of an elevated blood glucose level.

A deficiency of insulin causes changes in the metabolism of glucose, which results in numerous physiological effects. In the liver the glycolytic enzymes are inhibited, the gluconeogenic enzymes are activated, and amino acids are used to form glucose. Consequently, additional glucose is liberated into the bloodstream. Without insulin, glucose is unable to cross the cell membranes into muscle and fat cells, and hyperglycaemia occurs. The blood glucose level eventually exceeds the renal threshold, and glucose is excreted in the urine. The most significant effect of elevated blood glucose level is dehydration of the tissue cells because the increased osmotic pressure in the extracellular fluids causes osmotic transfer of water out of the cells. In addition, the loss of glucose via the urine causes diuresis, because of the osmotic effect of glucose in the renal tubules. The result is extreme polydipsia.

The manifestations of diabetes mellitus vary according to whether the disorder is type 1 or type 2.

Type 1 diabetes mellitus

This form of diabetes mellitus can occur at any age from infancy up to about age 40. There is a sudden onset of signs and symptoms, which include weight loss, polyuria, polydipsia, fatigue, and the presence of glucose and ketones in the urine. Hyperglycaemia and dehydration accelerate the development of metabolic acidosis and, if untreated, can lead to coma and death.

Type 2 diabetes mellitus

This form of diabetes mellitus is more likely to occur after age 40. The signs and symptoms develop slowly and the individual is generally obese. Type 2 diabetes mellitus may often go undetected, as the signs and symptoms of fatigue, polyuria and polydipsia can be quite insignificant. Diagnosis occurs when the individual presents with another disease, which is a common complication of diabetes mellitus, such as a monilial infection, cataracts, degenerative changes in the blood vessels or peripheral neuritis.

The individual with diabetes mellitus is prone to a range of complications, especially if the blood glucose level is uncontrolled. Complications include:

- Hyperglycaemia
- Diabetic ketoacidosis
- Hyperosmolar nonketotic hyperglycaemia
- Retinopathy
- Neuropathy
- Cardiovascular and peripheral vascular disease
- Nephropathy
- Hypoglycaemia (imbalance of food, exercise and medications).

Diagnostic tests

Laboratory evaluation of the pancreatic islets is mainly concerned with levels of glucose in the blood and urine, as the hormones secreted by the islets regulate blood glucose levels. Urine is examined for the presence of glucose and ketones. When the serum glucose level exceeds the renal threshold, the excess glucose is excreted in the urine. As a result of increased lipolysis, excess ketone bodies accumulate and are excreted in the urine. Blood tests measure the body's use of glucose and include:

- **Glucose tolerance test.** This test evaluates glucose absorption after its oral or intravenous administration. The individual fasts overnight before the administration of glucose; glucose levels are then measured at intervals to diagnose diabetes mellitus
- **Fasting serum glucose test.** Also referred to as fasting blood sugar, this test measures glucose level after the individual has fasted for an 8-hour period; the blood glucose level is then measured. In diabetes mellitus, the absence or deficiency of insulin allows persistently high serum glucose levels above 7.8 mmol/L
- **Two-hour postprandial serum glucose.** This test provides information about the body's utilisation and disposal of glucose after a meal. An elevated blood glucose level is indicative of diabetes mellitus
- **Tolbutamide tolerance test.** An intravenous injection of the drug tolbutamide usually stimulates the secretion of insulin. Normally, after administration of the drug, the serum glucose level will fall rapidly and return to normal baseline levels in 3 hours. In diabetes mellitus there is a slow initial drop and a prolonged time to return to pre-set levels
- **Glycosylated haemoglobin (HbA_{1c}) test.** This test is performed to review the control of diabetes mellitus over the previous 2–3 months. Results reflect the average glucose level within erythrocytes rather than the serum glucose level. In diabetes mellitus it may be elevated to three times the normal level.

CARE OF THE CLIENT WITH AN ENDOCRINE DISORDER

Because of the complexity of the endocrine system and its interrelation with other body systems, dysfunction of any endocrine gland can have widespread effects. Most endocrine disorders result from over- or under-production of hormones; that is, either hyper-functioning or hypo-functioning of a specific gland. The manifestations and effects resulting from a glandular disorder therefore relate to the hormone the affected gland secretes.

Endocrine dysfunction has widespread effects, and the medical management and nursing care depends on the diagnosis of a specific disorder. When care is being planned, the nurse must consider the effects that the disorder may have on the individual, and any issues the individual may be coping with, such as:

- A major change in lifestyle — as a result of diabetes mellitus the individual may have to depend on lifelong medication and dietary modifications
- The prospect of facing major surgery; e.g., removal of the thyroid gland may be indicated in the presence of hyperthyroidism, goitre or carcinoma of a gland
- Alterations in nutritional status; e.g., weight gain often occurs in hypothyroidism, whereas weight loss is common in people with type 1 diabetes mellitus. Nutritional status may also be affected if the individual is experiencing anorexia, nausea or vomiting
- Alterations in fluid balance — excessive loss of fluid may occur in diabetes mellitus or posterior pituitary gland disorders. Loss of fluid may also occur if the individual has diarrhoea, as may be present in disorders such as hyperthyroidism and Addison's disease. Conversely, retention of fluid may occur in disorders such as Cushing's syndrome
- Discomfort — many endocrine disorders result in problems related to body temperature regulation. A person with hypothyroidism is very sensitive to cold, whereas an individual with hyperthyroidism is commonly intolerant to heat. Other factors that may cause discomfort include pruritus associated with hyperthyroidism or diabetes mellitus, and joint pain associated with acromegaly. Anxiety and nervousness associated with certain disorders such as hyperthyroidism may also cause discomfort as the individual is restless and finds it difficult to relax
- Reduced independence — extreme fatigue often accompanies endocrine disorders, and the individual may require assistance to carry out activities of daily living. Certain disorders (e.g. Cushing's syndrome or hyperparathyroidism) may be accompanied by central nervous system involvement. Altered states of awareness or consciousness will reduce the individual's level of independence
- Altered body image; e.g., as a result of hirsutism associated with suprarenal gland dysfunction, or as a

result of increased skin pigmentation with Addison's disease.

The plan of care that the nurse designs for a client should specifically address the need for comfort, psychological support, and maintenance of nutritional and fluid status. Clients should also be given information regarding self-help groups and should be encouraged to contact these organisations for further support and information.

CARE OF THE CLIENT WITH DIABETES MELLITUS

Diabetes mellitus affects a great number of the Australian population. Of the total population with diabetes, type 2 is more common than type 1. The main aims of management of the client with diabetes mellitus are to maintain the blood glucose level within an acceptable range and to implement measures to assist the person to live as normal a life as possible. Diabetes can be controlled at present, but not cured; management is therefore aimed at controlling it and preventing complications. Care of a client with diabetes involves regulating the blood glucose level by diet, exercise, and insulin or oral hypoglycaemic agents, preventing infection and monitoring blood and urine glucose levels. The overall aim for the individual is self-management of the disorder, which makes education of the client in all aspects of care an essential part of management.

Diet

Diet is an important aspect in control of both type 1 and type 2 diabetes mellitus. A dietitian works with the client to develop a well-balanced, healthy food intake. It is essential that the client gains understanding of the principles and can then modify and adapt the diet to meet demands experienced during illness, injury, emotional stress or major changes in lifestyle. The aims of the diet for a person with diabetes are to:

- Satisfy hunger
- Provide for normal growth rate in children
- Attain and maintain a desirable body weight
- Maintain the level of blood glucose within the normal range to prevent hypoglycaemia and hyperglycaemia
- Meet the individual's energy requirements
- Prevent the development of long-term complications associated with diabetes mellitus.

Alcohol should be limited, as it is high in sugar and may cause adverse reactions to some medications used in the treatment of diabetes mellitus. The dietitian will supply the individual with instructions for planning nutritious and varied meals within the prescribed limitations. The importance of regular meals and snacks is emphasised, particularly an evening snack to prevent nocturnal hypoglycaemia. The diet is continually evaluated and adjusted as required. When the individual is in hospital it is important that the nurse observes the amount of each meal eaten because if nutrients are not all consumed the person may experience hypoglycaemia.

Exercise

The amount of exercise required by the client should be estimated and planned to balance with the dietary intake and insulin. A well-planned program of regular exercise that is adjusted as necessary is beneficial in weight control, in its physiological and psychological effects, and in terms of blood glucose control. Exercise stimulates the uptake of glucose by muscle cells, lowering blood glucose levels and increasing the absorption of injected insulin. For these reasons, exercise can increase the likelihood of hypoglycaemia. To prevent hypoglycaemia after exercise, the individual needs to either increase the nutritional intake or decrease the insulin dosage. Education is essential for the client to gain understanding to correctly balance the level of exercise with dietary intake and insulin dosage under varying conditions.

Insulin

As insulin is essential for the normal metabolism of glucose, it is a major factor involved in the regulation of blood glucose levels. Many types of insulin are available and these may be short-, intermediate- or long-acting. The different types of insulin vary in the time of onset and the duration of action, and are selected according to the time of day, activity and nutritional intake. As soon as possible after diagnosis, the client is given instruction on insulin administration and care for the equipment required. They are also instructed on rotating injection sites around the abdomen and thighs to prevent tissue atrophy or hypertrophy at regularly used injection sites. The abdomen provides the fastest and most consistent rate of absorption and is an accessible site for the person to use.

Oral hypoglycaemic agents

Oral hypoglycaemic agents may be prescribed in the management of type 2 diabetes mellitus unresponsive to diet alone. The oral medications used in the treatment of diabetes mellitus act either by stimulating the pancreas to release insulin or by delaying or impairing glucose absorption from the bowel.

Preventing infection

People with diabetes mellitus are susceptible to infection as a result of impaired body defence mechanisms. Uncontrolled diabetes may result in a range of infections, whereas if blood sugar level is well controlled they are less susceptible. The person with diabetes is particularly at risk of developing urinary tract infections, fungal infections such as candida, and infected skin lesions. To minimise the risk of infection the person should understand the importance of good control of blood glucose levels, of maintaining a high standard of personal hygiene, and of avoiding unnecessary exposure to infection. The skin should be kept clean and free from excessive irritation, friction or pressure. All injuries to, or infections of, the skin, however minor, should be cleaned with a mild antiseptic solution and covered with a dressing.

Skin lesions of the feet commonly occur in people with poorly controlled diabetes mellitus. Such lesions result from, or are exacerbated by, impaired circulation and peripheral neuropathy. If a minor injury or lesion is undetected or untreated, ulceration and infection may develop. Care of the feet and prevention of foot lesions is therefore of prime importance. Care of the feet includes:

- Wearing well-fitting socks or stockings, and shoes. Socks should be made from natural fibre (e.g. wool or cotton) with care taken to avoid hosiery with seams under the feet
- Daily cleansing, drying and inspection of the feet. A mild soap is used and the feet should not be soaked for long periods. After washing, the feet should be patted dry rather than rubbed. Dry feet may be gently massaged with lanolin or oil to prevent fissures
- Consulting a podiatrist if corns or calluses need attention
- Trimming the toenails straight across, to avoid damage to the surrounding skin
- Keeping the feet warm but avoiding placing them close to heating devices, to prevent possible skin damage. If an electric blanket is used to warm the bed, it should be turned off before the person gets into bed
- Avoiding walking barefooted or on hot surfaces
- Performing foot and leg exercises to increase circulation
- Avoiding constrictive clothing (e.g. socks with elasticised tops) and crossing the legs, both of which may reduce blood flow
- Seeking immediate attention from the podiatrist or medical officer if there is any injury, colour change, infection or discharge of pus or blood.

Monitoring glucose levels

Although it is less accurate than blood glucose monitoring, urinalysis is still used by some people with diabetes to assess glucose levels. The person is educated in the technique of urine testing for both glucose and ketones. Blood glucose monitoring is performed by obtaining a drop of capillary blood, which is then applied to a reagent strip and read by one of the many types of glucometers available on the market. The aim of self blood glucose monitoring is to assist the person with diabetes to assume more autonomy in the management of the condition. The person is educated on the use of the glucometer, the appropriate times at which to perform the test and how to make adjustments to the insulin dose to attain a desirable blood glucose level. (See Chapter 24 for guidelines for measuring blood glucose levels.)

Complications of diabetes mellitus

Complications may develop rapidly or progress insidiously over years before they become evident. The two main complications that occur because of uncontrolled blood glucose levels are hypoglycaemia and hyperglycaemia.

Hypoglycaemia

Hypoglycaemia is an abnormally low blood glucose level and may be caused by too much insulin, too little food or delayed food intake, excess physical activity or vomiting. Hypoglycaemia develops rapidly and the early manifestations are hunger, pallor, sweating, tachycardia, yawning, nausea, blurred vision, slurred speech, confusion or irrational behaviour. If the hypoglycaemia is not corrected rapidly, the person will become comatose and, if the coma is prolonged, permanent brain damage or death may occur.

Mild symptoms can often be reversed by ingesting a simple carbohydrate, such as fruit juice or honey. People with insulin-dependent diabetes should ensure that they always have ready access to some form of carbohydrate that is easily absorbed, such as barley sugar or jelly beans. If the person is unable to ingest a carbohydrate substance, intravenous administration of glucose or glucagon will be necessary. Glucagon can also be administered subcutaneously or intramuscularly. The Somogyi effect is a complication that may follow a hypoglycaemic episode, and results in rebound hyperglycaemia. Management of this phenomenon involves lowering the insulin dosage.

Hyperglycaemia

Hyperglycaemia, also known as diabetic ketoacidosis, is an abnormally high blood glucose level and an accumulation of ketones in the blood. It may be caused by too little insulin, incorrect diet (e.g., too much carbohydrate), lack of physical activity or stress (with infection being a common stressor). If hyperglycaemia is not corrected, metabolic acidosis occurs, producing vasodilatation and hypotension. Severe acidosis, if untreated, results in coma and death. Hyperglycaemia develops gradually over a period of hours or days, and the early manifestations are thirst, anorexia, nausea, vomiting, abdominal pain, muscle cramps, polyuria and drowsiness. Deep rapid respirations (Kussmaul's breathing) develop in an attempt to control acidosis. Dehydration and electrolyte imbalance occur as a result of osmotic diuresis. Ketones and glucose are excreted in the urine, and the breath smells of ketones (sweet fruity odour).

Management of hyperglycaemia focuses on correcting the fluid and electrolyte imbalances and lowering blood glucose levels to normal. Intravenous fluids such as normal saline are administered together with intravenous short-acting insulin. After the initial decrease in blood glucose level, the insulin dosage is reduced and intravenous dextrose is administered. This allows the blood glucose levels to return to normal more slowly, and prevents the development of hypoglycaemia. If the client becomes comatose as a result of hyperglycaemia and ketoacidosis, care is directed at preventing the complications of unconsciousness.

Long-term complications

Long-term complications of diabetes mellitus involve various body tissues and systems.

Atherosclerosis

Atherosclerosis is a relatively common complication of diabetes mellitus, with coronary artery disease being the major complication. Myocardial infarction, cerebrovascular accident and renal failure are the major causes of death in people with diabetes. Peripheral vascular disease is often widespread, causing manifestations of peripheral ischaemia — cold lower extremities, intermittent claudication, diminished or absent pulses, ulcers, infection and gangrene. If vessels in a leg become occluded, amputation of the limb may be necessary.

Neuropathy

Neuropathy (inflammation and degeneration of the peripheral nerves) gives rise to disturbances of sensation such as tingling and numbness, particularly in the lower limbs. Another form of neuropathy is characterised by a decreased sense of position (proprioceptive disturbances) and diminished sensation to touch, pain and temperature. These sensory deficits increase the possibility of injury and increase the chance of injuries being unnoticed by the individual. Peripheral motor involvement results in muscle weakness and atrophy, which may lead to deformities, particularly of the feet (Charcot's arthropathy).

Retinopathy

Retinopathy is a disorder of retinal blood vessels, characterised by haemorrhages and leakage of blood and serum into the retina. Repeated vitreous haemorrhage may result in retinal detachment or blindness. Cataracts may also develop in the presence of diabetes mellitus.

Nephropathy

Nephropathy may occur over a period of many years, and few signs or symptoms occur until uraemia and oedema develop. Diabetic nephropathy is more likely to develop if diabetes is poorly controlled. Renal function is gradually impaired by glomerulosclerosis, and it may progress to chronic renal failure. Preventing and treating any condition that may impair renal function, such as urinary tract infections or hypertension, reduces the development of diabetic nephropathy.

Impotence

Impotence occurs in about half of all men with diabetes. In addition to the psychological causes of impotence, the condition is thought to be caused by damage to the nerve endings as a result of diabetic neuropathy. Diabetic neuropathy involving the nerves controlling reflex blood flow to the penis appears to result from persistently elevated blood glucose levels. Conversely, low blood glucose levels may be the most common cause of occasional impotence in men with diabetes. Controlling blood glucose levels may therefore help to prevent or alleviate the problem of impotence associated with diabetes.

Education

The person with diabetes mellitus has to learn to accept the condition and the resulting lifestyle changes that need to occur. They need to gain confidence in managing the condition, which requires learning a considerable amount of medical knowledge and technical skills. A well-planned education program helps alleviate anxiety, creates autonomy in management and results in well-managed clients. Involving family members and close friends in the education program also assists the individual. The aims of an education program are that the individual will:

- Accept the condition and understand the importance of good diabetic control
- Acquire the technical skills needed to monitor blood glucose levels and administer medications
- Understand the importance of diet, exercise and medications in maintaining blood glucose levels
- Recognise disturbances of blood glucose levels and the development of complications.

A person with diabetes mellitus should always carry a form of diabetic alert identification with them, such as a card, bracelet or medallion. This ensures that appropriate care will be administered if a medical emergency occurs.

Some nursing diagnoses relating to endocrine disorders are listed in Clinical Interest Box 39.3.

SUMMARY

Apart from the placenta, which is a temporary organ formed to produce hormones during pregnancy, the endocrine system is made up of a number of glands structurally located both independently and within other organs. Endocrine glands secrete chemical substances called hormones directly into the bloodstream. Each hormone has a specific purpose in the body. Each of the glands of the endocrine system is dependent on the other glands in the system to maintain homeostasis in the body.

Disorders of endocrine function can result from genetic defects, neoplasia, obstruction, trauma, autoimmune

CLINICAL INTEREST BOX 39.3
Nursing diagnoses relating to endocrine disorders

- Activity intolerance
- Anxiety
- Growth, risk for altered
- Growth and development, altered
- Infection, risk for
- Skin integrity, risk for impaired

reactions, infection, inflammation or hyperplasia. Diagnostic tests used to assess the functions of an endocrine gland include estimating serum hormone levels, urine tests, scanning and ultrasonography. Medical management and nursing care varies according to the specific disorder. The nursing care is designed to help clients meet all their needs, specifically the need for comfort, psychological support, nutrition and fluids.

Diabetes mellitus is a disorder of blood glucose regulation. Aspects of management of the disorder include diet, exercise, use of insulin or oral hypoglycaemic agents, preventing infection, monitoring blood glucose levels and preventing complications.

REVIEW QUESTIONS

1. What is the difference between tetany and tetanus?
2. Explain the difference between diabetes insipidus and diabetes mellitus.
3. List three situations that could instigate a thyroid storm, or thyroid crisis.
4. The parathyroid glands secrete parathormone. What is the action of this hormone?
5. What hormones are secreted by the pancreatic islets?
6. What is the name of the condition caused by hypoadrenalism?
7. Does gigantism occur before or after epiphyseal closure?
8. Where are the adrenal glands situated and which hormones do they secrete?
9. What is the function of antidiuretic hormone?
10. Describe the two types of diabetes mellitus.

CRITICAL THINKING EXERCISE

Louise, 46, is a community care worker who lives with her trusty Jack Russell, 'Cobber'. She has always maintained a busy lifestyle and has arrived at a medical clinic for assessment, concerned by the gradual onset of several symptoms. She complains of weight gain, an increase of 3.5 kg over the last 3 months. She also conveys to the nurse a feeling of generally 'slowing down', describing symptoms such as constipation, tiredness, an impaired memory and feeling cold despite the warm spring evenings. She speaks slowly, occasionally slurring her words.

On examination, the nurse records a bradycardia of 52 beats per minute, notes the client's dry skin, oedematose eyelids and enlarged tongue. What endocrine disorder is Louise likely to be suffering from?

Louise is started on medication with the aim of normalising her thyroxine levels. If these oral thyroid medications cause her to become hyperthyroid, what signs and symptoms would the nurse educate her to be aware of?

What further education will Louise require to help her cope with the diagnosis?

REFERENCES AND FURTHER READING

Huether SF, McCance KL (2008) *Understanding Pathophysiology*. Mosby, London

LeMone P, Burke KM (eds) (2000) *Medical–Surgical Nursing: Critical Thinking in Client Care*, 2nd edn. Prentice-Hall, Upper Saddle River, NJ

Marieb EN (2006) *Essentials of Human Anatomy and Physiology*, 6th edn. Benjamin Cummings, San Francisco

McDowell JRS, Matth DM (2007) *Diabetes: a Handbook for the Primary Healthcare Worker*. Churchill Livingstone, Edinburgh

Neighbors M, Tannehill-Jones R (2000) *Human Diseases*. Delmar Thomson Learning, Albany

Smeltzer SC, Bare BG (2000) *Brunner and Suddarth's Textbook of Medical Surgical Nursing*, 9th edn. Lippincott, Philadelphia

Thibodeau GA, Patton KT (2007) *Anatomy & Physiology*. Mosby Elsevier, St. Louis

ONLINE RESOURCES

Diabetes Australia: www.diabetesaustralia.com.au

Chapter 40
REPRODUCTIVE HEALTH

OBJECTIVES

- Define the key terms/concepts
- Describe the physiology of the male reproductive system
- Describe the physiology of the female reproductive system
- Examine strategies to promote wellness and maintain optimal reproductive and sexual health
- Consider alterations in health status that affect male and female reproductive systems
- Discuss factors that influence reproduction
- Describe major manifestations of reproductive system disorders
- Explain the purpose of diagnostic tests used to assess reproductive function
- Briefly describe disorders of the female and male reproductive systems outlined in this chapter
- Develop client management strategies for an individual with a reproductive system disorder
- Identify nursing responsibilities in relation to child sexual abuse
- Understand the physical and social implications of sexually transmitted infections

KEY TERMS/CONCEPTS

amenorrhoea
contraception
dysmenorrhoea
dyspareunia
endometriosis
erectile dysfunction
fibroids
gamete intrafallopian transfer (GIFT)
impotence
in vitro fertilisation (IVF)
infertility
myomectomy
Papanicolaou (Pap) test
prostate-specific antigen (PSA)
prostatitis
sexual dysfunction

CHAPTER FOCUS

This chapter explains reproduction and outlines conditions that affect the male and female reproductive systems. The anatomy and physiology of the reproductive system is outlined so that the nurse can recognise common variations and deviations from normal. Factors that contribute to wellness and the maintenance of optimal reproductive health are discussed. The role of the nurse is explored in a variety of primary, secondary and tertiary health care settings. Alterations in health status that occur during illness or disease are correlated with client management strategies.

The reproductive organs of men and women are structured to produce ova and sperm, facilitate fertilisation and create an environment that allows for the growth, development and birth of a baby. Both systems also produce hormones that influence the development of secondary sexual characteristics. The male reproductive system functions to produce, store and introduce mature sperm into the female reproductive tract. The female reproductive system produces ova, receives sperm and allows for fertilisation, implantation, development and birth of the baby. Female reproduction is governed by complex cyclic hormonal changes.

LIVED EXPERIENCE

Judy and her partner had been trying to have a baby for 10 years. They underwent 10 cycles of IVF. During that time Judy had three ectopic pregnancies and two miscarriages. She had two operations (microsurgery) to her fallopian tubes. On the 10th cycle, Judy and her husband decided that this was the final attempt. Judy was 39 years old and she knew that this was her only chance of having a child. Only one ovum was harvested but the IVF procedure was a success. The pregnancy had been achieved but at a great emotional cost to the couple.

Reflecting on the turbulence of the years Judy stated that the struggle to achieve a pregnancy had put a great strain on the couple's relationship. 'I wouldn't advise people to go through it to the extent that we did. You need to be in a very loving relationship where you do things together and you need to be financially stable. It can make or break a relationship. Men don't really talk about what they are going through. I felt that I went through a lot on my own.'

Judy spoke about the denial of infertility — her own and society's. 'I used to say that I didn't really want a child. I did, but it was a kind of defence mechanism. Other people would make comments like "Stop trying so hard, it will happen naturally." With no tubes?'

Judy, age 39

THE MALE REPRODUCTIVE SYSTEM

The male reproductive system (Figure 40.1) consists of essential and accessory organs. The essential organs, or gonads, are the testes. Accessory organs consist of a series of ducts or passageways, supportive sex glands and external structures.

ESSENTIAL ORGANS

The testes are two glands that lie suspended outside the body in the scrotum. First formed in the upper abdominal cavity, they gradually descend into the scrotum before birth. The temperature in the testes is about 1°C below normal body temperature, an important requirement for the normal production of sperm. Each of the testes is divided into 250–300 wedge-shaped lobes, each containing a coiled seminiferous tubule. The tubule consists of a central passageway inside a long duct. Sperm production (spermatogenesis) takes place inside the walls of the tubule. Specialised endocrine cells between the seminiferous tubules (interstitial cells) produce testosterone, the male sex hormone.

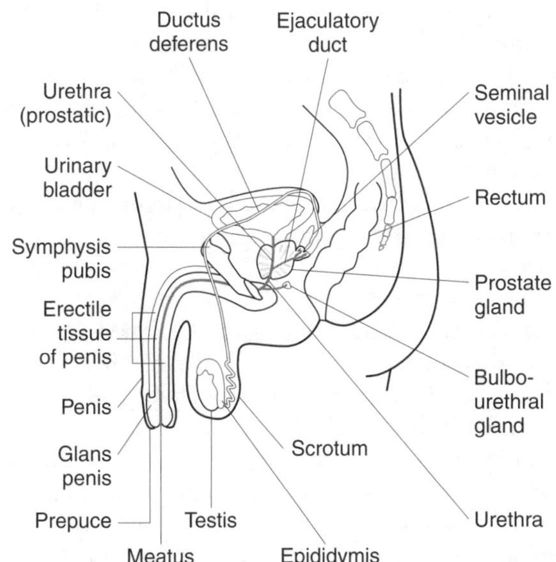

Figure 40.1 | The male reproductive system

SPERMATOGENESIS

Sperm cells, or spermatozoa (Figure 40.2), are produced continuously throughout life from puberty onwards under the influence of the hormones testosterone and follicle-stimulating hormone (FSH). The anterior pituitary gland secretes FSH. Sperm cells originate from primordial cells that appear in the embryo early in gestation but are not functional until puberty. Before puberty the testes produce stem cells called spermatogonia. These cells multiply by mitotic division. At puberty, under the influence of FSH, spermatogonia undergo both mitotic and meiotic cell division, which results in sperm production. A mature sperm consists of a head, mid-piece and tail. The head contains the nucleus, with its genetic material (DNA). The mid-piece contains mitochondria to provide energy for the rapid tail movements. The tail propels the sperm with a lashing movement through the female reproductive tract.

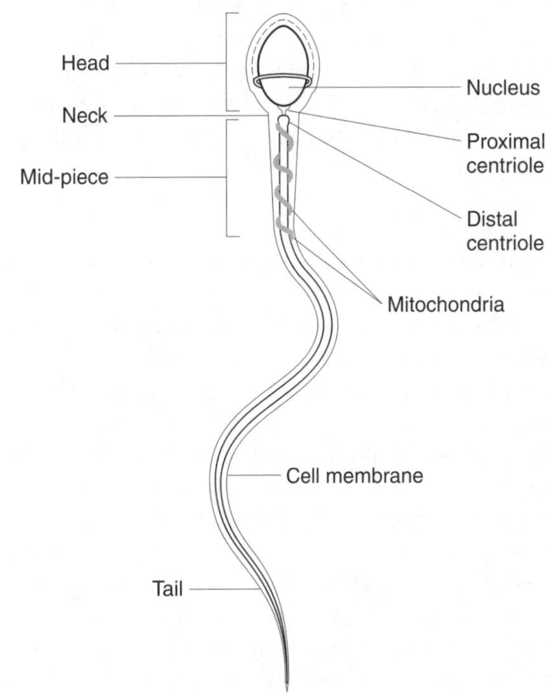

Figure 40.2 | The structure of a sperm cell

TESTOSTERONE PRODUCTION

During puberty, interstitial cells are activated by FSH and interstitial cell-stimulating hormone (ICSH), released by the anterior lobe of the pituitary gland. Testosterone is produced from puberty onwards for the remainder of the male's life. The chief function of testosterone is to stimulate the development of the male reproductive organs and the secondary sexual characteristics, including:

- Deepening of the voice, due to lengthening and thickening of the vocal cords
- Appearance of pubic, axillary and facial hair
- Increased activity of the sebaceous glands
- Broadening of the shoulders, due to increased bone density and a general increase in muscle mass
- Increase in the length and width of the penis, and genital pigmentation.

ACCESSORY ORGANS

The ductal system transports sperm from the testes to outside the body. It is composed bilaterally of the epididymis, the ductus (vas) deferens and ejaculatory duct. The urethra is the single passage for sperm to exit the body during ejaculation. The epididymis, a tightly coiled tube, about 6 m in length, is attached to the posterior portion of the testis. It provides a temporary storage site for immature sperm. Within the epididymis sperm mature and become fully functional.

The vas deferens is the tube that transports sperm from the epididymis to the ejaculatory duct. It passes up through the inguinal canal into the pelvic cavity, over the top and down the posterior side of the bladder. For most of its length it is suspended and contained within the spermatic cord. The vas deferens joins the duct from the seminal vesicle to form the ejaculatory duct. Each ejaculatory duct receives secretions from the seminal vesicles. Sperm and secretions pass through the ejaculatory duct, prostate gland and into the urethra. The urethra passes through the penis and is a passageway for both semen and urine.

ACCESSORY GLANDS

Two seminal vesicles, two bulbourethral (Cowper's) glands and the prostate gland produce secretions to nourish and support the sperm. The seminal vesicles are situated behind the bladder at the base of the prostate gland. They secrete a thick nutritive fluid that contributes to sperm motility and viability and makes up about 60% of the seminal fluid. Situated just below the bladder, the prostate gland encircles the upper part of the urethra. It secretes a thin, milky alkaline fluid that forms about 30–40% of the semen. Alkaline fluid protects against the acid environment of the female vagina and assists sperm motility. The bulbourethral glands are two pea-sized glands on either side of, and opening into, the urethra. They produce a small amount of mucus that neutralises the pH of any residual urine and lubricates the tip of the penis. Semen, or seminal fluid, is the fluid ejaculated by the male and consists of spermatozoa plus secretions from the accessory glands. Sperm are transported through the male reproductive system in semen. The average amount of semen ejaculated is about 3–5 mL, with each millilitre containing about 100 000 000 sperm.

EXTERNAL STRUCTURES

The penis and scrotum are the male external reproductive structures. The penis is a pendulous soft tissue structure attached to the walls of the pubic arch by muscles and ligaments. It has three columns of erectile tissue in the shaft, the central corpus spongiosum and the corpus cavernosa on either side. Skin covering the penis extends from its base to the glans penis, or tip, where it folds inwards and backwards on itself to form the prepuce, or foreskin. When erectile tissue becomes filled with blood during sexual arousal, the penis becomes enlarged, firm and erect. In the erect state the penis can be inserted into the female vagina. During ejaculation, sperm is transported through the male urethra into the vagina.

The scrotum, a thin-walled pouch of skin, is suspended from the groin. The interior is divided into two sacs, each of which contains a testis, an epididymis and a ductal system. Under normal conditions the scrotum hangs loosely, keeping the testes at a temperature suitable for sperm viability. When the external temperature is cold, or during tactile stimulation, the scrotum draws the testes closer to the body.

DISORDERS OF THE MALE REPRODUCTIVE SYSTEM

Many male reproductive disorders are developmental or age related. Abnormalities of the genitourinary system may be present at birth. Congenital or structural defects of the genitourinary tract can cause physical and psychological effects for a child. Both urinary and reproductive function can be compromised. Early corrective surgical treatment is necessary to minimise the possibility of these effects occurring. Nursing interventions aim to provide support for the child and family before and after surgery. The nurse can assist the child and family by educating them about procedures and allowing them time and opportunity to express any fears or concerns. Fact sheets that explain the condition without overuse of medical jargon can be given to parents to reinforce information given by the health care team.

Disorders of the male reproductive system are referred to as genitourinary disorders because of the shared anatomical structures of the urinary and reproductive systems. Common problems, which vary according to the type and severity of the disorder, include alterations in:

- Urinary elimination: the individual may experience alterations in the pattern of urinary elimination, related to urinary tract obstruction and retention. These include dysuria, difficulty in initiating or stopping the flow of urine or acute or chronic retention of urine

- Urethral discharge: this is most commonly associated with sexually transmitted diseases (STDs). Discharge may be thin or thick, scant or profuse, clear or mucoid, yellow, green or purulent
- Sexual dysfunction: sexual dysfunction includes impotence, premature ejaculation, dyspareunia (painful intercourse) and priapism (a state of constant erection not associated with sexual desire).

CONGENITAL DEFECTS

Hypospadias

Hypospadias is a congenital defect in which the urethral opening is on the underside of the penis or, in severe cases, on the perineum. The child is unable to urinate normally. Corrective surgery aims to extend the urethra to a normal position and restore normal reproductive and urinary function.

Epispadias

Epispadias is a congenital defect in which the urethra opens on the upper surface of the penis. Problems and nursing interventions are similar to those in hypospadias. Surgical correction involves penile and urethral lengthening.

Phimosis

Phimosis is narrowing of the foreskin, which may be retracted manually if mild, or by circumcision if severe.

Cryptorchidism

Cryptorchidism (undescended testes) is failure of one or both of the testes to descend into the scrotum. The condition is diagnosed by the absence, on palpation, of one or both of the testes in the scrotum. Inguinal hernias are found in about 50% of cases. Cryptorchidism is associated with an increased incidence of testicular cancer in later life. Surgical placement of the testes in the scrotum (orchiopexy) is performed to preserve sperm-forming cells that require a lower temperature than that of the abdomen. It is done at an early age to lessen concerns about body image.

CANCER OF THE TESTES

Cancer of the testes generally affects males between the ages of 15 and 40. Most cancers are of germ-cell origin. The aetiology of testicular cancer is unknown and therefore precludes preventive strategies being implemented. Hypotheses include early puberty, exposure to environmental oestrogens, occupational exposure and smoking. Known risk factors include a history of cryptorchidism, genitourinary abnormalities, a history of mumps orchitis, white race, high socioeconomic status and family history. Early diagnosis and improved treatment modalities have given a cure rate of over 90%. However, 50% are only diagnosed in the advanced stage, when the cure rate is about 70%. An early stage indicator is the presence of a smooth painless lump in the scrotum. Later metastatic symptoms include general abdominal and inguinal aching. Other metastatic symptoms include bowel or urinary obstruction and abdominal pain.

Diagnostic evaluation is based on physical examination, blood serum markers and scrotal ultrasound. Elevated levels of alpha-fetoprotein (AFP) and human chorionic gonadotrophin (hCG) are present in testicular cancer. Ultrasonography differentiates between a solid and a cystic lesion. Tests to detect potential metastases include chest X-ray and computerised tomography (CT) scans of the chest, abdomen and pelvis.

Management of the client depends on the type and stage of the disease. Chemotherapy is used to treat primary and metastatic tumours. Surgical intervention generally involves a unilateral orchidectomy to remove the testis, tunica and spermatic cord, and retroperitoneal lymph node dissection. Radiotherapy to lymph node pathways is often used after surgery.

Testicular cancer affects young, mostly well men during prime reproductive years. Some treatments can lead to infertility. Sensitivity to the individual's loss and fears about sexuality and mortality are key components of nursing management. The nurse can discuss possible sperm banking and reassure the client that surgery does not diminish virility. The client may be referred to support services outside the hospital and should be educated in testicular self-examination. It is recommended that he carry out periodic examinations, as there is an increased risk of a second tumour occurring.

INFECTIOUS AND INFLAMMATORY DISORDERS

Inflammation and infection of the urethra (urethritis) is generally caused by an ascending infection. A large number of cases are sexually transmitted and are discussed later in this chapter. Non-infective causes are associated with trauma secondary to urethral manipulation such as repeated cystoscopy.

In older men the main causes of epididymitis are bladder outlet obstruction and infection with urinary bacteria such as *Escherichia coli*. Clinical features include painful scrotal swelling, pain along the inguinal canal and vas deferens, a reddened scrotum, fever, chills, pyuria and bacteriuria. A midstream urine sample, urethral discharge culture and expressed prostatic secretions are collected to identify causative organisms. During the acute phase the client is encouraged to rest in bed with the scrotum supported to prevent traction on the spermatic cord, facilitate venous drainage and relieve pain. A scrotal support may be worn. Antibiotics and analgesics are administered. Intermittent ice packs or cold compresses may help decrease swelling and pain. The client is advised to avoid lifting, straining and sexual activity until the infection is completely resolved.

HYDROCELE

Hydrocele is a painless collection of fluid within the tunica vaginalis of the testis from defective or inadequate reabsorption of fluid normally produced within the testis. It causes swelling of the scrotum and may be associated with infections, trauma or tumours. The individual may experience a feeling of heaviness or pain associated with increased scrotal size and may feel embarrassed because of the appearance of the scrotum.

Ultrasound and transillumination are diagnostic tests used to differentiate between hydrocele and other causes such as tumours. If a hydrocele is present, transillumination will allow transmission of light through the scrotum. Treatment is not usually required unless there is compromised testicular circulation. However, a scrotal support can be worn to increase comfort.

VARICOCELE

Varicose veins of the spermatic cord within the scrotum are thought to be due to incompetent venous valves or obstruction of the gonadal vein. The client may experience a 'pulling' sensation, dull ache in the scrotum, pain and scrotal swelling. On palpation the scrotum feels like a 'bag of worms'. Untreated it can decrease sperm count and cause atrophy of the testicle, resulting in infertility.

Surgical treatment involves spermatic vein ligation. It is used to treat younger clients to prevent infertility, or when symptoms are painful. Nursing interventions postoperatively focus on client education and relief of pain and discomfort. Application of intermittent ice packs for the first few hours and wearing a scrotal support reduces oedema and increases comfort. Strenuous activities should be avoided until cleared by the surgeon.

DISORDERS OF THE PROSTATE GLAND

The prostate gland frequently becomes enlarged as a man ages. The three most common prostate problems are prostatitis, benign prostatic hyperplasia and prostate cancer.

Prostatitis

Inflammation of the prostate gland may be bacterial or abacterial. Often the cause is unknown. Bacterial causes are usually associated with *E. coli* urinary tract infections. Clinical manifestations include urinary symptoms of urgency, frequency, nocturia and dysuria. Bacterial prostatitis is characterised by sudden chills and a moderate to high fever. Pain in the perineum, rectum, lower back and during ejaculation are other symptoms. Diagnosis is based upon urine, urethral and prostatic fluid cultures. Digital rectal examination frequently reveals a tender swollen prostate.

Antibiotics and analgesics are administered for bacterial causes. Oral antispasmodic agents may provide relief from urinary frequency and urgency. The nurse can support the client with comfort measures such as salt baths to relax the muscles of the pelvic floor. Stool softeners can reduce pressure on the prostate gland and are given as prescribed. Fluids should be encouraged to mechanically flush out the urinary tract.

Benign prostatic hyperplasia

Benign prostatic hyperplasia (BPH) is enlargement of the prostate gland as a result of small non-cancerous growths inside the prostate that may be related to hormonal changes that occur with ageing. BPH usually does not affect sexual function but does affect urination. As the prostate enlarges it presses against the bladder and the urethra, blocking the flow of urine. Problems include difficulty initiating a urine stream or maintaining more than a dribble, frequency or urgency and nocturia. These problems can be highly distressing because of the embarrassment of hesitancy, frequency, soiling and smell.

Straining to empty the bladder can cause thickening of the bladder wall and loss of elasticity. This can lead to urinary tract infections and eventual renal failure. A completely blocked urethra is a medical emergency requiring immediate catheterisation. Other serious potential complications of BPH include bladder calculi, hydronephrosis and bleeding. Men with mild symptoms may simply be checked at regular intervals and treated if symptoms become worse. More severe symptoms require surgical intervention.

The type of surgery depends on the size of prostate, location of the enlargement, whether surgery on the bladder is also needed, and the client's age and physical condition. The most common surgical procedure is transurethral resection of the prostate (TURP), used in more than 90% of cases. Surgery relieves symptoms quickly, typically doubling the urinary flow within weeks. A fibre-optic scope is passed through the urethra to the prostate. Using either a tiny blade or an electric loop, the surgeon pares away the lining of the urethra and bits of excess prostate tissue to expand the passageway.

Postoperatively the individual is usually hospitalised for several days with a urinary catheter in situ to irrigate the bladder. TURP does not usually affect a man's ability to have an erection or an orgasm, since the nerves that control erection lie outside the prostate and are not touched by the operation. A more common side effect is dry or retrograde ejaculation, which occurs when the neck of the bladder fails to close properly during ejaculation. The result is that semen spurts backwards into the bladder rather than through the penis. Men who experience this side effect still have the sensation of an orgasm but are unable to ejaculate during intercourse.

Transurethral needle ablation (TUNA), which can be done with a local anaesthetic on an outpatient basis, uses radio-frequency energy delivered through needles to kill excess prostate tissue. A catheter that directs the needles towards the obstructing prostate tissue is inserted into the urethra. Some clinical studies have reported that TUNA improves the urine flow, with minimal side effects, compared with other procedures.

Researchers are working to develop BPH treatments that are more effective, less traumatic and have fewer side effects. These include using laser surgery, powerful electric currents and microwaves. Balloon urethroplasty and insertion of a stent into the urethra are other possible options.

Prostate cancer

Prostate cancer tends to grow slowly and may have metastasised before it is detected. Initially the man may be asymptomatic. When symptoms appear, they are often similar to those caused by BPH — difficulty urinating, a weak stream, a frequent urge to urinate, nocturia, painful or burning urination, and haematuria. Because prostate cancer tends to metastasise to the bone, bone pain, particularly in the back, can be another symptom. The major risk factor for prostate cancer is increasing age; more than 75% of prostate cancer cases are diagnosed in men aged 65 or older. Usually the younger the client the more aggressive the cancer.

Diagnostic tests include digital rectal examination, prostate-specific antigen levels, biopsy of the prostate, renal function tests and transrectal ultrasound. Prostate cancer may be treated by radiotherapy, chemotherapy, hormone therapy (palliative) or by open prostatectomy.

PROSTATE SURGERY—PROSTATECTOMY

Open prostatectomy may involve either a radical or partial procedure. A radical prostatectomy that removes the whole prostate is the treatment for cancer of the prostate. The incision is made through either the lower abdomen or the perineum. Impotence is a result of radical prostatectomy, as nerves and muscular tissue that function in penile erection are severed. When possible, nerve-sparing surgery is done to prevent this. The client is hospitalised for about 5–7 days. Partial prostatectomy, which leaves the posterior portion of the prostate intact, is used to treat BPH. The incision for a partial prostatectomy is usually through the suprapubic area of the abdomen. Open prostatectomy is used only when the prostate is extremely large.

Nursing management preoperatively requires establishment of adequate hydration and monitoring of the client's fluid status. Insertion of an indwelling or suprapubic catheter may be necessary to establish urinary output. Alterations in urinary elimination and pain and discomfort related to bladder spasms may have caused the client to limit fluids. The client should be encouraged to drink fluids freely. Bowel preparation may include drinking 2–3 L of a cathartic and an evacuant enema. Postoperatively the nurse should maintain bladder irrigation and drainage, and monitor for clots and haemorrhage.

The client is encouraged to talk about concerns related to urinary control and sexual functioning before discharge from the health care facility. Nurses working in this area need to adopt a holistic approach, including the man's partner in discussions if necessary. Nurses need to recognise that sexual activity does not necessarily stop with age, and nursing care planning and delivery should take account of this. Discharge education needs to take physical and psychosocial factors into consideration.

Discharge education

After a radical prostatectomy, an indwelling urinary catheter (IDC) may remain in situ for about 2 weeks. The client is taught how to manage the IDC at home. They need to maintain a high fluid intake to reduce the risk of clot formation, practise good perineal hygiene to decrease the risk of urinary tract infection, and recognise indicators of catheter blockage, dislodgement or urinary tract infection.

The client is advised that:

- Frequency and burning on urination are common after removal of the indwelling catheter but usually disappear within a few weeks
- Urinary incontinence can follow any type of prostate surgery
- Dribbling and cloudy urine may persist for a period of time
- Perineal exercises assist in regaining urinary control but this may take weeks to achieve
- Sexual functioning is not adversely affected by a simple prostatectomy, but retrograde ejaculation will be experienced
- Sexual activity may be resumed about 6–8 weeks after an open prostatectomy
- There are penile prostheses that may be used to achieve erection after a radical prostatectomy.

CANCER OF THE PENIS

Cancer of the penis is rare in Australia but is more common in south-east Asia, parts of Africa and in India. It is more likely to affect non-circumcised men aged over 60 and may be related to poor personal hygiene. The cancer occurs in the skin of the penis as a painless wart type growth or ulcer. Diagnostic tests include biopsy to confirm the diagnosis, chest X-ray, CT scan and lymph node biopsy to check for metastases. Surgery, internal and external radiation and chemotherapy are used alone or in combination to treat the condition. Surgical procedures can range from circumcision, laser or cryotherapy treatment to partial or total amputation of the penis.

The nurse can provide counselling and emotional support based on the needs of the individual. Education is offered about physical and psychological changes to sexual functioning. Awareness that the client may be affected by many different emotions, including anger, guilt, anxiety and depression, can assist management.

DISORDERS OF MULTIPLE CAUSE

Erectile dysfunction

Erectile dysfunction is defined as the inability to achieve and maintain an erection sufficient to permit satisfactory sexual intercourse. It may result from psychological, neurological, hormonal, arterial or cavernosal impairment or from a combination of these factors. The condition can be classified as psychogenic, organic, or mixed psychogenic and organic. Psychogenic factors may include performance anxiety, lack of arousability, relationship difficulties or mental health disorders such as depression and schizophrenia.

Organic causes of erectile dysfunction

Neurogenic

Decreased libido or difficulty initiating an erection can be due to diseases such as Alzheimer's or Parkinson's disease, cerebrovascular accident and cerebral trauma. In the case of spinal cord injury the degree of erectile dysfunction will depend on the nature of the injury.

Hormonal

A deficiency of androgens or an increase in prolactin secretion can both cause sexual dysfunction.

Vascular

Hypertension is associated with arterial stenotic lesions, while hyperlipidaemia is associated with athero-sclerosis. Both conditions prevent adequate blood supply to the penile artery. Cigarette smoking, diabetes mellitus and pelvic irradiation are other vascular causes of erectile dysfunction. Damage to the common penile artery may be due to blunt trauma to the pelvis or perineum.

Drugs

A variety of drugs is associated with erectile dysfunction, including antipsychotic, antidepressant and anti-hypertensive medications, and drugs that are antagonists to androgens, such as oestrogens and ketoconazole. Cigarette smoking is associated with vasoconstriction and has a contractile effect on the smooth muscle of the corpus cavernosa. Alcohol has varying effects according to the amount consumed. A small amount improves erection and decreases anxiety. Larger amounts can cause central nervous system depression and transient erectile dysfunction. Chronic alcoholism can lead to polyneuropathy and affect penile nerve function.

Systemic diseases and ageing

Sexual function declines with age even in healthy men. The period between sexual stimulation and erection increases, erections are less turgid and ejaculatory force and volume is less. About 50% of men with diabetes mellitus have erectile dysfunction. Other diseases that affect erectile function are chronic renal failure, angina, myocardial infarction and heart failure.

A thorough medical, sexual and psychosocial assessment should be undertaken. Urinalysis, full blood count, and fasting serum glucose, creatinine, cholesterol, triglycerides and testosterone are recommended laboratory tests. Treatment depends upon the cause. It can include a variety of drug therapies, which may be administered orally, transurethrally, or by subcutaneous or intracavernous injection.

ASSESSMENT AND DIAGNOSTIC TESTS

The client may be anxious or embarrassed about the physical examination and discussion of his sexual history. A calm insightful approach is required, as is preservation of the client's individuality and dignity throughout. Cultural and religious customs such as circumcision should be considered.

EXAMINATION OF EXTERNAL GENITALIA

Before the physical examination the client's genitourinary history is obtained. A history of urinary problems may be significant because of the anatomical relationship between reproductive and urinary systems. The external male genitalia and the inguinal canal are inspected for evidence of abnormalities such as penile discharge, tenderness, lesions, swelling, hard lumps or asymmetry. Abnormalities may indicate underlying disorders such as cancer of the testes or the presence of a sexually transmitted infection.

Testicular examination

Testicular self-examination (TSE [see Clinical Interest Box 40.1]) performed on a regular basis is the inspection and palpation of the testes to detect any changes. The testes are examined for size, shape, symmetry and texture. The earlier a change is discovered, the sooner it can be investigated and treated. It is important that the correct technique is taught to men in the target age group (15–40 years). Given that testicular cancer is most widespread in an age

CLINICAL INTEREST BOX 40.1
Client teaching — testicular self-examination

- Testicular self-examination is a quick and simple process. It is often easier after a warm bath or shower, when the skin of the scrotum is relaxed
- Both testes should be checked, one at a time. (Note: it is not unusual for one testis to be slightly larger than the other)
- Using the palm of your hand, support your scrotum. Try to become familiar with the texture and size of each testis. If there is any change to how it feels normally, see your local doctor
- Gently roll one testis between your thumb and fingers to feel for any lumps or swellings in or on the surface of the testis. Repeat with the other testis. A normal testis should be firm but not hard, and should have a smooth regular surface. The testes should be similar in shape, size and consistency
- Using your thumb and fingers, feel along the epididymis at the back of the testis. The epididymis is a soft, tightly coiled tube that carries sperm from the testis to the vas deferens. Check for any swelling in this area
- Even if you have had testicular cancer or are being treated, it is important to still perform a testicular self-examination, as there is about a 5% chance that a testicular cancer may develop in the other testis

group in which men are generally healthy, there may be limited openings to teach TSE. Health promotion and screening in primary care, such as well-man clinics, affords an opportunity for education. Nurses working in the areas of adolescent, student and sexual health are seen as strategic professionals in educating men about TSE. Occupational health nurses involved in work-based screening may also have valuable opportunities to discuss health issues with men.

INTERNAL AND SPECIMEN TESTING

Digital rectal examination

Rectal examination is performed to palpate the prostate gland. The examiner, usually a medical officer, inserts a gloved finger into the anus and palpates the prostate gland for size, shape and firmness. Prostatic secretions for laboratory analysis may be obtained by prostatic massage.

Prostate-specific antigen

Prostate-specific antigen (PSA) is a protein produced by cells of the prostate gland. It circulates in the blood and can be detected and measured with a relatively simple blood test. When the prostate gland enlarges, PSA levels rise. PSA levels can also rise if cancer develops. There is debate concerning whether the PSA test should be used for screening populations of men for prostate cancer in the same manner that breast screening is used to detect breast cancer. Increased levels of PSA do not necessarily indicate prostate cancer. Benign prostatic hyperplasia or prostatitis can also cause increased PSA levels. Only about one in three men with an increased PSA level who have a biopsy will be diagnosed with prostate cancer. Increased PSA testing over the last decade has led to an increase in the number of cases of prostate cancer detected, but no change to the mortality rate. This may be due to the length of time between diagnosis and death (10–15 years).

Transrectal ultrasound

A small probe that emits and picks up high-frequency sound-waves is inserted into the rectum. The reflected waves are detected and a visual image displayed on a monitor. The test does not provide sufficient information to make it a good screening tool by itself but is useful as a follow-up to a suspicious digital rectal examination or PSA test. It is also used to guide biopsies in sampling abnormal areas of the prostate, to estimate the volume of the prostate for calculating PSA density, and to situate radiotherapy implants.

Biopsy

Biopsy of the prostate gland may be performed to detect abnormal cells. A needle is inserted through the perineal skin and a quantity of prostate tissue is aspirated. Biopsy specimens of tissue are sent for cytological examination.

Urethral culture

A small swab is inserted 3–5 cm into the urethra to obtain a specimen for microbiological analysis.

Semen analysis

A sample of semen is obtained and the sperm examined for motility, morphology, quantity and quality.

Urological tests

A series of tests may be performed to evaluate the urinary tract. These include cystoscopy, intravenous pyelogram, urine flow studies, urogram and ultrasound.

Blood samples

Specific blood tests include hormone levels for infertility; alpha-fetoprotein (AFP) and human chorionic gonadotropin (hCG) for testicular cancer; and blood urea nitrogen (BUN), creatinine and urea to evaluate renal function.

NURSING INTERVENTIONS IN MALE REPRODUCTIVE HEALTH

Men have specific health needs, experiences and concerns related to their gender as well as their biological sex. This is a relatively new concept in medical and nursing literature. Psychosocial factors related to male health are poorly understood and frequently ignored by many health practitioners. Men engage in less healthy lifestyles and adopt fewer health-promotion strategies than women, for reasons that are complex. An awareness of men's health issues and poor health practices has led to the establishment of an international men's health movement — the International Society for Men's Health (www.ismh.org/). The aim of the movement is to increase awareness about current men's health issues and promote men's health initiatives.

A man with a reproductive system disorder may experience anxiety about sexual dysfunction, infertility, urinary problems and other implications of the disorder. He may suffer low self-esteem and encounter difficulties in accepting his condition and will often delay seeking health interventions. Nurses need to actively explore opportunities to promote health and to encourage and support men to make healthier lifestyle choices. To make appropriate health and lifestyle choices an individual must be provided with adequate information about his condition and its possible outcomes. He should also be offered opportunities to express his feelings, explore treatment options and, if necessary, be referred for sex counselling.

THE FEMALE REPRODUCTIVE SYSTEM

The female reproductive system functions to secrete hormones, produce ova, receive sperm and allow for fertilisation, implantation, development and birth of the baby. The female reproductive system (Figure 40.3) consists of essential and accessory organs. The essential organs, or gonads, are the ovaries. Accessory organs consist

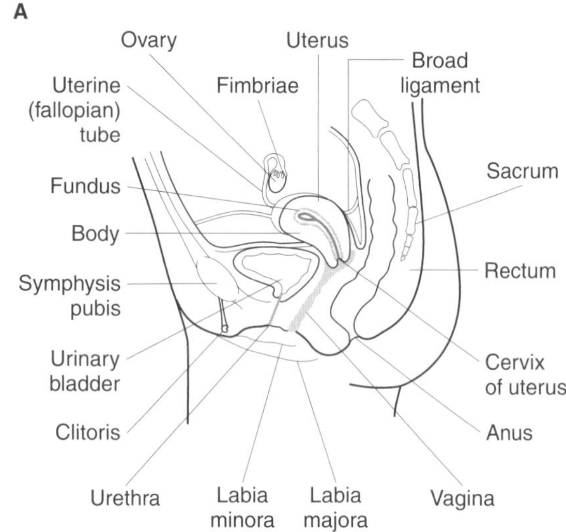

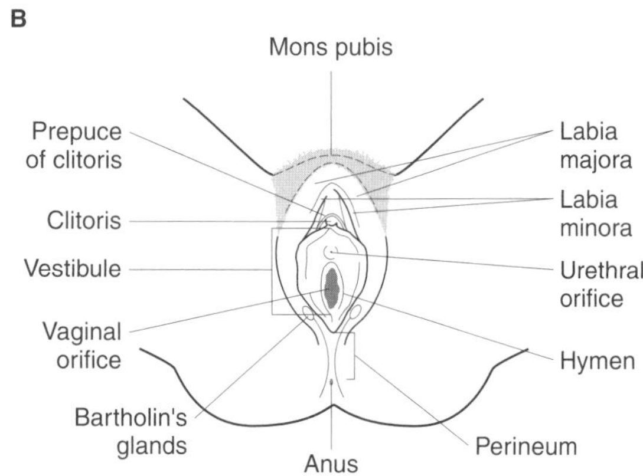

Figure 40.3 | The female reproductive system
A: Sagittal section of the female reproductive system **B**: External genitalia of the female

of a series of ducts, additional sex glands and external structures.

ESSENTIAL ORGANS

The primary sex organs of the female are the ovaries — two almond-shaped organs, one on either side of the uterus and attached by ligaments. Each is composed of an inner portion that contains nerves and lymph vessels, and an outer portion that contains follicles and ova. At birth a female has about two million ovarian follicles in the ovaries. Every follicle contains an immature female gamete called an oocyte. By puberty this number has reduced to about half a million primary follicles. The number decreases throughout the female reproductive years until about the age of 50 (menopause) when there are none. Only about 350–500 of the primary follicles will develop into mature follicles that release ova. Follicles that do not mature are reabsorbed by ovarian tissue.

OOGENESIS

The ovaries function to produce ova (oogenesis) and hormones. The cells of the developing ovarian follicle are stimulated to secrete oestrogen by follicle-stimulating hormone (FSH) from the anterior pituitary gland. Oestrogen enhances the growth and maturation of the follicle. As it matures, the follicle becomes distended with fluid and bulges onto the surface of the ovary. A sharp increase in the level of luteinising hormone (LH) from the anterior pituitary gland acts to trigger ovulation and the mature follicle ruptures to release an ovum. The ovum is released into the peritoneal cavity near the distal end of the uterine tube, where it is captured by the waving fimbriae. Usually one mature ovum is released each month. After ovulation the ovary undergoes structural and chemical changes. Under the influence of LH the ruptured follicle, or corpus luteum, secretes oestrogen and progesterone. If fertilisation does not occur the corpus luteum regresses to a non-functional state, the corpus albicans.

Production of ovarian hormones begins at puberty. Oestrogen influences the development of the female secondary sexual characteristics, including:

- Enlargement of the uterine tubes, uterus, vagina and external genitals
- Development of breasts
- Increased deposits of fat, particularly in the hips and breasts
- Widening of the pelvis
- Onset of the menstrual cycle
- Appearance of pubic and axillary hair.

Oestrogen also stimulates the lining of the uterus to prepare for a fertilised ovum.

The effects of progesterone are to:

- Promote the final preparation of the uterine lining to receive the fertilised ovum
- Inhibit contraction of the walls of the uterus
- Suppress further ovulation
- Stimulate the mammary glands to produce milk.

ACCESSORY ORGANS

Uterine (fallopian) tubes, each about 10 cm long, extend from either side of the upper uterus to the ovaries. The distal end of each tube curves over an ovary and fans out in a trumpet shape with finger like projections (fimbriae). An outer covering of peritoneum, a middle layer of involuntary muscle and an inner lining of ciliated mucous membrane make up the walls of the tubes. Ova are propelled through the tube by peristalsis and the sweeping action of cilia. Fertilisation of the ovum generally occurs in the distal one-third of the uterine tube.

The uterus is a hollow pear-shaped organ located in the pelvic cavity posterior to the urinary bladder and anterior to the rectum. It is suspended in the pelvis by a peritoneal fold (the broad ligament). Normally the uterus is in an anteverted position so that the upper portion rests on the bladder. The uterus consists of an upper rounded body and a lower narrow neck, the cervix. Above the point where the fallopian tubes enter is the fundus of the uterus. The walls of the uterus consist of an outer covering of peritoneum (perimetrium), a middle layer of thick involuntary muscle (myometrium) and an inner lining of mucous membrane (endometrium). The cervix is lined with mucus-secreting glands that provide lubrication. The functions of the uterus are to:

- Receive the fertilised ovum, which embeds itself in the endometrium
- Provide an optimal environment and nourishment for the fetus
- Expel the fetus at the end of pregnancy
- Shed the superficial layer of the endometrium if fertilisation of the ovum does not occur.

The vagina, an expandable passageway about 10 cm long, is situated between the urinary bladder and the rectum. It extends from the uterus to the vulva, where it opens to form the vaginal opening. The cervix projects into the upper part of the anterior vaginal wall. The vagina is acidic from menarche to menopause, and its surface moist from fluid secreted by the vaginal epithelium. Functions of the vagina are to receive the penis during sexual intercourse, provide a passageway for menstrual flow to leave the body, and provide a passageway through which the fetus is expelled from the uterus.

ACCESSORY GLANDS

Mammary glands (Figure 40.4) are accessory glands of the reproductive system. Their reproductive function is lactation. They are situated over the pectoral muscles and are attached to them by Cooper's ligaments. The breast is a complex structure composed of a glandular and ductal network, fat, connective tissue, fascia, blood vessels, nerves and lymphatic vessels. In the centre of the breast a pigmented area, the areola, surrounds the nipple. Each breast contains 15–20 lobes that radiate around the nipple and are separated from each other by adipose tissue. Within the lobes are lobules that contain clusters of milk-producing cells called alveoli. Lactiferous ducts drain the alveoli into openings in the nipple. Breast development at puberty is influenced by ovarian hormones.

EXTERNAL GENITALIA (VULVA)

The external genitalia consists of the mons pubis, labia majora, labia minora, clitoris, perineum, urethral and vaginal orifices, duct of Bartholin's gland and hymen. The mons pubis is a rounded pad of fatty tissue over the symphysis pubis that is covered by pubic hair after puberty. The labia majora are two rounded folds of tissue that shape the lateral boundaries of the vulva to form a protective covering. Their inner surface is smooth and hairless. Surrounded by the labia majora are the labia minora, two long thin folds of tissue. Their surface is smooth and does not contain hair follicles. The urethral and vaginal orifices are enclosed by the labia minora. The hymen, a membranous fold of tissue, surrounds and covers the vaginal orifice. It has an opening to allow menstrual flow to escape. It is usually ruptured when sexual intercourse first occurs. After rupture the hymen appears as irregular projections into the vaginal orifice.

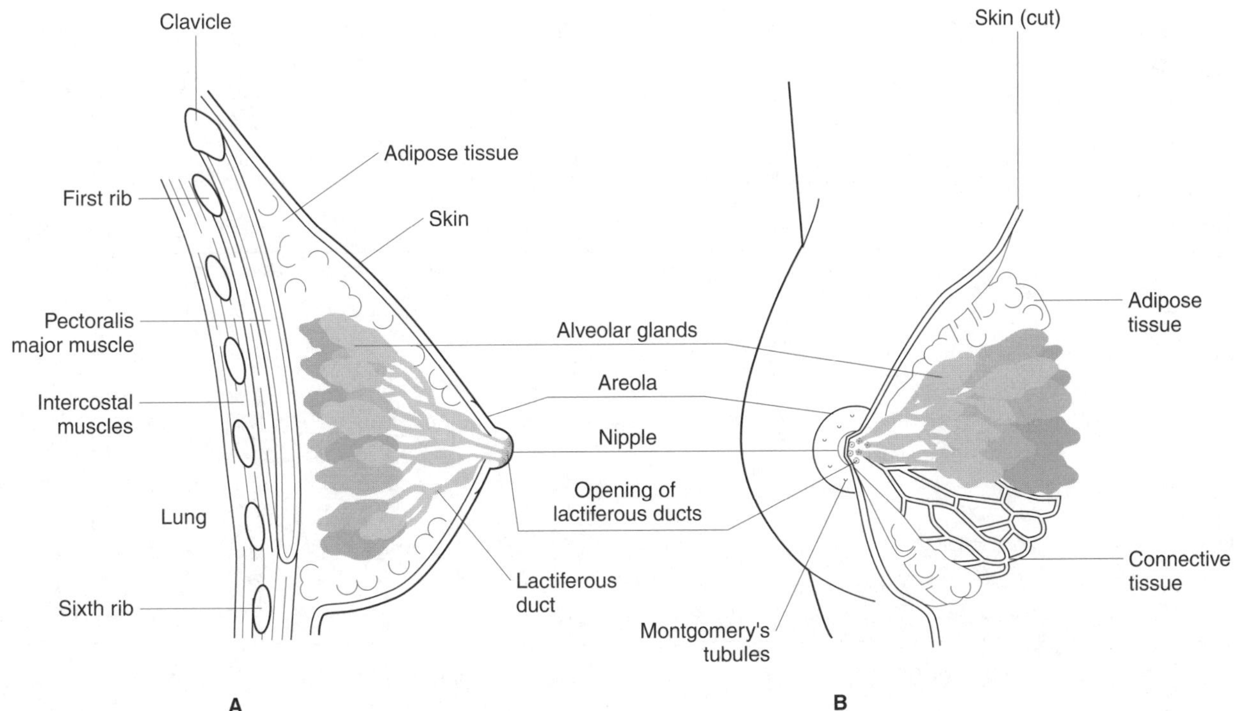

Figure 40.4 | The breast **A**: Sagittal section **B**: Anterior section

The clitoris is an area of erectile tissue about 5–6 mm in length and 6–8 mm in diameter situated between and partly covered by the anterior junction of the labia minora. It contains a large number of free nerve endings, which make it very sensitive to stimulation. Between the vaginal opening and the anus is a muscular layer covered with skin, the perineum.

Bartholin's glands, two small glands situated on either side of the vaginal orifice, secrete mucus to keep the vagina moist. Ducts from the glands open into the space between the labia minora and the vaginal orifice.

THE MENSTRUAL CYCLE

The menstrual cycle consists of a series of cyclic changes occurring at regular intervals, involving the reproductive organs. The average menstrual cycle is about 28 days but may vary from 24 to 35 days (Figure 40.5). It consists of the following three stages.

Days 1–5: Menstruation (menses)

Menstruation occurs if the ovum released during ovulation is not fertilised. The thickened enriched endometrium is not required and the superficial layer of cells, together with extra secretions and blood, is discharged from the uterus.

Days 6–14: Follicular stage and ovulation

After menses the endometrium is repaired under the influence of oestrogens produced by the growing follicles of the ovaries. Another ovarian follicle in the ovary ripens and the ovum begins to mature. The mature ovum ruptures through the surface of the ovary at about the 14th day (ovulation), and the ovum is discharged into the pelvic cavity. Ovulation occurs in response to a release of LH from the anterior lobe of the pituitary gland.

Days 15–28: Premenstrual (secretory) stage

The endometrium is once again prepared to receive a fertilised ovum. Rising levels of progesterone, and oestrogen produced by the corpus luteum, increase the blood supply to the endometrium. Progesterone also causes the endometrial glands to increase in size and to begin secreting nutrients into the uterine cavity.

Unless fertilisation occurs, the corpus luteum begins to regress and secretion of oestrogen and progesterone decreases. The decrease of ovarian hormones in the blood causes the blood vessels supplying the endometrium to go into spasm. When deprived of oxygen and nutrients, the endometrial cells begin to die, the endometrium is sloughed off, and the menstrual cycle begins again.

DISORDERS OF THE FEMALE REPRODUCTIVE SYSTEM

COMMON DISORDERS

Female reproductive disorders are frequently characterised by bleeding, pain, vaginal discharge, pruritus, urinary problems, and breast changes.

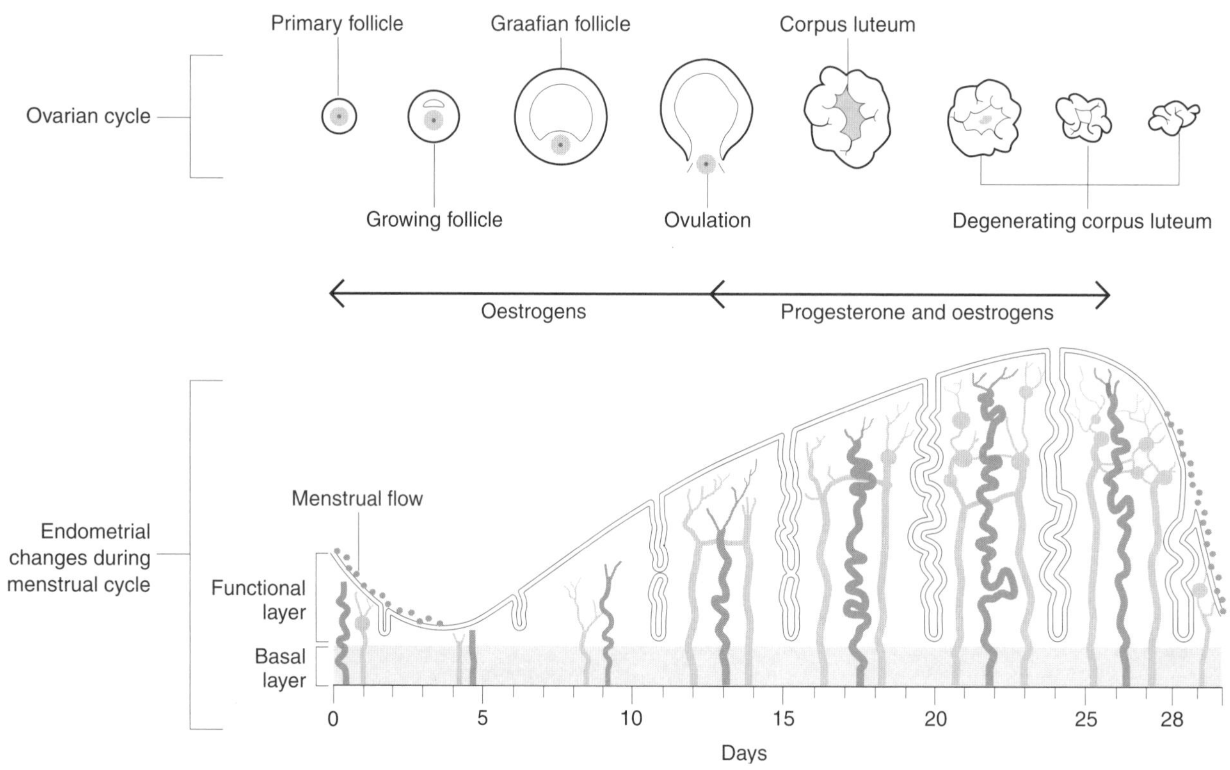

Figure 40.5 | The menstrual cycle

Bleeding

Amenorrhoea is absence of menstruation. It is normal before puberty, during pregnancy and after menopause. Secondary amenorrhoea generally results from anovulation due to hormonal dysfunction.

Excessive and/or prolonged bleeding (menorrhagia) is associated with erosive lesions, endometrial hyperplasia, bleeding disorders or neoplasms (tumours). Postmenopausal bleeding may result from the administration of oestrogen (hormone replacement therapy [HRT]), from an oestrogen-producing ovarian neoplasm, uterine hyperplasia or carcinoma, or vaginitis. Metrorrhagia, or intermenstrual bleeding, can occur at the time of ovulation, or it may be due to factors such as hormonal imbalance or neoplasms.

Pain

Dysmenorrhoea (painful menstruation) is the most commonly experienced type of pain in women. Usually perceived as intermittent, cramping lower abdominal pain, it can radiate to the back, thighs and groin. Some women may experience abdominal distension, painful breasts, headaches, nausea and vomiting. Dysmenorrhoea can be secondary to endometriosis, uterine fibroids or pelvic inflammatory disease (PID).

Abdominal or lower back pain occurring at times other than menstruation may be due to infection, inflammation or neoplasms. Intense lower abdominal pain of sudden onset may arise from torsion of an ovarian cyst or a ruptured ectopic pregnancy. If blood from the ruptured fallopian tube tracks to the diaphragm and stimulates the phrenic nerve, shoulder-tip pain may be evident.

Causes of pelvic pain include chronic inflammation, infection, pelvic congestion, ovulation, ovarian or uterine neoplasms, or ectopic pregnancy. Vaginal or vulval lesions are associated with local pain.

Pain associated with sexual intercourse (dyspareunia) is symptomatic of vaginal or vulval infections, endometriosis, neoplasms or PID. Decreased vaginal lubrication is a common cause of dyspareunia.

Painful breasts may be caused by congestion, inflammation, hyperplasia or neoplasms.

Vaginal discharge

Normal vaginal discharge is clear or white. Deviations from normal include an offensive odour or a change in character or amount of discharge. Vaginal and vulval irritation and pruritus may also be present. The most common cause of abnormal vaginal discharge is infection of the vagina or cervix.

Pruritus

A distressing, itching sensation of the vulva, pruritus may be symptomatic of contact dermatitis or vaginal infection.

Urinary problems

The most common urinary problems associated with reproductive system disorders are dysuria and stress incontinence. Infection, cystocele, and pressure from a pelvic neoplasm are possible causal factors.

Breast changes

Deviations from normal include a discharge from the nipple, pain or tenderness in the breasts, the presence of lumps or masses, nipple inversion and dimpling of the skin.

DISORDERS OF EXTERNAL GENITALIA

Cancer of the vulva develops from premalignant hyperplasia, and is more common in elderly women. It is characterised by vulval pruritus, a history of chronic vulvitis, and the presence of raised grey–white patches on the vulva.

Infectious and inflammatory disorders

Vulvovaginitis is inflammation of the vulva and vagina. Because of their relative anatomical positions, inflammation of one generally causes inflammation of the other. Causes of vaginitis include infection, vaginal mucosal atrophy, vulval atrophy, chemical irritants and poor personal hygiene. Yeast infection results from the presence of *Candida albicans* in mucous membranes and on the skin. Under certain circumstances overgrowth and infection can occur. Predisposing factors include diabetes mellitus, pregnancy, broad-spectrum antibiotic therapy and the use of oral contraceptives. Clinical indicators include pruritus and a thick, white vaginal discharge. Haemophilus vaginitis is caused by the bacterium *Haemophilus vaginalis*. This type of vaginitis is generally mild, with less severe pruritus than occurs in other infections. Genital herpes and infections with *Chlamydia trachomatis*, *Trichomonas vaginalis*, *Gardnerella vaginalis* or *Neisseria gonorrhoeae* are STDs that are sometimes characterised by vaginitis.

DISORDERS OF THE INTERNAL REPRODUCTIVE ORGANS

Pelvic inflammatory disease (PID)

Pelvic inflammatory disease (PID) is any acute, subacute, recurrent or chronic infection of the uterus and uterine tubes that can extend into the pelvic cavity. PID has many causes, including infection with *Neisseria gonorrhoeae* and *Chlamydia trachomatis*. It can result from microorganisms normally present in the cervix and vagina that are not sexually transmitted. PID can vary from mild to severe, with salpingitis being the most common finding. Abdominal pain, menorrhagia, metrorrhagia, increased vaginal discharge, and slight pyrexia are other clinical findings. Treatment includes administration of antibiotics, analgesics and antipyretics. The woman should be assisted into a position of comfort to facilitate drainage of vaginal discharge. She is informed about the importance of regular perineal hygiene and assisted with perineal care if necessary. Perineal cleansing may be provided by pouring warmed solution over the vulva and perineum, and gently cleaning the area from front to back to avoid cross-contamination from the rectal area to the vagina and urethra. The area is gently patted dry and a clean pad applied. Any vaginal discharge or bleeding or offensive odour is noted. All women should be counselled about potential complications of PID, as these include chronic abdominal pain, ectopic pregnancy and infertility. The possible impact on fertility may be significant if the woman is planning to have children.

Benign or malignant tumours (neoplasms)

Benign ovarian tumours are a group of disorders that can develop in the ovaries and uterus and include cysts and fibromas. Depending on type, the tumour may contain fluid or solid material. There may be no symptoms until the tumour enlarges and presses on other structures, ruptures or becomes twisted. Large or multiple cysts may cause pelvic discomfort or abnormal uterine bleeding secondary to disrupted ovulation. Rupture or torsion causes abdominal pain, distension and rigidity.

Benign uterine tumours are called leiomyomas, or fibroids. They are the most common condition affecting the female reproductive system and occur in about a quarter of all women before age 40. Composed of smooth muscle cells and connective tissue, and generally multiple, they may be submucous, interstitial or subserous. While the precise cause is unknown, it is thought that formation of fibroids is hormonally influenced, as they tend to decrease in size or disappear after menopause. Many women do not have symptoms but others experience dysmenorrhoea, menorrhagia, a feeling of heaviness in the pelvic region, frequency of micturition and an enlarged irregular uterus. Medical treatment includes the use of non-steroidal anti-inflammatory drugs for pelvic pain. Hormone therapy can be used to control heavy bleeding. Fibroids are removed surgically through myomectomy or hysterectomy.

Advances in radiological techniques have resulted in an alternative technique to surgery. Arterial embolisation of uterine fibroids involves the radiologist occluding the vascular supply to the fibroids. Preoperative preparation requires counselling and education about possible postoperative pain, which is common after this procedure. Preoperative analgesia and sedation are usually administered, and vital signs, ECG and arterial oxygenation saturation are monitored throughout.

Uterine cancer may originate in the cervix or endometrium. Cervical cancer is one of the most common cancers in women and may be one of two types: squamous cell carcinoma or adenocarcinoma. Cervical cancer begins as a change in the epithelial covering of the cervix and, if not treated, eventually involves the epithelial layer. Invasive carcinoma extends beyond the surface, involves the body of the cervix, and may spread via the lymphatic system to surrounding structures. Clinical signs of cervical cancer do not appear in the early stages. Later manifestations are 'spotting' between menstruation, postmenopausal bleeding, bleeding after sexual intercourse or a brown vaginal discharge. See Clinical Interest Box 40.2 for information on the Australian government program for HPV vaccination.

CLINICAL INTEREST BOX 40.2
National HPV Vaccination Program

Starting in April 2007, the Australian government will be providing the new vaccine free to girls aged between 12 and 13 through the National HPV Vaccination Program on an ongoing basis. There will also be a two-year period where the vaccine will be provided free for girls and young women aged between 14–26 years.

- For girls in school, the program will start in April and parents will be asked to give consent for their daughters to participate in the program. By the end of 2008, all girls currently aged between 12–18 years will have had access to the vaccine in school. In some states and territories, the vaccination program may be staggered, so that some schoolgirls are vaccinated in 2007 and the rest in 2008.
- For young women who are not in school and are still under 27 years, GPs and community immunisation clinics will provide the free vaccine from July 2007 until the end of June 2009.

The vaccine will be given in a series of three injections, spread out over a six month period.
(Department of Health & Ageing (2007)

Endometrial cancer is less common and usually affects women over 50. Abnormal vaginal bleeding, which may initially present as a watery discharge, is a significant finding.

Ovarian cancer is difficult to detect in the early stages and so is often not discovered until metastases are present. Sometimes the woman may experience an increase in abdominal girth due to ascites. Women are being made more aware about the risks of ovarian cancer and it is high on the agenda of women's health issues.

Women who have malignant neoplasms may be treated by chemotherapy, radiotherapy, surgery or a combination of these treatments. Nurses who work in gynaecology oncology units need to provide gender-sensitive care as well as specialist cancer care.

Hysterectomy is the surgical removal of the uterus. It is carried out for a variety of gynaecological conditions. About 15% of hysterectomies are carried out for cancer of the uterus, ovaries or cervix. Other indications include conditions that have not responded to more conservative treatments. Dysfunctional uterine bleeding, menorrhagia, leiomyomas, endometriosis, PID and uterine prolapse can be treated by hysterectomy if other treatment has failed. Various surgical options are available, depending on the indications for surgery. Hysterectomy may be performed through the abdomen or vagina. Laparoscopic surgery is associated with a faster recovery time and fewer postoperative complications. Client interventions for different types of surgery are outlined in Table 40.1.

The client is informed about what the surgery involves — the structures that are to be removed and the structures that will remain intact. Specific education is related to the type of operative procedure. The woman should be aware of the presence of vaginal packs, indwelling urinary catheters, wound dressings or drainage systems in the postoperative period. She should be advised on postoperative strategies to prevent complications.

A vaginal pack may be inserted after a vaginal hysterectomy to control bleeding. It is generally left in place for 24 hours. The nurse assesses the client for vaginal fluid loss through the pack and for any difficulty voiding. As removal of a pack generally causes discomfort, a prescribed analgesic medication is administered before removal. Removal of the pack is documented and the client assessed for vaginal bleeding or discharge.

Specific bladder management may include caring for the client with an indwelling urinary catheter, bladder scanning to assess residual urine, and re-establishing a normal voiding pattern. After most major gynaecological surgery, the client's bladder is continuously drained via an indwelling catheter for 3–5 days to prevent pain, dysuria, distension and infection. After this time the catheter may be clamped for 3–4 hours then released. A schedule of clamping and releasing may be continued for 24–48 hours before removal of the catheter. This assists in re-establishing normal bladder sensation and function.

Some women may experience difficulty voiding after catheter removal because of oedema and discomfort associated with surgery. The amount of residual urine may be estimated using a bladder scanner immediately after the individual has voided. This technique is generally discontinued when the residual urine is less than 100 mL on two consecutive occasions. Alternatively, a suprapubic catheter may be used. The catheter is inserted at the time of surgery, and is not removed until the individual is voiding normally.

Specific bowel management is directed at preventing constipation. This is generally achieved by providing

TABLE 40.1 | TYPES OF HYSTERECTOMY

Surgery	Description of procedure	Client interventions
Total hysterectomy	Removal of uterus and cervix through a horizontal incision just above the pubic bone (bikini line). A vertical lower abdominal incision can be used if the uterus is bulky or there is a previous scar	Psychological preparation and education is essential for the women undergoing any type of hysterectomy. She may feel a loss of femininity and self-image and may no longer feel like she is a real woman. Many women feel that they will be altered sexually and will be less attractive to their partner. The nurse can offer support, discussion and counselling Postoperative interventions include wound management of the abdominal incision and care of an indwelling urinary catheter
Subtotal hysterectomy	The uterus is removed without removal of the cervix	As for total hysterectomy The woman should be educated about the need to continue regular Pap tests
Bilateral salpingo-oophorectomy (BSO)	Removal of the fallopian tubes and ovaries. May be carried out at the same time as hysterectomy. Healthy ovaries may be conserved in premenopausal women	As for total hysterectomy If ovaries are conserved the woman may still experience cyclic changes such as breast tenderness, bloating, irritability or depression. If ovaries are removed she will experience menopause and may require hormone replacement therapy (HRT)
Radical hysterectomy	Uterus, ovaries, fallopian tubes, broad ligaments, surrounding tissue, pelvic lymph glands and upper third of the vagina are removed. Healthy ovaries may be conserved in premenopausal women	As for total hysterectomy Counselling and support related to fear of death and dying as well as loss of reproductive capacity. Educate the client about cyclic hormonal changes if ovaries are conserved. Chemotherapy and radiotherapy may also be given before and/or after surgery
Vaginal hysterectomy	The uterus is removed through the vagina. Usually carried out for uterine prolapse. Contraindicated for malignancy or a bulky uterus. May be accompanied by vaginal repair to strengthen and repair vaginal walls	The woman may have a vaginal pack in situ for 1–2 days. She should be educated about management of a suprapubic catheter, including 'clamp and release' protocol and estimation of residual urine The importance of long-term regular pelvic floor exercises should be discussed and explained
Laparoscopic hysterectomy	The uterus is removed through keyhole incisions. The cervix is not usually removed	Less time is spent in hospital. Ensure client education about the need to continue regular Pap tests

adequate fluid and fibre intake, encouraging ambulation and by administering any prescribed medications.

Nursing management of a client after a hysterectomy may involve wound care and the prevention of post-operative complications. It is important that the woman is helped to realise that loss of part of the reproductive tract does not mean loss of femininity or sexuality. However, psycho-social interventions must incorporate sensitivity to the individual and cultural implications of the loss of child-bearing ability.

Before discharge from hospital the woman is educated about follow-up care that may be required. She is informed about what to expect after surgery and how to recognise deviations from normal. Any restrictions on activities, including sexual activity, are carefully explained.

CONDITIONS OF MULTIPLE CAUSE

Throughout their adult lives, many women are affected by a variety of benign disorders of the reproductive organs that are often painful and debilitating. The main symptoms experienced are dysmenorrhoea, dyspareunia, menorrhagia and chronic abdominal or pelvic pain. Investigations often reveal an underlying cause but in many cases there is no obvious medical reason. Most women with gynaecological symptoms can be treated with a range of medical and surgical interventions.

Premenstrual syndrome

This is a collection of symptoms that occur about 4–7 days before menstruation and which subside with the onset of menstruation. Although the precise cause is unclear, symptoms are related to transient fluid retention. Women may experience oedema of the legs and fingers, abdominal distension, breast tenderness, headaches and mood changes.

Endometriosis

Endometriosis is the presence of functioning endometrium outside the lining of the uterus, usually confined to areas in the pelvic cavity. The cause is unknown, but research suggests that some endometrium is expelled from the uterus into the pelvic cavity, at the time of menstruation. The principal indicators of endometriosis are pelvic pain and infertility. Women will seek interventions based on one or both problems. Medical treatments focus on altering the menstrual cycle through hormonal manipulation. The aim is to produce a pseudo-pregnancy, pseudo-menopause or persistent anovulation, thereby creating an environment in which the endometrium does not grow or is not maintained. The ectopic endometrial tissue will not be subject to the normal menstrual cycle stimulation and the pain associated with endometriosis will be diminished.

Surgical treatment is also widely used to treat endometriosis. The conservative option is removal of all obvious ectopic endometrial implants from the abdomen and pelvis. A laparotomy or laparoscopy is performed, with the latter approach having a lower cost and recovery time. Endometrial tissue is destroyed using a variety of techniques, including vaporisation or excision. Surgery to remove all endometrial tissue involves removal of the ovaries and sometimes the uterus. Treatment for endometriosis is aimed at the ectopic implants but the symptoms can be managed directly. Non-steroidal anti-inflammatory drugs have proved to be of benefit as first-line treatment. Surgical intervention to interrupt neural pathways for pain conduction may be of benefit in selected cases. Clinical Interest Box 40.3 looks at treatment of infertility associated with endometriosis.

DEGENERATIVE DISORDERS

Menopause

Menopause is not a disorder but a natural event — the result of declining ovarian hormone production and function, which usually occurs between age 45 and 55. Menopause is the cessation of ovarian activity and menstruation. It may result in uncomfortable symptoms for the woman. Some women have no symptoms, apart from a halting of menstruation, while others experience a variety of symptoms including irregular menstruation, hot flushes, night sweats, palpitations, vaginal dryness, tiredness, crawling sensation of the skin and mood changes.

After menopause a lack of ovarian hormones may lead to osteoporosis, stress incontinence and uterine prolapse. Symptom relief may be accomplished with hormone replacement therapy (HRT). However, some scientific studies have shown an increased risk of breast and ovarian cancer associated with HRT. Natural or complementary therapies such as phyto-oestrogens and isoflavones found in soy products, black cohosh, vitamin E, dong quai, liquorice, chaste tree berry, evening primrose oil and wild yam cream

CLINICAL INTEREST BOX 40.3
Treatment of infertility associated with endometriosis

The results of a meta-analysis of trials of drug therapy for infertility associated with endometriosis indicated that none of the medical therapies commonly used to treat infertility associated with endometriosis were any better than one another or even the placebos used in the trials. There appears to be no role for drug therapy in the treatment of infertility associated with endometriosis.

Endometriosis that is severe enough to cause distortion of the pelvis may be treated surgically. Although there are no randomised trials to support fertility outcomes, numerous uncontrolled trials have shown that pregnancies do occur after surgical treatment for severe endometriosis. For women with early-stage endometriosis a meta-analysis of non-randomised trials of surgical treatment for infertility suggested it may be of some value. In vitro fertilisation may be a more effective option for infertility associated with endometriosis than repeated surgical intervention.

(Olive & Pritts 2001)

(known as a natural progesterone cream) have been reported to give symptomatic relief. However, scientific evidence of their effectiveness is lacking.

Pelvic floor problems

Childbirth and conditions that lead to sustained increased intra-abdominal pressure cause stretching of the cardinal ligaments and the pelvic floor muscles. The bladder, bowel and uterus are not supported adequately and shift downwards. Uterine prolapse is collapse of the uterus through the genital tract. It is classified according to degree of prolapse. First degree is descent of the cervix to the vaginal opening. Second degree is protrusion of the cervix through the vaginal opening. Third degree (procidentia) is prolapse of the entire uterus through the vaginal opening. The uterus may ulcerate and become infected. Women will experience problems depending on the degree of prolapse, including backache, a 'bearing-down' sensation, cervical erosion, and bleeding and urinary difficulties.

Stress incontinence of urine, urinary tract infections and pelvic pressure are symptomatic of a cystocele, which is herniation of the posterior aspect of the bladder into the vagina. A rectocele is herniation of the rectum into the posterior vaginal wall. There is often a feeling of rectal fullness, faecal urgency and incomplete defecation.

Initial management aims to strengthen the pelvic floor. The woman is encouraged to perform pelvic floor exercises, which are isometric exercises involving a series of voluntary contractions of the pelvic floor muscles and perineum. Exercises are designed to strengthen the pelvic floor and to promote muscle tone. If performed regularly they also help to minimise stress incontinence of urine. The exercise regimen consists of tightening then relaxing the muscles surrounding the entrances of the vagina, urethra and anus. Generally the muscles should be tightened and held for 5 seconds, followed by 10 seconds of relaxation. Alternating tightening and relaxation are repeated several times at various intervals throughout the day. There are various devices that may be used in conjunction with pelvic floor exercises to retrain the muscles. Surgical intervention may be carried out if symptoms are causing distress for the woman. These include hysterectomy for uterine prolapse and surgical repair of the anterior or posterior vaginal walls (or both) for cystocele and rectocele.

TRAUMATIC DISORDERS

A fistula, which is an abnormal passage from an internal organ to the body surface or between two internal organs, may develop in the female reproductive tract. Most fistulae occur after trauma to the reproductive tract or bladder but may also be caused by infection, malignancy or radiotherapy. Fistulae may develop between the bladder and vagina and, less commonly, between the rectum and vagina or between the bladder and uterus. Leakage of urine or faeces into the vagina is distressing and uncomfortable for the woman. It may act as a consistent reminder of her condition. Constant soiling, odour and incontinence may lead to depression and social withdrawal. Urinary tract infections are common and compound urinary difficulties already present. Surgical repair may be indicated. Palliative care should address pain management and odour control to increase comfort and enhance self-esteem. Preservation of client dignity can be assisted by the use of age appropriate incontinence devices, changed regularly to reduce odour and decrease the incidence of skin breakdown.

ASSESSMENT AND DIAGNOSTIC TESTS

Anxiety or embarrassment about the physical examination and discussion of the client's sexual history necessitates an empathic approach by the nurse. The presence of a female nurse during an examination by a male health practitioner is mandatory in many health care facilities. Social and cultural considerations include the provision of clinics for specific groups such as adolescents or women from a non-English speaking background.

EXTERNAL EXAMINATIONS

Hysterosalpingogram

Hysterosalpingogram is a radiological examination performed to visualise the uterine cavity and uterine tubes. The procedure involves taking X-ray films as contrast medium flows through the uterus and uterine tubes.

Ultrasonography

Ultrasonography is the generation of high-frequency sound waves that are reflected to a transducer and converted into electrical energy to form images on a screen. Pelvic ultrasonography is to be used to evaluate symptoms of pelvic disease or to monitor a pregnancy.

Breast examination

Examination of the breasts, or breast familiarisation, is the best method of detecting early breast changes. By examining her breasts regularly, a woman is generally able to determine what is normal and to recognise any changes that occur. The earlier a breast lump or other change is detected, the sooner it can be investigated and treated. Although the presence of any breast lump is frightening, about 90% of lumps are not malignant. Breast examination should be performed after each menstrual period (or monthly after menopause). Breast self-examination can be carried out using the following steps:

1. Careful inspection, in front of a mirror, of each breast. Breasts are assessed for symmetry in size and shape, puckering or dimpling of the skin, retraction of the nipple and any nipple discharge. Breasts should be inspected with the arms by the sides, with the arms raised over the head, and thrusting the breasts forward with the hands on the hips
2. Methodical palpation of each breast in the shower and when lying down. Breasts are palpated using

a small circular movement to detect any lumps or thickening. The three patterns used in breast palpation are strips, quadrants, and circles. Whichever approach is used the entire breast, including the axillary tail, is thoroughly assessed. The woman lies down on a flat surface, with a small pillow or folded towel under the shoulder on the same side as the breast to be palpated.

The procedure is outlined in Figures 40.6 to 40.10.

Mammography

Mammography is a radiographic technique used to detect breast changes, particularly those not palpable on physical examination. It is recommended that all women aged 50–69 have a mammogram every 2 years. Recent research indicates that it may be beneficial to screen women from age 40.

Breast ultrasound

Breast ultrasound is used in several ways. Its most common application is to investigate a specific area of the breast when a problem is suspected. A palpable lump and/or an abnormality discovered on a mammogram can be further evaluated by ultrasound. It is especially helpful in

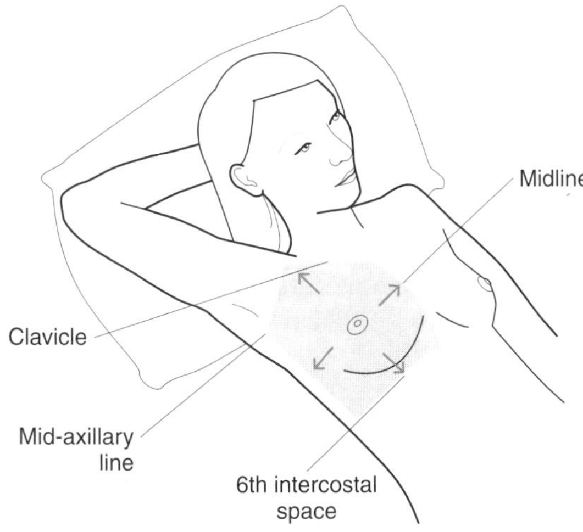

Figure 40.6 | Breast self-examination: boundaries of area to be examined

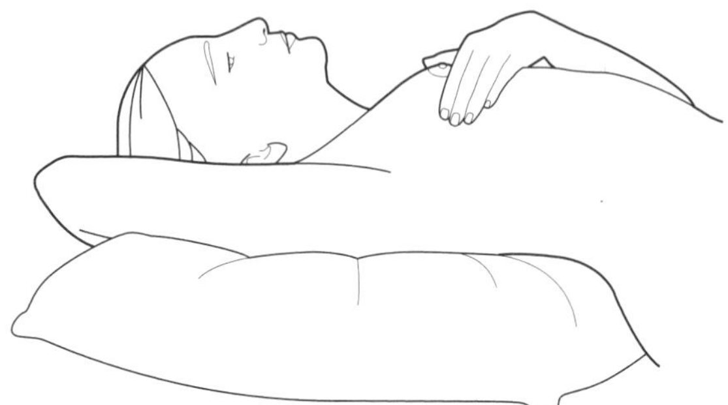

Figure 40.7 | Breast self-examination: lying down position

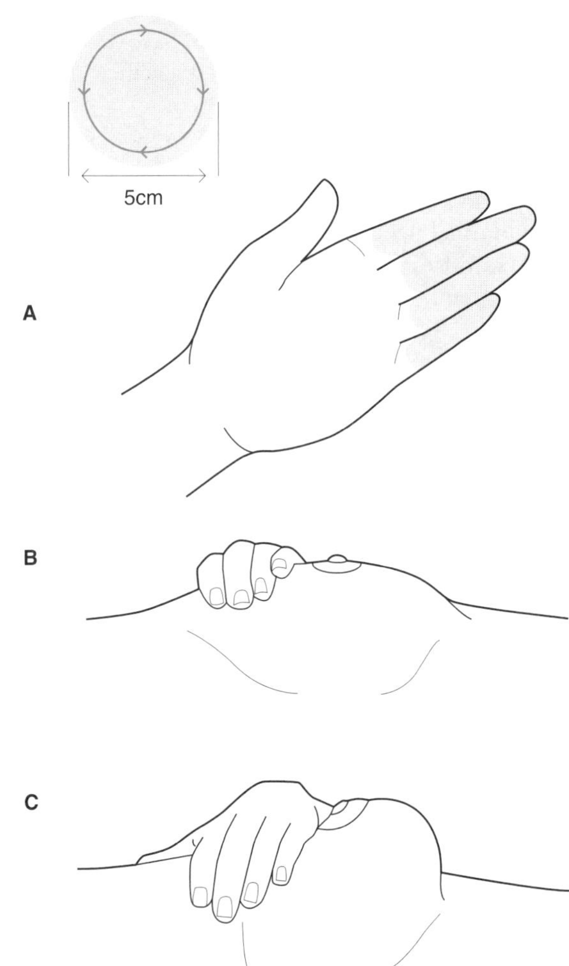

Figure 40.8 | Breast self-examination **A**: Area of fingers and circular movement used for palpation **B**, **C**: Both light and firm pressure should be used in palpation

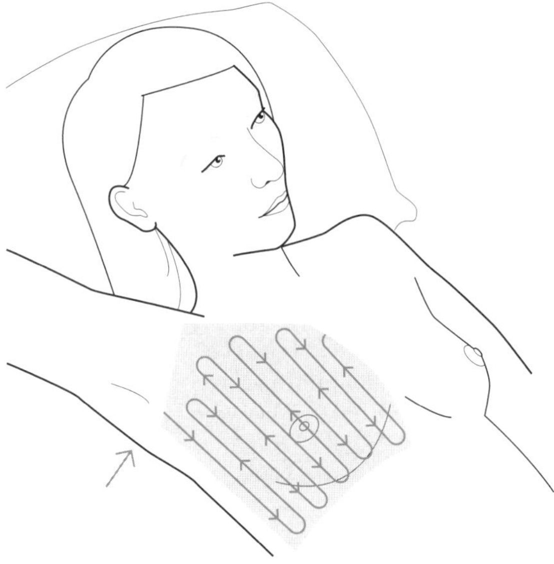

Figure 40.9 | Breast self-examination: vertical strip pattern of palpation. The large arrow indicates the starting point

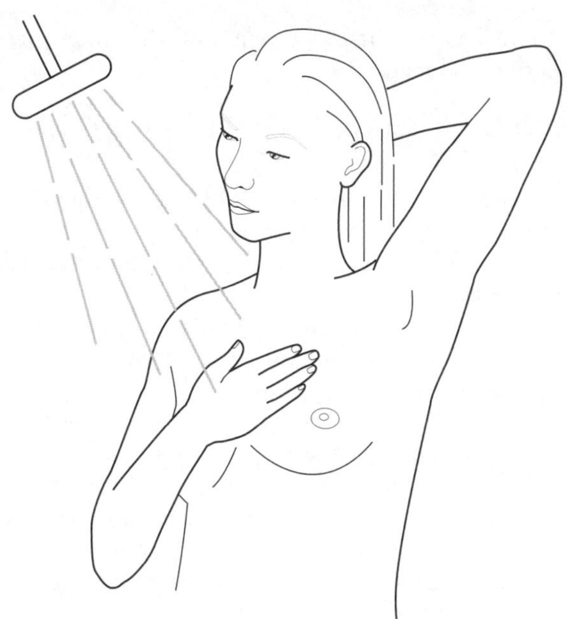

Figure 40.10 | Breast self-examination. Small firm breasts can be satisfactorily examined with a soapy hand while standing in the shower recess, with one arm raised on the side being examined

distinguishing between a fluid-filled cyst and a solid mass. Often it is the first study performed to evaluate masses in women under 35, whose mammograms can be difficult to interpret. It is ideal for studying breast abnormalities in pregnant women. Breast ultrasound is used to observe and guide a needle for several interventional procedures, including cyst aspiration, fine-needle aspiration, large-core needle biopsy and needle localisation before surgical breast biopsy.

INTERNAL EXAMINATIONS AND SAMPLING

Pelvic examination

Internal examination of the vagina and cervix may be performed manually or with the aid of a vaginal speculum. A bimanual examination enables examination of the uterus and ovaries for size, position, shape, tenderness and mobility. The examiner, usually a medical officer, inserts one or two gloved fingers into the vagina and the other hand is placed on the abdomen over the suprapubic area to palpate the ovaries and uterus. A speculum inserted into the vagina provides visualisation of the vagina and cervix and allows a sample of cells and secretions to be obtained.

Papanicolaou test

The Papanicolaou test (Pap smear) is performed to obtain a scraping of cervical cells. The exposed portion of the cervix is one of the most accessible parts of the female genital system for visualisation and diagnosis. Superficial cellular layers can easily be obtained as smears. Microscopic examination of the cells can determine the presence of abnormalities before symptoms of cancer appear. Changes may be due to acute or chronic inflammatory disease, benign tumours such as polyps and premalignant and malignant carcinoma. A vaginal speculum is inserted so that the examiner can collect some cells by gently scraping the cervix with a spatula, 'cytobrush' or a plastic paintbrush device. The cells are placed on a slide, sprayed with a fixative, stained and examined microscopically. Visual analysis by an experienced professional can reveal abnormalities with an acceptable degree of certainty. It is a standard tool in screening and cancer diagnostics. It is recommended that all women have an annual Pap test.

Colposcopy

A colposcope enables direct visualisation of the vagina and cervix. After inserting a vaginal speculum, the colposcope is positioned to provide illumination, magnification and biopsy of the tissue if indicated.

Cervical biopsy

A cervical punch biopsy is the removal of a small column of cervical tissue. The cervix is compared to a clock face and biopsy tissue labelled accordingly. Cone biopsy is the removal of a cone-shaped piece of tissue from the cervix. Possible complications after the procedure are haemorrhage and infertility due to the removal of mucus-producing glands, and the formation of scar tissue.

Laparoscopy

Laparoscopy is a surgical procedure performed to enable visualisation and exploration of the pelvic cavity and reproductive organs. After a general or local anaesthetic, the laparoscope is inserted through a small incision near the umbilicus. A second probe may be inserted through a suprapubic incision.

Diagnostic uterine curettage

Dilation of the cervix and curettage of the endometrium (D&C) enables samples of tissue to be obtained for cytology. Usually a general anaesthetic is administered before the medical officer inserts a series of graded dilators to stretch the cervix. After dilation, the uterine cavity is systematically scraped to obtain tissue.

Breast biopsy

Aspiration and biopsy of suspicious breast lesions may be performed to confirm or rule out malignancy. Aspiration involves removal of fluid or tissue from a breast lump using a syringe and needle. Biopsy involves excision of part of the lump or the whole lump.

NURSING INTERVENTIONS IN FEMALE REPRODUCTIVE HEALTH

Health promotion and preventive measures in the area of women's health have resulted in national breast and cervical screening programs. Target groups are identified and accessed using different methods, including mail-outs and mass media channels. Information and education is available in many languages through state, territory and Federal health departments. Women are encouraged and supported to access primary health programs through women's health centres, family planning clinics, sexual health centres, and adolescent and student clinics. Prevention of sexually transmitted diseases (STDs) and unplanned pregnancies through education, counselling and provision of suitable contraceptives are some of the roles of the nurse working in a primary care setting.

The reproductive system is concerned with both reproduction and sexuality. A woman who has a reproductive disorder may experience anxiety about the effects on future reproductive function, femininity and sexuality. Such anxiety can have a significant effect on the woman's body image and self-concept. Some will experience relief that a problem such as prolonged heavy bleeding is being rectified. In other cases women may experience feelings of loss and grief because of the treatment outcome, such as no longer being able to have children. To assist the client it is essential that she is provided with adequate and accurate information. She should be informed about the physiological effects of the specific disorder on menstruation, elimination, reproductive ability and sexual activity. The nurse should reinforce the medical officer's explanation about any implications on the individual's lifestyle and ensure that the information is understood. It may also be necessary to provide information about fertility control and prevention of STDs.

BREAST DISORDERS

Breast disorders are generally treated by specialist physicians and surgeons, not gynaecologists. Benign breast disease includes fibroadenomas, intraductal papillomas, cystic hyperplasia and chronic mastitis. Fibroadenomas are mobile, round, firm painless lumps that occur most often in younger women. Intraductal papilloma produces a serous or sero-sanguinous nipple discharge, and occurs most often in women aged 35–45.

Cystic hyperplasia and chronic mastitis are collectively referred to as fibrocystic disease. A painful mass decreases and increases in size in relation to the menstrual cycle. The mass is generally firm, mobile, regular in shape and is most often present in the upper outer quadrant of the breast. Fibrocystic disease usually regresses after menopause as levels of ovarian hormones decrease.

Breast cancer is the most common cancer in women and, although it usually affects women over age 50, it can also affect much younger women. Manifestations include increased size of a breast, changes in the shape of a breast, a palpable mass, dimpling of the skin, nipple retraction or ulceration and nipple discharge. Pain is not a common symptom.

It needs to be pointed out that breast cancer does not exclusively occur in women, and that men too are susceptible to breast cancer.

CARE OF THE CLIENT WITH A BREAST DISORDER

Any surgical procedure involving the breast can significantly affect body image, depending on the worth the woman places on her breasts as parts of her femininity and sexuality. Benign breast disease may be treated surgically or non-surgically and may have only a temporary or minor affect on the individual. Malignant breast disease can have a devastating impact.

Breast cancer usually develops in the epithelial breast tissue, more often in the upper outer quadrant. The epithelial cells undergo hyperplasia, which may progress to carcinoma in situ and invasive carcinoma. Cancer of the breast can spread, via the lymphatic system and bloodstream, to various sites in the body. Treatment may include any, or a combination, of:

- Surgery, lumpectomy or mastectomy
- Chemotherapy
- Radiotherapy
- Hormone therapy.

Breast surgery

The type of surgery will depend upon the characteristics and staging of the tumour. The two main options are breast-conserving surgery (lumpectomy), in which only the tumour is removed from the breast (usually followed by radiation therapy to the remaining breast tissue); and mastectomy, or removal of the whole breast (which may be followed by radiation). For invasive breast cancer, both these procedures may also be accompanied by axillary lymph node dissection. Systemic treatments such as hormonal therapy, chemotherapy, or both, may follow either approach.

Mastectomy

In a 'simple' or 'total' mastectomy, the surgeon removes the entire breast but does not take out any axillary lymph nodes. The pectoral or chest wall muscles are left intact. A total mastectomy is appropriate for women with ductal carcinoma in situ (DCIS) and for women seeking prophylactic mastectomies; that is, breast removal to prevent any possibility of breast cancer occurring.

A modified radical mastectomy removes the entire breast and includes axillary dissection, in which the axillary lymph nodes in the underarm area are also removed. Most women who have mastectomies have this surgical procedure.

Radical mastectomy includes removal of the entire breast, all axillary lymph nodes, and chest wall muscles under the breast. Although common in the past, radical mastectomy is now rarely performed because modified radical mastectomy has proven to be just as effective and less disfiguring. A radical mastectomy is recommended only when cancer has spread to the chest wall muscles.

Before surgery the client is informed about whether breast

reconstruction is a viable option. Breast reconstruction after mastectomy involves the creation of a breast mound and reconstruction of a nipple and areola. It may be performed at the same time as the mastectomy, or several months later. Most surgeons prefer the latter approach, as immediate reconstruction increases the risk of complications and may have a poorer cosmetic result. Care of the client undergoing a mastectomy involves preoperative preparation, emotional support, promotion of comfort and prevention of complications.

Preoperative preparation

In addition to preoperative physical preparation, it is essential that the client is provided with adequate information and emotional support. Contact with a person who specialises in breast prostheses, and with a woman who has had a mastectomy, provides a valuable opportunity for the client to discuss the implications of surgery. The woman must be able to discuss all possible physiological and psychosocial implications, for example:

- Loss of functional breast tissue
- Decreased movement and oedema of the arm on the affected side
- Disfigurement
- Fear of death
- Difficulty in adapting to altered body image
- Relationships and sexuality
- Need for a support system
- Available breast prostheses.

The nurse should provide sufficient opportunities for the client to express her fears, and should answer any questions and act as a liaison between members of the health care team. Breast prostheses are available in a range of styles. Generally a soft lightweight prosthesis is provided while the incision is healing and until all tenderness has disappeared. Commercial breast forms are available from a variety of sources, and the client may need to view a number of different styles before finding one that best meets her needs.

Postoperative care

Physical postoperative care includes providing pain relief, promoting comfort, care of the wound, prevention of complications, exercise instruction and continued emotional support.

Exercise instruction

Post-mastectomy exercises are started immediately after surgery to prevent shortening of muscles, contracture of joints and loss of muscle tone and to reduce any oedema in the arm on the affected side. Range-of-motion (ROM) exercises are performed for short periods three or four times daily. The client is encouraged to resume self-care activities as soon as possible to retain mobility and independence. Most health care institutions provide a leaflet that illustrates a range of post-mastectomy exercises which should be continued after the client is discharged.

Emotional support

Continued emotional support is vital in the postoperative period. As a member of a multidisciplinary team, the nurse can assist the client to adjust to surgery and an altered body image. The woman may take several days before she feels able to view the incision, and the nurse must remain sensitive to the client's feelings. It is important for the nurse to realise that the client's feelings of grief are a normal response to loss of a body part. In dealing with her feelings of loss and anxiety, the client may utilise mental defence mechanisms such as denial or anger. The nurse can assist the client to come to terms with the implications of a mastectomy by ensuring that she understands the information given to her and by providing opportunities for her to discuss her anxieties. The woman may appreciate the opportunity to talk with another woman who has had a mastectomy and who is able to offer advice and answer questions based on personal experience.

Before discharge from hospital the woman should be given information on the need to continue with exercises, and any follow-up treatment. She may be provided with a temporary breast prosthesis and given information on where to obtain a permanent prosthesis if one is required. She is also informed about the importance of performing regular breast self-examination of the unaffected breast.

REPRODUCTIVE SYSTEM HEALTH AND ILLNESS

Working in the area of reproductive health requires an understanding of the anatomy and physiology of the reproductive system to identify common variations and deviations from normal. The nurse is aware that normal variations exist in reproductive structure and function throughout the life span. The age at which males and females reach puberty, begin sexual activity and make decisions about family planning is governed by developmental, physiological, psychological, social, religious, economic and environmental factors.

Nurses actively promote reproductive and sexual health through client teaching, education and health promotion strategies. Client teaching is implemented through educating clients about normal developmental changes that occur throughout the life span (Table 40.2). The client is taught how to recognise deviations from normal to assist in early detection and treatment of disease. Benign conditions of the reproductive system are frequently age related or associated with ageing and may not require intervention unless they are troublesome to the client. Reproductive malignancies such as testicular cancer can occur as early as adolescence but have a high cure rate if detected and treated early in the course of the disease. Risk factors for STDs and cervical, breast, testicular and prostate cancer are identified and discussed. Strategies to prevent or minimise risk factors are suggested. Successful approaches must be feasible and able to be integrated into an individual's lifestyle.

TABLE 40.2 | COMMON REPRODUCTIVE CHANGES RELATED TO AGEING

Female	Client teaching	Male	Client teaching
Ovaries smaller and thinner. Decreased oestrogen levels	Discuss hormone replacement therapy (HRT) and complementary therapies if indicated	Increase in size of prostate	Educate the client about the need for regular prostate examinations and availability of prostate-specific antigen (PSA) testing
Decreased size of uterus and vagina		Decreased testosterone levels. Decreased amounts of facial and pubic hair	
Decreased vaginal secretions. Vagina dry and less elastic. Painful intercourse (dyspareunia)		Decreased circulation	
Vaginal tissue is more fragile, more alkaline, and more susceptible to infection	Suggest use of oestrogen creams or vaginal lubricant when indicated	Longer time taken to achieve erection	Inform the client about normal age-related changes. Educate the client about the effects of conditions such as hypertension and diabetes mellitus on sexual function
Decrease in amount of breast tissue	Promote good perineal and personal hygiene. Note presence, character and amount of any vaginal discharge	Decreased rate and force of ejaculation	Allow for verbalisation of concerns. Discuss the use of medication, techniques or devices that may assist the client

HEALTH PROMOTION

Health promotion is not confined to the health sector, but nurses and other health professionals do have a significant role to play. They have a responsibility to advocate for clients to have equitable access to health education and screening. Health-promotion strategies and programs should be adapted to local needs, taking into account social, cultural and economic structures.

BreastScreen

A health screening program that is adapted to local conditions is BreastScreen Australia, a joint federal–state/territory-funded program aimed at screening women aged between 50 and 69 for breast cancer. It provides a free service to clients. Screening for well women who have no symptoms of breast cancer is provided through a network of fixed and mobile services at over 500 locations across Australia. Women who have regular mammograms every 2 years can halve their risk of dying from breast cancer. Women over 40 are eligible for screening. Although some research recommends regular screening for all women in their 40s, there is insufficient evidence to recommend population-based screening for all women under 50.

The role of the nurse is to inform and educate clients about screening mammography. The advantages and limitations of the procedure are discussed. Women are advised to have a screening mammogram every 2 years between age 50 and 69. Younger women from age 20 should be educated in the technique of breast familiarisation, carried out monthly. Breast examination by a health care professional is recommended as a health screening component when women present for regular Pap smears.

Pap smear

Cervical cancer is one of the most preventable and curable of all cancers. It is estimated that most cases of squamous cell carcinoma could be prevented if cell changes were detected and treated early. The Pap smear is performed to obtain a scraping of cervical cells and is currently the best available screening tool for preventing the development of cervical cancer.

In 1991 Australia began what is now known as the National Cervical Screening Program. This joint federal–state/territory-funded program recommends and encourages women to have Pap smears every 2 years throughout their lives. States and territories maintain cervical cytology registries. Women automatically go on the register unless they specifically ask to be excluded. Confidential records and results are retained on a database. Reminders are sent to women on the register when Pap tests are overdue. Clinical Interest Box 40.4 provides information on client teaching in relationship to Pap smear testing.

Health professionals play an important role in encouraging women to have a Pap smear. The incidence of cervical cancer increases with age but the screening rate is low among older women. Women aged 55–70 participate in

CLINICAL INTEREST BOX 40.4
Client teaching — Pap smears

- All women who have ever had sex need to have regular Pap smears, including those who no longer have sex
- Women should have their first Pap smear around age 18–20 or a year or two after first becoming sexually active, whichever is the later. They should continue at 2-year intervals until about age 70
- Explain that a Pap smear is not a test for cancer but that it can differentiate between normal and abnormal cells. Pap smears are the best way for a woman to reduce her risk of developing cervical cancer
- Talk to women about registering on the cervical cytology register so that a reminder can be sent if a Pap smear is overdue
- Women who have any unusual symptoms, such as unexpected bleeding, discharge or pains should see their doctor, even if their last Pap smear was normal

screening less frequently than younger women. Primary health nurses can target this group and raise community awareness by actively promoting testing through education, discussion groups and appropriate and culturally sensitive literature.

Testicular cancer

Testicular cancer is a disease that predominantly affects young men. Men can be taught to examine their testes on a regular basis from age 15 onwards. Familiarisation with normal anatomical structures can assist in early identification of changes that may need investigation.

CONTRACEPTION

There are numerous methods of birth control available that act by preventing ovulation, preventing fertilisation or preventing successful implantation and development of a fertilised ovum. It is the individual's responsibility to obtain information about availability and suitability of the various methods. Contraception may be viewed as a preventive health measure. It protects against unplanned pregnancies and, depending upon the method used, may be effective in preventing STDs. Choices for men are limited at present to the condom, or permanent prevention such as vasectomy. Research to find a widely accepted male hormonal equivalent to the female oral contraceptive pill continues.

For most women, selecting and using a method of contraception is a significant decision. Choices about birth control are possible because of safe and available methods of contraception. Clinical Interest Box 40.5 provides current statistics relating to reproduction in Australia. No perfect contraceptive method exists but there are many good ones with both advantages and disadvantages. Selection of contraceptive method may be based on cultural or religious beliefs, individual health, effectiveness, cost or availability factors.

CLINICAL INTEREST BOX 40.5
Reproduction — choices

- Reproduction is influenced by physiological, psychological, social, religious, economic and environmental factors. Choices about family planning are available, including the choice not to have children
- Since 1901 Australia has experienced two long periods of fertility decline: from 1907 to 1934, and from 1962 to the present. Fertility peaked in 1961 when the total fertility rate reached 3.5 babies per woman
- By 1966 the total fertility rate had fallen to 2.9 babies per woman. Changing social attitudes, in particular a change in perception of desired family size, facilitated by the availability of the oral contraceptive pill, led to this decline
- During the 1970s the total fertility rate dropped again, falling to 2.1 babies per woman in 1976, where it has remained. This fall has been linked to the increasing participation of women in education and the labour force, changing attitudes to family size, lifestyle choices and greater access to contraceptive measures and abortion
- The proportion of women remaining childless has increased over time in all age groups. For women aged 25–29 in 1981, 35% were childless, while 59% of women of the same age in 2001 were childless. In 1981, 8% of 40–44-year-old women were childless. By 2001 this had increased to 13% of women

(Australian Bureau of Statistics 2003)

Birth control methods may be classified as:

- Mechanical barriers
- Chemical barriers
- Natural (ovulation)
- Intrauterine devices
- Hormonal contraceptives
- Sterilisation.

The types, advantages and disadvantages of various contraceptive methods are outlined in Table 40.3.

DISORDERS OF REPRODUCTION

INFERTILITY

Infertility is defined as the inability to conceive after one year of regular intercourse without contraception. It may be caused by anatomical, functional or psychological factors. Infertility may originate in the male or female or in both, and occurs in about equal proportion in both sexes. In many instances, no cause can be determined.

Male factors

In males the most common cause of infertility is the inadequate production of viable sperm. Many factors can affect the production, transport or ejaculation of sperm.

Sperm production can be disrupted by a variety of conditions such as abnormalities of the testes. Cryptorchidism or orchitis of the testes will interfere with sperm production. Excessive heat or wearing tight clothing can cause an increase in the temperature of the testes and inhibit

TABLE 40.3 | CONTRACEPTIVE METHODS

Type	Description	Advantages	Disadvantages/side effects	Convenience	Protection from STDs
Male condom	Sheath made of latex or polyurethane Provides a barrier between the sperm and ova	Condoms offer protection against STDs Used only as required High level of effectiveness Easy to use	Irritation and allergic reactions May break May alter feeling and sensitivity during intercourse May affect spontaneity Pregnancy may result if not used correctly	Applied immediately before intercourse Readily available; no prescription needed	Protects against all
Female condom	Sheath made of polyurethane Provides a barrier between the sperm and ova	Condoms offer protection against STDs Do not interfere with the menstrual cycle Used only as required High level of effectiveness Easy to use	Irritation and allergic reactions May break May alter feeling and sensitivity during intercourse May affect spontaneity Pregnancy may result if not used correctly	Applied immediately before intercourse No prescription needed	May give some protection
Diaphragm/cap	Diaphragm: thin, soft latex dome-shaped device that fits between vagina and pubic bone Cap: Smaller latex or silicone device that fits over the cervix	Do not interfere with the menstrual cycle	May slip out of position May alter feeling and sensitivity during intercourse Possible irritation from the material May affect spontaneity Pregnancy may result if not used correctly	Applied any time before intercourse Reusable devices Must be left in place for 6 hours after intercourse Fitted by health professionals	None
Spermicides	Spermicidal preparations in foam, creams, jellies and vaginal suppositories Block the passage of sperm and render sperm inactive	Do not interfere with the menstrual cycle Highly effective when used with a mechanical barrier Help to provide vaginal lubrication	Used alone, without a mechanical barrier, contraceptive failure is high May result in irritation of mucous membranes	Available without prescription	None
Natural methods	Based on abstinence from sexual intercourse during the fertile phase of the menstrual cycle Methods include: rhythm/calendar, temperature measurement, cervical mucus observation	No disruption to menstrual cycle Safe, easy and effective if practised correctly	Unreliable if menstrual cycles are irregular Infection may alter temperature pattern Needs practice to assess cervical mucus variations	All methods require considerable motivation and self-discipline Requires frequent monitoring of body functions	None
Intrauterine device (IUD)	Device inserted into the uterus to prevent pregnancy IUS (intrauterine system) releases low dose of hormone daily	No disruption to the body's hormonal system Continuous contraceptive coverage. High level of effectiveness IUS completely reversible	Increased menstrual bleeding, abdominal cramps, low back pain May be expelled from the uterus Risk of PID*, infertility, ectopic pregnancy if contraceptive failure	One time insertion May remain in place for up to 10 years depending upon type	None

TABLE 40.3 | CONTRACEPTIVE METHODS—cont'd

Type	Description	Advantages	Disadvantages/side effects	Convenience	Protection from STDs
Hormonal oral contraceptive (combined pill)	Combination of oestrogen and progestogen. Inhibits ovulation	High level of effectiveness Regular menstruation, reduced menstrual bleeding Protects against ovarian and endometrial cancer, PID	Nausea, weight gain, fluid retention, breast tenderness, break-through bleeding, mood changes, loss of libido. Rarely, cardiovascular disease, including thromboembolism and hypertension	Must be taken daily regardless of frequency of intercourse Requires prescription	None. Some protection from PID
Hormonal oral contraceptive (minipill)	Contains progestogen only Prevents thickening of the endometrium so implantation is unlikely Alters composition of cervical mucus	High level of effectiveness Reduced menstrual discomfort Protects against ovarian and endometrial cancer, PID	Menstrual disturbances, weight gain, breast tenderness	Must be taken daily regardless of frequency of intercourse Requires prescription	None. Some protection from PID
Hormonal injection	Long-acting progestogen in injectable form. Inhibits ovulation, changes endometrial lining and cervical mucus	Continuous contraceptive coverage	Menstrual disturbances, weight gain, breast tenderness	One injection every 3 months Requires prescription	None
Hormonal implant	Long-acting progestogen in implant form. Made up of matchstick-size rubber rods implanted under skin of upper arm	Continuous contraceptive coverage	Inflammation or infection at site of implant Menstrual disturbances Weight gain Breast tenderness	Effective for up to 5 years Requires prescription Implanted by health care provider as minor surgical procedure	None
Morning-after pill	Combination of oestrogen and progestogen in high doses Emergency measure after unprotected intercourse	High level of effectiveness Provides birth control if mechanical barriers failed during intercourse, if unprotected intercourse occurred, or if the woman forgot to take a contraceptive pill	Nausea Spotting or bleeding a few days later	Should be taken within 72 hours May require prescription	None
Sterilisation	Vasectomy for the male, tubal ligation for the female. Both methods are designed to prevent fertilisation	Generally effective and safe. Does not disrupt the normal menstrual cycle or sexual feelings	Should be considered as an irreversible process. Slight failure rate. Minor discomfort after surgery	One-time surgical procedure	None

*PID = pelvic inflammatory disease

sperm production. Hormonal dysfunction of the anterior pituitary gland or hypothalamus will affect testicular function. Autoimmune factors may also be implicated. Diseases such as coeliac disease, diabetes mellitus and alcoholism may prevent normal spermatogenesis.

Transport of sperm through the male reproductive tract can be impeded by adhesions, structural weaknesses or obstruction. Congenital or acquired anatomical factors that prevent sperm being ejaculated include obstruction of the duct system by injury, infection or tumour. Ejaculation of sperm may be impaired by diseases that alter the autonomic response, by psychosexual factors, or by systemic diseases such as diabetes mellitus.

Female factors

The most common cause of female infertility is related to ovulation problems. Irregular menstrual cycles or amenorrhoea may signal problems with ovulation. Stress, diet or rigorous athletic training are lifestyle factors that can affect hormonal balance. More serious causes are due to tumours of the pituitary gland. Structural abnormalities, endometriosis or scarring of the uterine tubes due to PID will prevent fertilisation and implantation. Treatment depends on the cause, so a full medical and sexual history has to be obtained. Diagnostic tests may be ordered for either the male or the female or both.

Assessment of infertility

The man's assessment will first concentrate on evaluation of the quality of the sperm, their number, shape and movement. Tests to exclude infection, hormonal imbalance or structural abnormalities may also be ordered. X-rays are taken if damage to the vas deferens is suspected. Sperm may be tested to see if it can swim through a sample of the woman's fertile vaginal mucus (also used to test the quality of the woman's mucus).

The first step in assessing the woman is to determine if she is ovulating. This may be done by testing basal body temperature and by examining cervical mucus. Diagnostic tests include:

- Blood tests for hormone levels
- Ultrasound of ovaries to check for ovulation
- Hysterosalpingogram to check patency of uterine tubes
- Laparoscopy to check for disease of tubes or ovaries
- Endometrial biopsy to check if lining is normal
- Sperm antibody tests.

TREATMENT OPTIONS

Treatment will depend upon the cause. Most infertility cases (80–90%) are treated with drugs. For women, medication may be prescribed to stimulate hormones. Multiple births occur in 10–20% of births where fertility drugs have been taken. Surgery is more rarely used to correct anatomical barriers to fertilisation.

Assisted reproductive technology

For some couples the use of assisted reproductive technology (ART) is their only option to achieve a pregnancy. Many of these methods are very costly, both financially and emotionally.

Artificial insemination by donor (AID). Donor sperm is inserted into the vaginal canal of the woman.

In vitro fertilisation (IVF). Medication is given to stimulate the woman's ovaries. Ova are harvested from the ovaries and placed on a culture dish with the man's sperm. About 2 days later, two or three fertilised ova are transplanted into the uterus to increase the chances of a successful pregnancy. Donor egg IVF uses donated ova when the women has ovarian disease or carries a genetic defect. Excess embryos may be frozen if the woman wishes to have another child in the future.

Gamete intrafallopian transfer (GIFT). Based on IVF, the fertilised ova are placed into a functioning fallopian tube.

Intracytoplasmic sperm injection. A relatively new procedure for men with sperm quality problems. In this procedure a single sperm is injected into an ovum to produce an embryo.

Nurses who work with essentially healthy people who are infertile need to be sensitive to their concerns and anxieties. Couples often rely on the nurse for support during their treatment. They frequently feel stigmatised by their experience of infertility. Education about infertility and treatment options available should be provided by knowledgeable and skilled practitioners.

SEXUAL ABUSE

Sexual abuse is a significant problem in Western society. It can occur at any age and to anyone regardless of social or ethnic background. Females experience sexual abuse more often than males but the incidence of abuse in males is also a significant issue. For any person who has been sexually abused there are commonly extensive physical and emotional effects. It is important for nurses to explore physical and psychological wellbeing when taking a sexual history and to be mindful of the prevalence of domestic violence and sexual abuse that often occurs at the hands of partners, ex-partners or other family members. It may be happening currently or may be part of a client's past experience. When abuse is recognised the nurse has a responsibility to instigate the necessary supports. A person who has been raped may need to work through the experience and may need ongoing help before being able to resume comfortable intimate relationships. Family therapy may be indicated in cases of incest or other abuse.

SURVIVORS OF TORTURE AND TRAUMA

Australia and New Zealand have large numbers of refugees, some of whom have been subjected to torture and trauma, including that of a sexual nature, as prisoners in their country of origin. Some, it has been claimed, may even have suffered such abuse in Australia's refugee detention centres (Skeers 2001). According to leading international human rights organisations, torture is practised in 90 countries around the world (Frase-Blunt 2003). Examples of sexual abuse include male and female rape, genitals being burned with cigarettes or boiling water and beatings of women, resulting in miscarriage. Nurses need to be aware that the trauma and torture can cause a range of permanent physical effects and even more devastating psychological effects lasting for many years after the event.

Nurses may be treating survivors of torture and not be aware of it. Clients may have language barriers or may not want to share this sensitive information. Things that happen in hospital can trigger memories of abuse that may cause severe anxiety or aggressive responses. This may happen, for example, when the nurse asks a client who has survived torture or trauma to undress or have a suppository administered. Nurses need to keep awareness of the possibility of torture and trauma in their minds when dealing with migrants or refugees from countries where such atrocities may have occurred. More information on working effectively with survivors of torture or trauma is available from specialist associations in each state and territory of Australia and in New Zealand; for example, in Australia there is the New South Wales Service for the Treatment and Rehabilitation of Torture and Trauma Survivors (STARTTS) and in New Zealand there is the Auckland Refugees and Survivors (RAS) Centre.

CHILD SEXUAL ABUSE

When the nurse knows about or suspects abuse of a child there is a legal requirement (mandatory reporting) in most states and territories of Australia and an obligation in New Zealand for the nurse to report to the relevant child protection agency. Notifying a child protection agency is the first step in the process of providing support and protection.

There is no standard profile to identify a person who has experienced sexual abuse, but a combination of clinical signs and symptoms and/or a pattern of behaviour or injury can arouse suspicion. It is the role of the nurse to be mindful of cultural practices (e.g., female circumcision) and certain disease processes that may result in variations from the normal. It is important for the nurse to be aware of the symptoms of sexual disturbance in children. There are many indicators, both physical and behavioural. Some of the more common physical indicators are:

- Vaginal or penile discharge
- Offensive odour, indicating genital infection
- Blood on underwear
- Pain or itching of the genital or anal areas
- Difficulty or discomfort sitting or walking
- Evidence of injury around genital or anal areas
- Pain when urinating or having bowel motions
- Foreign bodies in the vagina, rectum or urethra
- Frequent unexplained health problems.

Some of the more common behavioural symptoms are:

- Difficulty sleeping, waking up distressed, screaming or shaking, nightmares
- Reluctance to participate in activities previously enjoyed
- Negative change in performance at school
- Unexplained periods of panic, which may be caused by flashbacks to the abuse
- Regressing to behaviours too young for the stage of development for age (e.g. reverting to wetting the bed, thumb sucking)
- Drawings that show sexual acts
- Abnormal knowledge of sexual matters or unusual number of questions about human sexual activities
- Engaging in persistent sexual play with friends, toys or pets
- Showing unusually aggressive behaviour towards family members, friends, toys or pets
- Persistently overly interested in own genitals
- Loss of appetite or other eating problems or unexplained gagging
- Unusual fear of a certain place or location.
- Reluctance to be alone with a certain person, or fear of returning home
- Acts of self mutilation such as a child sticking or cutting themself
- Substance abuse.

In recent years concern about psychological damage to children resulting from exposure to sexual material on the internet has become an issue. Children who have been harmed by viewing pornography may present with a variety of behaviours, including excessive curiosity about or over-preoccupation with sexuality. Children in this situation may inappropriately expose their genitals to others or engage in a sudden high level of masturbation (see the Enough is Enough website at www.protectkids.com).

The most effective way to limit the damage caused by sexual trauma is firstly by prevention and secondly by early intervention. This is facilitated by education of parents and those in contact with children. Education is a primary role of community health nurses, who include school nurses and occupational health and safety nurses, but all informed nurses can participate in education and prevention measures.

The nurse dealing with clients who may have been sexually abused are advised to:

- Take any claim of abuse seriously
- Praise children or any client for talking about what has happened
- Control personal feelings of disgust or abhorrence
- Report suspicion or knowledge of child abuse to the relevant authority
- Ensure that a medical officer experienced in detecting and treating physical abuse is contacted
- Ensure that an experienced therapist is contacted to

work with the client and/or family to help with the psychological impact.

SEXUALLY TRANSMITTED DISEASES (STDs)

Sexually transmitted diseases (STDs) are infections or infestations that can be transferred from one person to another through sexual contact. People most at risk of contracting STDs are those who practise sex with multiple partners, but anyone having sex outside of a long-established and monogamous relationship can become infected with an STD. Sexual contact includes kissing, vaginal, anal, oral and oral–anal sex and the use of sexual aids such as vibrators. Some STDs can be transmitted by other means. STDs can be passed from a mother to her baby during pregnancy or during the birth process. Human immunodeficiency virus (HIV) and hepatitis are blood-borne viruses that are also present in other body fluids. Transmission can therefore occur whenever there is an exchange of body fluids.

Infection is caused by the transmission of microscopic organisms such as viruses, bacteria or parasites. Some STDs are caused by larger organisms, such as lice or mites. Table 40.4 identifies the causative organisms and major routes of transmission of some STDs common in Australia and New Zealand.

Some STDs are relatively harmless and easily treated but others are dangerous and life threatening. The symptoms of STDs vary with each type but there are some common signs. Nurses alert to the symptoms of STDs would be prompted to explore the sexual history of clients reporting any of the following:

TABLE 40.4 | SEXUALLY TRANSMITTED DISEASES COMMON IN AUSTRALIA AND NEW ZEALAND — CAUSATIVE ORGANISMS AND ROUTES OF TRANSMISSION

STD and responsible organism	Main route of transmission
Viral infections	
Genital herpes (herpes simplex type 2 [HSV-2]) virus	Direct skin–skin contact with infected site during vaginal, anal or oral sex
Genital warts (human papilloma virus [HPV])	Vaginal, anal or oral sex
Hepatitis B (hepatitis B [HBV] virus)	Vaginal, oral and especially anal sex Contaminated drug needles Skin pierced by contaminated medical instruments Contaminated blood or blood products
Human immunodeficiency virus infection–acquired immune deficiency syndrome (HIV–AIDS) (HIV virus)	Vaginal, oral and especially anal sex Contaminated drug needles Infected blood or blood products Transmitted from infected mother to infant in utero, during birth or while breastfeeding
Bacterial infections	
Bacterial vaginosis — common but not a true STD (caused by variety of bacteria of the vagina)	Believed to be due to changes in the vagina during and after sex
Chlamydia (*Chlamydia trachomatis*)	Vaginal and anal sex
Gonorrhoea (*Neisseria gonorrhoeae*)	Vaginal, anal or oral sex
Syphilis (*Treponema pallidum*)	Vaginal, anal or oral sex
Non-specific urethritis (NSU). Caused by a variety of organisms (any inflammation of male urethra not caused by gonorrhoea is classed as NSU)	Vaginal, anal or oral sex
Fungal infections	
Thrush (candidiasis) (*Candida albicans*)	Vaginal infection can be spread sexually
Protozoal infections	
Amoebiasis and similar conditions (parasites such as *Giardia lamblia*)	Anal or oral–anal sex
Trichomoniasis (*Trichomonas vaginalis* parasite)	Sexual contact but also possibly by contact with infected objects (survives on items such as washcloths)
Parasitic infestations	
Pubic lice ('crabs') (*Phthirus pubis* lice)	Any intimate contact — not necessarily sexual
Scabies (*Sarcoptes scabies* mites)	Any intimate contact — not necessarily sexual

- Itchiness, burning or discomfort in the genital or anal area
- Pain or discomfort during urination or sexual activity
- Unusual discharge of fluid from the vagina or penis
- Blisters, sores, ulcers, warts, lumps or rashes anywhere in the genital or anal area.

Some STDs may be asymptomatic. It is not uncommon for there to be a lack of symptoms in women with gonorrhoea or chlamydia, for example, and this can present a serious danger, as PID can occur, resulting in damage to the fallopian tubes, a risk of ectopic pregnancy or infertility.

Some STDs start with mild symptoms that may be ignored until they disappear. Syphilis, for example, manifests in three separate stages: primary, secondary and tertiary. If it is ignored in the early primary and secondary stages when symptoms are mild but highly infective, the carrier may transmit the disease to other people and be faced with possible fatal heart and brain damage when the illness returns in the dangerous tertiary phase. The full course of syphilis can take several years and can be fatal. Table 40.5 outlines the stages, signs and symptoms of syphilis.

DIAGNOSIS

A medical officer will use the results of swabs and blood tests to confirm which STD is causing problems. It is not uncommon for a client to have more than one STD at the same time.

Some nursing diagnoses relating to STDs are listed in Clinical Interest Box 40.6.

TREATMENT

When diagnosed early many STDs can be treated effectively. Those caused by bacterial infection can be treated with antibiotics, although some bacteria have become resistant to the drugs in common use and now respond only to newer, more potent types of antibiotics. When treatment is not instigated early, permanent damage may already have occurred to body organs. For example, human papillomavirus (HPV) infection, responsible for genital warts, is also linked to cervical and other genital cancers (refer to the National HPV Vaccination Program in Clinical Interest Box 40.2). Of the STDs transmitted to newborns, some can be cured easily but others can cause permanent disability or death: HIV is one of the latter.

CLINICAL INTEREST BOX 40.6
Nursing diagnoses related to sexually transmitted diseases

- Anxiety
- Pain
- Rape trauma syndrome
- Self-esteem disturbance
- Sexual dysfunction
- Sexuality patterns, altered

HUMAN IMMUNODEFICIENCY VIRUS (HIV)

HIV infection may be treated with combination therapies to reduce the amount of virus being reproduced in the body. It is recognised that HIV eventually results in acquired immune deficiency syndrome (AIDS), commonly about 10 years after infection but in some cases up to 17 years later. HIV and AIDS weaken the body's immune system, allowing opportunistic infections to cause serious health problems. Some common opportunistic infections are listed in Table 40.6.

The client with HIV–AIDS can present with a variety of complex needs at any stage of the illness and requires careful nursing assessment. Sexuality issues include concerns with effects on relationships, the ability to find an accepting partner, the risk of transmission and the impact on decisions about parenting. The client with HIV or AIDS is encouraged to maintain a healthy lifestyle and many find alternative therapies helpful with this. Clients are also treated with antiviral drugs. The drug therapy aims

TABLE 40.5 | STAGES, SIGNS AND SYMPTOMS OF SYPHILIS

Stages	Signs and symptoms
Primary stage	Chancre — painless open sore on penis or in vagina, rectum or throat. Can also occur on hands. May take as long as 3 months after infection to develop Nearby lymph nodes may be enlarged Chancre clears up within a few weeks
Secondary stage	Generalised non-itchy rash may appear 2–6 months after primary chancre disappears. Palms of hands and soles of feet may be affected by the rash Thin white sores may appear on mucosa of mouth and throat and around genital area and anus Headache, fever, painful joints, anaemia and alopecia may occur Symptoms may disappear after 3–12 weeks and reappear later
Tertiary stage	Symptoms may develop soon after secondary symptoms vanish or not for several years Lesions (gummae) appear on skin, bone, mucous membranes, upper respiratory tract, stomach and liver Cardiovascular and neurological impairment

TABLE 40.6 | COMMON OPPORTUNISTIC INFECTIONS IN HIV–AIDS

Infection	Description
Candidiasis (thrush)	Fungal infection of the mouth, throat or vagina
Cytomegalovirus (CMV)	Viral infection causing eye disease that can lead to blindness
Herpes simplex	Virus infection causing oral herpes (cold sores) or genital herpes — more frequently and more severely than in people without AIDS
Mycobacterium avium complex (MAC or MAI)	Causes recurring fevers, general malaise, problems with digestion and serious weight loss
Pneumocystis carinii pneumonia (PCP)	Protozoal infection that can cause fatal pneumonia
Toxoplasmosis	Protozoal encephalitis
Tuberculosis (TB)	Bacterial infection that attacks the lungs and can cause meningitis. Any person with HIV who tests positive to exposure to TB should be treated

to promote repair of the immune system and increase the ability to fight infection. Side effects of the medication can cause unpleasant symptoms until a suitable combination of drugs is determined. Currently there is no cure for AIDS. Nursing care is focused on maintaining normality and quality of life: research is focused on the development of improved treatment and a preventive vaccine.

The impact of STDs on sexual and general health is enormous. It is easier to prevent infection than treat it, and prevention needs to be the concern of all health professionals.

PREVENTION OF SEXUALLY TRANSMITTED DISEASES (STDS)

Avoiding infection means responsible sexual behaviour. The only absolutely certain way to avoid infection is not to have sex. Nurses can reinforce, especially to young clients, that they should never feel that they have to have sex if they don't want to. Nurses can also promote and educate people about safer sex practices. Safer sex reduces the risk of STD infection, particularly from major STDs, but the risk is not completely eliminated. For example, protection by use of condoms provides some protection against HIV and gonorrhoea, but they are less effective in protecting against trichomoniasis and chlamydia and provide virtually no protection against HPV, the cause of genital warts. This is because any intimate contact may spread some STDs.

Education about safer sex practices includes discussing choices about:

- Limiting activity to sensual caressing, massage and mutual masturbation
- Having sex with only one person in a monogamous relationship (the nurse providing education needs to stress that being safe means knowing that neither partner has or will have any other sexual partners and that both are uninfected)
- Insisting on tests for STDs before engaging in sexual activity with a new partner
- The use of good-quality latex condoms, with knowledge of how to use them safely and effectively
- Not allowing drugs or alcohol to impair judgment.

Education about the prevention of STDs also includes stressing the need for:

- Prompt treatment of any infection
- Investigation and treatment of anyone who has had sexual contact with an infected person
- Avoiding sexual activity during the infective stage of the disease
- Avoiding sexual contact with a person known to be, or suspected of being, infected
- Those engaging in sexual activity with other than reliable sexual partners to have periodic health checks and tests for STDs, regardless of other preventive measures employed
- Advising sexually active women to have a Pap smear every 2 years
- Advising that the full course of any prescribed antibiotics must be taken
- Implementing the recommended blood and secretion precautions as effective infection control measures (see Chapter 25 for guidelines).

Nurses have a responsibility to promote the reduction of incidence of STDs and so limit the distress they cause. A knowledgeable and skilled nurse will successfully encourage clients to discuss STDs, will inform about modes of transmission and treatments, and will ensure that at-risk clients will recognise the manifestations of STDs if and when they occur. The education that nurses are often in a position to relay helps disseminate accurate information. This can increase the number of clients that seek early medical advice, and so reduce the damaging physical and psychological effects of STDs.

SUMMARY

The purpose of both the male and female reproductive systems is reproduction of the human species. The reproductive role of the male is to manufacture and deliver sperm to the female reproductive tract. The female role is to produce ova, receive sperm and, after fertilisation (the fusion of a spermatozoon and an ovum to form one cell) development and birth of the baby. Female reproductive capacity is governed by complex cyclic hormonal changes.

The male reproductive system consists of external and internal structures. The testes, or male gonads, are concerned with the production of sperm and the hormone, testosterone. Testosterone's chief function is to stimulate the development of the male reproductive organs and the secondary sexual characteristics.

Common male reproductive system disorders include urinary problems, urethral discharge and sexual dysfunction. Tests used to assist or confirm the diagnosis of male reproductive system disorders include rectal examination, testicular examination, biopsy, semen analysis and renal function studies.

The female reproductive system also consists of external and internal structures. The ovaries, or female gonads, are concerned with the production of mature ova and the hormones, oestrogen and progesterone. Oestrogen's chief function is to stimulate the development of the female reproductive organs and the secondary sexual characteristics. Progesterone plays a major role in the menstrual cycle by promoting the final preparation of the uterine lining. The functions of the uterus are to receive the fertilised ovum, provide a suitable environment for the developing fetus, expel the fetus at the end of pregnancy, and shed the superficial layer of endometrium if fertilisation of the ovum does not occur. The menstrual cycle consists of a series of changes in the endometrium, as it responds to changes in the levels of ovarian hormones in the blood.

Common female reproductive system disorders include pain, bleeding, vaginal discharge, pruritus, urinary problems and breast changes. Tests used to assist, or confirm, the diagnosis of female reproductive system disorders include pelvic examination, colposcopy, laparoscopy, breast examinations, radiography and ultrasonography, biopsy and cytology.

A woman who has a reproductive disorder may experience anxiety about the effects on future reproductive function, femininity and sexuality. Such anxiety can have a significant effect on the individual's body image and self-concept. Nursing management of the individual with a reproductive disorder includes providing care for diagnostic tests, providing psychological support, perineal and vaginal care, and meeting elimination needs.

Choices concerning reproduction are influenced by physiological, psychological, social, religious, economic and environmental factors. In Australia the birth rate is declining due mainly to changing social attitudes and the availability of contraception.

Nurses who work in the area of sexual and reproductive health should be aware of cultural and religious beliefs as well as individual sexual practices and preferences. As health professionals they are actively involved in promoting reproductive and sexual health in a variety of health care settings. Nursing management of the individual with a disorder of the male or female reproductive system requires an acute awareness of the importance of providing psychological support as well as skilled clinical interventions.

REVIEW EXERCISES

1. What is the function of the male and female reproductive systems?
2. Describe the process of spermatogenesis.
3. What hormones are produced by the ovaries after the onset of puberty?
4. Outline the events of the menstrual cycle.
5. What two diagnostic tests would be performed initially in a male with symptoms of an enlarged prostate gland?
6. Describe the nursing management of a client after a transurethral prostatectomy.
7. Outline three bleeding abnormalities associated with female reproductive disorders.
8. What factors need to be taken into consideration when discussing methods of contraception with a client?
9. What are six signs that might indicate that a 6-year-old girl has been sexually abused? What are your nursing responsibilities when you believe sexual abuse has occurred?

CRITICAL THINKING EXERCISES

1. Con, 66, has been admitted for a transurethral resection of the prostate gland. Previously Con had been admitted through the emergency department with acute urinary retention. Explain the physiology of benign prostatic hypertrophy and how the two events above are linked.
2. Hans, 34, has been diagnosed with testicular cancer after discovering a hard lump in his left testicle. He is married and does not have any children. What information can the nurse give about his condition, treatment options and future fertility?
3. Indirha, 40, has had a modified radical mastectomy for cancer of the right breast. She returns to the ward with a vacuum drain in situ and intravenous therapy in progress. What specific nursing care is required for Indirha in the early postoperative period?
4. You are allocated to care for Debbie, a 14-year-old girl who had an appendicectomy late yesterday. The surgeon has told the nursing staff that he suspects she may be pregnant, although she has denied this to him. Today while you are helping Debbie with her hygiene she reveals to you that she likes going out with different boys, is sexually active and has been for over a year. She tells you that, just before she came into hospital, one boy that she liked finished the relationship they were having because she told him she was a bit late with her monthly period. Consider your role as an Enrolled Nurse (EN) and how you might best facilitate helping Debbie. Consider what you might do in relation to her possible pregnancy, knowledge about birth control, her sexual practices and risk factors for STDs.

REFERENCES AND FURTHER READING

Australian Bureau of Statistics (ABS) (2003) *Australia Now Year Book 2003*. ABS, Commonwealth Government of Australia, Canberra

Barber DA (2000) Fertile Field. *Nursing Standard*, 14(26): 77
Brown K (2000) *Management Guidelines for Women's Health Practitioners*. FA Davis, Philadelphia
Cates W, Steiner M (2002) Dual protection against unintended pregnancy and sexually transmitted infections: what is the best contraceptive approach? *Sexually Transmitted Disease*, 29(3): 168–74
Department of Health & Ageing (2007) *The National HPV Vaccination Program*. Online. Available: http://www.health.gov.au/cervicalcancer [accessed 5 June 2008]
Frase-Blunt M (2003) *Healing Deep Wounds: Program at Bellevue/NYU Provides Care for Torture Survivors*. AAMC Reporter. Online. Available: http://www.aamc.org/newsroom/reporter/jan03/healingdeepwounds.htm [accessed 4 June 2008]
Konkle-Parker D (2000) The regulatory and immune systems and the client with HIV. In: Hoeman P (ed.) *Rehabilitation Nursing Process. Application and Outcomes*, 3rd edn. Mosby, St Louis
Lue TF (2000) Drug therapy: erectile dysfunction. *New England Journal of Medicine*, 340(24): 1802–13
Marieb E (2006) *Essentials of Anatomy and Physiology*, 6th edn. Benjamin Cummings, San Francisco
Olive D, Pritts E (2001) Drug Therapy: Treatment of Endometriosis. *New England Journal of Medicine*, 345 (4): 266–75
Skeers J (2001) *Reports Reveal Systematic Abuse in Australia's Refugee Detention Centres*. World Socialist Web Site. Online. Available: http://www.wsws.org/articles/2001/dec2001/refu-d11.shtml [accessed 4 June 2008]

ONLINE RESOURCES

Andrology Australia. Prostate disease — PSA test: www.andrologyaustralia.org/prostate/psa.htm
Breastcancer.org: www.breastcancer.org
BreastScreen Australia: www.breastscreen.info.au
Cancer of the Cervix — Fact Sheet: www.gcsau.org/qcgc/cervix/fact_sheet.asp
Enough is Enough: www.protectkids.com
IVF Australia: www.ivf.com.au/htmlpages/treatment.html
MayoClinic.com: www.mayoclinic.com/invoke.cfm?id=HQ01409
The British Menopause Society: www.the-bms.org
The Cancer Council of Australia: www.cancer.org.au
The Cancer Council of New South Wales: www.nswcc.org.au
The Clinical Information Access Program: www.ciap.health.nsw.gov.au
The International Society for Men's Health: (www.ismh.org/)
The Jean Hailes Foundation: www.jeanhailes.org.au
University of Colorado Health Sciences Centre, Breast Imaging Centre. Breast ultrasound teaching files: www.uchsc.edu/uh/radiology/bus_tf
Urological Cancer Organisation: www.uco.org.au/cpinfo.html

Chapter 41

NEUROLOGICAL HEALTH

OBJECTIVES

- Define the key terms/concepts
- Describe the structure of the nervous system
- Describe the position of each part of the nervous system
- Describe the functions of the nervous system
- State the pathophysiological influences and effects associated with disorders of the nervous system
- Describe the major manifestations of nervous system disorders
- Briefly describe the specific disorders of the nervous system outlined in this chapter
- State the diagnostic tests that may be used to assess nervous system function
- Assist in planning and implementing nursing care for the individual with a nervous system disorder

KEY TERMS/CONCEPTS

absence seizure
aneurysm
aphasia
apraxia
ataxia
aura
cephalalgia
cerebrovascular accident (CVA)
chorea
decerebrate
decorticate
dysphasia
generalised seizure
hemiparesis
hemiplegia
hydrocephalus
neuralgia
neuritis
paraplegia
quadriplegia
spina bifida
status epilepticus
transient ischaemic attack (TIA)

CHAPTER FOCUS

The workings of the human brain, and indeed the entire nervous system, has both fascinated and mystified scientists for centuries. The knowledge that has been uncovered has enabled health care professionals to make more accurate assessments of clients, allowing implementation of safer and more effective treatments. While application of this knowledge has significantly improved the expected outcomes for many clients affected by disorders of the nervous system, there is still much research to be carried out to fully explain the workings of this intricate system.

The nervous system is responsible for the coordination of all other systems. It provides a network for communication within the body, and between the body and its environment. The brain is informed of events occurring both within and outside the body by nerve impulses that originate at a large number of sensory receptors. The receptors, which may be nerve endings, single specialised cells, or a group of cells forming a sense organ, convert the energy of a stimulus into impulses that pass to specific areas of the brain. An understanding of this complex and dynamic system underpins many aspects of client care, as almost all medical conditions can affect the human nervous system in some way.

LIVED EXPERIENCE

Here I was again, back in the doctor's office trying to find an answer. I honestly don't think I'm a wimpy sickly person — apart from the time I had really bad glandular fever when I was doing my final school year and seemed to be sick for so long I flunked out and had to repeat the entire year! Anyway, the last 12 months have reminded me of that time — I've just been so weak and lethargic. I actually went to the ophthalmologist and had my eyes tested because I started seeing two of everything! It is obviously stress; heaps of people have told me I took on too much — studying for my degree just after the wedding and while we are building the new house. But the other day when I collapsed in the kitchen because I couldn't feel my legs any more, Simon put his foot down and here we are to get the results of my MRI scan. I feel as if I am wasting everyone's time, I'm sure it's just stress . . . MULTIPLE SCLEROSIS! My whole world began to crumble . . .

Deborah, age 24

My God, Deb looked really upset when she heard about the MS. She just cracked up. But I'm sure she will be fine, always has been. I guess she will just need some vitamin tablets to get better, which will be good because next week we are going to be laying the driveway.

Simon, Deborah's husband

THE FUNCTION AND STRUCTURE OF THE NEUROLOGICAL SYSTEM

NERVOUS TISSUE

Neurons

Neurons (Figure 41.1) are the primary components of the nervous system. Functioning alone, or as units, neurons detect internal and external changes and initiate body responses needed to maintain homeostasis. Each neuron is composed of a cell body, with projections forming dendrites, and one long axon. The dendrites are short-branched fibres, which receive impulses and conduct them towards the cell body of a neuron. The axon, which may vary in length from miniscule to over a metre, conducts impulses away from the cell body of a neuron. Generally, a neuron has only one axon but many dendrites. Axons leave the grey matter and become the fibres of the white matter. Each axon has a covering called a neurilemma, and most have a fatty sheath, the myelin sheath. The myelin sheath protects and insulates the axon and increases the transmission rate of nervous impulses. Neurons are bound together by a special type of connective tissue called neuroglia.

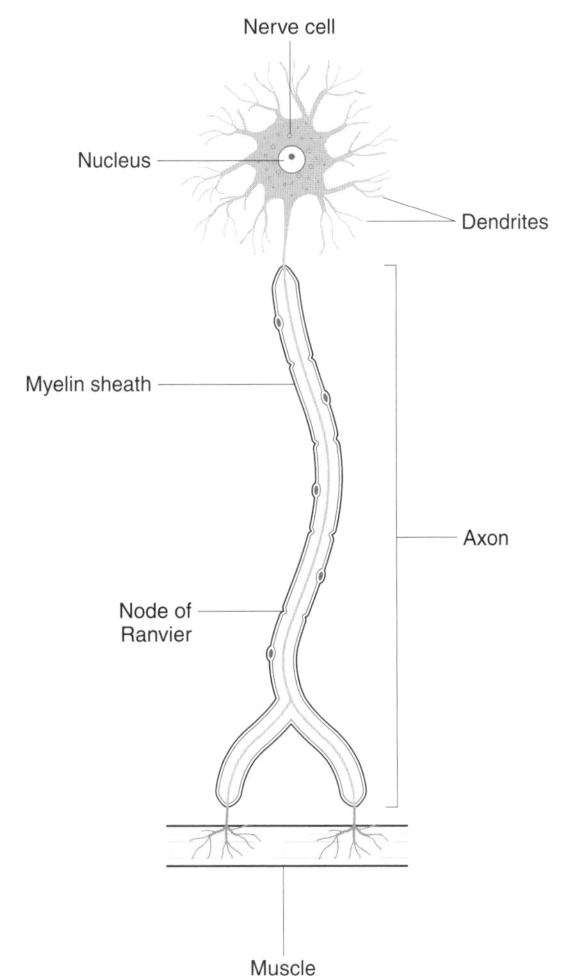

Figure 41.1 | A typical neuron

Neuroglia

The neuroglia includes many types of cells that support and protect the neurons. They play a role in regulating neuronal activity, and in providing neurons with nutrients. Neuroglia differ from neurons in that they are not capable of transmitting nerve impulses and never lose their ability to divide. The neuroglia are comprised mainly of two types of cells: astrocytes, cells with small cell bodies and processes like dendrites, which protect the neurons from harmful substances that may be in the blood by forming a living barrier between the capillary blood supply and the neurons; and oligodendrocytes, which have few processes and produce the myelin sheath around the processes of the neurons.

Functions of neurons

Neurons have two major functional properties: irritability and conductivity. Irritability is the ability to respond to a stimulus and convert it into a nerve impulse. Conductivity is the ability to transmit the impulse to other neurons, muscles, or glands. An impulse is a complex electrical and chemical signal transmitted along a nerve pathway in response to a stimulus. The speed of transmission varies with the size of the nerve fibre, and may be as much as 120 metres per second.

A synapse is the space between the terminal axon of one neuron and the dendrites of another. By means of a chemical substance (neurotransmitter) released by the axons, impulses are transmitted through this space from one neuron to another. Examples of neurotransmitters are acetylcholine and noradrenaline. Many different types of stimuli can excite neurons so that they become active and generate an impulse. Most neurons are excited by the neurotransmitters released by other neurons, but other stimuli can excite neurons. For example, sound excites some of the neuronal receptors of the ear, and pressure excites some cutaneous receptors of the skin. Receptors, or sensory nerve terminals, act as transducers, converting the energy of a stimulus into impulses that pass to the brain.

The nervous system can be divided into two primary divisions: the central nervous system, consisting of the brain and spinal cord, and the peripheral nervous system, consisting of nerves that connect the central nervous system with the body tissues.

THE CENTRAL NERVOUS SYSTEM

The central nervous system is composed of nervous tissue, which is commonly described as grey and white matter. Examination of a section of the brain reveals that it is grey on the outside and white on the inside. Microscopic examination reveals that the grey matter is composed of neuron cell bodies, and the white matter is made up of myelinated fibres.

The brain

The brain is a large organ weighing about 1.4 kg in the adult, held in position within the skull by membranes called the meninges. In most parts of the brain the outer portion, or cortex, consists of grey matter, while white matter forms the inner portion. The grey matter is convoluted to provide a greater surface area. The brain is divided into the:

- Cerebrum, comprising the left and right cerebral hemispheres
- Diencephalon, comprising the left and right thalamus and hypothalamus
- Brainstem, comprising the midbrain, pons varolii and medulla oblongata — the stalk-like section that connects the brain to the spinal cord
- Cerebellum.

The cerebrum

The cerebrum (Figure 41.2) is the largest part of the brain, filling the vault of the cranium from front to back. It is divided by fissures into the left and right hemispheres, and each hemisphere is further divided by fissures into four lobes:

1. The frontal lobe, responsible for voluntary motor function, motivation, aggression, personality, sense of smell and mood
2. The parietal lobe, which receives and evaluates sensory information
3. The temporal lobe, which receives input for smell and hearing and has an important role in memory
4. The occipital lobe, responsible for reception and integration of visual input.

The left hemisphere is usually associated with language, mathematical skills and reasoning. The right hemisphere is generally associated with skills such as artistic awareness and imagination. Within each hemisphere is a cavity called the lateral ventricle, which is concerned with the formation of cerebrospinal fluid.

The cerebrum is divided into several areas, some of which are sensory and some of which are motor areas. The sensory areas of each hemisphere receive and interpret sensations from the opposite side of the body, including touch, temperature, pain, pressure and an awareness of the position of the body in its environment. The motor areas of each hemisphere control all voluntary movement on the opposite side of the body. The centres of special sense are located in the various lobes, including the centres for hearing, speech, smell, taste and sight (Figure 41.3).

The functions of the cerebrum are therefore to receive and interpret impulses from the sensory organs, to initiate and control the movements of skeletal muscles, and to perform the higher levels of mental activity such as thinking, reasoning, intelligence, learning and memory.

The diencephalon

The thalami are two oval masses of grey matter that form the lateral walls of the third ventricle. Each thalamus is subdivided into a number of nuclei. Most sensory pathways

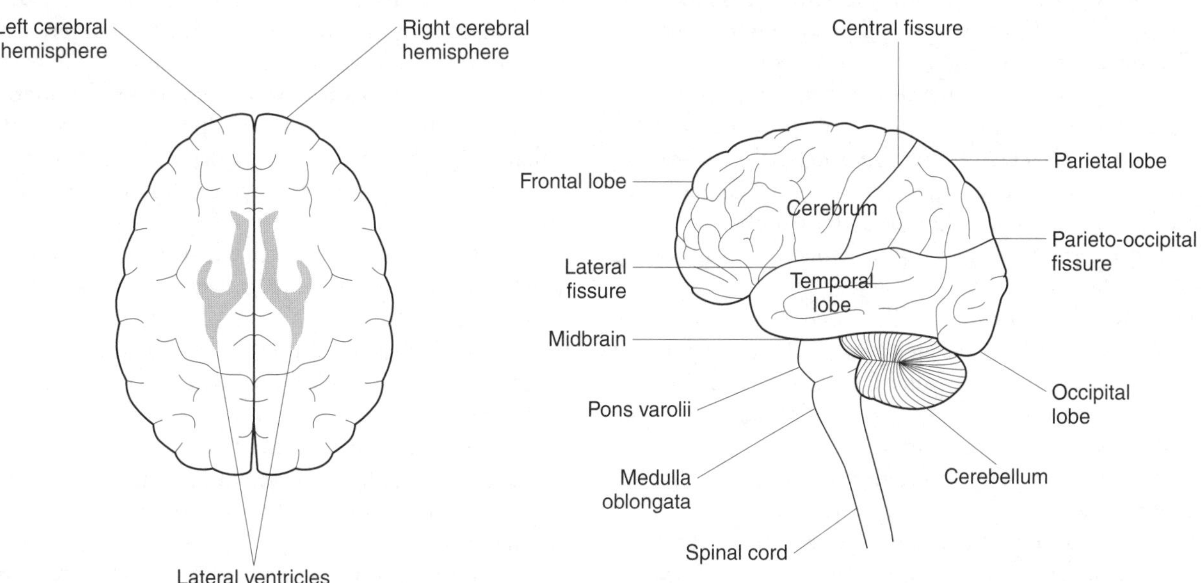

Figure 41.2 | The brain — cerebral hemispheres (left) and major structures (right)

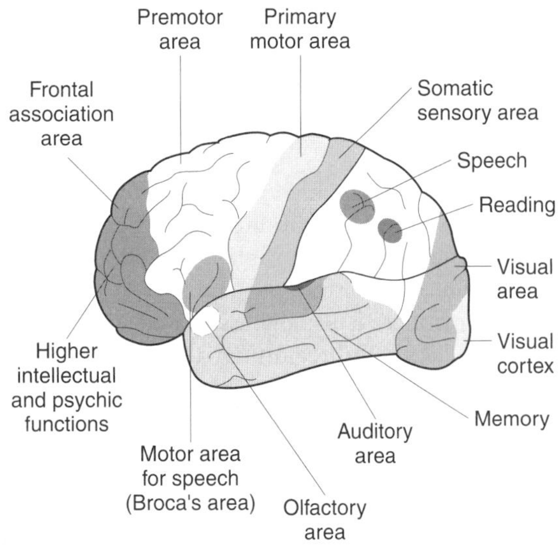

Figure 41.3 | The sensory and motor areas of the cerebrum

(except smell) synapse here. The thalamus plays a role in the control of somatic motor activity and also influences mood and strong emotions.

The hypothalamus lies beneath the thalami, and the pituitary gland is closely connected to it. The hypothalamus controls all the activities of the autonomic nervous system, which is described later in this chapter. The hypothalamus is important in controlling the endocrine system, as it regulates pituitary gland function.

The brainstem

The midbrain. The midbrain is a short narrow segment connecting the cerebrum with the pons varolii. It is composed primarily of ascending and descending fibre tracts. Its functions are to provide a pathway for impulses passing between the cerebrum and spinal cord, and to receive stimuli that initiate eye and postural movements.

The pons varolii. The pons varolii is about 2.5 cm long, lying anterior to the cerebellum and above the medulla oblongata. It contains two respiratory centres, the pneumotaxic centre and the apneustic centre. Its functions are to act as a relay station from the cerebrum to the cerebellum, and to modify the activity of the medullary respiratory centres through the pneumotaxic and apneustic centres.

The medulla oblongata. The medulla oblongata is about 2.5–3.0 cm long, lying between the pons and the spinal cord. It provides the link between the brain and the spinal cord and contains the cardiac, respiratory, vasomotor and reflex centres. Its functions are:

- To provide a pathway where nerve fibres to and from the brain cross over to the opposite side
- To control heartbeat (through the cardiac centre)
- To control ventilation (through the respiratory centre)
- To control constriction and dilatation of blood vessels (through the vasomotor centre)
- To initiate the reflex actions of swallowing, vomiting, coughing and sneezing (through the reflex centres).

The cerebellum

The cerebellum lies behind the pons and medulla and below the occipital lobes of the cerebrum. Like the cerebrum, the cerebellum is divided into two hemispheres that have shallow convolutions in their surface of grey matter. Its functions are coordination of muscular activity and regulation of muscle tone, and maintenance of balance and posture.

Blood supply to the brain

The carotid and the vertebral arteries supply blood to the brain. These arteries branch and join up again, forming a circle of arteries at the base of the brain called the circle of Willis. From here smaller cerebral arteries branch off to supply each region of the brain. Blood returns from the brain via the jugular veins to the superior vena cava.

The blood–brain barrier is a barrier that prevents or delays the entry of certain substances into brain tissue. The relatively low permeability of the capillaries supplying the brain means that some substances are either completely or partially prevented from gaining access to brain tissue. The blood–brain barrier thus acts as a protective mechanism, preventing substances such as bilirubin, which could disrupt brain function, from crossing the barrier.

The spinal cord

The spinal cord is a cylindrical structure that lies within a canal inside the vertebral column. It extends from an opening on the underside of the skull (the foramen magnum) to the level of the first or second lumbar vertebra. Below this level the vertebral canal is occupied by nerves from the lumbar and sacral segments of the cord; these constitute the cauda equina ('horse's tail'). The spinal cord, which is about 46 cm in length, consists of nervous tissue, with the white matter on the outside and the grey matter arranged roughly in an 'H' formation in the centre (Figures 41.4 and 41.5). The two anterior projections of grey matter are called the anterior horns, and the posterior projections are called the posterior horns. Sensory nerve fibres enter the posterior horns, and motor nerve fibres leave the anterior horns.

Leaving the spinal cord at intervals throughout its length are 31 pairs of spinal nerves. The functions of the spinal cord are:

- To receive sensory impulses from the tissues and convey them to the sensory areas of the brain via ascending (afferent) pathways
- To convey motor impulses from the brain to various parts of the body via descending (efferent) pathways
- To provide a pathway through which reflex actions take place.

A reflex action, or arc, is an automatic motor response to a sensory stimulus without conscious involvement (Figure 41.6). Most reflex actions are protective in nature and take place more quickly than voluntary actions. The structures involved in a reflex action are:

- A sensory organ (e.g. the skin) to receive the stimulus
- A sensory (afferent) nerve fibre to carry the impulse to the posterior horn of the spinal cord
- An association neuron in the spinal cord to receive the impulse and transmit it directly to the anterior horn
- A motor (efferent) neuron in the anterior horn to receive the impulse and transmit it to the motor organ
- A motor organ (e.g. a muscle) to receive and respond to the stimulus.

An example of a reflex action is when the hand comes into contact with a very hot object. The skin on the hand receives the stimulus of heat, and an impulse travels from the sensory nerve endings in the skin to the posterior horn of the spinal cord. From there, the impulse is transmitted to the anterior horn, then passed along the motor nerves to the muscles of the shoulder, arm and hand. As a result, the hand is pulled rapidly away from the source of heat before the brain has even processed the information. The brain may inhibit or exaggerate reflexes.

The meninges

The meninges are the three membranes that cover the brain and the spinal cord. The individual membranes are:

1. The dura mater (meaning 'hard mother') is the tough outermost layer. It consists of two layers of fibrous connective tissue, with one layer forming the periosteum covering the inner surface of the skull bones, and the other layer covering the brain and spinal cord
2. The arachnoid mater (meaning 'mother like a spider's web') is the middle layer. The name refers to the fact that it is so thin that, when viewed under a microscope, it resembles a spider's web
3. The pia mater (meaning 'gentle mother') is the delicate innermost layer. It adheres closely to the surface of the brain and spinal cord, dipping down

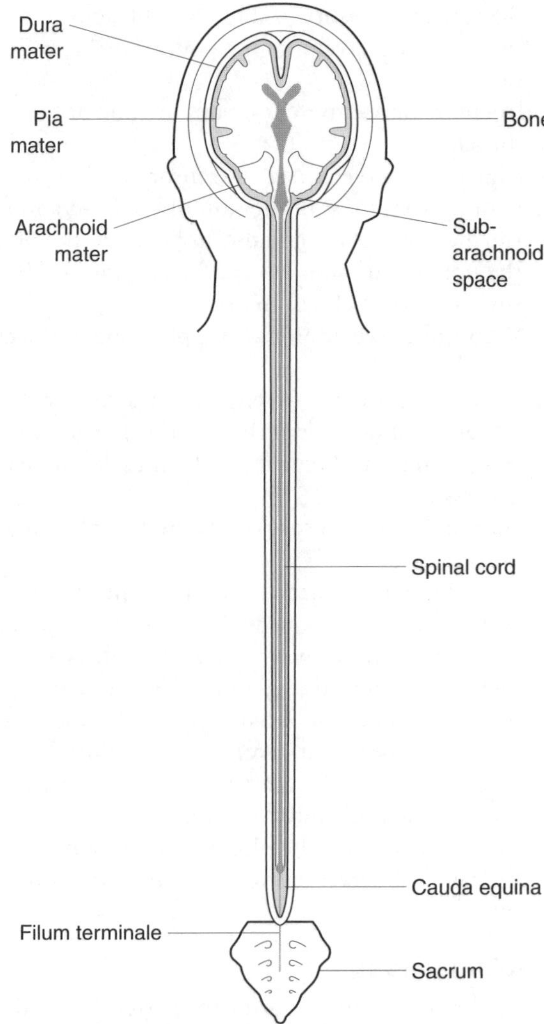

Figure 41.4 | Vertical section of the meninges and spinal cord

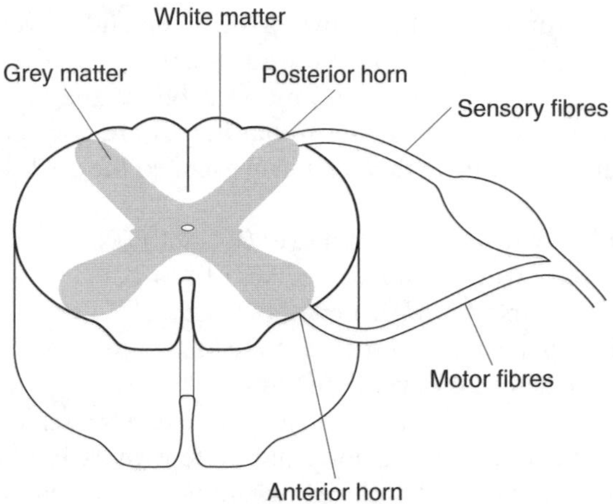

Figure 41.5 | Cross-section of the spinal cord

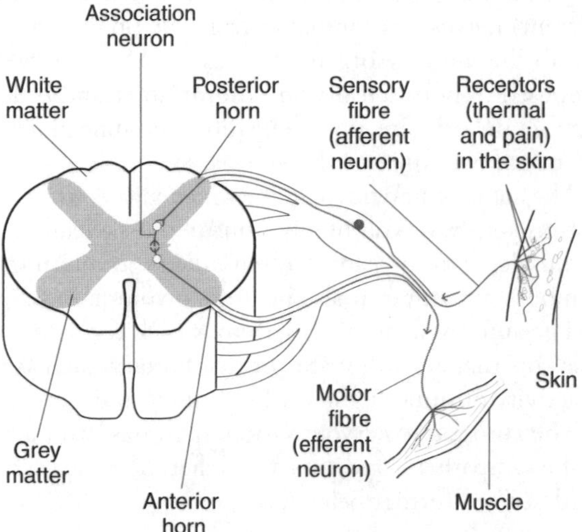

Figure 41.6 | A reflex arc

into all the convolutions and fissures. The pia mater is richly supplied with blood vessels that carry blood to the brain and spinal cord.

The subarachnoid space is the space between the arachnoid mater and pia mater, filled with cerebrospinal fluid in circulation. The functions of the meninges are to form a protective covering against physical injury around the brain and spinal cord, and to help secure the brain to the cranial vault.

Cerebrospinal fluid

Cerebrospinal fluid (CSF) is a clear watery fluid with a composition similar to plasma. It contains substances including water, glucose, sodium, chloride, potassium, protein and waste products such as urea. The CSF is formed from the blood and is produced by a combination of filtration and active secretory processes by the choroid plexus in the ventricles of the brain. CSF circulates in the subarachnoid space surrounding the brain and spinal cord. The total volume of the CSF is about 150 mL. The fluid is formed continuously in the ventricles at a rate of about 600–700 mL/day, and is reabsorbed into the blood at about the same rate. The normal CSF pressure when the body is horizontal is 5–10 mmHg. The functions of CSF are to:

- Form a protective cushion around the brain and spinal cord
- Maintain normal pressure around the brain and spinal cord
- Provide a medium for the exchange of nutrients and waste products between the bloodstream and the nervous tissue.

THE PERIPHERAL NERVOUS SYSTEM

The peripheral nervous system consists of the 12 pairs of cranial nerves that leave the brainstem, and 31 pairs of spinal nerves that leave the spinal cord. The peripheral nerves may be sensory, motor or mixed. Sensory (afferent) nerves carry impulses to the brain and spinal cord. Motor (efferent) nerves carry impulses from the brain and spinal cord to the muscles, organs and tissues. Mixed nerves are composed of both sensory and motor fibres and transmit impulses in both directions. The motor peripheral nervous system has two functional divisions:

- The somatic nervous system, which allows us to consciously, or voluntarily, control our skeletal muscles. This division is often called the voluntary motor system but it also includes involuntary reflexes
- The autonomic nervous system, which regulates events that are automatic, or involuntary, such as the activity of smooth and cardiac muscle and glands. The autonomic nervous system itself has two parts — the sympathetic and parasympathetic nervous systems (described further below).

The cranial nerves

Twelve pairs of cranial nerves leave the brainstem. The numbers (Roman numerals are the convention), names and functions of the cranial nerves are:

I. Olfactory nerve: sensory — the nerve of smell
II. Optic nerve: sensory — the nerve of sight
III. Oculomotor nerve: motor — supplies the muscle of the eye
IV. Trochlear nerve: motor — supplies one of the eye muscles
V. Trigeminal nerve: mixed — sensory fibres receive stimuli from most of the skin of the head and face, the membranes of the nose and mouth, the orbits, the upper and lower jaws and teeth; motor fibres supply the muscles of mastication
VI. Abducent nerve: motor — supplies one of the eye muscles
VII. Facial nerve: mixed — sensory fibres convey the sensation of taste from the anterior portion of the tongue; motor fibres supply the muscles of facial expressions
VIII. Auditory nerve: sensory — the nerve of hearing and balance
IX. Glossopharyngeal nerve: mixed — sensory fibres convey taste sensations from the posterior part of the tongue; motor fibres supply the pharynx
X. Vagus nerve: mixed — controls secretion and movement of the internal organs (e.g. oesophagus, larynx, trachea, heart, stomach, intestines, pancreas, spleen, kidneys and blood vessels)
XI. Accessory nerve: motor — supplies the muscles of the neck, and also the pharynx and larynx
XII. Hypoglossal nerve: motor — supplies the tongue muscles.

The spinal nerves

The spinal nerves project out of the vertebral canal, one pair emerging below each vertebra, and one pair emerging between the cranium and the first cervical vertebra. The spinal nerves are mixed nerves, containing both sensory and motor fibres. They allow for sensation and movement in peripheral parts of the body not supplied by the cranial nerves, such as skin, muscles, bones and joints of the trunk and limbs. The spinal nerves are arranged in groups according to their region of origin in the cord. There are:

- Eight pairs of cervical nerves (C1–C8)
- Twelve pairs of thoracic nerves (T1–T12)
- Five pairs of lumbar nerves (L1–L5)
- Five pairs of sacral nerves (S1–S5)
- One pair of coccygeal nerves.

In some regions the nerves divide immediately after leaving the cord. These then branch and unite with each other to form what is called a plexus (meaning braid). The major plexuses are:

- The cervical plexus, which supplies the muscles of the

neck and shoulders, and also gives rise to the phrenic nerves that supply the diaphragm
- The brachial plexus, which gives rise to the radial, median and ulna nerves, which supply the arm
- The lumbar plexus, which gives rise to the femoral nerve, which supplies the thigh muscles
- The sacral plexus, from which the sciatic nerve arises.

The sciatic nerve is the largest nerve in the body, running over the hip posteriorly down the back of the thigh to the knee where it divides into the peroneal nerve and tibial nerve.

THE AUTONOMIC NERVOUS SYSTEM

The autonomic nervous system is the division of the peripheral nervous system concerned with involuntary activity of the body. It supplies nerves to all the structures in the body that are not under conscious control. The autonomic nervous system consists of two divisions: the sympathetic and the parasympathetic nervous systems.

The sympathetic nervous system

The sympathetic nervous system arises from grey matter in the spinal cord from T1 through to L2. Sympathetic nerves then synapse in a chain of ganglia that lies on either side of the vertebral column, before reaching organs or tissues. A ganglion (plural ganglia) is a knot-like mass of cell bodies. Plexuses are formed by fibres from these ganglia; for example, the solar plexus lying behind the stomach and supplying the abdominal organs, and the cardiac plexus supplying the heart and lungs.

The parasympathetic nervous system

The parasympathetic nervous system consists of cranial nerves III, VII, IX and X and nerves that emerge from the sacral region of the spinal cord. The vagus nerve (cranial nerve X) is the largest autonomic nerve.

Functions of the autonomic nervous system

The functions of the autonomic nervous system are to control the movements of internal organs and the secretions of glands. The system provides dual control: the activity of an organ is stimulated by one set of nerves, and inhibited by the other set of nerves. This dual control achieves smooth rhythmic action of involuntary muscles and internal organs, maintaining a balance between activity and rest.

The sympathetic nerves are called adrenergic nerve fibres and release the neurotransmitter noradrenaline. These nerves can be affected by strong emotions such as anger, fear, or excitement, and have a stimulating effect on most organs. The effect resembles that produced by adrenaline, a hormone secreted by the adrenal glands. This effect is called the 'fright, fight or flight' effect, in which the body responds to a fright either by preparing to fight or by running away. The response of the body includes:

- Dilation of the pupils of the eyes
- Increased force and rate of heartbeat, increasing circulation
- Increased blood pressure and constriction of arterioles in the skin and abdominal organs to divert blood to all skeletal muscles, heart, lungs and brain
- Dilation of the bronchi to allow more oxygen to enter
- Slowing of digestion so that the digestive organs can receive a reduced blood supply, enabling blood to be diverted to vital structures
- Increased production of sweat by sweat glands
- A rise in blood sugar level, as the liver is stimulated to release more glucose for increased energy needs.

The parasympathetic nerves are called cholinergic fibres and release the neurotransmitter acetylcholine. These nerves tend to slow down body processes, so that the end result of the antagonistic action of each division of the autonomic nervous system is a balance between acceleration and retardation. After the 'fright' or stressful situation is over, the parasympathetic nervous system returns things to normal. The digestive organs receive more blood, the glands increase their secretions, the heartbeat is decreased and the blood pressure falls. The effects of sympathetic and parasympathetic stimulation on various body organs are compared in Table 41.1.

PATHOPHYSIOLOGICAL INFLUENCES AND EFFECTS OF DISORDERS OF THE NERVOUS SYSTEM

The pathophysiological changes that can disrupt normal function of part or all of the nervous system can be due to congenital or developmental disorders, infectious or inflammatory conditions, trauma, neoplasia, degenerative conditions, and metabolic or endocrine disorders. Any pathophysiological change is capable of causing various types and degrees of dysfunction.

AETIOLOGY OF NERVOUS SYSTEM DISORDERS

Congenital disorders

The central nervous system of the developing fetus is very vulnerable to damage. Factors that may cause nervous system damage include the passage of microorganisms and drugs across the placental barrier into the fetal circulation. Other factors that may cause nervous system defects and result in physical and intellectual deterioration include chromosomal abnormalities, metabolic disorders, cranial malformations and structural abnormalities. The central nervous system may also be damaged during the birth process; for example, by cerebral anoxia or cerebral haemorrhage.

Inflammatory and infectious conditions

Bacterial or viral infective processes affecting the central nervous system may result in the destruction of nervous tissue through the action of toxins released by the living microorganisms and from the material released from

TABLE 41.1 | EFFECTS OF SYMPATHETIC AND PARASYMPATHETIC STIMULATION

Organ	Sympathetic stimulation	Parasympathetic stimulation
Heart	Increases rate/strength of heartbeat Dilates coronary arteries to increase blood supply to the heart muscle	Decreases rate/strength of heartbeat Constricts coronary arteries to decrease supply of blood to the heart muscle
Bronchi	Dilates bronchi, allowing more air to enter the lungs	Constricts bronchi, limiting air intake
Digestive system	Decreases activity of the system and constricts digestive system sphincters Inhibits production of saliva	Increases peristalsis and relaxes sphincters Stimulates production of saliva
Urinary bladder	Relaxes bladder wall. Contracts internal sphincter muscle	Contracts bladder wall. Relaxes internal sphincter muscle
Eye	Dilates the pupil. Retracts the eyelids	Constricts the pupil. Closes the eyelids
Skin	Stimulates perspiration Stimulates smooth muscles attached to hair follicles, producing 'goose bumps'	No effect on sweat glands No effect on muscles/hair follicles

dead microorganisms, which stimulates the inflammatory process. Infection and inflammation of nervous tissue may result in altered behaviour, altered consciousness, and sensory or motor deficits.

Trauma

Trauma to the nervous system may result from elements within the system or from external forces. Trauma occurring from elements within the nervous system includes bleeding from an aneurysm or ruptured intracranial vessel; transient interruption of the cerebral blood flow, causing ischaemia; and occlusion of a cerebral blood vessel by a thrombus or embolus. The most common causative factors in these conditions are hypertension and atherosclerosis.

Trauma from external forces may be caused by a direct or an indirect injury. A direct acceleration brain injury occurs when the head is struck by a moving object, and a direct deceleration injury occurs when the head in motion strikes a stationary object. In an indirect brain injury, the traumatic force is transmitted to the head through an impact to another part of the body, such as the neck or buttocks.

In open head trauma, a penetrating injury damages the integrity of the skull and/or meninges and brain. Infection may occur, as the injury allows the entry of microorganisms. A closed head injury is non-penetrating, with no disruption to the integrity of the cerebral meninges. Closed head injuries can result in jarring, bruising or tearing of brain tissue, which can cause haemorrhage, cranial nerve damage and cerebral oedema. An important event in closed head injury is known as coup and contrecoup. The coup injury is cerebral bruising resulting from impact to the skull, and contrecoup refers to the rebound effect of the injury, the movement of the brain opposite to the site of impact.

The nervous system response to trauma, which may cause more damage than the actual injury, results in oedema, bleeding and increased intracranial pressure. These factors destroy nervous tissue by compression or restriction of the circulation.

The spinal cord may be damaged as a result of a crushing or penetrating injury, dislocation of the spinal column, prolapsed intravertebral discs or neoplasia. In addition to tearing of, and pressure on, the spinal cord tissues, damage may be caused by haemorrhage, oedema or disruption of the blood supply to the spinal cord.

Damage to the peripheral nerves may result in loss of sensory and/or motor function.

Neoplasia

Tumours of the nervous system, which may be either benign or malignant, cause symptoms related to pressure, destruction of nervous tissue, oedema and disruption of the blood supply. The neurological manifestations of a tumour affecting the nervous system depend on the location of the tumour and on its rate of growth.

Degenerative conditions

The causes of degenerative disorders of the nervous system are varied and involve atrophy of neurons and nerve fibres. The course of a degenerative disorder is generally gradual and progressive over many years. The effects of degenerative disorders include progressive muscular atrophy; impaired speech, chewing, swallowing and breathing; deterioration of intellectual capacity; impaired motor function; and dementia.

Metabolic and endocrine disorders

Nervous system dysfunction may result from the effects of certain metabolic and endocrine disorders. Some nutritional deficiencies may affect nerve cells, resulting in their damage or death. For example, degeneration of the posterior and lateral columns of the spinal cord may occur from the vitamin B12 deficiency of pernicious anaemia. Disorders of cortical function, leading to confusion or coma, may result from a deficiency of thiamine (vitamin B1).

Specific endocrine disorders such as hypothyroidism result in decreased metabolic rate, and hypothermia can develop. If the body temperature falls below 30°C, unconsciousness will result. Myxoedema coma is characterised by exaggeration of the signs and symptoms of hypothyroidism, with neurological impairment leading to loss of consciousness.

MAJOR MANIFESTATIONS OF NERVOUS SYSTEM DISORDERS

The manifestations of a nervous system disorder will vary depending on the type and severity of the disorder.

Headaches, or cephalalgia

Headaches are common in a variety of disorders and situations ranging from functional disturbances of blood vessels to tension and stress. In neurological disorders, headaches are one of the most common symptoms. Headaches can result from compression, traction, displacement or inflammation of the cranial periosteum, the dura mater, cerebral arteries or branches of the cranial nerves. Headaches may also occur as a result of tension within extracranial structures such as muscles, air sinuses and blood vessels. Headaches are commonly classified as vascular, tension or traction–inflammatory.

Vascular headaches

These include migraine, cluster headaches, hypertension headaches, and headaches resulting from temporal arteritis. Although the mechanisms of migraine are not completely understood, migraine appears to result from an inherited predisposition and seems to be precipitated by trigger factors such as stress, abrupt falls in oestrogen levels, low blood glucose levels and dietary intake. One theory is that migraine results from spasm of intracranial blood vessels and dilation of extracranial blood vessels. The classic characteristics of migraine headache include throbbing and a tendency for the attacks to be unilateral. Some attacks are preceded by a variety of visual disturbances, such as loss of half of the visual field, or flashing lights across the visual fields. Some individuals experience vertigo, nausea and vomiting.

Cluster headaches are a rapid succession of attacks over several days, followed by remission. Previously thought to be caused by histamine sensitisation, cluster headaches are now considered to have a vascular cause. Headaches associated with severe hypertension may be intense and similar to those caused by intracranial lesions. Temporal arteritis causes severe, throbbing headaches in the region of the temporal artery and is sometimes accompanied by visual loss.

Tension headaches

Tension headaches are caused by prolonged contraction (tension) of the neck, head or facial muscles. Tension headaches are frequently associated with psychological factors such as anxiety or depression. The pain tends to be bilateral and, unlike vascular headaches, is not throbbing in character.

Traction–inflammatory headaches

Headaches of this type are related to increased intracranial pressure, which causes irritation of, and traction on, blood vessels and the dura mater within the skull. Inflammation of the meninges (meningitis) can also result in severe headache. Headaches of intracranial origin related to increased intracranial pressure vary from mild to excruciating depending on the location and cause, such as a tumour, lesion or cerebral oedema.

Sensory changes

Sensory changes, which can result from disorders of the brain, spinal cord or peripheral nerves, include alterations in the sense of touch, pain, temperature sensitivity and the loss of a sense of position. The loss of these sensations may be partial or complete. Common sensory disturbances include neuritis and neuralgia. Neuritis, characterised by pain and tenderness along the path of a nerve, can progress to complete loss of sensory and motor function. Neuralgia is characterised by severe stabbing pain, and can be caused by a variety of disorders affecting the nervous system. Other sensory changes that may accompany nervous system disorders include a loss of taste or smell, visual changes and hearing loss.

Motor changes

Alterations in motor function include localised or generalised weakness, with difficulty in moving normally. Muscle tone may be abnormally increased or decreased. A pronounced increase in tone is referred to as rigidity. Spasticity of muscles is an increased resistance to passive stretch, with rapid flexion of a joint. Abnormal movements include:

- Twitching: localised spasmodic contraction of a single muscle group
- Tremor: rhythmic quivering movements resulting from involuntary alternating contraction and relaxation of opposing groups of muscles
- Myoclonus: spasm of a muscle or a group of muscles
- Dystonia: intense irregular muscle spasms
- Athetosis: slow, writhing involuntary movements of the extremities
- Chorea: involuntary, purposeless, rapid jerky movements
- Dyskinesia: involuntary twitching of the limbs or facial muscles.

Symptoms of ataxia, a condition characterised by impaired ability to coordinate movement, may be caused by a lesion in the spinal cord or cerebellum. Dizziness or vertigo, when the individual is unable to maintain normal balance in a standing or seated position, may also be related to a disorder of the nervous system. Unusual gait or stance may result from motor or sensory deficits caused by a disorder of the nervous system, such as Parkinson's disease. Paralysis, a symptom of motor disturbances, can occur in varying degrees with many nervous system disorders. Upper motor neuron lesions, in which the reflex area remains intact, generally cause spastic paralysis. Flaccid paralysis generally occurs in lower motor neuron lesions, which disrupt the reflex area.

Reflex changes

Reflex changes can provide evidence of damage to the nervous system. The absences of normal reflexes, or the presence of abnormal reflexes, generally indicate nervous system dysfunction. Reflexes are classed as either superficial (cutaneous) or deep tendon (muscle stretch). Superficial reflexes are elicited when a stimulus is applied to the skin surface or to mucous membrane. Deep tendon reflexes are elicited when a stimulus is applied to a tendon, bone or joint.

Altered awareness, personality or level of consciousness

A neurological disorder that results in altered brain structure may cause impairment of a person's cognitive functions. They may experience difficulty in being able to think, remember, reason or understand. The person may also be confused in that orientation to time, place and person is impaired. Signs of reduced alertness or responsiveness may also be shown. Brain damage, for example as a result of a head injury, can cause a confused state characterised by fluctuating disorientation and incoherence.

Cerebral impairment may also cause mood changes and/or inappropriate emotional responses. Diffuse brain damage such as that caused by a large cerebral infarction may result in emotional instability or lability (a tendency to show alternating states of happiness and sadness that seem to be inappropriate). The person may also show signs of emotional flatness or apathy, demonstrated by a reactive absence of emotions. Alternatively, the client may become euphoric.

Damage to the brain can also result in altered states of consciousness, ranging from drowsiness and difficulty in being aroused by normal stimuli, to coma. Further information on assessment of level of consciousness is provided later in this chapter.

Seizures

Seizures, which are paroxysmal events associated with sudden abnormal discharges of electrical energy in the neurons of the brain, may be secondary to central nervous system disease. Seizure disorders are described later in this chapter.

SPECIFIC DISORDERS OF THE NERVOUS SYSTEM

Disorders of the nervous system may be congenital or genetic, due to multiple causes, degenerative, infectious or inflammatory, immunological, neoplastic, obstructive or traumatic.

CONGENITAL DISORDERS

Structural congenital abnormalities include anencephaly, spinal cord defects and hydrocephalus.

Anencephaly

Anencephaly is the failure of normal development of the cranium and scalp. The precise cause is unknown, and babies with the disorder do not live.

Spinal cord defects

These include spina bifida, meningocele and myelomeningocele. These conditions are the result of incomplete closure of the neural tube during the first 3 months of embryonic development. Causes are thought to include maternal exposure to viruses, radiation and other environmental factors.

In severe forms, spina bifida involves incomplete closure of one or more of the vertebrae, causing protrusion of the spinal contents in an external sac. In spina bifida with meningocele, the sac contains meninges and CSF. In spina bifida with myelomeningocele the sac contains meninges, CSF and a portion of the spinal cord or nerve roots. Manifestations of congenital spinal cord defects vary and include a depression, dimple or tuft of hair on the skin over the spinal defect. The more severe defects cause neurological dysfunction such as paralysis of the legs, bowel and bladder incontinence and hydrocephalus.

Hydrocephalus

Hydrocephalus is an excessive accumulation of CSF within the ventricles of the brain. It may result from an obstruction in CSF flow or from faulty absorption of CSF. The condition can also occur after birth as a result of cerebral injury or disease. In infants, the obvious manifestation of hydrocephalus is abnormal enlargement of the head. Other characteristics include distended scalp veins, thin and fragile scalp skin, downward displacement of the eyes, a shrill high-pitched cry, irritability and abnormal muscle tone of the legs.

GENETIC DISORDERS

Hereditary genetic defects include muscular dystrophy, Huntington's chorea and neurofibromatosis.

Muscular dystrophy

Muscular dystrophy is a group of congenital disorders characterised by progressive wasting and weakness of muscles. Duchenne muscular dystrophy, which begins to manifest between the ages of 3 and 5 years, is the most common and severe form. Initially it affects the leg and pelvic muscles but there is progressive involvement of all voluntary muscles. Later in the disease, progressive weakening of cardiac and respiratory muscles results in heart or respiratory failure. Early manifestations of Duchenne's muscular dystrophy include a waddling gait, lordosis (increased curvature of the lumbar spine) and marked difficulty rising from a supine to a standing position. As the disease progresses, facial, oropharyngeal and respiratory muscles become involved.

Huntington's chorea

Huntington's chorea is a disorder in which degeneration of the cerebral cortex and basal ganglia causes chronic progressive choreiform movements and mental deterioration. Onset is generally in early middle age, and the individual gradually develops progressively severe choreiform movements and dementia. The movements usually begin slowly, with facial grimacing and jerking arm actions. Over time, the movements become frequent, erratic and violent, affecting the trunk and lower limbs. Dementia may be mild at first but eventually severely disrupts the personality.

Neurofibromatosis

Neurofibromatosis is characterised by a variety of congenital abnormalities and the condition is usually classified according to which parts of the nervous system are affected. In the peripheral form, multiple cutaneous and subcutaneous nodules of varying size occur. Subcutaneous nodules may attach to the peripheral portion of the nerve, causing pain or pressure and, rarely, sensory loss in the distribution of the affected nerve. Neuromas, which are an overgrowth of subcutaneous tissue, may reach enormous sizes and commonly affect the face, scalp, neck and chest. Neurological symptoms may appear if the tumours cause pressure on the brain or spinal cord.

DISORDERS OF MULTIPLE CAUSE

Cerebral palsy

Cerebral palsy comprises a group of neuromotor disorders resulting from prenatal, perinatal or postnatal cerebral hypoxia or damage. The incidence of cerebral palsy is highest in premature infants or in infants who have experienced a difficult birth resulting in cerebral damage. Causative factors include chromosomal abnormalities; prenatal factors such as maternal infections, exposure to harmful chemicals or malnutrition; perinatal factors such as premature birth or instrumental delivery causing cerebral anoxia; and postnatal factors such as trauma, infection or malnutrition causing cerebral damage.

The manifestations of cerebral palsy range from mild muscle incoordination to severe spasticity. The spastic form of the disorder is characterised by rapid alternating muscle contraction and relaxation, muscle weakness and underdevelopment, and muscle contraction in response to manipulation. The athetoid form of cerebral palsy is characterised by grimacing, writhing and jerking involuntary movements, which become more severe during stress. Ataxic cerebral palsy is characterised by disturbed balance, incoordination, muscle weakness and tremor. In addition to the range of motor deficits, the individual may experience sensory deficits such as speech, visual or hearing impairment. Intellectual disability accompanies cerebral palsy in about 40% of cases.

Cerebral aneurysm

A cerebral aneurysm is an abnormality of the wall of a cerebral artery that results in a localised dilation. If the aneurysm ruptures, blood enters the subarachnoid space or cerebral tissue. Causative factors include congenital defects in the arterial walls, sclerotic changes in blood vessels, hypertension and cerebral trauma. Manifestations of a cerebral aneurysm do not generally appear until the aneurysm ruptures. The most common symptom of rupture is the sudden onset of a severe headache, which may be accompanied by nausea and vomiting, motor deficits, visual disturbances and loss of consciousness. A cerebral aneurysm may be detected before it ruptures if the individual shows signs of oculomotor nerve compression, eyelid ptosis and a pupil that is sluggish or non-reactive.

Transient ischaemic attacks

Transient ischaemic attacks (TIAs) are recurrent episodes of neurologic deficit. The attacks, which may last from seconds to hours, are generally considered to be warning signs of an impending thrombotic cerebrovascular accident (CVA). The characteristics of a TIA, which may be caused by micro-emboli or arteriole spasm, are various symptoms of neurological dysfunction followed by a return of normal function. Symptoms include double vision, slurred or thick speech, unilateral loss of vision, staggering or uncoordinated gait, unilateral weakness or numbness, dizziness and falling because of leg weakness.

Trigeminal neuralgia

Trigeminal neuralgia is a painful disorder of one or more branches of the trigeminal nerve that produces paroxysmal attacks of excruciating facial pain. While the cause is often unknown, the disorder may be associated with other neurological conditions such as aneurysms, cerebral tumours or multiple sclerosis. The individual experiences excruciating burning pain, which generally occurs suddenly in response to a stimulus, such as a draft of cold air, drinking hot or cold fluids, brushing the teeth, or speaking or laughing. The frequency of attacks varies from many times a day to several times a month or year.

Intellectual disability

Intellectual disability is a syndrome of incomplete intellectual development associated with impaired learning and social adjustment. The causes include:

- Prenatal factors such as metabolic disorders,

chromosomal abnormalities, cranial malformation, maternal infections, malnutrition or anoxia
- Perinatal factors such as prematurity, anoxia or intracranial haemorrhage
- Postnatal factors such as cerebral injury, central nervous system infections, anoxia, neoplasms, degenerative diseases, cerebral haemorrhage, nutritional deficiencies and emotional deprivation.

Manifestations include poor motor development, impaired concepts of space and time, learning difficulties, inappropriate behaviour and difficulty with social interactions.

Peripheral neuritis

Peripheral neuritis (polyneuritis) is the degeneration of peripheral nerves, resulting in muscle weakness and atrophy, sensory loss and decreased or absent tendon reflexes. Causes include chronic intoxication (alcohol, arsenic, lead), metabolic and inflammatory disorders (diabetes mellitus, rheumatoid arthritis), nutrient deficiencies (thiamine), and infectious diseases (meningitis or Guillain–Barré syndrome). Manifestations usually develop slowly, beginning with leg pains and numbness or tingling in the feet and hands. As the disease progresses the individual experiences flaccid paralysis, muscle wasting, pain of varying intensity, and loss of reflexes in the legs and arms. Footdrop, ataxic gait and inability to walk will eventually occur.

Guillain–Barré syndrome

Guillain–Barré syndrome is characterised by an acute onset of ascending motor and sensory deficits, which are rapidly progressive. Although the precise cause is unclear, there is suggestion that the disorder may be viral or immunological in origin. About 50% of people with the condition experience a mild respiratory tract or gastrointestinal infection 1–3 weeks before the onset of polyneuritis. Manifestations include paraesthesia and weakness of the leg muscles, which extend to the upper body within 24–72 hours. Respiratory distress can result from diaphragm and intercostal muscle weakness, and the cranial nerves may become involved.

Bell's palsy

Bell's palsy is a disorder of the seventh cranial nerve that produces unilateral facial weakness or paralysis. An inflammatory reaction occurs in or around cranial nerve VII, resulting in nerve compression and the onset of flaccid facial paralysis. Factors responsible for the inflammatory reaction include infection, prolonged exposure to cold temperature, and local trauma. The seventh cranial nerve can also be affected by other conditions such as a cerebral tumour, meningitis or a middle-ear infection. Manifestations are unilateral facial weakness, which is sometimes associated with pain around the angle of the jaw or behind the ear. On the affected side the mouth droops and the individual is unable to wrinkle the forehead, close the eyelid, or smile. There may be excessive watering from the affected eye and drooling of saliva from the affected side of the mouth.

SEIZURE DISORDERS

Seizure disorders may be primary and idiopathic, or secondary and symptomatic of a central nervous system disorder. The most common type of seizure disorder is epilepsy. Seizures may be focal or partial, absence or generalised. Focal or partial seizures generally affect a specific body part, and the symptoms of an attack depend on the location of the cerebral focus. For example, the focal motor, or Jacksonian, seizure occurs from a lesion in the motor cortex or strip. Typically it causes stiffening or jerking in one extremity that is accompanied by numbness or tingling.

Absence, or petit mal, seizures last only a few seconds but may progress to generalised tonic–clonic seizures. They generally begin with a brief change in the level of consciousness, which is indicated by a blank stare, eyelid fluttering or head nodding, or a pause in conversation. The individual generally retains posture and returns to pre-seizure activity without difficulty. This type of epilepsy usually occurs in childhood and may continue into early adolescence.

Although seizures may result from a nervous system disorder, they may be caused by many other factors and are often idiopathic. The international classification of seizures is given in Table 41.2.

A generalised seizure is commonly referred to as a tonic–clonic, or grand mal, seizure or convulsion. This type of seizure usually consists of three phases:

1. Aura. The aura (which is not always experienced) is a warning of an impending seizure. An aura is a sensation (e.g. a specific taste or smell) experienced by the individual immediately before a seizure. The seizure commonly begins with a loud cry, which is caused by air being forced out through the vocal cords that are in spasm
2. Tonic–clonic (convulsive) phase. The individual then loses consciousness and may fall. The muscles become rigid, then alternate between episodes of muscle spasm and relaxation (tonus and clonus), resulting in jerky spasmodic body movements. Tongue biting, incontinence of urine, laboured breathing, apnoea and cyanosis may occur
3. Post-convulsive phase. The seizure generally stops within 2–5 minutes, when abnormal electrical conduction in the brain ceases. The individual regains consciousness but may be dazed and confused or fall asleep. Rarely, automatism may follow, and violence may be exhibited. Automatism is a state in which the individual exhibits mechanical, repetitive and undirected behaviour that is not consciously controlled.

Status epilepticus is a condition in which the individual experiences continuous seizures without regaining consciousness in between. It is generally accompanied by respiratory distress.

Figure 41.7 shows a sample nursing critical pathway

TABLE 41.2 | THE INTERNATIONAL CLASSIFICATION OF SEIZURES

I	**Focal or partial seizures** Simple (general, without an impairment of level of consciousness): • Motor, e.g. Jacksonian seizures • Sensory or somatosensory • Autonomic Complex (the spread of simple or partial to a generalised convulsive form such as temporal lobe or psychomotor)
II	**Generalised seizures (without a local onset, bilateral, symmetric)** • Absences (petit mal) • Tonic–clonic (grand mal) • Infantile spasms (convulsions) • Bilateral massive myoclonus • Clonic seizures • Tonic seizures • Atonic seizures • Akinetic seizures
III	**Unilateral seizures**
IV	**Unclassified seizures (when complete data are not available)**
V	**Classification of paroxysmal forms** • Benign febrile seizures • Convulsive equivalent syndrome • Breath-holding spells

for managing a client after a seizure, and Clinical Interest Box 41.1 provides an outline of teaching for home care of clients in relation to seizures.

DEGENERATIVE DISORDERS

Parkinson's disease

Parkinson's disease is a degenerative process of nerve cells in the basal ganglia and substantia nigra. The substantia nigra is an area in the basal ganglia considered necessary for motor control. Although the precise cause of the disorder is unknown, research has demonstrated that a dopamine deficiency prevents affected brain cells from functioning normally. Dopamine is a neurotransmitter that plays a role in the transmission of nerve impulses between synapses. Factors implicated in the development of Parkinson's disease include cerebral atherosclerosis and long-term therapy with drugs such as haloperidol and phenothiazine.

Manifestations of Parkinson's disease are related to disturbances of movement: tremor, muscle rigidity and dyskinesia. The most common initial symptom is tremor; for example, 'pill-rolling' movements of the fingers, and to-and-fro head tremors. Tremors are aggravated by fatigue and stress, and decrease when the individual performs a purposeful activity or is asleep. The person experiences difficulty in initiating voluntary movement and loss of posture control, so that walking is with the body bent

CLINICAL INTEREST BOX 41.1
Teaching for home care of clients affected by generalised seizures

Teaching must be planned around a systematic assessment of the needs of both the client and their significant others. Significant others need to be included so that they can learn seizure management, care and observations. The importance of safety and maintenance of a patent airway should be stressed. The following recommendations assist the client and significant others to adjust:

- Correct misconceptions, fears and myths about epilepsy
- Encourage both the client and their significant others to express their feelings
- Provide the name and location of community and national resources; for example, the Epilepsy Foundation of Victoria (www.epinet.org.au). Facilitate socialisation with others facing the same issues
- Stress the importance of follow-up care and keeping medical appointments
- Refer the client to employment or vocational counselling as needed
- Review any state and local laws that apply to people with seizure disorders. Usually a driver's licence can be reinstated after a 2-year seizure-free period and a letter from a medical practitioner
- Stress the importance of wearing a medical alert bracelet and carrying a medical alert card at all times
- Emphasise the importance of aura identification and plan action to take
- Emphasise the importance of taking anticonvulsant medication as prescribed, even when seizures no longer occur
- Avoid physical and emotional stress
- Help clients develop a positive focus on life
- In general, alcohol should be avoided and caffeine limited
- Discuss factors that may trigger a seizure (fatigue, abrupt stopping of medication, flashing video games).

CRITICAL PATHWAYS
For client post seizure
Expected length of stay 2 days

DATE:	Day 1 **Admission**	Day 2 **Discharge**	AM	PM	ND
Discharge planning	Family assessment if not previously complete Establish discharge objectives with client and family Determine discharge needs and support system with client and significant others Begin home care instructions	Complete family assessment Assess discharge objectives can be realistically achieved Implement referral to support services as required Ensure that home care instructions are understood			
Psychosocial	Assess level of anxiety Encourage expression of feelings and thoughts Provide information and ongoing support and encouragement to client and family Assess sleep patterns and provide measures that promote rest and sleep	Assess client's anxiety regarding discharge Encourage verbalisation of concerns Provide information and ongoing support and encouragement to client and family Provide measures that promote rest and sleep			
Investigations	CT scan EEG Blood chemistry profile Other tests as indicated to establish causative factors	Ensure that all investigation results are evaluated			
Observations	Mental status assessment hourly until stable Vital signs hourly until stable O_2 saturations Monitor for further seizures	Ensure that mental status and vital signs are normal Monitor for further seizures			
Assessments/ treatments	Assess urine and bowel elimination patterns and sleep patterns	Monitor urine and bowel elimination and sleep patterns			
Diet/hydration	Before offering food and fluids, assess return of gag and swallowing ability related to conscious level Ensure adequate hydration via most appropriate route Limit caffeine intake Implement any fluid restriction Provide nutritious food inclusive of all food groups when swallowing is adequate	Full liquids and diet as tolerated			
Safety/mobility	Assess safety needs and maintain appropriate precautions Nurse in lateral position until airway maintained Ambulate as client stabilises	Maintain appropriate precautions Progress to full ambulation			
Hygiene	Assist with hygiene as required	Assess that client is independent with hygiene			
Medications	Simple analgesics Implement alterations to antiepileptic medications as ordered PRN medications for further seizures	Monitor response to altered antiepileptic medications			
Referrals	Neurologist consultation	Arrange neurological follow-up appointments			
Education	Orientate client and family to room and routine Teach seizure management to client and family Use simple brief instructions Review plan of care	Finalise seizure management teaching to client and family Assess understanding of teaching Ensure that client understands new medication regimen Provide a written copy of discharge instructions			

Figure 41.7 | Sample nursing critical pathway for managing a client post seizure

forwards. The gait consists of short shuffling steps that are slowly initiated. Facial expression becomes mask-like, and the voice is commonly high-pitched and monotone. The person's intelligence is not affected.

Amyotrophic lateral sclerosis

Amyotrophic lateral sclerosis, which is the most common form of motor neuron disease, is a progressive degenerative condition that is generally fatal within 3–10 years after onset. The disease affects the upper and lower motor neurons of the central nervous system, resulting in progressive muscular atrophy, progressive bulbar palsy and upper motor neuron deficits. While the cause is unknown, the disease is thought to result from viral, metabolic, toxic, infectious and immunological factors. Manifestations include skeletal muscle weakness and atrophy and impaired speech, chewing, swallowing and breathing. The cause of death is commonly respiratory muscle weakness and bulbar palsy causing respiratory failure.

Alzheimer's disease

Alzheimer's disease is a progressive degenerative disorder that causes cerebral atrophy and dementia. Although the precise cause is unknown, several theories propose that the disorder may result from a genetic factor, immunological dysfunction, a toxin or a virus. Recent research has focused on the role of neurotransmitters and on the effect of a deficiency of acetylcholine in the brain as a cause of the condition. Manifestations of the disease generally occur in three stages:

1. Memory loss, decline in judgment and logic, disorientation, global aphasia, irritability, mood swings and agitation
2. Neglect of hygiene, inability to carry out deliberate voluntary movements (apraxia), inability to recognise the nature or use of objects (agnosia), repetition of a motor or verbal action (perseveration) and seizures
3. Marked dementia, unresponsiveness, aphasia and apraxia.

IMMUNOLOGICAL DISORDERS

Multiple sclerosis

Multiple sclerosis is a disorder characterised by progressive demyelination of nerve fibres in the spinal cord and brain. Patches of demyelination throughout the central nervous system result in varied neurological dysfunction. The cause is unknown, but the disease is thought to result from viral or immunological factors. Manifestations vary depending on the areas of the central nervous system that are affected. Some clients experience mild exacerbations, with long remission periods, while others have frequent relapses, with increasing residual deficits. The most common initial symptoms are fatigue, motor weakness and visual disturbances. Other characteristic changes include numbness and tingling sensations, intention tremor, gait ataxia, paralysis, urinary disturbances and emotional lability. Clinical Interest Box 41.2 provides a teaching plan for the client as well as their significant others.

CLINICAL INTEREST BOX 41.2
Teaching checklist — the client with multiple sclerosis

In formulating a teaching plan it is important that the client's significant others are included. The following aspects may be considered:

- Facilitate access to the Multiple Sclerosis Society of Australia (www.msaustralia.org.au)
- Ensure that the client understands the clinical course of multiple sclerosis. Dispel any myths
- Identify strategies to manage symptoms such as dysphagia or altered cognitive responses
- Plan strategies for preventing complications such as pressure ulcers or depression
- Identify coping strategies
- Identify strategies for minimising fatigue
- Explain how to prevent injury
- Discuss ways to adapt to sexual dysfunction
- Develop strategies to control bowel and bladder function
- Explain benefits of continued physical activity and exercise
- Identify ways to minimise immobility and spasticity
- Describe the medication regimen and possible adverse effects.

Myasthenia gravis

Myasthenia gravis is a chronic neuromuscular disorder that affects voluntary muscles and is characterised by fluctuating muscle weakness that is exacerbated by exercise. The disease is considered to be autoimmune in origin, resulting in an acetylcholine-receptor deficiency. The thymus gland is also thought to be involved in the disease because the gland is abnormal and remains active after puberty in clients with myasthenia gravis.

Manifestations include progressive weakness of certain voluntary muscles, with some improvement in muscle function after rest. The eye muscles are most commonly affected, with drooping of the eyelids (ptosis) and double vision (diplopia). Other affected muscles include those involved with facial expression, speech, chewing and swallowing. The client may experience problems with saliva, nasal regurgitation and choking. The shoulder and neck muscles may be affected so that the head tends to fall forward. Weakened respiratory muscles make breathing difficult and predispose the person to respiratory tract infections.

INFECTIOUS AND INFLAMMATORY CONDITIONS

Meningitis

Meningitis is inflammation of the meninges and can be caused by viruses, bacteria or fungi. The inflammation may involve one or all three layers of the meninges. Meningitis often begins when the causative organism enters the subarachnoid space, then the infection spreads because of the open communication over the brain's convexity. The accumulation of exudate from the inflammatory process over the convexities or in the ventricles can obstruct the flow of CSF. Aseptic meningitis is thought to occur from meningeal irritation resulting from encephalitis, leukaemia, lymphoma or the presence of blood in the subarachnoid space. The major manifestations of meningitis are severe headaches, pyrexia, irritability, neck rigidity, photophobia, and pain in the back and limbs. Other manifestations are alterations in mental status, altered levels of consciousness and restlessness. Vomiting may occur, and cranial nerve involvement causes visual disturbances, pupil abnormalities, strabismus and vertigo. There may be generalised seizures due to cerebral oedema.

Encephalitis

Encephalitis is inflammation of the brain tissue caused by viruses, bacteria, fungi or protozoans. Endemic encephalitis begins in a non-human host or reservoir from which the virus is transmitted to humans, for example, through mosquito bites. After the pathogen gains access to the central nervous system via the bloodstream or along nerves, the white matter and meninges develop non-suppurative inflammation, and diffuse cerebral oedema results. Initial manifestations are headaches, pyrexia, vomiting, malaise, and muscular aches and pains. These are often followed by alterations in the level of consciousness, confusion, motor and sensory deficits, hyperirritability and meningeal signs.

Brain abscess

A brain abscess is a collection of pus, usually occurring in the temporal lobes or the cerebellum. A brain abscess is accompanied by cerebral oedema and congestion. Most brain abscesses develop secondary to a primary source of infection such as mastoiditis or otitis media; or they may develop from a septic focus in the respiratory tract or, less often, from a pelvic or cardiac source. A small percentage result from a penetrating head wound such as a gunshot injury.

Manifestations include headache, pyrexia, vomiting, alterations in the level of consciousness, and partial or generalised seizures. Other features differ according to the site of the abscess and include motor, sensory and speech disturbances.

Myelitis

Myelitis is the term that applies to a group of infective and non-infective processes that affect the spinal cord. Myelitis can be due to viruses, occur secondary to meningeal inflammation or be of unknown aetiology. The most common viral diseases causing myelitis are poliomyelitis and herpes zoster. Manifestations include a sudden onset of motor paresis, accompanied by other neurological deficits such as loss of sensory and sphincter functions.

Herpes zoster

Herpes zoster is a viral disorder that causes inflammation of the posterior root ganglia. The condition develops from reactivation of the varicella virus, the virus responsible for chickenpox. There is also evidence of a relationship between herpes zoster and certain systemic infections, neoplasms and immunosuppressive therapy. Manifestations include mild to severe neuralgic pain in the affected nerve root distribution. The pain, which may be burning, tingling, dull or sharp, may occur with or be followed by skin reddening and eruption of vesicles. The vesicles become pustules and develop a crust within 1–2 weeks. If infection or ulceration accompanies the vesicles, permanent scarring may result.

Occasionally, herpes zoster involves the cranial nerves, especially the trigeminal or oculomotor nerve. Trigeminal involvement causes eye pain and, possibly, corneal damage and impaired vision. Oculomotor involvement may result in conjunctivitis or ptosis. Rarely, herpes zoster leads to generalised central nervous system infection. Post-herpetic neuralgia can persist for months or years, and the skin may remain hypersensitive to touch.

Poliomyelitis

Poliomyelitis is an acute infectious disease caused by one of the three poliomyelitis viruses, which generally enter the body through the mouth or nose, multiply in the bloodstream, and travel to the central nervous system. The viruses are then spread along neural pathways and destroy cells in the anterior horns of the spinal cord. The brainstem may also be damaged. The incidence of acute anterior poliomyelitis has decreased dramatically in the Western world since the introduction of vaccination in 1955.

The virus may cause only a minor illness, or there may be signs and symptoms of viral meningitis and paralysis. The extent of paralysis depends on the location of the affected neurons. The initial manifestations of paralytic poliomyelitis include pyrexia, headaches, vomiting, irritability and pains in the neck, back, arms and legs. About 5–7 days after onset, the individual experiences weakness of various muscles, paraesthesia, hypersensitivity to touch and resistance to neck flexion. If the disease affects the brainstem, the muscles involved in swallowing, chewing and ventilation are affected.

NEOPLASTIC AND OBSTRUCTIVE DISORDERS

Tumours of the nervous system may be benign or malignant, and primary or metastatic. Tumours may arise in the brain tissue, the meninges, the skull, in the peripheral and cranial nerves or in the spinal cord. Brain tissue (cerebral) tumours include astrocytomas and glioblastomas. Meningiomas usually arise from the arachnoid layer of the meninges and do not invade the brain. Skull tumours, which are rare, may be either osteomas (benign) or sarcomas (malignant). Peripheral and cranial nerve tumours include acoustic neuromas, schwannomas and neuroblastomas. Spinal cord tumours may be either extradural or intradural.

Manifestations of nervous system tumours are related to invasion or compression of surrounding neural structures. Brain tumours may produce symptoms as a consequence of increased intracranial pressure; for example, from cerebral oedema. The neurological manifestations of a brain tumour depend on the location of the tumour and on its rate of growth. The clinical features associated with a brain tumour include headaches, vomiting, papilloedema (swelling of the optic disc and distension of the retinal vessels), personality or behavioural changes, seizures, visual or hearing defects, dizziness, ataxia and hemiparesis. Manifestations of spinal cord tumours are related to spinal cord compression and include pain, paraplegia or quadriplegia, which may be slowly progressive or acute.

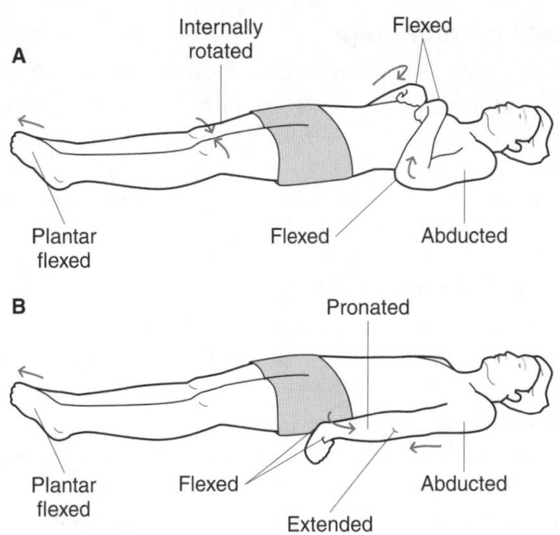

Figure 41.8 | Decorticate and decerebrate posturing
A: Decorticate rigidity **B**: Decerebrate rigidity

TRAUMATIC DISORDERS

Despite being well protected by bone, meninges and CSF, the brain and spinal cord are frequently injured. Serious cerebral or spinal cord damage can result from a variety of factors such as motor vehicle accidents, sports accidents and penetrating injuries such as gunshot wounds. Cerebral injury may be classified as concussion, contusion, laceration, haematomas and tentorial herniation.

Concussion

Concussion results from a blow to the head and is characterised by a loss of consciousness for less than 5 minutes and memory loss of events preceding and following the injury. Other features include headaches, confusion, dizziness, visual disturbances, vomiting and irritability.

Contusion

Contusion is bruising of the brain that disrupts normal nerve function in the bruised area and which may be associated with haemorrhage or oedema. Manifestations include drowsiness, confusion, behavioural changes, loss of consciousness, hemiparesis, unequal pupil response and decorticate or decerebrate posturing. With decorticate posturing the individual demonstrates hyperflexion of the upper extremities and hyperextension of the lower extremities (Figure 41.8A). With decerebrate posturing, both the upper and lower extremities are hyper-extended (Figure 41.8B).

Laceration

Laceration is tearing of the brain tissue, followed by intracerebral bleeding. Manifestations include prolonged unconsciousness, immediate neurological deficits and deterioration of the individual's condition.

Haematomas

Haematomas are collections of coagulated blood and, in the brain, may be epidural, subdural or intracerebral. An epidural haematoma results from haemorrhage in the epidural space between the skull and the dura mater. A subdural haematoma results from an accumulation of blood in the subdural space, between the arachnoid and dura mater. An intracerebral haematoma is a collection of blood within the brain tissue.

Manifestations of cerebral haematomas vary according to the location and whether the haematoma develops rapidly or slowly. Typically an epidural haematoma causes immediate loss of consciousness, followed by a lucid interval that eventually gives way to a rapidly progressive decrease in the level of consciousness. Accompanying features include hemiparesis, severe headaches, unilateral pupil dilation and signs of increased intracranial pressure (decreasing pulse and ventilation rate, increasing systolic blood pressure). Manifestations of a subdural haematoma may not occur until days after the injury. Common features include headaches, drowsiness, confusion, slow responses and seizures. Pupillary changes and motor deficits commonly occur. Manifestations of intracerebral haematoma include neck rigidity, photophobia, nausea and vomiting, dizziness, decreased ventilation rate and seizures.

Tentorial herniation

Tentorial herniation occurs when damaged brain tissue swells and herniates into the foramen magnum. This event constricts the brainstem, impairs vital centres and cranial nerves, and reduces the brain's blood supply. Manifestations include drowsiness, confusion, pupil dilation, neck rigidity, hyperventilation, bradycardia and decorticate or decerebrate posturing. Irreversible brain damage or death can occur rapidly.

Spinal cord damage

Spinal cord damage may occur from traumatic injuries as a result of motor vehicle or sports accidents, gunshot or stab wounds, or falls from high places. Fractures and dislocations can occur anywhere along the spinal column and, if the spinal cord is injured, may result in temporary or permanent damage.

Peripheral nerve damage

Peripheral nerve damage can result from pressure, compression, constriction or traction on a nerve, or as a consequence of skeletal fractures, lacerations or penetrating wounds. Nerve damage can also result from an injection of a toxic or metabolic substance into the nerve. The peripheral nerves most commonly injured are the radial, axillary and ulnar nerves and the brachial plexus. Manifestations include loss of motor function, loss of sensation and muscle atrophy. Depending on which nerve is damaged, there may be foot drop, wrist drop, limited range of motion, or paralysis.

DIAGNOSTIC TESTS

Specific tests may be performed for diagnostic purposes or to aid in evaluation of a client's condition.

THE NEUROLOGICAL EXAMINATION

The purpose of the neurological examination is to determine the presence or absence of disease in the nervous system by assessing cerebral, cranial nerve, motor, sensory and reflex function. Evaluation of cerebral function is performed by assessing the client's general behaviour and cognitive functions, such as orientation to time and place, concentration, memory, vocabulary and abstract reasoning. Evaluation of the cranial nerves involves assessing:

- The olfactory nerve: the sense of smell is tested by obstructing one nostril while testing the other. A variety of substances is placed near the unobstructed nostril and the client is asked to identify the odour of each
- The optic nerve: each eye is tested to assess visual acuity and visual fields. The fundus of each eye is assessed by ophthalmoscopic examination
- The oculomotor, trochlear and abducens nerves: these three nerves are generally tested together, as they supply the various muscles that rotate the eyeball. The ophthalmoscope is used during the assessment; the pupils are observed for size, shape and equality, and movement of the eyes is evaluated by requesting the client to follow a finger through the six cardinal areas of vision
- The trigeminal nerve: the sensory component of this nerve is tested with the client's eyes closed. Test tubes of warm and cold water are brought into contact with the skin of the face to check temperature perception. Touching the face with a wisp of cotton checks perception of light touch. Pain perception is evaluated either by applying pressure or by touching areas of the face with the point of a pin. The motor component of the trigeminal nerve is evaluated by asking the client to clench and unclench the teeth, and by observing their ability to open the mouth against resistance. The corneal reflex is assessed by lightly stroking the cornea with a wisp of cotton. If the corneal reflex is intact, the client will automatically blink
- The facial nerve: the sensory component of this nerve is assessed by placing sweet, salty, sour and bitter substances on various areas of the tongue, and asking the client to identify each taste. The motor component of the facial nerve is assessed by requesting the client to perform specific facial movements such as smiling, closing the eyes, pursing the lips and wrinkling the forehead
- The acoustic nerve: generally, unless the client has a history of vertigo, only the hearing branch of this nerve is assessed. A series of hearing tests is performed, and hearing in both ears is compared. For a more precise assessment of hearing acuity, a tuning fork is used
- The glossopharyngeal and vagus nerves: these nerves are usually tested together, as they are closely related both anatomically and functionally. A series of tests is performed to assess the gag and swallowing reflexes
- The spinal accessory nerve: this nerve is tested by evaluating the strength of the trapezius and sternocleidomastoid muscles; for example, by requesting the client to shrug the shoulders against resistance and by asking them to turn their head to one side and push their chin against the assessor's hand
- The hypoglossal nerve: the strength and movement of the tongue muscles are evaluated by testing the client's ability to protrude the tongue, and also by requesting them to push their tongue against a tongue depressor.

Evaluation of motor function

Evaluating motor function involves assessing the client's gait, posture, muscle strength and tone, balance and coordination. The assessor observes for abnormalities and compares the findings on both sides of the body for asymmetry.

Evaluation of sensory function

Evaluating sensory function involves assessing the client's ability to perceive various sensations with their eyes closed. Assessment includes testing of sensitivity to touch, pain, temperature, testing of joint motion and position, and assessment of discriminative function and vibratory sensation.

Evaluation of reflexes

Evaluation of reflexes involves testing the two types of reflex to assess the integrity of the motor and sensory systems.

The superficial reflexes

These include the upper abdominal, lower abdominal, gluteal and plantar reflexes. The abdominal and gluteal reflexes are evaluated by applying a stimulus to the skin surface; for example, stroking with a finger or pointed object and observing for muscle contraction. The plantar reflex is evaluated by stroking the sole of the foot, with one continuous movement from the heel to the toes. Normally, the big toe curls downwards in response to this stimulus. An abnormal response, Babinski's sign, when there is dorsiflexion of the big toe and fanning of the other toes, indicates upper motor neuron disease.

The deep tendon reflexes

These include the biceps, triceps, quadriceps and Achilles tendons. Deep tendon reflexes are elicited by using a percussion hammer and observing the response, as follows:

- The biceps reflex is tested with the arm partially flexed at the elbow and the palm down. When the hammer is applied to the biceps tendon, the elbow should flex
- The triceps reflex is tested with the arm partially flexed at the elbow and the palm directed towards the body. When the hammer is applied to the triceps tendon, the elbow should extend
- The quadriceps reflex is tested with the knee flexed. When the patellar tendon is struck with the hammer, the knee should extend
- The Achilles reflex is tested with the knee flexed. When the Achilles' tendon is struck with the hammer, the foot should plantar flex.

RADIOGRAPHIC EXAMINATION

X-ray

Plain X-ray films of the skull may be performed to detect fractures, to aid in the diagnosis of pituitary tumours or to detect congenital abnormalities. X-ray films of the spine may be performed to detect trauma to the vertebral column or to aid in the diagnosis of conditions that cause motor or sensory impairment.

Computerised tomography (CT) scan

Computerised tomography (CT) is commonly used to diagnose intracranial and spinal cord lesions. It is usually non-invasive but a contrast dye is sometimes administered to visualise blood vessels or to define lesions. The client lies on an X-ray table, with the head immobilised and face uncovered. The head is moved into the scanner, and a moveable frame revolves around it while X-ray films are taken. If a contrast agent is used the client may feel warm and experience a transient headache, a salty taste and nausea.

Myelogram

A myelogram involves fluoroscopy and radiography to evaluate the spinal cord and vertebral column after injection of a contrast medium into the subarachnoid space. A needle is inserted, most often in the lumbar area, into the subarachnoid space and about 10 mL of CSF is removed. Contrast medium is then injected through the needle and the client is positioned to allow the medium to flow through the subarachnoid space. A series of X-ray films are taken, after which the contrast medium may be either withdrawn or allowed to remain in the CSF. Water-soluble agents are allowed to remain, as they will eventually be excreted by the kidneys.

Angiography

Cerebral angiography involves injecting a radio-opaque contrast medium into an artery for radiological visualisation of the intracranial and extracranial blood vessels. Common injection sites are the carotid or femoral arteries, with X-ray films taken at various intervals after injection of the medium. Cerebral angiography may be performed using either local or general anaesthetic. Digital subtraction angiography is a computer-assisted radiographic procedure for visualising extracranial and intracranial vessels. The procedure is considered to be safer than cerebral angiography and involves injection of a contrast medium through a catheter into the superior vena cava. Cerebral vessels are visualised on a screen, and pictures taken.

Pneumoencephalography

Pneumoencephalography is performed infrequently since the advent of the CT scan. Pneumoencephalography allows radiographic examination of the cerebral ventricles after injection of air or oxygen into the subarachnoid space.

Magnetic resonance imaging (MRI)

An MRI is a non-invasive procedure in which the individual is placed in a strong magnetic field and is subjected to precise computer-programmed bursts of radio pulse waves. The sharpness and detail of the images produced assist diagnosis by providing identification of abnormalities, even before structural changes have occurred. MRI is contraindicated in clients with pacemakers, metallic aneurysm clips and some metallic prostheses.

Positron emission tomography (PET) scanning

PET scanning is a non-invasive nuclear imaging technique used to detect biochemical and physiological abnormalities. The client is injected with a nuclide that reacts with electrons and produces gamma-ray photons. A scanner detects the gamma rays and codes this data into a computer. The computer then reconstructs cross-sectional images of the tissues being examined. PET is not widely available.

Radionuclide scan

This test uses a camera or scanner to provide images of

the brain after administration of a radioisotope. The rays emitted by the radioisotope are converted into images that are displayed on a screen.

ELECTROENCEPHALOGRAPHY (EEG)

An electroencephalogram (EEG) is a recording of the electrical activity of the brain (brainwaves). Surface electrodes are attached to the scalp with a paste and transmit the brain's electrical impulses to a machine that records them as brainwaves on strips of paper. Brainwaves are recorded while the client is at rest, after hyperventilation, with photic stimulation, after a sensory stimulus and during sleep (see Clinical Interest Box 41.3).

CEREBROSPINAL FLUID ANALYSIS

A sample of CSF is generally obtained by lumbar puncture (Figure 41.9) or, less commonly, by cisternal puncture. A lumbar puncture may be performed for either diagnostic or therapeutic purposes. The diagnostic indications include:

- Measurement of CSF pressure
- Examination of CSF for the presence of blood or microorganisms
- Injection of air, oxygen or radio-opaque material to visualise parts of the central nervous system radiologically
- Evaluation for signs of blockage of CSF flow.

Therapeutic indications include introduction of spinal anaesthesia for surgery, and intrathecal injection of medications.

For the procedure the client assumes a lateral position, with their back curled and their knees flexed as close to their chest as possible. The head should be bent forward so that the chin touches their chest. After preparation of the site, the medical officer inserts a spinal needle with a stylus (a fine probe) between the third and fourth lumbar vertebrae into the subarachnoid space. When the stylus is removed, CSF should drip from the needle. If the lumbar puncture is being performed for diagnostic purposes, a manometer may be attached to the needle to measure CSF pressure. Samples of CSF are then collected for visual and laboratory examination. When the procedure is completed, the needle is withdrawn and an adhesive dressing applied over the puncture site.

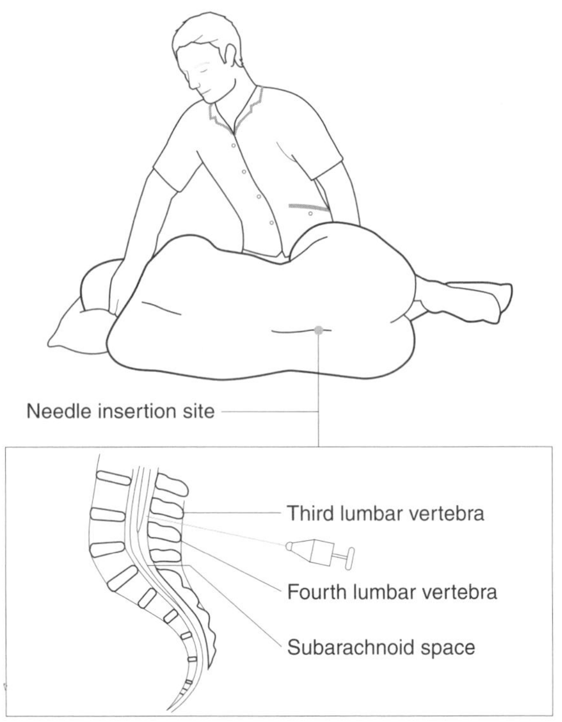

Figure 41.9 | Lumbar puncture, showing the position of the client and the insertion site

> **CLINICAL INTEREST BOX 41.3**
> **Care of the client undergoing an EEG**
>
> Client preparation
> - Explain the procedure to the client, emphasising the importance of co-operation
> - Withhold fluids, foods and medications (as prescribed) that may stimulate or depress brainwaves. These include anticonvulsants, tranquillisers, depressants and caffeine-containing foods (e.g. coffee, tea, colas and chocolate). Medications are usually withheld for 24–48 hours before the test
> - Help the client to wash their hair before the test
>
> Client and family teaching
> - The test takes about an hour
> - The test is painless and will be performed while the client sits in a comfortable chair or lies on a stretcher
> - The electrodes are applied to the scalp with a thick paste
> - During the test the client will first be asked to breathe in and out deeply for a few minutes, then to close their eyes while a light is flashed on them and, finally, to lie quietly with eyes closed
> - After the test, the nurse will help the client wash the paste out of their hair

Queckenstedt's test

Queckenstedt's test is sometimes performed as part of the lumbar puncture if an obstruction of the spinal subarachnoid space is suspected. While the lumbar puncture needle is in place, an assistant manually compresses both jugular veins for 10 seconds. The CSF pressure is read and recorded at 5-second intervals and again after release of jugular pressure. Normally, occlusion of the veins of the neck causes an immediate rise in spinal fluid pressure; if the vertebral canal is blocked, no rise occurs. The test is contraindicated if the client has increased intracranial pressure or cerebral bleeding, because brainstem herniation or further bleeding can occur.

Cisternal puncture

A cisternal puncture may be performed to obtain a sample of CSF when a lumbar puncture is contraindicated. A needle, with stylus, is inserted into the cisterna magnum and a sample of CSF withdrawn. Cisternal puncture is a potentially dangerous procedure because the needle is positioned close to the brainstem.

FURTHER INVESTIGATIONS

Echoencephalography (ECHO)

An echoencephalogram (ECHO) is a test that uses pulsating ultrasonic waves to indicate deviation of the cerebral midline structures. Since the advent of computerised tomography, echoencephalography is used infrequently.

Electromyography

This procedure involves recording the electrical activity of a muscle and peripheral nerve and may be performed to aid in diagnosis of neuromuscular disorders. Needle electrodes are inserted into the muscle to be examined, and recordings are made of the electrical activity of the muscle at rest and during contraction.

Nerve conduction studies

These studies involve application of an electrical stimulus to peripheral nerves, and measurement of their response by means of an oscilloscope.

Caloric testing for vestibular function

Caloric testing is a diagnostic procedure designed to evaluate the vestibular portion of the eighth cranial (acoustic) nerve. The underlying principle of the procedure is that thermal stimulation of the vestibular end organs with warm and cold water will elicit the oculovestibular reflex. This reflex, if intact, results in induced nystagmus and eye movement in response to cold or warm water irrigation of the external auditory canal. Each external meatus is irrigated for up to 3 minutes with both cold and warm water, with a pause of at least 5 minutes between irrigations. Irrigation with cold water should result in slow nystagmic eye movements on the same side, followed by rapid nystagmus to the opposite side. Irrigation with warm water should produce rapid nystagmus on the same side.

CARE OF THE CLIENT WITH A NERVOUS SYSTEM DISORDER

Although specific nursing actions and medical management vary depending on the disorder, the main aims of care are to:

- Promote a clear airway
- Maintain fluid and nutritional status
- Prevent and manage alterations in elimination
- Promote effective communication
- Promote safety
- Promote mobility
- Prevent complications of immobility
- Provide psychological support
- Assess neurological status
- Provide a suitable environment
- Provide pre- and post-diagnostic test care
- Promote rehabilitation and independence.

Each client presents specific nursing problems for which an individualised nursing care plan must be developed, implemented and evaluated.

PROMOTING A CLEAR AIRWAY

Disorders of the nervous system may affect the client's ability to breathe normally, to cough effectively, or to prevent the tongue from obstructing the airway. Altered levels of consciousness, decreased motor function or disrupted cranial nerve function may impair the client's ability to maintain a clear airway. To ensure a patent airway the client's nose, mouth and respiratory tract must be clear, allowing adequate oxygen and carbon dioxide exchange.

With a conscious client:

- The client should be assisted into a position that will promote effective breathing. A sitting or upright position provides better lung expansion, which improves breathing and lessens the risk of respiratory tract infection
- The client is instructed to take deep breaths hourly and to cough and expectorate mucus frequently. Chest physiotherapy (e.g. percussion) may be necessary to help mobilise secretions
- If the client's ability to chew and swallow is impaired, care must be taken when food, fluids or oral medications are being consumed
- Suction equipment should be readily available if the client is at risk of choking or unable to expectorate secretions effectively
- Active or passive range-of-motion (ROM) exercises and 2–4-hourly position changes help to mobilise respiratory tract secretions
- An adequate fluid input is provided to keep respiratory tract secretions moist.

With an unconscious client:

- The client should be nursed in a lateral recumbent position to promote drainage of secretions and to prevent the tongue from obstructing the airway. Positioning on alternate sides 2-hourly should be carried out to prevent pooling of secretions in the lungs
- Oronasopharyngeal suction should be performed to keep the upper airway free of accumulated secretions. Mouth and nasal care should be performed 2–4-hourly for the same purpose. (Information on oronasopharyngeal suctioning is provided in Chapter 38.)
- Chest percussion and postural drainage may be prescribed to help remove retained secretions, particularly if the cough reflex is impaired
- The individual may require mechanical assistance for adequate ventilation. A tracheostomy or endotracheal tube may be inserted and mechanical ventilation provided. (Information on tracheostomy care and

mechanical ventilation is provided in Chapter 38)
- Eye care is essential for the unconscious client. If the client's corneal reflex is absent, keep the eyes moist with artificial tears and protect the eye with a protective shield. These should be ordered by a medical officer.

MAINTAINING NUTRITIONAL AND FLUID STATUS

A client with a neurological disorder may have deficits that interfere with an adequate intake of food and fluid, such as:
- Altered level of consciousness
- Altered mental status
- Diminished or absent swallowing or gag reflex
- Inability to feed themself; for example, if there is paralysis of the arm(s)
- Fear of choking
- Paralysis of the muscles of mastication and/or the tongue
- Loss of appetite due to altered sensory function; for example, sight, smell, taste.

Information on assisting the client to meet nutritional and fluid needs is provided in Chapters 32 and 33. Specific nursing activities to assist the individual with a nervous system disorder include:
- Providing appropriate devices to facilitate the cutting and eating of food
- Ensuring that suction equipment is readily available should it be needed; for example, if the client's swallowing or gag reflexes are impaired
- Assisting the client who is unable to feed themself
- Placing the food into the unaffected side of the mouth if the client has any facial weakness. If able to feed themself, the client should be informed to feed in this manner
- Preparing food for the client who has motor deficits; for example, cutting meat, spreading butter, pouring fluids
- Redirecting the client's attention to eating if they become distracted or are unable to concentrate at mealtimes
- Assisting with the care of the client who is being provided with nutrition and fluids by alternative methods; for example, tube feeding or total parenteral nutrition
- Keeping a record of fluid input and output if the client has difficulty in feeding themself or swallowing or if they are receiving dehydrating medications or intravenous solutions to reduce or prevent increased intracranial pressure.

PREVENTING AND MANAGING ALTERATIONS IN ELIMINATION

Many disorders affecting the nervous system can result in constipation, retention of urine or incontinence. Factors that contribute to altered patterns of elimination include loss of sphincter control, diminished awareness of the need to empty the bladder or bowel, altered levels of consciousness, and impaired mental status, with resulting incontinence. (Information on the prevention and management of constipation, retention of urine and incontinence is provided in Chapters 32 and 33.)

PROMOTING EFFECTIVE COMMUNICATION

Disorders of the nervous system may affect the ability of clients to express themself verbally or non-verbally, and the ability to understand the spoken or written word. (General information on Communication can be found in Chapter 29.) The ability to communicate may be impaired by factors that include:
- Damage to the speech centres in the brain
- Damage to the temporal lobes, which hinders the perception and interpretation of stimuli
- Damage to the cranial nerves responsible for movement of the lips, tongue, pharynx and larynx
- Limited motor function that hinders non-verbal communication actions (e.g. facial expressions and gestures)
- Visual or hearing deficits
- Altered levels of consciousness or mental status.

The two major terms used to describe communication deficits are dysphasia (difficulty in communicating), and aphasia (loss of the ability to communicate).

Aphasia

Aphasia is subdivided into three major classifications.
1. Expressive aphasia (Broca's aphasia): inability to express oneself verbally or in writing. The degree of difficulty can range from mild hesitancy in flow of speech to limitation of expression to 'yes' and 'no'. The ability to understand the spoken and written word remains intact
2. Receptive aphasia (Wernicke's aphasia): inability to understand the spoken word. Although the client hears the sounds of speech, comprehension of speech is impaired. The client can speak but makes many errors when using words and is often unaware of the imperfect messages. The ability to comprehend the written word is also impaired
3. Global aphasia: a combination of both expressive and receptive aphasia. The client neither understands what they hear or read, nor can they convey their thoughts in speech or writing.

The loss or impairment of the ability to communicate is devastating and frustrating to the client and to their significant others, often resulting in fear and depression. Although the speech therapist will be the key person in the treatment of a client with a communication problem, the nurse must be aware of prescribed therapy so that it can be continued when the speech therapist is not with the client. The nurse should assume a calm, reassuring and supportive manner that conveys a sense of acceptance of the client's behaviour. Table 41.3 illustrates guidelines that can be used when working with a client with aphasia.

Communication with the unconscious client is very important because, although the client appears to be completely unaware of their environment, it is impossible to determine their awareness of any stimulus. Many clients have recovered from unconsciousness and given accurate details of events or conversations that took place in their presence while they were unconscious. Therefore the nurse should assume that some stimuli will penetrate the complexities of unconsciousness. Stimuli can be provided by talking to the client, by touch and by playing a radio or tapes. The client should be told what the nurse will be doing — orient the client to time, place and person and describe the surroundings. Coma arousal is a technique whereby the unconscious individual is continuously exposed to a variety of stimuli, such as sounds, touch and smells in an attempt to increase the level of consciousness.

PROMOTING SAFETY

The client with a nervous system disorder is often susceptible to injury because of factors such as impaired consciousness or awareness, reduced mobility, impaired motor and sensory functions and reflexes. The client is most at risk of skin breakdown, physical injuries or infection. (General information on meeting the client's need for safety is provided in Chapter 26.) This chapter addresses specific nursing activities that are implemented to promote the safety of the client with a nervous system disorder.

MAINTAINING SKIN INTEGRITY

The nurse should assess the client for potential skin problems and implement nursing measures to prevent skin breakdown from pressure, extremes of temperature, and physical trauma, as follows:

- The skin is kept clean and dried to prevent irritation and possible breakdown. Very dry skin should be lubricated with a suitable oil or cream to prevent cracking and breakdown
- A protective cream or lotion may be applied to the genital area and buttocks if the client is incontinent. Wet or soiled linen must be replaced immediately
- The client's position is changed every 2–4 hours to protect the skin from irritation and prolonged pressure. Pressure-relieving aids such as sheepskins may be used
- The skin is assessed every 2 hours for colour, temperature, dryness and the signs of impaired circulation. Any signs of skin breakdown are reported immediately so that appropriate actions can be implemented to prevent further deterioration
- Precautions must be taken to avoid injury to the skin by hot, cold, sharp or rough objects. The client is always moved correctly and gently to avoid damage to the skin.

PREVENTING PHYSICAL INJURIES

A client who has impaired motor, sensory or intellectual function must be protected from accidents and injuries. Protective measures include:

- Maintaining the bed in a low position when not providing direct care at the bedside
- Using alarms that are triggered when the client

TABLE 41.3 | ASSISTING THE APHASIC CLIENT

Expressive aphasia	Receptive aphasia
Stimulate conversation and ask open-ended questions	Speak slowly and distinctly, using a common vocabulary and simple sentences
Allow the client time to find the words to express themself	Stand within the client's line of vision, so that lip movements can be observed
Be supportive and accepting as the client deals with the frustration of finding the right words	Use simple gestures as an added cue
Accept self-expression (e.g. pointing or gestures)	Repeat or rephrase any instructions if they are not understood
Provide charts or books with pictures of common objects so that the client can point when they cannot say the word	Speak in a normal voice
Reassure the client that speech skills can be relearned, given time	Divide any tasks into small units, working with the client to accomplish the task
Give praise for achievements and progress	Use pointing and touch to express ideas Eliminate background distractions Give praise for achievements and progress

attempts unsafe activities (e.g. standing from chair unaccompanied)
- Accompanying the client when ambulating if they are unsteady or disoriented
- Providing walking aids and handrails as a means of support and to promote greater safety
- Providing an uncluttered environment and adequate lighting
- Placing the client's requirements, including the call bell, within reach
- Supervision of clients who are at risk of falling while performing the activities of daily living.

PREVENTING INFECTION

A client with a nervous system disorder that impairs mobility, motor function or level of consciousness is prone to infection. When a person is ill, the body's natural defence mechanisms are stressed and therefore less able than usual to resist the invasion of pathogenic microorganisms. The two most common types of infection that may occur are urinary tract infection due to urinary stasis or catheterisation, and respiratory tract infection resulting from inadequate lung expansion, pooling of secretions in the lungs, the presence of an artificial airway or mechanical ventilation.

Measures to prevent a urinary tract infection include ensuring that:

- The client receives an adequate fluid input
- Whenever possible, an external urinary drainage device or intermittent catheterisation is used rather than an indwelling catheter
- If an indwelling catheter is unavoidable, measures to prevent cross-infection are implemented. These measures include maintaining a sterile closed drainage system, performing meatal and perineal care, maintaining dependent drainage, maintaining strict aseptic care and using correct hand-washing technique, which is the most effective way of preventing cross infection. (Further information on maintaining an indwelling catheter is provided in Chapter 32.)

Measures to prevent a respiratory tract infection include ensuring that:

- When possible, the client is nursed in a sitting or upright position to promote maximal lung expansion
- The client performs 4-hourly deep breathing and coughing exercises
- If necessary, suction is used to remove oral and nasopharyngeal secretions
- Aseptic techniques are implemented when caring for an artificial airway.

PROMOTING MOBILITY AND PREVENTING THE COMPLICATIONS OF IMMOBILITY

Many nervous system disorders impair physical mobility through motor deficits, cerebellar dysfunction, alterations in sensory perception and changes in conscious or mental status. Prolonged lack of physical exercise and movement can lead to many complications, including pulmonary stasis, urinary stasis, venous stasis, decubitus ulcers, constipation and contractures. Impaired mobility varies from reductions in range of motion, or unsteady gait, to total immobility. Maintaining muscle tone and preventing orthopaedic disabilities are of prime importance when caring for a client with impaired mobility.

To prevent functional loss:

- Active or passive range-of-motion exercises should be performed every 4 hours
- The client should be repositioned every 2 hours to maintain correct body alignment. Weak or paralysed body parts must be carefully positioned to prevent deformity
- Specific exercises, such as lifting hand weights, may be prescribed to strengthen a weakened limb
- As soon as the client's condition permits, balancing and sitting exercises are implemented. If the client has been immobile for a prolonged period it is necessary to progress slowly to prevent orthostatic hypotension
- Once the client is able to balance and sit, transfer activities are started; for example, from bed to chair
- When the client is able to stand and balance in an upright position, ambulation is started
- For the client who is unable to ambulate, wheelchair mobility may be achieved.

The client's age, severity of illness, other neurological deficits, chronic conditions or complications contribute to progress. Client attitude and motivation are also important factors in regaining mobility. Frequent assessment provides evaluation of the client's needs so that rehabilitation can progress towards the greatest level of independence. Further information on preventing the complications of immobility is provided in Chapter 36.

PROVIDING PSYCHOLOGICAL SUPPORT

Many clients who have a nervous system disorder will suffer neurological deficits resulting in loss of independence, mobility, sensory function or speech. As a result, the client's body image and self-concept may be greatly altered and they may experience emotional lability, depression, anxiety, frustration or hostility. The client may undergo personality changes, which may be functional or organic in origin. They may require a lengthy period to regain what were once automatically performed skills involved in the activities of daily living, or they may have to come to terms with the realisation that some skills may never be regained. The emotional shock to a client who experiences paralysis can be devastating. The nurse has an important role in providing emotional and psychological support for the client and their significant others. Some of the key aspects related to supporting the client are as follows:

- During the period of dependence, it is important that dignity is preserved. Sensitivity is needed when dealing with any problems associated with loss of control (e.g. incontinence or loss of social restraint)
- Positive feedback should be provided for accomplishments no matter how minor they may appear
- Adequate information about the disease process and its management should be provided, and the client should be encouraged to participate in decision making regarding care
- Client needs should be anticipated to decrease frustration. As much self-care as practicable should be allowed, as a return to independence is the ultimate goal of care. The client's significant others should be allowed to be involved in care, if they so wish
- The client and their significant others should be encouraged to express their feelings and anxieties. If the client is experiencing a communication problem, appropriate methods of communicating should be developed. Time, patience and understanding are necessary to allow them to come to terms with the effects and implications of the disease
- The client should be encouraged to participate in activities of interest that will help to promote a feeling of self-worth. The occupational therapist and physiotherapist generally assist the client to find activities that interest them and that will also provide exercise for weak or paralysed muscles.

ASSESSING NEUROLOGICAL STATUS

Assessment is of prime importance in the care of a client with a neurological disorder. The nurse must recognise changes that indicate a change in condition, as changes can occur rapidly and dramatically or develop over a period of days or weeks.

INTRACRANIAL PRESSURE

Intracranial pressure is the pressure exerted by the CSF within the ventricles of the brain. However, it is more accurate to think in terms of intracranial 'pressures' rather than a single pressure, as the rigid skull is filled with brain tissue, intravascular blood and CSF. If any one of these three components increases in volume without a reciprocal change in volume of the other two, intracranial pressure will rise. Increased intracranial pressure affects the cerebral perfusion pressure, causing hypoxia, ischaemia, irreversible neurological damage and even death. Unless increased intracranial pressure is treated, the outcome will be herniation of a portion of the cerebrum through the tentorium, with pressure being exerted on the brainstem. The brainstem will then herniate through the foramen magnum, the only opening in the closed cranial vault.

Common causes of increased intracranial pressure include: space-occupying masses such as tumours, haematomas, abscesses or cerebral oedema; conditions that increase cerebral blood volume; and conditions that increase CSF. It is very important to identify early signs of increased intracranial pressure so that actions can be implemented to prevent or minimise irreversible brain damage. The manifestations of increased intracranial pressure include:

- Early signs and symptoms: deterioration in the level of consciousness (confusion, restlessness, lethargy), pupillary dysfunction, motor weakness such as hemiparesis and possible headaches
- Later signs and symptoms: continued deterioration in the level of consciousness (coma), possible vomiting, hemiplegia, decortication, decerebration, increasing systolic blood pressure, bradycardia and decreasing or irregular ventilations.

NEUROLOGICAL ASSESSMENT

Neurological assessment includes checking the level of consciousness, the pupils, motor function, sensory function and the vital signs. The frequency with which assessment is performed and documented depends on the client's condition and on the health care institution's policy. Table 41.4 outlines the procedure for performing a neurological assessment.

Level of consciousness

The level of consciousness is a most important factor in neurological assessment, providing valid information about changes in neurological status. Change can occur slowly over the course of many days, or it can occur rapidly in a few minutes or hours. The rapidity of change is an indicator of the severity of the neurological problem. The client's level of consciousness is evaluated by providing stimuli and observing the response. Sound and pain are the major stimuli used. Speaking to the client is the most common method of applying an auditory stimulus, while painful stimuli are reserved for the client with obviously decreased levels of consciousness. When spoken to, a fully conscious client should reply with an appropriate verbal response. A person with a decreased level of consciousness may respond in a puzzled way or may not respond at all, showing no response even when someone speaks directly into their ear.

Painful tactile stimuli

Painful tactile stimuli may be necessary to arouse the semi-comatose client. Painful stimuli can be provided by exerting firm digital pressure on the nail beds, the Achilles tendon or the gastrocnemius muscle. Response to painful stimuli can be classified into:

- Purposeful, when the client winces, pushes the assessor away, or withdraws the affected body part
- Non-purposeful, when the client may move the stimulated body part only slightly, or when the application of painful stimuli causes an extensor response (a contraction of muscles) only

TABLE 41.4 | PERFORMING A NEUROLOGICAL ASSESSMENT

Review and carry out standard steps in Appendix 1

Action	Rationale
Validate the medical orders in the patient record	Ensures correct procedure is about to take place
Explain the procedure to the client	Reduces anxiety and gains client's consent and cooperation
Critically think through your assessment data and problem solving, e.g. provide privacy, comfort measures, pain relief	Evaluating each aspect and its relationship to other data will help identify specific problems and modifications of the procedure that may be needed for the individual
Prepare equipment	
Locate and gather the equipment as indicated prior to beginning the procedure. You will need the following: • Sphygmomanometer, BP cuff, stethoscope • Thermometer • Watch with a second hand • Penlight and pupil gauge • Neurological observations sheet (Glasgow Coma Scale [GCS])	Ensures all equipment is at client's bedside to maximise efficiency, reduce apprehension on the client's part and increases the confidence in the nurse
Wash hands	Minimises the risk of cross contamination
Assess level of consciousness	Altered level of consciousness is a key indicator to brain function The nurse watches carefully for any response from the client If no response is gained, the client is spoken to, at first quietly, then more loudly Response is opening the eyes If there is no auditory response, gentle touch is used, then use a mildly painful stimulus
Assess the orientation of the client	The client who is able to respond is asked a series of simple questions e.g. identify themself, what month, season or year it is If the client is not orientated to person, place or time, ascertain their best verbal response. Scores on the GCS are confused, inappropriate words, incomprehensible sounds and no response
Assess motor response	Give client single response commands such as 'touch your nose', 'wiggle your toes' If they are unable to obey commands, apply a painful stimulus (pinching of the nailbed) and watch the response They may try to localise (push the stimulus away) or withdraw (move their hand/foot away from the stimulus) If no response is elicited score 1 Compare the right and left sides and upper and lower extremities. The *best* response is recorded
Assess pupillary activity	Pupil size is determined using the pupil gauge before the light reflex is used Pupil shape is determined as round, oval or drawn to indicate abnormality Pupil reactivity to light is assessed by bringing the penlight from the lateral side of the client's head towards the nose. Observe for pupil constriction and repeat with the other eye. Response is recorded as brisk, sluggish or fixed
Assess muscle strength and tone	Each extremity is assessed unless contraindicated The client is given clear commands such as 'squeeze my hands', 'push against my hands'. Compare both sides Response is recorded as normal, weak, minimal or no movement
Assess vital signs	Vital sign changes are late changes in brain deterioration. Initially vital signs are monitored every 15 minutes until stable then hourly or as per facility guidelines

TABLE 41.4 | PERFORMING A NEUROLOGICAL ASSESSMENT—cont'd

Action	Rationale
Documentation	
Report and document the procedure and any complications	The information gathered is documented on the Glasgow Coma Scale or neurovascular chart, where there are designated places for each of the observations Any change in the client's level of consciousness should be recorded in the client's progress notes and their doctor notified Documentation increases the communication between health care professionals and complies with legal requirements for reporting change

- Unresponsive: when the individual shows no sign of reacting to painful stimuli.

The Glasgow Coma Scale (Figure 41.10) was originally designed to assess the level of consciousness in people with head injuries but is now used in a variety of settings. It has gained increasing acceptance as an accurate and effective means of evaluating levels of consciousness. Using the Glasgow Coma Scale, a score of 15 reflects a fully alert, well-oriented person, while a score of 7 or less is considered to indicate coma. The lowest possible score of 3 is indicative of deep coma. As there are many adaptations of this scale, it is important that the nurse checks the scoring system, which changes with each chart.

GLASGOW COMA SCALE

Action	Response	Score
Eyes open	Spontaneously	(4)
	To speech	3
	To pain	2
	None	1
Best verbal response	Oriented	(5)
	Confused	4
	Inappropriate words	3
	Incomprehensible sounds	2
	None	1
Best motor response	Obeys commands	(6)
	Localised pain	5
	Flexion withdrawal	4
	Abnormal flexion	3
	Abnormal extension	2
	Flaccid	1
	Total score out of 15	

Figure 41.10 | The Glasgow Coma Scale

Evaluation of the pupils

Evaluating the pupils provides vital information about central nervous system function or dysfunction. The findings in one pupil are compared with the findings in the other, and the differences between the two pupils are documented. The pupils are assessed for size, shape and reaction to light. Normally the pupils are equal in size (average diameter of 3.5 mm), round, and they constrict briskly when light is shone into the eye. A pupil gauge may be used to estimate the size of each pupil. Abnormal responses of a pupil to light may be described as sluggish, non-reactive or fixed. Generally, any change in a pupil's size, shape or reaction is indicative of an intracranial change.

Assessment of motor function

Assessment of motor function usually focuses on the arms and legs, and the identification of significant changes is important for denoting improvement, stabilisation or deterioration in the client's condition. The techniques used to evaluate motor function depend on the client's level of consciousness. In the conscious client, the assessment can be made by observing motor responses to directions; for example, by asking the client to squeeze the assessor's hands. If the client is unconscious or is unable to provide accurate responses, the assessor must rely on observational skills to evaluate motor function.

Assessment of sensory function

Assessment of sensory function is described earlier in this chapter.

Assessment of the vital signs

Assessing the vital signs (Chapter 21) provides data concerning vital functions of the body. The client's temperature, pulse, ventilations and blood pressure are monitored and documented at a frequency that depends on their condition. Data from neurological assessments are documented according to the health care institution's policy. Many institutions use a special neurological assessment chart, similar to the one illustrated in Figure 41.10.

PROVIDING A SUITABLE ENVIRONMENT

The immediate physical environment should be adapted to meet the client's specific needs. Items should be arranged to promote safety; for example, adequate lighting, the call bell within easy reach, and the bed adjusted to a suitable height. If the person is experiencing sensory deprivation (a lack of sensory input from the environment), the nurse can provide multi-sensory stimuli. Sensory input can be provided by talking to the person, playing a radio or recordings of the voices of the client's significant others, by touch and by reality orientation. Reality orientation is a process of making the client aware of their environment, for example, the date, time, people, place and objects.

Conversely, the client may experience sensory overload, particularly if critically ill and the condition requires the use of equipment such as a mechanical ventilation or cardiac monitor, or if they are receiving the constant stimuli of nursing care. Sensory overload occurs when sustained multisensory experiences are perceived as confusing or irritating by the client. The manifestations of sensory overload are confusion, disorientation, restlessness, agitation, panic and possible hallucinations. Every effort should be made to control and moderate the intensity of stimuli, for example, reducing tactile and environmental stimuli.

When the client is to be discharged from hospital, the physical home environment should be evaluated and the delivery of any necessary equipment arranged so that the activities of daily living can be accomplished and independence maintained. The physiotherapist and occupational therapist arrange for the home use of ambulatory equipment and identify special needs and alterations in environment that could be beneficial to support the client's independence.

PROVIDING DIAGNOSTIC TEST CARE

Preparation of the client for, and care after, diagnostic tests is part of the nurse's role. The nurse must refer to the health care institution's policy manual for information about preparation of the individual for specific diagnostic tests. Preparation includes a general explanation of the procedure to reinforce the information provided to the client by the medical officer. Other preparation may include dietary or fluid restrictions, administration of prescribed medications, assisting the client into a specific position, skin preparation, and measurement of baseline vital and neurological signs.

Post-procedural care may include assessing vital and neurological signs, measuring and recording fluid input and output, administering prescribed medications and assessing the client for signs and symptoms such as headaches, back pain, neck rigidity, nausea or vomiting, elevated temperature or voiding difficulty.

PROMOTING REHABILITATION AND INDEPENDENCE

Rehabilitation is an integral part of care and is a dynamic process in which the client is assisted to achieve optimal potential. Throughout the client's illness, all care is directed towards the maintenance of optimal function and prevention of complications to promote as much independence as possible. Rehabilitation of a client with a nervous system disorder includes helping with relearning the activities of daily living, management of neuromuscular and impaired perception and communication deficits, bladder and bowel retraining, and educating the client and their significant others in preparation for discharge from hospital. (Information on rehabilitation is provided in Chapter 46.)

CARE OF THE UNCONSCIOUS CLIENT

Consciousness is defined as a state of awareness of self and the surroundings. Consciousness implies an ability to perceive sensory stimuli and to respond appropriately to them. Unconsciousness is defined as an abnormal state in which the client is unresponsive to sensory stimuli. There are degrees of unconsciousness that vary in length and severity, ranging from a brief episode of unconsciousness in the form of fainting, to a prolonged and deep coma.

CAUSES OF IMPAIRED CONSCIOUSNESS

Impaired consciousness arises from widespread damage to both cerebral hemispheres or from disruption of the reticular activating system in the upper brainstem. Loss of consciousness may result from a cerebral tumour, abscess, haemorrhage, haematoma, laceration, bruising or ischaemia, or from metabolic processes that depress or interrupt the function of both cerebral hemispheres; for example, hypoxia, hypoglycaemia or toxic agents.

Outcome of unconsciousness

The ultimate outcome of unconsciousness varies from full recovery of brain function, through a wide range of disabilities, to irreversible coma and death. The development of sophisticated monitoring techniques and life-support systems has increased the survival rate for comatose clients with severe brain damage. A small percentage of clients emerge from deep coma to a state of wakefulness without awareness, never regaining any recognisable mental function.

Persistent vegetative state

Persistent vegetative state is a term used to describe a chronic condition occurring after severe cerebral damage. It is characterised by intact autonomic functions, generally intact reflexes, presence of a sleep–wakefulness cycle, spontaneous eye opening to verbal stimuli, no localising motor responses to verbal stimuli, and no intact cognitive functions or awareness of self or of the environment.

Brain death

Brain death is a state of irreversible brain damage characterised by absence of cognitive functions and awareness of self and the environment, inability to maintain vital functions, and the absence of isoelectric activity on EEG. Brain death is a controversial legal, ethical and medical dilemma. Although there are no uniformly accepted criteria, the basic criteria for diagnosing brain death usually include:

- Apnoea
- Irreversible coma
- Absence of brainstem reflexes
- Isoelectric electroencephalogram (ECG)
- No spontaneous movements
- Evidence that brain dysfunction is the result of structural or metabolic disease, rather than the result of depressant drugs, alcohol, poisoning or hypothermia.

MANAGEMENT OF AN UNCONSCIOUS CLIENT

When a client is unconscious a high standard of care must be provided, with the objectives of maintaining and restoring body function and preventing complications. Medical management involves establishing a patent airway and providing adequate ventilation, controlling intracranial pressure and establishing the cause of unconsciousness and, if possible, reversing it. Nursing care of the unconscious client requires the following practices.

Maintaining a patent airway

With the absence of cough and swallowing reflexes, secretions accumulate in the posterior pharynx and upper trachea. An oral artificial airway may be sufficient to maintain patency, or tracheostomy or endotracheal intubation and mechanical ventilation may be necessary. To prevent airway obstruction:

- The client is positioned on alternate sides every 2–4 hours to prevent secretions accumulating in the airways on one side. The neck should be maintained in a neutral position
- Dentures and partial plates are removed
- Nasal and oral care is provided to keep the upper airway free of accumulated secretions and debris
- Oronasopharyngeal suction equipment may be necessary to aspirate secretions
- Chest percussion and postural drainage may be prescribed to assist in the removal of tenacious secretions.

Monitoring neurological function

The client's neurological signs are monitored at intervals determined by their condition. The results are documented and compared with previous assessments. Information on assessment of neurological function is provided earlier in this chapter.

Positioning

The client is generally nursed in a lateral position with a small pillow placed under the head and neck to maintain the head in a neutral position. The upper arm is positioned on a pillow to maintain the shoulder in alignment, and the upper leg is supported on a pillow to maintain alignment of the hip. The client's position is changed so that they lie on alternate sides every 2–4 hours. If hemiplegia is present the client may be positioned on the affected side for brief periods, but care must be taken to prevent injury to soft tissue and nerves, oedema, or disruption of the blood supply. Because vasomotor tone is decreased in the affected areas, such adverse effects can develop rapidly from improper positioning. If the correct position is maintained, secretions are able to drain from the client's mouth, the tongue is less likely to obstruct the airway, and postural deformities can be prevented.

Meeting hygiene needs

Care of the skin. This involves keeping it clean and dry, and protected from damage. Areas of the skin, particularly over the bony prominences, should be assessed regularly for the signs of impaired blood circulation and irritation that contribute to the formation of decubitus ulcers. Dry skin may be lubricated with a suitable cream or lotion to prevent cracking and breakdown, and a water-repellent substance may be used to protect the skin against excreta or perspiration. The male should receive a facial shave as part of his daily hygiene care, the client's nails are kept short and clean, and the hair is brushed, combed and washed as necessary.

Care of the mouth. This involves cleansing all areas at 2–4-hourly intervals to prevent a build-up of plaque, development of caries and development of a focus of infection. To prevent aspiration of fluid while oral hygiene is being performed, the client's head is turned to one side and suction equipment made available throughout the procedure. The lips are lubricated with a suitable water-based substance.

Care of the nose. This involves cleansing the nostrils to keep them free of dried mucus. Cottonwool-tipped applicators and saline solution may be used to remove mucus and dried crusts, and a thin coating of cream may be applied to the rim of the nostrils.

Care of the eyes. This involves swabbing the eyes with moistened cotton wool to remove secretions, the instillation of artificial tears (or antibiotic eye drops if prescribed), and protecting the eyes from corneal abrasions. If the eyelids do not close fully, the use of eye shields or pads may be necessary to protect the corneas. (See Chapter 42 for more information on care of the eye.)

Meeting nutritional and fluid needs

The nutritional and fluid needs of the client must be regularly assessed and met to maintain body function, support tissue repair and combat infection. The dietitian prescribes a nutritional program based on consideration of the individual's energy needs, requirements for tissue repair, loss of fluid, and basic life functions. Methods of administering nutritional and fluid support to the unconscious client include total parenteral nutrition, and enteral feedings administered via a nasogastric, nasojejunal or gastrostomy tube. Fluid input may be restricted to a specific amount of fluid in a 24-hour period. The purpose of fluid restriction is to control increased intracranial pressure by keeping the client slightly under-hydrated. As fluid input is correlated with output, an accurate input and output record must be maintained.

Meeting elimination needs

Because an unconscious client is incontinent, an external urinary drainage appliance or an indwelling catheter may be used to manage urinary drainage. Both methods are used to keep the skin dry, as urinary incontinence can quickly lead to skin breakdown. Urinary drainage devices also enable accurate calculation of urinary output. (Information on care of the client with a urinary drainage device is provided in Chapter 32.)

Constipation and faecal impaction are common complications in an unconscious client because immobility and lack of a normal diet inhibit peristalsis. A program is established whereby aperients and rectal suppositories are administered to promote regular bowel evacuation. The frequency of bowel actions and the amount and nature of the faeces are documented (see Chapter 33).

Promoting safety

Providing and maintaining a safe environment is of prime importance because an unconscious client is unable to perceive or react to safety hazards. (Information on promoting safety is provided in Chapter 26.) Clinical Interest Box 41.4 suggests alternative routes for measuring temperature when a client is in a state of altered consciousness.

Preventing complications

Because the unconscious client is not mobile, they are at risk of developing any of the complications associated with immobility (muscle contractures, decubitus ulcers, or venous, pulmonary or urinary stasis. Information on preventing these complications is provided in Chapter 36.

Providing sensory stimulation

The extent to which an unconscious client may be aware of what is happening to and around them cannot usually be determined; the nurse should therefore assume that the brain is receiving some sensory input. When the duration of coma extends into weeks or months, it may seem meaningless to keep explaining each activity to a client who gives no sign of comprehension. However, on regaining consciousness some clients have been able to describe accurately events that happened to and around them while they were unconscious. Although they were unable to communicate their feelings they were able to discriminate between the gentle caring manner of some people and the inattentive ways of others. Some clients have reported that they longed for someone to talk to them rather than about them.

The nurse should therefore act as though the client is conscious and demonstrate respect for them as a person. All activities should be explained to them, privacy during procedures should be ensured and they should be treated with dignity. Family members and friends should be encouraged to talk to and touch the unconscious client. They should be encouraged to perform certain activities for the client, such as combing the hair or applying skin lotion. Other sensory stimuli can be provided by playing a radio or tapes, or by placing perfumed flowers in the room.

Recovery from unconsciousness is a gradual process that tends to vary with each individual. Rehabilitation after a prolonged period of unconsciousness includes protecting the client from orthostatic hypotension. When able to tolerate a vertical position, an ambulation program is developed, unless neurological deficits make it unfeasible. (Information on rehabilitation nursing is provided in Chapter 46.)

CLINICAL INTEREST BOX 41.4
Altered consciousness and taking temperature

Temperature should never be taken orally in clients with altered conscious state. For an oral temperature reading to be taken safely and accurately, the client must be able to close their lips completely and understand the importance of not biting the thermometer. Measure temperature via the tympanic or axillary routes; of these, tympanic is more accurate and therefore preferred.

Management of the client with impaired motor function

Disturbance of motor function is common among clients who experience disorders of the brain, spinal cord or peripheral nerves, such as cerebral haemorrhage, spinal cord injury or peripheral neuritis. While this chapter addresses the care of a client who has experienced a CVA or a spinal cord injury, the principles of care can be applied to clients who experience impaired motor function from other causes. Some terms relating to impaired motor function are:

- Paresis: incomplete paralysis or muscle weakness
- Paralysis: loss or impairment of the ability to move part(s) of the body. Paralysis may be complete or incomplete, spastic or flaccid, symmetric or asymmetric, temporary or permanent
- Hemiplegia: unilateral paralysis, or paralysis of one side of the body. Because nerves cross in the pyramidal tract before descending to the spinal cord, damage to one side of the brain causes hemiplegia on the opposite side of the body
- Paraplegia: paralysis of the lower limbs and, sometimes, paralysis of the lower trunk and sphincters. Paralysis may be complete or incomplete, spastic or flaccid, temporary or permanent

- Quadriplegia (tetraplegia): paralysis of the arms and legs and of the body below the level of injury to the spinal cord.

CEREBROVASCULAR ACCIDENT (CVA)

Cerebrovascular accident (CVA) is one of the leading causes of death in the Western world, and each year many thousands of clients survive a CVA but are left with permanent disabilities. A CVA is a sudden impairment of cerebral circulation, which causes cerebral infarction. The two types of CVA are ischaemic and haemorrhagic. In an ischaemic CVA, cerebral blood flow is suddenly impaired by a thrombus or embolus. In a haemorrhagic CVA, the rupture of a cerebral blood vessel causes bleeding into the subarachnoid space or brain tissue.

Factors that increase the risk of a CVA include a history of TIA, atherosclerosis, hypertension, obesity, diabetes mellitus, cigarette smoking, elevated serum cholesterol and triglyceride levels, lack of exercise, use of oral contraceptives, coagulation disorders, dehydration, rheumatic heart disease and dysrhythmias. Manifestations of a CVA vary depending on the artery involved, and consequently the area of brain it supplies, and the severity of damage to cerebral tissue.

Table 41.5 lists the clinical features resulting from specific cerebral artery occlusion or rupture. If the CVA occurs in the left hemisphere, it produces symptoms on the right side of the body. If it occurs in the right hemisphere, the left side of the body is affected.

A thrombotic CVA, the most common type, is associated with atherosclerosis, which causes narrowing of the lumen of arteries. A thrombus forms in one of the cerebral arteries, occluding the vessel and resulting in cerebral ischaemia. An embolic CVA occurs when an embolus, which may be part of a thrombus, fat or other substance, is carried to the brain and occludes a cerebral blood vessel. A haemorrhagic CVA, which is often associated with hypertension, occurs when a cerebral blood vessel ruptures, spilling blood into the brain tissue. Rupture of an artery may result from a degenerative change in the arterial wall, or from an anatomical defect such as an aneurysm.

TABLE 41.5 | MANIFESTATIONS OF CEREBROVASCULAR ACCIDENTS ACCORDING TO VESSEL INVOLVED

Vessel	Manifestations
Middle cerebral artery	Hemiparesis or hemiplegia Aphasia Sensory impairment (same side as hemiplegia) Homonyous hemianopia Deterioration in conscious level from confusion to coma Headaches Inability to turn eyes towards the affected side Denial or lack of recognition of a paralysed extremity Possible Cheyne–Stokes breathing
Anterior cerebral artery	Hemiparesis or hemiplegia of leg and foot Paresis of the arm on the side of hemiplegia Gait dysfunction Expressive aphasia Mental status impairments: • Confusion • Amnesia • Perseveration • Short attention span • Apathy • Slowness Deviation of eyes and head towards the affected side Urinary incontinence
Posterior cerebral artery	Peripheral signs: • Homonyous hemianopia • Several visual defects • Memory deficits • Perseveration • Dyslexia Central signs: • Hemiplegia or hemiparesis • Diffuse sensory loss • Pupillary dysfunction • Nystagmus • Intention tremor
Internal carotid artery	Hemiparesis with facial asymmetry Parasthesia on same side as hemiparesis Hemianopia Repeated attacks of visual blurring or blindness in the ipsilateral eye Dysphasia (intermittent)

(Continued)

TABLE 41.5 | MANIFESTATIONS OF CEREBROVASCULAR ACCIDENTS ACCORDING TO VESSEL INVOLVED—cont'd

Vessel	Manifestations
Posterior inferior cerebellar artery	Dysphagia Dysarthria Loss of sensation on ipsilateral side of the face Loss of sensation on contralateral side of the body Horizontal nystagmus Ataxia Vertigo Ipsilateral Horner's syndrome (miotic pupils, ptosis and facial anhidrosis [inadequate perspiration]) Paralysis of larynx and soft palate
Anterior inferior cerebellar artery	Horizontal nystagmus Sensory impairment Deafness and tinnitus Facial paralysis Horner's syndrome Ataxia
Vertebral–basilar system	Dysarthria Dysphagia Vertigo Nausea Syncope Memory loss, disorientation Ataxic gait Double vision Tinnitus Nystagmus Facial paresis Drop attacks

Risk factors

Educational programs have been developed to inform the general public about CVA and prevention. Many factors have been identified as predisposing a person to a CVA and, by increasing public awareness, those at risk can seek medical advice to have any pre-existing conditions managed, thus reducing the risk of CVA. Risk factors include:

- A history of transient ischaemic attacks (TIA)
- Atherosclerosis
- Hypertension
- Family history of CVA
- Heart disease
- Diabetes mellitus
- Cigarette smoking
- Sedentary work with little exercise
- Obesity
- Elevated cholesterol and triglyceride levels.

Manifestations of a CVA

In all cases of CVA, areas of the brain are deprived of an adequate oxygen supply. If the blood supply is impaired for an extended period, the involved cerebral tissue may become necrotic, resulting in permanent neurological deficits. In instances of ischaemia, temporary neurological impairment may result. The particular type and degree of neurological deficits depend on the area of the brain involved (see Table 41.5). Table 41.6 lists a comparison of manifestations associated with right- and left-sided hemiplegia.

CARE OF THE CLIENT WHO HAS HAD A CVA

Medical management involves control of cerebral oedema and subsequent increased intracranial pressure, surgical intervention if indicated, and drug therapy; for example, thrombolytic medication such as tissue plasminogen activator (TPA) may be given to clients experiencing a non-haemorrhagic CVA. Nursing care of the client involves:

- Managing the acute phase
- Meeting basic needs
- Preventing complications
- Providing psychological support
- Promoting rehabilitation.

Care during the acute phase

The acute phase begins when the client is admitted, and continues until their condition is stable. Nursing care is directed towards maintaining a patent airway and monitoring vital and neurological signs.

Maintaining a patent airway. This involves positioning

TABLE 41.6 | MANIFESTATIONS OF HEMIPLEGIA

Right-sided hemiplegia (left CVA)	Left-sided hemiplegia (right CVA)
Aphasia — expressive, receptive or global	Spatial–perceptual deficits
Intellectual impairment	Tends to be distractible; impulsive behaviour
Slow behaviour	Appears to be unaware of deficits; poor judgment
Defects in right visual fields	Defects in left visual fields

the client on their side, administering oxygen as prescribed and suctioning secretions from the airway. Care must be taken when performing oronasopharyngeal suction, as suction applied for longer than 15 seconds at a time may increase intracranial pressure.

Recording fluid input and output. This information should be kept to monitor kidney function and to evaluate fluid and electrolyte balance.

Vital and neurological signs. These should be assessed frequently, for example every 15–30 minutes, to detect changes in the client's condition. Information on neurological assessment is provided earlier in this chapter. If the client is unconscious, the principles of care described previously should be incorporated.

Care after the acute phase

Detailed information about the nursing measures necessary to meet the client's basic needs for hygiene, safety, elimination, nutrition and fluids, psychological support, mobility and rehabilitation are provided elsewhere in this text. Assisting the client who is aphasic is described in Table 41.3, and Clinical Interest Box 41.5 provides some suggestions which can facilitate self-care after CVA.

The main aims of care for a client who has experienced a CVA are to:

- Assist in meeting hygiene needs
- Monitor vital and neurological signs
- Maintain muscle tone and prevent contractures
- Prevent skin breakdown
- Prevent venous stasis (thrombus and embolus formation)
- Prevent and manage alterations in elimination (e.g. incontinence, retention of urine, constipation)
- Maintain nutritional and fluid status
- Establish an adequate means of communication
- Promote reorientation of a confused client
- Enhance self-concept and body image
- Institute a rehabilitation program aimed at achieving an optimal level of independence.

Rehabilitation

Rehabilitation of the client begins on admission to hospital and continues for as long as necessary including after discharge home. In some health care institutions the client may be transferred to a rehabilitation unit after the acute phase of their illness. The focus of rehabilitation is directed at helping the client to relearn lost skills and to become as independent as possible. The client and their significant others are made aware of the plan and goals of the rehabilitative phase, and their active participation is encouraged. Recovery from a CVA is a slow process; therefore the nurse must provide support and positive feedback so that the client does not become discouraged. Rehabilitation of the client includes:

- Encouraging participation in their own care as much as possible
- Teaching them to perform the activities of daily living with regard to ways of compensating for any disabilities
- Teaching and assisting with performance of transfer activities (e.g. bed to chair)
- Assisting in the regaining of any lost communication skills
- Encouraging expression of feelings, to decrease anxiety and to allow for correction of any misunderstood information
- Developing a bladder and bowel retraining program (if necessary).

CLINICAL INTEREST BOX 41.5
Devices to facilitate self-care after CVA

The following list identifies useful items that may assist neurologically impaired clients to perform self-care more easily and safely after a stroke or other disorders.

Eating devices
- Plate guards to prevent food from being pushed off plate
- Wide grip utensils to accommodate weak grasp
- Non-skid mats to stabilise plates

Mobility aids
- Canes, walkers, wheelchairs
- Transfer devices such as slide boards and belts

Bathing and grooming devices
- Shower and bath chairs
- Electric razors with head at 90° to handle
- Grab bars, non-skid mats, hand-held shower heads
- Long-handled bath sponge

Dressing aids
- Velcro closures
- Elastic shoe laces
- Long-handled shoe horn

Toileting aids
- Raised toilet seat
- Grab bars next to toilet

(Further information on rehabilitation nursing is provided in Chapter 46.)

Planning for discharge

Discharge planning is directed at facilitating the transition from the health care institution to the home environment. Discharge planning involves assessing the client and the family, identifying specific needs, planning to implement ways of meeting those needs, and evaluating the discharge process and the results. After the client is discharged home, they and the family must have contact with support services, such as the district nurse, whom they can rely on for continued help and support.

SPINAL CORD INJURY

Injuries involving the spinal cord result most often from motor vehicle accidents, falls, sporting and industrial accidents, and firearm or stab wounds. Injuries to the vertebral column and spinal cord result from forces applied directly or indirectly to the head, neck or trunk. Apart from direct tearing of the spinal cord, the main damage is caused by haemorrhage, oedema and disruption of the blood supply to the cord. Additional compression can result if bony fragments or disc material press on the spinal cord.

Manifestations of spinal cord damage depend on the degree and site of the injury. Complete spinal cord transection causes a total loss of motor and sensory function below the level of injury. With cervical cord transection there is paralysis of all four extremities (quadriplegia/tetraplegia). There are varying degrees of arm and ventilatory paralysis, depending on the injury level. With thoracic cord transection, down to the level of the second lumbar vertebra, there is paralysis of the lower extremities (paraplegia). There is often some loss of intercostal muscle function and loss of bladder and bowel function. With transection in the region of lumbar vertebrae there is loss of a combination of sensory, motor, bowel and bladder function.

Complete cord transection results in immediate flaccid paralysis, loss of sensation and loss of reflexes below the level of injury. As paralysis subsides, reflexes usually return and flaccidity changes to involuntary spastic movements. Recovery of any motor or sensory function is rare when there has been complete paralysis of these functions for several days. With incomplete spinal-cord injuries, degrees of motor and sensory deficit below the level of damage vary. The client may experience temporary paralysis, with function returning when any oedema subsides.

Damage to the spinal cord and nerve roots results from:

- Compression by displaced bone or ligaments, extruded disc, or haematoma formation
- Excessive stretching, crushing, shearing or severance of neural tissue
- Swelling in response to bruising or compression
- Impaired capillary circulation and venous return.

There are four possible vectors (forces) that can be applied to the spinal column to cause injury:

1. Flexion: excessive flexion (hyperflexion) tends to produce compression of the vertebral bodies, with disruption of the posterior ligaments and the intervertebral discs. Hyperflexion injuries are caused by hyperflexion of the head and neck, as in sudden deceleration of a vehicle
2. Extension: excessive extension (hyperextension) usually causes fractures of the posterior elements of the vertebral column and disruption of the anterior ligaments. Hyperextension injuries are caused by hyperextension of the head and neck, as may occur in a rear-end vehicular accident
3. Rotation (lateral flexion): excessive rotation is most likely to produce rupture of the ligaments, fracture and fracture dislocation of the vertebral facets. Rotational injuries are caused by extreme lateral flexion or rotation of the head and neck
4. Compression: compression can result in fractures of the vertebral body and arch, and rupture of the supporting ligaments. Compression injuries are caused by vertical pressure as when a person falls from a height and lands on his feet or buttocks.

Classification of spinal cord injuries

Spinal cord injuries can be classified by the type of injury and by syndromes:

- Concussion: severe shaking of the spinal cord that causes temporary loss of function lasting about 24–48 hours
- Contusion: bruising of the spinal cord, which includes bleeding into the cord
- Laceration: an actual tear in the spinal cord
- Transection: severing of the cord — may be complete or incomplete
- Haemorrhage: bleeding into or around the cord. Escaped blood is an irritant to the delicate tissue
- Anterior cord syndrome: due to injury of the anterior part of the spinal cord and associated with flexion injuries and fracture dislocations of the vertebrae. Manifestations include loss of pain and temperature sensation and motor function below the level of the injury. The sensations of light touch, position and vibration remain intact
- Posterior cord syndrome: a rare syndrome in which the senses of position and vibration are involved
- Central cord syndrome: due to injury and/or oedema to the central cord in the cervical region (e.g. as a result of hyperextension injuries). Manifestations include a greater loss of motor function in the upper limbs (rather than the lower), bladder dysfunction and varying degrees of sensory impairment
- Brown-Séquard syndrome: results from open penetrating wounds that produce transverse hemisection of the cord. Manifestations include

TABLE 41.7 | SPINAL CORD INJURY — FUNCTIONAL LOSS

Level of injury	Motor function	Sensory function	Bladder/bowel function	Ventilatory function
C1–C4	Loss of all function from the neck down	Loss of sensation from the neck down	No bladder or bowel control	Loss of independent ventilatory function
C5	Loss of all function below the upper shoulders	Loss of sensation below the clavicles	No bladder or bowel control	Phrenic nerve is intact but the intercostal muscles are non-functional
C6	Loss of all function below the upper arms	Loss of sensation below the clavicles, but some arm and thumb sensation	No bladder or bowel control	Phrenic nerve is intact but the intercostal muscles are non-functional
C7	Incomplete quadriplegia. Loss of motor control to parts of the arms and hands	Loss of sensation below the clavicles but some arm and hand sensation	No bladder or bowel control	Phrenic nerve is intact but the intercostal muscles are non-functional
C8	Incomplete quadriplegia Loss of motor control to parts of the arms and hands	Loss of sensation below the chest and part of the hands	No bladder or bowel control	Phrenic nerve is intact but the intercostal muscles are non-functional
T1–T6	Loss of function below the mid-chest	Loss of sensation from the mid-chest down	No bladder or bowel control	Independent phrenic nerve function; some intercostal muscle impairment
T6–T12	Loss of function below the waist	Loss of sensation below the waist	No bladder or bowel control	No interference to ventilatory function
L1–L2	Loss of most control of the pelvis and legs	Loss of sensation to the lower abdomen and legs	No bladder or bowel control	No interference to ventilatory function
L3–L4	Loss of control of part of the lower legs and feet	Loss of sensation to part of the lower legs and feet	No bladder or bowel control	No interference to ventilatory function
L5–S5	Loss of control of parts of the hips, knees, ankles and feet	Loss of sensation to parts of the lower limbs, and perineum	May or may not be loss of bladder and/ or bowel control	No interference to ventilatory function

loss of pain and temperature sensation on the side opposite the injury, and loss of motor function, light touch, position and vibratory sensation on the side of the injury.

Manifestations of spinal cord injury

Generally, the degree of damage to the spinal cord at any level is described as incomplete or complete transection. Incomplete transection of the cord produces loss or impairment of sensation and motor function that reflects the specific nerve tracts that have been damaged. Complete transection of the cord results in permanent loss of voluntary movement, sensation, reflex and autonomic function below the level of injury.

Spinal shock

Spinal shock is an immediate response to an acute spinal cord injury and is the temporary suppression of reflexes controlled by the segments below the level of injury. After a period that may vary from hours to months, the spinal neurons gradually regain their excitability. Subsequent return of some function results from decompression of the cord as oedema resolves.

Functional loss from spinal cord injury

The different functions and dysfunctions associated with spinal cord injuries at specific levels are listed in Table 41.7. The effects of spinal cord injury on sexual response vary depending on the level and degree of injury. Sexual function is controlled by spinal levels S2, S3 and S4. Knowledge of the physiology of alterations in sexual response after spinal cord injury is incomplete, and significant individual differences exist. People with complete loss of sensation in the genitalia may still experience orgasm in response to sensations produced by stimulation of other areas of the body in which sensation is intact. Sexual pleasure can also be increased by psychological stimuli, such as memory, sight, sound and odour. Physical stimulation of the genitalia may produce reflex erection of the penis and vaginal lubrication, even though there is no sensory awareness of stimulation.

CARE OF THE CLIENT WITH SPINAL CORD INJURY

Management of the client at the scene of the accident is critical to the ultimate neurological outcome. The basic objectives of first aid management at the scene are to:

- Prevent death from asphyxia
- Prevent further spinal cord damage from torsion, flexion or extension of the unstable spine
- Transport the client rapidly and safely to an appropriate facility.

Subsequent management of the individual involves emergency department care, early management, post-acute and long-term management.

Initial management

On arrival of the client in the accident and emergency department, the medical officer assesses the client, and X-rays are taken to determine the extent of the injuries. The medical officer develops a plan of care that may include immediate surgery or a non-surgical approach with traction and immobilisation and insertion of a nasogastric tube, indwelling urinary catheter and intravenous infusion. Generally, glucocorticoid steroids are prescribed to reduce cord swelling.

Early management

After initial assessment and stabilisation of the client, they are admitted to the intensive care or spinal unit. A client with less severe injuries may be admitted to a general ward. Medical management will depend on the type of spinal cord injury and any associated injuries. Treatment may be surgical, non-surgical or a combination of both approaches. Surgical management may take the form of decompression laminectomy, fusion of vertebrae, open or closed reduction of fractures or dislocations, or the insertion of rods. Non-surgical management involves immobilisation of the spine (Figure 41.11) using skeletal tongs with traction, halo traction, a cervical collar, or a device designed to maintain thoracic or lumbar alignment, such as a fibreglass body jacket.

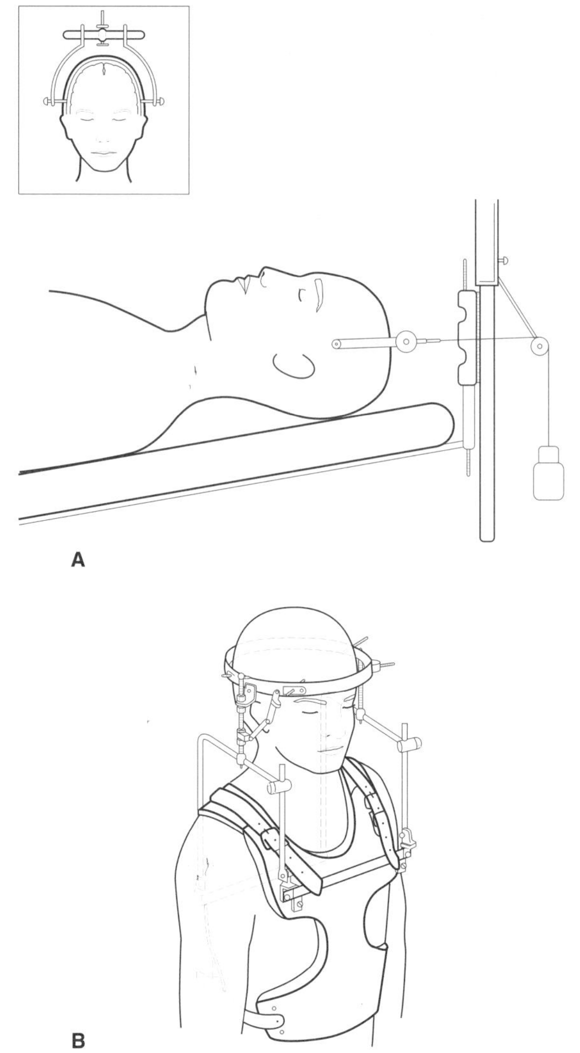

Figure 41.11 | Immobilisation of the spine
A: Cervical traction with tongs. The inset shows the position of the tongs on the bone structure of the skull **B**: Halo traction and vest

NURSING CARE OF THE CLIENT WITH A SPINAL CORD INJURY

Nursing management will vary according to the client's injury and whether a surgical or non-surgical approach is selected. However, the major aspects of care are directed towards maintaining respiratory function, immobilisation and alignment of the spine, preventing complications, meeting basic needs, providing psychological support, and rehabilitation.

Some nursing diagnoses relating to neurological health are listed in Clinical Interest Box 41.6.

CLINICAL INTEREST BOX 41.6
Nursing diagnoses related to neurological health

- Aspiration, risk for
- Communication, impaired verbal
- Disuse syndrome, risk for
- Injury, risk for
- Mobility, impaired physical
- Sensory/perceptual alterations
- Swallowing, impaired
- Unilateral neglect

Respiratory care

A client with a spinal cord injury can develop varying degrees of respiratory difficulty, depending on the level of spinal injury. The client will require a plan of care directed at preventing pulmonary complications. Intubation and mechanical ventilation will be required if there is impairment of respiratory muscle function. The program of care includes:

- Regular assessment for indications of inadequate ventilation
- Chest physiotherapy at least every 4 hours
- Maintenance of a patent airway
- Use of an incentive spirometer to promote lung expansion.

Immobilisation and alignment of the spine

After alignment of the spine has been achieved, immobilisation serves to maintain alignment and promotes healing at the site of injury. For most thoracic, lumbar or sacral injuries the client remains confined to bed, with the back positioned and supported to achieve hyperextension of the spine at the site of injury. A bed with a firm mattress and steel base and correctly positioned pillows are necessary to maintain the prescribed posture.

Skeletal traction

When the injury involves dislocation or fracture-dislocation of the cervical or high thoracic spine, skeletal traction is commonly used to accomplish alignment and immobilisation. Skeletal traction may be achieved by means of cervical tongs, such as Crutchfield tongs, or by the halo device (see Figure 41.11). The halo device may also be incorporated with the use of a body vest or jacket to stabilise the spine, thereby allowing the individual to be ambulatory. When skeletal traction is used, the client may be nursed on a firm mattress and fracture board, or on a special bed such as a Stryker frame.

After skeletal traction has been established, pain is decreased and the client's comfort is enhanced. Turning can be carried out using a special technique (as described in Chapter 7) to allow for skin care and a change of position. Alternatively, a client may be lifted in a Jordan frame for hygiene purposes. Management of the client in cervical skeletal traction includes:

- Checking the traction equipment every 2–4 hours to ensure safety and integrity of the treatment
- Inspecting, cleansing and dressing the pin sites according to the institution's policy (e.g. every 4–8 hours)
- Changing the client's position every 2 hours to prevent the complications of immobility. The 'log-rolling' technique or the Stryker frame is used to turn the individual to maintain the vertebral column in neutral position. (Information on the log-rolling technique is provided in Chapter 29.)
- Using various devices (e.g. pillows, a foot board, a cervical roll) to maintain good body alignment. When the client lies supine, the arms and legs are positioned in extension with support to maintain the feet in dorsiflexion. The hands are placed in a functional position and a cervical roll is used to maintain hyperextension of the neck. When the client is in a lateral position, the arms and legs are positioned in extension, and pillows are placed to support this position.

Preventing complications

Because prolonged immobility can lead to various complications, specific preventive measures must be implemented. (Information on preventing the complications associated with immobility is provided in Chapter 36.)

Meeting basic needs

Clients with impaired motor and sensory function require assistance to meet their needs for hygiene, safety, elimination, nutrition and fluids, temperature regulation and pain relief. (Information on assisting clients to meet these basic needs is provided in other chapters.)

Providing psychological support

A severe spinal cord injury has a devastating effect on the client and their significant others, and they will experience a range of emotional responses, from the time of injury and through the rehabilitation process. The client will have to adapt to the loss of motor function, and sensory deprivation, both of which severely threaten self-concept and body image. It is important that the nurse is aware of the impact that the injury has on the client's emotional and psychological equilibrium. The nurse must be sensitive to the emotional and psychological response of the client to the injury, and be supportive as they deal with the impact of the injury. The nurse can help to support the client by:

- Establishing a climate of trust
- Accepting behaviour, without being judgmental
- Encouraging expression of feelings
- Listening empathetically and attentively
- Allowing the client to make decisions and maintain control
- Providing information as necessary
- Supporting a positive self-concept and self-esteem
- Informing the client that it will take time to adjust to the disability.

Promoting rehabilitation

In most instances of spinal cord injury the client will require long-term rehabilitation. Rehabilitation after spinal cord injury is a lifelong process of learning to live with a disability. The client and family together with the health care team members contribute to the development of the rehabilitative plans. (Information on rehabilitation is provided in Chapter 46.)

SUMMARY

The nervous system is a complex system, responsible for communication within the body and between the body and its environment. It is divided into two primary divisions, the central nervous system and the peripheral nervous system.

Nervous tissue is commonly described as grey and white matter. The grey matter is composed of cells and the white matter is made up of fibres. Neurons are the primary components of nervous tissue, which are bound together by neuroglia. Neurons have two functional properties, irritability and conductivity. This means that neurons are able to respond to a stimulus, convert it into an impulse, and transmit the impulse to other neurons, muscles or glands. Impulses are transmitted through spaces, called synapses, between neurons.

The central nervous system consists of the brain and the spinal cord. The brain is a large organ composed of the cerebrum, diencephalon, brainstem and cerebellum. Each part of the brain has specific functions. The spinal cord lies within a canal inside the vertebral column, extending from the base of the skull to the first or second lumbar vertebra. The spinal cord receives sensory impulses, conveys motor impulses and is the centre through which reflex actions take place. The meninges are three membranes that cover the brain and spinal cord to protect them against physical injury. Cerebrospinal fluid is a clear watery fluid produced in the ventricles of the brain, which circulates in the subarachnoid space surrounding the brain and spinal cord. It protects the brain and spinal cord and provides a medium for the exchange of nutrients and waste products.

The peripheral nervous system consists of 12 pairs of cranial nerves and 31 pairs of spinal nerves. The nerves of the peripheral nervous system may be: sensory, carrying impulses to the brain and spinal cord; motor, carrying impulses away from the brain and spinal cord; or mixed. The motor nervous system is divided into somatic and autonomic nervous system divisions. The autonomic nervous system division is composed of the sympathetic nervous system and the parasympathetic nervous system. It is the section of the peripheral nervous system concerned with the involuntary activity of the body. Sympathetic nerves have a stimulating effect on most organs, while parasympathetic nerves tend to slow down body processes.

Normal function of the nervous system may be impaired as a result of congenital disorders, inflammatory or infectious conditions, trauma, neoplasia, degenerative conditions or metabolic and endocrine disorders. The major manifestations of nervous system disorders are headaches, sensory changes, motor changes, reflex changes, altered states of awareness or consciousness, and seizures. Disorders of the nervous system can be classified as those occurring from congenital or hereditary defects, from multiple causes, degenerative disorders, immunological disorders, infectious or inflammatory conditions, neoplastic or obstructive disorders, and trauma.

Diagnostic tests used to assess nervous system function include the neurological examination, radiographic examination, magnetic resonance imaging and electroencephalography. Care of the individual with a nervous system disorder includes promoting a clear airway, maintaining fluid and nutritional status, preventing and managing alterations in elimination, promoting effective communication, promoting safety, promoting mobility, preventing the complications of immobility, providing psychological support, assessing neurological status, providing a suitable environment and promoting rehabilitation.

REVIEW EXERCISES

1. What are the functions of the nervous system?
2. What are the pathophysiological changes that can disrupt normal function of the nervous system?
3. What are the common manifestations of nervous system disorders?
4. Which signs and symptoms are typically associated with Parkinson's disease?
5. Which diagnostic tests are most commonly used to aid in evaluation of nervous system disorders?
6. How can the nurse promote effective communication with the client affected by aphasia?
7. What are the aims of care when nursing an unconscious client?
8. What are the types of CVA? What are the risk factors? What are the manifestations?
9. Identify the major aspects of care when nursing a client with spinal cord injury.

CRITICAL THINKING EXERCISES

1. A client has been brought into the emergency department after a fall on his head at work. He says he was knocked out for about 10 minutes, but now seems alert and orientated. What type of injury is he most likely to have sustained? What discharge instructions would you give this client's family? How would you modify these instructions if this client lives alone?
2. A 19-year-old client has been admitted to the rehabilitation ward after complete transection of his spinal cord at C7 level, in a motor vehicle accident. What motor and sensory function would you expect the client to have? The client says he is looking forward to learning to use special equipment. Do you think his emotional response is appropriate? How would you respond? What elimination issues may emerge? How would you deal with these?
3. Mr Green, 57, has recently been diagnosed with early-stage Parkinson's disease. Mrs Green is quite concerned about the progression of the disease — whether Mr Green can still be employed, if he can be left alone for several hours at a time, and what medications he will be required to take. How would you respond to her concerns? Is there other information that would be helpful to the Greens? How can they find more information about Parkinson's disease?
4. Mr Hong is a 50-year-old police constable. He has been troubled by recurrent atrial fibrillation, and treated with an anticoagulant. Mr Hong was on a ladder cleaning the gutters of his house when he fell and hit his head. Although shaken, after his wife made him a cup of tea and after a short rest, he felt well enough to continue with his task. However, over the next few days, Mrs Hong began noticing several behavioural changes in her

husband. He seemed vague and forgetful at times. Finally, when she found him urinating in the freshly set fireplace, he was convinced to seek medical assistance. An MRI showed a subdural haematoma. Mr Hong was booked in for evacuation of the clot via burr holes. His surgery was highly successful and Mrs Hong was most grateful that she could confidently set her fire.

Before surgery, the nurse taking care of Mr Hong made the following nursing diagnoses:

- Risk for injury related to confusion secondary to increased intracranial haemorrhage
- Self-care deficit: bathing/hygiene related to decreased level of consciousness
- Sleep pattern disturbance related to frequent assessments and loss of sleep.

Describe the nursing interventions, with rationales, that may be planned in response to the above nursing diagnoses.

REFERENCES AND FURTHER READING

Ankner GM (2007) *Case Studies in Medical –Surgical Nursing*. Thomson Delmar Learning, Clifton Park, NY

—— (2008) *Medical–Surgical Nursing*. Thomson Delmar Learning, Clifton Park, NY

Brunner LS, Suddarth DS (2000) *Textbook of Medical-Surgical Nursing*, 9th edn. JB Lippincott, Philadelphia

Huether SF & McCance KL (2008) *Understanding Pathophysiology*. Mosby, London

Lemone P, Burke KM (2000) *Medical Surgical Nursing*, 2nd edn. Prentice-Hall, Upper Saddle River, NJ

Marieb E (2006) *Essentials of Human Anatomy and Physiology*, 6th edn. Benjamin Cummings, San Francisco

Neighbors M, Tannehill-Jones R (2000) *Human Diseases*. Delmar Thomson Learning, Albany

Seeley R, Stephens T, Tate P (2001) *Anatomy and Physiology*, 5th edn. McGraw Hill, New York

Thibodeau GA (2008) *Structure and Function of the Body*. Mosby, St Louis

ONLINE RESOURCES

ABC Online. Health Matters Library: www.abc.net.au/health/library

Epilepsy Foundation of Victoria: www.epinet.org.au

Multiple Sclerosis Society of Australia: www.msaustralia.org.au

National Institute of Neurological Disorders and Stroke: www.ninds.nih.gov

Parkinson's Australia website: www.parkinsons.org.au

The Better Health Channel: www.betterhealth.vic.gov.au

Chapter 42
SENSORY ABILITIES

OBJECTIVES

- Define the key terms/concepts
- Describe the position of each special sense organ
- Describe the structure of each special sense organ
- Describe the physiology of taste, smell, sight and hearing
- Describe the factors affecting sensory function of the special sense organs
- Describe the major manifestations of disorders of the eye and ear
- Briefly describe the specific disorders of the eye and ear outlined in this chapter
- Describe diagnostic tests that may be used to assess eye and ear function
- Assist in planning and implementing nursing care for the client with altered sensory function

KEY TERMS/CONCEPTS

ageusia
anosmia
cacogeusia
chemoreceptors
convergence
diplopia
dysgeusia
hyperopia
hypogeusia
hyposmia
myopia
otalgia
ototoxicity
parosmia
presbycusis
presbyobia
proprioceptive
refraction
tinnitus

CHAPTER FOCUS

The sensory abilities of taste, smell, touch, sight and hearing enable the client to receive stimuli that facilitate interaction and provide information about the environment. Perception of sensory stimuli has its origin in the five special sense organs, which are specially adapted for the reception of specific stimuli — tongue (taste), nose (smell), skin (touch), eyes (sight) and ears (hearing and maintenance of balance). Receptors in the sense organs pick up stimuli from the environment and transmit this information to the brain via pathways in the nervous system. In the brain the information is processed and interpreted. A person's senses are essential for growth, development and survival. Sensory stimuli give meaning to events in the environment. Any alteration in the individual's sensory function can affect their ability to function within the environment. Alterations in sensory function may lead to dysfunctions of sight, hearing, smell, taste, balance and coordination.

As the eyes and ears are the two major structures by which an individual receives information about the external environment, this chapter focuses mainly on the care of these organs. The eye is the means by which light, reflected from objects, travels to the retina so that an image is formed. Nerve endings in the retina transmit electrical impulses along the optic nerve to the brain for interpretation. The ear is the means by which soundwaves are collected and amplified. Nerve endings in the inner ear transmit electrical impulses along the auditory pathways to the brain for interpretation. The auditory system is also responsible for maintenance of balance.

LIVED EXPERIENCE

Well, I must admit, it has made a big difference to my life. Joan was right and in a way I'm pleased she pushed me into action. I was just missing out on so many things. I could see her frustration and now realise that the answer was a simple hearing test and a hearing aid. I was too proud to be labelled 'disabled' so I struggled on for the last couple of years with my deteriorating hearing only catching the end of phrases, blaring the television out and picking up on a bit of lip-reading. No doubt my 40 years of working in the timber mill until my retirement and the fact that I'm now 76 years old are both contributing factors to my hearing loss. Of course, the biggest bonus is that the grandchildren hardly notice the hearing aid and now I can hear them and enjoy their little concerts they perform for me when they come to visit Grandpa.

Bill, aged 76

I have never been so frustrated in my life as I was with Bill. It was obvious he couldn't hear properly and had some silly notion in his head that he would look disabled with a hearing aid. We had so many arguments and disagreements because he didn't hear whole conversations and would assume what was being said. I got so tired of repeating myself continually.

Joan, age 71, Bill's partner

COMPONENTS OF THE SENSORY EXPERIENCE

THE TONGUE (TASTEBUDS)

The sensory receptors for taste are the taste buds. They are widely scattered in the oral cavity, with most concentrated over the surface of the tongue (Figure 42.1) and a few found on the soft palate and inner surface of the cheeks. They are chemoreceptors that respond to substances present in food and generate nerve impulses that are transmitted to the brain for interpretation. The upper surface of the tongue is covered with small projections (papillae) some of which contain a taste bud. Each taste bud consists of sensory and supporting cells situated in the epithelium and opening into the surface through a small gustatory pore. Between the cells of the taste bud lie the ending of afferent nerve fibres derived from several cranial nerves. Taste buds on the anterior two-thirds of the tongue connect with fibres of the facial (seventh cranial) nerve. Taste buds on the posterior one-third of the tongue are associated with the fibres of the glossopharyngeal (ninth cranial) nerve, while pharyngeal taste buds send impulses to the brain via the vagus (tenth cranial) nerve.

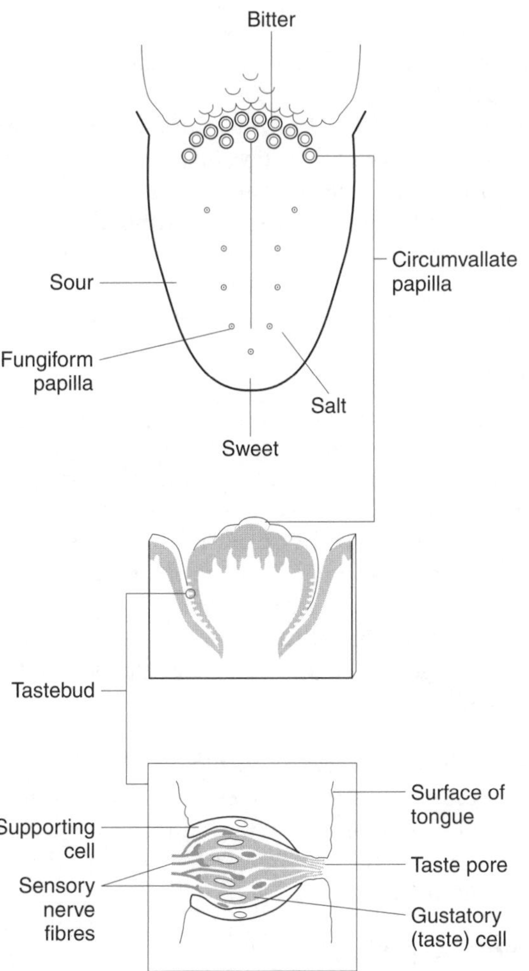

Figure 42.1 | The location and structure of the taste buds in the tongue

These taste buds can differentiate among sweet, salty, sour and bitter stimuli. The tip of the tongue is most sensitive to sweet and salty substances, the edges of the tongue are most sensitive to sour substances, and the back of the tongue is most sensitive to bitter substances. Substances must be in solution (saliva) so that they can enter the opening in a taste bud, and stimulate the nerve ending. Molecules pass into solution on the surface of the tongue then combine with the surface membranes of the receptor cells. Transmitter substances are released, which evoke action potentials on the sensory nerve fibres. Fibres from the seventh, ninth and tenth cranial nerves carry the taste impulses via the brainstem to an area of the cerebral cortex where the taste is experienced.

The sense of taste is intricately linked with the sense of smell, and the sense of taste depends on stimulation of the olfactory receptors. Both senses have a protective function; for example, in detecting substances that may be harmful. Interruption to the transmission of taste stimuli to the brain may cause taste abnormalities. Taste abnormalities may result from trauma, infection, vitamin or mineral deficiencies, neurological or oral disorders and the effects of drugs. Because tastes are most accurately perceived in a fluid medium, mouth dryness may interfere with taste. Alterations in taste may include ageusia (a complete loss of taste), hypogeusia (a partial loss of taste), dysgeusia (a distorted sense of taste) and cacogeusia (an unpleasant taste).

THE NOSE (OLFACTORY RECEPTORS)

The specific receptors for the sense of smell are the olfactory receptors. They are chemoreceptors that respond to airborne chemicals and generate impulses that are transmitted to the brain for interpretation. The olfactory receptors are situated in the mucous membrane lining the upper part of the nose (Figure 42.2). When these receptors are stimulated by chemicals they transmit impulses along the olfactory nerve to the brain. These receptors adapt quickly when exposed to an unchanging stimulus, which means that the client can become accustomed to an odour when constantly exposed to it.

Permanent alterations in the sense usually result when the olfactory neuroepithelium or part of the olfactory nerve is destroyed. Permanent or temporary loss can occur from inhaling irritants such as acid fumes that paralyse nasal cilia. Conditions such as ageing, Parkinson's disease and Alzheimer's disease may alter the sense of smell. Alterations in smell include anosmia (a total loss of sense of smell), hyposmia (an impaired sense of smell) and parosmia (an abnormal sense of smell).

There is a close relationship between the sense of smell and the sense of taste, and therefore they are not always distinguishable. The sensations of smell and taste play an important part in stimulating the secretions of digestive juices.

The nurse plays an important role in promoting the sense of taste and stimulating the sense of smell when caring for a client with altered sensory function. Client education regarding good oral hygiene practices will enhance taste perception, and discussing with the client what foods are the most taste appealing. If taste perception is improved, food intake and appetite will also improve. Taste perception is increased when foods are seasoned. The client's sense of smell can be stimulated by pleasant aromas such as flowers, perfumes and food.

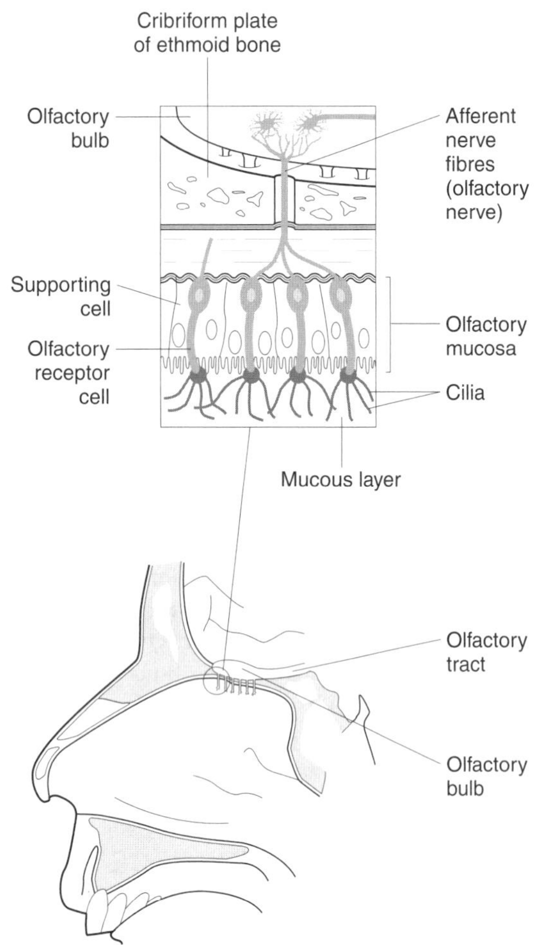

Figure 42.2 | The location and structure of the olfactory receptors in the nose

THE SKIN AS AN ORGAN OF SENSATION

The skin is an important sensory organ that allows us to receive information about our external environment. Distributed widely in the dermis of the skin are sensory receptors called cutaneous receptors, which are stimulated by heat, cold and touch, including pressure. Sensory neurons carry impulses from these receptors to the brain where the sensation is interpreted. The nurse can help stimulate altered sensory function by discussing with the client the introduction of touch therapy. This may include such things as touching arms, back rub and brushing of hair.

THE EYES

Sight, or vision, is a special sense that allows us to interact and experience our environment. The eyes allow us to see by providing a pathway for visual stimuli to reach the brain. Vision is the result of light rays being received by the eyes and transmitted by the optic nerve to the brain, where they are interpreted. The eyes are located within the orbits of the skull, one on either side of the nose. The ciliary artery and cental retinal artery, which are branches of the ophthalmic artery, supply arterial blood to the eye.

THE EARS

The ear is specially adapted as the organ of hearing but it is also concerned with sense of position, balance and equilibrium. Hearing is a complex mechanism in which the ears receive soundwaves and convert them into nerve impulses. The nerve impulses are transmitted by the acoustic (eighth cranial) nerve to the brain, where they are interpreted. The externally visible portion of each ear is located on the lateral surface of the head on each side. The remaining parts of each ear are embedded in the bone of the skull beneath.

SENSORY ALTERATIONS

People become accustomed to certain sensory stimuli and, when these change markedly, the individual may experience discomfort. Factors that contribute to alterations in behaviour are as follows.

Sensory deprivation

Sensory deprivation is thought of as a decrease or lack of meaningful stimuli. Because of reduced stimulation, a person becomes more acutely aware of the remaining stimuli and often perceives these in a distorted manner. The individual often experiences alterations in perception, cognition and emotion (Clinical Interest Box 42.1).

Sensory overload

Sensory overload generally occurs when a person is unable to process or manage the amount or intensity of sensory stimuli. Factors that can contribute to sensory overload are:

- Pain, dyspnoea and anxiety
- A noisy health care setting, intrusive diagnostic studies, contacts with many strangers
- Nervous system disturbances, certain medications.

Sensory overload can prevent the brain from ignoring or responding to specific stimuli. The clinical signs of sensory overload are listed in Clinical Interest Box 42.2.

Sensory deficits

A sensory deficit is impaired reception, perception, or both, of one or more of the senses. Impaired hearing and sight are sensory deficits. When only one sense is affected, other senses may become more acute to compensate for the loss. However, sudden loss of eyesight can result in disorientation. When there is a gradual loss of sensory function, people often develop behaviours to compensate for the loss; for example, a person with gradual hearing loss in the right ear may unconsciously turn the left ear towards a speaker. Clients with sensory deficits are at risk of both sensory deprivation and sensory overload (Kozier et al 2000).

CLINICAL INTEREST BOX 42.1
Clinical signs of sensory deprivation

- Excessive yawning, drowsiness and sleeping
- Decreased attention span, difficulty concentrating, decreased problem-solving ability
- Impaired memory
- Periodic disorientation, general confusion or nocturnal confusion
- Preoccupation with somatic complaints such as palpitations
- Hallucinations or delusions
- Crying, annoyance over small matters, depression
- Apathy, emotional liability

(Kozier et al 2000: 890)

CLINICAL INTEREST BOX 42.2
Clinical signs of sensory overload

- Complaints of fatigue, sleeplessness
- Irritability, anxiety, restlessness
- Reduced problem-solving ability and task performance
- Increased muscle tension
- Scattered attention and racing thoughts

(Kozier et al 2000: 891)

Factors affecting sensory function

A range of factors affect the amount and quality of sensory stimulation, including a person's developmental stage, culture, level of stress, medications, illness and lifestyle. These are outlined in Clinical Interest Box 42.3.

ASSESSING SENSORY FUNCTION

Nursing assessment of sensory-perceptual functioning includes:

- Nursing history: Clinical Interest Box 42.4 gives some examples of interview questions to elicit data about the client's sensory-perceptual functioning
- Mental status, including level of consciousness, orientation, memory and attention span
- Physical examination — the client's specific visual and hearing abilities; perception of heat, cold, light touch and pain in the limbs; and awareness of the position of body parts
- The client's environment — assess for quantity, quality and type of stimuli
- Social support network — the degree of isolation a person feels is significantly influenced by the quality and quantity of support from family and friends (Kozier et al 2000).

THE EYE

STRUCTURE OF THE EYE

The eye is a spherical structure (Figure 42.3) about 2.5 cm in diameter, consisting of three principal layers.

The outer layer

The outer fibrous layer consists of the sclera and the cornea, which is a transparent structure continuous with the sclera. About five-sixths of the outer surface is made up of a tough white opaque fibrous layer (sclera), while the cornea comprises the anterior one-sixth. Both the sclera and the cornea consist of layers of collagen fibres. In the cornea, the fibres are regular in size and arrangement, which

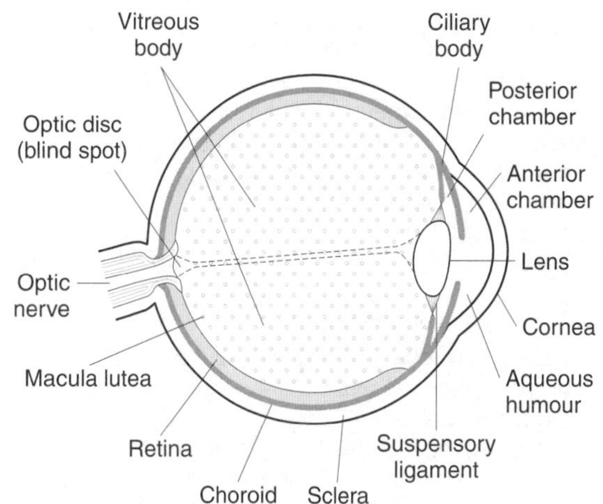

Figure 42.3 | The eye

CLINICAL INTEREST BOX 42.3
Factors that influence sensory function

Age

- Infants are unable to discriminate sensory stimuli. Nerve pathways are immature
- Visual changes during adulthood include presbyopia (inability to focus on near objects) and the need for glasses for reading (usually occurring from age 40–50)
- Hearing changes, which begin at age 30, include decreased hearing acuity, speech intelligibility, pitch discrimination and hearing threshold. Tinnitus often accompanies a hearing loss as a side effect of drugs. Older adults hear low-pitched sounds the best but have difficulty hearing conversation over background noise
- Older adults have reduced visual fields, increased glare sensitivity, impaired night vision, reduced accommodation and depth perception, and reduced colour discrimination
- Older adults have difficulty discriminating the consonants (*f, s, th, ch*). Speech sounds are garbled and there is a delayed reception and reaction to speech
- Gustatory and olfactory changes include a decrease in the number of taste buds in later years and reduction of olfactory nerve fibres by age 50. Reduced taste discrimination and reduced sensitivity to odours are common
- Proprioceptive changes after age 60 include increased difficulty with balance, spatial orientation and coordination
- Older adults experience tactile changes, including declining sensitivity to pain, pressure and temperature

Medications

- Some antibiotics (e.g. streptomycin, gentamicin) are ototoxic and can permanently damage the auditory nerve; chloramphenicol can irritate the optic nerve. Narcotic analgesics, sedatives and antidepressant medications can alter the perception of stimuli

Environment

- Excessive environmental stimuli (e.g. equipment noise and staff conversation in an intensive care unit [ICU]) can result in sensory overload, marked by confusion, disorientation, and the inability to make decisions. Restricted environmental stimulation (e.g. with protective isolation) can lead to sensory deprivation. Poor-quality environmental stimuli (e.g. reduced lighting, narrow walkways, background noise) can worsen sensory impairment

Comfort level

- Pain and fatigue alter the way a person perceives and reacts to stimuli

Pre-existing illness

- Peripheral vascular disease can cause reduced sensation in the extremities and impaired cognition. Chronic diabetes mellitus can lead to reduced vision, blindness or peripheral neuropathy. Strokes often produce loss of speech. Some neurological disorders impair motor function and sensory reception

Smoking

- Chronic tobacco use can cause the taste buds to atrophy, lessening the perception of flavours

Noise levels

- Constant exposure to high noise levels (e.g. on a construction job site) can cause hearing loss

Endotracheal intubation

- Temporary loss of speech results from insertion of an endotracheal tube through the mouth or nose into the trachea

(adapted from Potter & Perry 2008)

CLINICAL INTEREST BOX 42.4
Interview to assess a client's sensory-perceptual functioning

Visual

- How would you rate your vision (excellent, good, fair or poor)?
- Do you wear eyeglasses or contact lenses?
- Describe any recent changes in your vision.
- Do you have any difficulty seeing near or far objects?
- Do you have any difficulty seeing at night?
- Have you ever experienced blurred vision, double vision, spots moving in front of your eyes, blind spots, light sensitivity, flashing lights or halos around objects?
- When did you last visit an eye doctor?

Auditory

- How would you rate your hearing (excellent, good, fair or poor)?
- Do you wear a hearing aid?
- Describe any recent changes in your hearing.
- Can you locate the direction of sounds and distinguish various voices?
- Do you experience any dizziness or vertigo?
- Do you experience any ringing, buzzing, humming or crackling noises or fullness in the ears?

Gustatory

- Have you experienced any changes in taste (e.g. difficulty in differentiating sweet, sour, salty and bitter tastes)?
- Do you enjoy the taste of foods as you did previously?

Olfactory

- Have you experienced any changes in smell?
- Do things (foods, flowers, perfumes, etc) smell the same as previously?
- Can you distinguish foods by their odours and tell when something is burning?
- Have you experienced any changes in appetite? (Changes in appetite may be related to an impaired sense of smell.)

Tactile

- Are you experiencing any pain or discomfort?
- Have you experienced any decrease in your ability to perceive heat, cold or pain in your limbs?
- Do you have any numbness or tingling in your extremities?

Kinaesthetic

- Have you noticed any difficulty in perceiving the position of parts of your body?

(Kozier et al 2000: 892)

accounts for its transparency. The cornea functions as a refracting and protective layer through which light rays pass en route to the brain.

The middle layer

The middle pigmented vascular layer is composed of three structures: the choroid, the iris and the ciliary body. The choroid is a layer of tissue that lies between the sclera and the retina. It is composed largely of blood vessels, and contains highly pigmented cells that absorb light and prevent it from being reflected within the eyeball.

The iris is a pigmented circular membrane between the cornea and the lens, and gives the eye its colour. Sphincter and dilator muscles within the iris regulate the central aperture (the pupil). By either dilation or constriction of the pupil, the amount of light entering the eye is regulated. The pupil appears black because light rays entering the eye are absorbed by the choroid and are not reflected.

The ciliary body is a thickened area of the choroid, lying anterior to the choroid extending to the root of the iris. A circular array of fibres stretches from the ciliary body to the lens, to hold it in place. The ciliary body controls focusing of the lens and contains glands that secrete aqueous humour.

The innermost layer

The innermost layer is a thin structure called the retina. The retina lines the inner wall of the posterior portion of the eyeball and is comprised of a number of layers. The two main layers are the pigmented layer (the outermost layer of the retina, lying next to the choroid, and whose cells contain melanin) and the rod and cone layer, which lies next to the pigmented layer and is highly sensitive to light.

Rods and cones (specialised nerve endings) are distributed as a tightly packed mass throughout the retina, except at a point where the ganglionic fibres converge to form the optic nerve. This area, which is about 1.5 mm in diameter, is termed the optic disc. Since it possesses no photosensitive cells it is also known as the 'blind spot'. The prime function of rods and cones is to absorb light. Rods can be stimulated by dim light and allow perception of shapes and movement in dim light. Rods also provide far peripheral vision. Cones are specialised for fine visual discrimination and colour perception. There are three types of cones: one type responds mostly to blue light, another to red light, and the third type responds to green light.

In the centre of the retina is an oval yellowish area, the macula lutea. In the centre of the macula lutea is a small depression, the fovea centralis. Because the photosensitive cells are more exposed to light here than over the rest of the retina, visual acuity is at its highest.

Extraocular structure — accessory structures

Extraocular, or accessory, structures of the eye are portions of the eye outside the eyeball. These structures consist of the eyebrows, eyelids, eyelashes and lacrimal apparatus. The eyeball is anchored into position by several structures, including the extraocular muscles, the conjunctiva and the eyelids. The eyeball is surrounded and protected by a bony orbit, the eyebrow ridge and some fatty tissue. The eyeball is lubricated by the lacrimal glands.

The extraocular muscles bring about rotational movements of the eyeball. The muscles arise from the orbit and consist of four rectus muscles, which are attached to the sclera, and two oblique muscles. The oblique muscles are arranged so that, for part of their length, they lie around the circumference of the eyeball. The eyebrows and eyelashes are short coarse hairs that shade the eyes and protect the eyes from dust and sweat. The eyelids consist of connective tissue covered by skin, and lined with mucous membrane. The lining is reflected over the eyeballs, and is called the conjunctiva. The eyelids protect the eye from foreign bodies and excessive light as well as distributing tears by blinking.

The lacrimal apparatus (Figure 42.4) consists of the lacrimal gland, which is situated over the eye at the upper outer corner and secretes tears, which constantly wash over the conjunctiva. Tears leave the gland via several small ducts, and pass over the front of the eye eventually draining into the lacrimal sac, which is the expanded end of the nasolacrimal duct. Tears are secreted on to the anterior surface of the eyeball and are spread over it by the blinking movements of the eyelids. An antimicrobial substance in tears protects the eyes against microorganisms. Excess tears drain down the nasal cavity. The lacrimal glands are stimulated in response to chemical and mechanical irritants, thus producing tears to wash away irritants. Tears may also be produced as a result of emotion such as sadness, or happiness.

The refractive media

The refractive media are the transparent parts of the eye, and have the ability to bend light rays at the surfaces of two transparent media. The refractive media are the cornea, the

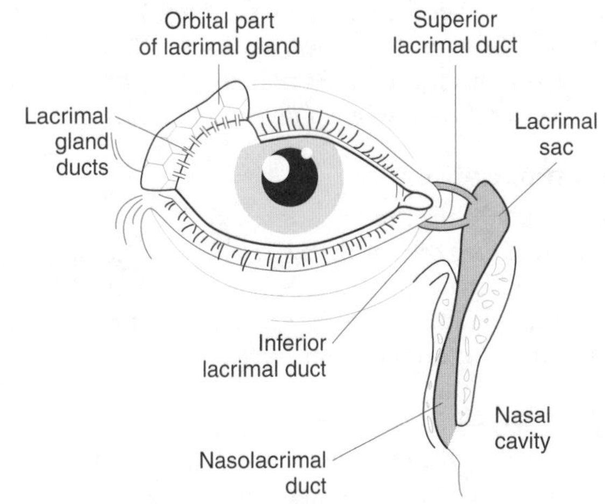

Figure 42.4 | The lacrimal apparatus of the eye

lens, the aqueous humour and the vitreous humour. The cornea functions as a refracting and protective layer through which light rays pass en route to the brain.

The lens is a transparent, biconvex encapsulated structure suspended from the ciliary body posterior to the iris. The lens is an elastic structure and this allows its shape to change when the eye is focused. The function of the lens is to refract (bend) light rays and to focus them on the retina.

Aqueous humour is a clear watery fluid that fills the cavities around the lens. These cavities are called the anterior and posterior chambers. Aqueous humour is derived from the plasma in the capillaries of the ciliary body, and passes into the posterior chamber. It then passes forwards through the pupil to the anterior chamber, where it is absorbed into the ciliary veins. The rate of secretion and reabsorption is balanced so that intraocular pressure is regulated. Aqueous humour serves as a refractory medium and provides nutrients to the lens and cornea.

Vitreous humour is a clear jelly-like substance that fills the intraocular space from the posterior lens to the retina. Because it does not regenerate, any significant loss of vitreous humour; for example, as a result of injury to the eye, may distort other ocular structures. Vitreous humour helps maintain the shape of the eyeball, helps keep the retina in position, and helps with the refraction of light rays.

THE PHYSIOLOGY OF SIGHT

Light travels from its source to various objects, where it undergoes reflection. This reflected light can then travel towards the eye, where it passes through the cornea, aqueous humour, the lens and the vitreous humour, before forming an image on the retina. Nerve endings in the retina transmit electrical impulses along the optic nerve to the brain. A coordinated process of refraction, accommodation, regulation of pupil size and convergence makes normal binocular vision possible.

Refraction

Refraction, or bending of light rays, occurs as the light waves pass through the cornea, aqueous humour, the lens and the vitreous humour. At the lens the light is bent so that it converges at a single point on the retina.

Accommodation

Accommodation is the process whereby the curvature of the lens is altered so that the eye is able to focus light from objects at different distances. As an object moves closer to the eye the curvature of the lens increases so that the image remains in focus on the retina.

Regulation of pupil size

The diameter of the pupil influences image formation, and the muscles of the iris respond to changes in light intensity. An increase in light intensity initiates constriction of the pupil, whereas a decrease in light intensity causes dilation of the pupil. Adjustment of pupil size therefore regulates the amount of light entering the eyes. Too much light may damage the retina, and too little light fails to stimulate it.

Convergence

Convergence is the medial movements of the two eyeballs so that they are both directed towards the object being viewed. Convergence allows light rays to fall and stimulate two identical spots on the retinas, resulting in the perception of a single image.

After an image has been formed on the retina by the processes of refraction, accommodation, regulation of pupil size and convergence, light impulses are converted into nerve impulses by the rods and cones. The light breaks down the photosensitive chemicals in either rods or cones, which stimulates electrical impulses to the brain for interpretation.

Nerve impulses travel from the retina along the optic nerve. The optic nerve emerges from the back of the eyeball and passes to the optic chiasma, an area at the base of the brain. At the optic chiasma the left and the right optic nerves come together, and one half of the fibres then cross to the opposite sides of the brain. The fibres then form the left and right optic tracts, which continue to the visual area of the brain in the occipital lobes. Here, further processing occurs so that the image is given meaning.

DISORDERS OF THE EYE

FACTORS AFFECTING SENSORY FUNCTION

Normal function of the eye can be altered by a variety of pathophysiological factors, including those that are congenital, degenerative, infectious, neoplastic or traumatic. The effects may be mild and temporary, severe or permanent. Disorders of vision include alterations in visual acuity, ocular movement, accommodation, refraction and colour vision.

Congenital factors

Eye function may be altered by a variety of conditions that are genetically determined, most of which lead to progressive visual impairment, pain or blindness. Congenital factors may cause refractive errors, motor anomalies, clouding of the lens or cornea, or optic atrophy. Other abnormalities, although not genetically determined, may be contracted by the fetus in utero or soon after birth.

Degenerative factors

Degeneration of the eyes is a normal part of the ageing process, or degenerative alteration may occur secondary to disease such as diabetic retinopathy. Degenerative alterations include loss of lens transparency, arteriosclerosis of vessels supplying structures of the eye, and the development of plaques on the cornea. All can affect vision with varying degrees of severity.

Infectious factors

The external eye structures may be infected by bacterial, viral or fungal microorganisms, while infection of the eyelid causes a stye. A corneal ulcer may result from bacterial, viral or fungal infections.

Neoplastic factors

Benign or malignant tumours may occur in the eye, eyelid or orbit. Tumours may destroy important structures and/or interfere with normal function. Neoplasms may obstruct vision, displace the lens, cause retinal detachment, obstruct the drainage of aqueous humour or displace the eye.

Traumatic factors

Trauma to the eye may have short- or long-term effects, depending on the extent and type of injury incurred. Contusions, abrasions, burns and perforations may all lead to pain, scarring, infection and impaired vision or blindness.

MAJOR MANIFESTATIONS OF EYE DISORDERS

The major manifestations of disorders that affect the eye are changes in vision, pain or discomfort, excessive production of tears or dryness, and discharge.

Changes in vision

Visual acuity refers to the ability to see things clearly. The most common problem of the eyes is a decrease in visual acuity. Myopia, also known as nearsightedness, means the client can see objects that are close but those at a distance are blurred. A client with hyperopia, or far-sightedness, can see objects at a distance clearly but those close are blurred. Presbyobia is a form of hyperopia that begins in middle age. The lens becomes firm and loses its elasticity; as a result, the ageing lens loses its ability to properly focus light rays and near objects appear blurred. This condition can be treated with the use of reading glasses or bifocals. People may also state that they are experiencing 'halos', which are coloured rings encircling bright lights, caused by alteration in the ocular media. Small moving spots or flecks seen before the eyes are commonly called floaters, and may be due to the ageing process as the vitreous material degenerates. Floaters may also be caused by retinal laceration, diabetic neuropathy or hypertension. Visual changes also include double vision, or diplopia. Photophobia may be caused by inflammation of the cornea or the iris and ciliary bodies.

Pain

Pain or discomfort may range from mild aching, to irritation, to severe pain or sensations of pressure. Pain may be worse at certain times of the day, or it may be aggravated by bright light. Keeping the eyelids closed by applying an eye pad, may relieve pain associated with infections, foreign bodies or corneal injuries. Burning or itching is frequently caused by inflammation of the eyelids or conjunctiva from infection or irritation.

Lacrimation

Excessive production of tears may be caused by irritation of the conjunctiva or cornea, or of the iris by photophobia. Excessive tears can also result from obstruction of the lacrimal drainage system. Dryness of the eyes may be caused by a variety of conditions, such as hypofunction of the lacrimal glands, or it may be part of the ageing process.

Discharge

A mucopurulent drainage from the eyes usually indicates a bacterial infection such as conjunctivitis. The drainage may be accompanied by inflammation and crusting of the eye margins.

SPECIFIC DISORDERS OF THE EYE

Congenital disorders

Strabismus

Strabismus is a condition of eye deviation in which the eyes fail to look in the same direction at the same time. The eyes may have an uncoordinated appearance and the person may experience diplopia. Congenital strabismus is an anomaly in which there is a defect in the position and fusion ability of the two eyes. The condition is usually easily observed and, in addition to crossed eyes, the client may squint, tilt the head, or close one eye to improve vision.

Ptosis

Ptosis, drooping of the upper eyelid, may be unilateral or bilateral. Congenital ptosis results from the failure of the levator muscle in the upper eyelid to develop. Manifestations are usually very obvious; the lid appears smooth and flat, and the client may tilt the head back to compensate if the lid droops over the pupil.

Degenerative disorders

Cataract

A cataract is a clouding of the lens of the eye. Cataracts generally develop bilaterally, with each progressing independently, with the exception of congenital and traumatic cataracts. Causes include the ageing process, inflammation, malignancy, metabolic factors, toxins, heredity and trauma. Manifestations generally begin with a decrease in visual acuity. The client complains of not being able to see clearly. They may also complain of blurred vision, glare and a decrease in colour perception. As the cataract progresses, the pupil appears milky white. Surgical removal of the cataract from the lens is indicated when activities of daily living are affected. Figure 42.5 outlines a sample critical pathway for a client having a cataract extraction.

CRITICAL PATHWAY
for cataract extraction with placement of intraocular lens
Expected length of stay Overnight

	Day 1 (Preoperative)	Day 1 (Postoperative)	Day 2	Day 3
Pre-admission	Client verbalises understanding of procedure and expected outcomes Obtain informed consent			
Discharge planning	Client understands importance of going home to a supportive environment. Client to arrange own transport home Client and family informed of approximate discharge time		Notify family of discharge time Transport arranged Follow-up appointment arranged	
Psychosocial	Client given opportunity to express concerns	Family given opportunity to ask questions	Client looking forward to going home	
Investigations	FBE/U&E CXR ECG BSL if diabetic Urinalysis			
Observations	Baseline vital signs recorded Baseline weight recorded	Vital signs Discharge from eye	All observations within normal limits	
Assessments/ treatments	Contact lenses/prosthesis identified. Removed or in situ	Dressing dry and intact	Eye toilets attended Minimal eye discomfort	
Diet/hydration/ elimination	Client able to verbalise fasting requirements Adequate hydration before fasting	Fluids tolerated Nil nausea/vomiting Normal diet		
Safety/mobility	Assess safety needs and implement appropriate precautions	RIB/client mobilising safely	Independent and safe	
Hygiene	Client showered	Self-care	Self-care	
Medications	Normal medication Preoperative eye drops as ordered	As ordered	Eye drops as ordered	
Client needs	As required	As required	As required	
Referrals			Surgeon review Others	
Education	Client understands expected postoperative outcomes as discussed	Explain reason for eye shield Client understands expected postoperative outcomes	Client demonstrates understanding of discharge instructions	

Figure 42.5 | Critical pathway for cataract extraction with placement of intraocular lens

Macular degeneration

This is degeneration of the macular area of the retina. The most common cause of the degeneration is ageing. This disease is the leading cause of visual impairment in clients aged 50 and over. Manifestations include loss of central vision, and activities that require fine detailed vision becoming impossible. The disease usually develops slowly and painlessly, and both eyes are generally affected. Vision may be improved in some cases by laser surgery. Generally blindness does not occur.

Infectious disorders

Stye

A hordeolum (stye) is a localised staphylococcal infection of a sebaceous gland of the eyelid. This gland is the base of a hair follicle or eyelash. Manifestations include localised inflammation, swelling and pain.

Blepharitis

Blepharitis is inflammation of the eyelid margins. It may be caused by bacterial infection or an allergic reaction to smoke, dust or chemical. Seborrhoea, a disorder of the sebaceous gland, may also cause blepharitis. Manifestations include itching, burning, redness of the eyelid margins, chronic conjunctivitis and yellow purulent discharge crusts on the lashes.

Conjunctivitis

This is the inflammation of the conjunctiva and may be caused by excessive exposure to wind, sun, heat, cold, allergens or chemicals, or by bacterial, viral or fungal infection. Manifestations include itching, burning, excessive tearing and pain. Allergic conjunctivitis may cause considerable swelling.

Trachoma

Trachoma is a chronic form of kerato-conjunctivitis that causes permanent damage to the cornea and, if untreated, can result in blindness. The condition results from infection by *Chlamydia trachomatis* and is associated with poor personal and community hygiene and lack of available clean water. There is a high incidence of trachoma among Australian Aboriginal people. Manifestations, which may not become apparent for many years, are similar to those for severe conjunctivitis. There is corneal inflammation and scarring, due to the eyelids turning inwards, which causes the lashes to rub against the cornea. Severe corneal scarring may result in blindness.

Keratitis

Keratitis is inflammation of the cornea and is frequently caused by trauma or infection. It usually affects only one eye, and frequently presents as a secondary infection to an upper respiratory tract infection involving cold sores (herpes simplex infection). Manifestations include opacity of the cornea, irritation, excessive tearing, blurred vision, redness and photophobia.

Orbital cellulitis

This is an acute infection of the orbital tissues and eyelids that does not involve the eyeball. The condition is generally secondary to infection of nearby structures. If orbital cellulitis is not treated, the infection may spread to the sinuses or the meninges. Manifestations include unilateral eyelid oedema, inflammation of the orbital tissues and eyelids, pain, impaired eye movement and purulent discharge from indurated areas.

Neoplastic disorders

Benign or malignant tumours may arise in the tissues surrounding the eye, but neoplasms of the eyeball are rare.

Choroidal melanoma

A choroidal melanoma is a malignant tumour of the middle of the eyeball. The major symptom is visual distortion. There is generally no pain unless glaucoma develops.

Retinoblastoma

Retinoblastoma is a congenital hereditary neoplasm that develops from retinal germ cells. It is the most common malignancy of the eye in childhood. Manifestations include diminished vision, strabismus, retinal detachment and an abnormal pupillary reflex. The tumour grows rapidly and may invade the brain and metastasise to distant sites.

Traumatic disorders

Abrasions

Abrasions are superficial scratches on the eyelid, conjunctiva or cornea. Corneal abrasions may be caused by foreign bodies or over-wearing of contact lenses. Manifestations include excessive tearing, pain, a sensation of something in the eye and photophobia.

Lacerations

Lacerations may involve the eyelids or the eyeball. Lacerations of the eyeball may lead to intraocular infection, cataract formation or loss of vision. Manifestations of a lacerated eyeball include severe pain and shock.

Contusions

Contusions of the eyeball involve a bruising injury in which intraocular damage occurs. The injury may result in bleeding into the anterior chamber (hyphema) or into the vitreous of surrounding tissues. Contusions generally result from a severe blow to the eye, such as from a fist, golf or squash ball. Manifestations include impaired vision, pain, bruising of the tissues surrounding the eye, and blood in the anterior chamber.

Foreign bodies

These may enter the conjunctiva or cornea, or they may penetrate and perforate the eyeball. Examples of foreign bodies that gain entry include eyelashes, dirt, small particles of metal, dust and glass. Manifestations include irritation, pain, excessive tearing and photophobia.

Burns

Burns to the eye may result from exposure to chemicals, radiant energy or high temperatures. The extent of damage to the eye depends on the duration of exposure and the causative agent. Manifestations include extreme pain, excess tearing, photophobia, inflammation or destruction of tissue, and visual impairment.

Disorders of multiple causes

Glaucoma

Glaucoma is a condition in which the intraocular pressure is abnormally increased so that it causes atrophy of the optic nerve and loss of vision. Glaucoma occurs in various forms: primary open-angle, primary closed-angle, secondary, congenital and absolute. Generally speaking, glaucoma progresses slowly and may or may not be symptomatic. It rarely affects clients under age 40. The condition may be caused by over-production of aqueous humour or obstruction to the outflow of aqueous humour, both of which result in accumulation of fluid and a rise in intraocular pressure. Manifestations of primary open-angle glaucoma are gradual and progressive; the client is unable to perceive changes in colour and experiences blurred vision and persistent aching eyes. Manifestations of primary closed-angle glaucoma occur suddenly. The client experiences intense pain, loss of vision, nausea and vomiting. The affected eye appears red, and the pupil is fixed, dilated and unresponsive.

The manifestations of secondary glaucoma are similar to those of the primary form depending on the cause. Congenital glaucoma is a rare disorder generally associated with other anomalies, and manifests as a large-diameter cornea. Absolute glaucoma is the end result of any uncontrolled glaucoma resulting in blindness. Clinical Interest Box 42.5 provides information on glaucoma prevention and preservation of sight.

Nystagmus

Nystagmus refers to constant involuntary movement of the eyes. The client may not be aware of the movement. Movements are usually rhythmic and may be horizontal, vertical, circular or a mixture of these. One or both eyes may be affected. Nystagmus may result from brain tumours, alcohol abuse, disease and congenital defects. Diseases include Ménière's syndrome and multiple sclerosis. Treatment involves treating the underlying cause. Congenital nystagmus is often permanent.

Retinal detachment

In this condition the sensory portion of the retina separates from the pigment epithelium of the choroid. The condition is usually unilateral and may be spontaneous or follow trauma. Predisposing factors include myopia, absence of the lens, and retinal detachment. Manifestations include the appearance of a shadow, or 'curtain', spreading across the field of vision, floaters, blurred vision and gradual painless loss of vision.

CLINICAL INTEREST BOX 42.5
Glaucoma prevention and preservation of sight

Routine eye screenings are recommended for early detection of glaucoma. Although it cannot at this time be predicted, prevented or cured, in most cases glaucoma can be controlled and vision preserved by early diagnosis. The client needs to be aware that certain prescription and over-the-counter medications can cause increased intraocular pressure and should not be taken without consulting their doctor. The client who has experienced an episode of acute angle-closure glaucoma is taught about the risks, warning signs and management of future attacks. Clients need to understand the importance of lifetime therapy and periodic eye examinations with intraocular measurement in controlling the disease and preventing blindness. The nurse should assess the client's compliance with routine health screening.

Refractive errors

These are a group of visual problems that include myopia (nearsightedness), hyperopia (far-sightedness), presbyopia (lack of focusing power) and astigmatism (asymmetric focus). Refractive errors may be genetically determined or caused by disease or injury. Manifestations include headaches, reduced visual acuity and ocular discomfort.

HEALTH PROMOTION

The nurse is in a key position to educate clients and their families about the ways by which eyesight can be protected and preserved for children. For adults, screening of visual function is imperative to detect problems early. Regular eye examinations are important, especially for clients with a family history of eye disorders and for clients who are more vulnerable to ocular complications such as diabetes mellitus. Recommended screening guidelines are structured on the basis of age. People under 40 years of age should have periodic eye checks as needed. Those aged 40–64 should have a complete eye examination every 2 years, and those aged 65 years and over should have a complete eye examination every year. Examination of the eyes is also recommended if a client experiences any disturbances of vision, pain, sudden appearance of floaters, photophobia, purulent discharge, trauma to the eye, or pupil irregularities. Prevention of eye infection includes washing the hands before touching the eyes, and not sharing eye make-up, eye drops or ointment.

Education is particularly important for clients involved in high-risk occupations and activities. Client education should focus on strategies for prevention and first aid measures. Teach clients what immediate care to give to prevent permanent loss of sight, such as immediately flush the eye with copious amounts of water if a chemical splash occurs. Prevention of injury includes wearing eye protection when working with chemicals or when the eyes may be exposed to dust, wood, metal or glass fragments. Protective eye wear should also be worn during recreational or sporting activities in which sticks or balls may contact the eye, such as squash. Excessive exposure to strong sunlight or sunlamps should be avoided, as these may damage the eyes. A common form of cataract, which can result from frequent exposure to intense sunlight, can largely be prevented if sun hats and good quality sunglasses are worn.

Prevention of eye fatigue includes using adequate illumination when reading or writing, resting the eyes often during prolonged use, and reducing screen glare when using a visual display unit. The nurse needs to inform the client and family of the importance of follow-up treatment and stress the importance of complying with prescribed activity restriction to prevent further eye damage. Clinical Interest Box 42.6 provides information on preventive screening for children.

CLINICAL INTEREST BOX 42.6
Childhood preventive screening

The most common visual problem during childhood is refractive error, such as nearsightedness. In early childhood, parents may be alerted to a visual problem by reduced eye contact from their infant or the infant's failure to react to light. Recommended screening guidelines are usually structured on the basis of age, and preventive screening occurs in pre-school-age children (ages 4–5 years), where the nurse's role is one of detection and referral.

At school entry (age around 5 years):

- examine eyes and observe for fixation, following, nystagmus, strabismus
- test visual acuity
- test hearing, perform otoscopy on children failing audiometry to determine appropriate action
- address parental concerns regarding vision & hearing.

(Department of Human Services 2008)

DIAGNOSTIC TESTS

Tests used to diagnose eye disorders may be classified as subjective, objective or special procedures. Subjective tests require oral responses from the client that must be interpreted by the examiner. Objective tests are those in which the examiner obtains precise measurements or directly visualises the interior of the eyes.

Subjective eye tests

Visual acuity test. A visual acuity test evaluates the client's ability to distinguish the form and detail of an object. Visual acuity is measured by the use of a Snellen chart. The client is required to read letters on this chart from a distance of 6 metres. Generally, the smaller the symbol the client can identify, the sharper their visual acuity.

Colour vision tests. These evaluate the client's ability to recognise differences in colour. The most common colour vision tests use plates made up of patterns of dots of the primary colours, superimposed on backgrounds of randomly mixed colours. A client with normal colour vision can identify the patterns.

Accommodation tests. Accommodation tests evaluate the ability of the eyes to adjust to the curvature of the lenses. The examiner may perform this test by questioning the client concerning their visual acuity, while placing trial lenses before their eyes. Alternatively the test can be performed using an ophthalmoscope.

Visual field tests. These tests evaluate the functions of the retina, optic nerve and optic pathways. The client's peripheral and central visual fields are assessed when the examiner moves an object from outside the field into the field, on a radial line, until the client states that they can see the object. Tangent screen examination detects visual field loss. In this examination, a screen is used and test objects from 1–50 mm in size are placed on the screen. Each eye is individually tested for visualisation of the objects.

Objective eye tests

Intraocular pressure. Intraocular pressure is assessed using a tonometer. A topical anaesthetic is instilled and the examiner places the tonometer on the apex of the cornea to determine pressure in the eye. An alternative method involves the use of an 'air-puff' tonometer that does not contact the eye. Tonometry serves as a valuable screening test for early detection of glaucoma.

Ophthalmoscopic examination. This involves the use of an ophthalmoscope to view the interior structures of the eye. The ophthalmoscope examines the fundus, or interior aspect, of the eye, allowing magnified examination of the optic disc, retinal vessels, macula and retina.

Slit-lamp examination. A slit lamp allows the examiner to visualise in detail the anterior segment of the eye. Before the examination, dilating eye drops (mydriatics) may be instilled. The client sits with their chin on a rest and their forehead against a bar attached to a lamp. Slit-lamp examination helps determine corneal abrasions, keratitis and cataracts.

Fluorescein staining. Fluorescein staining is a technique in which staining the eye's surface with dye provides a better view of the anterior portion of the eye. The test is generally performed when the conjunctival or corneal abrasions are suspected. Surface defects absorb more dye than normal areas.

Special procedures for assessing the eye

Fluorescein angiography. This involves rapid-sequence photographs of the fundus after intravenous injection of a contrast medium. Fluorescein angiography records the appearance of blood vessels inside the eye.

Culture. A culture to determine the microorganism causing an ocular infection may be obtained by passing a sterile swab over the conjunctival surface.

Computerised tomography (CT). CT of the orbit may be used to detect abnormalities such as intraocular foreign bodies or retinoblastoma. Contrast dye is injected and the eyeball is scanned.

Ocular ultrasonography. This involves the transmission of high-frequency soundwaves through the eye, and measurement of their reflection from ocular structures.

Vetrasonography. Vetrasonography can identify abnormalities that are undetectable through ophthalmoscopy, and may be used to locate intraocular foreign bodies.

CARE OF THE CLIENT WITH AN EYE DISORDER

While the general care of the client with a disorder of the eye is directed towards helping them to meet their needs, the three main aspects of care are maintaining a safe environment, client education and providing local eye care.

Maintaining a safe environment

Any visual impairment or loss renders the client susceptible to injury; therefore the nurse has a responsibility to protect the client from environmental hazards. These hazards may include such things as low levels of lighting, poor colour contrast or badly positioned furniture. The nurse should describe the layout of the room to the client. If the client is ambulant the nurse should encourage them to locate the various pieces of furniture so that they become familiar with their position in the room. Leave furniture and personal belongings in the same position in the room. Ensure that any doors are either fully closed or open, as a visually impaired client can easily be injured if a door is left ajar.

Client education

Education involves assisting the client to adjust to a visual impairment. The nurse should initially describe to the client the alteration to visual function that has occurred. The client who is experiencing visual loss that is either temporary or permanent needs assistance to adjust to the physical and psychosocial implications. Care of the client includes encouraging independence in the activities of daily living, and encouraging the client to express reactions and feelings to their visual loss. The visually impaired client may lose the ability to observe body language and the reading and writing components of communication. It is important for the client to be able to interact with people whom they encounter. Communication methods may also be taught to family members and significant others.

Key aspects related to assisting the visually impaired client

- Encouraging as much self-care as possible. The client who is experiencing recent visual impairment may need assistance until they adjust to their condition. A client who has been visually impaired for some time will probably have developed considerable self-reliance. The nurse should always consult the client when uncertain whether assistance is required.
- Address your client by name and identify yourself, visitors or others in the room. This avoids frightening the client and assists them in knowing who is in the room. It is also important to knock before entering and to inform them when you are about to leave the room.
- Speak to the client in the same manner as you would a fully sighted person. The nurse must suppress the urge to speak more loudly than usual, which people often do when conversing with a visually impaired client. There is no need to exclude words such as 'look' and 'see' from normal conversation.
- Any visual aids that the client uses (Table 42.1) should be kept in close proximity. The client should have easy accessibility to the call bell if required.
- The client should be encouraged to maintain an interest in the outside environment through listening to the radio or television and discussing newspaper items.
- Provide full descriptions of people, places and things.
- Provide items that can compensate for diminished vision, such as bright non-glare lighting, large-print books, talking books, telephones with enlarged buttons and a clock with numbers and hands that can be felt.
- At mealtimes it may be necessary for the nurse to describe the position of foods on the plate (such as, peas are at 9 o'clock, potatoes at 12 o'clock, pumpkin at 3 o'clock and chicken at 6 o'clock).
- It is of particular importance to thoroughly explain any procedure or treatment before it is started. Whenever possible, if it will not affect sterility, the client should be allowed to feel any items used during a procedure.
- Provide contrasting colours; for example, non-white crockery and brightly coloured telephones, handles, borders or edges allow familiar objects to become more visible. Coloured tape, paint or nail polish can be used to colour-code appliance dials.
- Painting the edge of stairs with bright paint can help the client distinguish the edge of the step more clearly.
- Informing the client when they are approaching stairs or steps, remembering to let them know whether they are up or down.
- When walking with the client, the nurse should walk slightly ahead and let the client take their elbow. This technique enables the client to sense the direction they are walking towards. The nurse should encourage the use of handrails while ambulating and warn the client of any hazards as they are approached.
- Cultural aspects of care should always be taken into account when caring for a client who has impaired vision.
- On discharge, review specific hazards in the home with the client and family. Assessment must be made of both indoor and outdoor living arrangements. Clients' living quarters should not be altered after they have become familiar with placement of furniture.
- Discuss with the client and family that progress will be slow and that they may need to seek support from outside agencies. Encourage families to explore community resources available to clients with partial or total loss of vision, and the rehabilitation programs available to them.

Local eye care

Various nursing procedures involving the eye should be performed in accordance with the policies of the health care institution. General principles that should be followed in all ophthalmic procedures include:

- Explaining what you are going to do
- Ensure that the client is sitting or lying with their head well supported
- Ensure that there is adequate lighting; lights should never be allowed to shine directly into the client's eyes
- Wash hands thoroughly before and after the

TABLE 42.1 | AIDS FOR THE VISUALLY IMPAIRED

Aid	Description
Magnifiers	Hand-held or standing magnifiers can be used to enlarge print, or for fine detail
Enlarged print	Large-print books, magazines and newspapers may be borrowed from the local library
Talking books	Tapes of books may be available on loan from agencies for the blind or from public libraries
Telephone aids	Special dials are available for telephones in both large print and braille
Braille	The braille system of writing and printing uses tangible points or dots, which the individual feels and 'reads' with the fingertips
Optical-to-tactile converters	Consist of devices that convert vision into tactile sensation, by reproducing the outline of a letter on a tactile screen
Canes	A variety of canes is available (e.g. a white, or collapsible cane) which helps the individual to locate obstacles in the environment. Laser canes also locate objects and can identify changes in the region from as far away as 6 metres
Guide dogs	Trained dogs allow greater mobility and independence for the visually impaired person. The individual holds a U-shaped handle, which is attached to a harness on the dog. Communication between the two takes place through the movements of the harness. When a guide dog is working (i.e. when it is in harness) other people should not approach or pat the dog without the handler's permission, as the dog may become distracted

procedure and wear disposable gloves to prevent cross-infection
- Use gentle unhurried movements and refrain from exerting any pressure on the eye
- Avoid all sudden movements
- Avoid touching the cornea with the fingers or equipment, to prevent corneal damage
- Use aseptic technique. When only one eye is infected or inflamed, the unaffected eye must receive attention first to prevent cross-infection
- Ensure that, if an eye pad is to be applied, the eyelid is closed firmly to avoid corneal abrasion.

Application of eye pads

A light eye pad may be applied to prevent further injury after trauma to the eye or to avoid eye damage after administration of a local anaesthetic. Before the eye pad is applied the client is asked to close their eyelid firmly. The pad should be applied so that the eyelid cannot be opened. Pressure should not be applied, unless the medical officer has prescribed it. The eye pad is secured into position using hypoallergenic tape, placing the tape diagonally from forehead to cheek.

Cleansing the eyelids

It may be necessary to cleanse the eyelids before applying a compress, before removing or inserting an artificial eye, before instilling drops or ointment, or to remove discharge from the margins of the eyelids. A suggested technique for eyelid cleansing is outlined in Table 42.2. The equipment required includes:

- A sterile dressing pack
- Extra sterile cotton wool swabs
- Sterile solution (e.g. 0.9% sodium chloride or sterile water, warmed to body temperature)
- Receiver for soiled swabs
- Disposable gloves if infection is present
- Towel.

Eye irrigation

Irrigation is a technique performed to flush secretions, chemicals or foreign bodies from the conjunctival sac. Chemical injuries to the eye require flushing the conjunctival sac with copious amounts of solution. It may be necessary to cleanse the eyelids before irrigation; for example, if there is excessive discharge or crusting. A suggested technique for eye irrigation is outlined in Table 42.3. The equipment required includes:

- Sterile container or pre-packed eye wash supplied in a disposable container
- Receiver
- Sterile cotton wool swabs
- Sterile solution (e.g. 0.9% sodium chloride warmed to body temperature)
- Bag for soiled swabs
- Towel.

Instillation of drops and ointment

Eye drops or ointment that may be prescribed include those that combat infection, dilate or constrict the pupil, act as a local anaesthetic, stain the cornea, reduce inflammation or reduce intraocular pressure. Eye drops or ointment are instilled only when they have been prescribed by a medical officer, and the nurse who is instilling them must follow the nursing regulations and policies regarding the administration of medications. Key aspects regarding the use of ophthalmic medications include:

- Ensuring that a Registered Nurse (RN) checks the name, strength and amount of drops or ointment to be instilled. The nurse must also check the time and

TABLE 42.2 | TECHNIQUE FOR CLEANSING THE EYELIDS

Action	Rationale
Review and carry out the standard steps in Appendix 1	
Explain the procedure and ensure privacy	Reduces anxiety
Starting with the less affected eye, assist the client into a recumbent position, with the head tilted towards the side	Minimises the risk of accidental infection from the other eye. Facilitates performance of the procedure
Place the equipment in a convenient location and ensure adequate lighting	Facilitates performance
Wash and dry hands thoroughly	Prevents cross-infection
Place a towel under a kidney dish beside the client's cheek. Observe eyelid for abnormalities	Provides a receiver for excess lotion and used swabs
Using sterile technique, open sterile pack and add sterile solution and extra swabs	Reduces risk of infection
Perform procedural hand wash and don gloves	Reduces risk of cross-infection
Beginning with the less affected eye, ask the client to close the eye	Reduces the risk of solution entering the lacrimal duct or contaminating the other eye
Moisten swabs and cleanse eyelids, from inner canthus to outer canthus, using each swab once only. Use swabs to gently dry the eyelids	Prevents cross-infection
If necessary, cleanse the lid of the other eye, after repositioning the head	Both eyes may need treatment
Assist the client into a comfortable position	Promotes comfort
Remove and attend to the equipment appropriately	
Wash and dry hands	Prevents cross-infection
Report and document the procedure	Appropriate care can be planned and implemented

frequency of administration and into which eye the medication is to be instilled. The expiry date on the container must also be checked, and the medication is discarded if the expiry date has passed

- Ensuring that a separate container of drops or ointment is supplied for each individual. Single-dose packaging is preferred, as contamination of the medication is likely to occur if the container is used repeatedly
- Using the container correctly. To prevent cross-infection, eye drops are supplied in a squeeze bottle with a nozzle top through which the drops are delivered.

(The technique for instilling eye drops and ointments is outlined in Chapter 30.)

Eye prostheses

Two types of eye prosthesis are contact lenses and the artificial eye.

Contact lens

A contact lens is a small plastic disc that is positioned on the cornea and held in place by surface tension. A client who has a refractive error, for example astigmatism, may wear contact lenses in place of glasses. A variety of lenses is available including hard, soft, gas permeable, extended wear, daily wear and disposable. It is important to know that all lenses require care and must be removed periodically to prevent corneal damage and eye infection. Client education is required regarding proper lens care; for example, daily-wear lenses should be removed overnight for cleaning and disinfection. Only the recommended solutions should be used for cleaning, soaking and storing lenses. Wetting lenses with contact lens solution before insertion minimises any discomfort. The hands should be washed and dried before inserting or removing lenses. Table 42.4 describes the insertion and removal of contact lenses.

Artificial eyes

An artificial eye may be inserted after surgical removal of an eye. Clients with artificial eyes have had enucleation of an entire eyeball. An artificial eye may be removed, the socket cleaned and the eye replaced. Alternatively, the prosthesis may remain in the socket permanently. Most clients prefer to care for their own eyes but there may be times when assistance from the nurse is required. When a prosthesis is removed from the socket it is placed in warm normal saline for cleansing. Table 42.5 describes the insertion and removal of an artificial eye.

THE EARS

Hearing is a special sense that allows us to experience the world in which we live by providing a pathway for sounds to reach the brain. The ear is specially adapted as the organ

TABLE 42.3 | TECHNIQUE FOR EYE IRRIGATION

Action	Rationale
Review and carry out the standard steps in Appendix 1	
Explain the procedure and ensure privacy	Reduces anxiety
Assist the client into a recumbent position, with the head tilted towards the affected side	Prevents the solution running either over the cheek into the other eye or out of the affected eye and down the side of the nose
Place a towel under the head on the affected side and across the neck. Place a kidney dish against the client's cheek and ask the client to hold it in position	Prevents solution from flowing down the neck
Wash and dry hands thoroughly and put on gloves	Prevents cross-infection
Pour irrigating solution into the undine or open the container of eye wash. Gently hold the eyelid open with one hand	The client will instinctively try to close the eye
Hold the spout of the undine or the container 2.5 cm away from the eye	If the undine is held too high, fluid will flow at increased pressure, causing discomfort and possible damage to the eye
Pour a little solution over the cheek first	Accustoms the client to the feel of the solution
Direct the flow of solution from the nasal corner outwards	Because the head is tilted, the stream of irrigating solution will flow over the eyeball and prevent contaminating the other eye
Avoid directing the stream forcefully onto the eyeball, and avoid touching the eye's structures	Prevents discomfort and damage to the eye
Ask the client to look up and down and to either side while irrigating	Ensures that the whole area is washed
When the eye has been thoroughly irrigated, ask the client to close the eyes, and use a new swab to dry the lids	Promotes comfort
Make the client comfortable	Promotes comfort
Remove and attend to the equipment appropriately. Remove gloves and wash and dry hands	Prevents cross-infection
Report and document the procedure	Appropriate care can be planned and implemented

TABLE 42.4 | INSERTING AND REMOVING A CONTACT LENS

Insertion	Removal
Review and carry out the standard steps in Appendix 1	
Wash and dry the hands	Wash and dry the hands
Place the lens on the tip of an index finger	With the individual looking up, the lens is slid down off the pupil with an index finger
The lids are held apart with the other hand	The lens is gently squeezed with the thumb and index finger and lifted off the eye
With the individual looking straight ahead, the lens is placed over the cornea	Alternatively, the lens is removed using a small rubber suction extractor
Releasing both eyelids, the individual blinks to centre the lens over the pupil	

of hearing but it is also concerned with sense of position, balance and equilibrium. Hearing is a complex mechanism in which the ears receive soundwaves and convert them into nerve impulses. The nerve impulses are transmitted by the acoustic nerve to the brain where they are interpreted. The externally visible portion of each ear is located on the lateral surface of the head on each side. The remaining parts of each ear are embedded in the bone of the skull.

STRUCTURE OF THE EAR

Each ear (Figure 42.6) can be divided into three areas: the external, middle and inner ear.

The external ear

The external ear consists of the auricle (pinna) and the external auditory canal. The auricle consists of a piece of elastic cartilage with a number of associated ligaments

TABLE 42.5 | INSERTING AND REMOVING AN ARTIFICIAL EYE	
Insertion	**Removal**
Review and carry out the standard steps in Appendix 1	
The hands are washed and dried	The hands are washed and dried
The socket is cleansed with warm sodium chloride 0.9% solution	The individual assumes a comfortable sitting or lying position
The prosthesis is moistened	With the individual looking up, the lower lid is gently drawn down. The lower lid is depressed with an index finger to raise the edge of the prosthesis
With the individual looking up, the prosthesis is inserted under the upper lid	With the individual looking down, the prosthesis is expelled from beneath the upper lid
The lower lid is pulled down until the prosthesis slips in behind the lid to rest in the lower fornix	The prosthesis is grasped between the thumb and index finger, and lifted out
The individual blinks gently, and a check is made to ensure correct position of the prosthesis	

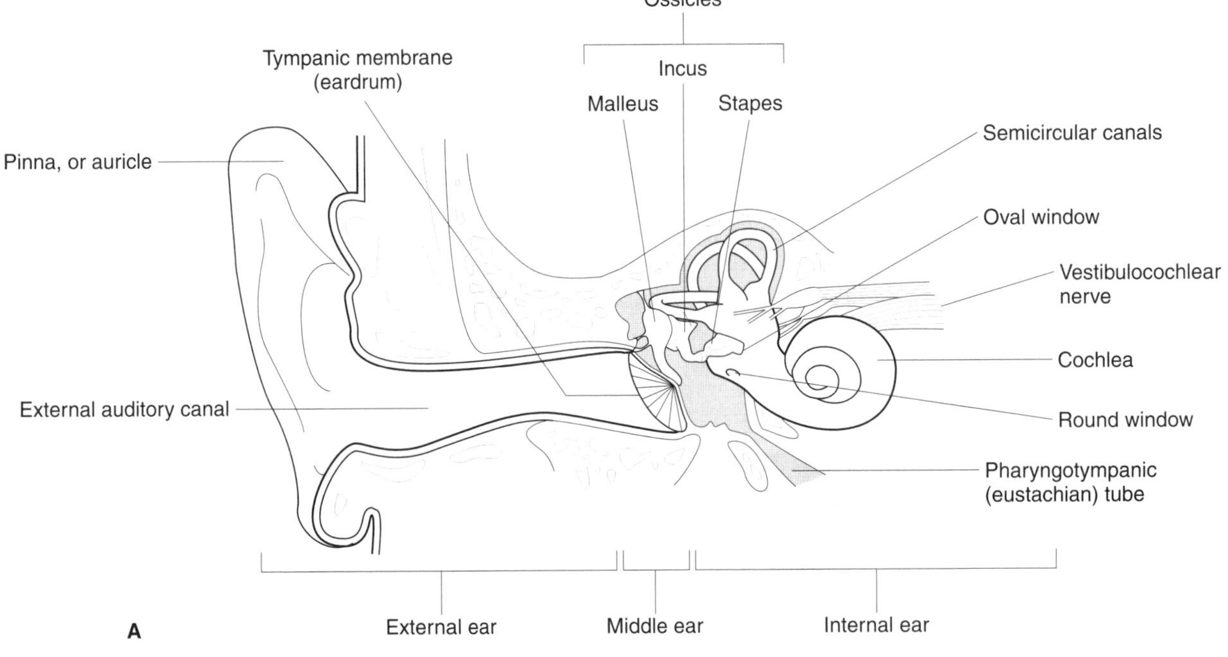

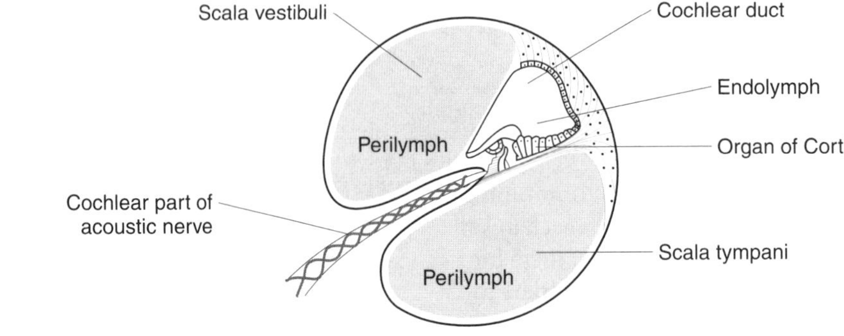

Figure 42.6 | The ear **A**: The parts of the ear **B**: A section of membranous cochlea showing the organ of Corti

and muscles, and has a small amount of adipose tissue in the earlobe. The skin of the auricle is covered with fine hairs and is continuous with the skin lining the external auditory canal. The external auditory canal is an S-shaped canal about 2.5 cm long. It extends from the auricle to the tympanic membrane (eardrum). The skin lining the canal contains glands that produce cerumen (wax) that protects the lining from damage and keeps dust particles away from the eardrum. The tympanic membrane lies between the external ear and the middle ear. It is a semi-transparent sheet consisting of three layers. The outermost layer consists of hairless skin, the middle layer is connective tissue and the innermost layer is continuous with the mucous membrane lining of the ear.

The middle ear

The middle ear, or tympanic cavity, is a small chamber within the temporal bone. Three small bones, or ossicles, lying in the middle ear transmit sound from the tympanic membrane to the oval window. Because of their shapes, the bones are named the malleus (mallet), the incus (the anvil) and the stapes (the stirrup). The malleus is attached to the tympanic membrane; the stapes is attached to the oval window; and the incus articulates with the other two ossicles. The three ossicles are attached to the wall of the middle ear by ligaments. The auditory tube (or eustachian tube) connects the middle ear with air from the nasopharynx. It is about 3–6 cm long and is lined with mucous membrane. Normally the tube is flattened and closed at the pharyngeal orifice, but swallowing or yawning opens it briefly.

The inner ear

The inner ear consists of a bony cavity within the temporal bone known as the osseous labyrinth. It is lined with periosteum and filled with a fluid called perilymph. The three divisions of the osseous labyrinth are the cochlea, the vestibule and the semicircular canals. The cochlea is a spiralling bony cavity, which resembles the shell of a snail. It houses the organ of Corti, the receptor organ for hearing. The vestibule lies between the cochlea and the semicircular canals. It contains structures responsible for maintaining equilibrium during movement of the head. The semicircular canals consist of three canals (in each ear), arranged at right angles to each other. They are filled with endolymph (the fluid inside the membranous labyrinth of the ear) and contain specialised nerve endings that are stimulated by the movement of the endolymph. The semicircular canals assist the body to adjust to changes in direction. The movement of fluid in this area can cause the client to experience a feeling of dizziness.

The membranous labyrinth is a membrane consisting of three layers, and lies within the osseous labyrinth. In the areas where it is not attached to the osseous labyrinth it is surrounded by perilymph. The fluid contained within the membranous labyrinth is known as endolymph. Part of the membranous labyrinth is concerned with hearing, and part is concerned with the position of the head in space. The ear is responsible for hearing and maintenance of equilibrium.

THE PHYSIOLOGY OF HEARING

Hearing is a sense that enables sound to be perceived. Soundwaves are collected and directed by the auricle into the external auditory canal, where they pass through and cause the tympanic membrane to vibrate. They then pass through the middle ear by vibration of the ossicles, and into the internal ear. From the internal ear, soundwaves are transmitted to the brain, via the acoustic nerve, for interpretation. Perception of sound involves interpretation of pitch and intensity. The entire process of hearing involves the following steps:

- Movement of air molecules causes a soundwave to form
- The soundwave travels through the air to the auricle, which directs it into the external auditory canal
- The soundwave enters the auditory canal and comes in contact with the tympanic membrane, causing it to vibrate
- The vibrations are transferred to the ossicles, which begin to vibrate, and the soundwave is transmitted across the middle-ear cavity to the oval window and into the fluid-filled internal ear
- The soundwaves set the cochlear fluids into motion. The receptor cells are stimulated, and the soundwaves are transmitted along the acoustic nerve to the temporal lobe of the brain for interpretation.

Two qualities of sound, pitch and intensity, are important in the interpretation of sound. Pitch is related to the frequency of the soundwave. A high-frequency sound stimulates the neurons supplying the cells near the base of the cochlea. Low-frequency sounds stimulate neurons nearer to the apex of the cochlea. Intensity is related to the loudness of sound and is measured in decibels (dB). A loud sound causes the nerve endings to be stimulated at a greater rate than does a softer sound. The intensity of normal conversational speech is about 60 dB, and a decibel level of 160 can cause bursting of the tympanic membrane.

MAINTENANCE OF EQUILIBRIUM (BALANCE)

Two structures within the internal ear — the semicircular canals and the vestibule — work together to help the individual maintain balance or equilibrium. Components of the semicircular canals alert the brain to rotational movement, and components of the vestibule alert the brain to gravitational movement. Movement of fluid in the canals gives a constant flow of information about body position and the speed and direction of any body movement. This information is used to coordinate movements and to maintain balance.

DISORDERS OF THE EAR

FACTORS AFFECTING SENSORY FUNCTION

Normal function of the ear can be altered by a variety of pathophysiological factors, including those that are congenital, degenerative, infectious, obstructive, neoplastic or traumatic.

Congenital factors

Congenital alterations, which may be either hereditary or acquired, include structural malformations that can lead to hearing loss or deafness, disorders resulting from maternal infection during pregnancy or trauma incurred during pregnancy or delivery or before maturity.

Degenerative factors

Degenerative changes in the bones and joints of the ossicles can result in conductive hearing loss, while narrowing of blood vessels to the inner ear can result in tinnitus, vertigo or hearing loss. Gradual sensorineural hearing loss can result from a decrease in the number of hair cells and nerve fibres in the auditory system as a consequence of the ageing process.

Infectious factors

Microorganisms can cause external, middle- or inner-ear infections, all of which result in pain and varying degrees of conductive hearing loss.

Obstructive factors

Obstruction of the auditory system, which may result in conductive or sensorineural hearing loss, includes impacted cerumen, foreign bodies, oedema and neoplasms. An obstruction can impede the passage of soundwaves, cause an imbalance of pressure on either side of the tympanic membrane or it may disrupt the transmission of sound to the inner ear.

Neoplastic factors

Neoplasms, which may be benign or malignant, can affect the external, middle or inner ear. The effects of a neoplasm include pain, discharge, vertigo, tinnitus and hearing loss.

Traumatic factors

Trauma to the external ear includes bruising, lacerations and frostbite. Trauma to the head can result in fractures of the temporal bone, dislocation of the ossicles, rupture of the tympanic membrane and damage to the auditory nerve. Trauma can lead to vertigo, tinnitus, nystagmus, pain, bleeding and hearing loss. Hearing loss can also result from sudden exposure to a loud explosive sound or from continued exposure to loud noise.

MAJOR MANIFESTATIONS OF EAR DISORDERS

The major manifestations of ear disorders are pain, discharge, tinnitus, vertigo, nystagmus and hearing loss.

Pain

Earache (otalgia) is a common manifestation of many ear disorders. Middle-ear pain associated with otitis media is often described as deep seated and throbbing. If the external ear is infected or inflamed, the client may experience pain and tenderness. Earache may also be referred from other parts of the body via various cervical or cranial nerves, as occurs with tonsillitis.

Discharge

Discharge from the ear (otorrhoea) is generally associated with infections of the middle ear. Purulent or haemopurulent discharge may drain from the middle ear through a perforated tympanic membrane. Otitis externa may be accompanied by profuse discharge and irritation of the pinna.

Tinnitus

Tinnitus, which may be constant or intermittent, describes a noise in the inner ear. Noises such as ringing, buzzing, hissing or roaring are due to irritation of hair cells in the organ of Corti. Causes include pressure from cerumen on the tympanic membrane, pharyngotympanic tube obstruction, otitis media, otosclerosis, Ménière's syndrome and tumours.

Vertigo

Vertigo is a sensation of spinning. The person may feel as if their head is spinning or as if the room is spinning around them. Causes of vertigo include trauma, tumours, inflammation, degeneration of the maculae in the inner ear, Ménière's syndrome and pharyngotympanic tube obstruction.

Nystagmus

Nystagmus is involuntary rhythmic movements of the eyes. The movements may be horizontal, vertical, rotary or mixed. Jerking nystagmus, characterised by faster movements in one direction than in the opposite direction, may be a manifestation of certain disorders of the inner ear, although it can be caused by other factors such as neurological disorders. Nystagmus may also be induced by introducing cold or warm water into the external auditory canal.

Hearing loss

Impaired hearing or deafness may be conductive, sensorineural or a combination of both these types.

Conductive hearing loss. This results from disturbances of the sound transmission mechanism of the external or middle ear, which prevents soundwaves from reaching the inner ear. Conductive hearing loss or deafness can result from impacted cerumen, foreign body in the ear canal, middle-ear infection, ruptured tympanic membrane, otosclerosis, pharyngotympanic tube obstruction, neoplasms or barotrauma (injury due to pressure).

Sensorineural hearing loss. Sensorineural (perceptive or nerve) hearing loss results from disturbances of the inner-ear neural structures, or nerve pathways leading to the brainstem. Sensorineural hearing loss or deafness can result from hereditary or de novo genetic factors, acoustic trauma, infection, neoplasms such as acoustic neuroma, advanced otosclerosis, haemorrhage or thrombosis of the cochlear vessels, and Ménière's syndrome.

Mixed hearing loss. Mixed hearing loss combines aspects of both conductive and sensorineural hearing loss.

SPECIFIC DISORDERS OF THE EAR

Disorders of the ear and auditory system may be classified as congenital, degenerative, infectious, neoplastic, traumatic or resulting from multiple causes.

Congenital disorders

Congenital disorders may be caused by a genetic defect or may result from prenatal trauma or toxicity. Some of the disorders affect the cosmetic appearance only, while others result in varying degrees of hearing loss. Congenital disorders include partial or total absence of the external ear (atresia), protruding ears, fused or absent ossicles, and malformation of the cochlea.

Degenerative disorders

Presbycusis is a slowly progressive bilateral hearing loss resulting from physiological changes of ageing. It results from a loss of hair cells in the organ of Corti and causes sensorineural hearing loss, usually of high-frequency tones. Manifestations include gradual progressive hearing loss, which may be accompanied by tinnitus and dizziness, depression or irritability.

Infectious disorders

Otitis externa. Otitis externa, which may be acute or chronic, is inflammation of the external ear canal and auricle. The most common causative organism is *Streptococcus pyogenes*, although *Proteus vulgaris*, *Staphylococcus aureus*, *Candida albicans* and *Aspergillus niger* may be responsible for infection. Predisposing factors include swimming in contaminated water, abrasion of the ear canal from inserting sharp or small objects to clean the ear, exposure to irritants, and constant use of earphones or ear plugs. Manifestations include otalgia which is exacerbated on chewing or opening the mouth, lymphadenopathy, pyrexia, regional cellulitis, offensive smelling discharge, pruritus and partial hearing loss.

Otitis media. Otitis media, which may be acute or chronic, is inflammation of the middle ear. Causative organisms include *Haemophilus influenzae*, pneumococci, and beta-haemolytic streptococci. Predisposing factors include the wider, shorter and more horizontal pharyngotympanic tube in infants and children; anatomical abnormalities such as cleft palate; and respiratory tract infection. Manifestations include severe otalgia, pyrexia, hearing loss, dizziness, nausea and vomiting. If the tympanic membrane ruptures, there is often purulent discharge from the ear canal.

Mastoiditis. Mastoiditis, which may follow otitis media, is infection and inflammation of the air cells of the mastoid antrum. Predisposing factors include chronic otitis media and untreated acute otitis media. Manifestations include aching and tenderness in the area of the mastoid process, swelling behind the ear, pyrexia and purulent discharge from the ear canal.

Neoplastic disorders

Acoustic neuroma. An acoustic neuroma is a benign tumour arising from the eighth cranial nerve and occurring within the internal auditory canal. As the tumour grows the cochlear branch of the eighth cranial nerve becomes involved. Manifestations include tinnitus followed by an increasing high-frequency hearing loss. As the tumour increases in size, symptoms of other cranial nerve involvement occur, such as trigeminal pain and loss of taste in part of the tongue. Nystagmus and ataxia may occur.

Traumatic disorders

Abrasion. Because of its vulnerable position, the external ear may sustain abrasion of the canal, burns, or contusions of the pinna. Foreign bodies may be inserted into the canal and become lodged, or insects may fly into the ear, causing irritation.

Perforated eardrum. A perforated tympanic membrane may be caused by a variety of factors, such as the introduction of a sharp object to clean the canal, unskilled irrigation of the auditory canal, middle-ear infection, trauma to the head or sudden exposure to loud noise. Most traumatic perforations heal spontaneously, but a perforated tympanic membrane results in scarring and renders the client susceptible to chronic ear infections and hearing loss. Manifestations include sudden severe pain inside the ear, loss of hearing, tinnitus and bleeding.

Barotrauma. Barotrauma is injury caused by changes of air pressure to the wall of the pharyngotympanic tube and mucous membrane of the middle ear. It is caused by failure of the pharyngotympanic tube to open sufficiently, resulting in unequal pressure between the middle ear and the atmospheric pressure. It may occur during take-off or landing in planes, or during deep-sea diving. Manifestations include severe pain, decreased hearing, tinnitus and vertigo.

Noise-induced hearing loss. This condition develops gradually as a result of continued exposure to environmental or industrial noise. Acoustic trauma is sudden hearing loss from brief exposure to a high-intensity sound at close range, such as gunshots. Manifestations of noise trauma include hearing loss, tinnitus and a feeling of fullness within the ear.

Ototoxicity. Ototoxicity is a toxic reaction to medications or chemicals that can damage the auditory and/or vestibular system. Auditory damage may be permanent, whereas vestibular damage may be reversed after the drug therapy is discontinued. A variety of substances may result in ototoxic reactions, including diuretics, alcohol, lead, carbon monoxide, aspirin and antibiotics. Manifestations include bilateral hearing loss, tinnitus, vertigo and ataxia.

Disorders of multiple causes

Otosclerosis

Otosclerosis is a disorder in which the spongy temporal bone becomes a dense sclerotic mass, eventually immobilising the stapedial footplate and causing a conductive hearing loss. Although no definite cause has been identified, heredity is a significant factor. Females have a higher incidence of the disorder than males. Manifestations are slowly progressive and include bilateral conductive hearing loss and mild tinnitus.

Ménière's syndrome

Ménière's syndrome is a disorder of the inner ear that results from over-production or decreased absorption of endolymph. The resulting dilation of the membranous labyrinth can progress to herniation and rupture. Manifestations are exacerbations and remissions of three symptoms — vertigo, tinnitus and sensorineural hearing loss. During an acute episode the client may experience nausea and vomiting, sweating, giddiness, nystagmus and ataxia.

HEALTH PROMOTION

The nurse is in a key position to educate clients about the ways by which hearing can be protected and preserved:

- Regular hearing examinations are important for the early detection of hearing problems, especially for children, whose ability to learn can be impaired by hearing defects
- Regular screening is also important for the client over age 65 because the ageing process is commonly accompanied by degenerative ear changes. Recommended preventive screening should be carried out for all ages as needed
- Prevention of trauma to the ears includes client education, such as the importance of never putting small or sharp objects into ears
- Excessive cleaning of the ear canal is contraindicated, as it removes the cerumen, which has a protective function
- Protection of the ears from contamination by water when swimming or diving is particularly important if the client has experienced ear infections
- Infections that could involve the ear (e.g. upper respiratory tract infections) require adequate treatment
- Protecting the ears from damage by noise. Prolonged exposure to noise levels greater than 85–90 dB causes cochlear damage. People working in areas of high noise levels are required to wear protective devices such as earplugs or earmuffs. Exposure to loud volume from live music, stereo equipment and headphones should be avoided
- The nurse assesses the client's compliance with routine health screening.

DIAGNOSTIC TESTS

Tests used to assist in the diagnosis of ear disorders assess auditory or vestibular function.

Auditory tests

Otoscopic examination. Otoscopic examination is the direct visualisation of the external auditory canal and the tympanic membrane through an otoscope (auroscope). Otoscopy is performed to detect foreign bodies or cerumen in the external canal, or to detect external and middle-ear pathology. Tuning forks detect hearing loss and provide information as to the type of loss:

- The Weber test determines whether the individual lateralises the tone of the tuning fork to one ear
- The Rinne's test evaluates air and bone conduction in both ears
- The Schwabach test compares the individual's bone-conduction response with that of the examiner, who is assumed to have normal hearing.

Audiometry. Pure tone audiometry is the testing of each ear separately for air conduction via earphones, and for bone conduction via a vibrator placed on the mastoid bone. The faintest point at which the individual hears the tone is called the hearing threshold level. Comparison of air and bone thresholds can suggest a conductive, sensorineural or mixed-type hearing loss.

Speech audiometry tests the client's ability to understand and discriminate sounds. Two-syllable words are presented through earphones to measure how loud speech must be before it is heard.

Speech discrimination testing measures the client's ability to distinguish phonetic elements of speech and thus understand what is heard. The examiner presents one-syllable words through earphones.

Impedance audiometry evaluates middle-ear function by measuring the flow of sound energy into the ear, and the resistance to that flow. The objective is to determine the resistance (impedance) or flexibility (compliance) of the tympanic membrane.

Vestibular tests

Electronystagmography. Electronystagmography (ENG) evaluates vestibular function by measuring the effect of the semicircular canals on the ocular muscles. Electrodes are positioned at precise points on the face and eye, with movements in response to specific stimuli recorded on a graph.

Caloric tests. Caloric tests compare the nystagmus produced by warm and cold stimulation in each ear. Each ear is irrigated with water to stimulate mild vertigo and nystagmus. No response indicates that the labyrinth is non-functional.

Other tests used to diagnose ear disorders include cultures of secretions to detect the source of an infection, and radiological examination of the temporal bone.

CARE OF THE CLIENT WITH AN EAR DISORDER

While the general care of the client with a disorder of the ear is directed towards helping them to meet their needs, the three main aspects of care are maintaining a safe environment, client education and providing any prescribed local ear care.

Maintaining a safe environment

Any hearing impairment renders the client susceptible to accidents and injury. Any environment can heighten or reduce sensory stimulation. The nurse must assess the client's environment in the health care setting as well as assisting the client and the family to identify hazards in the home environment, and recommend appropriate adaptations. Clients with vestibular disorders are at risk of losing balance and falling. Clients with proprioceptive problems may lose balance easily. It is important to ensure that bathrooms have a non-skid surface in the shower and bath, grab bars are installed, and that the nurse provides family education regarding supervision of the client when ambulant, to minimise the risk of falls.

Client education

The client who is experiencing hearing loss that is either temporary or permanent needs assistance to adjust to the physical and psychosocial implications. Communication is a key component of assisting the client with impaired hearing. Initially the client may withdraw by avoiding communication or socialisation with others to cope with the hearing loss. This can lead to social isolation and low self-esteem. The nurse should encourage the client to discuss feelings of fear and frustration with their family members. Clinical Interest Box 42.7 provides an overview of hearing aid care and client education.

Key aspects related to assisting the hearing-impaired client

- Reduce background noise. Attract the client's attention before speaking.
- Stand directly in front of the client or, if in a group setting, arrange semicircular seating. This enables the client to see facial expressions, body gestures and to read lips. Vision becomes a primary sense for the client who is hearing impaired. The nurse should avoid covering the mouth while speaking.

CLINICAL INTEREST BOX 42.7
Hearing aid care

A hearing aid helps capture, amplify and funnel sound waves to the auditory nerve in a client with sensorineural hearing loss. Hearing aids are delicate and must be protected from heat, moisture and breakage. The manufacturer's guidelines for instructions specific to the client's hearing aid should be read by the client and/or family members. The aid is turned on to be certain it is working, then the ear mould is gently inserted into the ear canal. Once the mould has been inserted, the individual adjusts the volume. The tube, if fitted, is placed over the ear and attached to the battery device. Key aspects related to care of aids include:

- Ensuring that the ear mould and tubing are not blocked by wax or moisture. The hearing aid may be wiped with a soft tissue to remove any oils or waxes
- Keeping the aid dry and away from high temperatures (e.g. direct sunlight)
- Removing the aid before the client showers or washes their hair
- Switching off the aid when it is not in use
- Checking the battery and replacing it when necessary. Ensure that the battery is inserted correctly
- Checking that the hearing aid is switched on when in use and that the volume is adjusted
- Investigating the cause of any 'whistling', which can result in embarrassment and annoyance. Causes of whistling include a poorly fitting ear mould, ear mould incorrectly positioned, cracked or broken tubing, and the volume turned up too high
- Notifying the audiologist or hearing-aid specialist if the aid is malfunctioning.

Research has resulted in the development of an implantable device to improve hearing — the cochlear implant. A cochlear implant is an electronic device that is surgically implanted. The device picks up environmental sounds and converts them to electrical impulses, which are relayed to an implant receiver. Direct electrical stimulation to the nerve fibres of cranial nerve VIII sometimes enables profoundly deaf clients to hear some sounds.

- Communication can be improved by employing non-verbal cues to help convey the meaning of your conversation; for example, facial expressions, hand gestures, pointing and writing.
- Allow the client time to insert, or adjust, any hearing aid before you speak.
- Speak clearly and more slowly than usual but avoid exaggerated lip movements and shouting. Shouting distorts sound and is painful to the wearer of a hearing aid.
- Rephrase your words if the client has not understood. It may be helpful to write out the message if you remain uncertain whether the client has understood.
- Encourage the hearing-impaired client who has a speech disorder to communicate verbally. If you do not understand their communication, do not pretend

to have done so. The client should be encouraged to repeat the sentence or to use other words and gestures to get the message across.
- Use items that are available from organisations such as the Deafness Foundation (http://www.deafness.org.au/). Such organisations provide packaged kits to health care institutions, designed to assist hearing-impaired clients and staff. The kit generally includes adhesive stickers, discs, cards and information sheets.
- Other assistive devices may be required, such as sound lamps in which the light responds to sounds, telephones and alarm clocks with enhanced noise or flashing lights (Table 42.6).
- Cultural aspects of care should always be taken into account when caring for the client who has impaired hearing.
- On discharge the nurse should encourage the client and their family to explore community resources available to people with partial or total loss of hearing, and rehabilitation programs that provide assistance in performing the activities of daily living.

Local ear care

Various nursing procedures involving the ear should be performed in accordance with the policies of the health care institution. The general principles should include explaining the procedure to the client, ensuring the client is sitting or lying with their head well supported, and ensuring adequate lighting. The nurse should wash hands thoroughly before and after the procedure to prevent cross-infection. Warm solutions and ear drops to body temperature, as hot or cold temperatures stimulate the inner ear, causing vertigo and sometimes nausea and vomiting. Place cotton wool or packing in the ear canal only if they have been prescribed, as obstruction of the canal may cause a pressure increase against the tympanic membrane. Nursing diagnoses related to conditions of the eyes and ears are listed in Clinical Interest Box 42.8.

CLINICAL INTEREST BOX 42.8
Nursing diagnoses relating to conditions of the ears and eyes

- Adjustment, impaired
- Communication, impaired verbal
- Injury, risk for
- Mobility, impaired physical
- Self-care deficit, bathing/hygiene
- Self-care deficit, dressing, grooming
- Self-care deficit, toileting
- Self-esteem disturbance
- Sensory/perceptual alterations
- Social isolation
- Thought processes altered

(adapted from Potter & Perry 2008)

Ear irrigation

The ear may be irrigated (Figure 42.7) to cleanse the external canal or to remove a foreign body or wax. As irrigation has the potential for causing damage, it is performed only by health professionals skilled in the technique. Irrigation is never performed if the tympanic membrane is ruptured, as this could cause further damage and infection. If the irrigation is performed to remove wax it may be necessary to instil a cerumenolytic agent, such as Cerumol aural drops, for at least 30 minutes beforehand. These have the effect of softening and loosening the wax. A technique for ear irrigation is outlined in Table 42.7. The equipment required includes:
- Aural syringe
- Large kidney dish
- 500 mL of irrigating fluid warmed to body temperature
- Cotton wool swabs or gauze squares
- Towel
- Auroscope.

Instillation of ear drops

Ear drops that may be prescribed include those that combat infection and those that soften wax. Ear drops are instilled

TABLE 42.6 | AIDS AVAILABLE TO HEARING-IMPAIRED CLIENTS

Aid	Description
Hearing aid	Device that receives speech and environmental sounds through a microphone, and amplifies sound. Various styles including those worn in the ear canal, behind the ear, on the arm of spectacles, and in the form of a transmitter that is attached to the clothing (body aid). Some styles may be used with an induction coil for use with television, telephone and radio
Modified telephone	Telephone fitted with volume control and induction coil
Radio and television	Used in conjunction with headphones, induction coils, infra-red and FM transmitters
Telephone typewriter	Device fitted to a telephone whereby a caller's message is typed and translated into a written message, which is either displayed on a screen or printout
Captioning devices	Added to a television set, these devices display captions or subtitles at the bottom of the screen. Not all television programs are coded for this service
Hearing dog	Dog trained to respond to specific sounds (e.g. door bell, telephone, a baby's cry) and to alert the hearing-impaired person to the source of the sound

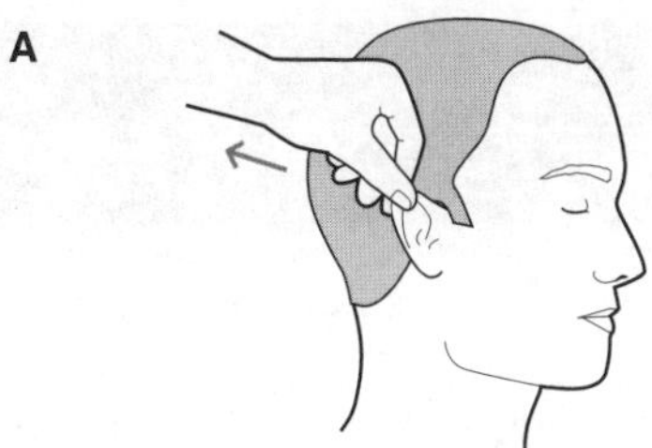

Adult: pull the ear up and back

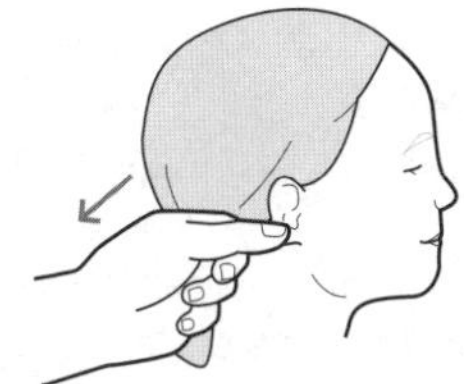

Child: pull the ear down and back

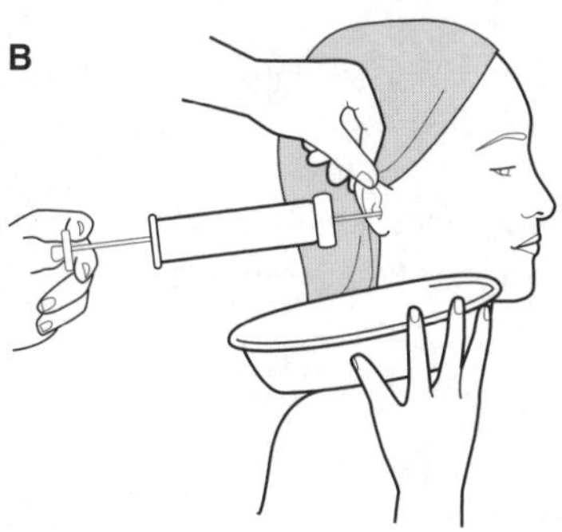

Insertion of the ear syringe

Figure 42.7 | Irrigating the ear
A: Note that the direction of pull is different for adults and children **B**: Insertion of the ear syringe

only when they have been prescribed by a medical officer, and the nurse must follow the nursing regulations and policies regarding the administration of medications. Key aspects regarding the use of otic medications are the same as those for using ophthalmic medications. (A technique of instilling ear drops is outlined in Chapter 30.)

SUMMARY

The special sense organs are those that contain receptors that pick up stimuli from the environment and transmit impulses to the brain for interpretation. The special sense organs that allow us to obtain information about the environment are the tongue, nose, skin, eyes and ears. Through these organs we experience taste, smell, touch, sight and sound.

The tongue contains taste buds that respond to substances in food and generate nerve impulses that are transmitted to the brain for interpretation. Taste buds are capable of detecting sweet, sour, salty and bitter tastes when substances are in a solution. Olfactory receptors in the mucous membrane lining the upper part of the nose are stimulated by chemicals and transmit impulses to the brain, where smell is interpreted. The sensations of taste and smell are closely related, and both play an important part in stimulating the secretion of digestive juices.

The skin, as one of its several functions, allows the perception of touch. It is therefore an organ of sensation, as it contains receptors that transmit impulses to the brain, where the sense of touch is perceived.

Sight is the result of light rays being received by the eyes and transmitted to the brain for interpretation. Each eye receives light from the environment and forms images on the retina, which converts them into nerve impulses, which in turn are transmitted to the visual centres of the brain.

A coordinated process of refraction, accommodation, regulation of pupil size and convergence makes normal binocular vision possible. The eyeballs are anchored into position by extraocular muscles and the conjunctiva, and are further protected by the bony socket, the eyebrow ridge and the eyelids. The lacrimal apparatus secretes tears and directs them onto the anterior surface of the eye, where they are spread over it by blinking movements of the eyelids.

Hearing is a complex mechanism in which the ears receive soundwaves and convert them into nerve impulses. The nerve impulses are transmitted to the brain for interpretation. Perception of sound involves interpretation of both pitch and intensity. Structures contained in the internal ear help the client to maintain balance.

The special sense organs enable the individual to interact and experience the environment. When caring for a client with sensory alteration it is important for the nurse to ensure that the client maintains the ability to interact and respond safely to their environment.

REVIEW EXERCISES

1. What is the term for a complete loss of taste?
2. List the five special sense organs.
3. What is the term for an abnormal sense of smell?
4. What is the medical term for double vision?
5. What is the medical term for nearsightedness?
6. What is the medical term for far-sightedness?
7. Name a common eye disorder that occurs with ageing.
8. What is the medical term for buzzing or ringing in the ear?
9. Which membrane lies between the external ear and the middle ear?
10. What is the slow but gradual loss of hearing common in the older adult called?
11. Name two types of hearing loss.

CRITICAL THINKING EXERCISES

1. Dianne, 51, has worked in the bridal boutique since she was 17. It was where she did her apprenticeship in dressmaking and design. She now specialises in intricate design and embroidery and is highly sought after by

TABLE 42.7 | TECHNIQUE FOR EAR IRRIGATION

Action	Rationale
Review and carry out the standard steps in Appendix 1	
Explain the procedure to the client and ensure privacy	Reduces anxiety
Assist the client to assume a sitting position, with their head tilted slightly forward and towards the affected side	Facilitates entry of the irrigating fluid into the ear canal
Place the towel over the client's shoulder and request the client to hold the kidney dish close to their head under the affected ear	Prevents irrigating fluid running down the back of the neck
Wash and dry hands thoroughly and wear gloves	Prevents cross-infection
Wipe the auricle and meatus of the canal with a swab moistened with the irrigating fluid	Avoids introducing debris into the ear canal
Draw up irrigating fluid into the syringe and expel any air. The fluid should be warm	Avoids introducing air into the canal. Cool water is very uncomfortable and causes dizziness and nausea
Pull the auricle upwards and backwards. For a child, the earlobe is pulled downwards and backwards	Straightens the ear canal
Place the tip of the syringe just inside the meatus and direct a slow, steady stream of fluid against the roof of the ear canal	Directing the stream upward prevents forcing debris further into the canal, and prevents injury to the tympanic membrane. The stream of fluid must be slow and with low pressure to avoid rupture of the tympanic membrane, causing pain and vertigo
Observe the client for signs of pain or dizziness. If either occurs, stop the procedure	The client may experience pain if too great a force is used. Dizziness may occur if the fluid is not at body temperature
When the syringe is empty, remove it and inspect the return flow in the kidney dish. Refill the syringe and continue the irrigation until the return flow is clear or the obstruction has been removed	Assess the effectiveness of the procedure
Remove the syringe and inspect the ear canal with the auroscope (otoscope)	Assess the canal for cleanliness
Encourage the client to tilt their head towards the affected side	Facilitates drainage of any residual fluid and debris
Dry the client's auricle and neck	Promotes comfort
Remove and attend to equipment appropriately. Remove gloves and wash and dry hands	Prevents cross-infection
Report and document the procedure	Appropriate care can be planned and implemented

her clientele. She loves her work but is feeling anxious because she is starting to have difficulty when sewing the tiny seed pearls and finishing the fine detail on the bridal dresses. She has noticed she is able to see better if she holds the material away from her, but this is awkward because there is so much material to handle. What do you think is probably occurring with Dianne's eyesight? What would be your advice to her?

2. Andrew has recently returned from living overseas for 2 years and this was the first visit to his grandfather since his return. He knocked on the door but there was no answer; he could hear the television blaring from inside so he knew someone was home. When his grandfather finally realised Andrew was at the door he was thrilled to see him because he has few visitors these days. While talking to his grandfather Andrew noticed that he would only respond when he was looking directly at or standing close to him, otherwise his grandfather seemed to ignore what was being said. What would be your advice to both Andrew and his grandfather to help improve communication?

REFERENCES AND FURTHER READING

Ankner GM (2008) *Medical–Surgical Nursing*. Thomson Delmar Learning, Clifton Park, NY

—— (2007) *Case Studies in Medical–Surgical Nursing*. Thomson Delmar Learning, Clifton Park, NY

Crisp J, Taylor C (eds) (2005) *Potter & Perry's Fundamentals of Nursing*, 2nd edn. Elsevier Australia, Sydney

Department of Human Services (2008) *Children Youth and Families*. *Maternal and Child Health Service Program Standards*. Online. Available: http://www.cyf.vic.gov.au/document_links/10_appendix_3 [accessed 5 June 2008]

Huether SF, McCance KL (2008) *Understanding Pathophysiology*. Mosby, London

Kozier B, Erb G, Berman AJ, Burke K (2000) *Fundamentals*

of Nursing: Concepts, Process and Practice, 6th edn. Prentice-Hall, Upper Saddle River, NJ
LeMone P, Burke KM (2000) *Medical Surgical Nursing*, 2nd edn. Prentice-Hall, Upper Saddle River, NJ
Marieb E (2006) *Essentials of Human Anatomy and Physiology*, 67th edn. Benjamin Cummings, San Francisco
Neighbors M, Tannehill-Jones R (2000) *Human Diseases*. Delmar Thomson Learning, Albany
Potter PA, Perry AG (2005) *Fundamentals of Nursing*, 2nd edn. Mosby, St Louis
—— (2008) *Fundamentals of Nursing*, 7th edn. Mosby, St Louis
Thibodeau GA, Patton KT (2007) *Anatomy & Physiology*. Mosby, St Louis
Thompson J, McFarland G, Hirsch J, Tucker S (2002) *Mosby's Clinical Nursing*, 5th edn. Mosby, St Louis
Waugh A (2001) *Ross and Wilson's Anatomy and Physiology in Health and Illness*, 9th edn. Churchill Livingstone, London

ONLINE RESOURCES

Better Hearing Australia: www.betterhearing.org.au
Deafness Foundation: http://www.deafness.org.au/
Vision Australia Foundation: www.visionaustralia.org.au

Chapter 43

PALLIATIVE CARE

OBJECTIVES

- Define the key terms/concepts
- Outline the philosophy of palliative care
- Understand the importance of a multidisciplinary approach to treatment
- Identify the attributes required of a palliative care nurse
- Identify a range of physical symptoms that may occur in the dying client
- Discuss the importance of nurturing hope
- Explain the dimensions of spirituality in relation to dying
- Identify ways to care for the carers

KEY TERMS/CONCEPTS

empathy
honesty
hospice
multidisciplinary team
palliation
prognosis
spirituality

CHAPTER FOCUS

The nurse working with people who have advanced illness is part of a multidisciplinary team necessary to maintain quality of life for clients and their families. Quality of life depends very much on the attitude and skill of the nurse. The role of the nurse is not only to care for the physical body but also to establish a genuine caring and honest relationship that facilitates psychological and spiritual wellbeing. In having the most frequent contact with clients and often the deepest relationships of all involved professionals, the nurse is privileged to journey with clients while helping to bring their lives to an end with hope, peace and dignity.

LIVED EXPERIENCE

The nurse suggested the rose and the candle and the nice pink sheets on the bed. Mum looked so peaceful and she died while her favourite Frank Sinatra CD played quietly. I am so glad the nurse prepared me for how it would be. I never thought I would cope, but I did, and Mum would have been proud of me.

Alison, age 21

THE PHILOSOPHY OF PALLIATIVE CARE

Palliative care is about caring for people who have an illness that is not responsive to curative treatment. The focus is not to cure but to 'palliate' — to relieve symptoms so as to keep the person with the illness comfortable. This involves the control of pain and other symptoms without hastening or postponing death. It aims to support clients and families to ease the physical, emotional and spiritual distress that are often present with an incurable illness. Throughout this chapter the term 'family' is used to represent all people identified by the client as being significant to them. Family therefore includes partners, relatives, friends, neighbours and anyone else providing support. Palliative care involves grief and bereavement support for family that extends throughout and beyond the duration of the illness.

WHAT IS INVOLVED IN PALLIATIVE CARE?

The provision of high quality palliative care means that clients and families need access to support from a coordinated team of specialised health care professionals. The team includes medical officers, nurses, allied health workers, counsellors, chaplains and volunteers. The knowledge and expertise of the multidisciplinary team combines to help people live as fully as possible within the increasing limits of the illness. Clients and their families are encouraged to take an active part in the planning and delivery of care.

Palliative care aims to help clients and their families feel in control of the treatment and quality-of-life decisions, including the decision about where care will be provided. Palliative care can be provided in the person's own home, a specialist in-patient hospice unit, an aged-care residential unit, a hospital or other health care facility.

WHAT IS AN IN-PATIENT HOSPICE UNIT?

An in-patient hospice unit is a place where specialist health professionals care for people with incurable illnesses. Clients often come to a hospice in the last stages of illness and remain until death occurs, or they may be admitted for assessment and relief of pain or other distressing symptoms and then return home. Sometimes clients are admitted for a period of respite care. Respite care may be used to provide a break for a family carer, as a time to evaluate and stabilise a client's troublesome symptoms, or in some cases to provide a period of 24-hour-a-day support for a client who is experiencing emotional distress such as unresolved anger or high levels of anxiety. The aim of an in-patient hospice unit is to provide expert care in a calm environment that is as home-like as possible. Palliative care units in busy mainstream hospitals are not always able to provide the same calm atmosphere as a hospice. Clinical Interest Box 43.1 provides an example of when an in-patient palliative care unit can help.

CLINICAL INTEREST BOX 43.1
Elaine's story

When the specialist told me I had the secondary tumours in my liver and in my lungs, my head just started to spin — I was laughing, then crying, but I felt like running away. My mum was with me — she just sat there with tears pouring down her face. We've been through hell and back, Mum and me, first with the surgery and the chemotherapy, then the pain and nausea, and then me being so weak. I've lost everything to this cancer — my looks, my job and my hopes of ever getting married or being a mum myself. I can't do much for myself now and until I came into the hospice I was feeling so down, so weak and useless. I feel better about myself now, emotionally stronger. The nurses make me feel that I matter, and I am happy to be here until the end because I feel I will matter until the very last moment.
(Elaine, aged 27, 6 weeks before dying of metastatic breast cancer)

HOME-BASED CARE

Many people express the desire to die at home, and some health care services provide personnel and equipment to enable this wish to be fulfilled. When a person prefers to die at home, the nurse may be involved in assisting family members in providing care. The nurse may also be required to provide counselling and teaching services; for example, teaching a family member how to sponge the person in bed or how to assist them safely to a commode. When nurses are permitted within their scope of practice to administer medications, they may also be required to teach relatives how to do so.

A home care program may be provided by a community palliative care service that, in addition to medical and nursing care, offers a wide range of other supports. These include counselling, dietary advice, loan of equipment, physiotherapy, occupational therapy, relaxation and music therapy, bereavement support and pastoral care. Many of these supports are offered at a day centre or, if the client is unable to attend, in the home. Trained volunteers play an important role in providing various forms of assistance, including respite for family members and bereavement support.

WHO CAN RECEIVE PALLIATIVE CARE?

Anyone who has an illness that is not responsive to curative measures can receive palliative care, regardless of age, gender, class, culture, race and religion or belief system. Most people receiving palliative care have cancer, but some have progressive chronic neurological problems such as motor neurone disease or multiple sclerosis. Others have acquired immune deficiency syndrome (AIDS), Alzheimer's disease or end-stage heart, lung or kidney failure. As the concept of palliative care is developing, more specialist palliative care teams are caring for people with illnesses other than cancer. Palliative care measures are also implemented for residents living in aged-care facilities who are in the last stages of life. Clinical Interest Box 43.2 provides an example of how

CLINICAL INTEREST BOX 43.2
Gerontology — an Enrolled Nurse's experience of palliative care

Last week I was with Vera when she died. Her only living relative, her sister, was too frail to come, and I wanted to be there with her. The other nurses took on extra work so that I could do that — we do it for each other so we can give special attention to our residents when they are dying. It is the policy here that no resident dies alone. I like that. Where I worked before I saw too many residents left to die on their own and it was so clinical and uncaring. Here we have a kit ready for palliative care residents. We have a cassette player, aromatherapy, a special bedside light with a pink globe and we always pick flowers from the garden. We make it special; the soothing atmosphere we create makes it easier on us nurses and it helps relatives too.
(Sue, an Enrolled Nurse working in aged care)

palliative care may be implemented in the residential care environment.

CULTURAL DIFFERENCE IN PALLIATIVE CARE

Those providing palliative care in a multicultural society require sensitivity to difference in the way people from various cultures understand issues surrounding death and dying. For example, pain and suffering, and quality and meaning of life, may be interpreted quite differently cross-culturally and intra-culturally (D'Avanzo 2008; Kirkwood 1998). Sometimes judgments and care decisions are influenced by the nurse's personal cultural values. It is important to avoid making assumptions about the client's wishes by asking the client what is preferred in relation to all treatment, care and quality-of-life activities. For example, death is a taboo subject for many Muslims, therefore grief counselling is not well accepted and may be perceived as an invasion of privacy (Kirkwood 1998).

WHEN DOES PALLIATIVE CARE BEGIN?

Palliative care is provided after it is acknowledged that curative measures are no longer appropriate. This may be early in the disease when the person is experiencing difficulty with symptoms that need to be relieved, or it may be later in the disease as death approaches. The timing of when palliative care measures are put into place is the choice of the client and varies from person to person.

EXPERIENCES AND RESPONSES IN PALLIATIVE CARE

Palliative care affirms life and regards dying as a normal process. All care is therefore aimed at relieving pain and other symptoms. The client may have symptoms that relate to physical, emotional or spiritual concerns and may be desperately seeking help simultaneously on all of these fronts (Old & Swagerty 2007). Physical comfort is the first priority and essential if palliative care work is to be effective in the other areas (Keubler, Berry & Heidrich 2002). Many clients experience several different physical symptoms at the same time. Pain and weight loss are two of the most common symptoms, but not all people with terminal illness experience pain (Kaye 1998).

PAIN

Pain is the symptom most feared by people with a life-threatening illness. This fear is justified because two-thirds of clients with advanced cancer, for example, experience significant levels of pain (McCaffery & Ferrell 1997). However, modern pain management means that clients receiving good palliative care can and should remain virtually pain free throughout their illness (World Health Organization 2008). Nursing measures such as careful positioning and repositioning, and gentle exercise or support for painful body parts play an important role in providing relief from pain and physical discomfort.

Medication is the primary method of controlling pain and many other physical symptoms. Surgery, radiotherapy, nerve blocks (injection of anaesthetic agent close to a nerve to cause temporary or permanent blockage in transmission of pain) and chemotherapy may also be used to palliate pain and/or prolong life in some circumstances (Kaye 1998; Keubler, Berry & Heidrich 2002). However, the burden of chemotherapy treatment and the resulting side effects frequently mean that stopping chemotherapy in favour of other palliative treatment methods is a welcome relief to clients and families.

Special physiotherapy techniques such as ultrasound and laser therapy can also be helpful in managing pain. Complementary therapies, such as massage, aromatherapy and guided imagery, can also be very valuable and are often combined with medical and nursing care to enhance the effectiveness of pain-relief measures, to reduce anxiety and to improve sense of wellbeing (McCabe 2001).

Medication to control pain

While not all dying clients experience pain, it is a significant symptom for many. Analgesics, ranging from paracetamol through to slow-release morphine and other related opiates, are central to treatment. Recent advances in pain-reduction techniques have seen the introduction of some drugs, including analgesics, in the form of skin patches.

Pain stems from a variety of sources, including bone, nerve root, viscera and soft tissue (Farrer 2002). For example, AIDS often results in the unsheathing of myelin fibres, causing nerve root pain, and pressure from a tumour on an organ capsule may cause visceral pain. Expert assessment of what is causing the pain affects the type of medication that will be most helpful. Most often a combination drug therapy is needed. Non-steroidal anti-inflammatory drugs, anticonvulsants and corticosteroids, in addition to analgesics, are some of the drugs used in combination therapy (Kaye 1998; Keubler, Berry & Heidrich 2002; Foyle &, Hostad 2007). The right combination of medications for each client depends on good communication between the client, family, medical and nursing staff and the expertise of the palliative care team. It is a core skill of the palliative care nurse to assess each aspect of pain and monitor it frequently. (Chapter 35 provides further information on the management of pain.)

Most pain can be controlled completely or kept at a level acceptable to the client (Kaye 1998; Keubler, Berry & Heidrich 2002; Foyle & Hostad 2007). Sometimes, for a variety of reasons, clients are reluctant to admit to the extent of their pain. People interpret their pain according to their life experiences, values and beliefs. Some people view the admission of pain as a sign of weakness, others prefer to deny it is there because increasing pain might mean the condition is getting worse. Some people are fearful of opiate drugs and may refuse to take morphine because they believe it is addictive or that it will not be effective later on when they need it most; others may believe that it will hurry their death. None of these things are true when morphine is taken to relieve pain and it is prescribed correctly. The nurse has an important role in developing a trusting relationship with the client and explaining the facts about morphine or other medications to allay fears.

PROMOTING PHYSICAL EASE

Nursing interventions are planned after holistic assessment of the client's needs has been undertaken. This assessment incorporates sensitive exploration of physical, psychological, social and spiritual concerns. The team approach is essential in meeting these multiple complex needs, but the nurse plays a crucial part in providing physical comfort. The needs of a dying person are complex but none can be addressed effectively unless the client is physically comfortable. Each client generally has a combination of physical concerns. In addition to acute or chronic pain, the dying process is often accompanied by a combination of symptoms causing discomfort. Some of the more common symptoms include:

- Weight loss
- Pain
- Anorexia
- Dyspnoea
- Cough
- Constipation or diarrhoea
- Weakness and fatigue
- Nausea and vomiting
- Insomnia
- Incontinence
- Sore and/or dry mouth
- Hiccups
- Pruritus (itching)
- Diaphoresis (sweating)
- Confusion and restlessness (Kaye 1998; Keubler, Berry & Heidrich 2002; Foyle & Hostad 2007).

For many of these symptoms, physical comfort is enhanced by nursing actions such as effective skin and mouth care and careful skilled moving and positioning. Weakness and fatigue can be minimised by sensible coordination of nursing care activities. However, many clients have co-existing symptoms such as pain, nausea or dyspnoea that exacerbate tiredness and frequently it is the combined efforts of nursing care, medical treatment and complementary health care therapies that bring relief.

Maintaining physical comfort depends on continuous reassessment of the client's needs because physical changes can occur particularly quickly in advanced illness. For example, pain can escalate rapidly and, because of fatigue, immobility, inadequate nutrition or emaciation, pressure ulcers can develop in a very short time. During all phases of care the nurse continually reassesses the situation while assisting the client to retain independence. When independence is no longer possible the nurse continues to provide the physical care in a manner that preserves self-esteem and dignity. (Physical care of the dying client is discussed in Chapter 14.)

HOLISTIC CLIENT-CENTRED CARE

Excellence in care of the physical body is paramount, but nursing care needs to be holistic. Nursing care that is focused too much on tasks objectifies the dying person. Client-centred care facilitates empowerment, choice, control, dignity and self-respect. These things can only happen when there is a genuine, caring and honest relationship between the nurse and the client. Being genuine and honest with the client is vital but sometimes difficult. As no one knows what it is like to be dying until they are faced with it personally, there are times when the nurse may not know what to say. The nurse who responds, 'I don't know what to say to that,' and can remain with the client in a shared comfortable silence is promoting an honest and genuine relationship (Stein-Parbury 2005). It is better to be honest than respond with a trite, inappropriate comment. Clinical Interest Box 43.3 provides an example of honest and open communication between a nurse and a client.

A genuine relationship is one that allows open and honest talk of death, not avoidance of it. It allows the client

CLINICAL INTEREST BOX 43.3
Genuine caring and honesty in a nurse–client relationship

Jack was subdued and thoughtful while the nurse gave him his wash in bed, then he said quietly, 'This isn't going to improve, I'm not going to get better. I'm not going to see my children grow up.' The nurse replied, 'Yes, Jack, that's right, and that must be terribly sad for you to think about.'

Nurses who are not experienced in working with dying clients can find acknowledging such statements very difficult, but responding in this honest way acknowledges Jack's sadness and demonstrates that the nurse understands his fears and feelings. This may assist Jack to feel comfortable discussing other aspects of his approaching death and his experience of dying with the nurse if and when he feels the need to do so.

to express feelings of sadness, and thoughts and beliefs about what is coming. The genuine relationship is also about the nurse knowing when the client wants to forget about dying and would rather talk about other things. It is about the nurse knowing when to simply sit and hold a hand, and being prepared to go away when not needed or wanted. The genuine honest relationship needs to be based on professionalism and a strong knowledge base about clinical care, but also about death and the process of dying. For example, it is important for nurses working in palliative care to understand the process of adjustment and to recognise that anger is not necessarily a personal attack but likely to be an expression of grief (Lockhart 2007; West 1996). (Chapter 14 provides explanations of the grieving process in relation to dying clients and their families.) A holistic client-centred approach in palliative care means that the nurse's knowledge base needs to include knowing how to explore clients' feelings and how to respond empathically to emotional needs.

PSYCHOLOGICAL WELLBEING

One of the most important aspects of psychological wellbeing is nurturing hope in clients and relatives. The client who has trust in the nurse and the palliative care team can hope for expert management of symptoms; the client who has supportive relationships can hope for comfort on the journey being faced. Nurses are in a key position to foster the client's hope for a better day tomorrow or the hope that a goal will be achieved (eg, the goal of living until a special event, such as a wedding or birth in the family, has taken place). The fostering of hope is at the heart of good palliative care (McIntyre & Chaplin 2002).

Nurturing hope is one important aspect of supporting psychological and spiritual wellbeing (see Chapter 11) but the nurse needs to explore other aspects of how the client is feeling, and this can be very challenging. It is helpful for nurses to seek out extra training to assist them with approaching and dealing with emotionally laden topics. There are some areas that nurses may find difficult to deal with, including responding to the difficult questions clients ask about diagnosis and prognosis, and responding to the anger and denial that clients and their families may demonstrate. Effective sensitive communication is the most important aspect of caring for the dying (see Chapter 29 for further discussion of communication skills). With effective and sensitive communication the nurse can be open and honest when answering the client's questions and discussing matters of psychological importance, such as what the future holds for the client, and any fears that may be associated with the journey the client is facing. It may be that, to meet the client's psychological needs, the nurse will need to seek the help and expertise of other team members, such as a visit from a member of the clergy. It should not be forgotten that psychological wellbeing can often be enhanced by the appropriate use of humour and discussion of everyday issues to maintain normalcy when the client and/or family indicate that 'being normal' is what is wanted at any particular time. (See Chapter 13 for further discussion relating to the therapeutic use of humour.)

Often the people closest to the client will want to do what they can to help that person during the illness and at the time of death. The sense of psychological wellbeing that family members experience depends in part on the relationship they maintain with the dying person, and believing that they have contributed well to the care. The nurse can promote this sense of wellbeing by gratefully accepting help with care measures such as the client's nutrition, bathing and toileting. When a client is being cared for at home, the nurse should teach family members how to undertake care measures skilfully and safely. This empowers the relatives and enables care to be provided effectively at times when the nurse is not there.

The nurse can facilitate relatives maintaining a close relationship with the dying person right up until the time that death occurs. It is helpful to reinforce that, although the sense of touch may be diminished, the client is still likely to be able to feel the pressure of touch and find comfort in this. It is also often helpful to tell family members that hearing is usually not diminished and it is best to speak to the dying person in a normal way. Even if the person appears to be unaware of their surroundings and not responding, everyone should be advised to assume that the hearing is still intact. It may be comforting for the dying person to be able to hear recognised voices or some favourite pieces of music, and relatives may take comfort in providing this solace for their loved one. When the dying person is unable to speak, the nurse, by example, can help family members feel comfortable in continuing to speak to the person even though there is no ability to reply (Ferrell & Coyle 2006; Kinghorn & Gamblin 2002; Old & Swagerty 2007).

Empowering relatives in this manner means that they may develop a strong sense of having done all they could for their loved one, which may help sustain them through the grieving process after their loved one dies. (See Chapter 14 for further information concerning psychological care of the dying and care of the bereaved.)

SPIRITUAL WELLBEING

The spiritual dimension of each person is unique. For some people it may be connected to personal religious beliefs and practices. If the rituals and practices are followed the person is more likely to feel spiritually fulfilled, but if they are not observed the person may feel worried and anxious and suffer spiritual distress. The spirituality of those who do not believe in a specific god or who do not have a particular faith relates more to their sense of who and what they are and the purpose of their existence (Smith 2002). Nurses caring for people confronted with death may find them searching for understanding of these issues.

The spiritual dimensions of dying clients may be reflected in a search for meaning in life or in their suffering or in their relationships with others. It may be reflected in a need for hope, love or a sense of forgiveness (Clinical Interest Box 43.4). Not all dying people experience the same needs, nor do they feel them with equal intensity. The nurse with expertise will be sensitive to the spiritual needs of each client and will implement actions to help those needs to be met. Some people meet spiritual needs through the rituals and sacraments of organised religion, others may find help from reading, music, art, meditation, guided imagery or other sources.

As with any aspect of caring for the dying client, it is the responsibility of the health care team in collaboration with the client to identify the person best suited to help with spiritual concerns. It may be the nurse but it may be a friend, a hospital chaplain or a pastoral care worker. It may be that the nurse helps the client identify the person they would like to speak to, and the nurse may then arrange the initial meeting. Palliative care facilities normally have lists of appropriate contacts.

A nurturing, supportive and caring relationship can help the dying client feel valued and safe, and this fosters increased ability to tackle the adjustment to impending death, a component of spirituality. Therefore the nurse who creates a calm atmosphere and attends sensitively to the dying person's basic bodily needs in a way that communicates respect, compassion and understanding will contribute to a sense of spiritual ease (West 1996). (Chapter 11 provides further information about spiritual caring.)

SUPPORT FOR THE NURSE

Care of the dying is one of the most challenging tasks nurses face. It can be very satisfying but it can be demanding and stressful, and nurses need a network of support to help them cope with the demands. Supports that can help range from personal relaxation activities to professional workplace supports such as specialist education and training, critical incident reflection, clinical supervision and counselling (Lockhart 2007; Setch 2002).

CLINICAL INTEREST BOX 43.4
Case study — spiritual distress

Mrs Owen was diagnosed with lung cancer and had accepted that there was no further curative treatment for her. She had been in the hospice for a week when she began having panic attacks. She had not spoken much to anyone and when she did she was often rather aggressive. After several weeks of not saying much she finally revealed to one nurse that she had an affair with her husband's brother. She was Catholic and believed that she was facing retribution for her sins, which meant that she would be sent to purgatory after death. Although Catholic she had not been to church for many years and was quite hostile towards the Catholic doctrine. Even so, her fear of retribution was entrenched. When suggested, she strongly refused the offer of having a priest visit. Over a period of time she talked through the issues with the nurse, who supported her in finding a priest who was empathic towards her. After only two visits from the priest, her anxiety reduced, her fears settled and she had no further panic attacks.
(adapted from Smith 2002: 118)

SUMMARY

Palliative care is a speciality area of nursing. Nurses are valuable members of the multidisciplinary palliative care team needed to provide for the complex needs of dying individuals and their families. Palliative care takes place in many different settings, but most people who have a choice prefer to die at home. Palliative care is provided within the philosophy that dying is a natural process and that dying people should be empowered to live life as fully as possible within the growing limits of their illness. The palliative care team aims to help meet physical, psychological and spiritual needs that arise during the client's journey towards the end of life and to support the client's family as they participate in the experience.

Nursing the dying can be extremely rewarding. When palliative care is administered successfully the nurse shares in a privileged journey with the dying client and the family up to and beyond the time when the client, free from pain and anguish, reaches the end of life peacefully and with dignity.

REVIEW EXERCISES

1. State three major functions of a palliative care team.
2. Describe how you could provide a warm, caring environment for a dying resident in an aged-care facility.
3. List five physical symptoms associated with incurable illness.
4. What nursing actions could help an emaciated client whose pain is controlled but who cannot get physically comfortable in bed?
5. Describe five ways you can promote a sense of wellbeing in the partner of a dying client in the acute-care hospital setting.

CRITICAL THINKING EXERCISES

1. In what ways does the culture in busy acute-care hospitals impact on the experience of clients who are dying? How does it impact on their family members? How might nurses improve the circumstances for dying clients and their families in this setting?
2. The specialist has just told you that you have a brain tumour that is inoperable and not curable. Reflect on your own values, attitudes and beliefs and consider what changes would happen in your life as a result of this prognosis. What would you need to help you cope? If you were living in a rural area 2 hours' drive from the nearest city, would the health service meet your needs?
3. Joe, 72, has lung cancer. He has been admitted to the hospice today. He has been a frequent visitor to the hospice day centre over the last few months, and several staff members have noted his positive attitude and how well he seems to have been coping physically and emotionally. Joe's condition has deteriorated now

and he is not expected to live for more than a few more days. He is alert but extremely agitated at the moment. Margaret, his wife, can't understand this anxiety because he has been so calm throughout his illness. She and his three daughters are finding his agitation very distressing. Consider factors that may be related to Joe's anxiety. How would you explore his agitation with him? What other health professionals may need to be consulted?

REFERENCES AND FURTHER READING

Berger AM, Shuster JL, Von Roenn JH (2006) *Principles and Practice of Palliative Care and Supportive Oncology*. Lippincott, Williams and Wilkins, Hagerstown, MD

Brown Jr E (2007) *Supporting the Child and the Family in Paeditaric Palliative Care*. Jessica Kingsley Publishers, London

D'Avanzo C (2008) *Mosby's Pocket Guide to Cultural Health Assessment*, 4th edn. Mosby Elsevier, St Louis

Farrer K (2002) Pain control. In: Kinghorn S, Gamblin R (eds) *Palliative Nursing: Bringing Comfort and Hope*. Baillière Tindall, Edinburgh

Ferrell B, Coyle N (2006) *Textbook of Palliative Nursing*, 2nd edn. Oxford University Press, New York

Firth P, Luff G, Oliviere D (2005) *Loss, Change and Bereavement in Palliative Care*. Open University Press, Berkshire UK

Foyle L, Hostad J (2007) *Innovations in Cancer and Palliative Care Education*. Radcliffe Publishing, Abingdon, Oxford

Kaye P (1998) *Symptom Control in Hospice and Palliative Care*. Hospice Education Institution, Essex

Keubler K, Berry P, Heidrich D (2002) *End of Life Care: Clinical Practice Guidelines*. WB Saunders, Philadelphia

Kinghorn S, Gamblin R (eds) (2002) *Palliative Nursing: Bringing Comfort and Hope*. Baillière Tindall, Edinburgh

Kirkwood N (1998) *A Hospital Handbook on Multiculturalism and Religion*. Moorehouse, Harrisberg

Lockhart SJ (2007) *Of Secrets, Sorrows, and Shame: Undergraduate Nurses' Experiences of Death and Dying*. Unpublished Masters Thesis. Faculty of Education: The University of Melbourne

Macleod S (2007) *The Psychiatry of Palliative Medicine: the Dying Mind*. Radcliffe Publishing, Abingdon, Oxford

McCabe P (ed.) (2001) *Complementary Therapies in Nursing and Midwifery: from Vision to Practice*. Ausmed Publications, Melbourne

McCaffery M, Ferrell BR (1997) Nurses' knowledge of pain assessment and management: how much progress have we made? *Journal of Pain and Symptom Management*, 14(3): 175–88

McIntyre R, Chaplin J (2002) Hope: the heart of palliative care. In: Kinghorn S, Gamblin R (eds) *Palliative Nursing: Bringing Comfort and Hope*. Baillière Tindall, Edinburgh: 129–45

Old JL, Swagerty D (2007) *A Practical Guide to Palliative Care*. Lippincott, Williams and Wilkins, Hagerstown, MD

Olson M (1997) *Healing the Dying*. Delmar, Albany

Parker J, Aranda S (1998) *Palliative Care: Explorations and Challenges*. MacLennan and Petty, Sydney

Pfund R (2007) *Palliative Care Nursing of Children and Young People*. Radcliffe Publishing, Abingdon, Oxford

Setch F (2002) Looking after yourself. In: Kinghorn S, Gamblin R (eds) *Palliative Nursing: Bringing Comfort and Hope*. Baillière Tindall, Edinburgh: 257–70

Smith M (2002) Spiritual issues. In: Lugton J, Kindlen M (eds) *Palliative Care: the Nurses Role*. Churchill Livingstone, Edinburgh

Stein-Parbury J (2005) *Patient and Person: Interpersonal Skills in Nursing* . Elsevier/Churchill Livingstone, Sydney

West R (1996) Nursing the spirit. *Australian Nursing Journal*, 4(1): 34–35

World Health Organization (2008) *Cancer Pain Relief and Palliative Care*. Report of a WHO Expert Committee Technical Report Series No 804. WHO, Geneva. Online. Available: www.who.int/bookorders/anglais/detart1.jsp?sesslan=1&codlan=1&codcol=10&codcch=804-29k [accessed 31 May 2008]

Chapter 44

PERIOPERATIVE NURSING

OBJECTIVES

- Define the key terms/concepts
- Describe the nature of the operative experience and outline the phases it entails
- Describe the general physiological, psychological and local responses to surgical intervention
- Describe the various classifications of surgical procedures
- Assist in planning and implementing preoperative and postoperative nursing care for the client who requires surgical intervention
- According to specified role and function, perform associated surgical nursing activities, such as caring for a surgical wound drainage system or removing sutures and staples safely and accurately

KEY TERMS/CONCEPTS

anaesthesia
intraoperative
perioperative
postoperative
preoperative
surgery

CHAPTER FOCUS

Perioperative nursing encompasses the care of a client who is undergoing a surgical procedure. Care takes place from the time the decision is made to have surgery, through to recovery from the procedure. Throughout the perioperative period it is essential that there is a flexible multidisciplinary team approach to ensure continuity of client care from admission, throughout the surgical experience to recovery at home. It is important for the nurse to be familiar with the types of surgery a client is likely to undergo in order to plan and implement adequate and individualised care and to provide appropriate psychological support. This chapter provides an overview of the perioperative period, which comprises the preoperative, intraoperative and postoperative phases as well as the specific physiological and psychological support that each phase requires.

LIVED EXPERIENCE

When I went to the operating suite to have my surgical procedure I was frightened, I was naked except for an ill fitting gown that was open down the back and I didn't know what results the operation would reveal. I felt like I had no control, my husband wasn't able to be with me, I found the situation overwhelming. I'm a Registered Nurse, I work in the perioperative environment everyday, but this day I was the patient. It was me who looked to the nurse for a smile, a touch, an explanation. When caring for my patients I reflect on my experience and ensure that my patients are cared for with the same professionalism, compassion and respect that I needed.

Sharon Ward, Registered Nurse

PERIOPERATIVE CARE

Perioperative nursing encompasses a wide variety of nursing functions related to the clients' surgical experience throughout the perioperative period. This period is divided into three phases: preoperative (before), intraoperative (during) and postoperative (after). Perioperative nurses are Registered Nurses (RNs) and Enrolled Nurses (ENs) who fulfil the following roles: circulating nurse (scout), instrument nurse (scrub), anaesthetic and post anaesthesia recovery nurse. The responsibilities of these nurses are specialised and multifaceted. The principal aim is to ensure that holistic, clinically effective, evidence-based care and support is given to the client throughout their perioperative experience. The perioperative nurse provides this care alongside other members of the multidisciplinary team, in an environment that is challenging, changing and fast paced. The nurse acts as the clients advocate and provides continued effective communication with the client, their significant others and the surgical team. The nurse undertakes efficient assessment and intervention, maintains accountability for their own practice, documents care and emphasises client safety in all phases (Crisp & Taylor 2005; Woodhead & Wicker 2005; Farrell 2003).

In Australia professional standards, guidelines and policy statements for perioperative nursing are set by the Australian College of Operating Room Nurses (ACORN). ACORN's ongoing focus is the improvement and standardisation, education and support of perioperative nursing care (Hamlin 2006).

SURGERY

Undergoing surgery is an experience that is unique to the individual; a client faces numerous stressors when confronting surgery. The anticipation of having a surgical procedure may incite fear and anxiety. Some clients associate having surgery with pain, disfigurement, loss of independence and even death. It is important for the perioperative nurse to quickly establish rapport with clients, listening to them so that their concerns are heard and relieved. Surgical procedures are classified according to risk, urgency or purpose (Crisp & Taylor 2005, Farrell 2003).

CLASSIFICATIONS OF SURGERY

Risk

Surgery is categorised as major or minor dependent on the degree of risk to the client.

- Major surgery comprises an increased degree of risk, it may be complicated or prolonged, vital organs can be involved, large blood losses could occur and post operative complications are more probable.
- Minor surgery usually involves a small amount of risk and has few complications.

Urgency

The urgency of surgery is dependent on whether the surgery is classified as an emergency or an elective procedure.

- Emergency surgery is performed to preserve the client's life, body part or body function
- Elective surgery is based on the client's choice, it is usually planned weeks or even months in advance, and it is not always essential and may not be necessary for health. Elective surgery is classified into categories which are dependent on urgency:
  - Category 1: Urgent cases — surgery within 30 days is desirable for a condition that could potentially quickly deteriorate to the extent where it might become an emergency.
  - Category 2: Semi-urgent cases — surgery within 90 days is desirable for a condition, pain, dysfunction or disability which is unlikely to deteriorate quickly or become an emergency.
  - Category 3: Non-urgent cases — surgery within 12 months is used as a guide for treatment of conditions causing minimal or no pain, dysfunction or disability, is unlikely to deteriorate quickly and does not have the potential to become an emergency (Department of Human Services 2005).

Purpose

Surgery is performed for a variety of reasons:

- Diagnostic — surgical exploration that allows the surgeon to confirm a diagnosis; tissue may be removed for further diagnostic testing
- Ablative — excision or removal of a diseased body part
- Constructive — restores lost or reduced function resulting from congenital abnormalities
- Reconstructive — restores appearance or function to tissues that are traumatised or malfunctioning
- Cosmetic — performed to improve the client's personal appearance
- Palliative — alleviates or reduces the intensity of disease symptoms, will not cure the disease. (Crisp & Taylor 2005)

RESPONSES TO SURGICAL INTERVENTION

There is a degree of risk with any surgical procedure. Various factors and conditions increase a client's risk during surgery. Knowledge of the risk factors allows the nurse to appropriately plan client care. Some of these risk factors include:

- Age — very young and very old clients are at risk during surgery due to their physiological status being immature or declining. See Table 44.1 Physiological factors that place older adults at risk during surgery
- Nutrition — the need for adequate nutrition is intensified by surgery; normal tissue repair and resistance to infection is dependant on sufficient nutrients
- Obesity — the bariatric (obese) client is at an

increased surgical risk due to reduced ventilatory and cardiac function. Diabetes, hypertension, coronary artery disease and congestive heart failure are common in the bariatric population. They are also susceptible to wound infections and poor wound healing, due to the structure of fatty tissue which contains deficient blood supply
- Fluid and electrolyte balance — the body responds to surgery as a form of trauma, the more extensive the surgery the more severe the stress. The degree of fluid and electrolyte imbalance is influenced by the severity of the stress response evoked.

Physiological responses

In response to surgical invasion, the body mobilises defences to maintain homeostasis. Most of these mechanisms are generally favourable to survival and healing. If, however, the mechanisms are prolonged or uncontrolled, they may contribute to the development of complications. Table 44.2 outlines the physiological responses to the stress of surgery.

Local responses to tissue injury

After injury, local inflammatory reactions occur to promote healing. A surgical incision, even though created under sterile and controlled conditions, still constitutes injury or insult. The inflammatory response begins with the creation of a surgical wound, and the normal sequence of tissue replacement and wound healing must occur to ensure tissue recovery. The physiology of wound healing involves a specific sequence of events and is discussed in Chapter 37, as are influences on healing, and the specific care of wounds.

Psychological responses

As a result of psychological stress related to surgical intervention, the individual may experience changes in mood and/or behaviour, including:

TABLE 44.1 | PHYSIOLOGICAL FACTORS THAT PLACE OLDER ADULTS AT RISK DURING SURGERY

Alterations	Risks	Nursing implications
Cardiovascular system		
Degenerative change in myocardium and valves	Reduced cardiac reserve.	Assess baseline vital signs. Recognise the longer time period required for heart rate to return to normal following stress on the heart, and evaluate the occurrence of tachycardia accordingly (Eliopoulos 2004).
Rigidity of arterial walls and reduction in sympathetic and parasympathetic innervation to heart	Alterations predispose client to postoperative haemorrhage and rise in systolic and diastolic blood pressure.	Maintain adequate fluid balance to minimise stress to the heart. Ensure blood pressure level is adequate to meet circulatory demands.
Increase in calcium and cholesterol deposits within small arteries; thickened arterial walls	Predispose client to clot formation in lower extremities.	Instruct client in techniques for performing leg exercises and proper turning. Apply elastic stockings, sequential compression devices (SCDs). Administer anticoagulants as prescribed by health care provider. Provide education regarding effects, side effects and dietary considerations.
Integumentary system		
Decreased subcutaneous tissue and increased fragility of skin	Prone to pressure ulcers and skin tears.	Assess skin every 4 hours; pad all bony prominences during surgery. Turn or reposition at least every 2 hours.
Pulmonary system		
Rib cage stiffened and reduced in size	Reduced vital capacity.	Instruct client in proper technique for coughing, deep breathing and use of spirometer.
Reduced range of movement in diaphragm	Greater residual capacity (volume of air is left in lung after normal breath) increases, reducing amount of new air brought into lungs with each inspiration.	When possible, have client ambulate and sit in chair frequently.
Stiffened lung tissue and enlarged air spaces	Alteration reduces blood oxygenation.	Obtain baseline oxygen saturation; measure as indicated throughout perioperative period.

(Continued)

TABLE 44.1 | PHYSIOLOGICAL FACTORS THAT PLACE OLDER ADULTS AT RISK DURING SURGERY—cont'd

Alterations	Risks	Nursing implications
Renal system		
Reduced blood flow to kidneys	Increased risk of shock when blood loss occurs.	For clients hospitalised before surgery, determine baseline urinary output for 24 hours.
Reduced glomerular filtration rate and excretory times	Limits ability to eliminate drugs or toxic substances.	Assess for adverse response to drugs.
Reduced bladder capacity	Voiding frequency increases, and larger amount of urine stays in bladder after voiding. Sensation of need to void often does not occur until bladder is filled.	Instruct client to notify nurse immediately when sensation of bladder fullness develops. Keep call light and bedpan within easy reach. Toilet every 2 hours or more frequently if indicated.
Neurological system		
Sensory losses, including reduced tactile sense and increased pain tolerance	Decreased ability to respond to early warning signs of surgical complications.	Inspect bony prominences for signs of pressure that client is unable to sense. Orient client to surrounding environment. Observe for nonverbal signs of pain.
Decreased reaction time	Confusion after anaesthesia.	Allow adequate time to respond, process information and perform tasks. Institute fall precautions.
Metabolic system		
Lower basal metabolic rate	Reduced total oxygen consumption.	Ensure adequate nutritional intake when diet is resumed, but avoid intake of excess calories.
Reduced number of red blood cells and haemoglobin levels	Ability to carry adequate oxygen to tissues is reduced.	Administer necessary blood products. Monitor blood test results and oxygen saturation.
Change in total amounts of body potassium and water volume	Greater risk for fluid or electrolyte imbalance occurs.	Monitor electrolyte levels, and supplement as necessary. Cardiac monitoring (telemetry) as needed.
Impaired thermoregulatory mechanisms	Cold operating rooms; exposure of body parts during procedure, IV fluids, medications.	Ensure careful, close monitoring of client temperature; provide warm blankets; monitor cardiac function; warm IV fluids.

(Potter & Perry 2008)

TABLE 44.2 | PHYSIOLOGICAL RESPONSES TO THE STRESS OF SURGERY

Response	Purpose
Increased peripheral vasoconstriction and blood coagulation	Prevents excessive blood and fluid loss
Increased rate and strength of heart beat, and dilation of the coronary arteries	Maintains cardiac perfusion and oxygenation
Increased reabsorption of sodium ions from the kidneys, causing retention of sodium and water	Maintains blood volume, blood pressure and cardiac output
Decreased peristalsis in the gastrointestinal tract	Reduces metabolic activity which is non-essential in the short-term emergency
Relaxation of smooth muscle that promotes dilation of the bronchioles	Improves gas exchange and tissue oxygenation
Increased breakdown of protein	Increases the availability of amino acids for repair of tissues
Proliferation of connective tissue	Promotes wound healing
Increased circulation of glucose and mobilisation of stored fat	Provides required energy
Increased basal metabolic rate	Provides required energy and nutrients for the tissues

- Anxiety, which may be related to the procedure itself, or to associated factors, including changed social circumstances, loss of independence or privacy, separation from family/support people, financial hardship or prolonged recovery time
- Depression
- Fear — anticipated pain, concern of mutilation or decreased function, dread of death, panic of waking up under anaesthetic
- Grief — associated with loss of health or a body part, self-image change, altered function or presence of a scar
- Anger
- Impaired judgment
- Reduced willpower
- Inability to concentrate and/or remember
- Intolerance of noise and other stimuli
- Emotional unpredictability
- Aimless non-productive activities.

(Chapter 13 provides information concerning how the nurse can help clients who are exposed to stress.)

PREOPERATIVE CARE

The preoperative phase begins when surgical intervention is first considered, and ends when the individual is transferred to the operating table. This phase may be of short duration if the client is taken directly to an operating room from the emergency department or transferred soon after admission to a surgical unit.

The duration depends on a number of factors, such as the amount of time required to prepare the client adequately for surgery. The preoperative phase may begin with the individual as an outpatient in a designated pre-admission clinic, where preoperative investigations are undertaken prior to the client's procedure.

In Australia it is now common practice for an individual, depending on the type of surgery to be performed, to be admitted for same-day surgery. In this instance the client is admitted in the early or late morning depending on if the client is on the AM or PM theatre list. The client is prepared for and undergoes surgery, is recovered from the anaesthetic, is cared for in the Day Surgery Unit (DSU) after the procedure, and is discharged home on the same day. Clients undergoing surgery who will require in-patient care are also, in most cases, admitted through the DSU as a day of surgery admission (DOSA). DOSA clients are taken to theatre from the DSU and are taken to the ward from the recovery room. DOSA clients require comprehensive preparation and teaching about home recovery. Follow-up at home (often by telephone) must be available for continuity of care to occur. Day-stay surgery is suitable for less complex surgical procedures, or invasive techniques for which some anaesthesia is required (e.g. endoscopy). These units are staffed by RNs and ENs.

Day surgery is now well established throughout Australia, in both the public and private sectors. Currently up to 60% of all procedures are undertaken as day patient procedures. At present, day surgery is widely practised; in over 240 freestanding day surgery centres, many large public hospitals and over 320 private hospitals around Australia have designated DSUs in place (Australian Day Surgery Council 2004). The advantages to the client and their relatives include considerable reduction in cross-infection risk compared with clients who remain in hospital; decreased risk of thrombo-embolism associated with early ambulation; less anxiety for the client as an overnight stay in hospital is avoided, particularly in the instance of children where minimal separation from parents is beneficial, and for the older client who may become disorientated when subjected to unfamiliar surroundings for extended periods of time. The client will have a quicker return to normal activities with less time off work, less stress for their relatives, a saving in time, travel and in some cases a need for accommodation required to visit an in-patient in hospital (Australian Day Surgery Council 2004).

Another trend is that overall length of stay in hospital after surgical procedures is decreasing. With this practice of earlier discharge comes the implication that clients may go home with complex medical and nursing needs and will require suitable follow-up with visiting nurses, or involvement in a 'Hospital in the Home' or a 'Rehabilitation in the home' program.

The overall aim of preoperative preparation is to ensure that the individual is in the best physical and psychological condition possible before undergoing surgery. It is essential to gather appropriate data concerning the client's health status through the taking of baseline observations and a detailed and accurate nursing history. Nursing assessment is based on the data collected and includes the identification of actual and potential problems that may be faced by the individual throughout any phases of the perioperative period. Although certain aspects of preoperative preparation are similar for most surgical procedures, other factors are specific, depending on the individual client's condition and on the type of operation to be performed.

Preoperative preparation generally consists of:

- Providing information
- Teaching activities (e.g. deep breathing and coughing techniques and leg exercises)
- Examination of the individual by the anaesthetist and surgeon
- Performing laboratory tests and diagnostic studies
- Gaining the individual's informed consent
- Preparation of the individual both psychologically and physically.

PROVIDING INFORMATION

Initial assessment of each client's knowledge base should be undertaken; even if the person's past surgical experiences are extensive. The client needs to be informed about all pre- and postoperative procedures and care because knowledge and understanding promote feelings of being in control, and a sense of control helps to relieve anxiety. Research has demonstrated that preoperative education has resulted in positive improvements on the levels of fear, anxiety and pain experienced by clients (Joanna Briggs Institute 2000). The information given to clients and, as appropriate, to their significant others should include:

- Preoperative procedures to be performed, and the reasons for them; for example, restriction of food and fluids, cessation of smoking, or preparation of the operation site
- Immediate preparation; for example, insertion of an intravenous (IV) cannula, the administration of pre-medication and the induction of anaesthesia, and what sensations may be experienced
- Details of the recovery phase in the Post Anaesthetic Care Unit (PACU) before returning to the DSU or the ward
- Postoperative situations to be expected; for example, the presence of an IV infusion or wound drain, and why these are necessary
- Postoperative activities; for example, deep breathing and coughing, early mobilisation, and why they are important
- Anticipated pain or discomfort, and options for how this will be managed
- Any additional information specific to the operation to be performed.

The information must be provided in such a way that the individual can understand it, and it should be repeated if necessary. This is essential, as anxiety about hospitalisation and/or the surgical procedure may influence the client's ability to process and retain information. The most helpful teaching program is designed so that all clients receive the same information.

TEACHING ACTIVITIES

Preoperative teaching can help to reduce anxiety and stress, and teaching specific activities that the individual can undertake to promote their own recovery gives them a positive role to play. In some cases the client may visit a specialty postoperative area; that is, an Intensive Care Unit (ICU) as familiarity with environments that will be encountered during or after surgery may help reduce the stress associated with the surgical experience.

Preoperative teaching of activities involves instructing the client how to perform deep breathing and coughing techniques, leg exercises and how to move and change position. The person is informed how important these activities are in the prevention of postoperative complications and is encouraged to practise them so that the techniques will be familiar when they are necessary postoperatively. Some clients will have postoperative pain relief medication administered by a self-operated infusion pump. This is called patient-controlled analgesia (PCA). Clients who are expected to return from surgery with a PCA will need to understand the purpose of the pump and will require preoperative education about how to use the device correctly. This teaching is generally the role of an RN, but the EN caring for a client using a PCA will need to monitor that the client is using it correctly and that pain relief is effective.

Deep breathing and coughing techniques

Deep breathing and coughing techniques are performed to facilitate gas exchange and expectoration of accumulated mucus. The client assumes a sitting position and takes several deep breaths followed by a short breath and cough. Alternatively, the client may be taught to take a deep breath, hold it for 2–3 seconds, then cough several times while exhaling. The client is informed that if coughing is likely to be painful, for example, due to a thoracic or abdominal incision, the provision of analgesia and external support (placing the hands over the incision, or splinting with a pillow) reduces pain and therefore may help facilitate coughing and deep breathing.

Leg exercises

Leg exercises are performed to stimulate blood circulation thereby prevent venous thrombosis. The client is instructed how to bend the knees and contract the hamstring and quadricep muscles, and how to dorsiflex and plantarflex the feet (see Chapter 36). Such exercises also act to prevent general muscle stiffness and soreness.

Moving and changing position

Moving and changing position helps to prevent complications such as skin breakdown and deep vein thrombosis. The nurse should inform clients that they will be assisted to move if they are unable to do so independently, or if special restrictions will be in place. If specialised techniques are required to facilitate movement in the postoperative period such as the use of a rolling or turning frame after total hip replacement, an opportunity to practise these techniques should be provided in the preoperative phase.

PHYSICAL EXAMINATION

The anaesthetist and a medical officer each perform a thorough physical examination of the client. The anaesthetist pays particular attention to the client's cardiovascular and respiratory systems to evaluate the general level of function and to identify any problems that may cause difficulty during induction or maintenance of anaesthesia, such as an upper airway abnormality, which may make placement of an endotracheal tube difficult, or a spinal condition which may hinder regional anaesthesia. The anaesthetist also evaluates possible sites for peripheral or central venous cannulation. After assessing the client, the anaesthetist may prescribe any preoperative medications deemed necessary to be administered prior to surgery.

LABORATORY TESTS AND DIAGNOSTIC STUDIES

Laboratory tests and diagnostic studies help detect any risk factors or possible issues. Specific tests and studies performed depend on the client's condition and on the nature and complexity of the operation. Ideally, diagnostic tests are carried out with sufficient time before the scheduled procedure to allow for correction of any detected problems.

Tests can include:

- Blood type and cross-match, for procedures in which significant blood loss is anticipated or possible
- Arterial blood gas and pH, to check respiratory function and oxygenation
- Blood urea nitrogen, to check renal function
- Full Blood Examination (FBE)
- Prothrombin and/or plasma thromboplastin time, clotting factors, especially if the client has been on anticoagulant therapy
- Serum electrolytes, including sodium and potassium levels
- Liver function studies
- Chest X-ray
- Electrocardiogram
- Pulmonary function studies
- Urinalysis.

INFORMED CONSENT

Before an operation is performed, the client must give informed consent which should be freely given without coercion. Informed consent involves the surgeon providing the client with enough information to understand the nature and consequences of the proposed procedure and informing the client about the facts and possible risks relating to the surgery concerned, in terms that ensures understanding by the client. The client then consents, in writing, to have the operation. The surgeon and the client must both sign a consent form, an important part of the documentation process that formalises the client's agreement to undergo surgery. The nurse is not responsible for obtaining the individual's consent, but the nursing role includes checking that informed consent has been obtained and making appropriate notifications if this is found not to be the case. In some agencies, nurses are asked to witness consent forms, but the act of witnessing only verifies that this is the person who signed the consent, and that it was given voluntarily. It does not relate to the client's actual knowledge or understanding of the procedure. (Further information on informed consent is provided in Chapters 3 and 4.)

PSYCHOLOGICAL PREPARATION

To minimise anxiety and prepare the client psychologically for the proposed procedure, the nurse must ensure that all relevant information is provided. People generally experience anxiety when they are facing the unknown, and anxiety is usually reduced somewhat when accurate and relevant information is supplied. The nurse must ensure that the client and the significant others are given opportunities to ask questions and to express any concerns they may have. It is important for the nurse to recognise that procedures that seem relatively minor or routine may not appear that way to clients or to their significant others. The prospect of any surgical intervention raises many fears about body image alteration, loss of control, pain or even the possibility of death. Some of the many factors that the client may be worried about include:

- What will happen while they are unconscious?
- Whether the surgeon will start the operation before the anaesthetic is effective
- Fear of experiencing severe pain
- Length of hospital stay
- Who will care for their family or pets?
- How long it will be before it is possible to return to work.

The family or significant others may also be worried, especially if the diagnosis is questionable or the outcome of the surgery is difficult to determine. If they choose to remain in the hospital while the operation is being performed, the nurse should ensure that they know where the waiting area is located and where they can obtain refreshments. If they prefer to remain at home they should be given an indication of what the notification process is; for example, if the surgeon will contact them after the procedure, what time, whom and when they can call to obtain information.

PHYSICAL PREPARATION

Ideal surgical conditions include a client who is haemodynamically stable, with no current clinical infection, and with well controlled pre-existing medical conditions. Depending on the individual's condition and the type of operation to be performed, specific measures may be implemented to minimise or eliminate any identified risks. For example, a client with breathing problems may be required to undergo active therapy such as incentive spirometry (inhalation into a specially designed spirometer, to achieve maximum inspiratory capacity and reduce risk of pulmonary consolidation), or elimination of pulmonary secretions by postural drainage (the use of positioning to drain secretions from specific segments of the lungs). An individual with dehydration or poor nutritional status may be admitted for some time before surgery so that fluid and nutritional deficiencies may be corrected. A specific diet may be prescribed, such as low fibre before bowel surgery. A person with potential for infection may be administered prophylactic antibiotics prior to the operation. Other preoperative measures may include comprehensive preparation of the gastrointestinal tract, and preparation of the skin. Table 44.3 lists medical conditions that increase the risks of surgery. Physical preparation may also include cessation or modification of certain medication administration; for example, aspirin and

TABLE 44.3 | MEDICAL CONDITIONS THAT INCREASE RISKS OF SURGERY

Type of condition	Reason for risk
Bleeding disorders (thrombocytopenia, haemophilia)	Increase risk of hemorrhaging during and after surgery.
Diabetes mellitus	Increases susceptibility to infection and impairs wound healing from altered glucose metabolism and associated circulatory impairment (Furnary 2003). Stress of surgery often causes increases in blood glucose levels.
Heart disease (recent myocardial infarction, dysrhythmias, congestive heart failure) and peripheral vascular disease	Stress of surgery causes increased demands on myocardium to maintain cardiac output. General anaesthetic agents depress cardiac function.
Obstructive sleep apnoea	Administration of opioids increases risk of airway obstruction postoperatively. Clients will desaturate as revealed by drop in O_2 saturation by pulse oximetry.
Upper respiratory infection	Increases risk of respiratory complications during anaesthesia (e.g. pneumonia and spasm of laryngeal muscles).
Liver disease	Alters metabolism and elimination of drugs administered during surgery and impairs wound healing and clotting time because of alterations in protein metabolism.
Fever	Predisposes client to fluid and electrolyte imbalances and may indicate underlying infection.
Chronic respiratory disease (emphysema, bronchitis, asthma)	Reduces client's means to compensate for acid–base alterations (see Chapter 41). Anesthetic agents reduce respiratory function, increasing risk for severe hypoventilation.
Immunological disorders (leukaemia, acquired immune deficiency syndrome [AIDS], bone marrow depression, and use of chemotherapeutic drugs or immunosuppressive agents)	Increases risk of infection and delayed wound healing after surgery.
Abuse of street drugs	Persons abusing drugs sometimes have underlying disease (HIV, hepatitis) that affects healing.
Chronic pain	Regular use of pain medications often results in higher tolerance. Increased doses of analgesics are sometimes necessary to achieve postoperative pain control.

HIV, Human immunodeficiency virus.
(Potter & Perry 2008)

other anti-coagulant drugs. Cessation of smoking should also be encouraged.

Preparation of the gastrointestinal tract

Gastrointestinal activity is slowed down by stress, sedation, general anaesthesia and the inactivity associated with surgery. Depression of gastrointestinal activity predisposes the individual to retention of food and fluids and therefore to abdominal distension and/or vomiting. It also contributes to postoperative constipation or faecal impaction. Before any abdominal surgery, particularly surgery that involves the intestines, it is necessary to ensure that the bowel is empty and cleansed, as this enables a clear operative view and reduces the risk of contamination and postoperative infection. Preparation of the bowel may include dietary modification, the administration of bowel preparations taken orally (i.e. Picolax, Fleet), rectal suppositories or an enema.

A period of fasting in which all oral foods and fluids are withheld aims to prevent and alleviate gastrointestinal problems. Allowing sufficient time for gastric emptying decreases the risk of regurgitation and subsequent pulmonary aspiration of gastric contents whilst the client is anaesthetised. It also reduces the possibility of postoperative nausea and vomiting. An extended period of fasting is not advocated, as it may result in fluid and electrolyte imbalances, especially in children and the elderly. Depending on the client's condition and the type of surgery, the preoperative fasting period for an adult is generally 6–8 hours. For a child this may be reduced to perhaps only 2–3 hours. The surgeon and/or anaesthetist determine the length of time the client is to fast. Minor surgical procedures using local anaesthetics are often performed without imposing any dietary or fluid restrictions. Fasting times are documented and handed over between nurses verbally. This is especially important if the client is a child or an adult who is confused.

Preparation of the skin

The skin to be incised is cleansed before surgery minimising the number of microorganisms on the skin and therefore reducing the risk of contamination and infection of the wound. Cleansing is generally achieved by the individual showering prior to coming to day surgery, or if on the ward, before going to theatre. Traditionally, extensive removal of hair from the skin by shaving has been an accepted practice. Current research has demonstrated that no hair removal, clipping the hair, using electric razors or depilatory cream are associated with lower infection rates than the traditional method of using a blade for shaving. Research has also demonstrated that shaving several hours before surgery allows time for bacterial colonisation of microscopic skin nicks or cuts. The trend therefore is to remove the hair immediately before surgery, often in the operating room. Some authorities state that, unless hair near the operative site is thick enough to interfere with the surgery, it is preferable not to remove it at all (Joanna Briggs Institute 2003). In the operating room, when the client is anaesthetised, the operation site is swabbed with an antiseptic, usually providone–iodine, using sterile gauze squares or pads. Skin patch testing for allergy to iodine-based substances may be carried out preoperatively.

Administration of medications

If a client takes prescription or over-the-counter medications, the surgeon or the anaesthetist may temporarily discontinue the medications before surgery or adjust the dosages. Certain medications have implications for the surgical client, creating greater risks for complications, as is illustrated in Table 44.4.

It is important for the nurse to be aware of the medical officer's instructions regarding administration of medications in relation to the surgical procedure. It will be decided that any medications that the client has routinely been prescribed be either administered or withheld on the day of surgery. If the individual is fasting, the medical officer may order that any prescribed medications are administered by the intramuscular route or, if given orally, with a very small quantity of water only. It is common that medications for treating cardiac conditions and hypertension will continue to be administered despite the fasting condition, but it is essential that orders be verified.

Preoperative medications (pre-medications) may be prescribed for administration in the period immediately before the operation. Pre-medication is no longer considered essential and is now often omitted or prescribed only when indicated for a specific reason. Indications include the need to allay anxiety, reduce secretions (salivary, gastric and bronchial), to decrease the risk of postoperative nausea or to provide prophylactic analgesia and/or sedation

TABLE 44.4 | MEDICATIONS WITH SPECIAL IMPLICATIONS FOR THE SURGICAL CLIENT

Drug Class	Effects During Surgery
Antibiotics	Antibiotics potentiate (enhance action of) anaesthetic agents. If taken within 2 weeks before surgery, aminoglycosides (gentamicin, tobramycin, neomycin) may cause mild respiratory depression from depressed neuromuscular transmission.
Antidysrhythmics	Antidysrhythmics (e.g. beta blockers such as metoprolol [Lopressor]) can reduce cardiac contractility and impair cardiac conduction during anaesthesia.
Anticoagulants	Anticoagulants, such as warfarin (Coumadin), alter normal clotting factors and thus increase risk of haemorrhaging. Discontinued at least 48 hours before surgery. Aspirin is a commonly used medication that alters clotting mechanisms.
Anticonvulsants	Long-term use of certain anticonvulsants (e.g. phenytoin [Dilantin] and phenobarbitone) alters metabolism of anesthetic agents.
Antihypertensives	Antihypertensives, such as beta blockers and calcium channel blockers, interact with anaesthetic agents to cause bradycardia, hypotension, and impaired circulation. They inhibit synthesis and storage of norepinephrine in sympathetic nerve endings.
Corticosteroids	With prolonged use, corticosteroids, such as prednisone, cause adrenal atrophy, which reduces the body's ability to withstand stress. Before and during surgery, dosages are often temporarily increased.
Insulin	Clients' need for insulin changes after surgery. Stress response and intravenous (IV) administration of glucose solutions often increase dosage requirements after surgery. Decreased nutritional intake often decreases dosage requirements.
Diuretics	Diuretics such as furosemide (Lasix) potentiate electrolyte imbalances (particularly potassium) after surgery.
Nonsteroidal antiinflammatory drugs (NSAIDs)	NSAIDs (e.g. ibuprofen) inhibit platelet aggregation and prolong bleeding time, increasing susceptibility to postoperative bleeding.
Herbal therapies: ginger, gingko, ginseng	These herbal therapies have the ability to affect platelet activity and increase susceptibility to postoperative bleeding. Ginseng is reported to increase hypoglycaemia with insulin therapy.

(Potter & Perry 2008)

(Bryant et al 2003). Most commonly, if pre-medication is required it is administered orally, approximately 1 hour before transfer to theatre. The nurse should be familiar with common pre-medications, their purpose, side effects and contraindications. Any medication must be administered in accordance with nursing regulations and the employing agency's policy.

PREPARATION OF THE CLIENT IMMEDIATELY PRIOR TO SURGERY

Although preparation during the 1–2 hours preceding an operation may vary slightly depending on the individual and type of operation, preparation generally involves various standard procedures. These include:

- Measuring and documenting height and weight. Knowledge of the individual's weight (mass) enables drug dosages based on body weight to be calculated accurately. It is also useful for comparison as progress is monitored postoperatively, especially in relation to assessment of fluid balance status
- Measuring and documenting vital signs. Any deviation from previous results must be reported immediately and documented, as abnormalities may result in postponement of the operation. These preoperative measurements serve as a baseline for comparison as the individual's progress is monitored postoperatively
- Requesting the client to pass urine to prevent distension of the bladder during surgery. Particularly during abdominal or pelvic surgery, distension predisposes the bladder to trauma. The time the client last passes urine is documented on the preoperation form
- Urinalysis, which is generally performed and documented. Any abnormalities must be reported immediately. As the kidneys excrete most drugs from the body, any sign of kidney dysfunction is significant
- Ensuring that the individual is not wearing any nail polish, lipstick, talcum powder or other cosmetics that could interfere with assessment of skin colour (i.e. pallor and cyanosis) or circulatory and oxygen saturation status
- Jewellery, hairpins, prosthetic devices, spectacles, contact lenses or hearing aids are removed and stored safely. If diathermy is used during the operation, any metal object being worn could result in the passage of electrical current to the individual and, consequently, burns. Each health care agency has its own policy regarding the wearing of wedding rings; for example, a ring may be left on and secured in position with adhesive tape.
- Whether any dentures or plates are left in the client's mouth depends largely on the anaesthetist's instructions. Usually dentures are left in situ, but partial plates or bridges are removed before surgery, as they may be dislodged during endotracheal intubation. It is important to check the presence of any loose teeth for the same reason.
- General hygiene and comfort needs are attended to by ensuring that appropriate clothing is worn and assisting the client to dress if necessary. Generally a plain cotton open-back gown with tie-tapes is worn. A disposable paper cap is also worn to cover the client's hair, and some facilities also provide disposable paper undergarments worn under the gown. In some agencies a red identification band is worn if the client has any known allergies
- Checking that the client's identification bands (usually two) are correct and in situ. It is also important to check all documents that will accompany the client to the operating room.

Each health care facility has its own pre-operative forms and checklist. Usually the information to be entered includes:

- The client's full name, age and unit record (UR) number
- The operation to be performed
- Latest vital signs and weight
- Time the client last ate, drank and voided
- Results of urinalysis
- Whether any dentures, partial plates or any other prosthetic devices (e.g. pacemaker) are in situ
- Details of any specific skin preparation
- Details of any known allergies
- The client's informed consent
- Details of any medications withheld or administered on that day, including the pre-medication.

It is important to ensure that the RN has administered any prescribed preoperative medications. These are administered when all the other preparations have been completed and at the time ordered by the anaesthetist, such as 30–60 minutes before operation. After the medications have been administered the client is advised not to get out of bed, as the medication may cause drowsiness. As a safety measure, and with appropriate client explanation, the side rails on the bed may be raised, the call bell or signal device placed within easy reach, and the individual should be allowed to rest quietly.

In many paediatric units it is policy to apply a local anaesthetic patch to the skin on the back of both hands approximately 1 hour before the need to establish IV access. This is usually the application of a product called EMLA (eutectic mixture of local anaesthetic) that has the ability to penetrate unbroken skin (Bryant et al 2003).

Furniture in the room should be arranged so that the client can be transferred easily onto a trolley if this is the mode of transport; for example, moving the over-bed table and locker away from the bedside. Many agencies transfer clients to theatre on their beds, as this reduces the number of transfers for the client or the need for manual handling. Some facilities walk their able clients from day surgery or the ward to the operating suite.

TRANSFER TO THE OPERATING ROOM

When the theatre orderly or escort arrives, the nurse should assist with the transfer of the client to the operating theatre. The client's privacy and warmth are considered and they are made as comfortable as possible. It is usual policy in the acute-care setting that the side rails on the bed are raised to promote safety while the client is in transit, and the nurse accompanies the client from day surgery or the ward to the operating suite. The nurse must ensure that the relevant documents (medical and nursing history, test results, X-rays) are taken with the client to the operating suite. During transit the nurse should be close to, and have full view of, the client so that it is possible to observe them constantly and provide psychological support. On arrival at the operating suite, the nurse hands over the care of the client, and the appropriate documentation, to the receiving operating room staff, usually a nurse. Client identity is verified, both verbally and by identification band and medical records, the checklist is completed ensuring that the client has a valid consent with them as they enter the theatre complex.

INTRAOPERATIVE PERIOD

Perioperative nurses undertake a variety of roles within the operating suite these include the circulating (scout) nurse, instrument (scrub) nurse, anaesthetic nurse, and recovery room (PACU) nurse. The circulating nurse is responsible for the documentation and management of all accountable items opened onto the sterile field. The scout supports the instrument nurse by being aware of the requirements of the surgical team and makes certain all supplies are deposited on to the surgical field aseptically. The circulating nurse performs the surgical count with the instrument nurse, and undertakes other responsibilities including patient positioning, client safety issues, specimen collection, provision of equipment, and being the communication link between theatre staff and those outside. The role of circulating or instrument nurse may be undertaken by an EN or RN, however if the circulating nurse is an EN the instrument nurse must be an RN and vice versa.

The instrument nurse is the one who assumes primary responsibility and accountability for all items used during the surgical procedure. The instrument nurse sets up all sterile instruments and supplies, and hands instruments to the operating team anticipating their needs. Nursing practices and interventions in the intra-operative phase also include establishing personal contact and supporting the client emotionally in the highly technical environment of the operating room. Protocols relating to the promotion of individual safety are another area of paramount importance, as during surgery, and particularly under anaesthesia, clients are unable to protect themselves from many sources of possible harm.

All personnel who enter the theatre complex wear clean scrub outfits, hair covers and shoe covers, with further sterile gowns, gloves, masks and eye protection during procedures. Strict surgical asepsis is mandatory throughout the surgical area, and all persons in the operating room must be alert to possible contamination of sterile items. Staff must consider their responsibilities in relation to the spread of infection and restrict or modify working if they have an upper respiratory or skin infection (ACORN 2006). See Chapter 27 for further information on the control and prevention of infection, surgical scrub and surgical asepsis.

Anaesthetic and PACU nurses are often referred to as perianaesthesia nurses. The anaesthetic nurse provides primary support to the anaesthetist and the client immediately prior to the surgical procedure carrying out client assessment and preparation, assists the anaesthetist during intubation and the administration of the anaesthetic, helps during the operation and assists with waking the client from the anaesthetic. The anaesthetic nurse works under the direct supervision of the anaesthetist and is responsible for the preparation of the required equipment, monitoring and pharmacology. Immediately following the procedure the client is transferred to the PACU where they are cared for by the PACU/recovery room nurse. The PACU nurse is responsible for airway assessment and management, client observations, identification and prompt correct action of surgical or anaesthetic complications. Postoperative pain and nausea management, accurate documentation of care and administration of medication as ordered are also roles of the PACU nurse. All these roles work collaboratively together with the individual roles dependent upon each other to work as a multidisciplinary team that aims to provide evidence-based best practice and optimal client outcomes (ACORN 2007, Drain 2003).

The anaesthetic nurse will notify the DSU or the ward that theatre is ready for the client. The client is brought to a pre-operative holding bay or anaesthetic room where it is identified that they are the correct client, any allergies are highlighted, fasting status is determined and the consent form is checked. The anaesthetist will insert an intravenous (IV) cannula and may give the client some medication to relax them; they are then transferred into the operating room and onto the operating table. ECG, blood pressure and oxygen saturation monitoring is applied, the client is positioned, padding to prevent injury to nerves and to minimise pressure over bony prominences is strategically placed and safety straps secured to maintain the client's position. Draping and preparation for surgery commences, ensuring the correct operation site is prepared.

It is important that the client is correctly positioned according to the procedure being performed. Common positions used for surgery are:

- Supine — client is flat on their back, heel supports are generally used to prevent pressure on the individuals' heel and calves, most common surgical position
- Trendelenburg — supine with a head down tilt, generally implemented for lower abdominal surgery

- Reverse Trendelenburg — a head up tilt, used for head and neck, ear, nose and throat procedures
- Lithotomy — supine with the legs raised and feet placed in stirrups, the lower end of the table is removed, often used for gynaecology and lower bowel operations
- Lateral — used to position the client on their side, small gel pads and pillows are placed between the legs, restraint straps keep the legs secure; a pelvis support is attached to the table, usually in the region of the client's stomach; a lateral support is placed in the client's back and a gutter arm support is used for the arms. Common position for nephrectomy, thoracic and lumbar spine surgery.
- Prone — client is placed face down on their front, head positioned to one side, pillows placed under chest, sacrum and legs, the body is supported with straps and the arms are supported with boards. Usual placement for spinal procedures (Woodhead & Wicker 2005).

INDUCTION OF ANAESTHESIA

In most cases, an operative procedure requires some degree and type of anaesthesia, but not all procedures require a full general anaesthetic. There are different means by which anaesthesia can be achieved. Factors influencing the choice of anaesthetic include the nature of the surgery (length and complexity of operation), the client's status (pre-existing medical conditions), anatomical and physiological conditions, and to some degree client preference.

Anaesthetics can be classified as general anaesthetics, regional anaesthetics and local anaesthetics.

General anaesthetic

General anaesthesia promotes unconsciousness, absence of sensation, loss of reflexes and muscle relaxation. Administration is primarily by IV injection, inhalation, or a combination of both. The four components of general anaesthesia are amnesia, analgesia, muscle relaxation and unconsciousness. Ventilation during general anaesthetic is separated into spontaneous or controlled. Clients whose ventilation is controlled have usually been administered muscle relaxants.

The three phases of general anaesthetic are induction, maintenance and emergence.

1. Induction — begins when the anaesthetic agents are administered and ends when the client is ready for positioning, prepping or incision. Intubation occurs during this phase.
2. Maintenance — continues from the end point of induction until the procedure is nearly complete. This phase is sustained with titrated doses or continuous infusion of IV drugs, or inhalation of anaesthetic gas.
3. Emergence — begins when the individual starts to emerge from anaesthesia and ceases when the client is ready to be transferred from the operating room to PACU. Extubation is usually carried out during emergence.

Commonly used anaesthetic gases and drugs are shown in Table 44.5.

Regional anaesthetic

Regional anaesthesia is a form of local anaesthesia; it results in loss of sensation to an area, by blocking the conduction of nerve impulses to and from specific sites in the body. The anaesthetist injects an anaesthetic agent around nerves thereby anaesthetising the area those nerves supply. The effect is dependent on the type of nerve concerned. Motor nerves are less readily blocked as they are the largest fibres and their myelin sheath is the thickest. Sensory fibres are intermediate and the smallest fibres with minimal covering are the sympathetic and pain nerves which are the most easily blocked. With these methods of anaesthesia the client is often awake during the procedure, but the area targeted for surgery is without sensation.

With regional anaesthesia there is no loss of consciousness, therefore considerations should be made for the fact that the client can still feel pressure and hear sound. The nurse must be sensitive that the environment is quiet and therapeutic, no unnecessary inappropriate conversation regarding the client, their diagnosis or the procedure being performed. Dependent on the operation being performed the anaesthetist may administer mild sedation to relieve anxiety or dull the individual's awareness of their surroundings. Regional anaesthesia is administered by infiltration and local application, including:

- Spinal (intrathecal) anaesthesia: is an injection of local anaesthetic into the cerebrospinal fluid (CSF) within the subarachnoid space at the lumbar level. The extent of anaesthesia can be from the xiphoid process down to the feet. Distribution up or down of the anaesthetic agent is influenced by the amount of fluid injected, the speed at which it was injected and client positioning. Spinal anaesthesia is frequently used for surgical obstetrics, lower extremity, lower pelvic and lower abdominal procedures.
- Epidural anaesthesia: local anaesthetic is injected into the epidural space, via an inserted catheter allowing a continuous infusion or intermittent boluses to be delivered. Epidural anaesthesia is frequently used in obstetric procedures and for postoperative pain relief.
- Caudal block anaesthesia: injection of a local anaesthetic into the caudal (sacral) portion of the spinal canal
- Peripheral nerve block anaesthesia: injection of a local anaesthetic into a specific site, such as the brachial plexus, to block a group of sensory nerve fibres.

Local infiltration

Local infiltration anaesthesia is the injection of an anaesthetic solution into the tissues at the incision site. Loss of sensation occurs at a targeted site e.g. a skin lesion or

TABLE 44.5 | COMMONLY USED ANAESTHETIC GASES AND DRUGS

	Common uses	Advantages	Disadvantages
Inhalation Gases			
Air	Maintenance with O_2; laser surgery near airway	less support of combustion than N_2O	No anaesthetic qualities
Oxygen (O_2)	Essential for life	Can slightly increase O_2 available to tissues in low cardiac output states	Can cause retinopathy in premature infants
Nitrous oxide (N_2O)	Maintenance; frequently for induction	Rapid induction and recovery; additive effects to other anaesthetics	No relaxation; can depress myocardium
Desflurane	Maintenance in short cases	Rapid emergence; good relaxation; 0.02% metabolised	May cause transient increased HR and decreased BP, airway irritation; requires heated vapouriser
Isoflurane	Maintenance	Good relaxation	Increased HR; slightly Irritating odour
Sevoflurane	Induction and maintenance	Rapid induction and emergence, good relaxation; ~5% metabolised	Metabolite (compound A) is nephrotoxic in rats; effect in humans is unknown.
Opioid Analgesics			
Morphine sulphate	Perioperative pain; Pre-medication	Inexpensive; duration of action 4-5 hr; euphoria; Good cardiovascular stability.	Nausea and vomiting; histamine release; postural; decrease in BP
Alfentanil	Surgical analgesia in Ambulatory clients	Duration of action 0.5 hr; used as bolus or infusion	–
Fentanyl	Surgical analgesia; epidural infusion for postoperative analgesia	Good cardiovascular stability; duration of 0.5 hr	–
Remifentanil	0.25–1 mcg/kg/min infusion for surgical analgesia; small boluses for brief intense pain	Easily titratable; metabolised by blood and tissue esterases; short duration; good cardiovascular stability	Expensive; requires mixing
Depolarising muscle relaxants			
Succinylcholine	Intubation; short cases	Rapid onset; short duration	Requires refrigeration May cause fasciculations Postoperative myalgias and arrhythmias, increased serum potassium with burns, tissue trauma, paralysis and muscle diseases; slight histamine release.
Nondepolarising muscle relaxants – intermediate onset and duration			
Atracurium	Intubation; maintenance of relaxation	No significant cardiovascular or cumulative effects; good with renal failure	Requires refrigeration; slight histamine release
Cisatracurium	Intubation; maintenance of relaxation	Similar to atracurium	No histamine release
Mivacurium	Intubation; maintenance of relaxation	Short acting; rapid metabolism by plasma cholinesterase; used as bolus or infusion	Expensive in long cases
Rocuronium	Intubation; maintenance of relaxation	Rapid onset (dose-dependent); elimination via kidney and liver	Vagolytic; may increase HR
Vecuronium	Intubation; maintenance of relaxation	No significant cardiovascular or cumulative effects; no histamine release	Requires mixing

(Continued)

TABLE 44.5 | COMMONLY USED ANAESTHETIC GASES AND DRUGS—cont'd

	Common Uses	Advantages	Disadvantages
Nondepolarising muscle relaxants – longer onset and duration			
Pancuronium	Maintenance of relaxation	–	May cause increased HR and BP
Intravenous anaesthetics			
Diazepam	Amnesic; hypnotic preoperative medication	Good sedation	Prolonged duration
Ketamine	Induction; occasional maintenance (IV or IM)	Short acting, client maintains airway; good in small children and burns clients	Large doses may cause hallucinations and respiratory depression
Midazolam	Hypnotic, anxiolytic; sedation	Excellent amnesic; water soluble; (no pain with IV injection); short acting	Slower induction than thiopental
Propofol	Induction and maintenance; sedation with regional anaesthesia or MAC	Rapid onset; awakening in 4–8 min	May cause pain when injected
Thiopental	Induction	Induction	May cause laryngospasm.
Local anaesthetics			
Bupivicaine	Epidural, spinal or local infiltration	Good relaxation; long acting	Overdose can cause cardiac collapse
Anticholinergics			
Atropine	Block effects of acetylcoline; decreases vagal tone; reverse muscle relaxants; treat sinus bradicardia	Increased HR; suppresses salivation, bronchial and gastric secretions	Depresses sweating; may cause dry mouth, flushing dizziness, CNS symptoms
Glycopyrrolate	Similar to atropine	Slightly increases HR; does not cross blood–brain barrier; can increase gastric pH	Prolonged duration of effects
Cholinergic agent			
Neostigmine	Reverses effects of nondepolarising neuromuscular blocking agents	Prevents breakdown of acetylcholine by inhibiting acetylcholinesterase	–

(adapted from Rothrock 2007)

a wound requiring sutures. Local anaesthesia is commonly used for minor procedures in DSUs or doctors' surgeries. Surgeons may infiltrate local anaesthetic to an operative area to enhance postoperative pain relief.

Anaesthetic agents may also be applied topically, as a cream, spray or drops applied to the skin or mucous membranes. Common local anaesthetic agents for infiltration, injection or for topical use include lignocaine, bupivacaine and procaine (Crisp & Taylor 2005; Farrell 2003; Drain 2003).

POSTOPERATIVE CARE

After completion of the operation the client is transferred to PACU, which is located within the operating theatre complex. The client is accompanied by the anaesthetist who will hand over to the PACU nurse the client's general condition, the operation performed and the type of anaesthesia used for the procedure and any complications encountered during the surgery and anaesthesia. Immediate assessment of the client's airway, heart rate, respirations, temperature and oxygen saturations are performed and recorded and blood loss is noted. Once these initial observations have been made it is essential to systematically assess the client, either head to toe or by systems: central nervous system (CNS), cardiovascular system (CVS), respiratory system (Resp), gastrointestinal tract (GIT), urinary function, wounds, drain tubes, fluid management, skin integrity and pallor. The client is not transferred back to the ward until fully awake, conscious and alert, motor and sensory functions have begun to return, vital signs are stable, pain is controlled, and there are no immediate complications from the anaesthetic or surgery. A verbal handover is given by recovery-room staff to day-surgery or ward staff receiving the client, including any allergies, anaesthetic, analgesic and antiemetic drugs administered, details of the procedure, post operative orders, as well as any other information relating to the client's condition.

PREPARATION OF THE CLIENT'S DAY SURGERY OR WARD ENVIRONMENT

While a client is in the operating suite, the day surgery or ward nurse prepares the client's bed area ready for their return. As discussed earlier, in many agencies it is common practice for clients to be transferred to theatre on their beds. The remaining linen, including the top bedclothes, are folded into a pack and stored in the bed area, which enables them to be unfolded over the client quickly and with minimal disruption on return to the ward. Generally, one pillow is placed at the head of the bed, and the remaining pillows are placed in a convenient location in the room (see Chapter 29 for further information concerning making an operation or surgical bed). If the patient is a day surgery client they will return to the DSU on a trolley.

The furniture in the room should be arranged to provide easy access for equipment; for example, the bed may be positioned away from the wall, and the over-bed table and locker should be positioned away from the bedside. The equipment required in the room will depend on the type of operation that was performed, but generally includes:

- Oxygen and suction apparatus
- IV therapy pole
- Postoperative assessment forms (i.e. a chart for frequent observations)
- Equipment for assessing the client's vital signs
- Covered emesis bowl
- Hangers or holders for drainage bags.

IMMEDIATE GENERAL POSTOPERATIVE CARE AND ASSESSMENT

When clients are transferred back to the DSU or the ward, an appropriate position is selected depending on their condition and the type of operation. Initially, this is often a lateral position, to promote a clear airway while the client is still recovering from the anaesthetic. (Chapter 27 provides information on alternative positioning that may be necessary.) The upper bedclothes are placed over the client to promote maintenance of body temperature and comfort. If an IV infusion is in progress, the bag of solution is suspended on a pole or stand, and the infusion is assessed to determine whether it is flowing at the prescribed rate. The client's arm, in which the IV cannula is inserted, is positioned so that there is no obstruction to the tubing. Any drainage bags, such as urinary or wound-drainage bags, are placed in a holder or hanger and positioned to facilitate drainage by gravity.

Early postoperative assessment of the client involves monitoring and documenting:

- Level of consciousness — although some drowsiness and disorientation is normal after a general anaesthetic, it should be possible to rouse the individual by verbal stimuli or touch. Orientation to person, place and time gradually return. Inability to rouse the individual should be reported immediately. After local or regional anaesthesia, it is important to monitor for the return of normal sensation and movement to the anaesthetised area. Generalised restlessness should also be reported, as it may be due to a change in the level of consciousness; or may be associated with pain, discomfort, respiratory difficulties or haemorrhage. It is important during the early postoperative phase that details of the client's condition and diagnosis should not be inappropriately discussed, as the client may be able to hear, even if not fully awake
- Colour — report any significant changes to the individual skin colour (e.g. extremely pale or cyanosed)
- Vital signs — any deviation from previous readings of temperature, pulse, respirations, oxygen saturation or blood pressure is reported immediately. If ordered, oxygen therapy is administered and monitored
- Presence of discomfort or pain — as individuals recover from the effects of anaesthetic, they may begin to feel pain. The level of pain experienced may vary according to the type of anaesthesia used; for example, after a spinal anaesthetic the operative area may still feel relatively numb until several hours after the procedure. The presence of any discomfort or pain must be assessed and reported immediately so that appropriate pain-relieving measures can be implemented
- Wound dressing — in the immediate postoperative period, assessing for haemorrhage is a major responsibility of the nurse. Both the dressing and the bed linen under the client should be checked for evidence of haemorrhage; an increase in blood staining on the dressing, or a sudden increase of blood in a drainage tube or bag, must be reported immediately. Body cavities that have had a surgical pack inserted (i.e., nasal or vaginal packs) also require close observation
- Urinary catheters — if the client has an indwelling catheter, the nurse must monitor the urinary output carefully. Absence of, or decreased amount of, urinary output must be reported; similarly, any unexpected presence of blood in the urine needs to be documented and reported.

SUBSEQUENT POSTOPERATIVE CARE

The overall aim of the postoperative nursing phase is the return of the individual to an optimal level of functioning and independence. Postoperative care is directed towards assisting the client to meet specific needs for oxygenation and circulation of blood, comfort, nutrition and fluids, elimination, movement and exercise, hygiene, psychological support, protection and safety. The nursing care plan (see

Table 44.6) identifies the importance of continuously assessing vital signs and the need for early frequent detection of postoperative complications.

Assessing respiratory and circulatory needs

In the initial postoperative period, the frequency with which the individual's vital signs are monitored depends on their condition. Generally, vital signs are assessed and documented every 30 minutes for the first 4 hours, then 1-hourly for 4 hours, then every 2–4 hours if the condition is satisfactory. If the client's condition is unstable, observations may be monitored more frequently for a longer period of time. Assessment is also made of colour and breathing to observe for the manifestations of any respiratory tract complications. Mucus secretions can accumulate, leading to pneumonia, bronchitis or atelectasis. Throughout the postoperative recovery, the individual is also at risk of thrombophlebitis and pulmonary embolus. During this period deep breathing, coughing and if possible leg exercises and early ambulation are encouraged to decrease the possibility of the above complications occurring.

Comfort needs

Client comfort can be promoted by ensuring that a suitable position is assumed. Unless contraindicated, the individual is encouraged and assisted to assume a semi-upright position. This position promotes adequate lung expansion, and assists urinary or wound drainage by gravity. Pillows are arranged to provide adequate support, without restricting movement. If the client is unable to move independently, the nurse must assist the client to change position every 2–4 hours. Regular administration of analgesia and assessment of pain levels, the prevention of nausea, tension on the surgical wound and bladder distension will all help to provide client comfort. With adequate comfort and pain relief the individual is able to rest and perform postoperative activities and exercises, all of which act to enhance recovery.

Nutritional and fluid needs

Because of the effects of stress and general anaesthesia on the gastrointestinal tract, in the initial postoperative period the individual may experience nausea and/or vomiting and be unable to tolerate oral fluids or food. Food and fluids are generally withheld until normal gastrointestinal functioning has returned, as made evident by the presence of bowel sounds and the passing of flatus. Until this has occurred, the individual receives fluids and nutrients intravenously. In some instances eating and drinking are contraindicated for an extended period, or the individual may require extensive nutritive therapy to rebuild tissue after the trauma of surgery. In such cases, hyperalimentation using parenteral nutrition may be indicated (see Chapter 33). After minor or uncomplicated surgical procedures, clients may be able to tolerate sips of fluid within a short time. If sips of fluid are tolerated, and there are no contraindications, clients progress to free fluids, then to a normal diet. Day surgery

TABLE 44.6 | A POSTOPERATIVE CARE PLAN

Postoperative care plan				
Date	**Nursing diagnoses**	**Client outcomes**	**Nursing interventions for 24–48 hours after surgery**	**Signed**
	Respiratory depression related to anaesthesia and subsequent narcotic pain relief	Early detection of hypoventilation	Record respiratory rate (specify) and maintain clear airway Position client in accordance with postoperative orders/needs	
	Pain due to surgery	Pain to be of a level acceptable to the client	Perform pain assessment on return to ward and at regular intervals (e.g. each time vital signs are recorded) Report unrelieved pain to RN and monitor effects of analgesics administered Assist client to a more comfortable position Monitor PCA (patient-controlled analgesia)	
	Potential for wound infection due to surgical incision	Prevent infection and promote wound healing	Dressing to remain intact until (specify date) Redressing to be performed as ordered using aseptic technique Observe wound for signs of infection. Report indications of infection promptly Monitor temperature 4/24 and report elevation promptly	

(Crisp & Taylor 2005; Carpenito 2001; Heath 1995)

clients are encouraged to eat and drink once they are fully awake and can tolerate sips of water.

Elimination needs

Generally, early ambulation and the intake of adequate fluids stimulates micturition. Some individuals may experience difficulty in passing urine, for example due to pain or the embarrassment or difficulty of having to use a bedpan or urinal. It is important to observe urinary output on an ongoing basis. If retention of urine or inadequate emptying of the bladder occurs, it may be necessary for the client to have a urinary catheter inserted. The need for catheter insertion is based on data collected using bladder scanning techniques, and medical orders following consultation. To re-establish normal bowel function the client is encouraged to ambulate as soon as possible and to consume adequate fluids and dietary fibre, although, as described above, oral fluids and food are initially withheld until normal intestinal peristalsis returns.

Movement and exercise needs

Postoperative exercises are started soon after the client's return to the ward. The nurse should encourage deep breathing and coughing and leg exercises to be performed at 2–4 hourly intervals. These exercises are best continued until the individual is fully ambulant. Mobility and activity are gradually increased as the person's condition improves. Initially, postural hypotension and dizziness may be experienced when getting out of bed. Allowing the client to gradually raise their head position, then sit on the edge of the bed and dangle their legs, then after a few minutes assisting them to get out of bed slowly, generally reduces these symptoms (Christensen & Kockrow 2003). The individual should be encouraged to ambulate a little more each day and should be informed of the benefits of ambulation.

Ambulation:

- Facilitates deep breathing and so prevents respiratory complications
- Stimulates the circulation of blood, thus preventing vascular complications
- Improves muscle tone and strength
- Aids in the elimination of waste from the bladder and bowel
- Reduces the risk of skin breakdown and decubitus ulcer formation
- Improves morale.

Hygiene needs

Until the individual is able to fully attend to their own personal hygiene needs, the nurse assists. Once the client has recovered from the major effects of the anaesthetic, the face and hands are washed, hair is brushed and mouth care provided. The client is assisted to get dressed into their own nightwear, and any soiled or damp bed linen is changed. In the initial postoperative period when the client is not having any oral fluids, frequent mouth care should be provided preventing dryness, soreness or cracking of the tongue and lips. When able, the client is encouraged to resume responsibility for personal hygiene needs. The nurse may be required to assist with a shower or bath and should be available to supervise activities to promote safety.

Psychological needs

Psychological support is provided by keeping the client informed, allowing expression of concerns about progress, change of body image, impact of surgery on lifestyle; and by encouraging visits from family and friends. Self-esteem is enhanced with increasing independence and should be encouraged; by allowing resumption of responsibility for own personal care, without endangering safety or recovery, the client may feel more empowered. Whenever possible, the client should be given a choice in care and in timing of activities and events. It is important that the client understands the expected time-scale to full recovery and how any problems will be managed should they arise. All procedures and activities and their rationales should be fully explained.

The nurse may need to help the client and significant others to develop effective coping strategies. Coping methods may include:

- Obtaining additional information to deal with a situation more effectively
- Trying out various ways of solving a problem, to see which one is most helpful
- Talking over a problem with someone who has been in a similar situation
- Engaging in an activity that is relaxing and of interest, such as reading or listening to music.

Protection and safety needs

In the postoperative period the nurse must implement measures to protect the client from hazards in the environment. This is essential both initially, when conscious state may still be compromised and the ability to respond is diminished, and later, when changes in function may require individual adjustments when carrying out activities of daily living. (See Chapter 26 for further information about the safety and protection of clients.)

WOUND CARE

Care of a surgical wound is directed towards promoting healing and preventing infection. Wounds are described as healing by first, second or third intention:

- First intention healing occurs when wound edges are brought together; for example, a sutured surgical incision. Granulation tissue is not obvious
- Second intention healing occurs when wound edges cannot be brought together; for example, a gaping wound. Granulation tissue fills in the wound until re-epithelialisation takes place and a large scar results
- Third intention healing occurs when wound closure

is delayed for a few days so that an infected or contaminated wound can be debrided. Closure of contaminated wounds is usually delayed until all layers of wound tissue appear healthy, usually within 4–10 days (see Chapter 37 on wound healing).

Influences on wound healing

Healing is governed not only by the condition of a wound itself, but also by factors intrinsic to the individual, such as nutritional status. Healing is further influenced by the efficiency of blood circulation to the area. The most common causes of delayed healing of a surgical wound are poor circulation and infection. Healing is also delayed if the client's immune system is impaired; for example, advanced age, irradiation, autoimmune system disorders, or immunosuppressive drugs. External factors such as excessive strain on the incision, for example from inappropriate or overactivity, can delay union of wound edges. Poor circulation reduces the supply of oxygen and nutrients to the wound site; and the presence of infection, pus, or dead tissue in a wound inhibits complete healing (Marieb 2002).

Wound healing generally takes place within 7–10 days, although the time for normal healing depends on several factors:

- The extent of tissue damage
- The amount of stress and tension placed at the incision
- The extent to which the wound edges have been approximated
- The individual's age and general condition.

Promotion of healing

To promote healing, a range of general measures may be implemented. These include:

- Maintenance of adequate nutritional status. Provision of a diet that contains adequate kilojoules, protein, vitamins C and A, iron, and zinc
- Promoting adequate oxygenation of the tissues. Deep breathing and coughing exercises and early ambulation to promote full lung expansion will enhance oxygenation of the blood
- Encouraging adequate blood circulation to the area, promoting transport of substances required for healing and combating infection. Adequate blood volume can be maintained by ensuring sufficient fluid intake and a suitable level of exercise and mobility can stimulate circulation
- Restricting movement of the area in the early stages of healing. If strain is placed on a wound, the newly formed granulation tissue may tear. The surgical wound area should be stabilised, rested and supported.

Wound management

Surgical wounds are covered with specific dressings when the client returns to the ward. These dressings are usually left intact until the client is reviewed by the surgeon. If leakage appears on the original dressing it is important to reinforce the dressing and report and document the leakage immediately. If wound drainage is present and copious and potential exists for skin excoriation, a drainage bag or pouch may be placed over the wound to protect the skin. Before application of the pouch, an adhesive skin barrier such as a pectin wafer is placed on the surrounding skin. The pouch is placed over the draining area and secured to the barrier using gentle digital pressure. The principles of application and care relevant to a wound drainage pouch are similar to those that apply to stomal appliances. Several factors must be considered in the selection of surgical dressings, such as the client's skin condition, allergies, the type and site of the wound, the amount of wound exudate and the availability of various dressings.

Dressing changes

In relation to a closed surgical wound, when and how often dressings are changed depends on the surgeon's orders, the health care facility's protocol and on the type of dressing used. The ideal surgical wound has edges that are well approximated and secured, and tissue layers that have also been appropriately sutured. Often an adhesive film dressing with a central non-adherent pad (Airstrip, Cutifilm) will be used to cover a sutured incision. Client apprehension may be high at the time of initial dressing removal, and may be related to the size and appearance of the wound and issues concerning scarring. The nurse needs to provide appropriate support at this time. Once the original dressing has been removed and the wound inspected, it may be ordered that the wound remains uncovered, or perhaps that wound edges be given simple reinforcement and support with hypoallergenic strips of paper tape (Steristrips). If a dressing is to be changed, sterile equipment and aseptic techniques are used to prevent cross-infection, even though the wound has been surgically closed. (Guidelines for dressing changes using aseptic procedure are outlined in Chapter 37.)

Drainage tubes

At the time of the operation, the surgeon may place a drainage tube through a separate 'stab' incision near the principal wound. A drainage tube acts to promote healing by providing an exit for blood, serum, and debris that may otherwise accumulate and result in postoperative swelling, pain, or infection and abscess formation. The type of drainage tube inserted depends on the site and extent of the wound. A drainage system may be covered with an adhesive collection bag (i.e., non-suction drain), may be connected to intermittent suction, or may be a self-contained disposable drainage system that supplies its own vacuum suction.

When a non-suction drainage tube (e.g. Yates drain) is inserted, a sterile safety pin is usually passed through the tubing just above skin level to prevent the drainage from slipping back into the incision. A gauze dressing is placed between the pin and the skin. Alternatively, the drainage tube may be secured in position by one or two sutures. An absorbent dressing may be placed over the drainage tube to collect exudate, or a pouch or bag may be applied to the surrounding skin for drainage collection.

A closed-wound drainage system consists of tubing sutured at the skin edge and connected to a vacuum suction unit (e.g. Bellovac, Provac, Exudrain). The unit is always positioned below wound level to promote drainage by gravity. There should be no kinks in the system or excessive tension on the tubing. Using standard infection-control precautions (see Chapter 25), the container is emptied as necessary. The vacuum in the container needs to be re-established each time the container is emptied, following the manufacturer's instructions. An absorbent dressing may be used to protect the drain exit site. While the system is in situ, it is important to observe both the system and the client. Although it is important to observe the amount and nature of the drainage, it is also important to observe the client's pain levels in relation to the drainage tube, skin condition surrounding the tube, and to monitor the client's temperature for early signs of infection.

It is the nurse's role to observe and note the location of any drainage tubes, the character of drainage and, if there is a collection device, to measure and document the volume of the drainage. Any sudden change in the amount of drainage, or leakage at the tube entry site, should be reported, as this may indicate a blockage in the drainage tube or bleeding (Crisp & Taylor 2005). Client education regarding the drainage system and its workings is essential. The length of time a drain tube remains in situ depends on several factors, such as the nature of the surgery, the anatomical area involved, and the amount of drainage. It is expected that initial drainage is bloodstained (perhaps heavily), and that over subsequent days the drainage will become lighter and more serous.

Prior to removal of a non-suction drainage tube the nurse may be asked to rotate and shorten it a small amount each day for several days, preventing the body tissues becoming adhered to the tube, and to promote healing from beneath to the skin surface. The technique for shortening a tube should follow the employing agency's procedure manual. Suction drain tubes are removed without prior shortening. Removal of a drain tube involves removing all retaining sutures, rotating the tube, then steadily and gently withdrawing it minimising discomfort. If the tube is attached to a suction device, the nurse must discontinue suction before removal of the tube, as per agency policy or manufacturer's directions. Generally, suction is discontinued to avoid damaging the tissues as the tube is being withdrawn, and to decrease pain. The amount of total drainage postoperatively must be documented on the client's fluid balance chart and the time of removal should also be recorded.

Sutures and clips

When surgery has been completed, the operative area is closed in separate layers; that is organ, muscle, fat and skin. The wound edges are approximated and held together by sutures, clips or staples. Usually a single line of sutures or clips is sufficient for skin closure. In some instances, tension (large, reinforced) sutures are also required to ensure closure and to provide additional support for the wound. Suturing methods include intermittent and continuous. With intermittent (interrupted) suturing, the surgeon ties and cuts each individual suture. Continuous suturing is a series of sutures with only two knots; one at the beginning and one at the end of the suture line. The manner in which the suture crosses and penetrates the skin determines the method of removal (see Chapter 37 for the clinical guidelines relating to suture removal).

When healing has progressed well, sutures, clips and staples are removed usually within 7–10 days after insertion. However this is dependent on the area of the body involved and the vascularity of the area. The wound is checked for union of the edges before sutures or clips are removed. Sometimes alternate sutures or clips are removed one day, and the remaining removed the next day. The most important principle in suture removal is never to pull the visible portion of a suture through underlying tissue, as pulling the exposed portion of the suture through tissues may lead to infection. It is also important to ensure that all sutures have been removed, and that there is no opportunity for retention of suture material. The nurse may be required to perform this procedure if it is within the specified role and function and institutional policy permits.

Sutures are generally removed using a disposable sterile blade or stitch-cutter, and staples or clips are removed using a sterile staple extractor/remover. It is easiest to lift the suture at the knot, raise it up off the skin, and cut the suture as close to the skin as possible. Ensure safety with the stitch-cutter by cutting away from the client, and pull out the suture to the opposite side at which it was cut. Supporting the skin edges with forceps may be appropriate. It is not always necessary to cleanse or swab the suture line before suture removal. This is indicated if there is dried blood or exudate present or if sutures are hard to see. Cleansing the incision gently with gauze swabs and normal saline may be necessary after suture removal, if oozing has occurred as a result of the removal. Agency guidelines and standard precautions should always be followed when undertaking such procedures.

POSTOPERATIVE DISCOMFORTS AND POTENTIAL COMPLICATIONS

During the postoperative period the nurse must assess the individual for the manifestations of various discomforts associated with surgical intervention, and potential complications. The nursing care plan should include any actual and potential problems, the goals, objectives or expected outcomes of the planned interventions and nursing measures to prevent, minimise or manage them. The nurse must know how to prevent complications and recognise the onset of discomforts or complications. Any manifestations or changes must be reported immediately. Table 44.7 lists some postoperative discomforts and potential problems.

PREPARATION FOR DISCHARGE

Discharge planning commences in the preoperative phase and is continually reviewed throughout the postoperative period until the client is discharged from the health care facility. The nursing care plan during this time is developed and implemented with the ultimate goal of returning the individual to an optimal level of functioning and independence. Before discharge the person and/or their significant others should understand how to meet any specific postoperative needs. The nurse may be required to demonstrate any techniques that are to be performed at home, such as dressing changes. (See Chapter 26 for more detail on the discharge process.)

The nurse must ensure that the person knows how to care for any wound that is present, whether there are any dietary or activity restrictions, whether any special exercise program is to be followed, or if and how prescribed medications are to be administered. The person should be informed of the date and time to visit the surgeon for a postoperative check. It may be necessary to notify the domiciliary nursing service if the client requires ongoing assistance; for example, wound care.

The day surgery client is discharged once they have fully woken from anaesthetic, have tolerated diet and fluids and have voided. They are discharged into the care of a friend or family member, as they are unable to drive, drink alcohol, or be left alone for the next 24 hour period. The DSU nurse will contact the client the next day to follow up on their progress and answer any concerns they may have.

SUMMARY

Surgery is a form of intervention whereby the surgical team operates to remove, repair, reconstruct or replace body tissues or organs. Surgical procedures may be classified as elective, essential, emergency, diagnostic, exploratory, curative, palliative, major or minor. Surgery imposes physiological stress on all the body systems, and psychological stress on the client and their significant others. Perioperative nursing encompasses the provision of a wide variety of nursing functions related to the client undergoing surgery and throughout their perioperative experience. Preoperative care is directed towards ensuring that the individual is in the best physical and psychological condition possible to undergo surgery. Preoperative care involves providing information, teaching activities, physical examination of the individual, the performance of laboratory tests and diagnostic studies, checking that informed consent has been obtained, and preparing the individual physically and psychologically.

The types of anaesthetic used during surgery are classified as general, regional or local. General anaesthetic agents are administered intravenously or by inhalation and promote unconsciousness, analgesia, amnesia and muscle relaxation. Local, or regional, anaesthetic agents are administered through infiltration or by topical application; their action blocks the conduction of nerve impulses to and from specific sites in the body.

Postoperative care includes: the immediate care of the client emerging from anaesthetic; the preparation of each client for their return to the ward or DSU; immediate assessment of the client's condition, and assisting clients to meet their needs for oxygen and blood circulation; comfort, nutrition and fluids, elimination, movement and exercise, hygiene, psychological support, protection and safety. Care of a surgical wound is directed towards promoting healing and preventing infection. Wound management may involve dressing the wound, care and removal of any drainage tubes, and removing sutures or clips. Throughout the post-operative period the client is prepared for discharge with the ultimate goal of returning to an optimal level of wellness, functioning and independence.

REVIEW EXERCISES

1. State five different reasons for surgery.
2. What are four significant factors that can affect the degree of risk in a client facing major surgery?
3. Identify six possible psychological responses that you, the EN, may find in a client with diabetes who is facing a below-knee amputation of their left leg.
4. Outline what is involved in the preoperative preparation of a surgical client and identify 10 items on the preoperative form that you should check.
5. Identify three types of anaesthesia.
6. State what action you would take if a client's surgical wound dressing was damp with blood.
7. State what action you would take if 6 hours after returning to the ward after surgery, a client's urinary catheter drainage was 20 mL.

CRITICAL THINKING EXERCISES

1. Mrs Schofield, an otherwise well 85-year-old woman, is admitted after a fall for repair of a fractured hip. Outline the possible postoperative complications that may be seen in the older client undergoing this type of surgery and what you, as an EN, can do to help minimise the risks of complications occurring with Mrs Schofield. Identify the discomforts and difficulties Mrs Schofield is likely to experience in the first 24 hours after surgery, and outline the nursing interventions you will implement to assist her.
2. You are asked to prepare a room for the return of a client from surgery after an abdominal hysterectomy. The client will have IV therapy and may have a urinary catheter and a wound drain in situ.
   (a) What supplies do you need?
   (b) How would you arrange the room?
   (c) When the client returns to the ward, how often will you need to take vital signs?

TABLE 44.7 | POSTOPERATIVE DISCOMFORTS AND POTENTIAL PROBLEMS

Condition	Manifestations	Causes	Prevention	Management
Nausea and/or vomiting	Pale, cool, damp skin. Sensation leading to the urge to vomit. Vomiting	Effects of anaesthetic agents, inadequate preoperative preparation, apprehension, sensitivity to medications	Adequate preoperative preparation (e.g. fasting; withholding oral fluids and food until gastrointestinal function has returned)	Withholding oral fluids and food, administering antiemetic medications, promotion of physical and psychological comfort
Abdominal distension	Sharp abdominal pains, swollen abdomen, inability to pass flatus	Increased production of gas in the intestines and reduced peristalsis, causing stasis of the bowel contents	Early ambulation	Encouraging ambulation; passage of a rectal tube to release flatus
Paralytic ileus	Abdominal pain and/or distension, no passage of flatus, nausea and vomiting	Absence of intestinal peristalsis related to the trauma of surgery, especially handling during bowel surgery	Withholding oral fluids and food until normal gastrointestinal function has returned	Insertion of nasogastric tube and aspiration of gastric contents; withholding of all oral fluids and food; administration of fluids intravenously; early mobility as able
Urinary retention	Suprapubic discomfort or pain, suprapubic distension, inability to void; bladder ultrasound confirms urinary volume	Pain, micturition reflex depressed by anaesthetic agents (especially spinal or epidural), anxiety or fear of pain	Early ambulation, relief of anxiety and pain	Encourage increasing ambulation; assistance to assume a natural voiding position; providing sensory stimulation (e.g. the sound of running water); ensure adequate fluid intake; catheterisation if other measures fail
Constipation	Abdominal discomfort and distension, 'gas' pains, nausea	Disruption of normal diet; reduced mobility; reduced fluid intake; depressive effects of anaesthetic agents and/or medications, especially narcotics, including codeine	Early ambulation, return to diet high in fibre as soon as possible, ensure adequate fluid intake	Increase dietary fibre and fluid intake, encourage increasing ambulation, administration of stool-softeners or rectal suppositories if necessary
Pain	Restlessness, 'guarding' the wound, verbal expression of pain, pale damp skin, rapid pulse	Tissue trauma, anxiety	Provide adequate analgesia, promote physical and psychological comfort	Provide psychological support; promote physical comfort, i.e., positioning; administer adequate analgesic medications
Shock	Hypotension; weak rapid pulse; restlessness; pale, cool damp skin; diminished urinary output	Reduction in the volume of circulating blood, physiological reaction to trauma	Avoid and relieve pain and fear, prevent reduction of circulating blood volume	Restoration of blood volume to normal, relieve pain and/or anxiety, administer oxygen, administer prescribed medications, maintain normal body temperature, place the individual in the recumbent position, possibly elevate feet

(Continued)

TABLE 44.7 | POSTOPERATIVE DISCOMFORTS AND POTENTIAL PROBLEMS—cont'd				
Condition	**Manifestations**	**Causes**	**Prevention**	**Management**
Haemorrhage (a) reactionary	Bleeding (obvious or concealed) within the first 24 hours after surgery; manifestations of shock	Dislodgement of clots from the cut ends of small blood vessels, or displacement of a ligature from a large blood vessel, as the blood pressure returns to normal		Arrest the bleeding. Combat shock. Individual may need to return to the operating room to have the haemorrhage arrested
Haemorrhage (b) secondary	Bleeding that occurs 7–10 days after the operation	Infection that weakens blood clots or erodes blood vessel walls	Prevent infection	Treat infection, arrest the bleeding, combat shock
Hypoxia	Tachycardia, tachypnoea, pallor or cyanosis, lethargy and decreased responsiveness, confusion, agitation	Ventilations depressed by anaesthetic agents or medications, resulting in poor oxygenation of the blood, airway obstruction	Maintain a clear airway, promote adequate lung ventilation, administer oxygen if necessary, monitor vital signs frequently	Promote adequate oxygenation and tissue perfusion
Atelectasis (lung collapse)	Diminished breath sounds, increasing dyspnoea, pyrexia	Collapse of a portion of the lung due to obstruction of part of the bronchial tree, (e.g. a plug of mucus or inhaled secretions or vomitus)	Maintain a clear airway, encourage regular deep breathing and coughing exercises, early ambulation	Promote adequate lung expansion, administer oxygen if necessary, administer prescribed medications
Pneumonia	Dyspnoea and cyanosis, pyrexia, tachycardia, limited chest expansion on the affected side(s)	Accumulation of secretions in the lung(s)	Maintain a clear airway, encourage regular deep breathing and coughing exercises, incentive spirometry, early ambulation	Promote adequate lung expansion, administer oxygen if necessary, administer prescribed medications
Thrombophlebitis	Calf tenderness; pain in the leg, perhaps increased when the foot is dorsiflexed; oedema and inflammation of the leg; pyrexia	Venous stasis related to inadequate mobility, reduced volume of circulating blood or damage to the veins by pressure or injury	Encourage leg and foot exercises; early ambulation, and use of antiembolic stockings; avoid pressure on back of legs, i.e., no crossing legs; administration of prescribed anticoagulants; ensure adequate fluid intake	Anticoagulant therapy, bed rest with legs elevated, antiembolic stockings applied, perhaps administration of fibrinolytic substances
Pulmonary embolism	Sudden onset of dyspnoea, severe chest pain, and cyanosis; urgent desire to defecate; sudden circulatory collapse and death	Blockage of one of the pulmonary arteries by a blood clot, air or fat	Prevent the development of deep vein thrombosis, administration of prescribed anticoagulants, maintain normal blood volume	Administer oxygen and prescribed medications (anticoagulants), emergency resuscitation if required, emergency embolectomy may be performed

TABLE 44.7 | POSTOPERATIVE DISCOMFORTS AND POTENTIAL PROBLEMS—cont'd

Condition	Manifestations	Causes	Prevention	Management
Wound infection	Pain, tenderness, redness and swelling around the wound, purulent wound discharge, pyrexia, tachycardia	Invasion of the wound by pathogenic microorganisms	Practise aseptic techniques, using sterile equipment	Administer prescribed medications (e.g. antibiotics, analgesics; prevent cross-infection)
Wound dehiscence (breakdown or rupture of wound closure)	Leakage of haemoserous fluid from the wound, separation of wound edges, with appearance of loops of intestine at abdominal wound surface	Poor tissue healing, which may be related to malnutrition, obesity, anaemia, wound infection, premature removal of sutures or clips, or stress on the unhealed incision (via excessive coughing or straining)	Prevention, management of malnutrition and anaemia, delay removal of sutures and clips until there is good union of wound edges, avoid stress on incision	Combat shock; cover wound with sterile moist saline dressing; do not attempt to reinsert intestinal loops; provide psychological support; prepare the individual for return to theatre

(d) What else will you assess? How often will you conduct these other assessments?

3. Identify the preoperative information and teaching you would provide for a client who is having elective endoscopic surgery to remove his gall bladder (cholecystectomy).

REFERENCES AND FURTHER READING

Anderson K, Anderson L, Glanze (1997) *Mosby's Medical, Nursing, and Allied Health Dictionary*, 5th edn. Mosby, London

Australian College of Operating Room Nurses (2006) *ACORN Standards for Perioperative Nursing*. ACORN, Adelaide

Australian Day Surgery Council (2004) *Day Surgery in Australia: Report and Recommendations of the Australian Day Surgery Council of Royal Australasian College of Surgeons, Australian and New Zealand College of Anaesthetists and the Australian Society of Anaesthetists.* Online. Available: www.surgeons.org/content/NavigationMenu/FellowshipandStandards/AustraliaDaySurgeryCouncil/Day [accessed 17 October 2007]

Brown F (2002) Enrolled Nurse Instrument Nurse: Why Not? *ACORN Journal* 15(4): 23

Bryant B, Knights K, Salerno E (2003) *Pharmacology for Health Professionals*. Elsevier, Sydney

Carpenito L (2001) *Handbook of Nursing Diagnosis*. Lippincott, Williams and Wilkins, Philadelphia

Christensen B, Kockrow E (2003) *Adult Health Nursing*, 4th edn. Mosby, St Louis

Crisp J, Taylor C (eds) (2005) *Potter & Perry's Fundamentals of Nursing*, 2nd edn. Elsevier Mosby, Sydney

Department of Human Services (2005) *Elective Surgery Access Policy*. Thaker Print, Blackburn Victoria

Drain C (2003) *Perianaesthesia Nursing A Critical Approach*, 4th edn. Saunders, St Louis

Farrell M (2003) *Smelrzer & Bare's Textbook of Medical Surgical Nursing*, Australian and New Zealand edn. Lippincott, Williams and Wilkins: Philadelphia

Hamlin L (2006) Setting the Standard: The Role of the Australian College of Operating Room Nurses — Part 1. *ACORN Journal* 19(1): 29–36

Heath HBM (1995) *Potter and Perry's Foundations in Nursing Theory and Practice*. Mosby, London

Joanna Briggs Institute (2000) Knowledge Retention from Pre-operative Patient Information. *Best Practice Information Sheet*, 4(6). Blackwell Science, Asia

—— (2003) *The Impact of Preoperative Hair Removal on Surgical Site Infection*. Best Practice Information Sheet, 7(2). Blackwell Science, Asia

Marieb E (2002) *Human Anatomy and Physiology*, 5th edn. Benjamin Cummings, San Francisco

McGarvey H, Charmbers M, Boore J (2000) Development and definition of the role of the operating department nurse: a review. *Journal of Advanced Nursing*, 32(5): 1092–1100

Potter PA, Perry AG (2005) *Fundamentals of Nursing*, 6th edn. Mosby, St Louis

—— (2008) *Fundamentals of Nursing*, 7th edn. Mosby, St Louis

Potter PA, Perry AG (2008) *Fundamentals of Nursing*, 7th edn. Mosby, St Louis

Rothrock J (2007) *Alexander's Care of the Patient in Surgery*,13th edn. Mosby Elsevier, St Louis

Simpson P, Popat M *Understanding Anaesthesia*, 4th edn. Elsevier Butterworth Heinemann, London

Woohhead K, Wicker P (2005) *A Textbook of Perioperative Care*. Elsevier Churchill Livingstone, Edinburgh

Chapter 45
MENTAL HEALTH

OBJECTIVES

- Define the key terms/concepts
- Understand the continuum of mental health and mental illness
- Identify factors that influence the development of mental health
- Reflect on the causes and impact of stigma on people with mental illness
- Understand the roles of the mental health nurse and the mental health team
- Gain an overview of the care issues involved when clients experience anxiety, depression, aggressive, self-destructive, hyperactive or confused behaviour
- Become aware of some of the basic legal and ethical issues in the field of mental health nursing

KEY TERMS/CONCEPTS

constructive coping mechanisms
deinstitutionalisation
destructive coping mechanisms
empowerment
mental health
mental illness
myths
self-concept
stigma
stress
theoretical models

CHAPTER FOCUS

Mental health (psychiatric) nursing is a specialised field of nursing. A variety of educational programs is aimed at preparing nurses to work specifically and effectively with clients who have mental health disorders. A nurse who has not undertaken a course specific to mental health nursing may be required to assist in caring for a client with a mental illness. The nurse may be required to work in a psychiatric unit or ward within a general hospital, or to assist in caring for a client who has been admitted to a general medical or surgical ward with a physical illness but has a concurrent mental health problem. It is therefore important that every nurse has a basic understanding of mental health, mental illness, and the principles of care related to clients who are experiencing a disturbance in mental wellbeing. It is not the aim of this chapter to provide the reader with comprehensive knowledge and skills to care for clients with mental health disorders. Rather, this chapter aims to introduce nurses to the basic concepts of mental health nursing, some of the theoretical frameworks that underpin psychiatric care and to raise awareness of some legal and ethical issues that confront mental health nurses. The texts and online resources listed at the end of this chapter are sources of more detailed information.

LIVED EXPERIENCE

It was like being down in a deep black pit. When the nurses told me things would get better I didn't believe them. But I did get better and now I know the warning signs and I have been helped to gain skills that I can use to stop me going deep into that pit ever again. I will always be prone to depression but I can control my negative thinking now. I just think it was such a waste that I had depression for so many years before I was empowered to control it.

Jason, diagnosed with clinical depression at age 39

Perhaps the most important aspect of understanding mental illness is being able to define the difference between mental illness and mental health. This first section aims to help nurses gain an understanding of mental health and mental illness and the factors that impact on both.

CONCEPTS OF MENTAL HEALTH AND MENTAL ILLNESS

WHAT IS MENTAL HEALTH?

The concept of mental health is difficult to define, as mental health is much more complex than merely the absence of a mental illness. There are numerous definitions of what constitutes mental health. It has been defined as a state in which people are able to cope with, and adjust to, the recurrent stresses of everyday living in an acceptable way (Watkins 2001). It has also been defined as a satisfactory adjustment to one's life stage and situation (Ebersole & Hess 2001), and it has been defined as relating to feelings of happiness, contentment and personal satisfaction with life's achievements, as well as with feelings of optimism and hope (Fontaine & Fletcher 1999; Stuart & Laraia 2001). For most people the feelings associated with mental health will be present sometimes and not others and will vary in intensity at different times. According to this view, then, mental health is a state that can change frequently and that can fluctuate according to specific circumstances. Ebersole & Hess (1985) capture the concept of fluctuation in this definition:

> Mental health is like a violin with strings of interaction, behaviour, affect (mood) and intellect. All of this together may produce a pleasant or stimulating melody, or they may be discordant and irritating. The tune constantly changes. No one is entirely mentally unhealthy and no one is fully mentally healthy at all times.

Some attributes considered to be indicators of mental health can be assessed by a mental health nurse. These include the person having:

- A positive self-concept and a sense of purpose in life
- Ability to laugh and feel pleasure
- Ability to form relationships, to love and feel loved
- Ability to feel empathy towards others
- Ability to be creative and productive
- Capacity to cope with conflicting emotions
- Ability to live without undue fear, guilt or anxiety
- Willingness to accept responsibility for own actions
- Feeling and being in control of own behaviour
- Ability to think clearly, use good judgment and reason logically
- Ability to have an accurate perception of reality (Varcarolis 2006).

Figure 45.1 illustrates some of the characteristics of mental health.

DEVELOPMENT OF MENTAL HEALTH

According to Shives (2005) the factors that influence the development of mental health relate to three main areas: inherited characteristics, nurturing during childhood and life circumstances.

Inherited characteristics

It is believed by some theorists that the ability to maintain a mentally healthy and positive outlook on life is in part connected to a person's genetic make-up, just as inherited defective genes are thought to predispose particular people to illnesses such as schizophrenia and depression.

Nurturing during childhood

Nurturing during childhood relates primarily to the relationships that develop between children, their parents and their siblings. It is thought that positive relationships, those that promote feelings of being loved, secure and accepted, facilitate the development of children into mature and mentally healthy adults. It is thought that negative relationships may result when children experience maternal deprivation, parental rejection, serious sibling rivalry and early communication failures, are more likely to result in a poor sense of self-worth and a lower level of mental health (Shives 2005). The quest for a sense of self begins in childhood; children who have positive nurturing experiences are more likely to have a stronger sense of identity than those who have negative nurturing experiences (Watkins 2001).

Life circumstances

Life experiences can influence mental health from birth onwards. Positive life experiences include pleasurable times and success at school and with friends, a good job, financial security and good physical health. Negative experiences include poverty, poor physical health, unemployment and unsuccessful personal relationships (Shives 2005).

Different people will react to childhood experiences and life circumstances in different ways. Some, despite negative circumstances, will develop positive strategies for coping and will not become mentally ill. Generally it is people who have not achieved a strong sense of identity who are more prone to mental illness (Watkins 2001). Perhaps this is most clearly understood when considering the mental health of Indigenous populations. It is not difficult to imagine how the effects of colonisation, the removal of children from their families, the loss of traditional lifestyle and cultural practices and the resulting social disruption may impact negatively on mental wellbeing. It is generally understood that the difficulties involved in belonging and adjusting to two different cultural contexts can make it difficult to establish a strong sense of identity. The difficulties faced by Indigenous people have led to some serious mental health concerns. For example, there are worrying levels of depression, substance misuse, self-harm, harm to others and suicide in Aboriginal people in Australia that are at higher rates than in the non-Indigenous population (Australian Bureau of Statistics [ABS] and Australian Institute of Health and Welfare [AIHW] 2003).

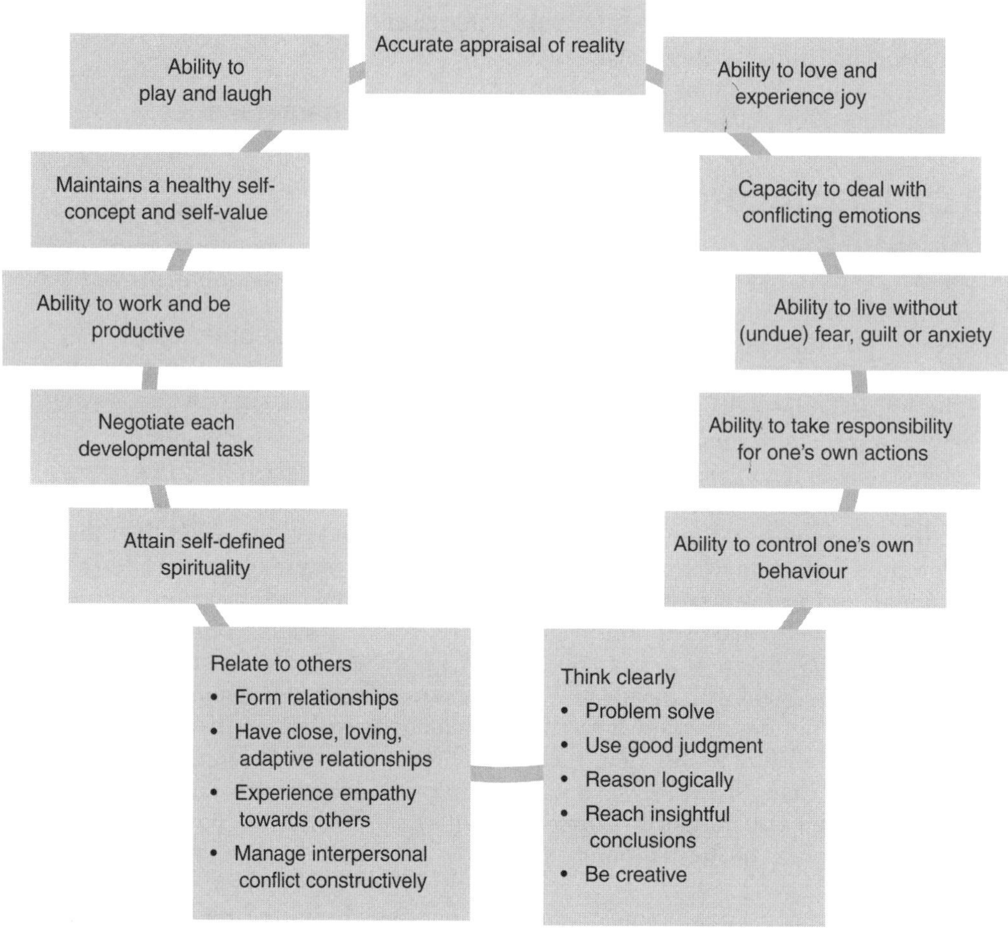

Figure 45.1 | Characteristics of mental health *(Varcarolis 2006)*

Nurses working with Indigenous people can better empathise and not negatively judge behavioural signs of mental ill-health if they recognise that it often stems from deep mental anguish and spiritual sorrow relating to the effects of European invasion (Brown 2001).

WHAT IS MENTAL ILLNESS?

Just as it is difficult to arrive at a precise definition of mental health, so too is it difficult to succinctly define mental illness because it is often related to what a given society considers is normal or acceptable behaviour and, as with mental health, mental illness is a matter of degree.

What society considers is normal

People tend to evaluate the behaviour of others based on their own social, cultural, ethical and behavioural standards. Therefore, behaviour that is regarded by one person as acceptable and normal may be perceived by another person as totally unacceptable. In addition, what is accepted as normal in a society may change over time. For example, homosexuality was at one time considered a diagnosable clinical mental disorder (Stevens 2001). When a person's behaviour is in question it is appropriate to ask 'Who is qualified to decide whether this behaviour is acceptable or not?' and 'What is the meaning and relevance of this behaviour in relation to the context in which it is occurring and to the person's society, religion and culture?'

In every society and cultural group there are different interpretations of certain behaviours and events. For example, in Western psychiatric terms, visual or auditory hallucination (people seeing or hearing things that no one else does) are viewed as abnormal and a sign of mental illness, whereas in some cultures these happenings are viewed as experiences of symbolic and spiritual importance and those experiencing them may be revered as visionaries as opposed to being perceived as mentally ill (Varcarolis 2006; Fontaine & Fletcher 1999).

A matter of degree

Anxiety, fear, anger, sadness and the need to be alone are feelings commonly identified in mental illness but they are normal feelings experienced at different levels of intensity by most people at various times. Depending on the intensity of the emotions, people may not feel as mentally healthy as they do at other times but will not necessarily be classified as mentally ill. It is when the feelings are exaggerated and extend over longer periods of time than deemed normal that the person is likely to seek professional help and be diagnosed as having a mental illness. For example, a diagnosis of a depressive disorder is likely when sadness or feelings of being 'down in the dumps' become deep, long-lasting feelings of despair that the person cannot escape from without professional help. Mental illness or mental disorder are therefore terms used to designate changes from normal mental functioning that are sufficient to become, and be diagnosed as, a clinical disorder (Weir & Oei 1996). Broadly, mental illness can be defined as a state in which an individual exhibits disturbances of emotions, thinking and/or action, but it can be defined in a multitude of ways. Clinical Interest Box 45.1 provides a range of definitions of mental illness.

CLINICAL INTEREST BOX 45.1
Definitions of mental illness

- Mental illness is a term that refers to all the different types of mental disorders. These include disorders of thought, mood or behaviour that cause distress and result in a reduced ability to function psychologically, socially, occupationally or interpersonally (Mayo Foundation for Medical Education and Research 2002)
- A disease that causes mild to severe disturbances in thought and/or behaviour, resulting in an inability to cope with life's ordinary demands and routines (National Mental Health Association [USA] 2008)
- A disorder causing abnormal behaviour more often than in most people (Shives 2005)
- Psychopathology exhibiting frequent irresponsibility, the inability to cope, being at odds with society and an inaccurate perception of reality (Shives 2005)
- The absolute absence or constant presence of a specific behaviour that has social implications regarding its acceptance (Shives 2005)
- The American Psychiatric Association's Diagnostic and Statistical Manual of Mental Disorders (DSM) is a classification system for mental illness. In the fourth edition (DSM-IV), mental illness is defined as being a clinically significant behaviour or psychological syndrome or pattern that occurs in an individual and that is associated with present distress (e.g. painful symptom) or disability (i.e. impairment in one or more areas of functioning) or with a significantly increased risk of suffering death, pain, disability, or an important loss of freedom. In addition, this syndrome or pattern must not be merely an expectable culturally sanctioned response to a particular event, for example, the death of a loved one. Whatever its original cause, it must currently be considered a manifestation of a behavioural, psychological or biological dysfunction in the individual. Neither deviant behaviour (e.g. political, religious or sexual) nor conflicts that are primarily between the individual and the society are mental disorders unless the deviance or conflict is a symptom of a dysfunction in the individual, as described above (American Psychiatric Association 2002)

There is no clear line that divides mental health from mental illness; the two grade into one another. Table 45.1 provides some areas of comparison between the two but it should be noted that, while these are general traits that mentally healthy or mentally ill people tend to share, different types of mental illness manifest with different effects and with different levels of intensity. In addition, mentally healthy people may experience more than one type of mental dysfunction at different periods in their lives.

Symptoms of mental illness occur on a continuum and range from minimal to severe. A person usually receives a diagnosis of having a mental illness when the level of mental distress causes them to seek professional help or when others in society perceive that they need professional psychiatric help. It is important to recognise that, in relation to the differences between mental health and mental illness, there is a 'grey' area into which all individuals may enter from time to time. Those with a severe and long-term psychiatric disorder may dip back into relative mental health and reality-based living for a while and, similarly, sometimes the stresses of everyday living are so overwhelming that the most well-adjusted 'normal' person may experience marked irrational thoughts, feelings and actions. Therefore, as in the case of physical illness such as diabetes, heart disease or cancer, anyone can develop a mental illness. A mental illness is not the fault of the person affected, and the cause may be related to a combination of biological, psychological and sociocultural factors.

SIGNS AND SYMPTOMS OF MENTAL ILLNESS

Symptoms of mental illness include changes in personal habits, social withdrawal and changes in mood and thinking. While particular symptoms occur with specific disorders, there are warning signs that indicate the presence of a mental health problem. Clinical Interest Box 45.2 provides examples of early warning symptoms of mental illness that may occur in children, adolescents and adults. (For details concerning the symptoms associated with specific disorders, refer to texts dedicated to mental health or psychiatric nursing such as those listed at the end of this chapter.)

WHO IS MOST AT RISK OF DEVELOPING A MENTAL ILLNESS?

Anyone can develop a mental illness but some groups of people in society are particularly at risk. Clinical Interest Box 45.3 identifies groups of people at greater risk of mental illness.

Many people from all age groups and of different social, educational and cultural backgrounds cope with highly stressful events and accumulative stressors. (Factors relating to the ability to cope with stress are described and discussed in Chapter 13.)

TABLE 45.1 | AREAS OF COMPARISON BETWEEN MENTAL HEALTH AND MENTAL ILLNESS*

Attribute	The mentally healthy person	The mentally ill person
Self-concept	Accepting of self and others. Able to develop talents and potential to fullest extent Adequately in touch with self and able to use the personal resources identified Acknowledges personal strengths and limitations	Poor self-image, low sense of self-worth and unable to recognise talents, so cannot achieve personal potential Lacks confidence and feels inadequate Tends not to recognise personal strengths and limitations
Relationships	Able to form close, meaningful and lasting relationships. Can communicate emotions and can give and receive Can accept authority Can share with people and grow from the experiences These factors often mean the presence of a strong social support network that aids coping in times of stress	Inability to cope with stress can result in disruption, disorganisation, inappropriate responses and unacceptable behaviour that make it difficult to meet the expectations of others in work or social environments. This means that there may be an inability to establish or maintain meaningful relationships. These factors may result in a limited social support network
Outlook on life	Optimistic and positive view, sense of purpose and satisfaction	Tends to a pessimistic negative view of present and future
Coping and adaptation	Able to tolerate stress and return to normal functioning after stressful events. Can cope with feelings such as frustration and aggression without becoming overwhelmed	Can feel overwhelmed by even minor levels of stress and may react with maladaptive behaviour
Judgment/decision making	Uses sound judgment to make decisions and is able to problem solve	May display poor judgment and avoid problems rather than attempting to solve them
Characteristics/traits	Can delay gratification	May feel an urgency to have personal wants and needs met immediately and may demand immediate gratification
Level of functioning	Accepts responsibility for own actions Can function effectively and independently	May act irresponsibly, be unable to accept responsibility for own actions and may blame others for outcomes May exhibit dependency needs because of feeling inadequate
Perceptions	Able to differentiate between what is imagined and what is real because can test assumptions by considered thought. Can change perceptions in light of new information	May be unable to perceive reality

(Shives 2005; Stuart & Laraia 2001; Varcarolis 2006)
*It should be noted that these are general points only. Different types of mental illness manifest with different effects and, while there are traits that mentally healthy people tend to share, many mentally healthy people may experience several areas of dysfunction at different periods in their lives. Mental illness may occur as a temporary inability to cope; it may occur episodically with long periods of mental health in between; or it may occur as a chronic condition that is constantly present.

CLASSIFICATION OF MENTAL DISORDERS

There are more than 200 classified forms of mental illness. These include:

- Cognitive disorders (e.g. dementia, delirium)
- Substance-related disorders (e.g. alcohol abuse or dependence, drug abuse or dependence)
- Anxiety disorders (e.g. phobias, panic disorder, obsessive disorder)
- Schizophrenia and other psychotic disorders (e.g. paranoid or catatonic-type schizophrenia)
- Mood disorders (e.g. depression, bipolar disorder [mixed mood])
- Personality disorders (e.g. antisocial personality disorder, dependent personality disorder)
- Sexual and gender identity disorders
- Eating disorders
- Sleep disorders
- Impulse-control disorders.

(Refer to mental health, psychiatric nursing texts for more information concerning specific psychiatric disorders.)

MEDICAL DIAGNOSES

The American Psychiatric Association's *Diagnostic and Statistical Manual of Mental Disorders (DSM)* is a respected and influential classification system under which a

CLINICAL INTEREST BOX 45.2
Warning signs and symptoms of mental illness

People may have one or two of these or other symptoms at any one time. This does not necessarily mean there is cause for alarm, but it is advisable they be assessed professionally. A combination of multiple symptoms is a strong signal that professional assessment and help should be sought as soon as possible.

In younger children
- Decline in standard of performance in school work or activities that does not pick up again over time
- The child is not managing or coping with tasks as expected at their developmental age
- Suggestions from teachers that there may be a learning difficulty, a behavioural problem or a problem making friends
- Hyperactivity
- Persistent crying, waking at night, or nightmares
- Persistent disobedience or aggression
- Frequent temper tantrums
- Excessive anxiety (e.g. preoccupation with fears of burglars, barking dogs, parents getting killed)
- Constant fighting with other children, and reports from school of the child being 'angry or disruptive'
- Refusal to go to school
- Refusal to go to bed, inability to sleep, or a need to sleep with, or close to, parents
- Decreased interest in playing
- The child tries to stimulate themself in various ways (e.g. hair pulling, rocking of the body, head banging)
- The child constantly says things that indicate low self-esteem (e.g. 'I'm dumb', 'I never do anything right', 'No one likes me', 'I'm too skinny', or too fat, too tall, too ugly, etc)
- The child is preoccupied with fire, or sets fires

In older children and adolescents
- Frequently asks or hints at the need for help
- Fears or phobias that interfere with normal activities
- Substance misuse
- Change in sleeping/eating/hygiene habits
- Isolating self from others excessively
- Involved in beating up others
- Inability to cope with problems and usual daily activities
- Excessive complaints about physical aches and pains
- Defiance of authority, truancy, theft and/or acts of vandalism
- Intense fear of weight gain
- Frequent outbursts of anger
- Demonstrates ritualistic behaviours (e.g. preparing for bed, a meal, or going out) using routines that are exact, precise and never vary
- Provocatively sexual behaviour that is not appropriate
- Participates in mutilating or killing animals
- Persistent and prolonged low mood (a major concern, especially if accompanied by poor appetite or thoughts and talk of death or signs of self-mutilation)

In adults
- Confused thought processes
- Prolonged periods of sadness/low mood and apathy
- Feelings of extreme highs and lows
- Persistent irritability
- Excessive anxiety/worrying
- Unrealistic or excessive fears
- Strange or grandiose ideas
- Social withdrawal
- Marked changes to eating/sleeping/hygiene or other habits
- Strong feelings of anger/outbursts of violent behaviour
- Increasing inability to cope with usual activities of everyday life
- Denial of anything being wrong even in light of obvious problems
- Numerous unexplained physical ailments
- Substance misuse
- Delusions or hallucinations
- Thoughts/talk about suicide or homicide (professional help needed immediately)

(National Mental Health Association (USA) 2008; American Psychiatric Association 2004)

mental illness is determined according to the symptoms experienced and the clinical features of the illness. There are many categories of classification but mental illness is mainly classified within the following areas:

- Thought disorders, such as schizophrenia, which disrupt the ability to think and perceive things clearly and logically and can impair a person's perception of reality
- Mood disorders, which affect how a person feels and can result in persistent low mood (depression) or cycles of low mood and euphoria (bipolar disorder)
- Behavioural disorders, which involve people acting in potentially destructive ways, including eating disorders such as anorexia nervosa and bulimia
- Mixed disorders, which have components of two or more of the other categories (Mayo Foundation for Medical Education and Research 2002).

Diagnosis according to the DSM (4th edition) has the benefit that clients may feel great relief when they have a diagnosis that helps them make sense of what is happening to them, and a medical diagnosis can guide clinical treatment. But this diagnostic system has a disadvantage in that a diagnosis can also be a label that has negative connotations; for example, a label of schizophrenia or a personality disorder is associated with significant social stigma. Diagnostic labels describe certain types of behaviour but they indicate very little about the nature or causes of the experience.

NURSING DIAGNOSES

Mental health nurses develop nursing diagnoses in response to the client's experience, emotions and behaviours. Nursing care responds holistically to the client's biological, psychosocial, spiritual and environmental needs and specifically addresses the client's feelings and behavioural responses to

CLINICAL INTEREST BOX 45.3
People at risk of mental illness

Anyone can develop a mental illness, but people at particular risk include:

- Adolescents: adolescents face a period of enormous physical, psychological and social change. Some adolescents may not have sufficient resources to cope with the demands placed on them at this challenging stage of life and to complete the developmental tasks necessary to move successfully from adolescence to adulthood. Erik Erikson's theory of personality development (Erikson & Erikson 1997) is one that is useful to explore in relation to life stages and developmental tasks
- New parents: new parents face a multitude of stressors (things that trigger a stress response) as well as many pleasures connected with a new baby. Stressors may include conflict over the acceptance of the pregnancy, transition from being a couple to being parents, loss of financial income, a baby's constant demands, and anxiety about the infant's welfare
- Women: women face factors such as a disadvantaged status in society, internal conflict arising from decisions about whether to pursue a career, become a home-maker or try to achieve both, or being subjected to domestic violence or abuse. These are social factors that may possibly predispose some women to mental illness
- Older adults (male and female): older adults may face many stressors, including loss of work role status because of retirement, reduced income, fear of declining physical and mental abilities, relocation, death of a partner and/or friends and siblings of similar age. The effect of these multiple losses may accumulate and leave some older adults at risk of mental illness
- Refugees and migrants: these people may experience a grief reaction on leaving their homeland, friends and family to live in a country where the cultural practices, values and beliefs are different and where they may be considered of low status and worth. It may be difficult for some migrants to work successfully through their grief because of language barriers, the stress from job and financial uncertainty, and lack of support from relatives and friends left behind. Some refugees and migrants may experience problems of adjustment, isolation and loneliness, each of which may contribute to mental illness. In some cases refugees have experienced torture and trauma in their country of origin, which creates a high risk of developing a post-traumatic stress disorder (Griffiths et al 2003)
- Physically or intellectually impaired persons: factors such as isolation, lack of meaningful relationships, social restrictions caused by disabilities, poor self-esteem, and negative stigmatising community attitudes towards people with disabilities are all aspects of experience that can elevate the risk of mental illness, particularly anxiety and depression (Dewer & Barr 1996)

CLINICAL INTEREST BOX 45.4
Examples of nursing diagnoses used in mental health nursing

- Impaired social interaction: insufficient or excess quantity or ineffective quality of social interactions
- Ineffective coping: inability to form a valid appraisal of the stressors, inability to use available resources
- Chronic low self-esteem: long-standing negative feelings about self or own capabilities
- Self-care deficit: impaired ability to perform or complete activities of daily living (e.g. hygiene, toileting, nutrition)
- Imbalanced nutrition, less than body requirements: intake of nourishment insufficient to meet the body's metabolic needs
- Powerlessness: perception that one's own actions will not significantly affect an outcome; a perceived lack of control over a current situation
- Disturbed thought processes: disruption in cognitive abilities and activities
- Disturbed sensory perceptions: alteration in the amount or patterning of incoming stimuli accompanied by a diminished/exaggerated/distorted/impaired response to the stimuli (often used for clients who are experiencing delusions, hallucinations, or illusions or have impaired awareness of self/environment)
- Impaired verbal communication: diminished, delayed or impaired ability to understand or transmit verbal messages
- Dysfunctional grieving: prolonged unsuccessful use of strategies and responses by which people attempt to work through the process of grieving (see Chapter 14 for information concerning the grieving process)
- Risk for injury: potential for injury as a result of environmental conditions interacting with the client's adaptive and defensive resources
- Risk for self-directed violence; risk for other-directed violence; existence of the potential for an individual to be physically, emotionally or sexually harmful to self or others
- Risk for suicide: potential for self-inflicted life-threatening injury

(Fortinash & Holoday Worret 2003; Varcarolis 2006)

those feelings, many of which are common across several different medically classified conditions. Examples of some nursing diagnoses commonly used in mental health nursing are provided in Clinical Interest Box 45.4.

A mental disorder can be categorised as temporary, episodic or chronic, according to the way it manifests:

- Temporary: a temporary inability to cope; for example, a single experience of depression. The vague definition of 'a nervous breakdown' is a common non-medical term for this kind of isolated non-recurring illness
- Episodic: an illness that occurs episodically; for example, recurrent episodes of a disabling condition such as bipolar disorder (once known as manic

depression) or schizophrenia. While the condition is disabling when it occurs, the person affected can often enjoy a comparatively normal life for much, if not most, of the time

- Chronic: a constant disabling and unrelenting illness that is extremely challenging for the affected person and their families to deal with; for example, a chronic type of schizophrenia or bipolar disorder or irreversible dementia.

Although the use of the terms psychosis and neurosis to describe particular illnesses is no longer favoured, nurses need to be aware of the meanings associated with each as the terms are still used in some contexts. The terms are out of favour because symptoms ascribed to each condition can occur in the other, and this causes confusion. The term psychosis refers to disorders that are so marked and incapacitating that the person who is afflicted is out of touch with reality and lacks insight into the illness and the associated behaviours, which may be unusual or bizarre. Psychosis was the term traditionally used to describe disorders such as schizophrenia and bipolar disorder, in which the symptoms experienced were quite different to those experienced by other people and included delusions and hallucinations (Gibb & Macpherson 2000). (Clinical Interest Box 45.5 provides explanations and examples of delusions and hallucinations.)

Unlike people suffering from a psychotic disorder, those with what used to be termed a neurosis have insight into their condition. For example, a person who has an obsessive-compulsive disorder may experience persistent and

CLINICAL INTEREST BOX 45.5
Delusions and hallucinations*

Delusion: a fixed thought or belief that is not reality based or true, is not consistent with the person's level of education and development or cultural background, and is not amenable to reason. It is categorised as a thought disorder

Type	Example
Somatic delusions (a false belief involving a body part or function)	A young woman believes her body is rotting away from the inside, her heart is made of ice and is gradually melting because she doesn't deserve to live
Nihilistic delusions (false feeling that the self, others or the world is non-existent)	A client refuses to eat, saying there is no need for him to eat because he has no body
Delusions of persecution (oversuspiciousness: the person falsely believes themself to be the object of harassment)	A client believes the staff belong to a cult, are watching his every move and are out to get him. He is afraid to go to sleep for fear of what the staff might do to him
Delusions of control (false belief that one is being controlled by an external source)	A client believes her feelings, thoughts and actions are being controlled by aliens who send messages to her via the television, instructing her on what to do
Delusions of grandeur (exaggerated beliefs about personal importance or powers)	A client believes he is God and controls the universe
Delusions of self-depreciation (beliefs of unworthiness)	A client believes she is ugly and sinful, saying, 'I don't deserve to be loved — look at me — it shows that I am full of sin'

Hallucinations: sensory perceptions that are not founded on any external stimuli. They may involve any of the five senses. They are most commonly visual or auditory

Type	Example
Visual hallucination	A client tells you that he sees his deceased wife in different areas of his home
Auditory hallucination	A 16-year-old client tells you she hears voices in her head saying derogatory things such as, 'You are worthless, you don't deserve to live'
Gustatory (taste) hallucination	A middle-aged client with organic brain syndrome complains of a constant metallic taste in his mouth
Olfactory hallucination	A 30-year-old client states that she smells 'rotten garbage' in her bedroom although no one else can smell anything unusual or unpleasant
Tactile hallucination	A middle-aged woman undergoing symptoms of alcohol withdrawal reports feeling ants crawling all over her body although no ants are present

(Shives 2005; Fortinash & Holoday Worret 2003)

*Clients can experience delusions and hallucinations together. For example, a client may hear her dead daughter's voice, see her standing close by and be convinced that she caused her daughter's death despite of evidence to the contrary that her daughter died as a result of injuries received in a car accident when on holiday with a friend.

intrusive thoughts (obsessions) about personal cleanliness. To decrease the level of anxiety the person may wash his hands hundreds of times a day, even if his hands become red and raw (compulsion to act). When they are extreme, such thoughts and acts may be so unusual and disrupt the person's life to the degree that to the observer the person is mentally ill. Unlike those experiencing a psychotic disorder, the affected person is aware that the behaviour is abnormal (there is insight into the behaviour and the illness). Despite their condition, people who have what was once classified as a neurosis can often continue to function in society, whereas a person who is psychotic cannot function effectively (Gibb & Macpherson 2000).

THEORETICAL MODELS AND CAUSATION OF MENTAL ILLNESS

Historically the medical profession was prominent in the care of people with mental illness and as a result there has been, and still is, a strong focus on identifying physical causes of mental illness. However, others have looked at psychological, sociocultural, interpersonal and human development factors and there are now many theoretical models used to explain the presence of a mental disorder. Mental health nurses select concepts from the various relevant models that best explain the client's behaviours, problems and needs. They then draw on these concepts as a basis for client assessment and then for planning, conducting and evaluating care (Varcarolis 2006). The following provide very basic examples of a small selection of theoretical models. To work effectively in the area of mental health, however, nurses need a deep and sound understanding of a wide range of models.

THE MEDICAL, OR BIOLOGICAL, MODEL

This model explains mental illness as being caused by physiological malfunction in the body. Physical causes can be separated into acquired and non-acquired factors. Acquired causes include head injury, cerebral infection and substance misuse. Non-acquired causes include genetic transmission, electrical conductivity changes in the brain, or alterations to the production and/or activity of neurotransmitters (Gibb & Macpherson 2000). There is evidence to support biological explanations. For example, studies indicate that depression and schizophrenia may be linked to abnormal neurotransmitter function, and that genetic factors may be linked to both (Kennedy & Mitzeliotis 1999; Varcarolis 2006). A medical approach to treating mental illness tends to focus primarily on medication and sometimes includes electroconvulsive therapy (ECT), both of which aim to correct chemical imbalance in the body believed to be caused by abnormal neurotransmitter function in the brain. Emil Kraepelin (1856–1926) is a theorist associated with the origins of the medical model.

PSYCHOLOGICAL AND PSYCHODYNAMIC MODELS

The psychoanalytical model, first conceptualised by Sigmund Freud (1856–1939), is possibly the most well-known model in this group. Freud's model viewed human personality as developing predominantly within the first 5 years of life and focused mostly on unconscious, non-rational and instinctual parts of human behaviour (Varcarolis 2006). Freud attributed disrupted behaviour in the adult to developmental tasks that were not accomplished successfully at earlier developmental stages. For example, within this theoretical framework a mental illness may be linked to a failure during adolescence to move successfully from dependence on parents to independence. Freud's mode of treatment was psychoanalysis, which aimed to bring unconscious problems to conscious awareness.

Carl Jung (1875–1961), Melanie Klein (1882–1960) and Erik Erikson (1902–1994) are some of the theorists that have expanded on Freud's thinking about the nature of human development and behaviour. Erikson's theory has provided nurses with a developmental model that encompasses the entire life span. Erikson studied healthy personalities and focused on human strengths as well as weaknesses, emphasising how people who failed to achieve developmental milestones at various life stages could rectify these failures at later stages (Varcarolis 2006).

It was Freud who identified the manner in which humans develop and used defence mechanisms to ward off anxiety that might otherwise be overwhelming and incapacitating (Varcarolis 2006). Defence mechanisms prevent conscious awareness of threatening feelings and can be a helpful response in adapting to stress, but their overuse can be a sign of maladaptation to stress and an indicator of mental ill-health. They are particularly relevant in understanding stress-vulnerability and stress-adaptation models of health and illness. Stress-vulnerability/adaptation models recognise that throughout life there is a need for everyone to adapt to change, for example, to adjust to school and then work life, to living with a partner, or to becoming a parent or a grandparent and then to retirement and perhaps the death of a spouse. The model views that some people find it more difficult than others to adapt to life's changes and to cope effectively with the stressors that change can bring. When life results in a stressful situation or there is an accumulation of multiple stressors, people who have been unable to develop and establish adequate coping skills and coping resources are at the highest risk of developing a mental illness. (See Chapter 13 for further information concerning these two theoretical models, the use of defence mechanisms and adaptation to stress.)

SOCIAL AND INTERPERSONAL MODELS

Social/interpersonal models draw attention to the impact of factors within a person's social environment on mental wellbeing. The basic concept is that negative social factors such as low status, low levels of support, isolation and poverty contribute to and increase the risk of developing mental illness such as depression (Gibb & Macpherson 2000).

Interpersonal models encompass the premise that internal conflict within one's personality and particular behaviours may be derived from unresolved conflicts within personal relationships, sometimes during early life experiences. This model also encompasses the premise that an individual's wellbeing is dependent on the amount of stress experienced and the effectiveness of personal coping strategies in dealing with that stress. Karen Horney (1885–1952), Harry Stack Sullivan (1892–1949) and Hildegard Peplau (1909–1999), a nurse theorist, are some of the important theorists who have conducted work related to social and interpersonal factors and mental health.

COGNITIVE BEHAVIOUR MODELS

Cognitive behaviour models stem from the assumption that behavioural responses are learned. Ivan Pavlov (1849–1936) developed the understanding of learned behaviours when he found that when a bell was repeatedly rung each time dogs were given food the dogs began to salivate just at the sound of the bell. This conditioned reflex was termed classic conditioning and is acknowledged as a form of learning that applies to humans, learning in which a previously neutral stimulus comes to elicit a given response through association. For example behavioural theorists would suggest that children who observe parents responding to every minor stress with anxiety would soon learn the response and would develop a similar pattern of behaviour (Stuart & Laraia 2001). According to the behavioural model, this early learning experience would be considered a significant factor in the cause of an anxiety disorder and limited constructive coping strategies in later life.

BF Skinner (1904–1990) added to behavioural theory by introducing the concept of operant conditioning. Operant conditioning refers to the use of reinforcers to motivate the repetition of particular behaviours. The use of positive reinforcement (the continual rewarding of desired behaviours) forms the basis of behaviour modification therapy used to help motivate clients to change undesirable behaviours. It has been effective for clients with phobias, alcohol addiction and a variety of other conditions (Varcarolis 2006).

Aaron Beck was one of the early founders of cognitive behaviour therapy (CBT), now a common and often very successful form of psychological treatment. It is based on the view that dysfunctional behaviour is linked to dysfunctional thinking, and that thinking processes are shaped by underlying beliefs. For example, the client with depression believes, 'I am no good at anything, I'm worthless, and nobody likes me'. Cognitive behaviour therapy is based on helping clients recognise, challenge and change dysfunctional thinking. (Chapter 13 provides further information about CBT.) Beck's work has primarily focused on helping people with depression but he has expanded the use of CBT to include working with people who have complex disorders such as borderline personality disorder and schizophrenia, and there are distinct signs of success (Fenichel 2000).

Mental health, like physical health, is clearly affected by a multitude of factors. Consequently, mental health nurses and psychiatrists are concerned with all the aspects of people's lives that distinguish them as human beings. The mental health nurse uses knowledge from the psychosocial and biophysical sciences, and theories of stress vulnerability, personality and behaviour, to develop a framework on which to base the art of nursing. The mental health nurse is an integral part of the interdisciplinary team required to meet the needs of clients who have a mental illness.

THE PROVISION OF CARE

THE MULTIDISCIPLINARY TEAM

Many people may be involved in assisting a person who is experiencing a disruption or potential disruption to their mental health. Mental health care commonly employs an interdisciplinary team approach to care management. The client's care, according to individual needs, is planned and implemented by a team composed of mental health nurses, psychiatric social workers, counsellors, clinical psychologists, general or specialist medical officers (depending on the client's physical status) and pharmacists. Additional team members may be required and, depending on individual needs, these may include: a dietitian; an occupational therapist; a recreational, art, music or dance therapist; complementary health care therapist; and a chaplain or other spiritual support person (Clinical Interest Box 45.6).

It should never be forgotten that the most important member of the team is the client, and often clients know what they need to promote their own recovery. Some clients have reflected on the times when they have been at their most vulnerable. For example, some clients who have experienced admissions to acute-care settings have identified that what they need most at times of severe mental distress is somewhere they can feel safe and supported, somewhere they can relax and calm down, and someone to be with them who will listen and really hear them (Watkins 2001). While the client may feel the need for medication, it is not appropriate or helpful to implement other therapeutic interventions, such as group therapy, recreational therapy or family therapy, until the client is feeling less distressed and can collaborate in decisions about what sort of interventions will be most helpful. Skilled helping involves actively listening to the client and working collaboratively with the client to achieve a process of recovery. (See Chapter 29 for information concerning active listening as a therapeutic measure.) The therapeutic process involves health professionals, including nurses, as facilitators who use their knowledge to help the client become more resourceful and self-reliant. This helping relationship needs to be a participative but never

CLINICAL INTEREST BOX 45.6
Some members of the health care team

- The psychiatrist: a physician whose specialty is mental disorders and who is responsible for diagnosis and treatment. A psychiatrist has the legal power to prescribe and to write treatment orders and, as such, is often the team leader
- The mental health nurse: a nurse with experience and expertise in clinical psychiatry, who promotes a holistic approach to care
- The clinical psychologist: a psychologist who has undertaken specialised education in the area of mental health and whose function includes applying and interpreting psychological tests and the implementation of specific therapies such as behaviour modification programs and sexual, marital or family therapy
- The psychiatric social worker: a social worker in the field of mental health, whose function includes assisting the client to prepare a support system that will help maintain their mental health on discharge into the community from an inpatient facility. A social worker may liase with employers, contacts in day-treatment centres, and those providing training and educational programs. The social worker may also assist the client to locate and access sources of financial aid and accommodation
- Occupational, recreational, art, music and dance therapists: according to their specialist areas of expertise, these various therapists assist clients to gain skills that assist them to cope more effectively, to gain or retain employment, to use leisure time in a way that promotes their mental wellbeing and to express their emotions in healthy ways

(Varcarolis 2006; Stuart & Laraia 2001)

a directive process (Watkins 2001). The model of helping relationships established by Carl Rogers (1961) and the model of skilled helping established by Gerard Egan (1994) are client-centred models of caring on which many mental health nurses can reliably base their therapeutic interactions with clients.

RESPONSIBILITIES OF THE MENTAL HEALTH NURSE

Mental health nursing may be described as an interpersonal process in which the nurse uses the presence of self, interpersonal communication skills and a knowledge of physiology, psychology and sociology to help clients in mental distress. A combined understanding of biological processes and psychodynamic processes is essential for the mental health nurse because many people with mental illness have a concurrent physical problem, and the two are often interconnected (Stuart 2001a).

Mental health nurses are very involved in psychiatric inpatient services and in community mental health services. They play a major role in education and health promotion, as well as in the provision of continuing care and counselling for people with mental health problems. For some experienced mental health nurses the role may include conducting specific psychological therapies such as cognitive behaviour therapy.

Nursing care aims to help clients cope with the experience of mental illness, prevent relapse and to promote a return to mental health through a successful rehabilitation program. The primary aims of mental health nursing (Watkins 2001) are to help individual clients to:

- Identify and clarify their needs and problems
- Create a better future for themselves (e.g. empower clients by developing self-help strategies)
- Create strategies to enable them to move forward (e.g. clients can become stuck in a particular way of responding to situations).

Rehabilitation is important for people who have been discharged from a psychiatric ward or unit. Some of these people need minimal support but others represent a population of chronically ill clients who return to hospital periodically over many years and require support in several different areas of their lives. The community mental health nurse and other members of the community mental health team may be involved in:

- Monitoring medication
- Individual and family therapy
- Crisis intervention
- Social skills training
- Medical care for concurrent physical problems
- Vocational training and support (Shives 2005).

FACILITATING DEVELOPMENT OF CONSTRUCTIVE COPING MECHANISMS

While the nurse's role in stress and stress management is explained in Chapter 13, some specific points need to be highlighted here. To recognise and deal with stress, individuals need to be provided with information about, and helped to recognise:

- Issues and events related to health and illness, and the importance of adhering to sound health practices (e.g. adequate nutrition, sleep, exercise and relaxation) as a way of promoting mental wellbeing
- The dimensions of potential stressors, possible outcomes, and their own established positive and negative coping mechanisms and their coping resources
- How to recognise their existing strengths and develop and maximise their abilities in problem solving, tolerating stress and dealing effectively with interpersonal relationships
- Where and how to gain access to additional coping resources (e.g. vocational training, support groups and counselling).

There is a wide variety of activities that clients may find helpful in promoting coping, but there is no one right or best activity. What works for one person may not work for another. Nurses have a responsibility to provide clients with information and options, but only the client can know what feels appropriate, so the choice of what activities to attempt or to become involved with should ultimately rest with the client. Clinical Interest Box 45.7 provides examples of positive constructive coping strategies, coping resources and negative destructive coping mechanisms.

THE NURSE'S ROLE IN EDUCATING THE PUBLIC AND REDUCING STIGMA

One particularly important facet of the community mental health nurse's role is educating the public about mental illness to reduce the stigma that for many mentally ill people is the biggest hurdle to overcome (Watkins 2001). There is a general lack of knowledge in the community about what constitutes mental illness and about the prognoses of mental disorders, which ensures that mental illnesses are often surrounded by mystery, misinformation and stigma (Weir & Oei 1996). Despite positive interventions in recent years, people suffering from mental illness remain among the most stigmatised, discriminated against, marginalised, disadvantaged and vulnerable members of society (Johnstone 2001). Clinical Interest Box 45.8 illustrates one person's experience of stigma.

Several myths about mental illness create fear of those affected and this fear serves to increase stigmatising behaviours and attitudes. For example, there is a widely held perception that people with mental illness are often out of control, unpredictable and may pose a threat. The truth is that most people with mental illness do not behave in this way; however, severe mental distress is often highlighted in the media, and this links images of dangerous behaviour with mental illness in the minds of the public (Watkins 2001). In addition, single, isolated and often very minor criminal acts committed by mentally ill people tend to be sensationalised by the media, contributing to negative stereotypes (Jewell & Posner 1996).

CLINICAL INTEREST BOX 45.7
Examples of positive constructive coping strategies, coping resources and negative destructive coping mechanisms

Positive constructive coping strategies

- Use of complementary therapies
- Leisure and recreational activities
- Yoga
- Physical activity
- Art and music
- Relaxation techniques
- Reading
- Adult education classes
- Walks in the countryside
- Prayer and religious contemplation
- Medication
- Slowing down
- Expressing feelings
- Keeping pets
- Keeping busy
- Disputing worrying thoughts
- Positive affirmation
- Talking with friends and family and/or mental health professionals
- Joining a self-help or service user group
- Keeping a journal
- Listening to talking books
- Finding out about my mental health problem
- Contacting the crisis team
- Helping others
- Having a socially valued occupation
- Taking respite breaks
- Getting enough rest
- Being listened to
- Understanding my symptoms
- Motivating myself
- Taking one day at a time
- Having a routine
- Having achievable goals
- Monitoring my symptoms
- Avoiding overloading myself

(Mental Health Foundation 1997)

Coping resources

- Economic assets
- Established abilities and skills
- Social supports
- Personal motivation
- Physical health, strength and energy
- Positive beliefs about self
- Established problem-solving and social skills
- Social and material resources
- Knowledge and intelligence
- Strong sense of identity
- Cultural stability
- A clear and stable system of values and beliefs
- An orientation towards preventive measures in health

(Stuart & Laraia 2001, Varcarolis 2006)

Examples of negative destructive coping strategies

- Always being submissive to others and so failing to get own needs met
- Excessive use of alcohol and/or other drugs or overeating (seeking comfort in substances)
- Promiscuity (seeking love and acceptance in a way that does not improve self-esteem)
- Overuse of defence mechanisms to cope with unacceptable or ambivalent feelings (see Chapter 13 for information about defence mechanisms). Defence mechanisms commonly used in a maladaptive manner (Stuart & Laraia 2001) include:
  - Regression: reverting to behaviour synonymous with earlier developmental stage (e.g. tantrums)
  - Projection: blaming others for what is happening
  - Denial: denying there is a problem (e.g. 'I am in control of my anger')
  - Rationalisation: avoiding dealing with an issue (e.g. 'What does a bit of shouting and banging matter? The children know I would never actually hit them')

CLINICAL INTEREST BOX 45.8
The stigma of mental illness

John was diagnosed with schizophrenia 2 years ago. Getting a diagnosis was such a relief, because then we knew what had caused such a big change in him. The nurses taught us about the illness and now, because we know what to look for, we pick up the early warning signs. He knows where to get help and most of the time he avoids a relapse.

John's pretty much in control of his illness now, but the thing that's upset him and us most is the way some people have treated him. He lost his part-time job in the supermarket and even one of his lecturers at college told him he should consider leaving his engineering course because of it. Even my own sister won't have him baby-sit his young cousins anymore. John now feels it is not safe to tell anyone about it. How do you think that makes him feel? If it was diabetes that made him ill I wonder if people would have reacted the same.
(Marjorie, mother of John, age 21)

The lack of accurate knowledge about mental illness that leads to fear, mistrust and sometimes violence against people living with mental illness and their families can also serve to:

- Lower the morale and self-esteem of people living with mental illness
- Prevent people with mental illness from admitting the problem and seeking professional help
- Prevent people with mental illness from gaining paid employment
- Limit the participation of people with mental illness in community activities and force them into a reclusive lifestyle
- Cause families and friends to turn their backs on the mentally ill person when support is most needed.

The picture is not always as dismal as this. Many mental health care users are themselves excellent ambassadors for people with mental illness. By calling themselves consumers or clients they have empowered themselves to become advocates for other people experiencing mental health disorders. Mental health care users or consumers now have a vital role to play in participating and planning the delivery of mental health services (Happell & Roper 2003). Consumer advocacy groups now exist in every state and territory of Australia to promote participation of consumers in planning, implementation and evaluation of mental health services. Accordingly, many consumers live and work within a local community, use the same facilities (e.g. shops, library, cinema, sports centres) as everyone else, are accepted by the people within the community and experience no harassment and attract no hostility from the local residents (Repper et al 1997). All nurses can play a part in highlighting and reducing stigma by:

- Acknowledging the person by using respectful language; for example, never referring to someone as a manic depressive, but rather referring to them as a person with a bipolar disorder
- Discouraging the use of disrespectful language; for example, terms such as schizo, lunatic, crazy, nut case or barmy. The nurse can advocate for people with mental illness by alerting someone to the fact that they are expressing a stigmatising attitude. Many people do this automatically without realising the hurt they are causing and the negative impact on the person with the illness or their family members
- Emphasising the person's abilities rather than their limitations
- Avoiding representing a successful person with a mental illness as superhuman.

In part it is the way people with mental disturbance were treated in the past that influences current perceptions of mental illness and the associated stigma. The next section provides a brief overview of historical perspectives relevant to understanding societal attitudes today.

HISTORICAL PERSPECTIVES AND MENTAL HEALTH CARE

In the past, when emotions, thoughts or actions were deemed to be abnormal, the terms madness and insanity were linked to those affected. Reasons for the perceived abnormalities were once attributed to a variety of factors such as the influences of magic, witchcraft, possession by the devil or evil spirits, loss of the soul or punishment by the gods. Healing methods included exorcism, magical ritual and incantation (Videbeck 2001). Later it was proposed that an imbalance of 'body humours' was responsible — body humours being blood, black bile, yellow bile and phlegm — and such imbalances were corrected by blood letting. During the medieval period, beliefs returned again to those connected with magic and demonology but also included beliefs that the moon influenced madness (lunacy). Some of those perceived as mad or lunatics were flogged, tortured and starved and those whose illness resulted in violent behaviour were shackled in prisons or put out to sea as a means of ridding them from civilised society. Fear and lack of knowledge resulted in significant cruelty.

In the late 19th and early 20th centuries, those with behaviours that were not manageable, who were misunderstood or were simply not acceptable in society were placed in custodial care inside large public mental hospitals or asylums. It can only be imagined how being confined and isolated inside large institutions might have caused feelings of abandonment and rejection. During this period physicians classified the symptoms of mental illness but had limited understanding of the sources of mental anguish (Wilson & Kneisl 1996).

Increased understanding of mental distress was promoted by the psychological, psychosocial and interpersonal theories to explain behaviour espoused by theorists such as Freud, Erikson and Stack Sullivan. The introduction of psychotropic drugs, such as chlorpromazine

(Largactil) in the 1950s helped staff members manage large numbers of clients with challenging behaviours, who were often accommodated in crowded conditions in the large institutions. In the 1990s (the time known as the decade of the brain) biological, scientific and technological concepts combined to expand on earlier understandings of mental illness. For example, advanced brain-imaging techniques now allow direct viewing of the structure and function of the living brain while it is functioning (Wilson & Kneisl 1996).

In the later part of the 20th century the negative impact of institutionalisation for people with mental illness was recognised. This recognition was in part the stimulus that shifted public policy to one of deinstitutionalisation and community-based care for people with mental illness. The push towards community-based mental health services also came from the Human Rights Movement and the philosophy of normalisation for people with disabilities of all kinds (Chapter 47 explains more about the principles of normalisation and people with disabilities). The discovery of psychotropic drugs in the 1950s also contributed to the current predominance of care in the community because these agents helped to modify challenging behaviours (Jewell & Posner 1996).

THE CURRENT SITUATION AND MENTAL HEALTH CARE

Mainstreaming of mental health care has resulted in the provision of psychiatric care to consumers in general hospitals with an inpatient psychiatric unit, hostels and other residential care facilities and sometimes in forensic centres for the mentally impaired who have committed crimes. However, mental health care is primarily provided in the community. Nurses may meet with clients in a variety of community settings, including:

- The client's home
- The client's foster home
- Community care units
- Special residential units
- Day and drop-in centres
- Boarding houses
- On the street (homeless clients).

Current health care policy promotes not admitting people to a treatment centre unless essential, and, when it is necessary for clients to be admitted to treatment centres, they are discharged back into the community as early as possible. Ideally, community-based mental health services provide appropriate networks of supports and resources for those who need it. The aim of service providers is to ensure that there are caring interventions aptly suited to assist each person to rehabilitate successfully and to cope well in society. The policy of community-based care has enabled many of those who once lived in psychiatric institutions to resettle successfully in the community and to be well supported.

Unfortunately, however, there are other instances in which the deinstitutionalisation process has not been supported with adequate community care. The result of this is that some people who experience mental ill-health have merely been relocated to substandard boarding houses or other semi-institutionalised accommodation, or face homelessness (Jewell & Posner 1996; Grigg et al 2004).

While there are still many problems for mentally ill people and health professionals to contend with and resolve, there is now more cause for optimism in relation to mental illness than in the past. Success rates for the treatment of many common mental disorders such as bipolar disorder, major depression and schizophrenia now equal or exceed the success rates for many other medical disorders (Goldberg 1998).

While this chapter does not aim to inform the nurse about the range of treatments available to assist clients with specific disorders, the next section provides a summary of possible nursing responses to some common emotional and behavioural problems that challenge clients with mental illness. The terminology used in mental health care, some of which is contained in the next section, is extensive and different from terms used in other areas of nursing. Some of the more common terminology is defined in Table 45.2.

CARE OF CLIENTS WITH SPECIFIC EMOTIONAL AND/OR BEHAVIOURAL CHALLENGES

This part of the chapter addresses some of the more common mental states that clients being cared for in non-psychiatric hospital settings may experience. Information is provided on caring for a person who is anxious, depressed, aggressive, displaying self-destructive behaviour, hyperactive, confused or disoriented.

THE CLIENT EXPERIENCING ANXIETY

Anxiety is an internal feeling usually experienced as an unpleasant or uncomfortable emotion and which is frequently associated with conflicts and frustrations. While a certain mild degree of anxiety can be beneficial when it stimulates motivation and energy, severe anxiety can be devastating and is the basis of many mental health disorders. Sometimes, in extreme anxiety, a person may experience panic attacks that result in markedly disturbed behaviour. The person may be unable to process what is happening in the environment and may lose touch with reality. During a panic attack behaviour may be erratic, uncoordinated and impulsive. Anxiety differs from fear in that anxiety attacks the person at a deeper level than fear, and the source of the anxiety may be unknown. Anxiety invades the very centre of a person's being. Severe anxiety is profound and persistent and can erode and destroy a person's sense of self-esteem and self-worth that contribute to a sense of being fully human (Varcarolis 2006).

Anxiety is experienced in a wide variety of situations and is generally the result of a threat to a person's self-esteem

TABLE 45.2 | TERMS ASSOCIATED WITH MENTAL ILLNESS

Term	Definition
Addiction	Physical or emotional dependence, or both, on a substance, such as alcohol or other drugs
Affect	Current, observable state of emotion, feeling or mood such as sadness, anger or elation
Aggression	Forceful behaviour that may be physical or verbal, as well as subtle manipulation
Akathisia	A condition of excessive restlessness that causes a person to move about constantly, fidget or pace. This can be a side effect of certain medications used in psychiatry
Anhedonia	Reduced or complete inability to feel pleasure from activities previously enjoyed
Amnesia	Loss of memory of events for a period of time that may range from a few hours to many years
Anxiety	A feeling of apprehension, dread or unexplained discomfort, associated with a sense of helplessness, arising from internal conflict
Apathy	Lack of feeling, emotion, concern or interest
Asylum	A place of safety or sanctuary; a refuge from the stresses of life. Historically the term asylum was associated with institutions that provided custodial care for people with a mental illness. Unfortunately, they were often associated not with the real meaning of asylum but with mistreatment and cruelty
Autism	Preoccupation with the self and inner experiences; a process of introspective thinking that is often rich in fantasy
Behaviour	Any human activity, either physical or mental. Some behaviour can be observed while other behaviour can only be inferred
Behaviour modification	A method of changing or controlling behaviour through the application of techniques based on the principles of classical conditioning
Bipolar disorder	A type of mood disorder that causes alternating periods of low and high moods; a combination of depression and mania
Body image	The conscious and unconscious attitudes a person has towards their body (e.g. feelings about size, function and appearance)
Catatonia	A state characterised by muscular rigidity and immobility (stuporose type) and which, at times, is interrupted by episodes of extreme agitation (excited type) and is usually associated with schizophrenia
Compensation	Process by which a person makes up for a deficiency in their self-image by strongly emphasising some feature of themself that they regard as an asset
Compulsion	An uncontrollable persistent urge to perform an act repetitively in an attempt to relieve anxiety. Compulsive behaviour often accompanies obsessions and may be directly linked to them
Confabulation	The fabrication of experiences or situations recounted in a plausible way to fill in and cover gaps in the memory. Used most often as a defence mechanism and most commonly by people with head injuries, dementia, amnesic disorders or alcoholism, especially those with Korsakoff's syndrome
Confusion	A cluster of abnormalities constituting disturbances of judgment, orientation, memory, affect and cognition
Coping mechanisms	Any effort directed towards stress management. They can be unconscious (defence) mechanisms that protect the individual against anxiety, or conscious attempts to solve a problem that is creating stress. (Information on defence mechanisms and stress management is provided in Chapter 13)
Deinstitutionalisation	A shift in the location of treatment from large public hospitals to community settings
Delusion	A fixed false belief resistant to modification. A delusion of grandeur is a false belief that one has great prestige, power or money, which may be manifested in the belief that the individual is a famous person. Delusions of persecution is an individual's belief that they are in danger, being harassed, are under investigation, or are at the mercy of some powerful force. A somatic delusion is a belief that one's body is changing and responding in an unusual way
Dementia	A mental disorder characterised by a gradual onset of usually irreversible cognitive impairments
Depression	A mood state that may be mild or short lived or more severe and persistent. The latter, a mood disorder, is characterised by extreme sadness, feelings of hopelessness, low self-worth and little or no conviction that things can ever improve
Disorientation	Lack of awareness of the correct time, place or person
Electroconvulsive therapy (ECT)	A therapeutic procedure in which an electric current is briefly applied to the brain to produce a seizure. This is used in treatment of severe symptoms that do not respond to other measures, most commonly used in the treatment of severe depression
Hallucination	A sensory experience that is not the result of an external stimulus; may be visual, auditory, tactile, gustatory or olfactory

TABLE 45.2 | TERMS ASSOCIATED WITH MENTAL ILLNESS—cont'd

Hyperactive	Excessively or unusually active
Illusion	Misperceptions and misinterpretations of real external stimuli; may be visual or auditory or, less commonly, olfactory or tactile
Labile	Subject to frequent or unpredictable changes: the term is commonly used with reference to emotions
Mania	A mood characterised by an intense feeling of elation or irritability, often accompanied by increased activity, rapid speech and poor judgment
Mood disorder	A group of disorders in which the predominant feature is disturbance in mood
Nervous breakdown	A non-medical term sometimes used by the public to describe an episode of overwhelming distress or depression
Obsession	A persistent thought, idea or impulse that cannot be eliminated from consciousness by logical effort
Obsessive-compulsive disorder	An anxiety disorder characterised by intense, unwanted and distressing recurrent thoughts (obsessions) and repeated behaviours (compulsions) that are beyond the affected person's ability to control
Panic attack	A period of sudden intense anxiety, often associated with feelings of impending disaster and accompanied by strong physiological symptoms, including shortness of breath, pounding heart or palpitations and dizziness
Paranoia	A serious personality distortion in which the person is markedly suspicious and mistrusting of others and may be convinced that they wish to harm him/her
Phobia	An intense fear of some situation, person or object, so that the danger is magnified out of proportion and may result in a panic attack
Psychosis	A state in which a person's mental capacity to recognise reality, communicate and relate to others is impaired. Delusions and hallucinations are often present
Psychotic	A person who is psychotic experiences delusions and hallucinations that cause disorganised thinking, unusual behaviours and a loss of touch with reality
Schizophrenia	A complex condition caused by brain dysfunction that results in hallucinations and delusions, distorted thinking and other disturbances
Suicidal ideation	Thoughts of suicide with an intention to end one's life
Tardive dyskinesia	A side effect of some antipsychotic medications that manifests with a variety of involuntary muscle movements including those that affect the face, jaw and tongue, the trunk and the extremities of the body. The involuntary movements are irreversible. They are also referred to as extrapyramidal side effects

or physical integrity. Threats to self-esteem include factors such as interpersonal difficulties, change in job status, social or cultural group pressures, a change in role, or confusion over one's identity. Threats to physical integrity include factors such as decreased ability to perform the activities of daily living, for example, as a result of injury or illness, or lack of basic requirements such as food, shelter and clothing. Mild and moderate levels of anxiety can alert the person to the fact that something is wrong and may be the stimulus to take appropriate action. Severe levels of anxiety interfere with problem-solving abilities, so that those affected have difficulty finding effective solutions to problems. For example, someone who experiences panic attacks may use unproductive relief behaviours to avoid the attacks from occurring, such as refraining from leaving the house to avoid the risk of a panic attack when driving the car, at work or at the supermarket. Unproductive relief behaviours perpetuate the cycle of anxiety (Varcarolis 2006).

Whether the source is known or unrecognised, anxiety can produce physiological responses, behavioural changes and emotional reactions. The type and extent of response depends on the level of anxiety experienced. Table 45.3 lists some physiological and other responses to different levels of anxiety. Emotional reactions are usually apparent in the person's descriptions of their experience. For example, they may state that they feel apprehensive, irritable, angry, depressed, helpless, on edge, unable to concentrate or remember things, or they may feel detached from events and the environment. The person may experience angry outbursts or a tendency to cry frequently.

Specific treatment and care of a person experiencing anxiety depends on the level of anxiety experienced and the effects on the individual, but generally interventions are directed towards reducing intense anxiety to a more manageable level and helping the person to develop self-help strategies to prevent overwhelming anxiety. Cognitive behaviour therapy (CBT), for example, helps clients develop strategies for controlling their anxiety and reducing the incidence of panic attacks. (Chapter 13 provides an explanation of how CBT can assist clients to control their level of anxiety.) Minor tranquillisers such as diazepam

TABLE 45.3 | PHYSIOLOGICAL AND OTHER RESPONSES TO ANXIETY

Mild anxiety	Moderate anxiety	Severe anxiety	Panic level of anxiety
Slight discomfort Attention-seeking behaviours Restlessness, irritability or mild agitation Mild tension-relieving behaviour (e.g. foot or finger tapping, lip chewing, hair twisting, fidgeting)	Voice tremors Change in voice pitch Difficulty concentrating Shakiness Repetitive questioning Loss of appetite Diarrhoea/constipation Memory impairment (e.g. interference with recall of events/facts) Chain smoking Increased use of alcohol or other substances Somatic (bodily) complaints (e.g. urinary frequency and urgency, insomnia) Increased respiration rate Increased pulse rate Increased muscle tension that may lead to backache or headache More extreme tension-relieving behaviour (e.g. pacing, banging hands on table, constant wringing of hands)	Feelings of dread or impending doom Confusion and bewilderment Purposeless activity, lack of coordination of movements and actions Worsening of somatic complaints (e.g. dizziness, nausea, headache, sleeplessness) Hyperventilation Tachycardia Elevated blood pressure Sweating Facial pallor Dry mouth Difficulty in breathing Withdrawal from interpersonal interactions Disturbances in sexual function Loud and rapid speech Intense tension-relieving behaviour that may include threats and demands	Feelings of absolute terror; fear that death may result Immobility or severe hyperactivity or flight Dilated pupils Chest pains/palpitations Severe dizziness Unintelligible communication or inability to speak Severe tremors Sleeplessness Extreme psychomotor activity may lead to exhaustion Severe withdrawal (e.g. agoraphobia) Hallucinations and delusions may occur and the person may lose touch with reality

(Shives 2005; Videbeck 2001)

(Valium), lorazepam (Ativan) and clorazepate (Tranxene) are sometimes prescribed to suppress the client's feelings of anxiety but, as medications do not cure the condition and there are problems with dependence, long-term use is not advocated (Healy 2002).

General care involves:

- Establishing and maintaining a trusting relationship
- Attempting to identify the cause (stressors) of the anxiety and encouraging the client to take effective action
- Facilitating open and honest communication about the client's anxiety and/or problems
- Identifying existing coping mechanisms and coping resources
- Discussing with the client ways of resolving conflicts
- Providing information about, and teaching, constructive coping strategies that can help to manage stress.

The most common coping mechanisms taught and encouraged (Schwecke 2003) are:

- Problem solving
- Assertiveness
- Positive self-talk
- Stress and anger management
- Communication skills
- Skills for establishing and maintaining relationships
- Conflict resolution
- Time management
- Community living skills.

In addition, strategies to help tolerate and decrease the effects of anxiety can be taught, although these address the effects rather than the cause of anxiety. These strategies include complementary therapies such as visualisation techniques, guided imagery, meditation and relaxation training.

An understanding of the types and levels of anxiety and defensive patterns of behaviour used in response to anxiety (Table 45.3) is basic to effective psychiatric nursing care. Hildegard Peplau is a nurse theorist whose conceptual model of anxiety provides a firm basis on which nurses can plan interventions for clients experiencing anxiety. Nurses would benefit from reviewing the work of Peplau (1971, 1991) and other psychiatric nursing texts to enhance their knowledge of the relationship between anxiety and mental illness and the range of treatment options available.

THE CLIENT EXPERIENCING DEPRESSION

Depression is an emotional state that most people experience at one time or another. It can manifest anywhere along a continuum from intermittent feelings of sadness to a persistent deep sense of unending despair accompanied by hallucinations and delusions (Shives 2005). At the onset of depression the mood begins with a feeling of sadness that may be described as 'feeling down in the dumps'. As depression worsens, sad feelings deepen until those affected feel gloomy and dejected much of the time. At this level of depression people may describe the experience with statements such as, 'I have no joy in my life anymore' or, 'I just feel unhappy'. For some people the depressed mood can deepen even further until there is a persistent feeling of utter desolation. Severely depressed people have a sense of hopelessness about the past and the present, and the future looks black and bleak. The heavy feelings of despondency, wretchedness and acute misery are relentless. People affected feel desperately low and worthless, and this experience is accompanied by a sense of despair so profound that they do not believe the feelings will ever lift (Fontaine 1999).

Feelings of sadness and even intense grief, such as might be felt at the death of a loved one, are normal reactions to the various losses encountered by most people during their lives. Sadness and depression in such cases may be transitory, with the person moving through a grieving process and recovering successfully after the loss (see Chapter 14 for information about normal response to loss and the grieving process). Sometimes recovery after a significant loss does not occur and the person moves into a level of persistent and severe depression that does not resolve without professional assistance. This would be termed dysfunctional grieving. In some cases sadness, moderate and severe depression can occur without the person affected being able to identify a particular trigger for the low mood. Depression caused by biochemical imbalance is an example of this (Shives 2005).

Feelings of depression are so common that depression is known as the 'common cold' of psychiatry. It can occur at any age, even in very small children. Children with parents diagnosed with a depressive disorder have a higher risk of experiencing depression than others, and certain events may predispose young people to develop depressive symptoms (Keltner & Jones-Warren 2003). These events include:

- Loss of parents through divorce
- Death of other individuals close to them (e.g. grandparents, siblings, other relatives or friends)
- Death of a loved pet
- Move to a new neighbourhood or town
- Academic difficulties or failure
- Physical illness or injury that entails a stay in hospital.

Depression has a wide range of signs and symptoms but even so some people are able to hide their depression from others. Clinical Interest Box 45.9 lists the common signs and symptoms of depression. For some people depression may also be accompanied by anxiety. Some people experience alternating moods of depression and elation that can be disruptive to their lives. The periods of elation may be accompanied by significant hyperactivity. Such conditions are categorised as bipolar affective (mood) disorders, whereas mood disorders that have only the one dimension of depression without periods of elation are termed unipolar (Videbeck 2001).

Care of a depressed client is directed towards firstly addressing immediate safety needs in those at risk of self-harm. This will require hospitalisation and frequent or constant observation of those so seriously depressed as to be actively contemplating suicide. Antidepressant medication,

CLINICAL INTEREST BOX 45.9
Signs and symptoms of depression

Signs and symptoms of depression vary according to the severity of the low mood but may include:

- Non-verbal cues (sad facial expression, crying, slumped posture)
- Disturbed sleep patterns (e.g. insomnia or sleeping for much longer periods than usual)
- Self-criticism and expressions of guilt feelings
- Low self-esteem that may result in thoughts of self-harm or self-destruction
- Indecisiveness and poor concentration
- Psychomotor retardation or marked reduced mental or physical activity (slow dragging gait, slowed speech pattern and slow, flat, lifeless, colourless verbal responses, lack of concern and apathy about maintaining personal appearance)
- Psychomotor agitation (some people with depression experience significant anxiety that may manifest as restlessness, pacing or constant walking or constant purposeless movements such as pulling at hair or wringing of hands)
- Appetite disturbance and marked loss of weight
- Loss of energy
- Loss of sexual libido
- Headaches, chest pains, gastrointestinal disturbances and other physical manifestations
- Increased consumption of substances such as nicotine, alcohol and non-prescribed drugs
- Anhedonia (inability to feel any pleasure when participating in activities that previously were pleasurable)
- Delusions and/or hallucinations.

Particular signs that may be associated with depression in children and adolescents include:

- Frequent, vague, non-specific physical complaints such as headaches, muscle aches, stomach aches or tiredness
- Frequent absences from school or poor performance in school
- Efforts to run away from home, or talk of this
- Outbursts of shouting, complaining, unexplained irritability or crying
- Complaints of being bored
- Lack of interest in playing with friends
- Reckless behaviour
- Extreme sensitivity to rejection or failure
- Increased irritability, hostility or anger
- Difficulty with relationships
- Substance misuse
- Fear of death.

(National Institute of Mental Health 2000; Varcarolis 2006; Keltner & Jones-Warren 2003)

CLINICAL INTEREST BOX 45.10
Strategies for promoting effective communication with clients who have depression

Acceptance

Spend time with the client and accept the person without judgement. People who have depression are not always able to express feelings and may express them through behaviour that is unusual or even bizarre. The nurse should be careful not to make or imply any criticism of the client's behaviour because people with depression have low self-esteem and are particularly vulnerable to feelings of disapproval that may be interpreted as rejection.

Openness and honesty

Because people with depression are less able than others to tolerate disappointment, the nurse should be truthful at all times and never make promises that for any reason might not be kept. Nor should the nurse offer false reassurance (see Chapter 29 for a full explanation of this).

It is important for the nurse to develop a trusting relationship with the client and this will only be achieved with honesty. For example, a client may wish to share something private with the nurse but not want the nurse to tell anyone else about what is disclosed. The nurse builds trust by telling the client that significant information will need to be shared with other members of the health care team. The client learns to trust the nurse as a professional whose main concern is shown to be the client's own best interest.

Empathy

Any attempts to cheer up a depressed client may be perceived as a failure to understand their feelings or difficulties. Inappropriate approaches such as this may cause the client to withdraw further from interactions and may increase their isolation and depression.

Empathy means facilitating the client to express feelings of pain and inner distress and to respond in a way that indicates recognition and understanding of that pain and distress (Chapter 29 provides information about therapeutic and empathic communication).

Tolerance

People with depression may be unable to make even the simplest decision (e.g. where to sit, what clothing to select and put on). The nurse needs to understand how low mood slows physical as well as mental responses and that the psychomotor retardation is part of the illness, not a deliberate act. It is impossible for clients with depression to 'shake themselves out of it' and it is not therapeutic to try to badger people with depression into activity. Tolerance is also required for clients with depression who experience psychomotor agitation.

Underlying anxiety in the depressed client may also manifest as hyperactivity or anger and hostility that may be directed towards the nurse. Clients sometimes shock themselves at the hostile and sometimes hateful things they say to others during periods of depression. It is a normal response for the nurse to feel some frustration and irritation or even anger towards clients at times, but the nurse must be mindful that the client's behaviour is an outward reflection of inner anguish and that to be therapeutic they must remain patient. To assist in this the nurse must reflect on, and implement, the strategies needed to maintain personal mental wellbeing. This may include discussing feeling responses to clients with a colleague.

(Shives 2005; Keltner & Jones-Warren 2003)

when necessary, is started immediately, but the symptomatic relief is not generally achieved for at least several days, and possibly up to 2–4 weeks after therapy starts. Other specific interventions include individual, family, group, cognitive and behavioural psychotherapy (Shives 2005; Keltner & Jones-Warren 2003). The major goals are to lift the client's mood, improve self-esteem, identify and reduce the impact of any major identified stressors, promote the development of constructive coping mechanisms, assist the client to regain interest and motivation in life and also to address any concurrent problems associated with physical health. General care involves:

- Establishing and maintaining a trusting relationship
- Helping the person, when the acute phase is resolved, to recognise and express emotions (e.g. through verbal and nonverbal communication)
- Helping the client to set realistic goals
- Encouraging the client to establish and maintain social contact and interpersonal relationships
- Encouraging visits by family or significant others, to reduce any feeling of isolation
- Promoting physical health and wellbeing (e.g. adequate exercise, sleep and nutrition)
- Providing information concerning measures that may reduce and help manage stress
- Identifying existing coping mechanisms and coping resources
- Assisting the client to develop and enhance constructive coping mechanisms, including decision-making and problem-solving skills.

People who are depressed are very vulnerable and this may be, in part, why they often withdraw and isolate themselves. This can make it very challenging for the nurse needing to establish effective communication. Clinical Interest Box 45.10 provides some strategies for promoting effective communication with clients who have depression.

Depression is a major problem in older adults and may also be accompanied by worry and anxiety. Symptoms of depression in the older age group are relatively common but often go undetected. This may be because sadness is considered a normal response to the losses associated with ageing, such as physical decline, loss of social role and loss of a spouse, and it may not be recognised when normal sadness and grief has developed into clinical depression requiring treatment. In addition the complexities of physical illness, the side effects of medication and the symptoms of dementia may combine with symptoms of depression, making diagnosis of what is happening complex and difficult (Keltner & Jones-Warren 2003). It is very important for nurses working with older clients, particularly those with dementia, to be alert for, and report, changes such as unusual expressions of sadness, voicing the wish to die, decrease in appetite, reduced enjoyment, loss of interest in activities, or other symptoms that may indicate the presence of depression. Clinical Interest Box 45.11 lists some issues relating to the mental health of older adults. Some key nursing interventions and principles of care that nurses should consider when working with clients who have depression are outlined in Table 45.4.

THE CLIENT EXPERIENCING FEELINGS OF ANGER AND HOSTILITY

Anger is a feeling experienced by most people at certain times. It generally occurs in response to fear, confusion or frustration. Anger often occurs in response to the anxiety a person feels when a threat is perceived. Most people have little difficulty in handling mild anger, which is experienced as annoyance and usually subsides quickly. Feelings of anger, disappointment and frustration may be expressed verbally or non-verbally, for example, by cursing or kicking a car when it won't start. When a person is very frustrated, such as when unable to attain an important goal, anger may

CLINICAL INTEREST BOX 45.11
Mental health issues in older adults

- The older person is vulnerable to emotional and mental stress from many losses, including the loss of a spouse, loss of social roles and resources, decreased income and loss of status and socialisation associated with paid employment
- Disorders common in the older population include depression, paranoid reactions and dementias
- Depression is the most common emotional disorder in the older population
- Paranoia may be related to depression and/or neurological disorders. It is also associated with sensory deficits and loneliness
- Of the dementias, the Alzheimer's type is the most common non-reversible dementia
- The risk of suicide increases with age, with men aged 75 and over being particularly vulnerable
- Family carers of people with dementia are more likely than other family carers to experience emotional health problems such as stress, exhaustion and depression

(Umstead-Raschmann 1995; Ashton & Keady 2000)

TABLE 45.4 | KEY NURSING INTERVENTIONS AND PRINCIPLES OF CARE FOR CLIENTS WITH DEPRESSION

Action	Rationale
Accept clients as they are and focus on their strengths	People with depression have low self-concept; this is the best approach to promote the return of a more positive sense of personal worth
Promote the client's own decision making; minimise dependency	Indecisiveness is a symptom of depression and can mean that clients struggle to make even the most basic decisions. The nurse needs to move the client towards independent decision making that is part of mental health
Avoid presenting clients with decisions to make when they are not yet ready to make decisions for themselves	At the height of a depressive illness it is best to simply present situations to the clients that do not require a decision; for example, 'It's time to come for lunch', 'It's time to have your shower', 'Here is a cup of tea'
Respond to hostility or anger therapeutically	Expressions of anger are often part of a depressive illness, possibly because the person has developed a previous pattern of containing any such strong feelings. Understanding the dimensions of the illness helps the nurse to focus on the issue at hand and assist clients to move towards more appropriate ways of expressing and dealing with their feelings
Spend time (brief but frequent) with withdrawn and isolative clients, even when this feels uncomfortable	Withdrawn clients remain aware of their surroundings and, even if they do not acknowledge the presence of the nurse or communicate in any way, they can be reassured by that presence. Spending time with the client communicates the client's worth as a person. It may be that the client will learn to be comfortable with the nurse and eventually initiate dialogue
Involve clients in activities in which they can experience success	People can feel good about themselves in many different ways. Accomplishment is one way to develop a sense of self-worth
Avoid reinforcing hallucinations or delusions	Confronting these symptoms tends to reinforce them. The best approach is for the nurse to state his or her view of reality and to begin discussing real people, situations and events

(adapted from Keltner & Jones-Warren 2003: 355)

become more intense. A person experiencing intense anger may try to disperse the unpleasant feeling through an angry outburst or an act of aggression. Occasionally a person may be so consumed by feelings of anger that they become violent and pose a threat to themself and to others nearby.

Nurses may encounter anger in the course of providing nursing care; for example, a person whose health is disrupted becomes frustrated, and frustration can lead to anger. Sometimes people express their anger through verbal or physical abuse towards others, including staff members. Therefore it is important that nurses are aware of the reasons why a person may be angry, of their own responses to outbursts of angry feelings, and of how to help an individual to express anger in an appropriate manner. Anger may be the result of various stressors. Some of the factors that may cause anger or aggression in people who are in hospital for any reason include:

- A feeling of loss of control and/or independence
- A sense of isolation from family and familiar environment
- A feeling of loss of identity or individuality
- Feelings of fear and discomfort because of inadequate privacy
- Anxiety about the possible outcomes of illness (e.g. altered body image).

Some of the specific risk factors leading to a potential for aggression in clients with mental illness have been identified (Watkins 2001) as including:

- A diagnosis of an illness with paranoid features (paranoia can lead to fears that induce aggressive acts aimed at defending against a perceived threat; for example, the belief that someone is plotting against you or trying to harm or kill you can lead to lashing out at that person defensively)
- Substance misuse
- Deterioration in family and/or social relationships
- A previous history of aggression or violence and declared threats of violence
- Developmental history of exposure to aggression and violence
- Non-adherence to a medication regimen
- Failure to learn to delay gratification of wants (e.g. extreme frustration when needs are not met immediately)
- Failure to learn alternative strategies other than aggressive responses
- Unresolved conflicts
- Hostility to authority
- Denial of aggressive behaviour
- Lack of remorse.

Aggressive outbursts may occur when a person is unable to find a solution to a problem that is causing fear, confusion or frustration. Aggressive action may be directed towards the person or object perceived as the source of the frustration, or at other persons or objects in the vicinity. Displacement is a defence mechanism whereby an individual discharges pent-up feelings, such as anger, on a person or object other than the one that aroused the feelings (Varcarolis 2006). Approaches for dealing with anger and hostile behaviour in the mental health care environment are outlined in Table 45.5. Nurses may apply the principles of these approaches, when necessary and appropriate, in any health care setting.

Preventing aggression and violence is important for

TABLE 45.5 | APPROACHES FOR DEALING WITH ANGER AND HOSTILE BEHAVIOUR IN THE MENTAL HEALTH CARE ENVIRONMENT

Action	Rationale
Accept the client but make it clear that certain behaviours are not acceptable	This is a non-judgmental approach that informs the client that they are accepted as a person but that certain aspects of their behaviour are not appropriate
Acknowledge the person's anger and their right to their feelings	This demonstrates respect and acceptance of the client
Allow expression of the anger in appropriate safe ways; for example, voicing angry feelings verbally, discharging anger in non-destructive acts (e.g. not damaging property or person)	Anger is self-limiting and it may be better to let it run its course than to forcibly try to stop an angry person. Attempting to stop the person's expression of anger can restimulate the aggressive feelings and lead to a continuance of displayed anger
Try to remain calm (self-talk and relaxation techniques such as deep breathing and muscle relaxation can help with this). Provide psychological containment by staying in the same calm 'gear' and avoiding any tendency to retaliate or placate	Retaliation or trying to placate an angry person can stimulate the client to higher levels of aggression. Clients need their feelings to be acknowledged and understood; retaliation and appeasing do not achieve this
Be aware of your body language — try not to communicate threatening non-verbal signals (e.g. keep your hands in a low position)	Raised hands may be interpreted as a threatening gesture, particularly by clients who are experiencing paranoia, confusion or disorientation and such a gesturing may be interpreted as indicating a failure to understand the client's feelings and point of view

TABLE 45.5 | APPROACHES FOR DEALING WITH ANGER AND HOSTILE BEHAVIOUR IN THE MENTAL HEALTH CARE ENVIRONMENT—cont'd

Action	Rationale
Do not try to defend the person or situation the client is feeling angry about	
Set limits and be firm and consistent in treatment approaches. Encourage the client to take control by raising awareness of options at times of angry feelings (e.g. time-out, walking/talking with nurse, medication). The client should also be aware of the outcomes if self-restraint is not demonstrated	A client at risk of aggressive outburst is helped to remain in control if limits on what is acceptable are clear and alternative options for dealing with feelings are provided; for example, exercise, informing and seeking help from a nurse or other therapist when feelings are surfacing
Later, when the client is calm, assist to explore the immediate cause of the anger and anything that precipitated the aggressive response	Recognition of triggers can assist with problem solving
Help the client engage in problem solving and exploring alternative ways of handling their feelings	Engaging the client in solving their own problems is empowering because it informs the client that they can take responsibility for their actions
Be supportive and provide positive feedback when the client controls hostile or aggressive behaviour	Positive reinforcement is a way of helping people to modify unwanted behaviour
Accept that some anger may be displaced or projected on to you	The defence mechanisms of displacement and projection serve to reduce the anxiety and the threat to self caused by the intense emotions. Understanding this helps the nurse to avoid taking the hostility personally
Don't take unnecessary risks. If a person's anger is not subsiding but is in danger of escalating into destructive or violent acts, take whatever action is necessary to protect yourself and others (e.g. remove yourself and others from the area, seek assistance from others)	Nurses have rights in relation to workplace safety (see Chapter 26). Apart from the risk of personal harm to the nurse or others, the client who causes harm can later feel devastated by what has happened. Such an occurrence can be extremely destructive to the person's self-esteem and to the therapeutic process
Debrief with colleagues after the incident and seek any additional support that you feel you require	Dealing with aggression is challenging and can be frightening. Debriefing is a way of relieving the associated stress and can serve to identify ways for nurses to reduce risks and improve responses in the future

(Watkins 2001; Shives 2005)

the wellbeing of clients and others. Assertive behaviour is one constructive way of dealing with anger. To be assertive is to stand up for oneself while taking into account other people's interests and feelings. It takes time to develop the ability to be assertive when people are in the habit of being subservient or responding to situations they are unhappy with by being aggressive. It is within the role of mental health nurses to conduct training for clients who will be helped by developing assertiveness skills.

THE CLIENT WHO IS AT RISK OF SELF-DESTRUCTIVE BEHAVIOUR

Self-destructive behaviour is that which results in physical harm and, sometimes, in the person's own death by suicide. Self-destructive behaviour includes self-mutilation and any form of suicidal activity.

Self-mutilation

Deliberate self-mutilation results from overwhelming mental distress and is the deliberate destruction of body tissue usually without conscious intent of suicide (Fontaine & Fletcher 1999). Self-mutilation may occur once or it may become repetitive. It may or may not be impulsive. It is a behaviour associated with a range of mental health disorders (Fontaine & Fletcher 1999) including:

- Childhood sexual abuse
- Borderline personality disorder
- Eating disorders
- Cognitive impairment disorders
- Obsessive-compulsive disorder
- Post-traumatic stress disorder.

Self-mutilation may involve skin cutting, severe skin scratching or burning, head banging, self-biting, eyeball pressing, tearing out hair, self-punching or inserting dangerous objects into body orifices such as the vagina or rectum. It may involve skin carving (words, designs, symbols), bone breaking or interfering with healing by picking at wounds. Very rarely, extremely serious acts of self-mutilation occur, such as eye enucleation or amputating fingers, toes or genital organs. Other behaviours that may be considered self-destructive include involvement in unsafe sex, irresponsible gambling or spending, substance misuse, driving recklessly and binge eating (Varcarolis 2006; Moller & Fontaine 1999). The reason for self-mutilation is not totally clear but various explanations are possible. It may be:

- A maladaptive coping mechanism that raises low self-esteem by denying helplessness or powerlessness
- A self-punishing act that helps relieve unconscious feelings of guilt
- Risk-taking behaviour that, when overcome, raises self-esteem
- A way to reconnect to feeling real and alive, as opposed to feeling empty or feeling nothing
- A way of releasing tension or anger
- Using physical pain to create distraction from emotional pain
- An unspoken request for nurturing and love
- A way of manipulating others.

There are three basic goals to helping clients manage self-harming behaviour:

1. To encourage communication about the behaviour. This may not be easy because such clients often feel shameful about their actions and so tend to be secretive about it. Non-judgmental, non-blaming and supportive communication entailing active listening helps the client to feel less isolated
2. To help decrease the client's negative self-criticism to reduce the sense of shame
3. To diminish the use of the maladaptive coping mechanism of self-mutilation by identifying and developing more constructive coping strategies (Moller & Fontaine 1999, Riley & Kneisl 1996).

The nurse working in the area of mental health is highly likely to encounter clients whose inner distress has caused them to self-mutilate; it is estimated to occur in about 24–40% of mental health clients (Moller & Fontaine 1999).

SUICIDAL BEHAVIOUR

Self-destructive behaviour may result from any stress a person perceives as overwhelming, and is commonly associated with low self-esteem. When the sense of self-worth is extremely low, self-destructive behaviour reaches its peak and it is at this point that the risk of suicidal behaviour is likely. Suicidal behaviour implies a loss of the ability to see oneself as being of any value or worth at all (Stuart & Laraia 2001). Some of the risk factors for suicide are identified in Table 45.6.

Risk assessment is a crucial intervention in estimating

TABLE 45.6 | SUICIDE RISK FACTORS

Variable	Risk categories
Age	Risk generally increases with age but also at particular risk are young men and young Asian females
Marital status	Higher risk in single, widowed, separated and divorced people. The death of a loved one is a particular risk factor in the older population
Gender	More common in men than in women (more women attempt suicide, more males succeed)
Physical health	Those experiencing chronic, debilitating, progressive or life-threatening illness Alcohol and drug misuse/addiction Sleep disorder/deprivation
Psychological health	Low self-esteem Depression Feelings of hopelessness Feelings of loneliness and abandonment ('nobody cares') Experience of significant loss Unrelenting and distressing hallucinations/delusions Command hallucinations (auditory hallucinations instructing the person to self-harm) Impulsiveness, hostility and aggression
Social health	Social isolation/exclusion or sense of alienation Poor level of social supports Conflict with supportive others Social upheaval (e.g. divorce, accommodation changes) Unemployment Poverty and poor living conditions (e.g. homelessness)
History	Suicide attempts in previous 12 months Family history of suicide Expressed intent Evidence of planning (e.g. has given away possessions, made a will, said goodbyes) Evidence of preparation; that is, has the means available (e.g. has a gun, has the pills) Early recovery phase in severe depression
Previous suicidal attempts	

(adapted from Ryrie 2000)

a person's intent to self-mutilate or end their own life, and a formal risk assessment should be conducted whenever there is any indication of the possibility of either, whether the client is in a general acute-care hospital, a mental health care facility, residential care or living in the community. Figure 45.2 illustrates one example of a suicide/self-harm

INPATIENT SUICIDE/SELF-HARM ASSESSMENT

Complete on admission if indicated by Risk Factor Assessment or any time when suicidal risk is suspected.

Directions:
1. Answer Section I.
2. Complete Section II by circling one of the three descriptors for each Key Factor that BEST describes the patient.
3. Complete Section III.
4. Add the points for each circled item in Sections I, II and III to obtain the total score.

I. Is the current admission precipitated by suicide attempt? Yes 2 No 1

II. Key Factors	High risk (1:1)	Moderate risk (q15min observation)	No Precautions
Contract for safety	Unwilling to contract OR Unable to contract because of impaired reality testing (hallucinations, delusions, dementia, delirium, dissociation) 2	Contracts but is ambivalent or guarded 1	Reliably contracts for safety 0
Suicide plan	Has plan with actual potential access to planned method 2	Has plan without access to planned method 1	No plan 0
Plan lethality	Highly lethal plan (gun, hanging, jumping, carbon monoxide) 2	Medium lethality of plan (sleeping pills, overdose of aspirin, barbiturates) 1	Low lethality of plan (superficial scratching, head banging, pillow over face, biting, holding breath) 0
Elopement risk	High elopement risk 2	Low elopement risk 1	No elopement risk 0
Suicidal ideation	Constant suicidal thoughts 2	Intermittent or fleeting suicidal thoughts 1	No current suicidal thoughts 0
Attempt history	Past attempts of high lethality 2	Past attempts of low lethality 1	No previous attempts 0
Symptoms (circle those that apply) hopelessness helplessness anhedonia guilt/shame anger/hostility impulsivity impaired problem solving	5–6 symptoms present 2	3–4 symptoms present 1	0–2 symptoms present 0
Current morbid thoughts (reunion fantasies, preoccupation with death, disturbing nightmares)	Constantly 2	Frequently 1	Rarely 0

III. RN's Subjective Appraisal of Patient's Reliability:

Pt replies not trustworthy; several non-verbal cues	4
Pt replies questionable, not trustworthy, at least one non-verbal cue	3
Pt replies trustworthy	0

Scoring Key:

High Risk Precautions (1:1)	=	10 or more
Moderate Risk Precautions (q15min observation)	=	4–9
Moderate Risk Precautions	=	4–9
No Precautions	=	0–3

Total Score ____________

Assessed by (RN): ____________

Date: ____________

Time: ____________

Figure 45.2 | An example of a suicide/self-harm risk assessment tool *(Stuart & Laraia 2004)* assessment tool. It should be noted that the successful use of an assessment tool involves the ability to establish effective open and honest communication with the client, and expertise in the art of therapeutic communication is perhaps the most important component of the mental health nurse's contribution to care. (See Chapter 29 for more information on therapeutic communication.)

The first priority in dealing with a person who is at risk of, or exhibits, self-destructive behaviour is to protect the person from harm. All dangerous or potentially dangerous objects that could be used in an act of self-harm must be removed from the individual's environment. This includes knives and other sharp implements, matches, glass, items of clothing such as belts, scarves or stockings or anything else that may be used by the client to inflict self-harm. Other approaches for dealing with self-harm and suicidal behaviour are outlined in Table 45.7. While it takes time and experience to become an accomplished mental health nurse, and the care and management of at-risk clients requires particular expertise, the principles of care, when necessary and appropriate, may be applied by others in any health care setting to protect clients.

Self-mutilation and suicide are complex issues, and a simple and very brief overview has been provided here. As people with depression and self-harming tendencies may be encountered in every area of nursing, it is recommended that nurses explore the issues further by accessing psychiatric or mental health nursing textbooks.

THE CLIENT WHO EXPERIENCES HYPERACTIVITY

Hyperactivity can be a manifestation of a variety of mental health disorders, caused by the misuse of certain substances such as cocaine and amphetamines (Chitty 2004), but is particularly associated with bipolar disorders. Bipolar disorders are a group of mood disorders that manifest with periods of depression and mania. The hyperactivity associated with mania is quite different to the normal exuberant activity engaged in by most people at various times. Hypomania is a clinical syndrome similar to, but not as severe as, mania, which is sometimes termed hypermania (Stuart & Laraia 2001). At one time people who experienced the mood cycles associated with bipolar disorders were said to have a manic–depressive illness.

Mania is characterised by excitability, optimism, marked hyperactivity, talkativeness and a decreased need for sleep. The symptoms vary in intensity. In the milder form, people can appear to have excess energy, they may present as the 'life and soul of the party', be able to work long hours and be very productive in work and leisure activities. If the symptoms increase to the most severe level, people may experience serious impairment in judgment that allows them to behave in ways not usually in keeping with their personalities. For example, a normally shy and quiet woman may become loud, dress in bright and gaudy clothing and become overtly sexually provocative; a normally sensible and frugal young man may run up huge and unmanageable debts on his credit card, drive his car at outrageously dangerous speeds and yell obscenities out of the car window as he narrowly misses other vehicles and pedestrians. Such dangerous and life-threatening behaviours may be of no concern to the affected person if they have psychotic symptoms, because delusional thoughts may make them believe that they are indestructible; for example, the young man above may believe that he is immortal because he is a new god come to save the world. Common symptoms associated with mania are summarised in Table 45.8. People who are experiencing the severe form of mania may need to be admitted to an inpatient unit for their own protection and for the protection of others.

Treatment includes firm limit-setting, seclusion (only when essential), cognitive therapy, counselling and chemical restraint (medication). Lithium is one drug that is effective in treating the symptoms of acute mania and in reducing or preventing recurrence of the mood swings associated with bipolar disorders. However, Lithium and other drugs often cause unwanted side effects and levels in the blood require strict monitoring to prevent Lithium toxicity. In addition, some of the feelings of elation and mania are enjoyed, so clients are understandably not always willing to take the medications that stop the feelings so drastically and they may seek alternative ways of controlling the illness. Nursing interventions vary according to the level of hyperactivity and include:

- Maintaining client safety and the safety of others
- Maintaining the client's biological normality (e.g. meeting rest, nutrition, fluid and elimination needs)
- Facilitating activities of daily living (e.g. meeting hygiene needs)
- Helping the client to regain and maintain self-control
- Preserving the client's dignity when behaviour is out of character and when it will be a source of embarrassment or humiliation when functioning more normally
- Reducing the amount of stimulation to which the client is subjected
- Providing a structured daily program that allows opportunities to expend energy in set activities (e.g. physical activity such as using an exercise bike or walking may help to drain excess energy).

The overall goals of care are to help the client establish constructive coping mechanisms and increase the client's satisfaction gained from interaction with the world (Stuart & Laraia 2001). To do this the mental health nurse must establish and maintain a trusting relationship with the client. Attempting to do this can be challenging and frustrating for the nurse, partly because particular unusual speech patterns are common in people experiencing episodes of mania that impact on the ability to communicate effectively, particularly when clients are in the acute phase of mania. The speech patterns associated with mania are listed in Clinical Interest Box 45.12.

TABLE 45.7 | APPROACHES FOR DEALING WITH SELF-HARM AND SUICIDAL BEHAVIOUR IN THE MENTAL HEALTH CARE ENVIRONMENT

Action	Rationale
Engage in an open exploration of suicidal ideas, including the frequency and intrusiveness of the thoughts, the planning and motivation	Open exploration is an essential component of identifying the level of risk of self-harm. Any statement that alludes to self-harm; for example, a threat or innuendo made by the client that they are thinking about harming themself should be taken seriously
Assess the risk factors	A formal risk assessment should be conducted whenever any risk of self-harm is detected. Risk-minimisation strategies appropriate to the level of risk identified should be put in place; for example, close observation, contractual agreement for the client to report to the nurse when thoughts of self-harm are likely to be acted on. Mental health care agencies usually have specific guidelines and policies for management of clients at risk of self-harm
Be with clients in a calm, accepting and empathic manner	Facilitates open and honest communication and the development of a therapeutic relationship
Engage in therapeutic conversation that facilitates the safe expression of distress and the identification of the underlying issues and concerns	Helps the client to identify the factors (stressors) responsible for wanting to commit acts of self-destruction and will inform as to the measures that are appropriate to facilitate the healing of mental anguish
Recognise the opportunity for learning, personal growth and positive change as a potential outcome of the client's present experience	Recognising that positive outcomes are possible stimulates a sense of hope in the nurse, which can be relayed to the client. Hope and realistic optimism facilitate recovery
Work collaboratively with at-risk clients, their significant others and other health professionals in assessing needs and planning care	Appropriate interventions may involve different areas of professional expertise; for example, recreational therapist, psychiatrist, dietitian, psychologist. The client's significant others need to be aware of the strategies required to maintain the client's safety, and their involvement can be supportive for the client
An appropriately qualified person should negotiate a risk-minimisation plan with the client and significant others	Risk-minimisation plans usually involve a contractual agreement, and this needs to be firm and clear. Nurses are advised to work with experienced staff in relation to these before attempting to implement them
Be clear about the client's responsibility for their own safety within the context of the plan	Clients need to understand that, within the contractual arrangement, control of the situation is theirs. This is empowering, but clients also need to feel supported in managing their feelings
The care plan must be clear to all staff working in the client's environment	It is a team responsibility to support and protect the client and facilitate the success of the contractual arrangement
Be clear about the availability of support when a person feels unsafe, and ensure the person understands the boundaries that apply	The client needs to be clear about who is available and when they can provide support, and the type of support that is possible. This ensures that the risk of inappropriate dependency on staff is reduced and the client's sense of responsibility in the situation is reinforced
Mobilise social support	Social support is important in maximising the client's coping abilities. It can also assist the client to increase self-esteem (e.g. by promoting relationships with others). For clients who are at risk but living in the community, arrangements may be made for another person to 'keep the means' (e.g. the client's medication), and for people to visit the client during times of the day when they are likely to be on their own
Engage in problem solving with the client	Helps maximise the client's constructive coping strategies and develop others
The nurse must be aware of personal and team responsibilities and accountability in relation to caring for at-risk clients	Client safety depends on staff fulfilling responsibilities. Responsibilities include knowing which clients are demonstrating an increasing risk of self-harm (e.g. increasing alienation), and which are showing signs of improvement (e.g. smiling, interacting with others). The nurse should be aware that signs of improvement can be misleading

(Watkins 2001; Kelly 2000)

TABLE 45.8 | COMMON SYMPTOMS ASSOCIATED WITH MANIA

Type	Symptoms
Affective (mood)	Elation or euphoria Expansiveness Humourousness (witty) Inflated self-esteem Intolerance of criticism Lack of shame or guilt
Physiological	Dehydration Inadequate nutrition Weight loss Reduced need for sleep
Cognitive	Ambitiousness Denial of realistic dangers Distractibility and poor attention span Flight of ideas (jumping from one train of thought to another without pause) Grandiosity (e.g. delusions of grandeur) Illusions Lack of judgment and impaired decision making (e.g. unable to evaluate realistic danger and consequences of actions) Looseness of associations Delusions
Behavioural	Irritability/argumentativeness/aggressiveness especially if thwarted in achieving what is desired Excessive spending when unemployed or broke and other forms of irresponsibility Grandiose acts that may involve excessive risk taking Increased motor activity and pressure of speech (extreme rapidity) Poor or bizarre personal grooming May wear bright and ornate clothing (reflect elevated mood) Sexual provocativeness and sexual hyperactivity that is often promiscuous Excessive involvement in pleasurable activities without regard for negative consequences (e.g. swimming in dangerous conditions, unprotected sexual activity with strangers)

(Stuart & Laraia 2001; Videbeck 2001)

CLINICAL INTEREST BOX 45.12
Examples of speech patterns associated with mania

Pressured speech	Rapid and accelerated speech that continues without pauses between words or sentences. The flow of rapid talking continues without regard to others who may be attempting to answer, intervene or add something
Clang associations	The stringing together of words that rhyme without regard to their meaning
Circumstantiality	Use of long irrelevant descriptions when trying to describe a person, situation or event. The account may include vast amounts of irrelevant and unrelated information and may include lots of repetition
Loose associations	Lack of a logical relationship between thoughts and ideas that renders spoken communication vague, unfocused (waffly) and diffuse (long-winded)
Flight of ideas	A nearly continuous flow of accelerated speech characterised by abrupt verbal skipping from topic to topic, usually based on chance associations between words
Tangentiality	Constantly diverging in mid-conversation to different and unrelated topics. When describing a situation, frequently losing the train of thought, and not completing descriptions of anything

(Stuart & Laraia 2004; Videbeck 2001; Shives 2005)

Some of the factors that present challenges to nurses in developing therapeutic relationships are that the client may:

- Have a brief attention span
- Find it difficult to be still, and need to be in perpetual motion
- Find it difficult to listen to others and constantly interrupt
- Appear unaware of verbal and non-verbal cues indicating that others wish to speak
- Continue with a constant stream of speech that is sometimes unintelligible

- Have confused thinking, with thoughts racing one after the other (this makes it difficult for the client to make connections between concepts and so when speaking they may jump rapidly from one subject to another)
- Have diminished awareness of personal space boundaries and tend to invade the 'intimate zone' of others (see Chapter 29 for information about personal zones)
- Have little understanding of how overpowering, excessive and confrontational their interactions can feel to others
- Test the rules and limits set for the therapeutic environment
- Be insistent on having their own way and may attempt to manipulate people, including the nurse, in order to achieve this
- Frequently insult staff or others, use foul or sexually explicit language, taunt and annoy others
- Be seductive towards the nurse (among others) (Fortinash & Holoday Worret 2004; Videbeck 2001; Varcarolis 2006).

Management includes setting clear limits on behaviour while being supportive but firm. Setting limits involves reinforcing that it is the behaviour and not the person that is rejected. For example, it is preferable to say, 'That sort of language is not accepted in this unit', rather than, 'You are so crude speaking like that'.

The nurse at all times needs to remain calm, speak clearly and explain what is required simply and firmly but in a caring manner. All staff must be aware of the limits and rules set for the client's behaviour, which must be constantly reinforced to assist the client to regain control of his behaviour. It must be remembered that behaviours that appear manipulative, fault finding or exploitative of others' vulnerabilities are the outward expression of inner turmoil, distress and often serious emotional need. Such behaviour is the client's way of trying to gain a sense of control at a time when they have no control of most aspects of their life; not even their own thoughts or feelings (Varcarolis 2006). Table 45.9 provides some approaches for dealing with hyperactivity associated with the manic phases of bipolar disorders, but the principles apply to clients experiencing excessive or uncontrolled hyperactivity from any cause.

Bipolar disorders and any disorder in which hyperactivity is a serious problem can be potentially devastating for clients and their families. It is an important part of the mental health nurse's role to ensure that everyone affected understands about the illness causing the behaviour, is aware of what can and cannot be done to control the illness, and what services and supports are available to help them to cope.

CLIENTS EXPERIENCING CONFUSION OR DISORIENTATION

A person may become confused or disoriented for a variety of reasons, including as a result of delirium, dementia or from the toxic effects of alcohol and some prescribed and non-prescribed drugs. The effect in each case is a significant marked change in cognitive abilities from the client's previous level of functioning. Cognitive functioning includes the mental processes of memory, reasoning, judgment, orientation, problem solving, decision making, the acquisition of knowledge and the ability to use and comprehend language. Some causes of cognitive dysfunction are reversible, others are not. Delirium, for example, is a syndrome that involves a disturbance to a person's state of consciousness, which is accompanied by changes in cognition, almost always due to an identifiable cause that can in most cases be rectified. Dementia, on the other hand, is a progressive, irreversible and disabling condition in which changes in cognitive function are caused by gradually increasing, permanent damage to the brain. The focus here is on caring for those with progressive dementia.

Dementia is one of the most common causes of confusion and disorientation, with over 162 000 people in Australia currently identified as having the illness. It is a disorder normally associated with older clients but, although the risk of dementia does increase with age, more than 6600 of those identified as having dementia are under age 65 (Access Economics 2003). Alzheimer's dementia (AD) is the most common form of the illness, but all types of dementia share similar symptoms and require similar interventions. The symptoms depend on the sequence in which areas of the brain are damaged by the disease process, so the progression of symptoms varies in different people. Symptoms change and increase in severity over the duration of the illness, which in the case of AD can be 3–20 years, the average span being 8 years (Access Economics 2003). Symptoms include:

- Gradual memory loss
- Increasing loss of language and communication skills
- Progressive decline in ability to perform routine tasks despite having intact physical functioning (in the early stages of dementia this may mean difficulty with coordination when preparing a meal or when shopping and handling money, or when driving a car. Later this extends to include difficulty with tasks such as dressing, eating, and bathing)
- Impaired judgment, abstract thinking
- Difficulty in concentrating and learning new information or skills
- Changes in behaviour (e.g. wandering, incessant walking, constant repetition of words, confabulation)
- Changes in personality and mood (up to two-thirds of people with AD have symptoms of depression, and about 20% exhibit aggression)
- Hallucinations and delusions (hallucinations are experienced by about 16% of people with AD, delusions by about 30%, and they are often paranoid in nature)
- Loss of initiative
- Altered sleep–wake patterns

TABLE 45.9 | APPROACHES FOR DEALING WITH HYPERACTIVITY ASSOCIATED WITH BIPOLAR DISORDERS (MANIC PHASE)

Action	Rationale
Use a firm and calm approach	This helps promote a therapeutic relationship and is reassuring for the client and provides structure and control for a client who is out of control
Use short concise explanations or statements	A short concentration span and confused thinking make it difficult for the client to absorb complex information
Remain neutral, avoid power struggles and value judgments	Avoids provoking hostility or combativeness. Client can use inconsistencies and value judgments as justification for arguing and escalating mania
Maintain a consistent approach; for example, provide a consistent and structured environment and keep expectations the same	This provides the framework that assists the client to regain a feeling of control. Clear and consistent limits and expectations minimise the potential for clients to manipulate staff or annoy others
Firmly redirect energy into appropriate and constructive channels, provide an outlet for physical energy in a non-stimulating environment; for example, use of a punching bag in a quiet area	Helps in establishing constructive mechanisms for coping with excess energy. Can help release pent-up hostility and relieve muscle tension
Decrease environmental stimuli whenever possible; for example, avoid loud music, noises, bright lights, and people	Limits distractions that can provoke agitation and escalate mania
Provide structured solitary activities — tasks that take minimal concentration are best. Avoid groups and stimulating activities	Solitary activities are best until distractibility is settled and the client is able to comfortably tolerate being part of a group
Spend one-on-one time with the client, especially when psychotic or anxious	Provides reassurance and gives the message that the client is a worthwhile person. As mania and hyperactivity settle, provides time for exploration of issues
Encourage frequent rest periods Provide high-calorie fluids and finger foods frequently throughout the day On a daily basis, monitor the client's sleep pattern, food and fluid intake, and elimination pattern (constipation is a common problem)	It is important that the client's physical wellbeing is maintained during the time they are not concerned with it themselves
Provide the client and the family with explanations and written information about the illness and the treatment plan (it is particularly important that the client and family understand the information concerning medication)	Information is important to promote compliance with treatment regimens and minimise the risk of recurrence of symptoms
Ensure client and family or significant others understand how to access the supportive services in the community	Knowing about community supports includes information about accessing help in a crisis, which can be reassuring. Information about support groups and activities aimed at prevention are helpful in promoting coping mechanisms and recovery

(adapted from Varcarolis 2000)

- Loss of bladder and bowel continence (usually later stage) (Access Economics 2003).

Caring for the client with dementia

Care interventions for clients with dementia are dependent on the client's abilities, and the focus of care should be on what the client can still do rather on abilities lost. General care interventions are listed in Clinical Interest Box 45.13.

Reality orientation is a form of rehabilitation used to orientate confused or cognitively impaired clients by promoting or maintaining their awareness of person, time and place. It is recognised as unrealistic to expect to orientate people in the later stages of dementia to present time reality, but some of the principles of reality orientation are appropriate and helpful (Ebersole & Hess 2001). Helpful aspects include:

- Calling the client by their preferred name every time they are approached
- Stating your name each time you start an interaction with the client
- Maintaining a normal day–night cycle; for example, opening curtains and blinds during the day and closing them at night and encouraging the client to

CLINICAL INTEREST BOX 45.13
Interventions appropriate for clients experiencing confusion or disorientation

Appropriate care for the confused or disorientated client includes:

- A safe, consistent, pleasant and familiar environment
- Freedom from physical/emotional/spiritual pain
- A calm, relaxed, caring and non-challenging atmosphere
- A stable and familiar staff
- Staff who have appropriate expertise and are compassionate
- Skilled communicators (expertise in communicating with cognitively impaired clients)
- Frequent and gentle touch
- Tactful use of humour
- Frequent contact and interaction with staff/family
- Contact with pets if desired (especially the client's own pets)
- Opportunities to socialise
- A structured individualised routine (as close to the client's familiar routine at home as is possible)
- The presence of the client's own familiar belongings (e.g. personal objects)
- Therapeutic activities/programs to promote cognitive stimulation (e.g. reminiscence therapy, music therapy)
- Nutritious diet/adequate hydration, including pleasurable snacks
- Adequate periods of rest and sleep
- High standard of hygiene/personal grooming
- Effective use of well-maintained visual/hearing/sensory aids
- Adequate daily exercise
- Access to a pleasant and safe outdoor area
- Maintenance of treatments ordered by the medical officer.

(adapted from Fortinash & Holoday Worret 2003: 244)

dress in their own clothes during the day, rather than in nightwear
- Leaving the furniture and the client's belongings in the same place, as rearranging objects in the environment adds to confusion
- Encouraging the client to wear their spectacles and/or hearing aids, as not wearing them adds to sensory confusion
- Maintaining a routine and a sense of order in daily activities
- Ensuring that the environment is designed to minimise confusion; for example, using distinctive colours or pictures on bathroom or toilet doors to help the confused person identify these areas, and ensuring adequate lighting in all areas to minimise the effect of shadows that might confuse perceptions of what is seen
- Using a notice board to display information about the date and place that is consistently maintained to give residents an opportunity to remain orientated to dates, times and important events.

Clients who have temporary confusion or who are in the early stages of dementia and are seeking to maintain orientation to time and place may benefit from the following interventions:

- Telling the person the date and time each morning and repeating the information as appropriate during the day
- Having the day and date displayed in large bold letters on a board and having the person change it accordingly each day
- Reminding the person of holidays, birthdays and other special events
- Providing cues to reinforce verbal information; for example, clocks with clear and large numbers, large calendars
- Discussing current affairs; for example, items in the newspaper or on television news.

A key to providing quality care is to find a way to connect with clients who have dementia. This is different to simply communicating, which can be one sided, with the nurse talking and the client largely passive. Connecting involves the nurse or other carer having to develop skills and spend time and effort establishing connection (Access Economics 2003). The use of validation therapy and reminiscence therapy promotes connection and they are highly appropriate for use with clients who have dementia (Sherman 1999; Feil 2002). (Issues concerning communicating effectively with clients who have dementia and the use of appropriate therapies such as validation and reminiscence therapy are outlined in Chapter 29.) Recreational, occupational and complementary therapies can also be therapeutic in promoting cognitive, sensory and physical stimulation and can provide opportunities for staff to connect with clients.

Managing challenging behaviours in confused clients

Many of the behaviours that people with dementia exhibit are a direct result of the illness and so need to be considered as 'normal' symptoms of the illness, rather than abnormal behaviours. Behaviours that fall into this category include aimless wandering, becoming lost, muddled actions and conversations, disturbances in sleep–wake cycles and, especially with some particular types of dementia (e.g. Picks disease), loss of emotional control and aggressive reactions (Sherman 1999). Other behaviours, such as unusual outbursts of physical or verbal aggression, dressing or disrobing publicly, or refusing to bathe, eat or attend activities previously enjoyed, can be due to a range of influences that can exacerbate the normal effects of the illness. The reason for the behaviour — the core of the problem — may be related to a variety of issues including:

- A change in the environment (e.g. too noisy, too busy, causing feelings of being overwhelmed)

- The person's physical condition (e.g. too hot or cold, clothing uncomfortable, pain or discomfort)
- Hallucinations or delusions (may create fear and anxiety)
- Provocation by another resident
- The way a particular staff member interacts with the person (e.g. being loud or bustling or rushing the person).

Whatever the client's behaviour, it is important for the nurse to respond quietly, calmly, confidently and kindly. This kind of response is often enough to modify the behaviour. The use of psychotropic medications for managing challenging behaviour is best avoided because these agents tend to have little effect on problem behaviour associated with dementia, particularly of the Alzheimer's type, and they may cause serious side effects more difficult to deal with than the behaviour itself (Sherman 1999). When behaviour is not acceptable the nurse should firmly let the person know that this is the case, and behaviour that is appropriate should be praised.

Care by staff who fully understand the effects of the dementia illness and have appropriate expertise in communicating with confused people is important to the client's sense of wellbeing, and it is clearly evident that disruptive behaviour is less likely in residential care settings when the principles of dementia care management are followed (Sherman 1999). The principles of dementia care management are outlined in Clinical Interest Box 45.13. It should be noted that, while many of these principles apply to caring for clients who are confused or disorientated from causes other than progressive dementia, the approach for reversible confusion or temporary disorientation may include strategies to assist the person with progressive dementia to remain orientated to reality. Other general nursing responsibilities for managing challenging behaviour are outlined in Clinical Interest Box 45.14.

Dementia is one of the most complex and disabling illnesses. It presents huge challenges to nurses and to the many family carers who tend loved ones with dementia at home. Table 45.10 provides a summary of some of the information that nurses need to know and some of the information that nurses need to teach to family carers.

Dementia care, while not always acknowledged as such, is a specialty area of nursing, requiring a high level of integrated skills. It is predominantly a disorder of the elderly, who often have multiple other concurrent health issues that the nurse must be knowledgeable about. Dementia clients are often not able to explain their feelings or their needs; the nurse therefore needs high-level observation and communication skills to provide quality care. The nurse also needs to be able to support the family carers of people with dementia, who are often devastated by what has happened to their loved ones.

This section briefly highlights some of the many issues relating to dementia care but it is recommended that nurses undertake specialist courses to enhance their knowledge and skills in this area. Organisations such as Alzheimer's Australia are available for up-to-date information relevant to people with dementia, their families and health professionals. Access details for the Alzheimer's Australia internet website is provided at the end of this chapter. All caring needs to be undertaken with understanding of the legal and ethical issues that relate to mental health nursing. The next section adds some specific points to the general legal and ethical principles impacting on nursing that are outlined in Chapter 3.

LEGAL AND ETHICAL ASPECTS OF MENTAL HEALTH NURSING

The provision of health care for individuals suffering from mental health disorders is governed by government mental health Acts. Each Australian state and territory has its own Act, as does New Zealand, and these Acts are periodically revised. The nurse who is involved in mental health nursing has a responsibility to be aware of the relevant current acts in the geographical area of their employment. Information about legal issues may also be accessed from government departments responsible for the health of the community such as the Department of Human Services (Victoria, Australia) or its equivalent in other states and territories.

Mental health Acts provide guidelines and directions regarding the provision of mental health care, for example criteria for determining criteria for admission to hospital, and regulations and requirements regarding the periodic review of individuals suffering from mental illness. The information here is based on the law as it relates to mental health clients in the State of Victoria, Australia, but the principles apply to laws across Australia and New Zealand.

LEGAL ISSUES RELATING TO INFORMAL AND FORMAL ADMISSION

Treatment in a mental health care facility or by a community mental health care team may take the form of informal or formal admission. Informal (voluntary) admission is when an individual chooses to receive treatment. Treatment may be at personal request or based on the advice of family or a health professional, and the client is able to withdraw from treatment or leave the health care facility whenever they choose.

Formal (involuntary) admission is when the request for admission comes from a source other than the mentally ill person, who is deemed incompetent to make an informed decision (see Chapter 3). An individual may be referred for admission if they pose a danger to themself or others or if they require treatment but are too confused or disorganised to seek voluntary admission. A medical officer completes a recommendation for admission form after examining the person. The admitting psychiatrist at the treatment centre then examines the person and decides whether or not to

CLINICAL INTEREST BOX 45.14
Nursing responsibilities for managing challenging behaviour

- Maintain a calm environment and respond to the situation calmly
- Remain neutral, do not attribute blame, never 'tell off' in a patronising manner or punish in any way
- Avoid the use of restraints, including chemical restraints, in particular physical restraints tend to increase agitation and confusion (see Chapter 26 for information about the use of restraints)
- Try to identify the cause
- Observe and keep a record of when the behaviour occurs, the type of behaviour, the client's mood, and where and with whom the behaviour occurs: this helps to identify triggers for the behaviour that in many cases suggest how the cause can be eliminated
- Assess the person
- Is there a physical or emotional trigger for the behaviour? Is the client or resident unwell, in pain, overtired, overstimulated, bored, anxious, embarrassed, or feeling ignored, misunderstood or patronised?
- Is the client or resident reacting to an unpleasant incident or is the behaviour associated with:
  - — a change?
  - — a disturbing memory?
  - — a particular person or occurrence?
  - — a situation or request that is culturally inappropriate?
  - — delusions or hallucinations?
  - — the memory of a traumatic past experience stimulated by the current situation?
- Consider all the facts together. Ask:
  - — does the behaviour always happen in the same place or in similar surroundings?
  - — is it new behaviour?
  - — how was this situation (e.g. daily shower) managed when the client lived at home?
  - — does it occur with a particular person in particular circumstances?
  - — is it connected with a particular staff member, relative, friend or other resident?
  - — what does the client say, if anything, about the behaviour?
  - — can the family carer provide any insights into the behaviour?
- Use a team approach to problem solving
- It may take time and several different ideas may need to be implemented before certain problem behaviours are resolved. If one nurse finds a successful intervention, this should be documented appropriately and shared with all team members

Redirection

Redirection involves distracting the client from the situation causing the behaviour. For example, the nurse may distract the client who is upset and shouting at another resident without obvious cause by saying, 'I don't know what's wrong but I think we should get away from here — let's go for a walk outside'. The client who is jumping up from the meal table and upsetting other clients by saying, 'this food is bad, it tastes like poison' may be directed if the nurse responds, 'I don't think things are right, come with me, you can leave that food, let's go and find something else to eat' or, 'You'd better leave that, let's get something else to eat later on — can you come and help me water the plants outside and then we'll eat later?'.

Triggers

The following example is an illustration of how identifying a trigger can help to reduce challenging behaviour and how different strategies may need to be tried until a successful way of stopping the behaviour is found.

Mrs Lamb, 72, who has dementia and is living in a residential care facility, was generally happily confused but on some days would be very agitated, pace about, bang on tables and sometimes swear and shout out abuse such as, 'get away you cow' at the top of her voice. On these days she would often start crying for no apparent reason and the staff found it difficult to console her or to establish what was upsetting her. On the last two occasions of being so upset, she became physically aggressive and even succeeded in biting one of the nurses.

After keeping a detailed record of when and where the behaviour occurred it was realised that it was on certain days of the week that corresponded with when a particular nurse was on duty. This was a surprise, as the nurse was respected for her compassion and skill in dementia care nursing, but it was soon confirmed that the challenging behaviour was definitely triggered by the nurse's presence. It was only after consulting with Mrs Lamb's sister that the cause became clear. The nurse bore a close resemblance to a next-door neighbour who had reversed her car over and killed Mrs Lamb's much adored labrador dog over 40 years previously.

The problem was discussed at a team meeting. It was decided that the nurse should not be responsible for Mrs Lamb's personal care and that she should attempt to reinforce her own identity with Mrs Lamb. When the nurse next came on duty she wore her hair differently and made a point over the next few weeks of consistently introducing herself and showing Mrs Lamb her name badge. She managed to tell Mrs Lamb about herself, she even used photographs of her family, her home and her holidays to assist the process of trying to reinforce her real identity. This seemed to be effective on most occasions, although Mrs Lamb sometimes continued to respond with agitation and aggression towards the nurse she believed had killed her pet dog.

Not knowing what else to do as Mrs Lamb one day yelled at her, 'get out, dangerous bitch' the nurse quickly said, 'I'm so sorry, I was so careless, I never meant to hurt your dog. I am so sorry, please forgive me.' With this, Mrs Lamb acknowledged the apology with a firm quick nod of the head, walked to her chair and with a sigh sat down. This seemed to settle what for Mrs Lamb may have been unfinished business. The nurse continued to use this approach whenever Mrs Lamb was agitated and eventually the agitation and aggressive response to the nurse stopped.

(Sherman 1999; Ebersole & Hess 2001; Videbeck 2001)

TABLE 45.10 | INFORMATION FOR NURSES AND FOR CLIENTS WITH DEMENTIA AND THEIR FAMILY CARERS

Information that nurses need to know	Information that nurses need to give people with dementia, and their family carers
• Short-term memory loss is a primary symptom in the early stages of dementia of the Alzheimer's type. Memory loss later becomes global and affects short- and long-term memory • Certain medications, especially in combination, can cause increased confusion and agitation • Safety in the home and in health care settings is a primary concern because clients with dementia are at increased risk of falls and other injuries from the combination of sensory effects, memory loss and age-related factors • Clients may be unable to communicate pain or emotional distress; the nurse needs to assess clients regularly and monitor closely for physical and mental concerns, including concurrent depression, which can exacerbate the symptoms of dementia • Sundowning syndrome (evening agitation associated with a busy time of day and resulting from client fatigue) may lead to challenging behaviours. Planned activities for clients are helpful in preventing agitated behaviour at this time • A structured environment with minimal changes is critical because it reduces client anxiety, confusion and agitation • Clients with AD may occasionally confabulate (attempt to fill memory gaps with unrelated information), which is not considered lying • Clients who confabulate may need gentle validation of their sense of what is true, or they may be gently redirected to another topic because confronting them with reality may result in confusion and distress • Intake of nutritional supplements, herbs and over-the-counter medications may interfere with the client's prescribed medications • Clients cared for at home may resist outside help and place undue demands and stress on the family carer • Stressors that can provoke client anxiety or confusion should be identified and modified or avoided as much as possible (e.g. loud music, cluttered rooms) • Potential elder abuse may be a result of family carer strain, and clients and carers need to be evaluated if abuse is suspected. Carers need to be made aware of all available supports and respite services in the community to reduce strain when people with dementia are cared for at home • Access current resources available on the Internet and in the library	• Teach clients (in the early stages of the illness) and their families about the disorder and explain the progression of the illness and prognosis so that expectations are realistic. Clients with dementia (especially those with young-onset disease) can choose and plan what they want to do with their lives in light of their prognosis, and can deal with any legal matters while cognition allows (e.g. make a will, advance directives) • Teach the family carers actions and precautions to reduce the client's risk for falls or other injury (see Chapter 26) • Instruct the family how to observe for non-verbal signs of pain and discomfort (e.g. groaning, cold clammy skin, holding body part, changed vital signs) • Teach the family about Sundowning syndrome and offer strategies to reduce fatigue, confusion and agitation (sometimes family carers themselves discover helpful strategies that they can pass on to professional carers, as the 24-hour/day care they provide often makes them experts in dementia management and care) • Teach the family about changes in condition (e.g. exacerbation of confusion, signs of depression) that are signs of health problems separate to dementia. Ensure awareness of who to contact for help and advice • Teach strategies that promote the client's existing memory and connectedness with others (e.g. validation, reminiscence, environmental cues, familiar songs, pictures, pets, etc) • Ensure awareness of correct medication regimen, possible side effects and importance of following the medical officer's directions for administration • Ensure awareness of discussing use of non-prescribed drugs (e.g. herbal remedies) with the medical officer to avoid side effects when combined with prescribed medications • Suggest that the client remain under care of one medical officer to provide consistent care and clear medication regimen. This avoids the risks of adverse drug interactions from incompatible medications and polypharmacy (multiple medications) • Teach the family about confabulation and stress that it is not lying, and that it is best to validate the person's belief of what is true. Stress that it can be distressing to challenge the person's view of reality. For example, if the person says they had egg, bacon and mushrooms for breakfast, it is best not to contradict them even if you are certain that they only had porridge • Teach to identify stressors (anxiety triggers) in the home environment, and offer realistic solutions • Explain the benefits of outside help when the help comes from skilled and reliable carers who can bond with the person with dementia • Encourage the family carer to take advantage of respite and other services that will reduce the strain of caring for someone with dementia. Encourage family members to share the caregiving responsibilities • Stress the importance of 'time out' for the family carer to recharge personal batteries, and the importance of maintaining their own health. This includes attendance to preventive strategies such as routine health checks, mammograms, flu injections etc • Inform family carers about how to access current information via the internet and libraries, and from agencies such as Alzheimer's Australia (there are Alzheimer's information centres in many areas of Australia and New Zealand, many of which offer client and family carer support groups, among other services. Many also offer educational programs for family and professional carers)

(adapted from Fortinash & Holoday Worret 2003: 245)

act on the recommendation by admitting the individual as a formal (involuntary) client, which means that the client may be given treatment deemed necessary whether or not they consent to the treatment.

In a crisis situation it may be a team of professionals based in the community, such as a crisis assessment and treatment team (CATT) that is called to assist. The team can request formal (involuntary) admission for a client but a medical officer must examine the client and sign the recommendation form as soon as possible. There are five criteria, all of which must be met to justify a person being admitted involuntarily. These are that:

1. The person must be mentally ill (mental illness is described in the *Victorian Mental Health Act 1986* as a medical condition that is characterised by a significant disturbance of thought, mood, perception or memory)
2. The person must need immediate treatment
3. The person must present a health or safety risk to themself or others
4. The person refuses or is unable to consent voluntarily to treatment
5. There is no less restrictive way of providing needed treatment.

As soon as a client no longer meets all five criteria they must be discharged from their involuntary status, or what is termed formal detention. There are strict guidelines governing who should review formal clients and how often they should be reviewed. Two psychiatrists must independently review formal clients on, or within 24 hours of, admission. All clients should be provided with a statement of rights on admission and given details of whom they can contact for support. Clients have a right to appeal against involuntary admission. The Mental Health Review Board reviews clients who appeal, but in any case automatically reviews formal clients on a regular basis.

TREATMENT ORDERS AND ISSUES OF CONSENT

Mental health clients who are admitted involuntarily to a mental health service are sometimes treated under a community treatment order (CTO) or a restricted community treatment order (RCTO) while living in the community. The CTO may require that the person lives in a particular place to facilitate treatment; the RCTO may stipulate which psychiatrist will provide treatment, where and how often treatment will be applied and how long the order will last. It may also stipulate other specific conditions under which the client may remain in the community while receiving treatment. All formal clients, whether treated in the community or in a hospital, are legally obliged to accept recommended treatment, and treatment can be enforced against the client's will if necessary. Even though this is the case it is in everyone's best interest for formal and informal clients alike to be given all relevant information connected with any treatment, and informed consent should be gained whenever possible. The right of formal and informal clients to seek a second opinion must be respected.

The mental health Acts in each state and territory have clear guidelines concerning issues such as informed consent to treatment, the way treatments may be implemented (e.g. electroconvulsive therapy) and the use of restraint, including the use of seclusion as a therapeutic measure (legal issues and the use of restraint and seclusion are discussed in Chapter 26). It is an offence to restrain or seclude someone if it is not conducted within the requirements of the mental health Act applicable to where the practice occurs, and the mental health service can be prosecuted and fined if an offence is committed. All consumers admitted to hospital under the Victorian *Mental Health Act 1986* (section 19A (1)) must have a treatment plan, the purpose of which is to provide a clear statement about the treatment and services to be provided to the consumer and to establish mutual expectations. The authorised psychiatrist must prepare, review on a regular basis and revise as required a treatment plan for each consumer.

LEGAL ISSUES AND ELECTROCONVULSIVE THERAPY

Electroconvulsive therapy (ECT) involves the client being given a light general anaesthetic and muscle relaxant medication. A regulated electrical current is passed through the brain until a seizure occurs (a therapeutic fit). This is sometimes referred to as shock treatment. A course of ECT involves a series of treatments. Informed consent must be gained whenever possible for any form of treatment, but there are some issues specific to ECT. The client can only consent to one course of ECT at a time. One course must not exceed any more than six treatments. No more than 7 days can pass between two treatments without the client's consent being sought again. The client's consent must be sought for each new course of treatment. ECT can be performed without consent on involuntary clients but only if set criteria are met. The criteria (Mental Health Legal Centre Inc 2000) are that:

- The ECT has clinical merit and is appropriate
- The benefits, discomforts and risks have been considered in the decision to perform ECT
- Other beneficial alternatives have been given due consideration
- Without ECT the client's physical or mental status will decline significantly
- All reasonable measures have been taken to contact the client's guardian or primary carer who can provide consent on behalf of the client.

Further information about ECT and the law can be located in mental health nursing texts, mental health Acts and at mental health legal centres. References and websites for accessing legal information are provided at the end of this chapter.

ETHICAL ISSUES AND DILEMMAS

Ethical issues and dilemmas abound in the area of mental health nursing. It is sometimes a challenge to balance the client's right to autonomy, the rights of others and the legal concepts relevant to nursing care. Some of the areas that may give rise to ethical concerns include:

- Informed consent/refusal of treatment
- Seclusion and other forms of restraint
- Client confidentiality versus the need to prepare/warn/protect other parties
- Client autonomy (self-reliance and choice issues) as opposed to paternalism
- Boundary issues in the nurse–client relationship.

Within these areas are situations that may give rise to the nurse experiencing conflicting or troublesome feelings. For example, enforcing medication or treatment that is refused, or needing to restrain a client by enforced seclusion, may give rise to feelings of guilt, concern or distaste. Or the nurse may be torn between a client's right to confidentiality and the importance of informing a family carer about a client's diagnosis, such as HIV (human immunodeficiency virus) infection, or of the risk of violence if the client has voiced threats when they do not want their diagnosis, feelings or voiced intentions revealed.

It can also be discomforting and confusing trying to balance establishing and maintaining a trusting and helping relationship while maintaining the appropriate professional boundary with certain clients, and this can cause ethical dilemmas, particularly for nurses new to psychiatric nursing (Horsfall et al 1999). Nurses must practise within professional codes of practice and the law, and consistently remain aware of the ethical principles of beneficence (do good), non-maleficence (do no harm), autonomy (client self-determination) and those of justice, fairness and equity when caring for clients. (These principles are outlined in Chapter 3.) Whenever ethical concerns arise where the decisions about what to do are not clear, nurses should openly raise and discuss the issues with colleagues. Stuart (2001b) recommends that nurses should take certain steps and consider the answers to particular questions when faced with ethical dilemmas. These suggestions are listed in Table 45.11. Nurses considering a career in mental health nursing are advised to access further information concerning ethical issues in mental health care.

SUMMARY

Many Enrolled Nurses (ENs) may wish to follow a career in the specialty area of mental health nursing, and those who remain in other fields may be required to assist in the care of individuals experiencing mental illness; for example, when they are being cared for in general hospitals or in residential care facilities.

There is no clear dividing line between mental health and mental illness; rather, mental wellbeing is represented on a continuum and no one is entirely mentally unhealthy or fully mentally healthy at all times. The ability to remain mentally healthy depends on a wide range of interrelating factors, including those that are physiological, psychological

TABLE 45.11 | STEPS AND QUESTIONS IN ETHICAL DECISION MAKING

Steps	Relevant questions
Gathering background information	Does an ethical dilemma exist? What information is known? What information is needed? What is the context of the dilemma?
Identifying ethical components	What is the underlying issue? Who is affected by this dilemma?
Clarification of agents	What are the rights of each involved party? What are the obligations of each involved party? Who should be involved in the decision making? For whom is the decision being made? What degree of consent is needed by the patient?
Exploration of options	What alternatives exist? What is the purpose or intent of each alternative? What are the potential consequences of each alternative?
Application of principles	What criteria should be used? What ethical theories are subscribed to? What scientific facts are relevant? What is the nurse's philosophy of life and nursing?
Resolution into action	What are the social and legal constraints and ramifications? What is the goal of the nurse's decision? How can the resulting ethical choice be implemented? How can the resulting ethical choice be evaluated?

(Stuart 2001b: 208)

and sociocultural. There are many theoretical models to explain the development of mental illness, on which mental health nurses base their clinical practice. These include the biological (medical) model, psychological/psychodynamic, social/interpersonal, cognitive-behavioural and stress vulnerability/adaptation models.

Mental illness can be diagnosed and formally classified according to the presenting symptoms. A diagnosis can guide treatment but also places a label on the person that can be a source of stigma, and stigma can be one of the most difficult aspects of mental illness for clients to cope with. It is a primary role of the mental health nurse to educate the public about mental illness to reduce stigmatising attitudes, which are in part based on historical factors.

Mental health nurses, who work as members of a multidisciplinary team, develop nursing diagnoses and focus care on the feelings of clients and the behavioural manifestations of mental distress that they display. The development of a trusting, helping relationship is essential to being able to work therapeutically with mentally unwell clients and in promoting the healing process. Assisting clients to develop constructive coping mechanisms is an important component of the therapeutic relationship, as is supporting effective rehabilitation of clients living in the community, where currently most mental health care takes place.

This chapter has not provided detailed information about mental illness but it has provided a brief overview of some issues, and some suggestions appropriate to the care of clients who are anxious, depressed, aggressive, self-destructive, hyperactive or confused. Throughout the chapter there has been an emphasis for the nurse interested in working in the wonderfully challenging area of mental health nursing to access further information about manifestations of mental anguish, models of care and the legal and ethical issues that relate to this dynamic field of nursing.

REVIEW EXERCISES

1. Explain what is meant by the mental health/mental illness continuum.
2. Identify three factors that impact on the development of mental health.
3. Identify four groups of people in society that are at particular risk of developing a mental illness and explain why.
4. Identify four early warning signs of mental illness in children, in pre-adolescents and in adults.
5. Explain the primary characteristics of thought disorders, mood disorders and behavioural disorders and give an example of each.
6. Define the terms hallucination, delusion and confabulation.
7. List and briefly explain three theoretical models on which mental health care nursing may be based.
8. Identify five different professional people who may be included in a mental health care multidisciplinary team.
9. Identify three primary functions of the community mental health nurse.
10. State two historical factors that promoted the move to deinstitutionalisation of people with mental illness.
11. Identify 10 interventions necessary to provide quality care for people with dementia in an aged-care residential facility. Consider the environment, the staff and nursing care activities.
12. What are the five criteria necessary for a client to be admitted as an involuntary client to a mental health care facility?

CRITICAL THINKING EXERCISES

1. You are caring for an 18-year-old client, Paul, who, while admitted for an appendicectomy on the medical surgical ward where you work as an EN, was also diagnosed as having clinical depression. He is being discharged tomorrow and will be returning home, where he lives with his mother and one sister. Paul has specifically told you that he doesn't want his mother or his sister or anyone else to be told of his diagnosis, but you and other nurses on your unit are worried about his mental status. Discuss the following with your colleagues:
   (a) What are the legal and ethical responsibilities of the nurse in this situation?
   (b) How might you approach discussing your concerns with Paul?
2. Mrs Clark is an 84-year-old woman who has dementia. She lives in a residential care facility where you work as an EN. Normally she is a smiling and contented lady who enjoys her meals, enjoys walking in the outside garden area and watching television. Recently she has been picking at her meals and eating very little and has been verbally abusive on several occasions when asked to get out of her chair and come for a walk. How would you attempt to identify the trigger for this change in behaviour? What are some of the areas you would assess in order to identify the problem?

REFERENCES AND FURTHER READING

Access Economics (2003) *The Dementia Epidemic: Economic Impact and Positive Solutions for Australia*. Prepared for Alzheimer's Australia by Access Economics, Canberra. Online. Available: www.alzheimers.org.au [accessed 1 June 2008]

American Psychiatric Association (1994) *Diagnostic and Statistical Manual of Mental Disorders*, 4th edn. APA, Washington DC

—— (2002) *Diagnosis: the DSM-IV Definition of Mental Illness*. Online. Available: www.psych.utah.edu/2002_fall_3250_01/Notes/9_12_Diagnosis.pdf [accessed 1 June 2008]

—— (2008) *Healthy Minds, Healthy Lives. What are the Warning Signs of Mental Illness?* Online. Available: www.healthyminds.org/warningsigns.cfm [accessed 1 June 2008]

Ashton P, Keady J (2000) Mental disorders of older people. In: Newell R, Gournay K (eds) *Mental Health Nursing:*

an Evidence-Based Approach. Churchill Livingstone, Edinburgh

Australian Bureau of Statistics (ABS) and Australian Institute of Health and Welfare (AIHW) (2003) *The Health and Welfare of Australia's Aboriginal and Torres Strait Islander Peoples*, 4th edn. ABS Cat No 4504.0. AIHW Cat No HHW–11. ABS, Canberra

Australian Health Ministers Advisory Council (1996) *National Standards for Mental Health Services*. Australian Government Publishing Service, Canberra

Australian Health Ministers (1992) *National Mental Health Policy*. Australian Government Publishing Service, Canberra

—— (1998) *Second National Mental Health Plan: 1998–2003*. Australian Government Publishing Service, Canberra

Australian Institute of Health and Welfare (AIHW) (2002) *Mental Health Services in Australia 1999–2000*. AIHW, Canberra

Beck CK, Rawlins RP, Williams SR (1988) *Mental Health–Psychiatric Nursing*, 2nd edn. Mosby, St Louis

Brown R (2001) Australian Indigenous Mental Health. *Australian and New Zealand Journal of Mental Health Nursing*, 10(1): 33

Chitty K (2004) Clients with mood disorders. In: Kneisl CR, Wilson HS, Trigoboff E (eds) *Contemporary Psychiatric-Mental Health Nursing*. Prentice Hall, NJ

Dewer A, Barr J (1996) Chronic illness. In: Clinton M, Nelson S (eds) *Mental Health and Nursing Practice*. Prentice Hall, NJ

Ebersole P, Hess P (1985) *Towards Healthy Ageing: Human Needs and Human Response*. Mosby, St Louis

—— (2001) *Geriatric Nursing and Healthy Ageing*. Mosby, St Louis

Egan G (1994) *The Skilled Helper: a Problem Management Approach to Helping*. Brooks Cole, Pacific Grove

Erikson E, Erikson J (1997) *The Life Cycle Completed*. WW Norton, New York

Feil N (2002) *The Validation Breakthrough: Simple Techniques for Communicating With People With Alzheimer's Type Dementia*, 2nd edn. MacLennan and Petty, Sydney

Fenichel M (2000) Concepts in practice: on therapy — a dialogue with Aaron T Beck and Albert Ellis. Reported highlights from the American Psychological Association 108th Convention, Washington DC, August 4–8. Online. Available: www.fenichel.com/Beck-Ellis.shtml [accessed 1 June 2008]

Fontaine KL (1999) Mood disorders. In: Fontaine KL, Fletcher JS, *Mental Health Nursing*, 4th edn. Addison Wesley, Menlo Park

Fontaine KL, Fletcher JS (1999) *Mental Health Nursing*, 4th edn. Addison Wesley, Menlo Park

Fortinash KM, Holoday Worret P (2007) *Psychiatric Nursing Care Plans*, 5th edn. Mosby, St Louis

Gibb R, Macpherson G (2000) A common language of classification and understanding. In: Thompson T, Mathias P (eds) *Lyttle's Mental Health and Disorder*. Baillière Tindall, Edinburgh

Goldberg RJ (1998) *Practical Guide to the Care of the Psychiatric Patient*. Mosby, St Louis

Griffiths R, Emrys E, Finney Lamb C (2003) Operation safe haven: the needs of nurses caring for refugees. *International Journal of Nursing Practice*, 9(3): 183–91

Grigg M, Judd F, Ryan L, Komiti A (2004) Rural and remote psychiatry: identifying marginal housing for people with a mental illness living in rural and regional areas. *Australasian Psychiatry*, 12(1): 36–42

Happell B, Roper C (2003) The role of a mental health consumer in the education of postgraduate psychiatric nursing students: the students' evaluation. *Journal of Psychiatric Mental Health Nursing*, June;10(3): 343–50

Healy D (2002) *Psychiatric Drugs Explained*, 3rd edn. Churchill Livingstone, Edinburgh

Horsfall J, Cleary M, Jordan R (1999) *Towards Ethical Mental Health Nursing Practice*. Australian and New Zealand College of Mental Health Nurses Inc, Greenacres, South Australia

Jewell K, Posner N (1996) A consumer focus. In: Clinton M, Nelson S (eds) *Mental Health and Nursing Practice*. Prentice Hall, Sydney

Johnstone MJ (2001) Stigma, social justice and the rights of the mentally ill: challenging the status quo. *Australian and New Zealand Journal of Mental Health Nursing*, 10(4): 200–10

Kelly S (2000) Suicide and self harm. In: Newell R, Gournay K (eds) (2000) *Mental Health Nursing: an Evidence-Based Approach*. Churchill Livingstone, Edinburgh

Keltner NL, Jones-Warren B (2003) Depression. In: Keltner NL, Schwecke LH, Bostrom CE (eds) *Psychiatric Nursing*, 4th edn. Mosby, St Louis

Kennedy W, Mitzeliotis C (1999) Schizophrenia and other psychotic disorders. In: O'Brien P, Kennedy W, Ballard K *Psychiatric Nursing: an Integration of Theory And Practice*. McGraw Hill, New York

Mayo Foundation for Medical Education and Research (2002) *Mental Illness: an Overview with a Mayo Clinic Psychiatrist*. Online. Available: www.mayoclinic.com/invoke.cfm?id=HQ01079 [accessed 1 June 2008]

Mental Health Foundation (1997) *Knowing Our Own Minds. A Survey of How People in Emotional Distress Take Control of their Lives*. Mental Health Foundation, London

Mental Health Legal Centre Inc (2000) *Patients' Rights: a Self-help Guide to the Mental Health Act*, 5th edn. MHLCentre, Melbourne. Online. Available: www.communitylaw.org.au/mentalhealth/ [accessed 1 June 2008]

Moller M, Fontaine KL (1999) Common clinical problems. In: Fontaine KL, Fletcher JS (1999) *Mental Health Nursing*, 4th edn. Addison Wesley, Menlo Park

National Institute of Mental Health (2000) *Depression in Children and Adolescents: a Fact Sheet For Physicians*. NIH Publication No 00-4544, September. Online. Available: www.nimh.nih.gov/publicat/depchildresfact.cfm [accessed 1 June 2008]

National Mental Health Association (USA) (2008) *Mental Illness in the Family: Recognizing the Warning Signs and How to Cope*. NMHA MHIC Fact sheet. Online. Available: www.nmha.org/go/information/get-info/mi-and-the-family/recognizing-warning-signs-and-how-to-cope.cfm [accessed 1 June 2008]

Peplau HE (1971) A working definition of anxiety. In: Bird SF, Marshal MA, *Some Clinical Approaches to Psychiatric Nursing*. The Macmillan Co, London

—— (1991) *Interpersonal Relations in Nursing: a Conceptual Framework of Reference for Psychodynamic Nursing*. Springer Publishing Co, New York

Repper J, Sayce L, Strong S (1997) *Tall Stories from the Backyard: a Survey of 'NIMBY' Opposition to Community Mental Health Facilities Experienced by Key Service Providers in England and Wales*. MIND (National Association for Mental Health), London

Riley E, Kneisl CR (1996) Suicide and self destructive behaviour. In: Wilson HS, Kneisl CR (eds) *Psychiatric Nursing*, 5th edn. Addison Wesley, Menlo Park

Rogers C (1961) *On Becoming a Person*. Houghton Mifflin, Boston

Ryrie I (2000) Assessing risk. In: Gamble C, Brennan G (eds) *Working with Serious Mental Illness. A Manual for Clinical Practice*. Baillière Tindall, Edinburgh

Schwecke LH (2003) Anxiety, coping and crisis. In: Keltner NL, Schwecke LH, Bostrom CE (eds) *Psychiatric Nursing*, 4th edn. Mosby, St Louis

Sherman B (1999) *Dementia with Dignity: a Handbook for Carers*, 2nd edn. McGraw Hill, Sydney

Shives LR (2005) *Basic Concepts of Psychiatric Mental Health Nursing*, 6th edn. Lippincott, Philadelphia

Smith P (1993) *So You Think You Are Going Crazy?* Dunmore Press, New Zealand

Stevens L (2001) *Does Mental Illness Exist?* Online. Available: www.antipsychiatry.org/exist.htm [accessed 1 June 2008]

Stuart G (2001a) Psychophysiological responses and somatoform and sleep disorders. In: Stuart G, Laraia T (eds) *Principles and Practice of Psychiatric Nursing*, 7th edn. Mosby, St Louis

—— (2001b) Actualizing the psychiatric nursing role: professional performance standards. In: Stuart G, Laraia T (eds) *Principles and Practice of Psychiatric Nursing*, 7th edn. Mosby, St Louis

Stuart G, Laraia T (2001) *Principles and Practice of Psychiatric Nursing*, 7th edn. Mosby, St Louis

—— (2004) *Principles and Practice of Psychiatric Nursing*, 8th edn. Mosby, St Louis

Umstead-Raschmann C (1995) *Age Specific Considerations: the Elder Client*. Online. Available: www.ihs.gov/MedicalPrograms/nursinged/files/handouts/elder.doc.html [accessed 1 June 2008]

Varcarolis EM (2000) *Psychiatric Nursing Clinical Guide: Assessment Tools and Diagnoses*. WB Saunders, Philadelphia

—— (2006) *Foundations of Psychiatric Mental Health Nursing: a Clinical Approach*, 5th edn. WB Saunders, Philadelphia

Videbeck SL (2001) *Psychiatric Mental Health Nursing*. Lippincott, Philadelphia

Watkins P (2001) *The Art of Compassionate Care*. Butterworth–Heinemann, Oxford

Weir D, Oei T (1996) Life stressors. In: Clinton M, Nelson S (eds) (1996) *Mental Health Nursing and Nursing Practice*. Prentice Hall, Sydney

Wilson HS, Kneisl CR (1996) *Psychiatric Nursing*, 5th edn. Addison Wesley, Menlo Park

ONLINE RESOURCES

AllPsych Online: www.allpsych.com/biographies (provides biographical information about some significant theorists in the areas of psychology and psychiatry)

Alzheimer's Australia: www.alzheimers.org.au (help sheets concerning every facet of dementia care are available. Recent reports, research and future conference details are also provided)

Australian and New Zealand College of Mental Health Nurses: www.anzcmhn.org (a variety of low-priced publications relating to all aspects of mental health nursing can be ordered from this site. *Towards Ethical Mental Health Nursing Practice* is one such publication that is focused specifically on ethical dilemmas in clinical mental health nursing)

British Psychological Society: www.bps.org.uk/documents/Rep03.pdf (extensive report by the Society that provides information about recent advances in knowledge that promote understanding of mental illness and in particular psychotic experiences)

Mental Health Legal Centre Inc (Vic): www.vicnet.net.au/~mhlc (home page for the Mental Health Legal Centre Inc in the State of Victoria. Provides information relating to all aspects of the law and mental health service user rights. A variety of informative publications can be downloaded from this site)

Victorian Government Department of Human Services: www.health.vic.gov.au/mentalhealth (contains broad amount of information about mental illness, clients' legal rights, and aspects of treatment)

Victorian Government Health Information: www.health.vic.gov.au/mentalhealth (useful web page from where a range of information can be accessed, e.g. clinical disorders, services, terminology in mental health)

Victorian *Mental Health Act 1986*: www.health.vic.gov.au/mentalhealth/mh-act/index.htm

Chapter 46
REHABILITATION NURSING

OBJECTIVES

- Define the key terms/concepts
- Recognise the terminology used in rehabilitation nursing to describe the client's level of functioning
- Explain the philosophy of rehabilitation
- Outline the functions of each member of the rehabilitation team
- Describe the process of adjustment to disability
- Assist in planning and implementing care for clients who require rehabilitation

KEY TERMS/CONCEPTS

adaptation
choices
client-centred goals
community
decision making
education
empowerment
independence
problem solving
team

CHAPTER FOCUS

Rehabilitation is a dynamic process which, to be effective, must occur as a collaborative process involving all members of the rehabilitation team, of which the client is the most important. Effective rehabilitation enables the individual to achieve optimal physical, emotional, psychological, social and vocational potential, to maintain dignity and self-respect. Rehabilitation empowers the individual to make informed choices about health care and achieve a level of wellness that is acceptable to that individual. The focus of this chapter is to introduce the nurse to the processes of rehabilitation and the many facets of rehabilitation that can be practised in any care setting.

LIVED EXPERIENCE

Denise had experienced a cerebrovascular accident. When the rehabilitation team sat down with her to set some client goals, what Denise wanted most was to get back to ballroom dancing. The team were a bit perplexed as to what to do, as Denise's stroke had been a very severe one and she had become quite despondent and depressed. Rob, her husband, was also experiencing depression and hopelessness. However, each team member was able to work toward this goal little by little. Short-term goals were set with Denise and Rob achieving small tasks first, which, altogether, would build toward the main goal. This empowered both Denise and Rob. Each small achievement was celebrated — first just standing, then taking a few steps, then walking the length of the ward corridor. Their moods lifted and progress was enhanced. Denise went home to continue her rehabilitation with the Rehabilitation in the Home Program and then as a Community Care client. Denise and Rob came back after only a few months to show the in-client rehabilitation program team that they had achieved the major goal and gave a demonstration of their ballroom dancing.

Isabella, Enrolled Nurse, rehabilitation unit

Rehabilitation is a complex process with a range of dimensions including: motivation; adaptation to change; coping with stress; adjustment to altered circumstances; body capabilities and/or appearance; and regaining independence and wellness.

AIMS AND CHARACTERISTICS OF REHABILITATION

The basic aim of rehabilitation nursing is to limit the effects of disability and handicap in clients with particular impairments. It begins with immediate care to minimise the effects of damage and to prevent complications in the stage immediately after an accident or the onset of illness. It continues through the time clients are receiving restorative care and it often necessitates helping clients to adapt to a permanently changed situation and a new kind of life. Rehabilitation nursing includes a wide range of activities that include working collaboratively with other members of a rehabilitation team to:

- Retrain physically damaged clients to walk again
- Retrain cognitively damaged clients to communicate effectively orally or in writing
- Help clients adapt to impairment in a way that enables them to care for their own needs, such as showering, dressing and eating and using ordinary toilet facilities
- Promote client abilities to manage ordinary everyday modes of travel
- Teach clients how to put on, remove and care for different types of prosthetic appliances, e.g., an artificial limb or eye (Hoeman 2008; Jester 2007).

Rehabilitation also takes place in the area of mental health nursing and includes minimising impairment in functioning and preventing relapse in clients who experience recurrent problems with mental ill-health. This can be achieved through an approach that includes community-based programs such as educational groups, vocational and skills training and halfway houses (Collins & Diego 2000). Clinical Interest Box 46.1 indicates the main characteristics of rehabilitation.

CATEGORIES OF INDIVIDUALS REQUIRING REHABILITATION

A person may experience a disability of acute or chronic onset at any stage of the life span. Rehabilitation programs may be developed and implemented in hospitals, other health care settings, and in the home, for an individual who is experiencing:

- Disturbance of musculoskeletal function as a result of injury, illness or surgical intervention (e.g. fractured femur, arthritis, amputation, joint replacement)
- Brain damage (e.g. following a cerebrovascular accident or head injury)
- Nervous system impairment (e.g. as a result of a spinal cord injury or disease such as multiple sclerosis)
- Impaired skin integrity (e.g. as a result of burns)
- Removal of a body part (e.g. a limb, mastectomy, laryngectomy, or hemicolectomy with subsequent colostomy)
- Cardiac impairment (e.g. after a myocardial infarction)
- Impaired renal function (e.g. renal failure requiring dialysis)
- Impaired bladder control (e.g. as a result of neurogenic bladder disorder)
- Respiratory impairment (e.g. as a result of obstructive disorders of the airways such as asthma or pulmonary emphysema)
- Impaired vision or hearing
- Chronic pain
- Substance abuse
- A psychiatric or emotional disorder (e.g. schizophrenia, depression, anxiety).

(Derstine & Drayton-Hargrove 2001; Flannery 2004; Hoeman 2008)

In many situations complete rehabilitation is achieved but in others complete recovery of function is not possible and the individual faces a permanent disability or impairment (see Chapter 47 for definitions of these terms). When this happens, individuals must be helped to accept, adapt to, and compensate for the existing impairment to establish an optimal level of independence and quality of life. Clinical Interest Box 46.2 provides an explanation of the term adaptation.

THE MEANING OF HABILITATION AND REHABILITATION

Habilitation, rather than rehabilitation, is a term that refers to the process in which a person who is born with

CLINICAL INTEREST BOX 46.1
Main characteristics of rehabilitation

- Reduction of disability and handicap
- Self-sufficiency and independence
- Empowerment
- Problem solving
- Client centred
- Holistic approach
- Educational process

(Smith 1999)

CLINICAL INTEREST BOX 46.2
Explanation of adaptation

Adaptation implies the ability to adapt oneself or to modify behaviour and expectations in line with changing circumstances. Adaptation is a mechanism that affects the whole being, physically, socially and psychologically, and is a necessary process of normal life. However, in times of trauma or when facing disability, individuals may find it beyond their capabilities to adapt to circumstances without professional assistance. For a clearer understanding of adaptation it is recommended that the reader refer to Sister Callista Roy's work *The Roy Adaptation Model* first published in 1984.

an impairment is helped to achieve optimal independence and function by learning new skills that empower them to make choices and have degrees of control. Long-term habilitation programs are necessary for individuals born with conditions such as spina bifida, Down syndrome, or intellectual or physical impairment.

One aspect of rehabilitation addresses chronic health problems and degenerative diseases. Although there may be no cure for such conditions, a rehabilitation program can improve the quality of life. In this sense rehabilitation is directed towards the maintenance of optimal function and prevention of complications, or towards retaining the greatest amount of function and independence that the client desires for as long as possible.

Rehabilitation begins at the onset of illness or accident and continues until it is decided by the client, in consultation with the rehabilitation team, that the optimal level for that particular individual has been attained. The rehabilitation process may extend over a period ranging from a few weeks to several months or years. Rehabilitation programs are conducted in a variety of settings, including acute care hospitals, specific rehabilitation institutions, day clinics, the home, and in the community (Pryor 2000).

PHILOSOPHY OF REHABILITATION

A philosophy is a broad statement of basic related principles, concepts and beliefs. A philosophy of rehabilitation offers a framework from which the rehabilitation process can be developed. Although rehabilitation teams devise their own philosophy, philosophies of rehabilitation are generally based on the premise that rehabilitation recognises the worth and uniqueness of the person as a valuable human resource, and that rehabilitation programs must be a major integral component of care offered by health services. Rehabilitation necessitates the participation and coordination of all health team members through constant communication with the client and significant others to develop a comprehensive rehabilitation plan acceptable to and agreed to by the client. The individual receiving rehabilitation must be viewed as an active team member, and the process must actively involve the family and significant others in the individual's life.

Rehabilitation is concerned with the whole person and includes the sociocultural aspects of the person's life, sexuality, family and home, job, vocation, religion and community role. Rehabilitation aims to achieve the highest level of empowerment and independence possible for the individual and is client and goal focused (Derstine & Drayton-Hargroves 2001; Hoeman 2008).

CLIENT-CENTRED GOALS AND EMPOWERMENT

Goal setting can be seen as a way to give control back to clients and make empowerment real. It is seen as a move away from the traditional medical model in which nurses tended to tell clients what to do, to one that focuses on health promotion, clients' abilities rather than disabilities, and wellness rather than illness. Empowerment is a process that enables groups or individuals to change after being given the skills, resources, opportunities and authority to do so (Rodwell 1996). Empowerment:

- Is a helping process
- Is a partnership that values self and others
- Involves mutual decision making using resources, opportunities and authority
- Confers freedom to make choices and accept responsibility (Rodwell 1996).

A partnership between team members and the client transfers power and builds on the client's self-esteem and self-worth. Often clients in rehabilitation experience feelings of poor self-esteem and a sense of worthlessness. They can be grieving for what they perceive as a loss of independence and lifestyle. Client-centred goals can assist in identifying what is important to that individual. The client may not always set the goals at the level the team believes they should be able to achieve. It is not effective use of resources if therapists aim for the client to walk 100 metres if the client only wants to walk around the house or only wants to be able to walk to the letterbox. The goals must be realistic and the client must have a desire to reach them.

The importance of the client feeling in control of what is happening, what is being planned and of decisions that affect their life cannot be emphasised strongly enough. This sense of control is facilitated when the client is involved in determining their own rehabilitation goals. Clinical Interest Box 46.3 provides an example of a formula for setting client-centred goals. It is important for nurses working in the area of rehabilitation to keep in mind that throughout the process of rehabilitation the client and the family are often facing markedly changed circumstances and may be struggling to adapt to what has happened.

ADJUSTMENT TO DISABILITY

The process of adjustment as it relates to disability is similar to that in dying (see Chapter 14 for further information

CLINICAL INTEREST BOX 46.3
Client-centred goal setting

- Subject — client is assumed subject unless otherwise stated
- Verb — desired behaviour
- Condition — environmental context/assistance/aids/strategies
- Criteria — measurable outcome; for example, 90% degree of accuracy, within a stated time limit, over a set distance
- Time frame — aim date

Example: Mrs Johnson will walk independently for 50 metres, using a four-point stick, from her front door to her letterbox safely by 15.7.04.
(MacPhail 1998)

on loss, grief and dying). Disability involves loss and is accompanied by an adjustment process as the individual and significant others learn to come to terms with the disability and its implications. The individual may experience loss of:

- Sensation
- Skin integrity
- A body part
- Ability to walk
- Use of an arm
- Bowel and/or bladder control
- Sexual function
- Ability to speak, read, write and comprehend
- Memory
- Ability to relate to other people and the environment
- Self-image, sense of self-worth, self-esteem, sexuality
- Independence.

The person whose disability has only occurred recently generally experiences four stages in adjustment during the rehabilitation process:

1. Acute disorganisation. The individual may express feelings of extreme anxiety, fear and disbelief that such an event has occurred
2. Assessment. The individual begins to assess what has happened and begins to recognise and identify changes in function and ability. The client may experience anger, depression, denial and bargaining. The individual may hope for a spontaneous recovery or a medical miracle, and tends to resist activities designed to help regain function with an impairment
3. Mourning. The individual continues to experience anger and depression; however, there is generally a new awareness of the losses involved. The individual begins to accept the changed probable future and no longer denies or ignores the disability. Eventually the client begins to participate more fully in the rehabilitation program.
4. Re-entry. The individual resolves the depression of the mourning process and begins to experience more positive feelings about self and the future. They recognise that the disability does in fact exist and are keen to find means to adapt their personal lifestyle to the disability.

It is important for nurses to understand that each client will have an individual timetable for adjusting and adapting to living with a disability. Thus, while some people adjust in a relatively short time, others will take much longer. There is no normal period of time before a person finally accepts and adjusts to a disability. It must not be forgotten that the family also goes through a process of grieving and adjustment. The rehabilitation team plays an important role as it supports the individual and family during the process of adjustment and adaptation (see Chapter 13 for information on adaptation to stress).

THE REHABILITATION TEAM

Effective rehabilitation involves client-centred care planning with the individual, family or significant others, and the whole health care team. The special needs of the individual determine the fields of expertise that are represented in the rehabilitation team. A multidisciplinary team is required and consists of members from various disciplines, each with a vital role to play. Clinical Interest Box 46.4 identifies some of the people who might be included in a multidisciplinary rehabilitation team. Who is included depends on the specific needs of individual clients; for example, a non-English speaking client would need an interpreter to be included.

MEMBERS OF THE REHABILITATION TEAM

The client

It is essential that the individual who requires rehabilitation be viewed as the pivotal team member. The other team members must help motivate the client to be actively involved in the rehabilitation process, however slow it may be. Unless the client is encouraged, a lack of motivation and cooperation with prescribed therapy may result. It

CLINICAL INTEREST BOX 46.4
Members of a multidisciplinary rehabilitation team

- The client
- The client's family/friend(s) or significant other(s)
- Nurse
- Case manager
- Counsellor (possibly an expert in grief and loss counselling)
- Physiotherapist
- Occupational therapist
- Speech therapist
- Social worker
- Dietitian
- Podiatrist
- Prosthetist/orthotist
- Psychiatrist
- Psychologist
- Chaplain or other religious/spiritual support person
- Teacher/educator (essential for children undergoing long-term rehabilitation)
- Medical officer (often the team's clinical director)

The team most often works to an interdisciplinary model, which means that there is an integrated and collaborative approach to identifying goals, which reduces duplication (particularly in goal setting) and conflict. There is some blending of roles and building of knowledge that goes beyond the original discipline. The interdisciplinary team involves members who are engaged in problem solving beyond the confines of their particular knowledge base. This particular model of a rehabilitation team broadens the capacity of the team to obtain the outcomes that the client wants (Hoeman 2002).

is important that each small achievement is positively reinforced (e.g. recognised, praised or rewarded). At all stages of rehabilitation, the rest of the team must consider the client's strengths and weaknesses and the social and cultural influences that affect adjustment to disability. The team must be aware of how the client perceives the illness and the impact of the disability that has occurred.

A disturbance of an individual's body image, for example, paralysis resulting from a cerebrovascular accident, is difficult to accept. The initial reaction is usually one of shock, followed by denial. As the individual gradually realises what has happened and the implications, the client may experience depression, anger or guilt, believing that life may never be the same again. Self-esteem and self-worth are threatened (see Chapter 14 for information concerning responses to loss). While there is inevitable dependency initially, the overall aim of rehabilitation is to help the individual regain optimal quality of life. The motivation of the individual is crucial, and it is essential that the client be regarded as the most important team member, who must be encouraged to participate actively in all aspects of the rehabilitation process. The individual must be involved in planning the personal rehabilitation program with the team. The client must learn in detail about the disability that has been experienced and ways of accomplishing the desired goals. The team must inform the client as to what options are available so that the person can choose the best options for a successful outcome.

The family or friends

The family, or significant others, are recognised as a potential support system for the individual. Members of the family are evaluated to determine their ability to help with the rehabilitation process. All families, or significant others, cannot contribute in the same way or to the same degree. In some instances the individual could return home and receive excellent care and support, while in other situations the family may be unable or unwilling to help care for the person. As each situation presents different problems, individual evaluation is essential.

The family, or significant others, need to understand and/or be involved with the rehabilitative goals that the individual develops with the team, and the methods selected to meet these goals. Partners, family members or supportive friends need to understand that their greatest contribution may be to allow the individual to be as independent as possible. This may be difficult for them at times, as their natural instinct may be to assist and 'do for' their loved one. In addition, those supporting the client can be instructed in how to assist with specific therapy, thus enabling them to feel that they are playing a vital role in rehabilitation.

It is important to understand that, when illness or disability occurs, family life is interrupted and altered. The effects of illness have significant implications for the family as well as for the individual. Plans for the rehabilitation process should, therefore, also address the needs of the family as well as those of the client. The nurse and the team must remember that a spouse or partner can become depressed if their loved one faces permanent lifestyle changes. It is important to inform the spouse or significant other that this is a normal reaction and encourage the person to seek assistance from a medical officer or team psychologist. Another concern with family occurs when ageing carers assisting relatives with disabilities in the home environment themselves become ill and are no longer able to provide care for their dependent relatives. People who have been cared for by their loved ones in the community for many years are sometimes suddenly faced with a crisis because that carer has become ill. This often limits the amount of support that the carer has for transition back into the community, and placement of the individual they cared for may be an issue if the carer cannot resume a level of functioning that enables a return to the role of carer.

The nurse

Rehabilitation nursing is a speciality area of practice requiring specialised knowledge, skills and attitudes. The goal of rehabilitation nursing is to assist people with disability and chronic illness in attaining maximal functional ability, maintaining optimal health and adapting to an altered lifestyle (Hoeman 2008). Nurses are in a prime position to promote these things because they spend more time with the client than any other member of the rehabilitation team, and therefore play a pivotal role in assessing, planning, implementing and evaluating care. A nursing assessment includes an evaluation of the extent to which the individual's physical and psychosocial needs are met.

The rehabilitation nurse develops a nursing care plan to meet the needs of the client, taking into account the person's goals, both short and long term. In many settings, nursing is the only component of the rehabilitation team represented throughout the entire 24 hours of each day. Nurses are therefore responsible for reinforcing the teachings of other team members, such as the physiotherapist and occupational therapist, throughout this time, so that there is continuity of the rehabilitation program. The rehabilitation nurse's role includes preventing complications that would impede the restoration of optimal functioning; therefore, attention to potential problems as well as actual problems is necessary.

The effective rehabilitation nurse understands the short- and long-term goals of the client and the rehabilitation program. The nurse has a pivotal role in the multi-disciplinary team and is aware of the need to liaise and communicate closely with all team members to achieve coordinated and effective outcomes for the client. This often means that the nurse's role needs to be flexible and amenable to change. The nurse requires a full understanding of the role and function of each team member and needs to recognise when to refer to the expertise of others as the client's needs indicate.

Individuals react and respond in various ways to personal health conditions and the rehabilitation program. The nurse must be able to assess accurately, monitor and educate the clients and their significant others throughout the process, so that the client's goals and the rehabilitation goals can be achieved successfully. The nurse works in a partnership with the client, assisting them to make informed choices and have control over the process. At times the nurse might find it difficult to empower the client, especially if the client is despondent and in the early stages of denial. It is essential that the nurse has time to build rapport and trust. Client advocacy is vital for this trust to develop. The nurse should be responsive to the client's rights and be able to advocate for the client in team discussions. The nurse's role involves being an educator not only for the client but also for the family, carers and other staff. This education will involve teaching rehabilitative techniques, preventing complications and promoting a healthy lifestyle. The nurse will act as a resource for information and clarification and know when to call in other professionals to assist.

Many clinical skills are employed when working as a rehabilitation nurse. Depending on the individual client, skills employed may include pain and continence management, preventing pressure sores and care and/or behaviour management. While the rehabilitation nurse needs to acquire excellent general nursing knowledge, there may be a necessity to refer to more advanced trained rehabilitation nurses specialising in neurological, orthopaedic, cardiac/pulmonary, oncology, renal, gerontic or paediatric rehabilitation nursing. The rehabilitation nursing team members between them commonly have a skill mix that meets the needs of the clients.

Rehabilitation nursing takes place in any specialty or clinical environment where the aim is to maximise independence and minimise the impact of disability and handicap in clients with particular impairments. Therefore, many nurses, including those who have not specialised in rehabilitation nursing, are involved in the rehabilitation process. However, should a nurse choose to make rehabilitation nursing a career focus, there are many different specialty areas of rehabilitation nursing, including orthopaedics, burns, spinal injury, head injury, amputation, cardiac and stroke rehabilitation (Jester 2007).

The case manager

The case manager is a relatively new member of the rehabilitation team and can be of any discipline. It is fast becoming a very popular role for the rehabilitation nurse with advanced training. The case manager develops a formal, written, comprehensive needs assessment that includes a formal review of evaluations performed by other members of the rehabilitation team. The case manager assists the client and the service provider in planning and program development that meets the needs identified and prioritised in the assessment. The case manager's role and function will vary depending on the practice setting. The case manager may be employed in an institutional setting such as a hospital or rehabilitation facility, or they may work in the insurance industry, such as the Transport Accident Commission or Health Insurance Organisation.

The physiotherapist

Physiotherapists evaluate the client's physical capabilities and limitations in a collaborative assessment process. The physiotherapist administers therapies designed to correct or minimise deformity, increase strength and mobility or alleviate discomfort or pain. The physiotherapist has a client-centred approach. Treatments include the use of specific exercises, heat, cold, aqua therapy and electrophysical therapy. A physiotherapist is also involved in educating the client and their family or significant others and other team members in correct methods of positioning, transferring and mobilising so that what is taught in therapy sessions can be carried over to day-to-day activities and reinforced by the nurse.

The occupational therapist

Occupational therapists are concerned with assisting the client to achieve independent performance in the activities of daily living. They also assess the need for, and provide, adaptive devices, for example aids such as specially designed cutlery which promote independence with meals. The occupational therapist usually assesses the client's home in preparation for transition back into the community. This is done in conjunction with the client and family on the pre-discharge home visit. Home modifications may be required as well as equipment to ensure that the home environment is safe and conducive to the client's independence level. Modifications may be minor, such as installation of a handrail, or major, such as structural alterations to enlarge space in a toilet and bathroom if a wheelchair or lifting machine needs to be accommodated.

The speech pathologist/therapist

Speech pathologists, otherwise referred to as speech therapists, are also involved in the client goal-setting process and are concerned with assessing, diagnosing and treating communication disorders, such as the formation and perception of speech, the ability to articulate words and to understand and initiate speech. As part of the rehabilitation process a speech therapist may be required to assist a person to relearn communication skills. Communication deficits present a real problem for affected clients, and much reassurance and counselling are often required. The client who cannot speak may feel hopeless and frustrated. Often, depending on the area of brain affected by a cerebrovascular accident, the client can understand fully but cannot articulate. Technical devices may need to be utilised to assist the client communicate to others. If both areas of the speech centre are damaged, global aphasia may occur, in which the person cannot speak or understand the spoken word. How to empower this client becomes a very real challenge.

CLINICAL INTEREST BOX 46.5
Videofluoroscopy — a diagnostic test to identify dysphagia

Videofluoroscopy is a modified barium swallow conducted by the speech pathologist and radiologist to determine the extent of dysphagia and to identify if the client is at risk of aspiration. The test allows for the viewing of the oral cavity, laryngopharynx and cervical oesophagus. The client swallows small amounts of a liquid puree or solid mixed with barium. As the client manipulates the bolus in the oral cavity and swallows, the fluoroscopic study is recorded on videotape. Videotaping of the swallowing study allows clinicians to have repeated viewing and slow-motion analysis.
(Hoeman 2008: 294)

A speech pathologist may also be involved in the management of an individual whose chewing and swallowing abilities are impaired, for example after a cerebrovascular accident. The speech pathologist liaises closely with the nurse, dietitian and family to achieve safe swallowing strategies for the client. In consultation with the client, a videofluoroscopy (see Clinical Interest Box 46.5) may be required to ascertain the level of the swallowing deficit. Often the client and family will resist the strategy of thickened fluids to prevent aspiration; therefore, in-depth education and counselling are required so that informed choices, including a full understanding of the risks, can be made. Ultimately it is the client's choice as to whether treatment strategies are followed.

The social worker

Social workers are concerned with counselling and assisting clients and their families who are experiencing personal problems as a result of illness or injury. A social worker acts as an advocate by liaising with existing community groups and resources, and assists the individual and the family to deal with social, domestic, financial and emotional implications of the illness or condition. The social worker engages in discharge planning and often accompanies the occupational therapist and client on the pre-discharge home visit. The social worker communicates with the community services that may be required to assist the client when discharged home or, if alternative placement is required, the social worker would assist in this process.

The dietitian

Dietitians are concerned with assessing nutritional needs and planning ways to meet those needs. As part of the rehabilitation process, the client may require specific dietary restrictions or modifications, and a dietitian collaborates closely with the individual to plan an appropriate diet. The dietitian also plays an important role in ensuring that all those involved with the individual's care understand the importance of a specific diet to the person's recovery.

The podiatrist

Podiatrists are concerned with assessing, preventing and treating disorders of the feet. As part of the rehabilitation process, a client may be required to relearn how to ambulate, for example, after a cerebrovascular accident. In order to mobilise, the feet must be in good condition, with no skin lesions or nail disorders, and the podiatrist plays an important role in maintaining the health and integrity of the skin and toenails. In collaboration with the client, the podiatrist determines appropriate footwear for safe mobilisation.

The prosthetist/orthotist

Prosthetists are concerned with assessing a client's need for a prosthesis, such as an artificial limb. After assessment, a prosthetist designs and supplies an appropriate prosthesis. Generally a temporary prosthesis is provided and trialled before a permanent one is supplied. Modifications to an existing prosthesis may be made by a prosthetist, who also checks at regular intervals to ensure that the prosthesis is meeting the client's needs. Some individuals may need to be fitted with splints or braces to correct deformities or provide added support. Such mechanical devices are called orthoses, and include braces for the neck, arm or leg.

The psychiatrist and psychologist

If the client is experiencing a psychiatric or emotional problem, either a psychiatrist or a psychologist is generally involved in the rehabilitation process. A psychiatrist is concerned with the causes, prevention and treatment of mental, emotional and behavioural disorders. A clinical psychologist is concerned with the causes, prevention and treatment of individual social problems especially in regard to the interaction between the client and the physical and social environment. A psychiatrist, clinical psychologist or neuropsychologist may be involved in the rehabilitation of an individual who is depressed as a result of the implications of the disability, or if behavioural problems result from the condition. The psychologist can also assist the rehabilitation team with strategies to manage clients who have behavioural disturbances that impact on the day-to-day rehabilitation process. These disciplines can also assist the family or significant others if problems of coping and adaptation are identified. Depression can be common in the client undergoing rehabilitation; family members are also vulnerable to depression.

The clinical director (medical officer)

The clinical director is commonly a medical officer specialised in rehabilitation medicine and often the first member of the team to encounter the client as a response to a referral for rehabilitation intervention. The medical officer is responsible for the medical and/or surgical management of the person and oversees the treatment that involves meeting the physical, emotional and social needs of the client. These needs must be satisfied to successfully restore the client's quality of life to maximum potential. The medical officer collaborates with all members of the team and is usually the team leader. They assess the client's health status regularly and explain the diagnosis and prognosis to the client and relatives. The medical officer often takes on the role of chairing the case conferences and other meetings, such as team and family meetings. Regular ward rounds are conducted by the medical officer, who also has an active educative role with team members, particularly for more junior medical members of the team.

CASE CONFERENCES AND TEAM MEETINGS

These meetings are held at regular intervals and are the forum where team members discuss the progress and problems of every individual who is undertaking rehabilitation. During these meetings the client's short- and long-term goals are discussed, with each member being aware of, and respecting, the roles of others in accomplishing these goals. Goals must be re-evaluated regularly with the client, so that the client and therapists can determine whether they are realistic and/or whether they have been accomplished. All goals should be set with specific time frames. Specific therapy goals are also set at these meetings. These therapy goals are compatible with the client's goals but are usually broken up into smaller attainable sequences, with time frames; for example, John will stand for 3 minutes, with the aid of the tilt table, three times tomorrow; John will increase time on the tilt table in increments of 2–3 minutes until standing for 10 minutes three times a day.

Each team member explains to the other members the procedures and techniques to be carried out. The proceedings are documented in terms that are meaningful and valid for all persons concerned. The client and/or family may or may not be present at the case conference, depending on the time limitations of the meeting and the individual health care facility's policy. Quite often a designated team member meets with the client and family before or after the meeting to discuss and inform and assist in the decision-making process. Family conferences can be conducted aside from the case conference, when more time can be given to the concerns of the client and family.

THE PROCESS OF REHABILITATION

The rehabilitation process involves assessing the client's rehabilitation potential, planning and implementing an appropriate program, and continuous evaluation of progress.

ASSESSMENT OF REHABILITATION POTENTIAL

Assessment of the client and a realistic evaluation of their rehabilitation potential is the first step towards planning a program. In some instances this can be a relatively simple process, while in others it is more complicated. For example, it is comparatively easy to assess the rehabilitation potential of a healthy young adult with a fractured femur, while it is more difficult to make an assessment in an elderly person with diabetes who has experienced a cerebrovascular accident. Assessment of each individual must take into account:

- The nature of the disability. Some conditions affect only isolated areas of the body, while others exert widespread effect. Some disorders cause progressive and diverse impairment of function
- The overall condition of the client and their ability to cope with a rehabilitation program. There may be other existing conditions that could influence the choice of rehabilitation measures; for example, chronic conditions such as arthritis or emphysema may restrict the person's ability to engage in active exercise
- The motivation of the client and the understanding of the situation. The client's motivation should stem from a realistic acceptance of the situation and should not be the result of over-optimism or a refusal to acknowledge limitations
- The client's home environment and the ability of the family or significant others to be supportive.

Physical and psychological assessment of the client is performed to evaluate functional state, so that a suitable program involving both short- and long-term goals can be set. Assessment includes evaluating muscle function, range of joint motion, body alignment and posture, neurological function, cardiopulmonary function, mood and cognition.

DETERMINING SHORT- AND LONG-TERM GOALS

Short-term goals of a rehabilitation program are those that may be achieved in a short period of time. For example, activities such as achieving a standing position, moving from a bed to a chair, managing meals independently, tying shoelaces or formulating a sentence may be set as short-term goals. Long-term goals are those that are expected to take much longer to accomplish and depend on success in achieving the short-term goals. These may include activities such as walking, managing to climb stairs, independence in the activities of daily living, or returning to employment.

The value of setting goals is that both the client and the team know what they are aiming for and will be able to identify when they have achieved a specific goal. As mentioned earlier, the client and family assist in the development of the goals and this assists in empowering the client and providing a degree of control. If realistic goals are to be set the entire rehabilitation team must be involved in the planning process and must meet frequently to re-evaluate the situation.

It may be difficult for a client to maintain a high level of motivation and they may think that little progress is being made and that the set goals are unattainable. They may view the rehabilitation program as tedious, boring, exhausting or painful. As a result, they may become depressed and discouraged. The nurse may help by:

- Being empathic about the situation, which involves trying to understand how the client is feeling
- Emphasising what progress has been made and expressing honest confidence in the person's ability to make further progress
- Spending as much time as possible with the person, particularly during activities in which active encouragement is required
- Ensuring that the client does not become over-tired or attempt to exceed the limits prescribed. Encourage the client to take one day at a time. Some days will be better than others
- Encouraging the individual to concentrate on achieving one goal at a time. An over-ambitious program may result in frustration and despair
- Encouraging the individual to express feelings. A relationship can be established by listening to the client. This creates a sense of trust so that the client feels able to express concerns and feelings to the nurse (see Chapter 29 for information concerning therapeutic communication skills).

NURSING ASPECTS OF REHABILITATION

A rehabilitation program is developed for each client. The nursing activities involved will depend on many factors such as the client's age, degree of independence and type of impairment. The overall purpose of rehabilitation is restoration of the individual to optimal functioning, or to assist the individual to adjust to a disability after an illness or injury. As a member of the rehabilitation team, the nurse provides support and assists the client to meet personal physical and psychological needs.

Regardless of the specific impairment, the philosophy and aims of rehabilitation remain the same. The nurse plays a key role in assisting the client to carry out the activities of daily living and must be aware that the ultimate aim is to achieve the goals that the client has developed with the team. The achievement of personal goals that the client has developed is one of the most important aspects of their rehabilitation. The main activities of daily living are identified as:

- Maintaining a safe environment
- Communicating
- Breathing
- Eating and drinking
- Eliminating
- Personal cleansing and dressing
- Controlling body temperature
- Mobilising
- Working and playing
- Expressing sexuality
- Sleeping
- Dying.

(Roper, Logan & Tierney 2000)

Depending on the client's disability and needs, a rehabilitation program is planned in which goals are set to assist the client to achieve independence in the activities of daily living. For example, in a program developed for a person who has experienced a cerebrovascular accident and subsequent hemiplegia, one specific long-term goal may be that the person is able to dress themself. For that goal to be achieved, short-term goals will be set, such as, 'The person is able to sit up in a chair'. The occupational therapist will be involved in teaching dressing and undressing techniques, and the nurse should understand the techniques the person is using so that the teaching of the occupational therapist can be reinforced in day-to-day activity. Continuity of care is vital for effective rehabilitation outcomes. It is destructive to the rehabilitation process for the nurse to take over when a client is attempting to dress themself; for example, doing up the buttons on a shirt when a client is making slow progress may save the busy nurse time, but it undermines the importance of the client's efforts and may deter the client from trying in the future.

Another important nursing function is preventing the complications of immobility which include:

- Decubitus ulcers
- Contractures
- Footdrop
- Venous stasis
- Pulmonary stasis
- Urinary stasis
- Constipation
- Postural hypotension
- Subluxation of a hemiplegic shoulder
- Psychological consequences such as boredom or depression.

(See Chapter 36 for further information concerning mobility.)

AIDS TO DAILY LIVING

There are numerous devices to help a person with a disability perform the activities of daily living. Such devices are invaluable, as they make a degree of independence possible. For example, there are long-handled shoe horns to promote independence with dressing (Figure 46.1), long-handled brushes to promote independence with hygiene (Figure 46.2) and devices to promote independence with meals (Figure 46.3) and drinking (Figure 46.4). Nurses should be familiar with the full range of aids available and should be capable of teaching the individual and their family the correct way to use them. A range of available aids is listed in Clinical Interest Box 46.6.

In most states and territories of Australia there are centres for independent living that provide a wide range of aids to assist with the tasks of daily living. A variety of community services is available to assist persons with disabilities to remain at home, including community health centres, day hospitals and day centres, drop-in centres, elderly/senior

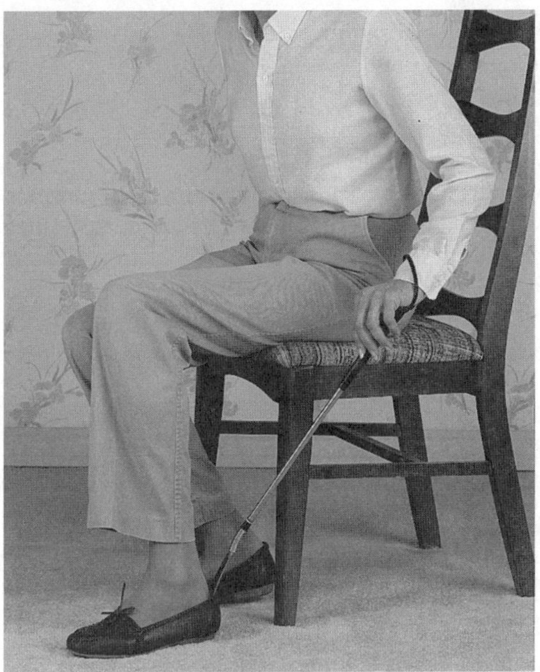

Figure 46.1 | Long-handled shoe horn *(Hoeman 2008. Reproduced courtesy of Sammons Preston, a Bissell Healthcare Co. Bolingbrook, IL)*

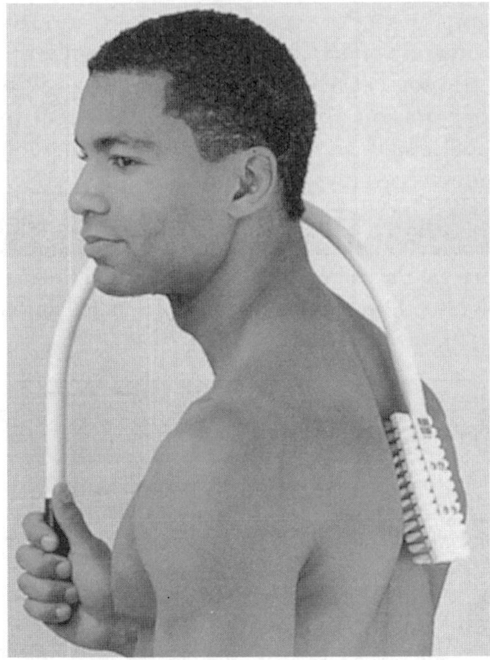

Figure 46.2 | Long-handled brush *(Hoeman 2008. Reproduced courtesy of Sammons Preston, a Bissell Healthcare Co. Bolingbrook, IL)*

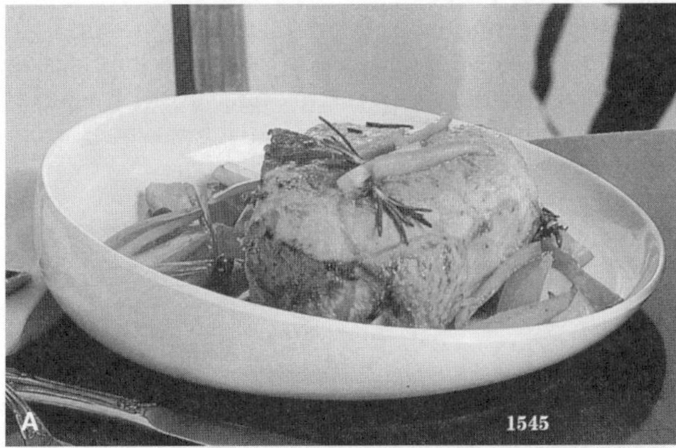

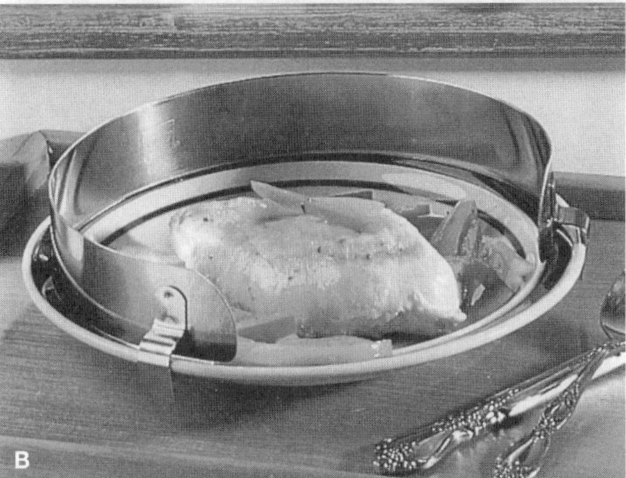

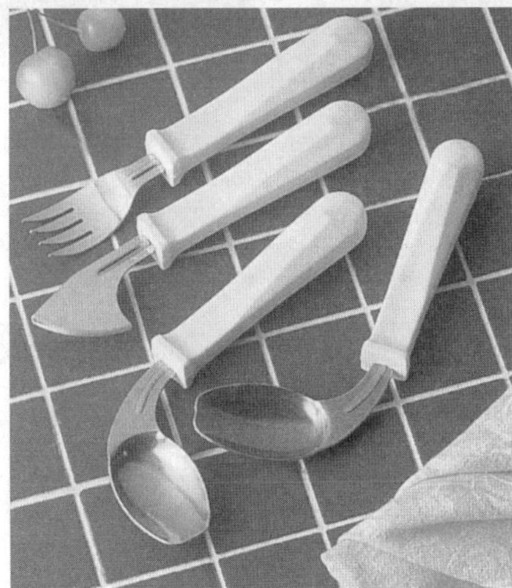

C

Figure 46.3 | Aids to promote independence with eating **A**: Scoop dish **B**: Food guard **C**: Easy-hold utensils (knife blade cuts in both slicing and rocking motions) *(Hoeman 2008. Reproduced courtesy of Sammons Preston, a Bissell Healthcare Co. Bolingbrook, IL)*

citizens clubs, self-help groups, home nursing services, Meals on Wheels and sheltered workshops. Nurses should be aware of the state/territory-specific social welfare services and agencies, most of which are listed in the telephone directory *Yellow Pages*.

DISCHARGE PLANNING

Discharge planning prepares the client for the transition to another setting, such as from hospital to home. The elements of the discharge planning process should begin on the day of admission. The overall goal of discharge planning is to promote continuous health care services to meet the individual's needs (see Chapter 24 for further information on discharge planning). An effective discharge plan depends on the resources available to the individual who is being rehabilitated. Available resources include:

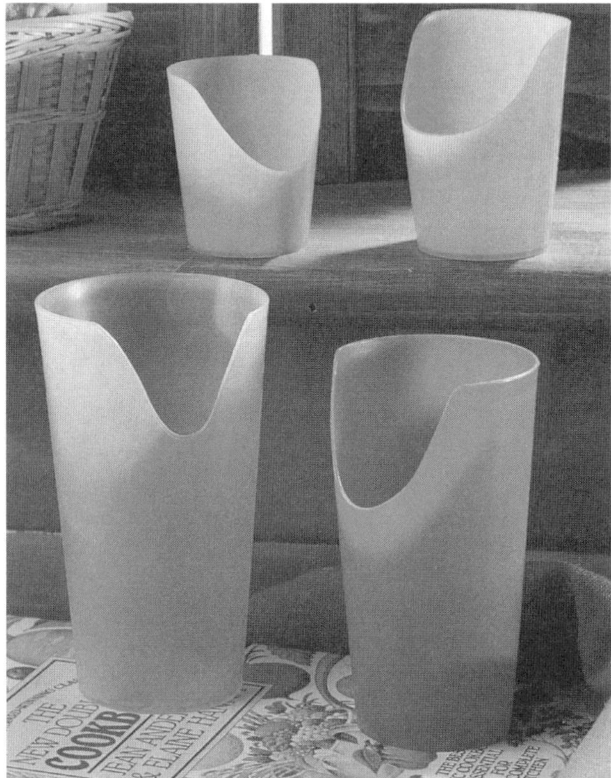

Figure 46.4 | Aids to promote independence with drinking. Tumbler with a special cut-out for the nose allows the client to drink without tipping the head back *(Hoeman 2008. Reproduced courtesy of Sammons Preston, a Bissell Healthcare Co. Bolingbrook, IL)*

- The family or significant others — the client's support systems
- Home care nursing
- Social and counselling agencies
- Volunteer community services
- Support and special interest groups; for example, Multiple Sclerosis (MS) Australia, Diabetes Australia, the National Cancer Council, the National Heart Foundation, Arthritis Australia
- Medical supplies and equipment
- Adaptation of the home environment for safety and optimal independence.

The client and the nurse, together with other team members, assist in coordinating and developing the discharge plan, using the steps of the nursing process to achieve the final plan.

SUMMARY

Rehabilitation is a dynamic process in which clients are helped to achieve optimal quality of life by increased function and independence, within the limits of their disability. A disability is any physical, mental, emotional or social impairment that limits a person's ability to carry out an activity in the usual manner.

Effective rehabilitation involves the client, family or significant others and professional members of the health care team. As part of the rehabilitation team, the nurse plays a vital role in helping the individual to meet physical and psychological needs as independently as possible. The rehabilitation process empowers the client to make informed decisions and choices about treatment modalities, care regimens and lifestyle options.

REVIEW EXERCISES

1. What are the main goals of a rehabilitation program?
2. What are the philosophical principles underlying any rehabilitation program?

CLINICAL INTEREST BOX 46.6
Aids to independent living

- Suction devices fitted to kitchen utensils, backs of nail brushes, etc, for the benefit of a person with the use of only one hand
- Boards with spikes to hold fruit or vegetables to be peeled, or bread to be buttered
- Face washers in the shape of a mitten, with a pocket to hold the soap
- Long-handled tongs for a person who is unable to pick items up by bending or stooping
- Dressing sticks with one end covered by foam rubber to grip the sleeve or shoulder of a garment, making it easier to don and remove
- Various devices to enable socks and stockings to be put on
- Overlapping adhesive fastenings (e.g. Velcro) on clothing for people unable to manage other conventional types of fastenings
- Long-handled shoe horns to make bending or stooping unnecessary (see Figure 46.1)
- Elastic shoelaces, which do not have to be untied when shoes are removed
- Cuffs, which when placed over the hand, hold a pencil, toothbrush or razor
- Easy-to-turn tap fittings
- Raised toilet seats
- Chairs with an ejector seat, which rises as the occupant leans forward
- Ramps to replace stairways
- Hand grips in bathroom and toilet areas
- Long-handled brushes to enable clients to perform their own hygiene activities (see Figure 46.2)
- Low-level fittings for occupants of wheelchairs (e.g. sinks, stoves, mirrors, light switches)
- Eating and drinking aids (see Figures 46.3 and 46.4)
- Walking aids

3. List three areas of assessment the nurse could be involved in when a rehabilitation program is being planned for a client who has experienced hemiplegia as a result of a cerebrovascular accident (stroke).
4. List three ways a rehabilitation nurse can assist in empowering the client who has lost the ability to speak but can understand.
5. List three areas of health education that might be helpful for the rehabilitation nurse to provide for an older client who has recently been diagnosed with Parkinson's disease.
6. List four roles within the rehabilitation team that the nurse may undertake.
7. List four settings in which the rehabilitation nurse may function, and identify six types of illness, condition or injury that clients might experience in which rehabilitation would be essential.

CRITICAL THINKING EXERCISE

Mr Richards, 49, has experienced a motor vehicle accident in which he suffered multiple fractures of both legs. He has worked hard during the restorative phase of his illness and is able to walk short distances with the aid of forearm crutches. Plans are in progress for his discharge home. His wife and two children, aged 9 and 11, live at the home. Because of financial pressures, Mrs Richards cannot give up her full-time paid work to care for him during the day.

1. Discuss the role and function of the nurse in planning for Mr Richards' discharge.
2. Identify the issues that Mr Richards might face on returning to the community.
3. What options might need to be discussed with the client and family in relation to decreasing the potential for falls or other injury when he returns to the community?
4. Describe three community services or other resources that could help to facilitate a successful community re-entry for Mr Richards.

REFERENCES AND FURTHER READING

Australasian Rehabilitation Nursing Association (ARNA) (2004) *Rehabilitation Nursing Competency Standards for Registered Nurses*. ARNA), Sydney

Collins AM, Diego L (2000) Mental health promotion and protection. *Journal of Psychosocial Nursing*, 38(1): 27

Davis S, O'Connor S (1999) *Rehabilitation Nursing Foundations for Practice*. Baillière Tindall in association with Royal College of Nursing, Edinburgh

Derstine B, Drayton-Hargrove S (2001) *Comprehensive Rehabilitation Nursing*. WB Saunders, Philadelphia

Dethmers F, Granthem P, Lee R, Pearson S, Sigmund-Orth E (1999) An interdisciplinary team approach in client rehabilitation. *Journal of the Australasian Rehabilitation Nurses Association*, 2(2): 12–19

Flannery J (2004) *Rehabilitation Nursing Secrets*. Elsevier, Sydney

Gibbon B (2003) The contribution of the nurse to stroke units in the United Kingdom. *Official Journal of the Australasian Rehabilitation Nurses Association*, 6(2): 8–13

Hitchcock JE, Schuber PE & Thomas SA (2002) *Community Health Nursing: Caring in Action*. Thomas Delmar Learning, New York

Hoeman SP (2002) *Rehabilitation Nursing. Process, Application & Outcomes*, 3rd edn. Mosby Year Book, St Louis

—— (2008) *Rehabilitation Nursing. Prevention, Intervention & Outcomes*, 4th edn. Mosby, St. Louis

Jester R (2007) *Advancing Practice in Rehabilitation Nursing*. Blackwell Publishing, Hoboken, NJ

Kearney PM, Pryor J. (2004) The International Classification of Functioning, (ICF) disability and health and nursing. *Journal of Advanced Nursing*, 46:2: 162–70b

Landry K, Lopez S Pratama, Y (2005) *Enabled in Words: The Real Lives, Real Victories of People With Disabilities*. Enabled Media Group Inc. Online. Available: www.enabledonline.com [accessed 4 June 2008]

MacPhail M (1998) Client centred goal setting research project: guidelines for data collection. Unpublished paper. Ballarat Health Services/Queen Elizabeth Centre Rehabilitation Services

Pryor J (2000) Creating a rehabilitative milieu. *Rehabilitation Nursing*, 25(4): 141–4

Pryor J, Smith C (2000) *A Framework for the Specialty Practice of Rehabilitation*. Rehabilitation Research and Development Unit, Australasian Rehabilitation Nursing Association (ARNA), Sydney

Rodwell CM (1996) An analysis of the concept of empowerment. *Journal of Advanced Nursing*, 23: 305–13

Roper N, Logan W, Tierney A (2000) *The Roper-Logan-Tierney Model Of Nursing Based on Activities of Daily Living*. Elsevier, Sydney

Smith M (ed.) (1999) *Rehabilitation in Adult Nursing Practice*. Churchill Livingstone, Edinburgh

Sondermeyer J (2002) Independent with an aid. A critical investigation into the language of recovery. *Official Journal of the Australasian Rehabilitation Nurses' Association*, 5(4): 7–11

World Health Organisation (2001) *The International Classification of Functioning: Disability and Health*. WHO, Geneva

ONLINE RESOURCES

Association of Rehabilitation Nurses: www.rehabnurse.org

Australasian Rehabilitation Nurses Association: www.arna.com.au

Ability First Australia: Disability Services: www.abilityfirstaustralia.com.au

Enabled: www.enabledonline.com

Chapter 47

BEHAVIOURAL AND SOCIAL ASPECTS OF DISABILITY

OBJECTIVES

- Define the key terms/concepts
- Understand the ways in which disabilities are classified
- Gain an overview of causative factors
- Recognise the impact of societal attitudes on the experience of having a disability
- Identify the community services available to support people with a disability
- Gain an understanding of what is required to competently assist in assessing, planning and providing care for a person with a disability
- Acknowledge the important role family carers play in supporting people with disabilities
- Identify health promotion strategies that serve to reduce the incidence of disability in society

KEY TERMS/CONCEPTS

choice
dignity
disability
equity and access
family carer
handicap
health promotion
impairment
inclusion
independence
normalisation
rights
segregation
social role valorisation
stigma

CHAPTER FOCUS

The disabilities that people live with range from minor to profound in severity, and many people live with multiple disabilities. They are extensively varied in type and cause and in the way they impact on a person's functioning. Historical factors influence society's responses to people with disabilities and, although there have been improvements in recent years, people with disabilities still face inequities in access to many things taken for granted by the general population. The current philosophy of care is based on the concepts of inclusion, normalisation and person-centred planning. The emphasis is on the importance of enabling a person with a disability, as far as possible, to live like any other person. This means that there must be services and provisions in the community that enable the person with a disability to pursue their personal interests in a positive way. There is also a strong emphasis on respecting the person with the disability, and their close family carers, as the primary authorities on what is desirable and important to the quality of life of the person with the disability. This chapter outlines the classification and causative factors of disabilities, explains the current philosophy of care and the important role of family carers. It also indicates some health promotion strategies to limit the incidence of disability in the future. The theme throughout is the need for nurses to recognise and promote the importance of successful integration into society and quality of life for all people with disabilities.

LIVED EXPERIENCE

Sheelagh, 27, has flexion deformities in both arms and legs. She also has epilepsy, is doubly incontinent and is mute. Plus she has difficulty eating and drinking. When I was told at handover that she had been admitted to our ward with an infected leg I thought, 'This is the limit, we are too busy here to cope with someone like her'. But Sheelagh has been here for 2 weeks and I will be sorry to see her leave. Her great smile and her wicked sense of humour has lifted the mood of everyone around her, including the other clients.

Faye, 23, Enrolled Nurse

CLASSIFICATION OF DISABILITY

Disability is the outcome of an impairment or change to a person's physical body or mental ability or the way that person is able to function. The impact of disability on a person's life is very much related to the social and physical environment in which that person lives, on cultural responses to disability and on the individual's psychological and physical condition. There are numerous types and causes of disability, so people with disabilities do not form a homogenous group. For example, people with learning disabilities, those who are visually, hearing or speech impaired and those with restricted mobility or other physical challenges all encounter barriers of different kinds that have to be overcome in different ways. Conditions that result in disability may be classified using two criteria: according to the type and cause, or according to the level of restriction incurred.

CLASSIFICATION ACCORDING TO TYPE AND CAUSE

This classification is made according to whether the disability is:

- Inherited: conditions genetically transmitted (e.g. Down's syndrome, spina bifida, muscular dystrophy, short stature)
- Congenital: conditions resulting from infection during the mother's pregnancy, or injury during or soon after birth (e.g. cerebral palsy)
- Acquired: resulting from accident, intentional injury, substance misuse or illness during life (e.g. amputation due to effects of diabetes or injury in a motor vehicle accident)
- Of unknown origin (e.g. some intellectual and behavioural disorders and mental health problems).

Clinical Interest Box 47.1 lists some causes of intellectual disabilities in children.

Disability may also be categorised as:

- Sensory (e.g. hearing or vision impairment)
- Physical (e.g. arthritis, amputation, spinal cord injury, acquired brain injury, multiple sclerosis, muscular dystrophy)
- Mental illness (e.g. dementia, schizophrenia, bipolar mood disorder)
- Intellectual (e.g. learning difficulties) (Gething 1997).

Clinical Interest Box 47.2 presents further information about intellectual disabilities.

With the help of appropriate education, training and support, people with intellectual disabilities can and do learn many new skills. The problem cannot be cured but most can lead independent or semi-independent lives (Gething 1997). Learning disability can be mild, moderate, severe or profound. One of the most important factors in caring for people with any learning disability is never to presume that they have reached their full potential of learning.

CLINICAL INTEREST BOX 47.2
Intellectual disability

People with an intellectual disability do not have a medical illness; rather, they find it more difficult to learn than other people, and for this reason the term 'learning disability' is frequently substituted. The extent of learning disability varies between individuals but often it is not that they cannot learn, but that they are just slower at doing so than the average person. People with learning disabilities also need more time to process information and to respond to it. The problem may have existed from birth, or it may be the outcome of an illness or injury during childhood development or at the time of adolescence. Generally it is agreed that learning disability comprises significant below-average intellectual functioning that coexists with below-average social functioning, and that this becomes obvious before age 18.
(Gates 2007)

CLINICAL INTEREST BOX 47.1
Causes of intellectual disabilities in children*

Numerous factors can cause intellectual disability but sometimes no specific cause can be identified. An intellectual disability may be either congenital or acquired. Causes of congenital disabilities include:

- Chromosomal abnormalities; for example, an extra chromosome 21, causing Down's syndrome; an additional X chromosome, causing Klinefelter's syndrome
- Inherited metabolic defects; for example, decreased phenylalanine hydroxylase, causing phenylketonuria (PKU)
- Maternal infections during pregnancy; for example, rubella or toxoplasmosis; maternal malnutrition
- Chronic maternal illness such as renal or cardiac disease
- Exposure to toxic agents; for example, drugs or environmental chemicals, during intrauterine life; exposure to high-energy radiation
- Premature birth, which may result in cerebral damage; birth injuries; for example, cerebral damage due to disruption of oxygen supply
- Drug misuse during pregnancy, including excess alcohol consumption and smoking.

Acquired intellectual impairment may result from:

- Malnutrition in infancy and early childhood
- The inability of the infant's body to metabolise, use or excrete products efficiently
- Illnesses that damage the brain, such as meningitis or encephalitis
- Injury or poisoning that damages the brain during infancy or early childhood
- Severe neglect or abuse by carers during infancy or early childhood; for example, sensory and social deprivation.

(Gething 1997; Watson 2003)
*This list is not exhaustive — it lists some of the more common causative factors only.

CLASSIFICATION ACCORDING TO LEVEL OF RESTRICTION

Disability can be further categorised according to the level of restriction it imposes on the individual. The Australian Bureau of Statistics (ABS) categorises restriction in relation to limitations on schooling or employment and 'core' activities of everyday living (self-care, mobility and communication). Self-care activities relate to bathing, showering, dressing, eating, using the toilet and managing incontinence. Mobility relates to moving around at home and away from home, getting into and out of a bed or chair and using public transport. Communication relates to understanding and being understood by others.

The level of restriction is categorised as profound, severe, moderate or mild, and determined according to the following descriptions:

- Profound: unable to perform a core activity or always needing assistance. This would apply to a person who has quadriplegia, for example
- Severe: sometimes needing assistance to perform a core activity. This might apply to a person with a condition such as schizophrenia or multiple sclerosis, which is characterised by episodes of remission and relapse
- Moderate: not needing assistance but having difficulty performing a core activity
- Mild: having no difficulty performing a core activity but using aids or equipment because of a disability. This might apply to a person who is an amputee, walks with the aid of a prosthesis, and uses a bath seat and support rails to shower (ABS 2001).

MULTIPLE DISABILITIES

Many people experience more than one disability; for example, many people with an intellectual disability also have at least one of the following:

- Impaired mobility
- Impaired motor control of hands
- Impaired speech, hearing or vision
- Seizures
- Lack of bladder and/or bowel control
- Emotional or behavioural challenges.

A client who has cerebral palsy may need assistance with self-care and have mobility challenges. The same client may also experience sensory difficulties as a result of hearing, vision or speech impairment (Buzio et al 2002).

COMMON TERMS

It is useful to have an understanding of the different terms used in relation to people with disabilities. The World Health Organization (WHO), in its *International Classification of Impairments, Disabilities and Handicaps (ICIDH)* of 1980, made a distinction between the concepts of impairment, disability and handicap. The WHO definitions are as follows:

- Impairment: impairment is any loss or abnormality of psychological, physiological or anatomical structure or function. Impairments are disturbances at the level of the organ, which include defects in or loss of a limb, organ or other body structure, as well as defects in or loss of a mental function. Examples of impairments include blindness, deafness, loss of sight in an eye, paralysis of a limb, amputation of a limb, mental retardation, partial sight, loss of speech or mutism
- Disability: disability is a restriction or lack (resulting from an impairment) of ability to perform an activity in the manner or within the range considered normal for a human being. It describes a functional limitation or activity restriction caused by an impairment. Disabilities are descriptions of disturbances in function at the level of the person. Examples of disabilities include difficulty seeing, speaking or hearing; difficulty moving or climbing stairs; difficulty grasping, reaching, bathing, eating or toileting
- Handicap: a handicap is a disadvantage resulting from an impairment or disability that limits or prevents the fulfilment of a role that is normal (depending on age, sex and social and cultural factors) for that individual. Examples of handicaps include being bedridden or confined to home, being unable to use public transport or being socially isolated (Wen & Fortune 1999).

THE INTERNATIONAL CLASSIFICATION OF FUNCTIONING, DISABILITY AND HEALTH

In May 2001, the World Health Organization (WHO) endorsed a new *International Classification of Functioning, Disability and Health (ICF)*. This new approach does not aim to classify people or disabilities. Rather it aims to identify and describe the full range of human functions and locate any disturbance to those functions on a continuum, regardless of the type or cause of disability. The classification identifies three dimensions in which these functions of the body operate:

1. **b** (body): body function and structure (physiological or psychological function and anatomical parts)
2. **a** (activities): activities at the individual level
3. **p** (participation): participation in society.

This new approach addresses the fact that these three dimensions may be affected by environmental (e) factors. The environmental component is a new and important addition to the classification process because it incorporates the context in which the disability is experienced; for example, the physical, social and attitudinal environment in which people with disabilities live their lives. Within this framework a person's functioning and disability are viewed as a dynamic interaction between health conditions, the environment and personal factors. Using a five-point numerical scale for each area assessed, findings are recorded as either facilitators or barriers to indicate the effect they have on the individual's functioning (Australian Institute of Health and Welfare [AIHW] 2008).

HISTORICAL BACKGROUND

INSTITUTIONAL TO COMMUNITY-BASED CARE

Many changes occurred during the 20th century that impacted on attitudes to disability all over the world. For the greater part of the last century, most people with disabilities lived in institutions. They were segregated from society and denied the rights of access to services and opportunities available to the rest of the population, such as education, work, sports and the arts. Among the institutions involved were mental hospitals, nursing homes and buildings that were designated to house people within specific disability groups. For example, there were hostels for groups of people with cerebral palsy, and for people who were blind. People who entered institutional care facilities often remained there for their entire lives.

SEGREGATION, STIGMA AND ABUSE

The segregation from the general community in the past is in part responsible for the lack of awareness and level of discomfort felt by many people towards those who are different because of a disability. It also accounts to some extent for the social stigma that continues to confront people with disabilities today. Enquiries revealed that, during the period of institutional care, many people with disabilities suffered abuse at the hands of those designated to provide care (Manthorpe 2003). Unfortunately, issues of various kinds of abuse from those associated with service provision and other members of the community continue to be a concern. In particular, those who require assistance with personal care activities such as washing and dressing are sometimes vulnerable to sexual abuse. Some people with disabilities are trained by their carers to be compliant, with the result that they are made to feel they have little control over what happens to their bodies (Sherry 2000). Nurses have a legal and moral obligation to report any instance of abuse that comes to their notice (this includes physical, psychological, emotional or sexual abuse). They also have a responsibility to promote confidence and self-assertiveness in those who are potentially vulnerable.

ACHIEVEMENTS

It was not until the United Nations introduced the Declaration of Rights of Disabled Persons in 1974 and then designated 1981 as the International Year of Disabled Persons that general awareness of this denial of basic human rights was raised globally, and a massive rethinking of attitudes towards people with disabilities was instigated. Countries all over the world were encouraged to provide equal access for people with disabilities (Disability Services Australia 2001).

A Decade of Disabled Persons (1982–1993) was declared and provided a time frame for the world to make the necessary changes to achieve equity and access for people with disabilities in all areas of life. As in many countries of the world, Australia and New Zealand responded by setting up particular government bodies and organisations to start the process of bringing about the required changes. For example, in New Zealand a Disability Strategy was implemented by the Ministry of Health (Manatū Hauora) in 2001. This involved government agencies implementing action plans to address issues for people with disabilities across all areas of concern, which are similar worldwide. People with disabilities in New Zealand are expected to maintain a key role in monitoring the effectiveness of the strategy and how it continues to be implemented today.

In Australia, many achievements have improved the lives of people with disabilities, especially over the last decade. Table 47.1 lists some examples of Australia's National organisations that continue to work towards addressing issues concerning the rights of people with disabilities. In addition to government bodies, many disability groups developed their own organisations to air their particular concerns and fight for their rights. Many such organisations operate at a national level. In Australia these include the National Council on Intellectual Disability, the Head Injury Council of Australia, Women with Disabilities Australia, The National Ethnic Disability Alliance and the Physical Disability Council of Australia (National Disability Services 2008).

During the Decade of Disabled Persons, in line with other countries, the Australian Government began a review of services for people with disabilities, resulting in the *Disability Services Act 1986*. This Act changed the focus of care away from big institutions and into the community, into homes or smaller more home-like environments. People with disabilities could now live independently at home, with support from a range of services. They may live at home, but be dependent on the assistance and care provided by a member of their family or significant other person (family carer). They may live in a house with other people with disabilities, assisted by a paid carer who may or may not be a nurse. Others may live in special accommodation units with the assistance of a team of care staff.

For people with disabilities, being part of the community is essential to wellbeing, so this move was of vital importance. Unfortunately the demand for appropriate community-based accommodation is not always met and some people with disabilities, even some who are young, find themselves forced to live in aged-care facilities that are ill-equipped to meet their needs and fail to provide the quality of life to which they are entitled.

THE PHILOSOPHY OF INCLUSION AND NORMALISATION

Governments made recommendations and introduced reforms that aimed to ensure protection and address equity

TABLE 47.1 | EXAMPLES OF AUSTRALIAN NATIONAL ORGANISATIONS CONCERNED WITH THE RIGHTS OF PEOPLE WITH DISABILITIES

Organisation	Role
Australian Human Rights Commission	Established in 1981 to promote and protect the rights of all Australians, including people with disabilities
Australian Human Rights and Equal Opportunities Commission (HREOC)	A new commission established in 1986, with more specific objectives: to eliminate discrimination against people with disabilities and to promote wider acceptance and inclusion of people with disabilities into the community
Disability Services Australia	Range of services, including daytime activity programs and support with accommodation to help bridge the gap between school and adult life
Australian Council for Rehabilitation of the Disabled (ACROD)	National industry association for disability services, influencing government legislation and funding to promote quality services for people with disabilities
ACE (Action for Carers and Employment)	National body representing the many state [and territory] organisations that provide employment assistance and support to people with disabilities in the regular workforce
Australian Institute of Sport (AIS)	Activities include a program to coach elite athletes with disabilities
Active Australia — Australian Sports Commission	Promotes active lifestyle for all Australians, including those with disabilities. Activities include an education program to train teachers and community leaders to run sports and other outdoor events suitable for people with disabilities
Australian Sport and Recreation Association for People with an Intellectual Disability (AUSRAPID)	National sporting body that promotes equal access to sport and recreational programs for people with intellectual disabilities
Other organisations that promote inclusion in sporting activities include Wheelchair Sports Australia, Cerebral Palsy — Australian Sport and Recreation Federation, Disabled Wintersports Australia, Riding for the Disabled Association of Australia, Australian Blind Sports Federation, Australian Deaf Sports Federation	
(Disability Services Australia 2001)	

and access issues for people with disabilities, and these have been incorporated into legislation, such as the *Disability Discrimination Act 1992* (Australia). The reforms include recommendations concerning equity of access to buildings, employment, education, transport and travel. They reflect the drive for the inclusion of people with disabilities, as opposed to the earlier model of segregation and exclusion. They also reflect the drive towards 'normalisation'. Normalisation does not mean trying to make everyone fit a definition of whatever is viewed as normal. It refers to providing services for people with disabilities that are the same or as close as possible to the same as those provided for others. It means providing whatever is needed to ensure that people with disabilities can participate in the activities of normal life (Gething 1997).

The new philosophy of care and provision of services to people with disabilities adheres to the concepts of inclusion and normalisation. It emphasises the importance of enabling a person with a disability, as far as possible, to live like any other person. Inherent in this concept is the belief that a person with a disability is entitled to participate in community life and to enjoy the same rights and privileges as others. The concept of normalisation is applied to the provision of community services and to the care of people with disabilities in residential facilities.

The principle of normalisation (also known as social role valorisation) stems from Wolf Wolfensberger's (1972) basic philosophy that socially valued roles for people with disabilities should be supported and defended because their social roles as individuals are at risk of being devalued. Having a social role includes being a member of a family, for example, son or daughter, brother or sister, aunt or uncle, parent or grandparent. There are many more social roles, and people with disabilities should be encouraged and assisted to hold them. Social roles include those associated with being:

- A home owner (e.g. rent/mortgage payer)
- An employee (e.g. wage earner, tax payer, union member, work colleague)
- A community member (e.g. library member, customer, neighbourhood watch member or voter).

The aim of promoting these roles is to maximise the rights of people with disabilities to participate in life, just like everyone else in the community.

Goals of social role valorisation

The major goal of social role valorisation is to create or support socially valued roles for people because, if a person holds valued social roles, they are highly likely to receive, or at least have the opportunity to receive, the good things in life that are available to others in that society (Wolfensberger 1992). There exists a high degree of consensus about what the good things in life are. These include, to mention only a few major examples:

- Home and family
- Friendship
- Being accorded dignity, respect and acceptance
- A sense of belonging
- An education
- The development and exercise of one's capacities
- A voice in the affairs of one's community and society
- Opportunities to participate in life
- A decent material standard of living
- Somewhere to live that is as home-like and normal as possible
- Opportunities for work and self-support.

Box 47.1 provides some examples of how the philosophical principles of inclusion and normalisation have been, or are still to be, implemented.

CONTINUING BARRIERS

The many changes that have occurred over the last 10–15 years have led to society taking a more accepting view of people who are different and less able than others than has occurred in the past, but there are still significant social barriers facing people with disabilities (Atherton 2003). Despite the changes, barriers still include those relating to gaining employment, travelling safely and establishing intimate relationships. Many able-bodied people still tend to feel uncomfortable interacting with people with disabilities, and such barriers may impact significantly on the way people with disabilities perceive and feel about themselves.

It is an important component of professional caring work to influence the environment in which people with disabilities live in order to break down the barriers. This can be achieved in many different ways, including by advocating to governments or councils; for example, to improve wheelchair access to a cinema, park or a sports complex. The nurse can also promote inclusion at an individual level. For example, when a client moves to new accommodation the community nurse may visit the local shop to explain to the staff how they can participate in enabling the client to complete shopping needs successfully.

Box 47.1 | Implementation of normalisation and inclusion principles

EDUCATION
- Significantly increased integration of children with disabilities into mainstream schools
- Arts, sports and recreation
- The Paralympics Arts Festival held in Australia in 2000 provided a forum for artists with and without disabilities to participate and display their skills across a broad range of events, including musical concerts, drama and art exhibitions
- The Paralympic Games conducted in Sydney in 2000 provided an opportunity for elite athletes with disabilities to participate and display their athletic skills
- The Special Olympics for people with intellectual disabilities also provided an opportunity to display athletic skills and provides a year-round training program

EMPLOYMENT
- Access to employment has improved as a result of stipulated requirements and government schemes
- Employers are required to modify workplaces to facilitate the employment of people with disabilities (e.g. purchasing special equipment, provide for wheelchair access) unless doing so causes unjustifiable hardship to the business
- Government funding is available to assist with modifications to some business workplaces
- Advertisements for jobs must not discriminate against or exclude a person with a disability from applying for the position provided that they have the ability to do the work

TRANSPORT
- In 2000 Australia's Commonwealth Government introduced standards and stipulated time frames in which all public transport would be converted to ensure full access for people with disabilities. Bus, train, tram, taxi, plane and ferry services must comply. Indications are that most types of public transport will be 55% accessible by 2010 and that the aim is for 90% accessibility by 2015 (Disability Services Australia 2001)

ACCESS TO BUILDINGS

The Building Code of Australia stipulates that buildings must be designed to facilitate access and meet the needs of people with a range of disabilities. Requirements include:
- Doorways wide enough for people using wheelchairs
- Appropriate toilet space and facilities
- Minimum lighting to meet needs of visually impaired people and those who communicate by sign language or lip-reading

ENTERTAINMENT
- Captioning: in 1982 the Australian Captioning Centre was established to provide captioning services for hearing impaired people. Captioning on film or television provides written on-screen messages about what is being said and what sound effects or music are happening. Australian legislation requires that captions are provided for news, current affairs and prime-time television programs. In 2001 captioning was introduced in major cinemas around the country, but not all films are yet captioned
- Holidays: a travel guide, Easy Access Australia, was published for people with disabilities in 1995. It provides details of accessible walkways, user-friendly accommodation, tourist attractions and where other appropriate facilities can be located

(Disability Services Australia 2001)

The nurse may accompany the client on one or two visits to role-model how the staff should interact with the client and to try to eliminate any negative or judgmental attitudes the client may otherwise have to battle.

Sometimes people who acquire a disability are confronted by prior judgmental attitudes they themselves held towards people with disabilities. Concerns about being similarly judged may be a source of high stress in the immediate aftermath of becoming a person with a disability (Thomas 1999). Nurses require great sensitivity when caring for people who have a recently acquired disability.

RESPONSES TO DISABILITY

UNIQUE MEANINGS OF DISABILITY

Individual people perceive and experience disability in quite unique ways relative to their circumstances. An injury to the leg that results in permanent inability to bend the knee might be a serious anxiety-provoking disability for a man who is a carpet layer by trade and has a family to support. The impact of the same disability on an elderly man who lives alone, spends most of his time watching television and rarely goes out of the house may be quite different; by comparison, he may be relatively unconcerned. For many people permanent disability is an integral part of their lives, but often not the most significant aspect, and sometimes adjustment is so successful that it is an almost insignificant aspect. Therefore, people who have a disability may not consider themselves handicapped (see Clinical Interest Box 47.3).

ADJUSTMENT

The way a person adjusts to disability (or disabilities) is broadly dependent on a range of factors that include:

- Length of time the person has had the disability
- Amount and quality of support (e.g. family)
- Schooling and level of education
- Own acceptance of disability
- How obvious the impairment is to others
- Whether the disability was congenital (present at birth) or acquired later
- The manner and timeliness of health service responses
- The nature of health service interventions and other supports (e.g. did they foster dependence or promote independence within the client?)
- The responses of other people (societal attitudes) (Gething 1997).

CLINICAL INTEREST BOX 47.3
The meaning of disability to Mary Brown

I have been without an arm since I was 13 years old — that's 40-odd years now. I don't need it. I have everything I need and I enjoy life. I have a job, I play darts and cards with my friends, I dance and I cook, even though I admit I use packet potatoes that don't need peeling, but that's OK with the family. Some people I know can't keep a relationship going, can't keep a job . . . pretty inadequate really. I consider them to have hidden disabilities that are much more troublesome than mine.
(Mary Brown, age 55)

It is important to recognise that adjustment to disability may be short and relatively uncomplicated, but commonly it can be a long and difficult process involving extensive rehabilitation and a process of grieving (Chapter 46 provides further information concerning rehabilitation; Chapter 14 provides information on the grieving process). While individuals respond differently, it is helpful to recognise that in the initial period after illness or accident, when clients are first facing disability, they may be extremely stressed. This stress may result in behaviours that the person does not usually display, including:

- Hostility or anger
- Rebelliousness (e.g. refusing care, refusing to get up or shower)
- Refusal to socialise, shunning visitors, even close family and friends (this may be due to embarrassment at changed appearance or abilities, or fear of rejection)
- Depersonalisation (avoiding or disowning self or parts of self, which may be demonstrated by a refusal to acknowledge, talk about or look at an altered body part such as a stoma, a stump, or a burned area)
- Refusal to participate in activities (Thomas 1999).

(Ways for the nurse to assist clients experiencing stress are discussed in Chapter 13. Chapters 29 and 45 have information concerning communication and relating to clients displaying challenging behaviour.)

PROVIDING CARE FOR CLIENTS AND THEIR FAMILIES

Nurses may provide care for clients with disabilities and their carers in any setting in which care is provided. These include:

- The client's own home
- Community houses
- Day or drop-in centres
- Day clinics
- Residential care facilities
- General hospitals
- Rehabilitation units
- Obstetric units (neonates born with a disability)
- Respite care accommodation

Nurses may encounter clients with disabilities who are hospitalised for totally unrelated reasons; for example, a client with epilepsy who needs an appendicectomy. Others may be in hospital to provide respite for a family carer (e.g. a client with multiple sclerosis) and some may have only just acquired the disability (e.g. hemiplegia as a result of a cerebrovascular accident). This means that nurses need to adapt the ways they communicate with and respond to clients according to the type of disability and the specific circumstances. Clinical Interest Box 47.4 provides some guidelines to aid the nurse caring for clients with disabilities.

Sometimes people with disabilities demonstrate behaviour that even experienced nurses find challenging to manage (Emerson 2001; Newman & Summerhill 2003; Mottram & Berger-Gross 2004). There are often complexities involved in managing challenging behaviours, and it is recommended that nurses refer to texts concerned specifically with this issue to enhance their knowledge and expertise.

PERSON-CENTRED PLANNING

Whenever the client with a disability is encountered, a careful individual nursing assessment must be undertaken, and this should always be from the perspective that clients are people first, and that their disability is second. Person-centred planning is based on respect for the dignity and desires of the person with the disability and on the

CLINICAL INTEREST BOX 47.4
Suggestions to aid relationships between nurses and clients with disabilities

Keep in mind that:

- In many cases the client and the family carer will know more about the disability than the nurse
- The person with a disability is the same as anyone else, just with particular needs associated with that disability
- Many difficulties that the person faces are likely to be more to do with societal attitudes than the disability itself
- It is best to concentrate on what the person can do rather than on the things they are unable to do
- It is best to let the person guide how and at what pace things should be done
- Self-responsibility should be handed over to people with disabilities as soon as they are ready

When communicating:

- Adapt your pace of communication to suit the other person and, when communication ability is impaired, allow time for responses
- Speak directly to the person — do not use another person (e.g. family carer) as a go-between
- Monitor how much input into the conversation the person with the disability has — be careful that you don't dominate the conversation
- Take the person's lead, pick up on what the person may prefer to talk about, or finds interesting or important. Be alert to signals and act on them; for example, in a person whose speech is impaired, eye movement towards an object may indicate that the object is wanted
- Ask the person what help is required; avoid automatically doing things for the person; do not insist on helping and do not assist without asking first
- Ask if unsure of how to behave towards the person; for example, if the person has an arm missing or has uncontrolled limb movements, how do they prefer you to place meals or other objects?
- Respond with understanding and good will if the person knocks something over or spills something; for example, a glass of water. Humour can also be helpful and, when used effectively, can minimise embarrassment
- Do not be overly concerned if you say something that feels inappropriate; for example, saying 'Do you want to hop into the shower now?' to a person who has a right leg amputation. Having a disability does not remove a person's sense of humour, and humour can relieve discomfort for both nurse and client
- Whatever the disability, always use age appropriate language; for example, speak to the adult person with intellectual or cognitive impairment in the same manner as you would any other adult (Chapter 31 provides further information on communicating with people who have hearing, visual or cognitive impairment)

Caring for people in wheelchairs

- Do not assume that the person in a wheelchair needs assistance
- Do not try to move the person or wheelchair without first gaining permission
- Do not hold on to the wheelchair unnecessarily. It is part of the person's body space and the person cannot step away from you
- Ensure you are familiar with how a wheelchair is pushed and manoeuvred before taking a person in a wheelchair out and about. This includes knowing how to get it up and down steps, how to tip it backwards, how to use the brake and how the armrests are removed (never lift a wheelchair by the arm rests — most are removable) and how it folds up. It is a useful exercise to practise pushing and manoeuvring a wheelchair with a person who does not have a disability sitting in it

Promoting confidence

- Reinforce that people with disabilities have the same rights as other people in their community and in society as a whole
- Reinforce that they have the right to have a say in all decision making that concerns their lives, their treatment and their general wellbeing
- Reinforce that it is appropriate to be assertive and persistent in defending their rights, and to be firm but polite when defending their rights to things such as access, independence or privacy

Encourage people with disabilities to:

- Feel comfortable about asking for assistance when needed and avoid apologising for what they cannot do
- Feel comfortable in communicating in whatever way is appropriate for them, and about having to repeat things that are not understood or about asking other people to repeat or re-explain things that are unclear
- Understand that many people have little knowledge of disabilities (e.g. the realities of cerebral palsy), and to be tolerant of and polite to people who are unsure of how to respond to them in social situations, or who offer help that is not needed
- Be prepared for times when they may feel anxious or depressed. Reinforce that such feelings are common and that help is available should they need it
- Try to create opportunities to instigate the person's contact with positive role models of others who have a similar disability. For example, it may be encouraging to a client who has recently become visually impaired to talk with a person who has adapted successfully to vision impairment. It may be helpful for people who are hearing impaired to meet with deaf people communicating avidly with sign language.

(Gething 1997; Ferris-Taylor 2003)

acknowledgement of the family carer and the person with the disability as the experts in relation to identifying needs and appropriate interventions. Person-centred planning incorporates the principles of inclusion and normalisation and involves helping to break down community barriers so that the person can participate in life as normally as possible and can achieve personal desired goals.

As explained previously, current attitudes towards the care of a person with a disability reflect the belief that such a person is entitled to the same rights and freedom as any other person in society. Regardless of whether an individual with a disability is able to remain at home or lives in alternative accommodation, the overall goal of care planning must be to enable the achievement of as much independence and autonomy as possible, and to maximise the full potential of that person's capabilities.

PROVISION OF SERVICES

The Federal, state and territory governments in Australia fund a range of services for people with disabilities and their family carers, including:

- Family support services such as respite care and community-based respite care
- Domiciliary support, such as help with cleaning, house and garden maintenance, and Meals on Wheels
- Personal care support
- Home modification and provision of equipment
- Independent living skills programs
- Pre-vocational training, vocational placement and employment support
- Social support, including recreational and culturally specific activities
- Community-based accommodation and support; for example, support available to people with a disability living at home or in other accommodation in the community
- Sexual counselling
- Education and training for carers and clients
- Behaviour management programs
- Specialist assistance from professionals such as psychiatrists, psychologists, speech therapists and occupational therapists
- Case management, providing individual support, advocacy and monitoring
- Client's disability allowance
- Carer's allowance (small regular financial payment to assist with additional expenses).

These services aim to assist people with disabilities to achieve as much independence as possible by promoting family and community acceptance and involvement, providing sufficient support services, and by offering a range of accommodation options.

As discussed earlier, there is now much greater acceptance of the importance of family living and of participation in community life than in earlier times. The wellbeing of people with disabilities depends on recognition of their rights, promotion of community acceptance, and the implementation of programs that appropriately promote education, provide training for employment, develop independent skills in activities of daily living and promote enjoyment of life. Professional support is primarily directed towards enabling a person with a disability to achieve as much independence as possible, through interventions that promote independent living and vocational capacities. Planning and implementation of appropriate educational and vocational programs is performed on an individual basis and takes into account any associated physical, sensory or emotional effects of the disabilities.

Basic principles that should guide the provision of services include:

- A collaborative approach between health professionals: the client and the family should be consulted to decide what is needed, what will be of most help and how that help should be implemented for maximal benefit
- Identification of client and family strengths and capabilities
- Recognition and confirmation of emotions.

These principles should be kept in mind when assessing, planning, implementing and evaluating care.

ASSESSMENT

Decisions about the most appropriate plan of care are made after individual assessment. A multidisciplinary approach to assessment is generally required. Depending on the age and type of disability the person is experiencing, assessment may involve:

- Teachers
- Medical officers
- Maternal and child health nurses
- Nurses specialised in disability and rehabilitation nursing
- Generalist nurses
- Social workers
- Psychologists
- Psychiatrists
- Occupational therapists
- Speech pathologists
- Dietitians
- Physiotherapists
- Geriatricians
- Paediatricians.

The purpose of assessment is to identify the abilities and specific needs of an individual so that appropriate care may be planned. The overarching goal is to ensure support that allows the person to live life as near to the life they desire as possible. The assessment process will consider all aspects of the person's life:

- Physical needs
- Health and medical needs
- Financial support
- Spiritual and emotional support needs

- Cultural needs
- Learning needs
- Behavioural support needs
- Need for meaningful work
- Recreation and leisure needs
- Transport issues
- Accommodation needs
- Support networks (family and community)
- Impact of the client's environment.

The team may assess the individual using a variety of methods, such as observation, interviewing and testing. A checklist may be used to help identify activities that can be performed independently by the individual, and those for which assistance is required. When assessment is complete, the team, collaboratively with the client or family carer, can plan the care to be implemented.

The extensive types of disability and the fact that many clients will have multiple disabilities means that, after the assessment process, nurses may determine a broad range of nursing diagnoses for each individual client. Clinical Interest Box 47.5 identifies some common nursing diagnoses related to the needs of clients with disabilities. The list is by no means exhaustive and not in any particular sequence. The degree of relevance and nursing response will vary with each client and each situation.

PLANNING AND IMPLEMENTING

Using the information obtained from the assessment process, a program is developed to meet the client's needs. Central to development of a program is the concept of helping the individual to achieve as much independence as possible. The stages of the program include:

- Clearly identifying the client's capabilities
- Establishing goals
- Identifying skills and abilities to be developed
- Determining the most effective teaching strategies
- Determining the most effective interventions to meet social, educational and other needs.

For any program to be successful the goals and the skills to be accomplished by the individual must be clearly expressed and understood by the client, family carers, and all the team members. Based on the principle that people with disabilities have the same rights as the rest of the community, the plan of care should focus predominantly on what the person can, rather than cannot, do. The goals of care relate to helping people to develop the following skills and abilities:

- Take part in activities and experiences that improve their quality of life
- Develop practical skills to live as independently as possible
- Develop the interpersonal skills necessary to form relationships
- Make choices and decisions about their own lives.

These principles and goals of care are the same regardless of age or where a client with a disability resides. Clinical Interest Box 47.6 provides principles that govern care in a residential setting.

CLINICAL INTEREST BOX 47.5
Nursing diagnoses related to the needs of clients with disabilities

Psychological needs
- Impaired adjustment
- Ineffective individual coping
- Self-concept disturbance (incorporating body image/self-esteem/role performance/personal identity)
- Hopelessness
- Powerlessness
- Altered sexuality pattern
- Impaired social interaction

Physical needs
- Impaired physical mobility
- Impaired verbal communication
- Self-care deficit (incorporating hygiene/dressing and grooming/toileting)
- Sleep pattern disturbance
- Altered patterns of elimination (incorporating urinary/bowel)
- Potential for impaired tissue integrity
- Potential for falls/injury

EVALUATION

Evaluation must be performed continuously to assess progress in achieving the goals of care. Continuous evaluation is also needed to identify whether there are potential risks that have not been considered previously and to confirm that safe, holistic care is maintained.

FAMILY CAREGIVING – IMPACT AND SUPPORT

RESPONSIBILITY — 24 HOURS A DAY

Family carers of people with disabilities, particularly when the disabilities are multiple or profound, provide care and

CLINICAL INTEREST BOX 47.6
Principles of care in a residential setting

- Encourage and teach the individual to be as independent as possible
- Allow the individual to exercise choice at every possible opportunity
- Recognise the individual's right to privacy
- Establish routines that promote a sense of security
- Provide regular and frequent opportunities (e.g. daily/weekly) for participation in social and leisure activities
- Provide regular and frequent opportunities for interaction with others
- Provide a physical environment that is as much like a comfortable home as possible
- Ensure that the environment is equipped with features that facilitate independence; for example, handrails, ramps, access to benches and equipment, adequate lighting

support for them around the clock, on call 24 hours a day. Unlike nurses, they do not get breaks between shifts. Even when respite is available, the responsibility is permanent, 7 days a week, often lifelong and often falling primarily on one family member (Brown 1996).

For many the responsibility begins with the birth of a child with a disability. Parents in this situation are faced with an unplanned lifetime of giving fulltime care that interferes with their ability to give as much time as they would like to their other children or to conduct their lives as previously planned. They are faced with coping with the situation as they deal with the grief associated with lost expectations about their baby and the future. For others it begins at the stage of life when caring responsibilities are expected to reduce; for example, the parent caring for an adolescent offspring who has an acquired brain injury or has developed serious mental illness. For many it begins in older age, when caregiving responsibilities are usually over and when personal health or stamina may be declining; for example, a spouse caring for a partner with Alzheimer's disease.

Families caring for adolescents face particular challenges impacting on daily life: internal factors such as changing family roles and relationships and external factors such as service discontinuity, where forfeiting of a desired alternative may be necessary. These challenges indicate that family routine in the adolescent years is dynamic rather than static. Families use multiple strategies to accommodate these challenges, which are underpinned by their beliefs, values and resources. Professionals working with families caring for an adolescent with disability need to be aware of these in order to support families effectively to sustain a meaningful family routine during the adolescent years (Schneider et al 2006).

THE IMPACT OF CARING: LIFESTYLE CHANGES AND LOSS

Whenever the carer role begins, it is often associated with great lifestyle changes and many losses, including:

- Loss of the ability to continue with a career or paid employment
- Loss of income and financial security
- Loss of status and socialisation that often accompanies a paid work position
- Lost hopes and dreams of what the future will bring
- Loss of freedom and socialisation
- Loss of a normal or expected relationship (e.g. loss of companionship or a sexual partner when physical and cognitive functioning are profoundly affected) (Funnell 1998).

Despite the seriousness of their situation, many people caring for family members with disabilities gain pleasure, a sense of satisfaction and feelings of personal fulfilment from the role they have undertaken (see Clinical Interest Box 47.7).

CLINICAL INTEREST BOX 47.7
Charlie's story

Charlie, 66, cares for his wife, Anna, who has multiple sclerosis. Charlie retired from work early, 12 years ago, to care for her at home. He has gradually adjusted, with the help of service providers, to her increasing dependency. Anna is now paralysed and can move her head, but not her limbs. She is no longer continent. Charlie bathes her every weekday, using a lifting machine, assists her with toileting, all meals (which he prepares himself) and takes her out, with her wheelchair, in a specially adapted van to enjoy trips to the zoo and the botanical gardens.

Charlie admits to getting very tired at times but has no regrets — he feels the role of carer has improved him as a person. 'I am a different person because of caring for Anna,' he says. 'It's shown up different areas of my life that needed changing, like my impatience and quick temper. I've had to change. It's been a teaching time, a time for reflection. I think I'm a much more caring person, I can put myself in other people's shoes, which I couldn't before.'

When Charlie and Anna were offered more professional assistance with Anna's hygiene and meals, Charlie declined, although Anna expressed concern for him. Charlie responded 'I want to do it — I feel I am repaying Anna for all the times I wasn't there for her and the kids in the early part of our marriage . . . and I feel good because I do things for her I never thought I'd be able to do, and I've earned her love and respect and the respect of my kids now.'

(Funnell 1998)

SUPPORT FOR PRIMARY (FAMILY) CARERS

It is essential that nurses and other professionals acknowledge and credit family carers as having the primary caregiving role, and carefully assess how to best enable and facilitate their ongoing coping abilities. Some family carers prefer to cope independently, some prefer a regular visit from a nurse or other team member, others may view such visits or other interventions as an invasion of privacy (Funnell 1998). Some simply need the reassurance of having a contact to call when information or assistance is needed. Others need a significant amount of support, particularly in managing challenging behaviours (Emerson 2001). The amount and type of support may vary over time but whenever and whatever services are implemented, such as personal care assistance for the dependent person or help with house cleaning, they should be determined in collaboration with the primary carer. There are key times when additional services or support may be needed. These include:

- At the time of diagnoses or identification of a disability
- During the care of a preschool child with a disability
- When educational needs and potential need to be determined or reviewed
- Before transition from child to adult services or from adult to aged-care services
- When the client is unwell
- When the primary carer is unwell

- When the client's general functioning declines and care needs increase (Wake 2003).

The opportunity for primary carers to take short-term breaks through the use of respite services should be integrated into care planning. Even though such breaks do not resolve the stresses and strains of full-time caring, they may have a positive influence on the ability of the primary carer to continue the carer role in the long term. However, some family carers feel guilty about putting a dependent loved one into respite care, and choose not to take much needed breaks, and sometimes demands for respite services exceed supply (Funnell 1998).

One of the significant issues facing primary carers is what will happen to the dependent loved one if they should get sick or die. This is particularly worrying for parents who have spent a lifetime caring for dependent children, particularly given the shortage of appropriate accommodation for people with disabilities. Whenever possible, a plan should be developed in advance to ease this worry, but this is not a simple matter. The current shortage of suitable accommodation options that sometimes already results in even young people with disabilities living in aged-care facilities is likely to worsen in the future. As the current older generation of family carers die, the demand for appropriate accommodation and care will increase significantly and there is a very real possibility that, unless action is taken now, many people with disabilities will be left without a suitable home and without appropriate care and support. It is the role of nurses to advocate for appropriate resources for people with disabilities.

Caring for people with profound or multiple disabilities and their carers is challenging, Careful assessment of needs, sensitive and timely interventions, respect for the client and acknowledgement and appreciation of the role of the primary carer are at the heart of excellent nursing care.

HEALTH PROMOTION: DISABILITY PREVENTION

While much can be done to improve the lives of people with disabilities, it is equally as important to minimise disability in the community as much as possible. Several strategies have been implemented with the aim of reducing the number of people who are born with or acquire a disability (Clinical Interest Box 47.8).

Prevention of disability needs to be a priority. Currently there is an estimated 3.9 million people in Australia (20% of the population) who live with one or more limitations to functioning (AIHW 2008). It is difficult to determine exactly how many of these disabilities were preventable. According to the AIHW, in 2007 10 000 people in New South Wales alone acquired a brain injury (AIHW 2007). This information puts the need for preventive educational programs into perspective. Brain injury is mostly acquired through:

- Road-, sport- or work-related injuries
- Misuse of drugs, including alcohol

CLINICAL INTEREST BOX 47.8
Strategies for health promotion/disability prevention

- Vaccinations have been promoted to prevent serious illness that can lead to a range of impairments; for example, vaccination against the rubella virus is important because maternal rubella in the early stages of pregnancy can cause congenital abnormalities
- Road safety campaigns and 'Swimsafe' campaigns have aimed to reduce the number of disabilities caused by road, diving and near-drowning accidents
- Safe-sex campaigns have aimed to reduce the incidence of AIDS and other disabling disorders
- 'Safety in the Workplace' and 'Safety in the Home' programs have aimed to reduce avoidable injuries to employees and children
- Anti-smoking campaigns have aimed to reduce the physical impairment caused by damage to the lungs and other organs by smoking
- Education of pregnant mothers about the dangers of smoking to the unborn infant have aimed to reduce the risk of brain damage and intellectual disabilities in children. Education programs for pregnant mothers have also focused on the importance of healthy nutrition and the elimination of alcohol and other drugs
- 'SunSmart' campaigns have aimed to reduce disability caused by skin cancer

- Lack of oxygen from near drowning or severe asthma attacks
- Cerebrovascular accident (stroke)
- Brain tumours
- Falls.

Maybe not all, but many of these causes of acquired brain damage, and the causes of other congenital or acquired disabilities, could be minimised by health and safety education programs and/or programs that promote and support a healthy lifestyle. An important role for nurses, particularly those working in community settings, is the prevention of additional illness in people with disabilities by ensuring their access to routine health screens. This is sometimes difficult, perhaps due to a physical disability preventing a person achieving the correct position for a particular health screen, such as a mammogram or a Papanicolaou test (Pap smear) for example. This does not mean that health screening should be put in the 'too hard basket'. Consultation between medical officers, radiographers, physiotherapists, nurses and especially the person with the disability is needed to establish a way in which tests can be successfully managed.

SUMMARY

A disability may be inherited, congenital or acquired, and the impact of the disability on a person's life varies between minor and profound. Many people live with multiple disabilities. The meaning of impairment is unique to each individual.

The focus of service provision has shifted from institutional to community based, with many people with disabilities living independently or semi-independently and many living at home supported by family carers. The philosophy of care is based on principles of inclusion and normalisation, recognising that people with disabilities are entitled to the same rights and freedoms as everyone else. Therefore the goal of professional carers is to assist people with disabilities to live as much as is possible like any other member of the community. This involves ensuring equality of access to education, employment, transport and travel, leisure activities and relationships with others. While a range of services are working to achieve this, people with disabilities still face stigma and social barriers.

Nurses work with clients who have disabilities in a wide range of settings and situations. Guidelines for promoting recognition of their rights and providing sensitive and appropriate care have been provided. A multidisciplinary approach to providing services is important, and consultation with the client and family carer is essential in the assessment process and in decisions about the supports to be implemented. Nurses and other professional service providers are advised to work with clients from the perspective that the person with a disability is a person first, and the disability is secondary, and to acknowledge and respect the vital role that family carers play in supporting people with disabilities living in the community.

Examples of preventive measures that can be implemented to help reduce the incidence of disability have been provided, as health promotion and disability prevention is a particularly important role for nurses and all health professionals. Nurses may like to consider undertaking further study in specific areas of disability nursing, including the areas of learning disabilities, head trauma or spinal injury, mental health, neurological disorders and dementia. Nurses are recommended to read more widely to expand understanding of the basic concepts raised in this chapter and to develop empathy and understanding of the many needs and issues that concern people with disabilities and their families.

REVIEW EXERCISES

1. Identify the ways in which disabilities may be classified.
2. Define the terms disability, impairment and handicap.
3. List three possible causes of (a) physical impairment and (b) intellectual impairment.
4. Explain what is meant by the term 'social role valorisation'.
5. Identify the types of support services available to people with disabilities living in the community.
6. Identify five barriers that people with disabilities may face in the community.
7. Identify measures that could reduce the number of people with disabilities in the future.

CRITICAL THINKING EXERCISE

Grace is 42 years old. When she was born she suffered a brain injury. Until now her parents have cared for her at home. Every day of her life her father has lifted her from her bed in the morning and carried her to a recliner chair in the lounge and later returned her to bed the same way. Each day her mother has prepared the food and assisted Grace with her meals. This has always been a lengthy process, as Grace has some difficulty controlling food that is put into her mouth. Between them Grace's parents showered her and assisted her with getting dressed each day and undressed again each evening. Sometimes this went smoothly but at other times Grace would resist and yell out. Grace was incontinent of urine and her parents fitted her with disposable pads every morning and changed them frequently during the day. They took care of her pressure areas that sometimes developed.

After she left school Grace began attending a day centre 3 days each week. She was taken there in a community bus specially designed to accommodate her wheelchair. Activity at the centre revolves mostly around the staff meeting the hygiene, toileting, medication, mobility and nutritional needs of the two dozen or more people with severe or profound disabilities who also attended. The staff reported that Grace spent a lot of her time there simply dozing.

On the days she was at home Grace had many things surrounding her that gave her pleasure. She had a box containing many different pieces of material. She enjoyed the feel of the different textures, especially the velvet and silk. Other times she held on to colourful toys and, although she had a profoundly limited vocabulary, she enjoyed television, music, being with her mother in the kitchen and sitting on the outside veranda watching people walk past the house. Many of the neighbours greeted her cheerfully.

Grace's parents have been anxious for some time about their future ability to care for her, but now Grace's mother has fallen and fractured her hip. Her father is exhausted and cannot manage to care for Grace alone. Grace has been admitted to a residential care unit, where most of the residents are elderly and have dementia. There is nowhere else available at the moment. With a group of colleagues, consider and discuss:

1. How Grace's mother and father may be feeling about this situation. What could be done to help them?
2. The impact of this move on Grace. How might she be feeling? How can staff help ease the transition to her new accommodation and situation?
3. What are Grace's rights? What are the risks to those rights being infringed?
4. What can staff do to ensure that her rights are not infringed?
5. How can staff create a stimulating and pleasurable environment for Grace?

REFERENCES AND FURTHER READING

Annison J (1996) *Disability: a Guide for Health Professionals*. Thomas Nelson Australia, Melbourne

Atherton H (2003) A history of learning disabilities. In: Gates B (ed.) *Learning Disabilities. Toward Inclusion*, 4th edn. Churchill Livingstone, Edinburgh

Australian Bureau of Statistics (2001) *Australian Welfare: the 5th Biennal Welfare Report*. AIHW Cat No Aus 24. ABS, Canberra

Australian Institute of Health and Welfare (AIHW) (2007) *Disability in Australia: Acquired Brain Injury*. Bulletin 55, December. Online. Available: www.aihw.gov.au/publications/aus/bulletin55/bulletin55.pdf

—— (2008) *The 8th Biennial Welfare Report*. AIHW cat no AUS 93. AIHW, Canberra. Online. Available: www.aihw.gov.au/publications/index.cfm/title/10527 [accessed 1 June 2008]

Bollard M (2002) Health promotion and learning disability. *Nursing Standard*, 16(27): 47–55

Brown P (1996) Caregivers — the invisible workforce: caregiver and gender issues. In: *Towards a National Agenda for Carers. Aged and Community Care Service Development and Evaluation Reports*. No 22: 68–84. AGPS, Canberra

Buzio A, Morgan J, Blount D (2002) The experiences of adults with cerebral palsy during periods of hospitalisation. *Australian Journal of Advanced Nursing*, 19(4): 8–14

Disability Services Australia (2001). *Life to Live*. Online. Available: www.dsa.org.au/life_site/text/timeline/index.html [accessed 1 June 2008]

Edwards SD (2005) *Disability: Definitions, Value and Identity* Radcliffe Publishing, Oxford

Emerson E (2001) *Challenging Behaviour: Analysis and Intervention in People with Severe Intellectual Disabilities*. Cambridge University Press, Cambridge UK

Ferris-Taylor R (2003) Communication. In: Gates B (ed.) *Learning Disabilities: Toward Inclusion*, 4th edn. Churchill Livingstone, Edinburgh

Funnell R (1998) For better or worse: caregiving husbands of wives with multiple sclerosis. Unpublished Master of Arts thesis, LaTrobe University, Bundoora, Vic

Gates B (ed.) (2006) *Care Planning and Delivery in Intellectual Disability Nursing*. Blackwell publishing, Edinburgh

—— (ed.) (2007) *Learning Disabilities: Toward Inclusion*, 5th edn. Churchill Livingstone, Edinburgh

Gates B, Wilberforce D (2003) The nature of learning disabilities. In: Gates B (ed.) *Learning Disabilities: Toward Inclusion*, 4th edn. Churchill Livingstone, Edinburgh

Gething L (1997) *Person to Person: a Guide for Professionals Working with People with Disabilities*, 3rd edn. MacLennan & Petty, Sydney

Holburn S, Vietze PM (2002) *Person Centered Planning: Research, Practice and Future Directions*. Paul H Brookes Publishing Company, Baltimore

Hunt R (2001) *NZ Government Action on Disability Strategy*. Online. Available: www.disabilityworld.org/07-08_01/gov/nz.shtml [accessed 1 June 2008]

Manthorpe J (2003) Accessing services and support. In: Gates B (ed.) *Learning Disabilities: Toward Inclusion*, 4th edn. Churchill Livingstone, Edinburgh

Markwick A, Parrish A (eds) (2003) *Learning Disabilities: Themes and Perspectives*. Butterworth–Heinemann, Edinburgh

Mottram L, Berger-Gross P (2004) An intervention to reduce disruptive behaviours in children with brain injury *Pediatric Rehabilitation*, 7(2): 133–43

National Disability Services (2008) Australian disability services website. Available: www.nds.org.au/national/default.htm [accessed 1 June 21008]

Newman DW, Summerhill L (2003) Working with an adult male with Down's syndrome, autism and challenging behaviour: evaluation of a programme of staff support and organizational change *British Journal of Learning Disabilities*, 31: 85–90

Parsons I (1996) *Duty of Care: Who's responsible? A Guide for Carers who are Supporting People With Disabilities*. Villamanta Legal Service, Geelong, Vic

Presant FP, Marshak L (2006) Helpful actions seen through the eyes of parents with disabilities. *Disability & Society*, 21(1): 31–45

Riches V (1996) *Everyday Social Interaction: a Program for People with Disabilities*. MacLennan and Petty, Sydney

Rivalland J (2000) Definitions & identification: who are the children with learning difficulties? *Australian Journal of Learning Disabilities*, 5(2): 12–16

Robinson GL (2002) Assessment of learning disabilities: the complexity of causes and consequences. *Australian Journal of Learning Disabilities*, 7(1): 29–39

Schneider J, Wedgewood N, Llewllyn G, McConnell D (2006) Families challenged by and accommodating to the adolescent years. *Journal of Intellectual Disability Research*, 50(12): 926–936

Seligman M, Darling R S (2007) *Ordinary families, Special Children*, 3rd edn. Guilford Press, New York

Sherry M (2000) *Hate Crimes Against People with Disabilities*. University of Queensland, School of Social Work. Online. Available: www.wwda.org.au/hate.htm [accessed 1 June 2008]

Thomas D (1999) The nurse as psychological support in rehabilitation. In: Smith M (ed.) *Rehabilitation in Adult Nursing Practice*. Churchill Livingstone, Edinburgh

Wake E (2003) Profound and multiple disability. In: Gates B (ed.) *Learning Disabilities: Toward Inclusion*, 4th edn. Churchill Livingstone, Edinburgh

Watson D (2003) The nature of learning disabilities. In: Gates B (ed.) *Learning Disabilities: Toward Inclusion*, 4th edn. Churchill Livingstone, Edinburgh

Wen X, Fortune N (1999) The definition and prevalence of physical disability in Australia. In: Australian Institute of Health and Welfare (AIHW) *World Health Organization 2001 International Classification of Functioning, Disability and Health (ICIDH-2)*. AIHW, Canberra

Wolfensberger W (1972) *The Principle of Normalisation in Human Management Services*. National Institute of Mental Retardation, Toronto

—— (1992) *A Brief Introduction to Social Role Valorisation as a High Order Concept for Structuring Human Services*. Training Institute for Human Service Planning. Leadership and Change Agentry (Syracuse University), Syracuse NY

World Health Organization (WHO) (2001) *The International Classification of Functioning: Disability and Health*. WHO, Geneva

ONLINE RESOURCES

Alzheimer's Australia: www.alzheimers.org.au (provides a wide range of information on all aspects of dementia)

Australian Department of Health and Aged Care: www.health.gov.au

Human Rights and Equal Opportunities Commission: www.hreoc.gov.au (information related to discrimination of all types)

Kidsafe — the child accident prevention foundation of Australia: www.greenweb.com.au/kidsafe (provides

information on ways to prevent disability caused by accidents to children)
Multiple Sclerosis Australia: www.msaustralia.org.au (provides a wide range of information on all aspects of MS)
Person Centered Practices: www.reachoflouisville.com/person-centered/whatisperson.htm (provides clear explanations and examples of person-centred planning for people with disabilities)
United Nations: www.un.org (information on human rights and international laws relevant to people with disabilities)
Victorian Government Disability Services: www.dhs.vic.gov.au/disability

Chapter 48
EMERGENCY CARE

OBJECTIVES

- Define the key terms/concepts
- State the aims and principles of emergency care
- Understand and overcome the barriers that commonly keep people from acting in an emergency situation
- Recognise and respond to different emergencies
- Follow the step-by-step plan of action for any emergency
- Provide care for injuries or sudden illnesses until professional medical help arrives

KEY TERMS/CONCEPTS

bystander
cardiopulmonary resuscitation (CPR)
danger, response, airway, breathing, compression, defibrillation (DRABCD)
external cardiac compressions (ECC)
primary and secondary survey
rescue breathing

CHAPTER FOCUS

Emergencies can happen at any time and, when confronted with an urgent situation, it is vital that the nurse is aware of the correct procedure to follow. In a health care facility the nurse is most likely to be the first person to be on the scene and needs to be able to recognise an emergency and respond appropriately. This emergency care chapter will prepare the nurse to make appropriate decisions regarding first aid care, and to act on those decisions.

LIVED EXPERIENCE

It was 9:30 pm and I was just doing the final paper work after a fairly busy evening in the Emergency Department when I heard a woman's voice screaming out 'someone help my baby'. I rushed into the waiting room to find a woman holding her baby in her arms. The baby was pale and floppy. I took the baby from her arms and went into the examination room. The baby was about 10 months old — the same age as my little girl, home safe and well in bed. It is always harder to work on someone if they remind you of a loved one — harder to dissociate from what you are doing. I had to suppress my 'mothering' response and work in a systematic manner. I pressed the emergency button, as I knew I needed help, and calmly began the mental checklist. Danger, response, airway, breathing and compression . . .

Karen Lawrence, RN

INTRODUCTION

First aid is the emergency care of a sick or injured person until medical aid is available or until the person recovers. The nurse may encounter an emergency situation in a health care facility, in the home environment or in a public place. Knowing what to do in an emergency situation may mean the difference between a person living and dying. An emergency situation within a health care facility may involve a patient, a visitor or a staff member. Under these circumstances lifesaving equipment and expert help are usually at hand, but prompt emergency care given by the person who is first on the scene may still save lives. Documentation of the incident will be required, and health care facilities provide incident and accident forms for this purpose. Information to be documented includes: details of the onset of the incident; the date, time and location; the emergency care provided; and the name of any person who witnessed the incident. The nurse attending the emergency must remain with the individual and summon assistance. If the incident occurs within a ward area, the nurse in charge must be notified immediately.

This chapter addresses some emergencies and the basic care that needs to be provided. For more detailed information, the nurse is advised to consult a current first aid text.

AIMS OF FIRST AID

First aid is given to a casualty in an emergency situation for five purposes:

1. To preserve life
2. To protect the unconscious casualty
3. To prevent the condition from worsening
4. To relieve pain
5. To promote recovery.

RECOGNISING AN EMERGENCY

An emergency is a situation requiring immediate action. Recognising an emergency is the first step in responding. You may become aware of an emergency because of certain things you observe (Australian Red Cross 1998), such as unusual noises, sights, smells, signs or behaviours.

UNUSUAL NOISES

Noises are often the first thing that may call your attention to an emergency. Some noises that may indicate that an emergency situation has occurred are:

- Noises that indicate that someone is in distress, such as screaming, yelling, moaning, crying and calling for help
- Alarming noises such as breaking glass, crashing metal or screeching tyres
- Abrupt or loud noises such as falling ladders, collapsing structures.

UNUSUAL SIGHTS

Unusual sights are things that look out of the ordinary, and can possibly go unnoticed by the unaware observer. These may include:

- An overturned saucepan on the floor
- A spilled medicine container
- A fallen chair
- Broken glass
- A stalled vehicle
- Fallen electrical cables (high voltage).

UNUSUAL SMELLS

Many smells are part of our everyday life, such as petrol fumes at a petrol station. You may become aware of an unusual smell in the workplace when smells are stronger than usual or are not easily identified or are unrecognisable. Remember to put your safety first if you find yourself in a situation in which there is an unusual or very strong smell, as many fumes can be poisonous.

UNUSUAL SIGNS AND SYMPTOMS

Certain signs and symptoms can indicate an emergency; for example, you may find a client collapsed on the bathroom floor or sliding out of their chair. Other signs and symptoms that may draw your attention to an emergency event are if the person:

- Is unconscious
- Has difficulty breathing
- Is clutching the chest or throat
- Is sweating
- Has an uncharacteristic skin colour.

UNUSUAL BEHAVIOUR

It may be difficult to detect whether someone's appearance or behaviour is unusual, especially if the person is unfamiliar to you. If an incident occurs within the ward environment, where the clients are familiar to you, this will be more easily recognisable. Some unusual behaviours include:

- Slurred or hesitant speech
- Being disorientated or confused
- Unexplained irritability
- Drowsiness.

Recognising that an emergency situation has occurred is the first phase in providing emergency care. It is worth mentioning at this point that these indicators may occur individually or together. For example, a person having a cerebrovascular accident may present with a headache alone or with a headache accompanied by weakness down one side and slurred speech.

RESPONDING TO AN EMERGENCY

In an emergency situation your involvement as a nurse may be critical, as staffing levels are frequently at a minimum and all personnel are called on to give assistance. In a health care environment, strict emergency protocol is laid out and should be firmly adhered to. When working as a nurse it is part of your responsibility to ensure that you are familiar with each facility's protocol. All the relevant information will be located in the facility's policy and procedure manuals, commonly located at the nurse's station, or electronically on the facility's intranet site.

BARRIERS TO ACTION

In a first aid situation you may be the only person available to assist the casualty. There are many ways to help, but to do this you must first make the decision to respond. Sometimes people do not respond to an emergency because they are unaware that a situation is occurring, and at other times they are reluctant to offer help for various reasons. These include:

- Presence of bystanders
- Uncertainty about the casualty
- Nature of the illness or injury
- Fear of disease transmission
- Fear of doing something wrong.

See Clinical Interest Box 48.1. However, the worst thing to do is nothing!

CLINICAL INTEREST BOX 48.1
Barriers to responding to an emergency

Presence of bystanders*
- Can cause confusion
- May cause you to feel reluctant to offer assistance
- Can endanger themselves and the casualty

Uncertainty about the casualty
- Uncomfortable touching a stranger
- Hesitant if the casualty is much older or younger than you
- Different race or gender
- Has a disabling condition
- Is a casualty of crime
- If the casualty is intoxicated

Fear of disease transmission
- In an emergency you will not know what infection risks are present
- Can occur through any cuts or skin abrasions
- Safest to assume that all body fluids can transmit infection between casualty and rescuer; however, disease transmission is very rare

Minimising the risk of disease transmission
- Intact skin
- Use of protective barriers such as disposable gloves
- Use goggles or wear glasses
- Wash thoroughly after giving first aid
- Seek medical advice as soon as possible if direct contact has occurred

Fear of doing something wrong
- Fear of making things worse
- If unsure what to do, call for an ambulance
- First aiders have nothing to fear if they act reasonably, with caution and follow accepted teaching and protocols (Australian Red Cross 1998)

* There are also positive aspects to the presence of bystanders: for example, you can ask them to call an ambulance, send them for blankets or other supplies, and they can meet and direct the ambulance to the scene, keep the area free of unnecessary traffic and help you to give care.

PRIORITIES OF ACTION IN AN EMERGENCY

The following four emergency action principles (Australian Red Cross 1998) should guide the nurse's actions in an emergency:

1. Survey the scene
2. Do a primary survey and check for life-threatening problems
3. Call emergency help
4. Do a secondary survey when appropriate, and care for additional problems.

Implementing these principles (Figure 48.1) provides safety for you and for others and ensures that critical care is given to those who need it.

Survey the scene

When it becomes apparent that an emergency has occurred and you decide to respond, you must ensure that the scene is safe for you and for others. Take the time to look at the scene and observe for anything that may pose a threat to

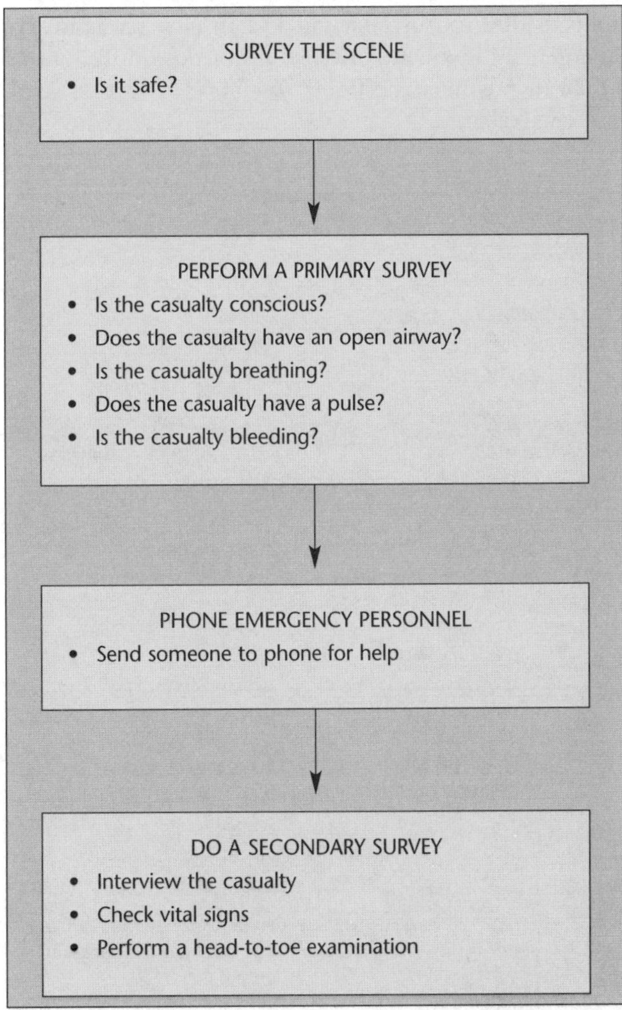

Figure 48.1 | Emergency action plan *(adapted from Australian Red Cross, First Aid, 1998)*

your safety and that of the casualty or other bystanders. If any dangers are evident, do not approach the scene — call emergency personnel immediately for help. If you decide that the area is safe, then proceed to perform the primary survey. Figure 48.2 shows the basic life support flow chart that should be followed when attending all emergencies.

Primary survey

In every emergency situation you must first look for conditions that are an immediate threat to the casualty's life. These are briefly mentioned here and will be discussed in more detail under 'Resuscitation'. Clinical Interest Box 48.2 lists some definitions the first aider must be familiar with. In the primary survey, check for:

- Conscious state
- Airway
- Breathing
- Circulation
- Severe bleeding.

Call emergency personnel

The emergency number to call for ambulance, fire or police is **000** in Australia and **111** in New Zealand. For emergencies involving bites, stings or poisoning, call **13 11 26** in Australia and **0800 764 766** (0800 POISON) in New Zealand.

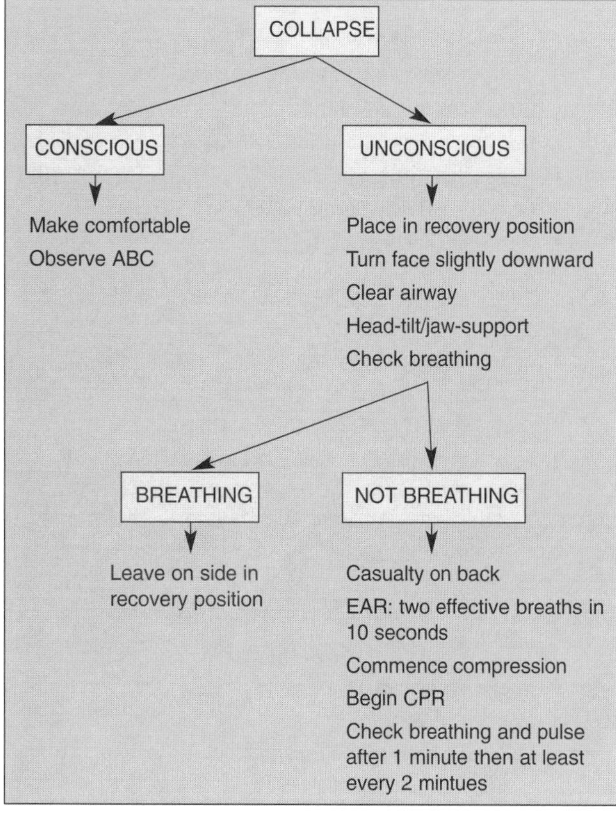

Figure 48.2 | Basic life support flow chart *(adapted from Australian Red Cross,* First Aid, *1998)*

CLINICAL INTEREST BOX 48.2
Definitions to know

BLS	basic life support
RB	rescue breathing
ECC	external cardiac compression
CPR	cardiopulmonary resuscitation
D	danger
R	response
A	airway
B	breathing
C	compression
D	defibrillation (if available)

Secondary survey

This is a systematic method of finding other injuries or conditions that may need care. The secondary survey has three basic steps:

1. Question the casualty and bystanders
2. Check vital signs
3. Do a head-to-toe examination (Dolan & Holt 2001).

RESUSCITATION

Resuscitation is the preservation of life by establishment and/or maintenance of airway, breathing and circulation. The objective of resuscitation techniques is to ensure adequate supply of oxygen to the brain, not only to preserve life but also to prevent the damage to brain cells that results from lack of oxygen (Australian Red Cross 1998). Clinical Interest Box 48.3 presents more detail on resuscitation.

RESCUE BREATHING

Rescue breathing is a method of breathing into a casualty's lungs in an effort to maintain adequate oxygen needed for survival. Rescue breathing is given to casualties displaying no signs of life.

> No signs of life = unconscious, unresponsive, not breathing normally, not moving
>
> (ARC 2006)

Figures 49.3, 49.4, 49.5 and 49.6 show the correct technique for ensuring effective rescue breathing.

Rescue breathing can be given:

- Mouth to mouth (most common method)
- Mouth to nose (performed in deep water)
- Mouth to nose and mouth (children aged < 2 years)

EXTERNAL CARDIAC COMPRESSIONS

When the heart stops beating, circulation of the blood stops. Performing external cardiac compressions (ECC) provides an artificial pumping mechanism, which when carried out effectively, distributes blood around the body. Figures 49.7 and 49.8 show the correct location of ECC on an adult and child. ECC provides an artificial blood circulation by exerting rhythmic pressure at regular intervals (Figure 48.9) compressing the heart between the sternum and the spinal column.

CLINICAL INTEREST BOX 48.3
Resuscitation

The central focus of resuscitation is the protection of the brain and heart from ischaemia, and the steps involved in resuscitation are systematic and implemented in order of priority. The principles of basic life support (BLS) include: (i) establishing and maintaining an airway; (ii) breathing; and (iii) circulation — the objective being to provide the brain and heart with an oxygenated blood supply. If a defibrillator is available, defibrillation is performed by attaching an AED (Automated External Defibrillator), and following the prompts (Australian Resuscitation Council [ARC] 2006).

Effective BLS techniques rely on rapid assessment of the situation and initiating procedures that facilitate and maintain an adequate supply of oxygenated blood to the brain before irreversible damage occurs.

Advanced life support (ALS) techniques include a range of therapeutic and technological interventions carried out by trained health personnel. These are not discussed here.

Basic life support

If a person collapses, the rescuer must assess the situation quickly, ensure the safety of the rescuer, casualty and bystanders, call for help, and start basic life support (BLS).

The level of consciousness is determined by the use of verbal and tactile stimuli. These stimuli should never reach a level that causes or aggravates injury, and infants and small children should never be shaken. The shoulders should be firmly grasped and squeezed to elicit a response. Verbal stimuli should also be used. If conscious, the person will respond. Allow the person to adopt a comfortable position and observe them closely for any changes in condition.

If there is no response to the stimuli, the person is unconscious and should be turned on their side. Help should be summoned. Anyone who fails to respond to touch or the spoken word is considered to be unconscious, and more vigorous efforts to obtain a response (such as painful stimuli) are not warranted.

The priorities of BLS are:

- Airway
- Breathing
- Compression.

Airway

The key to successful resuscitation is a clear airway. When an unconscious person is lying on their back, the lower jaw tends to drop, which causes the tongue to fall to the back of the pharynx and occlude the airway. The problem is compounded by relaxation of soft palate tissues and the epiglottis. In addition, an unconscious person is unable to swallow or cough, and any foreign material in the mouth or pharynx can contribute to obstruction of the airway. Simply turning the person on his or her side, and supporting the jaw, can often prevent death. This often relieves the obstruction, and gravity assists any foreign material to drain from the mouth. Visible material or debris that could be blocking the airway can be actively removed by sweeping a gloved index finger around the mouth.

Airway management

Airway assessment and management can take place with the person lying on his or her side or back. In many instances, lying on the side is preferable for the reasons stated above. However, because many cardiac arrests result from ventricular fibrillation, it might be appropriate to manage a person on their back to facilitate early defibrillation when a defibrillator is immediately available.

The steps involved in airway management include:

- Clear the airway: remove loose-fitting dentures and any visible foreign material from the mouth. Allow fluids or vomitus to drain by turning the face slightly downwards
- Open the airway: tilt the head backwards and support the jaw. The head is tilted backwards by placing one hand on the forehead and supporting the jaw at the point of the chin in such a way that there is no pressure on the soft tissues of the neck. This brings the jaw and tongue forwards, thus opening the airway. If it is suspected that the person has injured their neck or back, the head should not be moved; the jaw-thrust method to open the airway should be used (see next point)
- Jaw thrust: pressure is applied behind the angle of the jaw to thrust it forwards.

Recognition of airway obstruction

If the airway is partially or completely occluded, attempts to breathe result in:

- Flaring of the nostrils
- Use of accessory muscles, evidenced by sucking in of the soft tissues of the neck and upper chest, in-drawing of the chest and out-pushing of the abdomen
- Noisy and laboured respiratory efforts if the airway is partially obstructed, and no movement of air if completely obstructed
- Increasing peripheral and central cyanosis, particularly if obstruction is complete.

Note: There might be no attempt to breathe at all.

Breathing

Once the airway is open, the unconscious person's breathing should be checked. With an ear placed over the person's nose and mouth:

- look for movement of the chest and abdomen
- listen for the passage of air into and out of the mouth and nose
- feel for the escape of exhaled air on your face.

If breathing is abnormal or absent, turn the person on their back and perform rescue breathing by giving two initial breaths, observing for the rise and fall of the chest. If the chest does not rise and/or rescue breathing is not effective:

- Check the head-tilt and jaw-support technique to prevent an air leak
- Ensure that the breaths delivered are full inflations, approximately 1 second per inspiration.

If no signs of life, commence CPR.

Note: Distension of the stomach with air occurs if the breaths delivered are too hard or are delivered when the airway is partially obstructed. This can precipitate regurgitation and vomiting and can further compromise the airway.

Methods of rescue breathing include mouth-to-mouth respiration, mouth-to-nose respiration, mouth-to-stoma respiration and mouth-to-mask respiration.

CLINICAL INTEREST BOX 48.3
Resuscitation—cont'd

Compression
As the pulse check is no longer used to identify the need for chest compressions, CPR — rescue breathing and chest compressions — is given to all victims requiring resuscitation, that is, victims not displaying signs of life (ARC 2006):
- Ensure the person is on a firm flat surface
- Begin external cardiac compression (ECC) by locating the middle of the lower half of the sternum; the rescuer should visualise the 'centre of the chest' and compress at that point (ARC 2006)
  - — place heel of hand on the lower half of the sternum, and place heel of other hand on top of the first.
  - — interlock fingers of both hands and raise fingers
  - — do not apply pressure over the ribs, upper abdomen or bottom half of the sternum.

Position yourself vertically above the casualty's chest, and with straight arms, press down on the sternum (St John Ambulance 2007).

The end result is that the heel of one hand is lying on the long axis of the lower half of the sternum. The other hand is used to provide additional force, so that all pressure is exerted through the heel of the bottom hand.

Depth and rate of compression
The sternum should be compressed 4–5 cm (1–2 inches) with each compression. The rate of compression is approximately 100 times per minute. During ECC, the heel of the hand remains on the sternum.

Ratio of compressions to inflations
The compression/ventilation ratio is 2 breaths to 30 compressions (30:2), and this ratio applies regardless of the number of rescuers.

CPR is continued until the casualty shows signs of life (breathing, moving or responding), or until appropriate assistance arrives (ARC 2006).

Correctly performed, CPR can re-establish cardiac function, or at least maintain an artificial circulation sufficient to preserve neurological function until personnel trained in ALS arrive at the scene.

BLS for infants and children
BLS for infants (age < 1 year) and children (1–8 years) is essentially the same as for adults, with the following exceptions:

Airway
- Avoid over-extension of the head and neck when opening the airway, especially with infants

Breathing
- Infants: Obtain a firm seal over the mouth and nose and deliver a volume that is less than for a child but enough to ensure that the chest rises. Give 2 initial breaths, listen and feel for signs of air being expelled. Repeat sequence of 2 breaths. If no signs of life, commence CPR.
- Children: As for adults, maintain head tilt and chin lift, give 2 breaths, listen and feel for signs of air being expelled. Repeat sequence of 2 breaths. If no signs of life, commence CPR. (St John Ambulance 2007)

Compression
- Infants: Using two fingers, compress the sternum below the mid-point. Depth of compression is about one-third of the depth of the chest, at a rate of 100/minute
- Children: For children aged 1–8 years, use the heel of one hand to compress the sternum below the mid-point. For children older than 8 years, perform compressions as for adults. For children 1 year and older the depth of compression is about one-third the depth of the chest, at a rate of 100/minute.

Andrea Marshall (This is an edited version of the ARC Guidelines March 2008. For full details please visit the ARC website at http://www.resus.org.au/)'

Cardiopulmonary resuscitation management steps

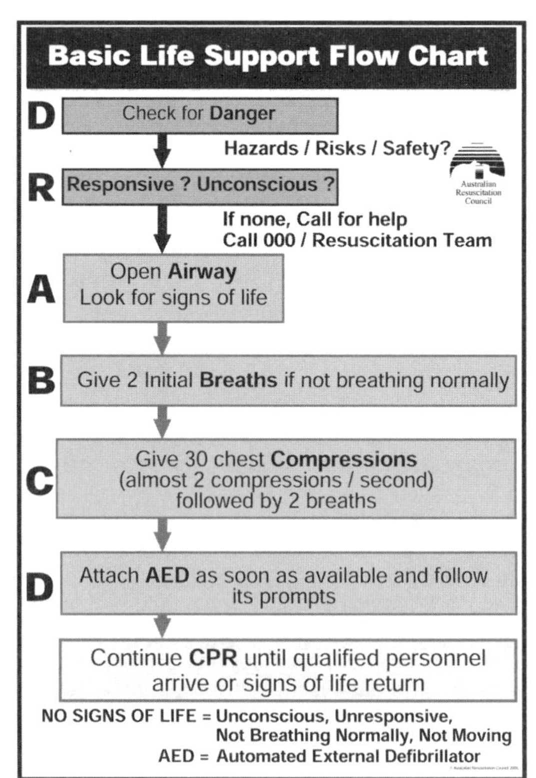

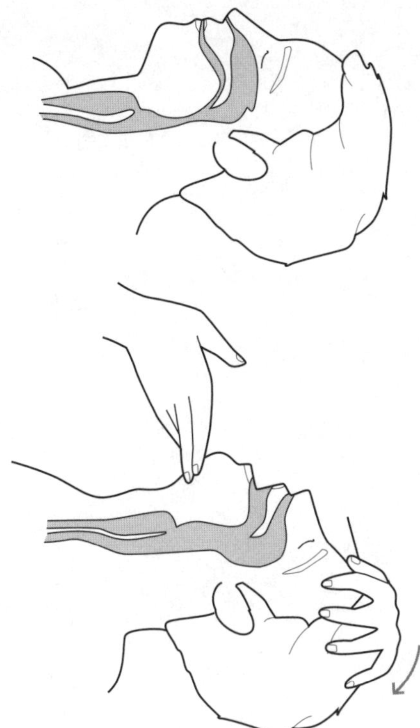

Figure 48.3 | Head lift in an adult

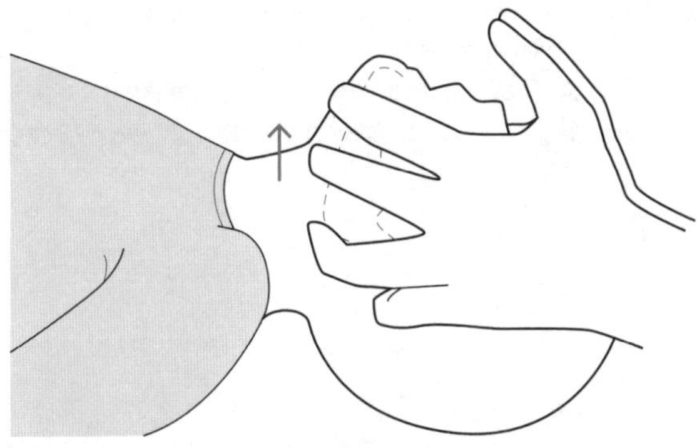

Figure 48.4 | Head lift in a child

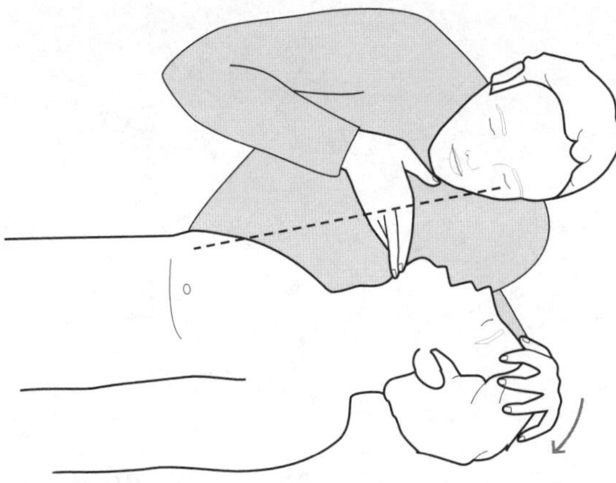

Figure 48.5 | Adequate ventilation in an adult

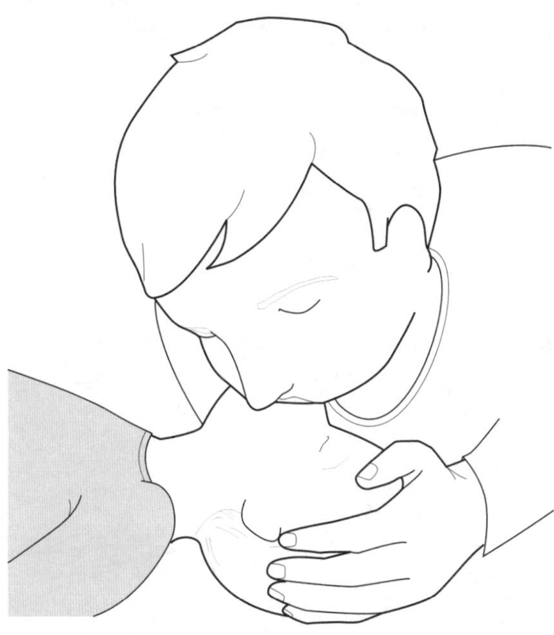

Figure 48.6 | Adequate ventilation in a child

CARDIOPULMONARY RESUSCITATION

Cardiopulmonary resuscitation (CPR) is the technique of rescue breathing with external cardiac compressions. As the pulse check is not used to identify the need for chest compressions, CPR — rescue breathing and ECC — are given to all casualties displaying no signs of life: unconscious, unresponsive, not breathing normally, not moving.

CPR consists of 30 compressions, followed by 2 ventilations (ratio of 30:2).

Interruptions to compressions should be avoided, however compressions must be paused to allow for ventilation (ARC 2006).

PRINCIPLES OF EMERGENCY CARE

Every emergency situation must be assessed, and appropriate measures taken in the sequence most logical for that particular situation. A variety of factors influences the actions taken and the order in which they are taken; for example, the presence of life-threatening circumstances, the availability of assistance, the location where the emergency occurs and the availability of transport. Clinical Interest Box 48.4 outlines the emergency response steps. The general principles of emergency care are:

- Check whether there is danger to self, the casualty or any bystanders. Proceed only if it is safe to do so
- Remain calm, as calmness and efficiency will help the casualty to feel more secure
- Assess the situation quickly and decide the order of priorities. Perform lifesaving actions first

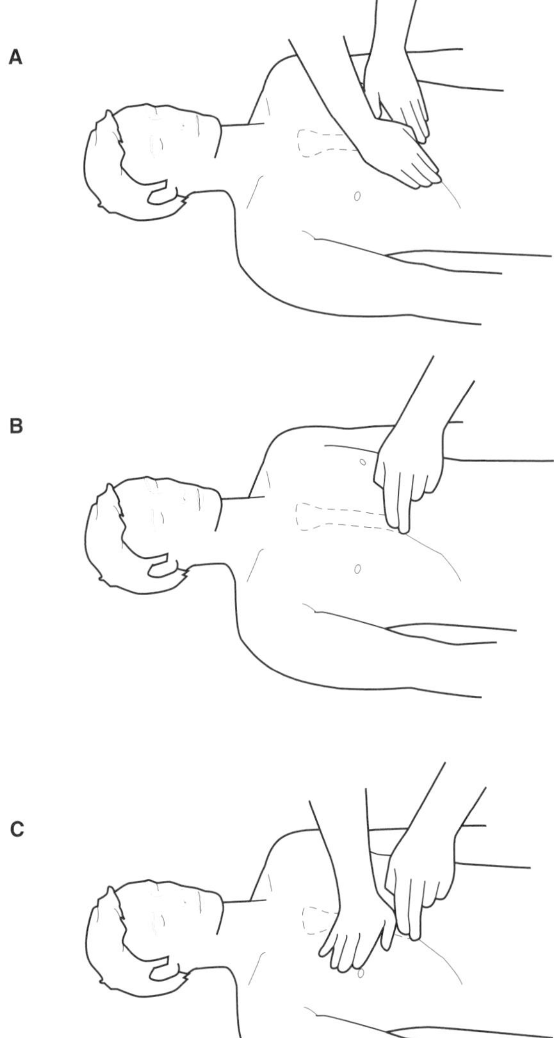

Figure 48.7 | Location of ECC point in an adult. Proper hand position for CPR
A: Finding the rib cage
B: Moving fingers along the rib cage to the notch
C: Placing the heel of the hand next to the index finger

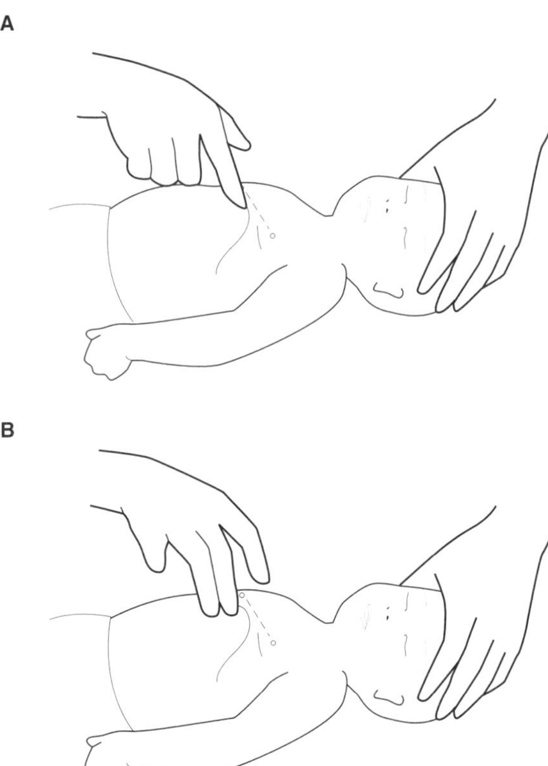

Figure 48.8 | Location of ECC point in a child. Locating hand position for infant chest compressions
A: Drawing an imaginary line between the nipples
B: Placing 2 fingers on the sternum about 1 finger-width below the imaginary line

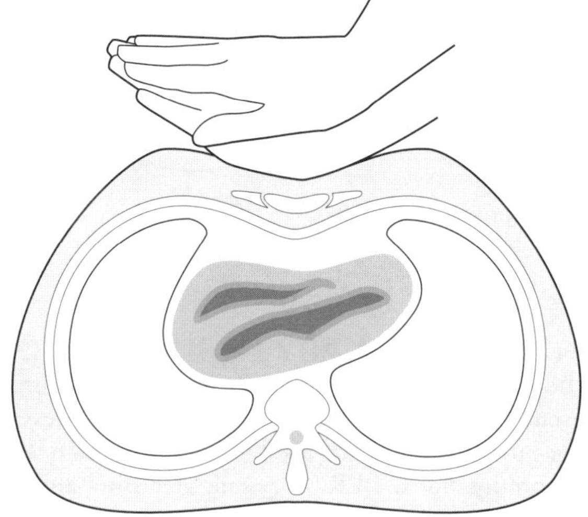

Figure 48.9 | Compressing the heart

- Remove the cause of the emergency or, if this is not practicable, remove the casualty from the cause
- Assess the casualty. Assessment is made of the individual's conscious state, airway, breathing and circulation
- Begin to manage the situation according to priorities decided on as a result of assessment
- Provide emotional support for a conscious casualty
- Keep the casualty lying down or in the position in which you found them, as any injury could be exacerbated if moved. Exceptions to this principle are when the casualty is unconscious and must be positioned to maintain a clear airway, or when resuscitation measures must be implemented
- Seek assistance from any helpers who are available
- Arrange for medical aid. Ask a bystander to telephone for an ambulance. Information provided to the

ambulance service should include your location, the number of casualties and the nature of the emergency
- Maintain the casualty's normal body temperature. Use coats or knitwear if a rug is not available
- Prevent bystanders from giving the casualty any food or fluids, as the ingestion of substances may cause harm or delay any surgical intervention that may be required
- Remain with the casualty and continue to provide physical and emotional care until medical assistance arrives
- Provide emergency personnel with information regarding your assessment of the casualty, and any care provided.

CPR should stop when:
- If the casualty shows signs of life: breathing normally, moving or responding.
- Trained or qualified help arrives and takes over
- A medical officer arrives and certifies that death has occurred
- The first aider is physically unable to continue.

CLINICAL INTEREST BOX 48.4
Emergency response steps

D — Danger
- Unconscious casualties cannot protect themselves from any danger
- If possible remove the danger from the casualty
- Otherwise remove the casualty and yourself from the danger

R — Response
- When it is safe to do so, determine the casualty's conscious level
- Ask firmly, 'Are you OK?' or, 'What happened?'
- If there is no response to voice, gently shake the casualty's shoulders
- If they respond, make them comfortable and observe ABC
- If they do not respond, move onto ABC

A — Airway
- Airways can become blocked by foreign bodies such as broken teeth, small objects or vomitus, or narrowed if the tongue slips back or the head tilts forward
- To clear the airway turn the casualty onto their side into the recovery position
- Sweep two fingers through the front of the mouth to remove any solid material

B — Breathing
- With the casualty still lying in the recovery position:
  — Look for movement of the lower chest and upper abdomen
  — Listen for the escape of air from the casualty's mouth or nose
  — Feel for movement of the lower chest and abdomen and for the escape of air from the casualty's mouth or nose

C — Compression
- Check the casualty for signs of life, (breathing, moving, or responding)
- Continually check the casualty's condition until medical aid arrives
- If the condition deteriorates; that is, the casualty becomes unresponsive, not breathing normally, ceases breathing, turn casualty onto back and commence CPR

D - Defibrillation
- Attach an AED (automated external defibrillator) if available, and follow the prompts

SPECIFIC EMERGENCY SITUATIONS

Emergency situations requiring first aid management include: shock, bleeding, exposure to extremes of temperature; respiratory, cardiac and neurological incidents; injuries to bones and joints; poisoning, bites and stings; and some mental health situations.

SHOCK

Shock is a condition in which tissue perfusion is inadequate to maintain the necessary supply of oxygen and nutrients for normal cell function and to remove the waste products of metabolism. It may result from inadequate cardiac function or a reduction in circulating blood volume. Shock may develop immediately, or progressively over several hours. If severe, shock may lead to collapse of the circulatory system and death. Clinical Interest Box 48.5 gives an overview of one situation in which shock may develop. Shock may be caused by one or a combination of factors, including:
- Haemorrhage
- Severe fluid loss (e.g. as a result of burns, diarrhoea or vomiting)
- Cardiac damage (e.g. heart attack)
- Excessive vasodilation as a result of injury to the spinal cord, severe pain, severe infection or certain poisons (Lough et al 2004).

Manifestations of shock

The manifestations of shock include:
- Rapid and weak pulse
- Rapid and shallow ventilations
- Low blood pressure
- Anxiety and restlessness
- Faintness, dizziness or altered conscious state
- Nausea and, sometimes, vomiting
- Pale, cold, moist skin.

The manifestations become progressively more evident as shock becomes more severe. The skin may become cyanosed and the casualty may become drowsy, confused or unconscious (Lough et al 2004).

Care for shock

When caring for a casualty who is experiencing shock, the nurse should:
- Prevent further injuries
- Check ABC

CLINICAL INTEREST BOX 48.5
Latex allergy

Latex is the milky sap of the rubber tree *Hevea brasiliensis*. It is treated with preservatives, accelerators, stabilisers and antioxidants to make a more elastic stable rubber. Reactions to products containing latex can be triggered by either the latex protein or an additive used in the manufacturing process.

Latex reactions can be classified into three different categories:

1. Irritation (non-allergic inflammation occurring when the skin is abraded)
2. Delayed hypersensitivity (non-IgE-mediated response to the chemical agents added during the manufacturing process)
3. Immediate sensitivity (IgE-mediated response to latex proteins).

Although the overall prevalence of latex allergy in the general population is only 1%, it is much higher (28–67%) in selected groups, such as:

- Patients with neural tube defects (spina bifida, myelomeningocele, lipomyelomeningocele)
- Patients with congenital urological disorders
- People who have undergone multiple surgeries or who have a history of allergy to anaesthetic drugs
- Health care, rubber industry or glove-manufacturing plant workers.

Five routes of exposure to latex proteins have resulted in systemic reactions:

1. Cutaneous (contact with moist skin)
2. Mucous membranes (mouth, vagina, urethra, rectum)
3. Internal tissue (during surgery and other invasive procedures)
4. Intravascular (exposure to anaesthesia equipment or endotracheal tubes)
5. Inhalation (exposure through the aerosolisation of glove powder).

It has been postulated that the latex allergen adheres to the cornstarch or powder and is released into the air with the manipulation of latex rubber gloves.

The American Academy of Allergy and Immunology has published guidelines for providing care to persons with latex allergy. All persons at risk for latex allergy should have a careful history and should complete a standardised latex allergy questionnaire. A history suggestive of reactivity to latex includes local swelling or itching after blowing up balloons, dental examinations, contact with rubber gloves, vaginal or rectal examinations, using condoms or diaphragms and contact with other rubber products. Other historical information that may suggest increased risk of latex allergy includes hand eczema; previous unexplained anaphylaxis; oral itching after eating bananas, chestnuts, kiwi fruit or avocados; and multiple surgical procedures in infancy. Patients at high risk should be offered clinical testing for latex allergy.

The patient with a latex allergy should be cared for in a latex-free environment; that is, an environment in which no latex gloves are used and there is no direct patient contact with other latex devices.

(Lough et al 2004. Data from Warshaw EM *Journal of the American Academy of Dermatology*, 39(1): 1; and Wai DME 1999 *Gastroenterological Nursing*, 22: 263)

- Control any external bleeding
- Help the casualty to become comfortable
- Maintain normal body temperature
- Elevate the legs to assist the return of blood, unless you suspect:
  - — Head, neck or back injuries
  - — Fractured bones in the legs or hips
  - — Heart attack or cerebrovascular accident
- Not give the casualty anything to eat or drink
- Advise the casualty not to smoke
- Call an ambulance as soon as possible.

If the casualty's condition deteriorates, unconsciousness may occur: if this happens, commence CPR.

BLEEDING

When bleeding occurs the brain, heart and lungs immediately try to compensate for blood loss to maintain oxygen flow to vital organs. Haemorrhage (bleeding) is classified according to the site and according to the type of blood vessel involved. Haemorrhage may be external and visible, or internal and concealed. External haemorrhage is usually obvious, although the source may not be immediately evident. Internal haemorrhage occurs into tissues, joints, organs or cavities within the body and is not visible, although it may be revealed if blood escapes through a body orifice (Newberry 2003). Blood may reach the surface of the body in:

- Haemoptysis, when blood is coughed up
- Haematemesis, when blood is vomited
- A melaena stool, which is black and tarry due to digested blood
- Frank blood from the rectum or anus
- Haematuria, when blood is present in the urine
- Vaginal bleeding
- Epistaxis (bleeding from the nostrils).

Manifestations of bleeding

Arterial haemorrhage is bleeding from a damaged artery. The blood is bright red in colour and the bleeding occurs in spurts, which coincide with the beats of the heart. Venous haemorrhage is bleeding from a damaged vein. The blood is dark red in colour and the blood flows steadily. Capillary haemorrhage is bleeding from damaged capillaries. A small amount of blood flows as a gentle ooze (Sorrentino 2004). The manifestations of bleeding are:

- Rapid and weak pulse
- Rapid and shallow ventilations
- Low blood pressure
- Anxiety and restlessness
- Faintness or dizziness

- Pale and clammy skin
- Thirst
- Loss of consciousness
- Escape of blood through a body orifice.

CARE OF BLEEDING

External bleeding is controlled by pressure, elevation and rest (Clinical Interest Box 48.6).

Applying direct pressure to a bleeding wound

Pressure controls bleeding by compressing the blood vessels leading to the wound and by retaining blood in the wound long enough for it to clot. A thick dressing is placed over the wound and manual pressure is applied. A firm bandage is applied over the dressing to maintain pressure. If a dressing is not available, apply direct pressure with the bare hand. If bleeding is profuse it may be necessary to grasp the sides of the wound and firmly squeeze them together. Elevate the injured part to decrease blood flow to it. This action is contraindicated if a fracture is suspected. Rest the injured part to lessen the demand for blood by the tissues and to prevent dislodgement of the forming clot. Place another dressing over the first if bleeding continues, and apply manual pressure. Do not remove a dressing, as this leads to dislodgement of the clot and further bleeding (Sorrentino 2004). Clinical Interest Boxes 48.6 and 48.7 describe the management of bleeding in general and management of specific types of bleeding, respectively.

CLINICAL INTEREST BOX 48.6
Care of bleeding

Controlling external bleeding
- Apply direct pressure
- Elevate the injured area
- Apply a pressure bandage
- Continue to monitor ABC
- Observe circulation below pressure bandage to ensure adequate circulation
- Apply pressure
- Apply pressure bandage
- Observe circulation

External bleeding with a foreign body
- Apply padding on either side of the object
- Build up padding, without putting pressure on the object
- Raise the injured area
- If the wound is on the head, chest or abdomen lay the casualty in the position of greatest comfort
- NEVER ATTEMPT TO REMOVE A FOREIGN BODY

Internal bleeding
- If you suspect internal bleeding, call an ambulance as soon as possible
- Prevent further injury
- Monitor ABC
- Place the casualty in a position of comfort
- Maintain normal body temperature
- Loosen restrictive clothing
- Keep the casualty still

Preventing disease transmission

Transmission of diseases can happen when attending to an emergency situation, but this is very rare. Most of the time you will be performing emergency care on people you know, for example, your family or friends, as these are the people that you spend most of the day with. However, it is important always to take steps to minimise the possible transmission of bodily fluids from casualty to carer. Some of the ways that this can be achieved include:

- Place an effective barrier between your skin and the casualty's blood, such as gloves or a clean folded cloth
- Wash hands thoroughly with soap and water immediately after providing care
- Avoid eating, drinking and touching your mouth, nose or eyes while providing care or before washing hands (Sorrentino 2004).

BURNS

The emergency care of burns is directed towards removing the casualty from the source of heat, cooling the burned area and preventing infection and shock:

- Remove the casualty from danger
- Extinguish burning clothing by smothering it with a blanket, rug, an item of clothing or by using water
- Hold the burned area under cold, gently running water for at least 10 minutes. For chemical burns, continue to flush the affected areas with water for 20 minutes
- Remove any jewellery (e.g. rings or bracelets) from the burned part before swelling occurs

CLINICAL INTEREST BOX 48.7
Management of specific types of bleeding

Epistaxis
- Keep the client sitting up
- Tilt head forward and encourage client to breathe through the mouth
- Apply finger and thumb pressure on soft part of nostrils below the bridge of the nose for 10–15 minutes
- Loosen tight clothes around neck
- Apply a cold compress to the back of the neck
- If bleeding continues after 20 minutes, seek further help
- After bleeding stops, advise casualty to rest and avoid blowing the nose

Abrasions
- Clean with warm soapy water
- Soak area (if possible) to remove grit
- Dry well with gauze
- Allow to air dry or cover with a non-adherent sterile dressing

Puncture wound
- Clean with warm soapy water
- Tetanus spores may be trapped deep in the wound
- Cover with a non-adherent sterile dressing
- Do not use an occlusive-type dressing
- Discover casualty's date of last tetanus booster

- Cut away clothing over the burned area but leave any clothing that is adhered to the skin
- In the event of scalding or chemical burns, remove clothing immediately, as it may retain heat or chemicals
- Cover the burned area with a sterile or clean non-adherent dressing (Brown 2001).

Clinical Interest Box 48.8 depicts the right and wrong steps to take in the emergency care of burn injuries. Clinical Interest Box 48.9 illustrates this with a common type of burn injury and its appropriate treatment.

HEAT EXHAUSTION AND HEAT STROKE

Heat exhaustion is due to an imbalance between heat gain and heat loss. Heat stroke may occur if the body's heat-regulating mechanism fails. People most at risk of either condition are the elderly, infants and those who are unsuitably clad when working or exercising in hot environmental temperatures (Lough et al 2004). Manifestations include:

- Exhaustion
- Nausea
- Thirst
- Faintness
- Shortness of breath
- Muscle cramps
- Lack of coordination
- Irritability or confusion
- Flushed and dry skin.

Emergency care of heat stroke involves:

- Moving the casualty to a cool place where there is circulating air
- Removing unnecessary clothing
- Sponging the casualty's body with cool water
- Providing cool oral fluids if the casualty is alert
- Seeking medical assistance
- Providing emotional support.

CLINICAL INTEREST BOX 48.8
Dos and don'ts of burn care

DO
- Cool burns by flushing with cool water
- Remove rings and jewellery
- Cover burn with a dry sterile dressing
- Take steps to minimise shock

DON'T
- Apply ice directly to the burn
- Remove pieces of cloth that stick
- Try to clean a full-thickness burn
- Break blisters
- Use ointments or oils on severe burns
- Use cotton wool or 'fluffy' materials

CLINICAL INTEREST BOX 48.9
Case study — burns

While on holiday, Katie was preparing to cook the evening meal. The hotplate in the unit where they were staying was electric and Katie was used to using gas at home. A few moments after turning the dial onto high, Katie wasn't sure if she had turned on the correct element. She placed the palm of her hand onto the element and immediately felt a searing pain in her hand and by reflex pulled her hand away instantly.

D — turn off element at switch
R — alert and conscious
A — clear
B — high respiratory rate
C — pulse present

Plan of care
- Katie rushed to the kitchen sink and ran cool water over her hand for 20 minutes
- Erythema and minimal, small intact blisters were evident
- Burn cream was applied and the wound covered with sterile dressing

FROSTBITE

Frostbite results from local freezing of body tissues, generally in the extremities. Severe frostbite may impair the blood supply to the limbs so badly that gangrene develops (Dolan & Holt 2001). Manifestations include:

- Numbness and tingling
- Insensitivity to touch
- Areas may appear waxy, white, mottled blue-white
- Firmness and coldness of the areas
- Possible blistering.

Emergency care of frostbite involves:

- Moving the casualty to a warm dry place
- Removing constricting garments or jewellery from the affected areas
- Re-warming the areas by applying body heat
- Covering blisters with a clean dry dressing
- Seeking medical assistance.

HYPOTHERMIA

Hypothermia is a condition caused by a loss of surface heat, followed by heat loss from the deep tissues and organs. Causes include prolonged immersion in cold water and prolonged exposure to cold environmental temperatures (Lough et al 2004). Manifestations include:

- Cool skin
- Slow pulse
- Slow and shallow breathing
- Apathy or confusion
- Unconsciousness.

Emergency care of hypothermia involves:

- Moving the casualty to a warm dry place
- Placing the casualty between blankets so that their body temperature can rise gradually
- Giving warm sweet drinks, if the person is conscious
- Seeking medical assistance urgently
- Placing the casualty in the coma position if they are unconscious.

The warming process should not be sped up by applying artificial heat, such as an electric blanket, hot-water bag or by immersion in warm water. This can cause a rapid drop in blood pressure, which may precipitate hypovolaemic shock (Dolan & Holt 2001).

RESPIRATORY EMERGENCIES

Respiratory emergencies can cause asphyxia, which is a severe state of hypoxia. Lack of oxygen, if not corrected, may lead to brain cell damage, altered consciousness, absent breathing, absent pulse and death (Oman et al 2001). Asphyxia may be caused by any factor that interferes with the exchange of gases in the lungs and tissues, such as:

- Drowning
- Electric shock
- Aspiration of vomitus
- Lodgement of a foreign body in the air passages
- Inhalation of toxic gas or smoke
- Oedema of the lining of the air passages
- Strangulation
- Asthma
- Chest injuries (e.g. flail chest)
- Cerebral injury or disease.

CHOKING

Choking occurs when the airway is totally or partially obstructed by swollen tissues or a foreign body. Manifestations include:

- Inability to speak, breathe, cry or cough
- Noisy breathing, wheezing or whistling
- Clutching at the throat
- Red or congested face
- Bulging neck veins
- Cyanosis
- Collapse and unconsciousness.

Total airway obstruction

For emergency treatment of a child or infant with total airway obstruction:

- Position the child face down with the head lower than the chest
- Give four back slaps between the shoulder blades (Figure 48.10)
- If there is no improvement give four lateral chest thrusts
- Observe ABC, and if no signs of life, commence CPR

For emergency treatment of an adult with total airway obstruction:

- Assist the casualty down to the floor
- Lie the casualty onto one side into the recovery position
- Give four back blows between the shoulder blades
- If there is no improvement give four lateral chest thrusts
- Observe ABC, and if no signs of life, commence CPR.

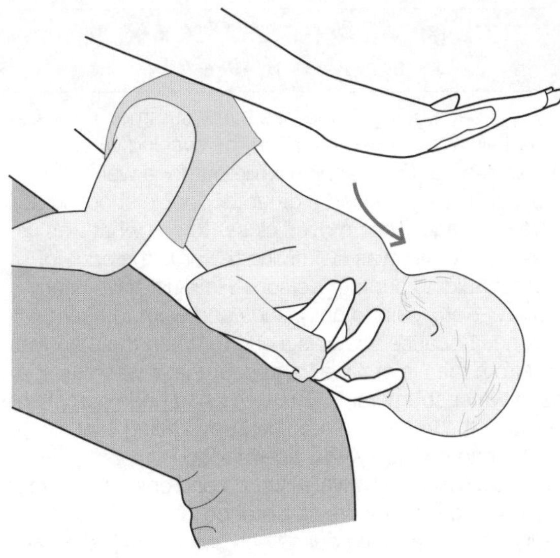

Figure 48.10 | Back slaps on a child *(Sorrentino 2004)*

Partial airway obstruction

If obstruction is partial the casualty will be able to breathe, speak, cry or cough. Treatment involves:

- Staying with the casualty until they have recovered
- Encouraging the casualty to cough
- If there is no improvement call 000 in Australia, 111 in New Zealand
- Observe ABC
- Note and record respiratory and heart rate.

DROWNING AND NEAR-DROWNING

Drowning stimulates various physiological responses, but the actual cause of death is asphyxiation. In any near-drowning or drowning event, the victim swallows water, some of which hits the larynx, causing intense laryngospasm. Hypoxia occurs and causes relaxation of the airways allowing water to be aspirated into the lungs as the victim becomes unconscious (Newberry 2003). Clinical Interest Box 48.10 depicts a near-drowning event and the related care provided. Care for near-drowning involves:

- Removing the casualty from the water if possible
- Observing ABC
- Calling for help
- Being prepared to perform CPR if necessary.

CARDIAC EMERGENCIES

Angina

Angina is a condition that occurs when the coronary arteries become seriously narrowed by disease and the supply of oxygenated blood to the heart becomes insufficient for the increased oxygen needed (Thibodeau & Paton 2003).

Manifestations of angina

Clients often describe the pain as constricting, squeezing or suffocating, usually occurring after exercise. Angina can

CLINICAL INTEREST BOX 48.10
Case study — near-drowning

Kerry had been going to the lake every summer for years and had always enjoyed a walk in the evening when the sun was setting. One evening while out for a walk with some friends they noticed a group of people shouting at the water's edge. They moved closer to see what was happening. A man was swimming towards the edge of the water holding another person. 'He must have nearly drowned,' Kerry said to her friends and went to offer assistance because she was a nurse. When the man was pulled from the water it was apparent that it wasn't just a case of water submersion. Both legs had been completely severed at the knee. The man had been riding a jet ski when he had collided with a speedboat.
D — remove man from water's edge and ensure bystanders move back to a safe working distance
R — incomprehensible sounds only, no words just moaning. Ask bystanders to call for emergency personnel
A — cleared
B — irregular, slow, shallow
C — skin pale, cool and clammy

Plan of care

- Ask bystanders to gather as many towels as possible
- No bleeding evident around traumatic amputation sites due to submersion in cold water and shock — injuries covered with the least fluffy towels
- Dry towels placed over the casualty to maintain temperature
- ABC continued to be monitored until arrival of emergency personnel

CLINICAL INTEREST BOX 48.11
Case study — myocardial infarction

Mr Thompson from next door is mowing his lawn when you get home from work. You notice he is sweating profusely and it is not a very hot evening. You wave and Mr Thompson waves back, then clutches his chest and falls to the ground.
D — move the lawn mower away from casualty and turn off
R — no response to verbal or tactile stimulation
A — upper dentures are loose and removed from casualty's mouth
B — no breath sounds, no chest movement. Call out to neighbours to alert emergency personnel. Commence rescue breathing
C — no signs of life: CPR started, ratio 30:2

Plan of care

- Continue CPR until emergency personnel arrive.

also be brought on by exposure to cold or emotional stress and is often of a short duration.

Management of angina

Emergency management of angina includes:

- Reducing the workload on the heart
- Encouraging the casualty to rest
- Keeping the casualty quiet and still
- Moving the casualty to a warm environment
- Removing constrictive clothing
- Observing ABC.

Myocardial infarction

A myocardial infarction (heart attack) occurs when disruption of the blood supply to the coronary arteries results in the death of part of the myocardium. Blood flow to the myocardium may be obstructed by atherosclerosis or thrombus formation (coronary occlusion). Damage occurs to the heart muscle when blood supply in the coronary arteries is blocked (Thibodeau & Paton 2004).

Manifestations of myocardial infarction

Clients can often confuse the pain with indigestion, as it ranges from discomfort to unbearable. The pain is often described as crushing, squeezing, tightness, aching, constricting or heavy, and is frequently around the central chest area, but may radiate to the back, shoulder, neck, jaw and arm. The client may have cool, pale and clammy skin, which are early signs of shock (Clinical Interest Box 48.11). One of the significant differences between angina and a myocardial infarction is that medication or rest does not relieve it.

Management of myocardial infarction

Emergency management of myocardial infarction includes:

- Keeping the casualty still
- Calling emergency help
- Obtaining information about the casualty's condition
- Assisting with prescribed medication
- Monitoring vital signs
- Be prepared to perform CPR if there are no signs of life

NEUROLOGICAL EMERGENCIES

Many neurological emergencies are related to head injuries. There are many causes of head injuries — road accidents, sporting injuries, falls and vascular-related incidents. A good understanding of the anatomy and physiology of the brain and related structures is vital in caring for clients with head injuries. (For further information on the neurological system, see Chapter 37.) Head injuries often result in unconsciousness, as may cerebrovascular accident, drug or alcohol overdose, fainting, poisoning or seizure disorders. The period of unconsciousness may last for a few minutes, as in fainting, or for much longer. The unconscious individual is unable to respond to external stimuli such as voice and touch (Dolan & Holt 2001).

General emergency care

As the unconscious individual is unable to communicate, maintaining a clear airway, and protection from danger are vital (Dillon 2003). Emergency care involves:

- Placing the casualty in the recovery position

- Ensuring a clear and open airway
- Seeking medical assistance
- If no signs of life, commence CPR
- Providing emotional support for relatives or friends who are with the individual.

SYNCOPE

Syncope (fainting) is a temporary loss of consciousness due to an inadequate supply of oxygen to the brain. Fainting may result from nervous shock, injury, standing still for a long time, or a sudden postural change. Manifestations are:

- Giddiness
- Blurred vision
- Weakness
- A 'hot and cold' feeling
- Yawning
- Pale, cold, clammy skin
- Slow and weak pulse.

Loss of consciousness follows.

Emergency care

Loss of consciousness may be prevented by prompt action to restore blood supply to the brain:

- Lie the individual down, with the head and body flat and the legs raised
- Loosen tight clothing
- Ensure a good supply of fresh air
- Encourage deep breathing
- Provide emotional support
- Allow the casualty to rest for a few minutes until they have fully recovered
- If the individual loses consciousness, place in the coma position
- Seek medical assistance if unconsciousness persists for more than a few minutes.

SEIZURES

Seizures are sudden attacks involving involuntary contraction of skeletal muscles due to disturbances of cerebral function. Three forms of seizure disorders are generalised tonic–clonic (grand mal) epilepsy, absence (petit mal) seizures and febrile seizures. Absence seizures do not usually require any emergency management (Oman et al 2001). (Information on possible causes of seizure disorders is provided in Chapter 37.)

Manifestations of tonic–clonic seizures

This type of generalised seizure generally follows a characteristic pattern:

1. An aura, the warning phase which signals an impending attack. This does not always occur, but may consist of a specific taste, smell or other sensation experienced by the individual. The casualty may give a characteristic 'cry' as air is forced out through the vocal cords, which are in spasm
2. The tonic stage, in which the individual loses consciousness. Muscle spasms occur, the individual becomes rigid and the teeth are tightly clenched. The face and neck become cyanosed due to a brief period of apnoea
3. The clonic stage, in which intermittent violent contractions of muscle cause jerky spasmodic movements of the body. Frothing at the mouth commonly occurs and there may be blood if the individual bites the tongue or the inside of the cheek. There may be loss of bladder and/or bowel control
4. The comatose stage, in which the muscles relax and the individual remains unconscious
5. The postictal stage, in which, on regaining consciousness, the individual may be confused or drowsy. In some instances the person performs actions that are repetitive and undirected (automatism); they are unaware that they are performing these actions (Oman et al 2001).

Emergency care of a seizure

During a seizure the objective is to protect the affected individual from injury. This can be achieved by:

- Moving harmful objects out of the way
- Not attempting to put anything in the person's mouth
- Loosening constrictive clothing and placing a folded towel or jumper under the head if the individual is lying on a hard surface
- Placing the person on their side when the convulsions begin to subside, to maintain a clear airway
- Treating any injuries resulting from a fall to the ground, or from the seizure
- Seeking medical aid if the person is not known to have epilepsy
- Allowing the individual to rest after the seizure
- Providing emotional support.

Manifestations of febrile seizures

Seizures are relatively common between the ages of about 6 months and 4 years. Seizures usually occur during temperature elevation rather than after prolonged rise. Febrile seizures may accompany upper respiratory, gastrointestinal or ear infections and 25–30% of children with simple febrile seizures have recurrence with subsequent infections (Newberry 2003). Manifestations are:

- Stiffness of the body
- Twitching of the limbs
- Arching of the head and back
- Rolling of the eyes
- Congestion of the face and neck
- Cyanosis of the face and lips.

Emergency care of febrile seizures

Emergency management of febrile seizures involves:

- Placing the child on the floor for safety

- Ensuring a clear airway by turning the child onto one side
- Loosening and removing any excess clothing
- Seeking medical assistance
- Reducing body temperature by moving to a cooler environment
- Providing emotional support.

SKELETAL AND SOFT TISSUE INJURIES

Skeletal and soft tissue injuries range in severity from life- or limb-threatening to self-limiting minor injuries. The aim of first aid management of skeletal and soft tissue injuries is to prevent movement at the site of injury so as to prevent further damage, to minimise pain and to prevent shock. (Information on injuries to the bones or joints, including causes, types and manifestations, is provided in Chapter 32.) The general aims are to:

- Sit or lie the casualty down and support the injured part in a position of comfort. Support the injured part in a slightly elevated position, if possible, to reduce swelling (Clinical Interest Box 48.12)
- Handle the injured limb gently and do not use force to position it, as this could cause further injury and pain
- Never attempt to re-align a fracture
- Cover any wounds with a sterile or clean dressing and control bleeding
- Seek medical assistance
- Only stabilise the fracture with a splint if the casualty has to be moved (remote or isolated area) (Clinical Interest Box 48.13)
- Provide emotional support (Dolan & Holt 2001).

If spinal or neck injuries are suspected the individual must not be moved, as movement could result in damage to the spinal cord. The ARC no longer recommends routinely rolling casualties onto their side to assess airway and breathing, except in cases of submersion or obstruction (ARC 2006). Spinal or neck injuries should be suspected if the casualty experiences back pain, altered sensation, loss of movement or feeling below the injury, manifestations of shock, breathing difficulties or loss of bladder and bowel control (Clinical Interest Box 48.14). General emergency care involves:

- Leaving the casualty where they are until expert assistance arrives
- Checking that the airway is clear and observing for signs of respiratory failure
- Placing a blanket or coat over the casualty
- Instructing the casualty not to attempt to move
- Providing emotional support
- Seeking medical assistance urgently (Walsh & Kent 2001).

CLINICAL INTEREST BOX 48.12
RICE

RICE stands for rest, ice, compression, elevation.

Rest
- Avoid any movement or activity that causes pain
- Help the casualty into a comfortable position
- If there are head, neck or back injuries, keep the casualty flat

Ice
- Apply a wrapped icepack after bleeding has been controlled
- The cold compress reduces swelling and eases pain

Compression
- Apply a firm bandage to give even pressure
- Use light padding under the bandage if pain is severe

Elevation
- This slows the flow of blood to the area and reduces the swelling
- Raise the injured area above the level of the heart
- Do not elevate if a spinal injury is suspected

CLINICAL INTEREST BOX 48.13
Case study — musculoskeletal injury

On a camping trip to a remote section of the Murray River, Sam walked along the home-made jetty to have a swim. The jetty was made of wood and was just slightly covered with water, making it extremely slippery. Sam felt his feet slip from underneath him and he fell backwards onto his outstretched hand. He immediately felt pain in his right wrist followed by tingling in his fingers.

D — wet slippery jetty. Ask Sam to carefully shuffle back along the jetty to the dry section

R — alert

A — clear

B — rapid and shallow respirations

C — fast full-bounding pulse. Skin pale and cool to touch

Plan of care
- Ask Sam if he can move his fingers (responded yes)
- Small area of swelling noted over the medial aspect of Sam's right wrist
- Tender to touch, minimal movement
- Capillary refill brisk and fingers cool (note: unaffected hand same temperature)
- Crepe bandage applied and arm elevated
- Ice from the esky wrapped in a towel and applied over swollen area
- Sam taken to local hospital for X-ray

SPRAINS AND STRAINS

A sprain is the stretching and tearing of ligaments and other soft tissue structures at a joint. A ligament is a fibrous band that holds bones together at a joint. A strain is the stretching and tearing of muscles and tendons. A tendon is a fibrous band that attaches muscle to bone (Dolan & Holt 2001).

Manifestations of a sprain or strain

Manifestations of a sprain or strain include:

- Pain
- Swelling
- Deformity

CLINICAL INTEREST BOX 48.14
Care of spinal injuries

Signs and symptoms
- Changes in the conscious state
- Severe pain or pressure in the head, neck or back
- Tingling or loss of sensation in the extremities
- Blood or other fluid in the ears or nose
- External bleeding from the head, neck or back
- Seizures
- Impaired breathing or vision
- Nausea and vomiting
- Persistent headache
- Loss of balance
- Partial or complete loss of movement in any body part

Emergency care
- Maintain airway
- If unconscious, turn into recovery position
- Minimise head and neck movement
- Monitor conscious state
- Control any external bleeding
- Maintain body temperature
- Call for medical assistance

(Australian Red Cross, *First Aid*, 1998: 264)

- Discolouration of the skin
- Inability to use the affected part
- Sound of a pop or snap at the time of injury.

Care of sprains and strains

Care of sprains and strains involves:
- Stopping all activity
- Observing the injured area for swelling, bruising and deformity
- Comparing one side of the body with the other to assess damage
- Touching the area to assess for warmth, tenderness and muscle spasm
- Seeking medical advice if the casualty cannot move the injured area
- Assessing the range of movement if they can move the injured part
- Seeking medical advice if there is a loss of power.

POISONING

Poisons are substances that damage cells and may destroy life when they are introduced into the body. Poisons may be solid, liquid or gaseous and they may enter the body by:
- Ingestion (i.e. via the mouth)
- Inhalation (i.e. via the lungs)
- Absorption (i.e. via the skin)
- Injection (i.e. via the intravenous, intramuscular or subcutaneous route).

Some poisons take effect immediately, while others cause delayed but rapidly progressing effects (Brown 2001).

Manifestations of poisoning

Depending on the type of poison, and the route by which it entered the body, some or all of the following may be present:
- Abdominal pain
- Nausea or vomiting
- Drowsiness or unconsciousness
- Burning pains from the mouth to the stomach
- Burns around and inside the mouth
- Breathing difficulty and/or cyanosis
- Headache
- Blurred vision
- Ringing in the ears
- Odours on the breath
- Contamination of the skin
- Injection or bite marks.

Emergency care for poisoning

Detailed information for the emergency management of specific poisons can be obtained by telephoning the nearest Poisons Information Centre (13 11 26 in Australia, 0800 764 766 in New Zealand) or by contacting the emergency department of the nearest hospital. General management depends on whether the casualty is conscious or not, and whether the substance was corrosive or not.

Unconscious casualty

Commence CPR immediately, seek urgent medical assistance.

Conscious casualty

For a conscious casualty it is essential to determine whether the poison taken was a corrosive or petroleum-based substance, or a non-corrosive substance. A corrosive substance is one that directly damages tissue by erosion; for example, oven cleaner, toilet cleaner, strong disinfectants, bleach and battery acid. Petroleum-based substances include petrol, kerosene, turpentine and diesel oil (Brown 2001; Newberry 2003).

Emergency care for poisoning involves the following:
- Survey the scene and ensure safety
- Remove the casualty from the scene if safe to do so
- Assess the casualty's ABC
- Care for life-threatening situations
- Look for containers and try to identify the poison
- Follow directions from the Poisons Information Centre
- Do not give anything to eat or drink
- Do not induce vomiting.

BITES AND STINGS

Australian snakes, spiders and marine creatures are among the most venomous in the world. Some of the most poisonous creatures are the:
- Brown snake
- Taipan
- Red-back spider
- Funnel-web spider

- Blue-ringed octopus
- Cone shell
- Stonefish
- Stingray
- Box jellyfish.

Manifestations of snake or spider bites

Manifestations of snake or spider bites include:

- Headaches
- Blurred or double vision
- Puncture marks on the skin
- Swelling and inflammation of the bitten area
- Nausea
- Faintness or giddiness
- Sweating
- Chest and/or abdominal pain
- Breathing difficulty
- Muscle weakness or spasm.

Emergency care of snake and spider bites

Emergency care of snake and spider bites involves the following:

- Keep the casualty at rest
- Apply a pressure-immobilisation bandage over the bitten area and around the limb. The bandage should be applied firmly and should cover as much of the limb as possible. Note that a pressure-immobilisation bandage is not applied in the management of red-back spider bite as this will increase the casualty's pain. Instead, a cold pack or compress is placed over the bitten area
- Splint the bitten limb. The splint should immobilise the entire limb, and be held in position with bandages
- Assess the casualty's ABC, commence CPR if no signs of life (see Clinical Interest Box 48.15)
- Seek medical assistance urgently
- Provide emotional support (Australian Red Cross 1998).

CLINICAL INTEREST BOX 48.15
Case study — Bee sting

At a family picnic, Tina was stung by a bee and within minutes complained of feeling unwell and being dizzy. She then collapsed to the ground.
D — remove picnic baskets, cutlery, etc, away from Tina
R — no response to verbal or tactile stimulation: call for emergency personnel
A — clear
B — no breath sounds present, no chest movement noted: two effective breaths given in 10 seconds
C — commence compressions

Plan of care

- Commence CPR, and continue until emergency personnel arrive
- Ask someone to locate the bee sting and carefully remove the barb

Emergency care of marine stings and bites

The emergency care of marine stings varies slightly depending on the cause of the sting. The following is a general overview of the emergency treatment (for more specific information refer to a current first aid text or call the Poison Information Centre; in all instances the casualty's ABC must be assessed, and CPR begun if there are no signs of life.

- Management of blue-ringed octopus stings and stone fish bites is the same as for snake bite
- Management of stonefish and sting ray stings involves removing any foreign body, bathing the area with warm water, and seeking medical assistance
- Management of box jellyfish stings involves flooding the stung area with vinegar for at least 30 seconds before applying a firm compression bandage over the area (Australian Red Cross 1998).

MENTAL HEALTH EMERGENCIES

A mental health emergency is any disturbance in the client's thoughts, feelings or actions for which immediate therapeutic intervention is necessary (Oman et al 2001). The nurse, however, is not trying to make a psychiatric diagnosis but rather assess the behaviours displayed by the client and prevent disruption from the surrounding area. Working with clients undergoing a mental health crisis involves patience, understanding and flexibility. There are many mental health conditions; the most frequently observed are anxiety, panic disorder, depression and schizophrenia. Regardless of presenting symptoms it is important to treat the client with empathy and respect while protecting them and others from harm.

Manifestations of mental health emergencies

Clinical features will depend to a certain extent on the type of mental health condition occurring (see Chapter 47 for more information on mental health and mental illness). However, any of the following suggest that a mental health situation may be occurring:

- Delusions: fixed false idea or belief held by the client
- Hallucinations: apparent perception of external objects not actually there
- Disorder of thoughts: the client may believe others are interfering with their thoughts or trying to control their minds
- Disturbance in speech: can vary, from irrelevant answers to being unable to string together a sentence
- Emotional disturbance: may be inappropriate (e.g. laughing at sad news or speaking without altered pitch)
- Motor disturbances: agitation, pacing or stupor (Dolan & Holt 2001; Newberry 2003).

Emergency care of the client with mental illness

Emergency care of the client with mental illness involves the following:

- A calm quiet manner
- Patience
- Do not provoke or make fun of the client
- Listen to the client's fears
- If possible, remove the client to a quiet place
- Call emergency personnel.

SUMMARY

First aid is the emergency care of a sick or injured person until medical assistance is available or until the person recovers. Emergency situations may be encountered in a health care facility, in the home environment or in a public place. It is the nurse's responsibility to become familiar with the emergency codes and policies of the health care facility in which they are employed. Emergency situations requiring first aid management include: shock; bleeding; exposure to extremes of temperature; respiratory, cardiac and neurological incidents; injuries to bones and joints; poisoning; bites and stings; and mental health situations. This chapter has addressed some of these emergencies and the basic care that needs to be provided. For more detailed information, the nurse is advised to consult a current first aid text.

REVIEW EXERCISES

1. List the five aims of first aid.
2. What are seizures and how are they classified?
3. A client falls out of bed and hits their head on the floor. What actions will you take?
4. What are the similarities and differences between angina and myocardial infarction?
5. What are hypothermia and hyperthermia? Describe the care for each.
6. What is the initial management of a casualty that you suspect has taken an overdose of a sedative?

CRITICAL THINKING EXERCISE

While driving home from work late one night you witness a panel van veer off the road, turn over and end up lying upside down on the grass on the side of the road. You turn around to drive back to the scene and observe another car pulling over. When you get out of the car you notice:

- One person is lying outside the car on the grass groaning
- Another person is trapped in the passenger side of the van
- Tools from the van are scattered around the area
- It is dark and your length of vision is limited.

1. What is your first response?
2. Who will you offer assistance to first?
3. What precautions will you take?
4. How can you utilise other bystanders?

REFERENCES AND FURTHER READING

Australian Red Cross (1998) *First Aid. Responding to Emergencies*. ARC, Melbourne

Australian Resuscitation Council (ARC) (2006) *Policy Statements on Cardiopulmonary Resuscitation*. ARC, Melbourne

Brown AFT (2001) *Emergency Medicine Diagnosis and Management*. Butterworth–Heinemann, Melbourne

Dillon PM (2003) *Nursing Health Assessment. Critical Thinking Case Studies*, 4th edn. FA Davis, Philadelphia

Dolan B, Holt L (2001) *Accident and Emergency Theory into Practice*. Harcourt Publishers, Edinburgh

Lough ME, Stacey KM, Urden LD (2004) *Priorities in Critical Care Nursing*, 4th edn. Mosby, St Louis

Newberry L (ed.) (2003) *Sheehy's Emergency Nursing Principles and Practice*, 5th edn. Mosby, St Louis

Oman KS, Koziol-McClain J, Scheetz LJ (2001) *Emergency Nursing Secrets*. Hanley & Belfus, Philadelphia

Sorrentino SA (2004) *Mosby's Textbook for Nursing Assistants*, 6th edn. Mosby, St Louis

St John Ambulance (2007) *First Aid Information Fact Sheets*. Online. Available: www.stjohn.org.au [accessed 12 June 2008]

Thibodeau GA, Patton KT (2003) *Anatomy and Physiology*, 5th edn. Mosby, St Louis

—— (2004) *Structure and Function of the Body*, 12th edn. Mosby, St Louis

Walsh M, Kent A (2001) *Accident and Emergency Nursing*, 4th edn. Butterworth–Heinemann, Oxford

ONLINE RESOURCES

Australian Red Cross: www.redcross.org.au
St John Ambulance: www.stjohn.org.au
The Australian Resuscitation Council (ARC): www.resus.org.au

Chapter 49

MATERNAL AND NEWBORN CARE

OBJECTIVES

- Define the key terms/concepts
- Describe the physiology of pregnancy
- Describe the physiological changes that occur during pregnancy
- Discuss the care of the pregnant woman during the pre/antenatal period
- State the stages of labour
- Explain the postnatal care of the woman
- Describe the care of the newborn

KEY TERMS/CONCEPTS

amenorrhoea
Apgar score
breast milk
colostrum
fetal heart rate
labour and birth
lochia
meconium
morning sickness
uterine enlargement

CHAPTER FOCUS

Maternity nursing involves the care of a woman during her pregnancy and labour, and the care of both the woman and her baby during and after birth. Although midwifery is a specialised profession, requiring the learner midwife to undertake a separate educational program, the nurse may be required to assist in the provision of maternity care. It is therefore important that the nurse has a basic knowledge of human growth and development, the processes of normal pregnancy and labour and an understanding of the immediate and subsequent care of the mother and the newborn infant.

LIVED EXPERIENCE

. . . once the baby was out, I was euphoric. It was like there was no one else in the labour ward but me and my baby. I was amazed at how quickly I forgot about the labour, and how tired I was just a few minutes ago.

Melissa, reflecting on the birth of her first baby

The birth of a baby follows a woman's pregnancy and the process of labour. The first part of this chapter focuses on the physiology of pregnancy and the indicators and methods of confirming pregnancy and pregnancy care, which includes preparing for the birth. Later, the four stages of labour, and nursing measures for mother and baby during the postnatal period, are explained.

PREGNANCY

Pregnancy (the gestational process) comprises the growth and development, within a woman, of a new individual from conception to birth. The average duration of pregnancy is 266 days after fertilisation of the ovum, or 40 weeks from the first day of the last normal menstrual period.

Pregnancy, which is a normal physiological function, produces changes in almost all the mother's body systems. Most of these changes are temporary and most are the result of hormone actions. These changes prepare the mother's body to protect the developing embryo and fetus, provide for the demands of the fetus, and prepare to feed the baby when it is born. Profound endocrine changes occur that are essential for maintaining pregnancy, normal fetal growth and postpartum recovery. The hormonal factors involved in pregnancy are listed in Table 49.1.

PHYSIOLOGICAL CHANGES

Adaptation to pregnancy involves all of a woman's body systems. The mother's physical response is assessed in relation to normal expected alterations. Women can experience varying signs that can signify pregnancy. The maternal physiological changes during pregnancy are listed in Table 49.2.

PSYCHOLOGICAL CHANGES

During pregnancy a woman's psychological status may alter; for example, she may experience anxiety and emotional liability. The pregnant woman's psychological status depends on many factors, including her basic personality, whether the pregnancy was planned and is desired, the strength of her social and family support systems, and her self-concept.

CONFIRMATION OF PREGNANCY

The signs of pregnancy are divided into three general groups: possible, probable and positive.

Possible indicators of pregnancy

Signs of possible pregnancy are those from which a definite diagnosis of pregnancy cannot be confirmed. Signs and symptoms during this stage can often be caused by other conditions. The indications of possible pregnancy are:

- Amenorrhoea
- Nausea and vomiting
- Breast enlargement and tenderness
- Frequency of micturition
- Quickening.

Amenorrhoea (the cessation of menses) in a sexually active healthy woman is often the first indication of pregnancy. However, other factors may cause amenorrhoea, such as eating disorders (anorexia nervosa, bulimia), excessive exercise or changes in metabolism and endocrine function.

The symptoms of nausea and vomiting, which can occur at any time of the day, are often referred to as morning sickness. Nausea often occurs between 6 and 14 weeks' gestation and is believed to be a result of large quantities

TABLE 49.1 | HORMONAL FACTORS IN PREGNANCY

Source	Hormone	Actions
Ovary	Oestrogens and progesterone during the first few weeks of pregnancy	Oestrogens influence: • Uterine growth • Breast growth • Water and sodium retention • Pituitary hormone release Progesterone influences: • Relaxation of smooth muscle • Relaxation of connective tissue • Secretory changes within the breasts • Development of the lactiferous ducts
Placenta	Oestrogens and progesterone when the placenta is fully developed	
	Placental lactogenic hormone	Promotes growth, stimulates development of the breasts and plays a role in maternal fat metabolism
	Relaxin	Has a relaxant effect, especially on connective tissue
Pituitary	Thyroid-stimulating hormone (TSH)	Stimulates release of thyroxine to maintain increased metabolism
	Oxytocin	Contraction of the uterus (at the end of pregnancy). Secretion of milk (after birth)
	Prolactin	Initiates and sustains lactation (after baby is born)
Parathyroids	Parathormone	Maintains normal calcium ion concentration
Adrenals	Adrenal hormones (e.g. glucocorticoids and aldosterone)	Increased secretion maintains increased metabolism

TABLE 49.2 | PHYSIOLOGICAL CHANGES IN PREGNANCY

Area of change	Description
Uterus	Increase in size to about 30 × 22 × 20 cm (at term) Increase in mass to about 1 kg (at term) Cervix becomes softer (in preparation for labour) A plug of mucus (the operculum) is formed by, and remains in, the cervix from the eighth week until labour begins The uterus forms into two segments; the lower segment is thinner and becomes soft and dilated towards the end of pregnancy Painless, irregular contractions (Braxton Hicks contractions) occur throughout pregnancy
Vagina	In early pregnancy, the vagina (and cervix) change in colour from pink to dark red/blue The amount of acidic vaginal secretions increases Thickness increases, due to venous dilation
Breasts	Increase in size and mass Nipples enlarge and become more prominent and darker in colour Areolae become darker Prominent sebaceous glands (Montgomery's tubercles) appear on the areolae at about 12 weeks Increased sensation and tingling Colostrum (the fluid secreted during pregnancy) can be expressed at 16 weeks
Skin	Darker pigmentation in the nipples and areolae, on the face (chloasma) and on the abdominal midline (linea nigra) Stretch marks may appear on the abdomen, breasts and buttocks Spider naevi (bright red lesions with minute radiating branches) may appear on the face and upper chest
Musculoskeletal system	Spinal curvature changes to compensate for the abdominal enlargement, resulting in arching of the back The symphysis pubis and sacroiliac joints become mobile and the pelvis becomes wider, due to softening of the connective tissue in preparation for labour
Urinary tract	Relaxation of smooth muscle causes the ureters to become dilated, elongated and kinked These changes may lead to stasis of urine and infection Frequency of micturition may occur in the early months, as the uterus occupies more of the pelvis Reduced muscle tone in the pelvic floor, and increased pressure from the growing fetus, may result in stress incontinence towards the end of pregnancy
Gastrointestinal tract	Hormonal and mechanical changes, e.g., increased hormonal levels and reduced intestinal motility, may result in morning sickness, gastric acid reflux and constipation
Cardiovascular system	Blood volume increases by 40–50% Cardiac output is increased because of increased blood volume Haemodilution (due to increased plasma volume) results in lowered haemoglobin level Coagulability of blood is slightly increased Reduced tone in blood vessels may result in varicose veins
Respiratory tract	Ventilation rate is increased to obtain the higher amounts of oxygen required
Basal metabolic rate (BMR)	In the second half of pregnancy, BMR increases by 15–25% to cope with the increased demands
Body mass	Increases by about 25% of the pre-pregnant weight. Weight gain is due to the growth of the uterus and breasts, the uterine contents, increase in maternal blood volume and interstitial fluid, and maternal storage of fats and protein

of placental hormones (progesterone, oestrogen, human chorionic gonadotropin [hCG] and human placental lactogen).

Breast enlargement and tenderness are a result of the placental hormones stimulating the breast ductal system in preparation for breastfeeding. Some women experience similar symptoms premenstrually and pregnancy is often overlooked for this reason.

Increased pigmentation of the skin occurs over the face (chloasma), breasts (darkening of the areolae) and abdomen (linea negra — a dark line extending from the umbilicus to the symphysis pubis).

Frequency of micturition occurs at the start of pregnancy and then again in the third trimester. In the first trimester the enlarging uterus competes for space in the pelvic cavity and exerts pressure on the urinary bladder. In the later stage of pregnancy the descending fetal part of the uterus moves into the pelvic cavity in preparation for birth.

Quickening is the result of fetal movement and is first perceived at 16–20 weeks' gestation. The sensation is felt by the mother and described as gentle fluttering in the lower abdomen (Leifer 2003).

Probable indicators of pregnancy

Abdominal uterine enlargement, the presence of Braxton Hicks contractions and a positive pregnancy test are indicators that a woman is probably pregnant. However, there may be other conditions or factors (uterine tumours, medications or premature menopause) that cause these events on very rare occasions.

Abdominal and uterine enlargement occurs around the 12th week of pregnancy. At this stage the fundus of the uterus can be located just above the symphysis pubis, and extends to the umbilicus between weeks 20 and 22.

Braxton Hicks contractions are irregular, painless uterine contractions that first occur in the second trimester. They are more pronounced in multiparas (women who have had more than one child) and can be mistaken for labour contractions.

A pregnancy test may be performed after the first missed menstrual cycle. Pregnancy tests use maternal blood or urine to determine the presence of the placental hormone human chorionic gonadotropin (hCG). A positive result from a pregnancy test is considered an indicator of probable pregnancy. Provided that they are carried out precisely according to the given instructions, home pregnancy tests based on the amount of hCG in the urine are capable of greater than 97% accuracy.

Professional pregnancy tests based on urine or blood serum are even more reliably accurate. The most highly reliable test is the radioimmunoassay (RIA), a technique in radiology that can accurately identify pregnancy as early as 1 week after ovulation. While attributed with high levels of accuracy, pregnancy tests cannot be classed as absolutely certain indicators because there are factors that may interfere with the reliability of test results. These factors include premature menopause, the effects of taking some particular medications (anticonvulsants or anti-anxiety drugs) and the presence of a malignant tumour or haematuria (Leifer 2003).

Positive indicators of pregnancy

The most positive sign of pregnancy is a growing and developing baby. The fetal heartbeat can be detected as early as 10 weeks' gestation using equipment such as a (tocograph) pelvic ultrasound (or Doppler device). This scan enables (allows) the examiner to detect and record the fetal heart rate and therefore confirm pregnancy. The Doppler can be used to listen to the baby's heart rate from 18–20 weeks gestation onwards.

Fetal body parts can be felt by an educated examiner (medical officer, obstetrician or midwife) from the second trimester onwards. This gives the examiner an indication of the position of the fetus, which is vital during the third trimester when discussing birthing options.

Estimated confinement date

The date when the baby is due (confinement date) may be calculated by dates, the height of the uterine fundus or using ultrasound. Calculation by dates to determine the estimated due date is made by ascertaining the first day of the last known menstrual period and adding 9 months and 7 days. Calculation by assessing the fundal height (Figure 49.1) is made by measuring the height of the uterine fundus from the symphysis pubis. As the uterus enlarges steadily and predictably, the date of confinement can be determined reasonably accurately. Calculation by ultrasound is made by using height frequency, short wavelength and soundwave reflections to visualise the size of the fetus.

MINOR DISCOMFORTS ASSOCIATED WITH PREGNANCY

The pregnant woman may experience one or a variety of minor disorders or discomforts, many of which are the result of increased secretion of hormones or pressure from the uterus and its contents on other body structures. Table 49.3 lists the potential discomforts and outlines guidelines that can be used to increase women's levels of comfort.

PRENATAL CARE AND PREPARATION

Prenatal (or antenatal) means before birth. The aims of prenatal care are to:

- Promote a healthy pregnancy and normal labour
- Promote the birth of a healthy, living baby
- Prepare the woman and her partner for labour and birth
- Detect and manage any complications.

Because of increased public education and awareness, a woman is likely to request prenatal care as soon as she thinks she may be pregnant. Prenatal care involves physical examination of the woman, discussion and education about the importance of diet, exercise, general hygiene, preparation for labour and her expected role as a mother (Bobak & Jensen 1993).

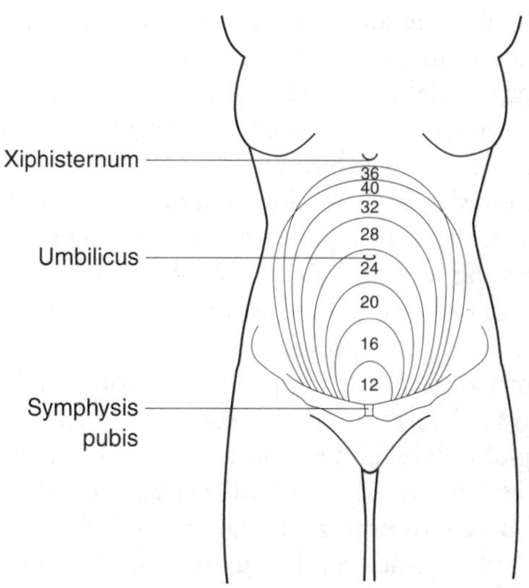

Figure 49.1 | Fundal height of the uterus

TABLE 49.3 | CLIENT EDUCATION: MANAGEMENT OF MINOR DISCOMFORTS DURING PREGNANCY

Discomfort	Management guidelines
Morning sickness	Small, frequent dry meals Fluids in between meals Something to eat, e.g., a dry biscuit, before getting out of bed in the morning Avoid fried and heavily spiced foods
Indigestion	Small frequent meals Avoid spicy foods if not used to them Elevate the head of the bed
Constipation	High-fibre foods Adequate fluids Exercise
Fainting	Avoid sudden postural changes Avoid constrictive clothing Avoid lying on the back during late pregnancy Avoid fatigue
Backache	Maintain correct posture Daily rest periods Wear low-heeled shoes Sleep on a firm surface (e.g. place a board under the mattress)
Varicose veins	Avoid long periods of standing Avoid constrictive clothing Elevate the legs whenever possible Wear supportive stockings Avoid sitting or standing with the legs crossed
Urinary tract infection	Adequate fluids Perineal hygiene measures (e.g. wiping from front to back after elimination)
Leg muscle cramps	Avoid standing for long periods Elevate the legs whenever possible Relieve symptoms by pulling upwards on toes
Haemorrhoids	Avoid constipation Relieve discomfort by applying cold compresses or icepacks

THE INITIAL MATERNITY CONSULTATION

The woman's initial consultation concerning her pregnancy may be with her general practitioner, obstetrician or, possibly, especially if she resides in a rural or remote area, a midwife. The first consultation involves obtaining a comprehensive health and social history, thorough physical examination, pelvic examination, and discussion on selecting where the woman wishes to give birth.

The physical examination includes checking the blood pressure, heart, lungs, palpating the abdomen and breasts and assessing weight, height, body build and skin colour. Samples of urine and blood are obtained and tested. Urine is tested to diagnose pregnancy and to detect the presence of abnormalities; for example, glucose or protein. Blood is tested to determine blood group and Rh factor status, haemoglobin level and the presence of rubella antibodies. It may also be tested to exclude certain disorders such as blood-borne viruses (e.g., human immunodeficiency virus [HIV] and hepatitis) and sexually transmitted infections (e.g., syphilis).

The pelvic examination may involve bimanual and speculum examinations to assess uterine size; to observe the cervix, vagina and perineum; and to estimate the pelvic capacity. A cervical smear and/or cervical swabs may be obtained if the woman has not had regular Papanicolaou (Pap) smears or if infection is suspected. This may be delayed until the woman has her 6 week post-birth check-up.

If pregnancy is confirmed, the obstetrician will discuss with the woman possible options regarding the birth. The woman may choose to give birth in a hospital, or in a birthing centre; she may also choose not to continue with the pregnancy (Leifer 2003).

Prenatal education may be provided by the obstetrician, midwives, or childbirth educators. The educational aspects of prenatal care are listed in Table 49.4.

SUBSEQUENT CONSULTATIONS

The frequency with which subsequent visits occur depend on the obstetrician and the needs of the woman, but the usual practice is to schedule visits every 4 weeks until 28 weeks, then every 2 weeks until 36 weeks, then weekly until birth.

TABLE 49.4 | PRENATAL EDUCATION

Aspect	Description
Diet	A balanced diet designed to meet the nutritional requirements of pregnancy: • An extra 600–800 kilojoules per day in the latter 6 months of pregnancy • An extra 500 mg of calcium per day in the last 4 months of pregnancy • An extra 3 mg of iron per day throughout pregnancy • Increased amount of vitamins, supplied by suitable foods rather than artificial supplements • Total daily intake of about 10 500 kilojoules
Exercise	Moderate exercise encouraged (e.g. a daily walk or swim). Some activities (e.g. vigorous athletics) may need to be avoided if the woman has a history of abortion or premature labour Prenatal classes educate the woman in specific exercises designed to prepare her for labour and birth
Rest	Fatigue should be avoided by obtaining sufficient sleep and by having numerous short rest periods during the day
Hygiene	Normal hygiene practices should be continued. Vaginal douching is to be avoided
Clothing	The woman is advised to wear comfortable non-constrictive garments, and shoes with low heels Maternity girdles are available, which provide support for just above the symphysis pubis and the lower back
Preparation for labour and birth	Education on childbirth and relaxation techniques are conducted on an individual or group basis by midwives, or physiotherapists. The woman's partner is also encouraged to attend the childbirth education program, which prepares the couple for labour and birth. The classes include instruction in relaxation techniques The couple is also informed of the physiology of labour and encouraged to discuss all aspects of pregnancy, birth and care of the baby
Manifestations of complications	The woman is advised to contact her obstetrician or the hospital immediately if there is: • Vaginal bleeding • Abdominal or 'menstrual-type' pain • Severe headaches • Drainage of fluid from the vagina • Excessive vomiting • Blurred vision • Difficulty in passing urine • Swelling of the hands, feet or face
Manifestations of labour	The couple are informed of the manifestations of the onset of labour: • Regular contractions • Vaginal 'show' (blood-stained mucus) • Drainage of amniotic fluid from the vagina (ruptured membranes)
Breasts	Maternity brassieres are designed to support the breasts as they increase in size and mass If the nipples are flat or inverted, nipple shields may be worn under the brassiere. The shields depress the areolae and allow the nipples to extend
Sexual activity	Sexual activity may be continued throughout the pregnancy, unless there is a risk of haemorrhage (e.g. from a malpositioned placenta [placenta praevia]) If the woman has a history of spontaneous abortion, she may be advised to avoid sexual intercourse during the first 3 months of pregnancy
Environmental hazards	Factors potentially harmful to the pregnancy should be avoided: • Smoking is linked to abortion, intrauterine growth retardation and perinatal death • Alcohol is linked to physical and mental fetal abnormalities and fetal growth retardation • Many drugs, prescribed and unprescribed, are linked to physical and mental fetal damage • Exposure to microorganisms (e.g. the rubella virus) in the first 3 months can result in fetal abnormalities • Immunisations generally should not be performed during pregnancy because of possible damage to the fetus • Exposure to radiation during the early weeks of pregnancy may inhibit normal cell division • Exposure to pesticides and other chemicals may result in fetal abnormalities

At each visit assessment is made of:

- Weight – only done at booking-in visit and later if indicated
- Blood pressure
- Urine (to detect the presence of protein, glucose, ketones) – only done at booking-in visit and later if indicated e.g. a health complication arises.
- Ankles, feet, hands (to detect the presence of oedema)
- Fundal height
- Fetal position and heartbeat.

Blood tests or other investigations, for example ultrasonic examination, may be performed as part of a medical officer's routine care or when other tests or physical symptoms indicate there is a need.

LABOUR

Labour is the process whereby the woman has uterine contractions to assist with her baby's birth. The process also include the vaginal birth of the placenta and membranes. Normal labour occurs spontaneously at about 40 weeks of pregnancy and lasts for up to 24 hours after onset. Factors that cause the spontaneous onset of normal labour include changes in hormonal levels, uterine distension, fetal pressure and a sudden reduction of intrauterine pressure when the membranes rupture (Leifer 2003). Labour is divided into four stages; Table 49.5 lists the characteristics of each stage. During labour the uterus contracts rhythmically to dilate and efface (take up) the cervix and push the fetus through the birth canal. After the baby is born the uterus continues contracting to aid in birth of the placenta and membranes.

Labour and childbirth are normal events, accompanied by a variety of emotions, such as excitement, fear, anxiety and anticipation. As the management of, and attitudes towards, labour and birth differ widely among different cultures, expectant women, obstetricians and midwives, practices are adjusted according to individual needs, knowledge and experience. The following part of this chapter addresses the general aspects of care and support throughout labour and birth.

THE FIRST STAGE

Care during the first stage involves monitoring the progress of labour, monitoring the condition of the woman and unborn baby (fetus), and promoting physical and psychological comfort. Progress of labour is monitored by assessing the strength, frequency and duration of contractions, by palpating the abdomen to assess the position and descent of the fetus, and by performing vaginal examinations only when deemed necessary to assess the degree of cervical dilatation and the position of the presenting part of the fetus. The condition of the woman and her response to labour are monitored by checking her vital signs, by observing urinary output and testing the urine for the presence of protein and ketones; and by observing her for the manifestations of fatigue, discomfort or pain.

The health of the unborn baby is monitored by assessing the fetal heart. As the fetal heart rate and rhythm is the main

TABLE 49.5 | STAGES OF LABOUR

Stage	Characteristics
First	Contractions occur at fairly regular intervals, from about every 10 minutes at the onset of labour to about every 2 minutes at the end of the first stage The cervix is effaced (raised up) The fetal head begins to descend in the pelvis The cervix is gradually dilated The membranes may rupture, and release amniotic fluid
Second	Strong contractions occur, lasting about 60 seconds and becoming expulsive, and the woman experiences a desire to bear down The woman uses abdominal muscles and the diaphragm to assist in pushing the fetus down the birth canal The muscles of the pelvic floor are displaced by the advancing fetal head The vagina is dilated, and the perineum is thinned and flattened by the advancing head The vulva and vaginal orifice bulge and the anus dilates as the head advances The baby is born
Third	After a brief period the placenta separates from the uterine wall Uterine contractions restart to expel the placenta and membranes Signs of separation and descent of the placenta are: • A small rush of blood from the vagina • The cord lengthens at the vulva • The uterus is firmly contracted and the height of the fundus drops to umbilical level
Fourth	In the 1–2 hours after birth of the baby and expulsion of the placenta and membranes, the uterus begins the process of involution. Involution is the return of the uterus to its normal size. The fourth stage of labour completes when the mother's body has returned to physiological stability

indicator of the baby's health, the heartbeat is regularly assessed during labour. The heart rate should remain between 120 and 160 beats per minute and the beat should remain strong and regular. Assessment may be performed by listening to the heart through a stethoscope placed on the woman's abdomen or by using a fetal monitoring device, such as electronic fetal monitoring (cardiotocograph). Fetal monitoring devices provide an audible and/or visual record of the fetal heartbeat.

Another way that the condition of the fetus is assessed is by observing the passage of 'liquor' draining from the woman's vagina. Normally the liquor remains clear and straw coloured, while green-tinged liquor indicates the presence of meconium. The passage of meconium (the dark green tarry substance formed in the fetal bowel) by the fetus while still in the uterus indicates that the fetus is physically distressed because of a period of fetal oxygen deprivation (Bobak & Jensen 1993).

Promoting comfort

Unless there are factors that may compromise the condition of the woman or her baby, the woman is encouraged to do whatever will contribute to her comfort. She may choose to walk around or may prefer to sit or lie down. The woman may like to engage in some form of activity, such as reading, watching television or listening to music. Some women find that frequent warm showers enhance their comfort, while others may prefer to have their partner or the midwife massage the abdomen and back.

During the first stage the woman may need to be encouraged and supported to use the relaxation techniques learnt in prenatal classes. She is encouraged to empty her bladder at least every 2 hours, as a full bladder can inhibit uterine action. The woman is also encouraged to consume frequent small amounts of clear fluids (e.g., 75 mL/h). Because the absorption of food is slowed down during labour and because there is the possibility that a general anaesthetic may be necessary, solid food is generally restricted during labour. The input and output of fluids are monitored to assess for the manifestations of the woman becoming dehydrated. Because the process of labour requires the expenditure of large amounts of energy, the woman may become fatigued. Fatigue is minimised by encouraging rest and relaxation and by relieving discomfort of pain.

Strong contractions may cause considerable discomfort, and the measures used to minimise and relieve discomfort will vary according to the needs and choices of each woman. Measures to relieve discomfort aim to reduce pain and tension without causing any harmful effects to the woman or baby. Measures include practising relaxation techniques, assuming the most comfortable position, back and abdominal massage, using music as a distractor and medications. Medications such as analgesics may be prescribed. Any medication administered must not cause harmful effects to the baby or retard the progress of labour. Analgesic medications may be administered by inhalation (e.g., nitrous oxide and oxygen), intramuscular injection (e.g. Pethidine) or intrathecal injection of local anaesthetic solution into the epidural space surrounding the spinal cord, from which the nerves supplying the uterus or cervix arise (epidural analgesia).

Throughout the first stage the midwife should provide emotional support and encouragement, and do all that she can to ensure that the labour is not a distressing experience.

THE SECOND STAGE

Although it may be accompanied by some anxiety, the second stage of labour signals the imminent birth of the baby. It concludes with the actual birth of the baby (Leifer 2003). Progress of labour and the condition of the unborn baby are monitored as in the first stage, but at more frequent intervals. During contractions the midwife and/or partner should offer encouragement. As the fetal head reaches the pelvic floor, most women experience the urge to push. Automatically the woman will begin to exert pressure downwards by contracting her abdominal muscles while relaxing her pelvic floor. This bearing-down reflex is an involuntary reflex response to the pressure of the presenting part on stretch receptors of pelvic muscles. The midwife then encourages the woman to push when the urge to push is felt, rather than giving a long prolonged push on command.

Research has shown that forced breath-holding by women for more than 5 seconds diminishes the perfusions of oxygen across the placenta, which results in fetal hypoxia to the baby. Between contractions the woman may wish to have her lower back massaged, and should be encouraged to rest. Small sips of fluid or ice chips should be offered to moisten her mouth, and the woman may wish to have her face wiped at frequent intervals. Labour is often hard and tiring work. The woman is encouraged to adopt the position in which she feels the most comfortable for the birth. Physical support may be needed to maintain the woman in a suitable position. She may wish to have her back supported by pillows, depending upon the position she adopts. Clinical Interest Box 49.1 provides a case study of the transitional stage of labour.

The birth

Birth of the baby may take place with the mother lying down, standing, squatting or kneeling. Some maternity units and birth centres are equipped to accommodate the woman and her partner in a home-like environment. During birth of the baby the obstetrician or midwife assists by gently controlling the emergence of the head to prevent perineal damage. In some instances an episiotomy (incision into the perineum to enlarge the vaginal opening) may be necessary. Sometimes the application of obstetric forceps to the fetal head may be necessary to assist in its passage through the birth canal.

During an uncomplicated birth, after the baby's head has cleared the vagina, the shoulders and the rest of the

> **CLINICAL INTEREST BOX 49.1**
> **Case study — Mandy and Tom**
>
> Mandy had been in labour for 12 hours and was physically and emotionally exhausted. We both had been awake for more than 24 hours. I felt helpless and thought that there was nothing I could do. The midwife encouraged me to continue massaging Mandy's back and thighs. Sometimes Mandy told me to stop and then to start massaging again. I kept thinking I must be doing something wrong. The midwife explained that this was normal behaviour and a woman's needs change frequently towards the end of the first stage. I remembered from our antenatal classes that this meant that Mandy must nearly be fully dilated and would start pushing soon. I reminded Mandy of this and together we seemed to find extra energy, knowing that we would soon meet our beautiful baby.
> (Tom, with his partner, at the birth of their first baby)

baby's body are gently pushed out. Immediately after birth, provided that everything is normal and as expected, the baby is generally placed on the mother's abdomen. The umbilical cord is clamped in two places and cut between the clamps (Leifer 2003). Although about 95% of babies present head first, a small number are born buttocks first (breech presentation). A caesarean birth is the birth of the baby through a surgical abdominal incision. A caesarean section may be indicated for a variety of reasons, including maternal or fetal distress or failure to progress in labour.

The second stage is completed when the baby is born, which is an emotional time for everyone involved in the birth process. The baby is placed on the mother's abdomen, and both she and her partner can look at and caress their infant. The obstetrician or midwife remains nearby so that the condition of both mother and baby can be monitored. It may be necessary to aspirate mucus from the baby's mouth to prevent inhalation. The midwife encourages the mother to initiate skin-to-skin contact with her baby where the baby is placed at her breast and encouraged to suckle. This is thought to help establish the attachment process between mother and baby, and suckling promotes uterine contractions, necessary for expulsion of the placenta (Bobak & Jensen 1993).

THE THIRD STAGE

During this stage the placenta and membranes are expelled, without touching the uterine fundus. In most settings, oxytocic medications such as ergometrine or syntometrine are given to promote uterine contraction and reduce the risk of postpartum haemorrhage. After expulsion the woman's vulva and vagina are swabbed clean so that the areas can be inspected for any lacerations or tears. Any laceration or episiotomy is repaired. A sterile vulval pad is applied to collect the vaginal discharge. The woman is assessed for signs of haemorrhage and for any adverse effects of the birth. To assist with involution (decrease in size of the uterus), the midwife will massage the uterine fundus through the abdominal wall to promote contraction and retraction. The placenta and membranes are assessed to see if they are normal and complete. If they are incomplete, there may be fragments retained in the uterus, preventing uterine contraction and providing a focus for infection (Leifer 2003).

THE FOURTH STAGE

The fourth stage of labour is the first 1–4 hours after birth of the placenta, or until the mother has regained physiological stability (Leifer 2003). During this time the midwife's role includes monitoring the mother for her emotional health and wellbeing, levels of pain, bladder function, blood loss and recovery from anaesthesia. The midwife also provides the initial care for the new baby. The role also includes providing emotional support that may be necessary for the mother, family or significant others. It should be acknowledged that not all mothers will have partners, not all will have the family support they may desire and this may be a time when particular sensitivity is required.

CULTURAL INFLUENCES ON BIRTHING PRACTICES

The needs and wishes of the woman during pregnancy, labour and the postnatal period may be influenced by her cultural background. This may be very different to that of the midwife, but must be understood and respected. Australia and New Zealand are multicultural societies, and providing for the many different cultural preferences of clients requires flexibility on the part of midwives and nurses. There are differing cultural beliefs of significant importance to clients concerning:

- Who should be present during the labour and birth
- Showering or bathing after birth
- What is considered an appropriate diet for a new mother
- How long and how much a woman should rest after the birth
- What should happen to the baby, e.g., when breastfeeding should begin, what clothing and adornments should be used
- Specific rituals and practices that promote healing of the body
- What should happen to the placenta (Rice 1994).

Cultural attitudes vary enormously across cultures. For example, in over 50 known cultures, including Filipino, Vietnamese, Korean and Mexican, it is not the cultural norm for women to give infants colostrum, and breastfeeding is delayed until the milk has come in (Crisp & Taylor 2005). In most South-East Asian cultures it is seen as essential that the woman is not exposed to anything cold after the birth, as this is believed to risk the onset of arthritis and bladder problems. Many people of Vietnamese culture believe that showering and washing the hair too soon after giving birth leads to recurring headaches and hair dropping out quickly in old age. Many people in Hmong culture believe that when a person dies they must collect the person's placenta (termed 'black jacket') and put it on the deceased so they can be allowed entry into heaven. For this reason a woman may be very anxious about what is happening to her placenta and may request that it be given to the family for burial at the woman's home (Rice 1994). Clinical Interest Box 49.2 provides examples of cultural preferences in women who are of Anglo-Saxon and South-East Asian descent.

When nurses understand the beliefs behind particular cultural practices, this reduces the risk of confusion and conflict concerning what the woman chooses to do during and after the birth of her baby. However, care should be taken not to generalise about what happens in particular cultures because attitudes, values, beliefs and practices can vary significantly even within each cultural group (see Unit 3). In addition, the process of assimilation into a new culture may alter traditional beliefs and practices. Clinical Interest Box 49.3 provides examples of traditional birthing practices in the Indigenous populations of Australia and New Zealand.

POSTNATAL CARE

The postpartum period is called the puerperium. Sometimes called the fourth trimester of pregnancy, the puerperium begins after childbirth and continues for the following 6 weeks (Leifer 2003). This is the time during which the changes to the woman's body brought about by the pregnancy gradually resolve. It is also a time of adjustment to changed responsibilities. Mothers generally return home within days of the birth, so it is important to provide as much help and education as possible before discharge. While this section focuses mostly on care in the birthing centre or hospital, the ongoing needs of the mother, baby and family should be considered so that support can be planned as necessary for the remainder of the puerperium.

After the third stage of labour is completed, the mother's immediate comfort is promoted by ensuring that any wet or soiled clothing is replaced, and by offering her a drink and snack. She and her partner should be allowed to spend time together with the baby. If the mother is exhausted she may appreciate being left to rest or sleep.

CLINICAL INTEREST BOX 49.2
Cultural preferences in women from Anglo-Saxon and South-east Asian descent

Women who are of Anglo-Saxon descent

Women in labour often (but not always):

- Tend to be stoic
- Like a partner or other support person to be present
- Participate actively
- Use complementary and alternative methods for pain management
- Drink and eat small quantities throughout the first stage of labour
- Welcome family and friends soon after the birth
- Breastfeed their baby with colostrum (do not wait until the milk comes in).

It is generally accepted that:

- Women hold their babies immediately after the birth
- Family and friends will be welcome to visit soon after the birth
- The woman will be active and return to full health and functioning quickly.

It is generally accepted that the partner:

- Provides support
- Encourages and assists with care of the woman, including comfort and hygiene measures and position changes
- Will want to be involved in postnatal care of the infant.

Women of South-East Asian descent

Women in labour often but not always:

- Prefer a female to conduct internal examinations and assist at the birth
- As a first choice prefer their mother or mother-in-law rather than their husband or partner to attend the birth (there is a traditional belief that if the husband attends, the birth will be difficult)
- Prefer to sit or squat to deliver the baby
- Fear caesarean birth because traditional beliefs say that if the body is cut open the soul may leave.

Traditionally the woman is viewed as in a state of being 'cold' after a birth because of blood loss. This is not physical coldness, but an imbalance of body humour — a humoral coldness — a concept that originates from the Chinese yin and yang views of health and illness. Postnatal care is focused on returning the body to balance, which means the woman must keep herself warm. This may mean that:

- The woman avoids even touching cold water and may not wish to shower or wash her hair for several days or weeks after the birth. Traditionally Vietnamese women had a sponge wash in bed for 1 month after the birth
- The woman eats only certain foods that promote heat and healing in the body. Beef, lamb and seafood are avoided, as are fresh salad and some sour fruits. In particular, cold drinks are avoided.

Other traditional beliefs include that:

- Women usually will not breastfeed until colostrum is replaced by breast milk
- Women may choose to eat very salty foods because this is seen to stimulate thirst, and drinking more water promotes milk production and reduces constipation
- Women may get upset if the baby is praised, e.g., 'Isn't he beautiful, he's so cute'. This is because many South-East Asian mothers believe that praising the baby attracts the attention of spirits, who may take the baby away with them, meaning that the baby will die
- The woman or someone else in the family may wish to place a silver necklace around the baby's neck before the cord is cut. In Hmong culture (predominantly Buddhist) this is believed to seal the baby's soul in the body. It is believed, traditionally, that if this does not happen the baby will have ill-health and will not thrive.

(Rice 1994)

CLINICAL INTEREST BOX 49.3
Cultural beliefs and childbirth of indigneous people in Australia and Aotearoa (New Zealand)

Birth is seen very much as 'women's business' in Aboriginal society. Much of the education has been traditionally undertaken through observation and involvement in the life of the extended family, with elders imparting specific knowledge as required. Traditionally men have not been involved during the pregnancy or the birth and appeared to play a minor role in baby care and child raising.

Much of this is changing as Aboriginal people move in from the bush to town living, and family support systems shrink. Western ideas are being embraced as young Aboriginal people seek inclusion in the wider Australian way of life. Many Aboriginal women now give birth in hospitals, often far from family and friends. The traditional women's business of childbearing seems to be breaking down in some places, as men accompany their partners during labour and birth in hospitals.

Traditionally Maori women in Aotearoa enjoyed full control over their birthing processes. With the help of a tohunga (priest), midwives and whanau (family), women controlled conception, abortion, birth and parenting. They followed the strict protocols of karakia (incantations), tapu (spiritual powers) and noa (blessing) (see Chapter 10). Most deliveries were in the squatting or standing position, with support if desired. There was no interference and, if problems arose, the most appropriate tohunga who specialised in that particular situation was called upon to resolve the problem. The placenta was buried by the appropriate person and when the pito (umbilical cord) had fallen off the infant, it too was appropriately buried or planted in a rock crevice or tree.
(www.ngamaia.co.nz)

CARE OF THE MOTHER

The degree of care required will depend on a variety of factors, such as where the birth occurred, how long the mother remains in the maternity unit or birth centre, whether the birth was full or preterm, if it was uncomplicated, whether there were multiple births, and whether there are any postnatal discomforts or complications. In addition, care must be adapted to meet any specific cultural needs. Postnatal care is directed at promoting the health of both mother and baby. Aspects of care include promoting:

- Adequate rest
- Reducing the risk of infection
- Freedom from discomfort or pain
- Establishing lactation and breastfeeding
- Promoting the mother's confidence in caring for her baby.

Assessment is made of the lochia, the vaginal discharge that occurs after birth. Lochia consists of blood and broken-down endometrium and is discharged for up to 3–4 weeks after birth. At first it is bright red in colour, then becomes pink, and ultimately presents as a colourless or white discharge. Lochia should not have an offensive odour or contain any blood clots; the presence of either indicates the possibility that products of conception have been retained in the uterus.

Perineal care involves daily showering to cleanse the area, and frequent changing of vulval pads. If a perineal tear occurred or if an episiotomy was performed, care may be needed to reduce discomfort and prevent infection around the area. Local care may involve the application of cold packs to the area, or sitz baths to which salt has been added. A soft cushion to sit on or lying on her side to feed may help to relieve perineal soreness, and analgesic medications such as paracetamol may be prescribed.

Fundal height is assessed by the midwife and documented each day to monitor involution of the uterus. It may be necessary to massage the fundus to promote uterine contraction. The height of the fundus decreases by about 1 cm each day until, by the 11th or 12th day it can no longer be palpated abdominally.

The breasts and nipples are assessed each day for any red areas, oedema, cracking or bleeding. Palpation of each breast detects any areas of hardness, which may indicate blocked milk ducts.

Postnatal exercises are started on the first day. They are designed to strengthen the pelvic floor and abdominal muscles. An instruction sheet illustrating the exercises to be performed is generally given to the mother and explained by the midwife (Wickham 2003).

A balanced diet, which provides adequate nutrients and fibre, is advised. In the hospital setting a dietitian may be responsible for accommodating special cultural needs in relation to diet but often family members will want to bring meals from home for the new mother. If the woman is breastfeeding, she should consume an extra 2500–4000 kJ/day above the requirements of pregnancy. This provides the extra energy required to produce milk. In addition to nutritional requirements, the lactating mother requires three litres of fluid a day.

The lactating mother is advised to avoid consuming foods that may effect her lactation and can upset the baby. This is very individual and may include highly spiced foods. The woman who wishes to breastfeed should also be advised of the substances known to be excreted in the breast milk. Substances that should be avoided or taken sparingly include:

- Nicotine
- Alcohol
- Caffeine
- Laxatives
- Anti-infective agents
- Sedatives.

MINOR POSTNATAL DISCOMFORTS

Some discomforts are associated with the postnatal period. These include after-pains, constipation, difficulty with passing urine and engorged breasts. After-pains are cramps that may occur for a few days after birth, as the uterine muscles contract during the process of involution. Mild pain-relief medication may be prescribed.

Constipation may result from inadequate fibre or fluid intake. The woman may also be afraid to go to the toilet post-birth as it may increase her levels of pain and discomfort. Increasing fibre in the diet and maintaining a high fluid intake is important and, if necessary, a stool-softening medication may be prescribed. Analgesia may also be given prior to the woman going to the toilet.

Difficulty in voiding may be experienced initially because of loss of bladder tone, bruising of the urethra, or perineal soreness. Some women may find that voiding in a bowl or bath of warm water eases the soreness. If the woman finds that this helps, she should be advised, as a precaution against infection, to wash the perineal area gently after voiding.

Engorged breasts may occur a few days after the birth because of increased blood supply to the breasts in beginning lactation. The breasts may become full, distended, hard and uncomfortable. The midwife should advise mothers that this is not unusual and that wearing a supportive nursing bra, even during the night, will help, provided that it is not too tight. Breastfeeding the baby at frequent intervals (2–3 hours if necessary) helps and promotes engorgement to diminish naturally. A qualified midwife or lactation consultant should be contacted to assist women who are concerned about breast engorgement.

BREASTFEEDING

Breastfeeding is the optimal method of feeding the baby. While most women will choose to breastfeed, there are others who, for a variety of reasons, will prefer not to. While it is important that a woman be advised of the benefits of breastfeeding, it is also important that she is not made to feel guilty if she chooses to bottle feed.

Lactation

During pregnancy, placental hormones, oestrogen, progesterone, hCG and placental lactogenic hormone stimulate the development of glandular tissue and ducts in the breasts. Colostrum is the fluid secreted by the breasts during pregnancy and during the first few days after birth. It is a thin, yellow serous fluid consisting of water, protein, fat, carbohydrates and immunologically active substances. When the placenta is expelled after birth of the baby, the anterior pituitary gland releases prolactin, which activates the mammary cells to produce and release milk (Leifer 2003).

Lactation depends on the maintenance of milk production and on the 'let-down' reflex, whereby milk is ejected from the breasts. The let-down reflex is stimulated by a neurogenic reflex, with oxytocin released from the pituitary gland in response to suckling, forcing milk out of the alveoli in the breasts. The let-down reflex, which generally occurs a short time after the baby begins to suck on the nipple, can also be stimulated when the mother sees, hears or thinks about her baby. Conversely, the reflex can be inhibited by anxiety, fear or tension.

Breastfeeding has advantages for both the mother and baby. Breast milk is free from microorganisms, is easily digested, contains all the essential nutrients necessary for the baby's development, and contains immunoglobulins and other substances that protect the infant from some infections while the immune system is under-developed. Breastfeeding aids involution of the uterus and is generally emotionally satisfying for the mother. Breastfeeding is also convenient and economical.

Management

Women are able to usually successfully breastfeed, with guidance and support from health care professionals. Initially a woman may require some assistance to ensure that the baby's mouth is correctly positioned over the nipple. The baby's 'seeking reflex' is initiated when its cheek touches the breast, and it will turn the face to find the nipple. A few drops of breast milk can be expressed onto the nipple to encourage the baby to take the nipple into its mouth. The nipple should be placed into the baby's mouth, over the tongue, and the lips should be in contact with the areola. The baby's mouth should remain wide open against the breast so that it covers a substantial part of the areolar. It is important that the baby is able to breathe freely while feeding.

When breastfeeding, the woman should position herself so that she is comfortable and able to hold the baby securely. The baby should also be comfortable, in a clean and dry napkin, with the arms remaining free. During the feed the baby should be sat up and de-winded if necessary. To detach the baby from the nipple, the mother should place a finger into the side of the baby's mouth to let air in to break the suction. Gentle detachment helps to prevent the development of sore nipples.

After the feed the baby is checked to ensure that it is clean and comfortable, and should then be placed in its cot without too much handling. To guard against possible regurgitation, and subsequent inhalation of milk, the baby should be placed on its side. The mother should ensure that her nipples are clean and dried. Expressed breast milk is rubbed into the nipple after the feed then allowed to dry, to protect them against soreness or cracking.

The baby is fed when hungry (demand feeding). Each baby is an individual and some may require breastfeeding as frequently as every 2 hours, while others will be content if they are fed every 3–4 hours. The length of time the baby feeds also varies. The baby and mother establish their own feeding routine, and the mother's milk supply adjusts according to demand.

Breast milk may be expressed, either manually or with a breast pump, if necessary. Expression may be necessary to relieve discomfort if the breasts are overfull, to help stimulate milk production, or to put breast milk into a feeding bottle; for example, if the baby requires feeding when the mother is temporarily unavailable. Expressed breast milk can also be provided by the mother if the baby is premature or ill and is unable to feed at the breast.

Breastfeeding difficulties sometimes arise for a variety of reasons:

- Maternal anxiety or frustration about breastfeeding
- Cracked nipples, which cause pain when the baby sucks
- Inverted nipples, which are difficult for the baby to grasp
- Breast engorgement, which prevents the milk from flowing readily
- Over-abundance of milk, which flows too quickly causing the baby to splutter and perhaps vomit
- Failure of the let-down reflex
- Inability of the baby to suck well enough at the breast.

Management of breastfeeding difficulties depends on the cause, but with time, patience and encouragement, most can be overcome. Organisations such as the Australian Breastfeeding Association and La Leche League New Zealand provide support and advice on how to prevent and deal with breastfeeding difficulties.

Artificial bottle feeding is the method of infant feeding women choose if not breastfeeding their babies. Artificial feeds are generally based on cow's milk, although other preparations are available, such as a soy-based formula. The formula selected will depend on the needs of the mother and the baby. Some formulae are expensive, others may not be readily available, or the baby may require a special formula, such as soy based or lactose free. Whichever formula is selected, the mother must know how to make it up, how to store it and how to care for the bottles and teats. This information is given by the midwife during the mother's stay in hospital.

IMMEDIATE CARE OF THE BABY

Immediately after the birth the midwife or obstetrician checks that the baby's airway is clear and that it is breathing normally. Ventilation is initiated in response to high blood carbon dioxide level, stimulating the respiratory centre in the medulla. In the first few breaths, air is drawn in to expand the alveoli in the lungs, thus oxygenating the blood. Because the newborn baby has a limited ability to regulate its body temperature in relation to the environment, care is taken to ensure that it does not become cold.

One minute after birth, and again at 5 minutes, the Apgar score estimation is performed. The Apgar scoring system gives an estimation of the baby's condition and is an indicator of whether special resuscitation measures are required. Table 49.6 illustrates the Apgar score chart. A total score of 10 indicates that the infant is in optimal condition; if the score is 6 or less the baby requires immediate attention. A score of 8–10 is normal, a score of 4–7 indicates that the infant's condition is moderately depressed, while a score of 0–3 indicates a severely depressed condition.

In a health care setting such as a hospital or birth centre, an identification band is placed on the baby's wrist or ankle for identification. This identification procedure must be performed before the baby is removed from the mother's bed; this is essential to prevent any later confusion about which baby belongs to which mother. The baby is weighed and measured and the information documented. It is recommended that every baby be given an intramuscular injection of vitamin K as a preventive measure against bleeding tendencies (see Clinical Interest Box 49.4).

CLINICAL INTEREST BOX 49.4
The role of vitamin K

Haemorrhagic disease of the newborn (HDN) results from low levels of vitamin K, causing excessive bruising, petechiae, prolonged bleeding and, if not treated, intracranial haemorrhage and death. In Australia, vitamin K prophylaxis is given to prevent HDN, almost exclusively by the intramuscular route.

Vitamin K is required for blood clotting and is produced by the intestinal flora. However, the bowel is sterile at birth and time is required for the intestinal flora to become established and produce vitamin K. The liver plays a large role in blood coagulation during fetal life and continues to function as such during the first few months after birth. Coagulation factors II, VII and X are all synthesised in the liver and activated under the influence of vitamin K.

A transient blood coagulation deficiency occurs between the second and fifth day of life and from there the levels of coagulation factors rise slowly over the first few months of life. However, the coagulation factors do not approach normal levels until 9 months of age or later. For this reason an artificial dose of vitamin K is routinely given to all newborns.

(Lawrence 1999)

TABLE 49.6 | APGAR SCORING

	Score		
Factor	**2**	**1**	**0**
Heart rate	Over 100	Less than 100	Absent
Respiration	Established and almost regular	Intermittent, gasping in character	Absent
Colour	Pink all over	Centrally pink, but with blue extremities	Cyanosed or pale
Muscle tone	Good (active movements)	Fair (some flexion of extremities)	None (completely limp)
Response to stimulation	Vigorous withdrawal	Minimal withdrawal	None

TABLE 49.7 | THE NORMAL NEWBORN

Anatomy	Characteristics
Head	Average circumference 35 cm Anterior fontanelle — no tension or depression Posterior fontanelle — palpable May be elongated from moulding as the skull bones glide over each other during passage through the birth canal
Face	Nose and cheeks may have tiny white spots (milia)
Skin	Normal colour for race May be covered with lanugo (fine downy hair) May be vernix (white, greasy protective substance) in the skin folds
Eyes	Dark blue; white sclera Blink reflex present
Thorax	Average circumference 34 cm Expands symmetrically with ventilations Breast tissue palpable in males and females
Abdomen	Prominent but not distended Moves up and down with ventilations Umbilical cord blue/white
Limbs	Symmetrical, warm, rounded Move freely Hands and feet may be slightly cyanosed
Back	Spine straight, intact, easily flexed
Genitalia	Male: large in relation to body, scrotum contains both testes, foreskin adheres to glans, urethral meatus central on tip of penis Female: prominent labia and clitoris, vaginal opening visible
Anus	Patent

An initial examination of the baby is performed soon after the birth so that any abnormal findings can be acted on as soon as possible. Table 49.7 outlines the findings expected in a normal newborn. The examination assesses the baby's ventilation, colour, muscle tone, reflexes, movement and the presence of any obvious abnormalities. Later on a more thorough examination is performed.

Subsequent care of the baby

Care of the baby in the period immediately after birth is directed towards keeping the baby adequately nourished, clean, warm and free from infection. Careful observation is necessary to detect any problems should they occur. In most health care agencies it is common practice for the baby to remain in the same room as the mother. This is termed rooming-in and enables the mother to care for the baby from the beginning. The mother gets to know, and gains confidence in caring for, her baby. The midwife is available to offer guidance and encouragement in all aspects of infant care.

Hygiene and skin care

Health care settings establish their own protocols for washing or bathing newborn babies (neonates). The baby is usually washed or bathed daily; a mild pure soap may be used. It is important that the infant's skin is kept clean and dry, with special attention being paid to the scalp, skin folds and genitals. The buttocks and groin area are washed with plain water or cleansed with a mild lotion each time a wet or soiled nappy is removed. A protective cream or lotion may be applied. Disposable or cloth nappies may be used. The mother may need some advice on how to fold and apply napkins.

The remnant of the cord is observed every time a napkin is changed, until it has separated and the umbilicus has healed. It is kept clean and dry and observed for any bleeding or signs of infection. The cord remnant separates from the umbilicus by a process of dry necrosis on day 6–8.

If the baby's fingernails are long, the infant may scratch their face and the scratches may become infected. Mittens may be worn to prevent the infant from scratching.

Elimination

After the first day (when the neonate may void only once or twice) urine is passed about 10–12 times per day. Any unusual colouration or odour must be reported to the medical officer. The baby's first bowel action consists of meconium, the dark green tarry substance formed in the intestinal tract during intrauterine life. When the baby begins to take milk, there is a gradual transition to the normal yellow stools of the neonate. Breastfed babies pass stools that are yellow to pale brown, soft and unformed. The stools of an artificially fed baby are yellow to pale green, firmer and have a distinctive odour.

Nutrition

The baby is fed when hungry. Frequent feedings, for example, every 2 hours, may be indicated if the baby shows signs of hypoglycaemia. In health care settings the neonate is generally weighed every second day to assess weight gain or loss. More frequent weighing is indicated if the birth weight was low or if the baby is losing excessive weight. A loss of up to 10% of the birth weight is normal in the first 3–4 days, then the baby should begin to gain weight. It is expected that the baby will be back to its birth weight within 7–10 days.

Infection control

The baby is protected from infection by normal hygiene practices, the most important aspect of which is washing the hands thoroughly before attending to the baby. Anyone with an infection is advised to limit close contact with the baby.

Temperature control

As the neonate's temperature-regulating centre is not fully functional, the baby must be protected from extremes of environmental temperature. This can be achieved by maintaining the room at an even, comfortable temperature, dressing the baby in suitable clothes and wrapping the infant in warm lightweight rugs.

NEONATAL DISORDERS

Only brief mentions of some of the disorders that can affect neonates are included here. For detailed information, the nurse should refer to a current paediatric text. Disorders may be minor and temporary, major and permanent, or life threatening. They include:

- Prematurity
- Low birth weight
- Jaundice
- Hypoxia
- Atelectasis
- Hyaline membrane disease
- Hypoglycaemia
- Persistent vomiting
- Birth injuries
- Congenital abnormalities.

SUMMARY

The nurse may be required to assist qualified midwives in the care of mothers and their newborn babies. This chapter has briefly outlined the basic knowledge that is essential for the nurse who undertakes this role. The processes of normal pregnancy, labour and birth and the postnatal care of the mother and her baby have been outlined. It is recommended that nurses gain an understanding of cultural differences in birthing beliefs and practices of the women they care for during and after the birth of their babies. It is also recommended that nurses access current paediatric textbooks to gain or enhance knowledge of neonatal care and disorders that may be encountered in the areas of maternal and child health nursing.

REVIEW EXERCISES

1. Indications of pregnancy are generally divided into three groups: possible, probable and positive. List four indications of each stage.
2. What are the minor discomforts of pregnancy and what are some of the nursing interventions that you could implement to help overcome these?
3. What are the four stages of labour? List nursing interventions that you could implement during each phase to promote client comfort and wellbeing.
4. Immediately after the birth of a baby an assessment is performed on the neonate. What is this called and what does it entail?

CRITICAL THINKING EXERCISES

1. You are caring for Gaylene, a 32-year-old woman who 3 days ago gave birth to her first baby. She tells you her breasts feel really heavy, tight and uncomfortable and the baby is not feeding properly.
   (a) What is the likely reason for this discomfort?
   (b) What might help to relieve the discomfort?
   (c) What advice would be appropriate in relation to promoting satisfactory breastfeeding?
   (d) What are your responsibilities as an Enrolled Nurse in this situation?
2. You are caring for Hong, a young woman who came to Australia from a refugee camp in Thailand a year ago. She gave birth to her first baby earlier today. The midwife has instructed her to get up and go and have a shower. Hong is crying and distressed and tells you that 'the midwife doesn't understand'.
   (a) What do you think might be the reason for Hong's distress?
   (b) How could this misunderstanding have been avoided?
   (c) What will you do now to relieve Hong's distress?
   (d) What other cultural issues need to be explored to ensure that care is culturally appropriate?

REFERENCES AND FURTHER READING

Bobak I, Jensen M (1993) *Maternity and Gynecological Care. The Nurse and the Family*. Mosby, St Louis

Crisp J, Taylor C (eds) (2005) *Potter & Perry's Fundamentals of Nursing*, 2nd edn. Elsevier Australia, Sydney

Lawrence K (1999) What is the optimal time for administration of intramuscular vitamin K to newborn babies? Unpublished Master of Health Science degree research

Leifer G (2003) *Introduction to Maternity & Pediatric Nursing*, 4th edn. WB Saunders, Philadelphia

Rice P L (1994) When I had my baby here! In: Rice PL (ed.) *Asian Mothers, Australian Birth. Pregnancy, Childbirth and Childrearing: The Asian Experience in an English Speaking Country*. Ausmed Publications, Melbourne

Sherblom Matteson P (2001) *Women's Health During the*

Childbearing Years. A Community-Based Approach. Mosby, St Louis

Wickham S (2003) *Midwifery Best Practice*. Elsevier Science, London

ONLINE RESOURCES

About Pediatrics: www.pediatrics.about.com
Active Birth Centre: www.activebirthcentre.com
Birth Psychology: www.birthpsychology.com
Childbirth.Org: www.childbirth.org
KidsHealth: www.kidshealth.org
La Leche League International: www.lalecheleague.org
NGA MAIA: www.ngamaia.co.nz
Online Birth Center: www.moonlily.com/obc
US Centers for Disease Control and Prevention: www.cdc.gov

Appendix 1

STANDARD STEPS FOR ALL NURSING PROCEDURES/ INTERVENTIONS

These are the essential steps that must be done consistently with each client contact in order to deliver responsible and safe nursing care.

BEFORE THE PROCEDURE

Step 1

- Check the order in the chart, client's nursing/ medical history
- Gather equipment/supplies
- Wash your hands

Step 2

- Check the client's identification
- Introduce yourself to the client and/or family
- Explain the procedure to the client
- Assess client to determine whether intervention is still appropriate
- Identify teaching needed and describe what the client can expect

Step 3

- Provide privacy
- Raise the bed to appropriate height
- Provide adequate lighting for the procedure
- Arrange supplies and equipment

Step 4

- Wash hands
- Put on gloves following standard precautions as appropriate
- Place on eyewear, mask and gown as appropriate

Step 5

- Mentally review the step of the procedure beforehand
- Discuss the procedure with your instructor/ supervisor, if required
- Confirm correct facility protocols

DURING THE PROCEDURE

Step 6

- Promote client independence and involvement if possible
- Assess client tolerance to the procedure

AFTER THE PROCEDURE

Step 7

- Dispose of sharps appropriately
- Remove gloves and wash hands

Step 8

- Make the client comfortable and inform them of how the procedure went, or of any results/values
- Restore the bed height and unit. Wash hands again

Step 9

- Record and document the procedure
- Report abnormalities as required

(from deWit [2005] *Fundamental Concepts and Skills for Nursing*, 2nd edn. WB Saunders, Philadelphia, reproduced with permission; and Elkin, Perry & Potter [2007] *Nursing Interventions & Clinical Skills*, 4th edn. Mosby Elsevier)

Appendix 2
UNITS OF MEASUREMENT

Base units

Physical quantity	Name of unit	Symbol
Mass	kilogram	kg
Length	metre	m
Time	second	s
Electric current	ampere	A
Temperature	kelvin	K
Luminous intensity	candela	cd
Amount of substance	mole	mol

Derived units

Derived units to measure other quantities are obtained by multiplying or dividing any two or more of the seven base units. Some of these have their own names and symbols. For example:

Physical quantity	Name of unit	Symbol	Base or derived units
Force	newton	N	$kg/m/s^{-2}$
Pressure	pascal	Pa	N/m^{-2}
Energy, work, heat	joule	J	N/m
Power	watt	W	J/s^{-1}

Prefixes used for multiples

Factor	Prefix	Symbol
10^{-12}	pico	p
10^{-9}	nano	n
10^{-6}	micro	μ
10^{-3}	milli	m
10^{-2}	centi	c
10^{-1}	deci	d
10	deca	da
10^{2}	hecto	h
10^{3}	kilo	k
10^{6}	mega	M
10^{9}	giga	G
10^{12}	tera	T

Comparative temperatures

Celsius (°C)	Fahrenheit (°F)	Celsius (°C)	Fahrenheit (°F)
100.0 (boiling point)	212	38.5	101.3
95	203	38	100.4
90	194	37.5	99.5
85	185	37	98.6
80	176	36.5	97.7
75	167	36	96.8
70	158	35.5	96
65	149	35	95
60	140	34	93.2
55	131	33	91.4
50	122	32	89.6
45	113	31	87.8
44	112.2	30	86
43	109.4	25	77
42	107.6	20	68
41	105.8	15	59
40	104	10	50
39.5	103.1	5	41
39	102.2	0 (freezing point)	32

- To convert readings on the Fahrenheit scale into Celsius, subtract 32, multiply by 5, and divide by 9. For example: 98 – 32 = 66 × 5 = 330 ÷ 9 = 36.6.
  Therefore 98°F = 36.6°C.
- To convert readings on the Celsius scale into Fahrenheit, multiply by 9, divide by 5, and add 32. For example: 36.6 × 9 = 330 ÷ 5 = 66 + 32 = 98.
  Therefore 36.6°C = 98°F.
- The term 'Celsius' (after the Swedish astronomer who invented the scale in 1742) is now being internationally used instead of 'centigrade', which term is used in some countries to denote fractions of an angle.

Capacity

The SI unit of volume is the cubic metre (m^3), but the litre (L) is more commonly used and accepted.

1000 microlitres (μL)	= 1 millilitre (mL)
1000 millilitres	= 1 litre (L)
1 cubic centimetre (cm^3)	= 1 millilitre
1 teaspoon	= 5 mL
1 dessertspoon	= 10 mL
1 tablespoon	= 15 mL
1 cup	= 250 mL
1 tumbler	= 285 mL

Weight

1000 micrograms (μg)	= 1 milligram (mg)
1000 milligrams	= 1 gram (g)
1000 grams	= 1 kilogram (kg)
1000 kilograms	= 1 metric tonne

Energy

A dietetic calorie is the amount of heat required to raise the temperature of 1 litre of water by 1°C and is equal to 4.184 kilojoules.

1 g fat will produce 38 kilojoules or 9 calories.

1 g protein will produce 17 kilojoules or 4 calories.

1 g carbohydrate will produce 17 kilojoules or 4 calories.

Appendix 3
TABLE OF NORMAL VALUES

Normal values for adults based on those obtained from major teaching hospitals. These reference ranges can vary, depending on the assay used in particular laboratories

Haematology	
Basophil granulocytes	0.01–0.1 $\times 10^9$/L
Eosinophil granulocytes	0.04–0.4 $\times 10^9$/L
Erythrocyte sedimentation rate (ESR)	0–10 mm/h
Haemoglobin (male)	13–18 g/dL
Haemoglobin (female)	11.5–16.5 g/dL
Leukocytes	4.3–10.8 $\times 10^9$/L
Mean corpuscular haemoglobin (MCH)	1.7–2.0 fmol
Mean corpuscular haemoglobin	32–36 g/dL
concentration (MCHC)	
Mean corpuscular volume (MCV)	76–96 fL
Monocytes	0.2–0.8 $\times 10^9$/L
Neutrophil granulocytes	3.5–7.5 $\times 10^9$/L
Packed cell volume (PCV) (male)	42–63 mL/dL
Packed cell volume (PCV) (female)	36–45 mL/dL
Plasma volume	45 ± 5 mL/kg
Haematology	
Platelet count	150–400 $\times 10^9$/L
Red cell folate	> 160 μg/L
Reticulocyte count	0.5–2.5% of red cells
Serum B12	160–925 ng/L
Serum folate	5–63 nmol/L (3–20 μg/L)
Total blood volume (male)	75 ± 10 mL/kg
Total blood volume (female)	70 ± 10 mL/kg
Coagulation	
Bleeding time (Ivy method)	2.5–9 min
Partial thromboplastin time (PTTK)	30–40 seconds
Prothrombin time	12–15 seconds
Biochemistry	
Acid phosphatase (phostatic)	<0.8 U/L
Alanine aminotransferase (ALT)	<30 U/L
Albumin	36–47 g/L

Biochemistry (cont'd)	
Alkaline phosphatase	30–100 U/L
Alpha-$_1$-antitrypsin	2–4 g/L
Alpha-fetoprotein	<10 kU/L
Amylase	<220 U/L
Angiotensin-converting enzyme	5.5–28 IU/L
Aspartate aminotransferase (AST)	5–40 U/L
Bicarbonate	23–31 mmol/L
Bilirubin	<18 μmol/L
Calcium	2.2–2.67 mmol/L (8.5–10.5 mg/dL)
Chloride	100–106 mmol/L (100–106 mEq/L)
Cholinesterase	7–9 U/mL
Copper	12–25 μmol/L (100–200 μg/dL)
Complement (total haemolytic)	150–250 U/mL
Creatinine	0.06–0.12 mmol/L (0.6–1.5 mg/dL)
Creatinine kinase (CPK)	<195 U/L
Ferritin	5.8–120 nmol/L (15–250 mmol/L μg/L)
Gamma glutamyl transferase (gGT)	10–40 U/L
Glucose	3–5.8 mmol/L
Glycosylated haemoglobin (HbA_{1c})	3.8–6.4%
Hydroxybutyric dehydrogenase (HBD)	40–125 U/L
Iron	10–30 μmol/L
Iron binding capacity (total)	42–80 μmol/L (250–410 μg/dL)
Lactate dehydrogenase	<150 U/L
Lead	1.8 μmol/L
Magnesium	0.7–1.1 mmol/L
Osmolality	275–295 mosmol/kg
Phosphate	0.8–1.4 mmol/L
Potassium	3.5–5.0 mmol/L
Protein (total)	61–84 g/L
Sodium	135–146 mmol/L
Urate	0.2–0.5 mmol/L

Biochemistry (cont'd)	
Urea	3–8 mmol/L
Vitamin A	0.5–2.1 μmol/L (0.15–0.6 μg/mL)
Vitamin D (25-hydroxy)	19.4–137 nmol/L (8–55 ng/mL)
Vitamin D (1,25-dihydroxy)	62–155 pmol/L (26–65 pg/mL)
Zinc	10–18 μmol/L
Blood gases	
Arterial PCO_2	4.8–6.1 kPA (36–46 mm Hg)
Arterial PO_2	10–13.3 kPa (75–100 mm Hg); for every year over 60, add 0.13 kPa
Arterial $[H^+]$	35–45 nmol/L
Arterial pH	7.35–7.45
Cerebrospinal fluid	
Pressure (adult)	50–200 mm water
Cells	0–5 lymphocytes/mm^3
Glucose	2.5–5.6 mmol/L
Protein	100–400 mg/L
Faeces (normal fat content)	
daily output on normal diet	<7 g
fat (as stearic acid)	11–18 mmol/24 h

Lipids and lipoproteins	
Cholesterol	<5.5 mmol/L
Triglyceride	<2.0 mmol/L
Lipoproteins HDL (male)	0.90–1.80 mmol/L
Lipoproteins HDL (female)	0.90–2.10 mmol/L
Lipids (total)	4.0–10 g/L (400–1000 mg/dL)
Urine	
Total quantity in 24 h	1000–1500 mL
Specific gravity	1.010–1.025
pH	4–8
Urine: average solids excreted in 24 h	
Calcium	<7.5 mmol
Copper	<1.1 μmol
Creatinine	8–16 mmol
5-Hydroxyindole acetic acid	<40 μmol
4-Hydroxy-3-methoxymandelic acid	<40 μmol
Hydroxyproline	0.08–0.25 mmol
Lead	0.14–0.40 μmol
Magnesium	3.3–5.0 mmol
Oestriol	varies widely during pregnancy (μmol)
Phosphate	15–50 mmol
Protein (quantitative)	<0.15 g
Urea	300–600 mmol

Appendix 4
COMMONLY USED ABBREVIATIONS

Abbreviations in use can vary widely from place to place. Each institution's list of acceptable abbreviations is the best authority for its records.

Abbreviation	Meaning
ABG	arterial blood gases
ABO	three basic blood groups
ACE	angiotensin-converting enzyme
ACTH	adrenocorticotrophic hormone
ADHD	attention deficit-hyperactivity disorder
ADH	antidiuretic hormone
ADL	activities of daily living
AF	atrial fibrillation
AFB	acid-fast bacillus
AIDS	acquired immune deficiency syndrome
AK	above the knee
ALS	advanced life support; amyotrophic lateral sclerosis
AMI	acute myocardial infarction
BK	below the knee
BMI	body mass index
BMR	basal metabolic rate
BP	blood pressure
BPH	benign prostatic hypertrophy
bpm	beats per minute
BSE	breast self-examination
Bx	biopsy
./c	with
CABG	coronary artery bypass graft
CAT	computed (axial) tomography
CCU	coronary care unit; critical care unit
CF	cystic fibrosis
CHF	congestive heart failure
CHO	carbohydrate
CI	cardiac index; cardiac insufficiency; cerebral infarction
CMV	cytomegalovirus
CNC	clinical nurse consultant
CNS	central nervous system; clinical nurse specialist
c/o	complains of/complaints of
COAD	chronic obstructive airways disease
COLD	chronic obstructive lung disease
COPD	chronic obstructive pulmonary disease
CPAP	continuous positive airway pressure
CPM	continuous passive motion
CPR	cardiopulmonary resuscitation
CSF	cerebrospinal fluid
CT	computed tomography
CVA	cerebrovascular accident
CVP	central venous pressure
CVS	chorionic villi sampling
CXR	chest X-ray
D&C	dilation (dilatation) and curettage
DIC	desseminated intravascular coagulopathy/coagulation
DKA	diabetic ketoacidosis
DM	diabetes mellitus
DNA	deoxyribonucleic acid
DNR	do not resuscitate
DOA	dead on arrival
DOB	date of birth
DOE	dyspnoea on exertion
DRG	diagnostic-related groups
DT	delirium tremens
DVT	deep venous thrombosis
EBP	evidence-based practice
ECG	electrocardiogram; electrocardiograph
ECHO	echocardiography
ED	emergency department
EEG	electroencephalogram; electroencephalograph
ENT	ears, nose and throat
ESR	erythrocyte sedimentation rate
ESRD	end-stage renal disease
F	fahrenheit
FEV	forced expiratory volume
FH, Fhx	family history
FSH	follicle-stimulating hormone
GI	gastrointestinal; glycaemic index
GP	general practitioner
GTT	glucose tolerance test

Abbreviation	Meaning
GU	genitourinary
Hb; Hgb	haemoglobin
HCT	haematocrit
HDL	high-density lipoprotein
HIV	human immunodeficiency (AIDS) virus
Hx; hx	history
ICP	intracranial pressure
ICU	intensive care unit
IDC	indwelling catheter
IDDM	insulin dependent diabetes mellitus (type 1 diabetes)
Ig	immunoglobulin
IM	intramuscular
IOP	intraocular pressure
IPPB	intermittent positive pressure breathing
IQ	intelligence quotient
IV	intravenous
IVP	intravenous pyelogram
K	potassium
KVO	keep vein open
lab	laboratory
LLQ	left lower quadrant
LMP	last menstrual period
LOC	level of consciousness; loss of consciousness
LP	lumbar puncture
MI	myocardial infarction
MRI	magnetic resonance imaging
MS	multiple sclerosis
MVA	motor vehicle accident
N	nitrogen
Na	sodium
NaCl	sodium chloride
N/A	not applicable; not available
NAD	no abnormalities detected; non-adherent dressing
NBM	nil by mouth
neg	negative
NG, ng	nasogastric
NICU	neonatal intensive care unit
NIDDM	non-insulin dependent diabetes mellitus (type 2 diabetes)
NS	normal saline
NSAID	non-steroidal anti-inflammatory drug
OR	operating room
OTC	over-the-counter
PACU	post anaesthesia care unit
Pap test	Papanicolaou smear
PCA	patient-controlled analgesia

Abbreviation	Meaning
PE	pulmonary embolism
PET	positron emission tomography
pH	hydrogen ion concentration (alkalinity and acidity in urine and blood analysis)
PID	pelvic inflammatory disease
PKU	phenylketonuria
PM	evening
PMT	premenstrual tension
PRN	as needed
PUO	pyrexia of unknown origin
PVC	premature ventricular contraction
PVD	peripheral vascular disease
qid	four times a day
RBC	red blood cell; red blood count
Rh	rhesus factor
ROM	range of motion
rpm	revolutions per minute
RUQ	right upper quadrant
R_x	treatment
SC	subcutaneous
SGOT	serum glutamic oxaloacetic transaminase
SIDS	sudden infant death syndrome
Sl	sublingual
SLE	systemic lupus erythematosus
SOB	shortness of breath
SG; sp.gr.	specific gravity
SR	sedimentation rate
s/s	signs and symptoms
Staph	Staphylococcus
stat	immediately (*statim*)
STD	sexually transmitted disease
Strep	Streptococcus
TB	tuberculosis; tubercle bacillus
TENS	transcutaneous electrical nerve stimulation
TIA	transient ischaemic attack
TPN	total parenteral nutrition
TPR	temperature, pulse and respiration
TURP	transurethral resection of prostate
Tx; Rx	treatment
UA	urinalysis
URI	upper respiratory infection
UTI	urinary tract infection
VSD	ventricular septal defect
WBC; wbc	white blood cell; white blood count
wt	weight
X-ray	Roentgen ray

(adapted from deWit 2005; reproduced with permission)

Appendix 5 DRUG CALCULATIONS

1. Oral medications (tablets, capsules)

$$\text{number required} = \frac{\text{dose required}}{\text{stock strength}}$$

Example 1

Mr Smith has been ordered ranitidine 300 mg. The stock strength of the drug is 150 mg per tablet. How many tablets would you administer?

$$\text{number required} = \frac{\text{dose required}}{\text{stock strength}} = \text{tablets}$$

$$\text{therefore, number required} = \frac{300\text{ mg}}{150\text{ mg}} = 2\text{ tablets}$$

that is, number required = 2 tablets

Example 2

A patient is ordered 0.25 mg of digoxin orally. The digoxin is available in tablets containing 125 mcg. How many tablets would you administer?

First, change both strengths to the same units: 0.25 mg = 250 mcg.

Then apply the above formula:

$$\text{number required} = \frac{\text{dose required}}{\text{stock strength}}$$

$$\text{therefore, number required} = \frac{250\text{ mcg}}{125\text{ mcg}} = 2\text{ tablets}$$

that is, number required = 2 tablets

2. Oral medications (liquids)

$$\text{volume required} = \frac{\text{dose required}}{\text{stock strength}} \times \text{volume}$$

Example

A patient is ordered 750 mg of erythromycin orally. The stock suspension contains 250 mg/5 mL. Calculate the volume to be administered.

$$\text{volume required} = \frac{\text{dose required}}{\text{stock strength}} \times \text{volume}$$

$$\text{therefore, volume required} = \frac{750}{250} \times 5\text{ mL}$$

that is, volume required = 15 mL

3. Parenteral administration

$$\text{volume required} = \frac{\text{dose required}}{\text{stock strength}} \times \text{volume}$$

Example 1

A patient is ordered 75 mg of pethidine for pain. The ampoule contains 100 mg in 2 mL. What volume would you administer?

$$\text{volume required} = \frac{\text{dose required}}{\text{stock strength}} \times \text{volume}$$

$$\text{therefore, volume required} = \frac{75}{100} \times 2\text{ mL}$$

that is, volume required = 1.5 mL

4. Calculation of infusion rates

Infusion rates

To determine intravenous infusion rates (mL/hr)

$$\text{rate (mL/hr)} = \frac{\text{volume (mL)}}{\text{time (hrs)}}$$

Example

A patient is to receive 1000 mL of normal saline over 8 hours. How many millilitres per hour should the pump be set at?

$$\text{rate (mL/hr)} = \frac{\text{volume (mL)}}{\text{time (hrs)}}$$

$$\text{therefore, rate (mL/hr)} = \frac{1000\text{ mL}}{8\text{ hrs}}$$

that is, rate = 125 mL/hr

Drops per minute

To calculate the drops per minute:

$$\text{drops per minute} = \frac{\text{volume (mL)}}{\text{time (minutes)}} \times \text{drip factor (drops/mL)}$$

Example 1

A patient is to receive 500 mL of normal saline over 6 hours (360 minutes). An IV set that delivers 20 drops per mL (that is, a drip factor of 20 drops/mL) will be used. Calculate the required drops per minute.

$$\text{drops per minute} = \frac{\text{volume (mL)}}{\text{time (minutes)}} \times \text{drip factor (drops/mL)}$$

$$\text{therefore, drops per minute} = \frac{500\ \text{mL}}{360\ \text{minutes}} \times 20\ \text{drops/mL}$$

that is, drops per minute = 27.7 drops/min

Example 2

An infant is ordered 150 mL of normal saline to run over 10 hours (600 minutes). The microdrip delivers 60 drops per mL (that is, a drip factor of 60 drops/mL). Calculate the required drip factor in drops per minute

$$\text{drops per minute} = \frac{\text{volume (mL)}}{\text{time (minutes)}} \times \text{drip factor (drops/mL)}$$

$$\text{therefore, drops per minute} = \frac{150\ \text{mL}}{600\ \text{minutes}} \times 60\ \text{drops/mL}$$

that is, drops per minute = 15 drops/min.

INDEX